Textbook of
Neuro-Oncology

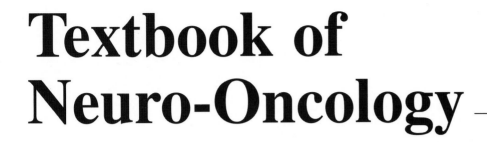
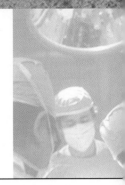

Textbook of
Neuro-Oncology

Mitchel S. Berger, MD

Professor and Chair of Neurological Surgery
Kathleen M. Plant Distinguished Professor of Neurological Surgery
Director, Brain Tumor Research Center
University of California, San Francisco, School of Medicine
San Francisco, California

Michael D. Prados, MD

Professor of Neurological Surgery
Charles B. Wilson Endowed Chair in Neurological Surgery
Director, Clinical Neuro-Oncology Program
Brain Tumor Research Center
University of California, San Francisco, School of Medicine
San Francisco, California

ASSOCIATE EDITORS

Ossama Al-Mefty, MD
Professor and Chair of Neurosurgery
University of Arkansas for Medical Sciences
Little Rock, Arkansas

G. Evren Keles, MD
Assistant Professor of Neurological Surgery
University of California, San Francisco,
    School of Medicine
San Francisco, California

Michel Kliot, MD
Associate Professor of Neurological Surgery
University of Washington School of Medicine
Seattle, Washington

Keith Kwok, MD
Visiting Research Scholar
University of Washington School of Medicine
Seattle, Washington

Paul C. McCormick, MD, MPH
Professor of Neurosurgery
The Neurological Institute of New York
Columbia-Presbyterian Medical Center
Columbia University College of Physicians and
    Surgeons
New York, New York

Andrew T. Parsa, MD, PhD
Assistant Professor of Neurological Surgery
Principal Investigator, Brain Tumor Research
    Center
University of California, San Francisco,
    School of Medicine
San Francisco, California

James T. Rutka, MD, PhD, FRCSC
Professor and Chair of Neurosurgery
Dan Family Chair in Neurosurgery
Director, The Arthur and Sonia Labatt Brain
    Tumour Research Centre
The University of Toronto
Toronto, Ontario, Canada

Raymond Sawaya, MD
Professor and Chair of Neurosurgery
Mary Beth Pawelek Chair in Neurosurgery
Director, Brain Tumor Center
University of Texas M.D. Anderson Cancer Center
Houston, Texas

ELSEVIER
SAUNDERS

ELSEVIER
SAUNDERS

The Curtis Center
170 S Independence Mall W 300E
Philadelphia, Pennsylvania 19106-3399

TEXTBOOK OF NEURO-ONCOLOGY   ISBN: 0-7216-8148-4

NOTICE

Neurosurgery is an ever-changing field. Standard safety precautions must be followed, but as new research and clinical experience broaden our knowledge, changes in treatment and drug therapy may become necessary or appropriate. Readers are advised to check the most current product information provided by the manufacturer of each drug to be administered to verify the recommended dose, the method and duration of administration, and contraindications. It is the responsibility of the treating physician, relying on experience and knowledge of the patient, to determine dosages and the best treatment for each individual patient. Neither the Publisher nor the authors assume any liability for any injury and/or damage to persons or property arising from this publication.

The Publisher

Library of Congress Cataloging-in-Publication Data

Textbook of neuro-oncology / [edited by] Mitchel S. Berger, Michael D. Prados. – 1st ed.
     p. ; cm.
  Includes index.
  ISBN 0-7216-8148-4
  1. Nervous system–Tumors. I. Berger, Mitchel S. II. Prados, Michael.
  [DNLM: 1. Brain Neoplasms. 2. Neoplasms, Neuroepithelial. 3. Peripheral Nervous System Neoplasms. 4. Skull Base Neoplasms. 5. Spinal Cord Neoplasms.   WL 358 T355 2005]
  RC280.N4T49 2005
  616.99'481–dc22   2004042996

Acquisitions Editor: Rebecca Schmidt Gaertner
Developmental Editor: Denise LeMelledo
Publishing Services Manager: Joan Sinclair
Project Manager: Cecelia Bayruns

Printed in China.

Last digit is the print number: 9 8 7 6 5 4 3 2 1

Contents

PREFACE

It takes an integrated multidisciplinary approach to provide the best care for patients with brain tumors, and in consulting with our colleagues on the patient-care team we've often been frustrated by the lack of an all-inclusive resource that provides a comprehensive picture of the multifaceted aspects of the challenges involved. In working with our colleagues doing basic science research into the causes and mechanisms of brain tumors, we have been impressed by their interest in the clinical details of translational therapies developed through their creative work. With the enthusiasm and support of the publisher, we were encouraged to outline a book intended for everyone curious to understand more about the varied clinical roles in the treatment of brain tumors and the basic biology and epidemiology of this most perplexing disease.

This book is intended for everyone on the medical team caring for patients with brain tumors, from the physicians who first suspect the diagnosis, to the neuroradiologists involved in diagnostic work-ups, to the medical specialists in neuro-oncology who monitor care, to radiation oncologists and neurosurgeons. It is a "Tumor Board in Print" where each specific type of brain tumor occupies a chapter in which all of the multidisciplinary specialists involved in treating that specific tumor are heard. We have also tried to make this a book for other members of the patient-care team, for residents and students interested in brain tumors, and in particular for basic scientists wanting to understand more about the clinical complexities of managing neuro-oncology patients.

To this end, we enlisted the aid of some of the most respected people working in the field. Ossama Al-Mefty, at the University of Arkansas, signed up to deal with tumors of the cranial base. Ray Sawaya, at the University of Texas M.D. Anderson Cancer Center, said he would take on the section on brain metastasis. Paul McCormick of the Columbia Presbyterian Medical Center and the Neurological Institute of New York agreed to help out with a section on tumors of the spinal axis together with Andy Parsa, who has since joined us in San Francisco. Michel Kliot, at the University of Washington School of Medicine in Seattle, agreed to edit the section on peripheral nerve tumors together with Keith Kwok. Jim Rutka, at the University of Toronto's Hospital for Sick Children, agreed to edit the section on pediatric neuro-oncology, and our colleague Evren Keles joined forces in editing the section on the treatment of intracranial tumors in adults. With this world-class team working with us, we felt we could produce a comprehensive text that would be useful for everyone immersed in or interested by the field of neuro-oncology. These section editors have done their part, enlisting a distinguished panel of specialists who have provided chapters that more than fulfill our optimistic hopes for this textbook. Together with our fellow editors, we hope you will find this volume both an interesting and useful resource.

Mitchel S. Berger, MD
Michael D. Prados, MD
Editors

CONTRIBUTORS

Joann Aaron, MA
Scientific Editor
Department of Neuro-Oncology
University of Texas M.D. Anderson Cancer Center
Houston, Texas
24: *Mixed Gliomas*

Emad T. Aboud, MD
Fellow, Department of Neurosurgery
University of Arkansas for Medical Sciences
Little Rock, Arkansas
52: *Epidermoid Tumors*

A. Leland Albright, MD
Professor of Neurosurgery
University of Pittsburgh School of Medicine;
Chief of Pediatric Neurosurgery
Children's Hospital of Pittsburgh
Pittsburgh, Pennsylvania
87: *Hypothalamic Hamartomas*

Kenneth D. Aldape, MD
Associate Professor of Pathology
University of Texas M.D. Anderson Cancer
    Center
Houston, Texas
24: *Mixed Gliomas*
27: *Astroblastoma*

Mubarak Al-Gahtany, MD, FRCSC
Clinical Fellow in Neurosurgery
The University of Toronto
Toronto Western Hospital
Toronto, Ontario, Canada
74: *Malignant Peripheral Nerve Tumors*
107: *Peripheral Nerve Tumors in Children*

Ossama Al-Mefty, MD
Professor and Chair of Neurosurgery
University of Arkansas for Medical Sciences
Little Rock, Arkansas
44: *Nonacoustic Schwannomas of the Cranial
    Nerves*
45: *Meningiomas*
46: *Meningeal Hemangiopericytomas and
    Sarcomas*
48: *Chordomas and Chondrosarcomas of the
    Cranial Base*
49: *Paragangliomas of the Skull Base*

Nabeel Al-Shafai, MD
Neurosurgery Resident
The University of Toronto
Toronto Western Hospital
Toronto, Ontario, Canada
97: *Choroid Plexus Tumors*

Christopher Ames, MD
Assistant Professor of Neurological Surgery
University of California, San Francisco,
    School of Medicine
San Francisco, California
69: *Benign Tumors of the Spine*

Lilyana Angelov, MD
Associate Staff
Department of Neurological Surgery
The Cleveland Clinic
Cleveland, Ohio
30: *Mixed Neuronal and Glial Tumors*

Edgardo J. Angtuaco, MD
Professor, Department of Radiology
University of Arkansas for Medical Sciences;
Chief, Division of Neuroradiology
University of Arkansas for Medical Sciences
45: *Meningiomas*
48: *Chordomas and Chondrosarcomas of the
    Cranial Base*

Henry E. Aryan, MD
Clinical Instructor of Neurosurgery
University of California, San Diego,
    School of Medicine;
Neurosurgeon
University of California, San Diego,
    Medical Center;
Children's Hospital Medical Center
San Diego, California
101: *Pediatric Skull Base Tumors*

Kurtis Ian Auguste, MD
Resident Physician
Department of Neurological Surgery
University of California San Francisco School of
    Medicine
San Francisco, California
40: *Hemangioblastomas*

Samer Ayoubi, MD, FRCS
Attending Physician
Damascus University School of Medicine;
Consultant Neurosurgeon
Al-Muwasat University Hospital
Damascus, Syria
44: *Nonacoustic Schwannomas of the Cranial
    Nerves*
46: *Meningeal Hemangiopericytomas and
    Sarcomas*

Matthew T. Ballo, MD
Associate Professor of Radiation Oncology
University of Texas M.D. Anderson Cancer Center
Houston, Texas
61: *Skull Base Metastasis*

Geoffrey R. Barger, MD
Associate Professor
Department of Neurology
Wayne State University School of Medicine;
Co-Chief, Neuro-Oncology
Karmanos Cancer Institute
Detroit, Michigan
35: *Medulloblastoma*

Fred G. Barker II, MD
Assistant Professor of Neurosurgery
Harvard Medical School;
Assistant Visiting Neurosurgeon
Massachusetts General Hospital
Boston, Massachusetts
20: *Pilocytic Astrocytoma*
34: *Pineoblastoma*

Gene H. Barnett, MD, FACS
Professor of Surgery
Cleveland Clinic Lerner College of Medicine;
Chairman
The Brain Institute
Cleveland, Ohio
30: *Mixed Neuronal and Glial Tumors*

Michael E. Berens, PhD
Senior Investigator
TGen, The Translational Genomics Research
    Institute
Phoenix, Arizona
3: *Animal Models*

Mitchel S. Berger, MD
Professor and Chair of Neurological Surgery
Kathleen M. Plant Distinguished Professor of
    Neurological Surgery
Director, Brain Tumor Research Center
University of California, San Francisco,
    School of Medicine
San Francisco, California
1: *Epidemiology of Brain Tumors*
9: *Surgical Strategies in the Management of Brain
    Tumors*
17: *Diffuse Astrocytoma*
28: *Gliomatosis Cerebri*
40: *Hemangioblastomas of the Central Nervous
    System*

Mark Bernstein, MD, FRCSC
Professor of Surgery
The University of Toronto;
Neurosurgeon
Toronto Western Hospital
University Health Network
Toronto, Ontario, Canada
22: *Subependymal Giant Cell Astrocytoma and
    Tuberous Sclerosis Complex*

Ratan D. Bhardwaj, MD
Neurosurgical Resident
The University of Toronto
Toronto, Ontario, Canada
94: *Pituitary Tumors in Children*

Asis Kumar Bhattacharyya, MBBS, MS, MCh
Fellow, Division of Neurosurgery
University of Toronto
Toronto Western Hospital
Toronto, Ontario, Canada
22: *Subependymal Giant Cell Astrocytoma and
    Tuberous Sclerosis Complex*

Juan M. Bilbao, MD
Associate Professor of Pathology
The University of Toronto;
Neuropathologist
Sunnybrook Hospital
Toronto, Ontario, Canada
80: *Lhermitte-Duclos Disease*

Mark H. Bilsky, MD
Assistant Attending, Department of Surgery
Memorial Sloan-Kettering Cancer Center
Cornell University Medical Center
New York, New York
71: *Therapeutic Options for Treating Metastatic
    Spine Tumors*

Devin K. Binder, MD, PhD
Chief Resident
Department of Neurological Surgery
University of California, San Francisco,
    School of Medicine
San Francisco, California
14: *Gene Therapy for Malignant Gliomas*

Deborah T. Blumenthal, MD
Assistant Professor of Neurology and Oncology
University of Utah
Huntsman Cancer Institute
Salt Lake City, Utah
54: *Small Cell Lung Carcinoma*

Robert J. Bohinski, MD, PhD
Assistant Professor, Department of Neurosurgery
University of Cincinnati;
Mayfield Clinic and Spine Institute
Cincinnati, Ohio
60: *Multidisciplinary Management of Patients with Brain Metastases from an Unknown Primary Tumor*

Melissa L. Bondy, PhD
Professor of Epidemiology
University of Texas M.D. Anderson Cancer Center
Houston, Texas
1: *Epidemiology of Brain Tumors*

Margaret Booth-Jones, PhD
Assistant Professor of Oncology and Psychiatry
H. Lee Moffitt Cancer and Research Institute
University of South Florida
Tampa, Florida
18: *Anaplastic Astrocytoma*

Donald E. Born, MD, PhD
Clinical Assistant Professor, Department of Pathology
University of Washington School of Medicine
Seattle, Washington
73: *Evaluation and Management of Benign Peripheral Nerve Tumors and Masses*

Kristin Bradley, MD
Assistant Professor of Human Oncology
University of Wisconsin School of Medicine
Madison, Wisconsin
10: *Basic Concepts Underlying Radiation Therapy*

Steven Brem, MD
Professor of Oncology, Neurosurgery, and Neurology;
Director of Neurosurgery;
Program Leader, Neuro-Oncology Program
H. Lee Moffitt Cancer Center and Research Institute
Tampa, Florida
18: *Anaplastic Astrocytoma*

William C. Broaddus, MD, PhD
Associate Professor of Neurosurgery, Anatomy and Neurobiology, Physiology, and Radiation Oncology
Virginia Commonwealth University;
Director of Neuro-oncology
Medical College of Virginia Hospitals;
Chief of Neurosurgery
Hunter Holmes McGuire VA Medical Center
Richmond, Virginia
38: *Fibrous Tumors*

Douglas L. Brockmeyer, MD
Associate Professor of Neurosurgery and Pediatrics
University of Utah School of Medicine;
Attending Neurosurgeon
Primary Children's Medical Center
Salt Lake City, Utah
104: *Spinal Column Tumors in Pediatric Patients*

Jeffrey N. Bruce, MD
Associate Professor of Neurosurgery
The Neurological Institute of New York
Columbia-Presbyterian Medical Center
Columbia University College of Physicians and Surgeons
New York, New York
33: *Pineocytoma*

Derek A. Bruce, MD, ChB
Professor of Pediatric Neurosurgery
George Washington University
Children's National Medical Center
Washington, D.C.
101: *Pediatric Skull Base Tumors*

John M. Buatti, MD
Professor and Head
Department of Radiation Oncology
University of Iowa Hospitals and Clinics
Iowa City, Iowa
58: *Intracerebral Metastatic Colon Carcinoma*

Ketan R. Bulsara, MD
Instructor of Neurosurgery
University of Arkansas for Medical Sciences;
Children's Hospital
Little Rock, Arkansas
45: *Meningiomas*

Eric C. Burton, MD
Assistant Professor of Neurological Surgery
University of California, San Francisco;
Neuro-Oncologist
University of California, San Francisco, Medical Center
San Francisco, California
17: *Diffuse Astrocytoma*

Thomas Carlisle, MD, PhD
Associate Professor, Clinical Internal Medicine
University of Iowa
Roy J. and Lucille Carver College of Medicine
Iowa City, Iowa
58: *Intracerebral Metastatic Colon Carcinoma*

James H. Carter, Jr., MHS, PAC
Assistant Clinical Professor of Surgery
Division of Neurosurgery
Duke University Medical Center
Durham, North Carolina
56: *Brain Metastases from Malignant Melanoma*

Steve Casha, MD, PhD
Neurosurgery Resident
The University of Toronto
Toronto Western Hospital
Toronto, Ontario, Canada
92: *Pediatric Meningiomas*

Soonmee Cha, MD
Assistant Professor of Radiology and Neurological Surgery
University of California, San Francisco, School of Medicine;
Attending Neuroradiologist
University of California, San Francisco, Medical Center
San Francisco, California
4: *Diagnostic Imaging*

Marc C. Chamberlain, MD
Professor of Neurology and Neurosurgery
University of Southern California Keck School of Medicine;
Co-Director of Neuro-Oncology
Norris Cancer Center
Los Angeles, California
36: *Adult Supratentorial Primitive Neuroectodermal Tumors*

Susan M. Chang, MD
Associate Professor of Neurological Surgery
University of California, San Francisco
San Francisco, California
16: *Clinical Trials*
28: *Gliomatosis Cerebri*
34: *Pineoblastoma*

Michael Y. Chen, MD
Resident
Virginia Commonwealth University;
Medical College of Virginia
Richmond, Virginia
38: *Fibrous Tumors*

Thomas Chen, MD, PhD
Associate Professor, Neurosurgery and Pathology;
Director of Surgical Neuro-Oncology
University of Southern California;
Staff Neurosurgeon
University of Southern California University Hospital;
Norris Cancer Hospital
Los Angeles, California
36: *Adult Supratentorial Primitive Neuroectodermal Tumors*

Terri Chew, MPH
Academic Coordinator, Neurosurgery Research
University of California, San Francisco
San Francisco, California
1: *Epidemiology of Brain Tumors*

John H. Chi, MD, MPH
Resident, Department of Neurological Surgery
University of California, San Francisco
San Francisco, California
72: *Intrinsic Metastatic Spinal Cord Tumors*
81: *Cerebellar Astrocytomas*

Dean Chou, MD
Assistant Clinical Professor of Neurological Surgery
University of California, San Francisco
San Francisco, California
70: *Malignant Primary Tumors of the Vertebral Column*

H. Brent Clark, MD, PhD
Professor of Neurology and Laboratory Medicine and Pathology
University of Minnesota Medical School;
Director of Neuropathology
Fairview University Medical Center
Minneapolis, Minnesota
32: *Dysembryoplastic Neuroepithelial Tumor*

Aaron A. Cohen-Gadol, MD
Neurosurgery Resident
Mayo Clinic
Rochester, Minnesota
64: *Spinal Meningiomas*

Benedicto O. Colli, MD
Division of Neurosurgery
Department of Surgery
Ribeirão Preto Medical School
University of São Paulo
Ribeirão Preto, São Paulo, Brazil
48: *Chordomas and Chondrosarcomas of the
    Cranial Base*

Ceasare Colosimo, MD
Professor of Radiology
Institute of Radiology
University of Chieti
Chieti, Italy
85: *Desmoplastic Infantile Ganglioglioma*

Joseph F. Costello, PhD
Assistant Professor of Neurological Surgery
University of California, San Francisco
San Francisco, California
2: *Molecular and Cell Biology*

Deborah L. Cummins, MD, PhD
Associate Professor of Clinical Pathology
University of Southern California
    Keck School of Medicine
Los Angeles, California
36: *Adult Supratentorial Primitive
    Neuroectodermal Tumors*

Lisa M. DeAngelis, MD
Professor of Neurology
Weill Medical College of Cornell University;
Chairman, Department of Neurology
Memorial Sloan-Kettering Cancer Center
New York, New York
41: *Lymphomas and Hemopoietic Neoplasms*

Franco DeMonte, MD, FRCSC, FACS
Professor of Neurosurgery and Head and Neck
    Surgery
University of Texas M.D. Anderson Cancer
    Center
Houston, Texas
50: *Carcinoma of the Paranasal Sinuses and
    Olfactory Neuroblastoma*
61: *Skull Base Metastasis*

Concezio Di Rocco, MD
Professor of Pediatric Neurosurgery;
Chief of Pediatric Neurosurgery
Catholic University of Rome
Rome, Italy
85: *Desmoplastic Infantile Ganglioglioma*

Eduardo M. Diaz, Jr., MD, FACS
Associate Professor;
Center Medical Director
Department of Head and Neck Surgery
University of Texas M.D. Anderson Cancer
    Center
Houston, Texas
50: *Carcinoma of the Paranasal Sinuses and
    Olfactory Neuroblastoma*

Peter B. Dirks, MD, PhD, FRCSC
Assistant Professor of Neurosurgery
The University of Toronto;
Staff Neurosurgeon
The Hospital for Sick Children
Toronto, Ontario, Canada
75: *Supratentorial Low-Grade Gliomas*
90: *Supratentorial Primitive Neuroectodermal
    Tumors*

Egon M.R. Doppenberg, MD
Chief Resident, Department of Neurosurgery
Medical College of Virginia
Virginia Commonwealth University Health
    Center
Richmond, Virginia
38: *Fibrous Tumors*

James G. Douglas, MD, MS
Associate Professor
Departments of Radiation Oncology, Pediatrics,
    and Neurological Surgery
University of Washington Cancer Center;
Chief, Division of Radiation Oncology
Children's Hospital and Regional Medical
    Center;
Co-director, University of Washington Gamma
    Knife Center
Harborview Medical Center
Seattle, Washington
35: *Medulloblastoma*

Christopher F. Dowd, MD
Clinical Professor of Radiology, Neurological
    Surgery, Neurology, and Anesthesia and
    Perioperative Care
University of California, San Francisco,
    School of Medicine
San Francisco, California
12: *Neurointerventional Techniques*

James M. Drake, BSE, MBBCh, MSc, FRCSC
Professor
The University of Toronto;
Chief of Neurosurgery
The Hospital for Sick Children
Toronto, Ontario, Canada
78: *Midbrain Gliomas*
92: *Pediatric Meningiomas*

Rose Du, MD, PhD
Resident, Department of Neurological Surgery
University of California, San Francisco,
    School of Medicine
San Francisco, California
95: *Craniopharyngioma*

David H. Ebb, MD
Instructor and Assistant Professor, Department of
    Pediatrics
Harvard Medical School;
Assistant Pediatrician
Pediatric Hematology-Oncology
Massachusetts General Hospital
Boston, Massachusetts
20: *Pilocytic Astrocytoma*

Said El-Shihabi, MD
Resident in Neurological Surgery
University of Arkansas for Medical Sciences
Little Rock, Arkansas
55: *Management of Central Nervous System
    Metastases from Breast Carcinoma*

Daryl R. Fourney, MD, FRCSC
Assistant Professor of Neurosurgery
University of Saskatchewan;
Director of Residency Training Program
Royal University Hospital
Saskatoon, Saskatchewan
50: *Carcinoma of the Paranasal Sinuses and
    Olfactory Neuroblastoma*

Allan H. Friedman, MD
Guy L. Odom Professor of Neurological Surgery;
Neurosurgeon-in-Chief
Duke University Medical Center
Durham, North Carolina
25: *Ependymoma*
56: *Brain Metastases from Malignant Melanoma*

Henry S. Friedman, MD
James B. Powell Jr. Professor of Neuro-Oncology;
The Brain Tumor Center at Duke
Duke University Medical Center
Durham, North Carolina
25: *Ependymoma*

Adam S. Garden, MD
Associate Medical Director
Head and Neck Center;
Associate Professor of Radiation Oncology;
Associate Radiation Oncologist
Department of Radiation Oncology
University of Texas M.D. Anderson Cancer Center
Houston, Texas
50: *Carcinoma of the Paranasal Sinuses and
    Olfactory Neuroblastoma*

Gary L. Gallia, MD, PhD
Neurosurgery Resident
Johns Hopkins University School of Medicine
Baltimore, Maryland
29: *Chordoid Glioma of the Third Ventricle*

Felice Giangaspero, MD
Professor of Histopathology
Department of Experimental Medicine and
    Pathology
University "La Sapienza"
Rome, Italy
85: *Desmoplastic Infantile Ganglioglioma*

Wayne M. Gluf, MD
Chief Resident, Department of Neurosurgery
University of Utah
Primary Children's Medical Center
Salt Lake City, Utah
104: *Spinal Column Tumors in Pediatric
    Patients*

Karen Goddard, MBChB, FRCP
Associate Professor of Radiation Oncology
University of British Columbia;
Radiation Oncologist
British Columbia Cancer Agency
Vancouver, British Columbia
103: *Epidural Spinal Tumors*

Ziya Gökaslan, MD, FACS
Professor of Neurosurgery, Oncology, and
    Orthopedic Surgery;
Director of Neurosurgical Spine Program
The Johns Hopkins Medical Institutions
Baltimore, Maryland
21: *Pleomorphic Xanthoastrocytoma*
70: *Malignant Primary Tumors of the Vertebral
    Column*

Ira M. Goldstein, MD
Assistant Professor
Department of Neurological Surgery
University of Medicine and Dentistry of New
    Jersey
Newark, New Jersey
67: *Spinal Cord Astrocytomas: Presentation,
    Management, and Outcome*

Robert Goodkin, MD
Professor of Neurological Surgery
University of Washington School of Medicine
Seattle, Washington
73: *Evaluation and Management of Benign
   Peripheral Nerve Tumors and Masses*

Fredric Grannis, MD
Assistant Clinical Professor
Department of Surgery
University of California, San Diego;
Staff Physician and Head
Section of Thoracic and Vascular Surgery
City of Hope National Medical Center
Duarte, California
53: *Brain Metastasis from Non–Small Cell Lung
   Cancer*

Abhijit Guha, MD, FRCSC, FACS
Professor of Neurosurgery
The University of Toronto;
Attending Neurosurgeon
University Health Network;
Co-Director and Senior Scientist
The Arthur and Sonia Labatt Brain Tumour
   Research Centre
The Hospital for Sick Children;
Alan and Susan Hudson Chair of Neuro-Oncology
The Hospital for Sick Children
Toronto, Ontario, Canada
74: *Malignant Peripheral Nerve Tumors*

Nalin Gupta, MD, PhD
Assistant Professor of Neurosurgery and Pediatrics
University of California, San Francisco,
   School of Medicine;
Chief, Division of Pediatric Neurosurgery
University of California, San Francisco, Medical
   Center
San Francisco, California
81: *Cerebellar Astrocytomas*
95: *Craniopharyngioma*

Van V. Halbach, MD
Clinical Professor
Department of Radiology, Neurological Surgery,
   Neurology, and Anesthesia and Perioperative
   Care
University of California, San Francisco,
   School of Medicine
San Francisco, California
12: *Neurointerventional Techniques*

Walter A. Hall, MD
Professor of Neurosurgery, Radiation Oncology,
   and Radiology
University of Minnesota Medical School;
Active Staff in the Clinical Service of
   Neurosurgery
Fairview University Medical Center
Minneapolis, Minnesota
32: *Dysembryoplastic Neuroepithelial Tumor*
59: *Gynecologic Malignancies*

Fadi Hanbali, MD
Assistant Professor of Neurosurgery and
   Orthopaedics Surgery
University of Texas Medical Branch
Galveston, Texas
61: *Skull Base Metastasis*

Marlan R. Hansen, MD
Assistant Professor of Otolaryngology
University of Iowa
Iowa City, Iowa
7: *Neurotology*

Cynthia Hawkins, MD, PhD, FRCPC
Assistant Professor of Pathology
The University of Toronto;
Neuropathologist
The Hospital for Sick Children
Toronto, Ontario, Canada
80: *Lhermitte-Duclos Disease*
91: *Dysembryoplastic Neuroepithelial Tumor*
100: *Langerhans Cell Histiocytosis*

Glenda Hendson, MBBCh, FRCPC
Clinical Assistant Professor of Pathology and
   Laboratory Medicine
University of British Columbia;
Pediatric Neuropathologist
Children's and Women's Health Centre of British
   Columbia
Vancouver, British Columbia, Canada
103: *Epidural Spinal Tumors*

Stephen John Hentschel, MD
Assistant Professor of Neurosurgery
University of Saskatchewan;
Neurosurgeon
Royal University Hospital
Saskatoon, Saskatchewan
103: *Epidural Spinal Tumors*

Randall T. Higashida, MD
Clinical Professor of Radiology, Neurological
   Surgery, Neurology, and Anesthesiology;
Chief, Division of Interventional Neurovascular
   Radiology
University of California, San Francisco,
   School of Medicine
San Francisco, California
12: *Neurointerventional Techniques*

Dominique B. Hoelzinger, MS
Research Assistant
Translational Genomics Research Institute
Phoenix, Arizona
3: *Animal Models*

John K. Houten, MD
Assistant Professor of Neurosurgery
Albert Einstein College of Medicine of Yeshiva
   University;
Director, Neurosurgery Spine Service
Montefiore Medical Center
Bronx, New York
67: *Spinal Cord Astrocytomas: Presentation,
   Management, and Outcome*

Creig S. Hoyt, MD
Theresa and Wane Caygill Professor and
   Chairman
Department of Ophthalmology
University of California, San Francisco
San Francisco, California
8: *Neuro-Ophthalmology*

Eugen B. Hug, MD
Professor of Radiation Oncology and Pediatrics
Dartmouth Medical School
Hanover, New Hampshire;
Chief, Radiation Oncology
Dartmouth Hitchcock Medical Center and Norris
   Cotton Cancer Center
Lebanon, New Hampshire
48: *Chordomas and Chondrosarcomas of the
   Cranial Base*

Muhammad M. Husain, MD
Associate Professor, Department of Pathology
University of Arkansas for Medical Sciences
Little Rock, Arkansas
49: *Paragangliomas of the Skull Base*

Laura F. Hutchins, MD
Professor of Internal Medicine
University of Arkansas for Medical Sciences;
Director of Hematology-Oncology
Arkansas Cancer Research Center
Little Rock, Arkansas
55: *Management of Central Nervous System
   Metastases from Breast Carcinoma*

W. Bradley Jacobs, MD
Resident, Division of Neurosurgery
University of Toronto
Toronto, Ontario, Canada
74: *Malignant Peripheral Nerve Tumors*
107: *Peripheral Nerve Tumors in Children*

John A. Jane, Jr., MD
Assistant Professor, Department of Neurosurgery
University of Virginia Health System
University of Virginia
Charlottesville, Virginia
47: *Pituitary Adenomas*

Abdul-Rahman Jazieh, MD, MPH
Associate Professor of Medicine and
   Environmental Health;
Associate Professor and Acting Division Director
Department of Internal Medicine, Division of
   Hematology and Oncology
University of Cincinnati College of Medicine
The Vontz Center for Molecular Studies
Cincinnati, Ohio
60: *Multidisciplinary Management of Patients with
   Brain Metastases from an Unknown Primary
   Tumor*

Jaque Jumper, MD
Clinical Fellow in Neuroradiology
University of California San Francisco
San Francisco, California
26: *Choroid Plexus Tumors*

Peter Jun, MD
Howard Hughes Fellow
Department of Neurological Surgery
University of California, San Francisco
San Francisco, California
26: *Choroid Plexus Tumors*

Tetsuo Kanno, MD
Professor, Department of Neurosurgery;
Director
Fujita Health University
Toyoake, Aichi, Japan
51: *Craniopharyngioma*

Bruce Kaufman, MD
Professor of Neurosurgery
Director, Division of Pediatric Neurosurgery
Medical College of Wisconsin;
Chief, Pediatric Neurosurgery
Children's Hospital of Wisconsin
Milwaukee, Wisconsin
82: *Brainstem Gliomas*

Brian D. Kavanagh, MD, MPH
Associate Professor
Department of Radiation Oncology
University of Colorado Health Sciences Center
Denver, Colorado
57: *Brain Metastases: Renal Cell Carcinoma*

G. Evren Keles, MD
Assistant Professor
Department of Neurological Surgery
University of California, San Francisco,
    School of Medicine
San Francisco, California
9: *Surgical Strategies in the Management of Brain
    Tumors*
17: *Diffuse Astrocytoma*
39: *Melanocytic Tumors*

John R.W. Kestle, MD, FRCS, FACS
Associate Professor of Neurology
University of Utah
Salt Lake City, Utah
86: *Pleomorphic Xanthoastrocytoma*

Sara H. Kim, MD
Attending Medical Staff
Glendale Adventist Medical Center
Glendale, California
36: *Adult Supratentorial Primitive
    Neuroectodermal Tumors*

Bette K. Kleinschmidt-DeMasters, MD
Professor of Pathology, Neurology, and
    Neurosurgery
University of Colorado Health Sciences
    Center
Denver, Colorado
37: *Lipomatous Tumors*

Michel Kliot, MD
Associate Professor
Department of Neurological Surgery
University of Washington School of Medicine
Seattle, Washington
73: *Evaluation and Management of
    Benign Peripheral Nerve Tumors
    and Masses*

Paul Kongkham, MD
Resident, Division of Neurosurgery
The Hospital for Sick Children
Toronto, Ontario, Canada
108: *Neurocutaneous Syndromes*

William E. Krauss, MD
Neurosurgery Consultant
Mayo Clinic
Rochester, Minnesota
64: *Spinal Meningiomas*

Ali F. Krisht, MD, FACS
Assistant Professor, Department of
    Neurosurgery
University of Arkansas for Medical
    Sciences
Director, Neuroendocrine Clinic and
    Cerebrovascular Clinic;
Chief of Service, Department of
    Neurosurgery
John L. McClellan Memorial Veterans Clinic
Little Rock, Arkansas
52: *Epidermoid Tumors*

Johan M. Kros, MD, PhD
Professor of Neuropathology
Department of Pathology
Erasmus Medical Center
Rotterdam, The Netherlands
23: *Oligodendroglial Tumors*

Abhaya V. Kulkarni, MD, PhD, FRCSC
Assistant Professor of Surgery
The University of Toronto;
Staff Neurosurgeon
The Hospital for Sick Children
Toronto, Ontario, Canada
100: *Langerhans Cell Histiocytosis*

Sandeep Kunwar, MD
Assistant Professor
Department of Neurological Surgery
University of California, San Francisco,
    School of Medicine;
Principal Investigator, Brain Tumor Research
    Center;
Co-Director, Pituitary Treatment Center
University of California, San Francisco
San Francisco, California
6: *Neuroendocrinology*

William J. Kupsky, MD
Professor of Pathology
Wayne State University School of Medicine;
Chief of Neuropathology
Detroit Medical Center
Detroit, Michigan
35: *Medulloblastoma*

Keith Kwok, MD
Visiting Research Scholar
University of Washington School of Medicine
Seattle, Washington
73: *Evaluation and Management of Benign
    Peripheral Nerve Tumors and Masses*

Robert D. Labrom, MBBS, MSc, FRACS
Senior Lecturer
University of Queensland;
Director of Pediatric Orthopaedic Surgery and
    Pediatric Spinal Surgeon
Royal Children's Hospital
Brisbane, Queensland, Australia
103: *Epidural Spinal Tumors*

Enrico C. Lallana, MD
Director of Medical Neuro-Oncology
Seacoast Cancer Center
Wentworth-Douglass Hospital
Dover, New Hampshire
41: *Lymphomas and Hemopoietic Neoplasms*

Kathleen R. Lamborn, PhD
Adjunct Professor
Departments of Neurological Surgery and
    Epidemiology and Biostatistics
University of California, San Francisco,
    School of Medicine;
San Francisco, California
16: *Clinical Trials*
28: *Gliomatosis Cerebri*

Jeffrey L. Laurent, MD
Resident, Department of Neurosurgery
University of Texas M.D. Anderson Cancer Center
Houston, Texas
47: *Pituitary Adenomas*

Edward R. Laws, Jr., MD
Professor of Neurosurgery and Medicine
University of Virginia Medical School
Charlottesville, Virginia
47: *Pituitary Adenomas*

Michael L. Levy, MD, PhD
Head, Division of Pediatric Neurosurgery
Children's Hospital of San Diego;
Co-Director, Residency Training Program
University of California, San Diego
San Diego, California
101: *Pediatric Skull Base Tumors*

Kevin O. Lillehei, MD
Professor, Department of Neurosurgery
University of Colorado Health Sciences Center
Denver, Colorado
37: *Lipomatous Tumors*
57: *Brain Metastases: Renal Cell Carcinoma*

Mark E. Linskey, MD
Associate Professor and Chair
Department of Neurological Surgery
University of California, Irvine
Orange, California
55: *Management of Central Nervous System
    Metastases from Breast Carcinoma*

Russell R. Lonser, MD
Staff Neurosurgeon
Surgical Neurology Branch
National Institute of Neurological Disorders and
    Stroke
National Institutes of Health
Bethesda, Maryland
68: *Spinal Cord Hemangioblastomas*

R. Loch Macdonald, MD, PhD
Associate Professor of Surgery and Radiation and
    Cellular Oncology
University of Chicago Hospitals
Chicago, Illinois
98: *Colloid Cysts in Children*

Cormac O. Maher, MD
Clinical Fellow, Department of Neurosurgery
Mayo Graduate School of Medicine;
Chief Resident Associate, Department of
    Neurosurgery
Mayo Clinic
Rochester, Minnesota
89: *Medulloblastoma*

Todd Mainprize, MD
Resident, Division of Neurosurgery
The University of Toronto
The Hospital for Sick Children
Toronto, Ontario, Canada
80: *Lhermitte-Duclos Disease*
91: *Dysembryoplastic Neuroepithelial Tumor*

Adam N. Mamelak, MD
Associate Professor
City of Hope Cancer Center;
Visiting Associate in Biology
California Institute of Technology;
Director of Neurosurgery
City of Hope Cancer Center
Duarte, California
53: *Brain Metastasis from Non–Small Cell Lung
    Cancer*

Timothy B. Mapstone, MD
Vice Chairman and Professor
Department of Neurological Surgery
Emory University;
Chief Pediatric Neurosurgeon
Children's Healthcare of Atlanta/Egleston
Atlanta, Georgia
83: *Dorsally Exophytic Brainstem Gliomas*

Charles Matouk, MD
Neurosurgical Resident
The University of Toronto
Toronto, Ontario, Canada
78: *Midbrain Gliomas*

Masao Matsutani, MD
Department of Neurosurgery
Saitama Medical School
Iruma-gun, Saitama, Japan
42: *Germ Cell Tumors*

Cordula Matthies, MD, PhD
Professor of Neurosurgery
Hannover Medical School;
Neurosurgical Attending
Klinikum Hannover Nordstadt
Hannover, Germany
43: *Acoustic Neuromas (Vestibular Schwannomas)*

J. Gordon McComb, MD
Professor, Department of Neurological Surgery
University of Southern California
    Keck School of Medicine;
Head, Division of Neurosurgery
Los Angeles Childrens Hospital
Los Angeles, California
102: *Tumors of the Skull*

Paul C. McCormick, MD, MPH
Professor of Neurosurgery
The Neurological Institute of New York
Columbia-Presbyterian Medical Center
Columbia University College of Physicians and
    Surgeons
New York, New York
62: *Spinal Axis Tumors: Incidence, Classification,*
    and Diagnostic Imaging
66: *Intramedullary Ependymomas*

Michael W. McDermott, MD
Associate Professor
Department of Neurological Surgery
University of California, San Francisco,
    School of Medicine
San Francisco, California
26: *Choroid Plexus Tumors: Choroid Plexus*
    Papilloma and Choroid Plexus Carcinoma
95: *Craniopharyngioma*

Patrick McDonald, MD, FRCSC
Assistant Professor of Neurosurgery
University of Manitoba;
Pediatric Neurosurgeon
Winnipeg Children's Hospital
Winnipeg, Manitoba, Canada
78: *Midbrain Gliomas*

Roger E. McLendon, MD
Professor of Pathology;
Chief of Neuropathology;
Director of Anatomic Pathology Services
Duke University School of Medicine
Durham, North Carolina
25: *Ependymoma*

Minesh Mehta, MBChB
Chair and Professor, Department of Human
    Oncology
University of Wisconsin School of Medicine
Madison, Wisconsin
10: *Basic Concepts Underlying Radiation Therapy*

Hal S. Meltzer, MD
Associate Professor of Neurosurgery
University of California, San Diego,
    School of Medicine;
Department of Pediatric Neurosurgery
Children's Hospital of San Diego
San Diego, California
101: *Pediatric Skull Base Tumors*

Thomas E. Merchant, DO, PhD
Chief, Division of Radiation Oncology
St. Jude Children's Research Hospital
Memphis, Tennessee
88: *Ependymoma*

Christina A. Meyers, PhD
Professor of Neuropsychology
University of Texas M.D. Anderson Cancer Center
Houston, Texas
15: *Functional Outcomes*

Rajiv Midha, MD, FRCS
Head and Chairman, Division of Neurosurgery
Department of Clinical Neurosciences
University of Calgary
Foothills Medical Centre
Calgary, Alberta, Canada
74: *Malignant Peripheral Nerve Tumors*
107: *Peripheral Nerve Tumors in Children*

Yuriko Minn, MS
Medical Student
Stanford University
Palo Alto, California
1: *Epidemiology of Brain Tumors*

Robert J. Morgan, Jr., MD
Assistant Clinical Professor of Medicine
University of California;
Professor of Oncology;
Staff Physician;
Director of Continuing Medical Education
City of Hope Comprehensive Cancer Center
Duarte, California
53: *Brain Metastasis from Non–Small Cell Lung*
    Cancer

Reed Murtagh, MD
Neuro-Oncology Program
H. Lee Moffitt Cancer Center;
Department of Radiology
University of South Florida
Tampa, Florida
18: *Anaplastic Astrocytoma*

Prithvi Narayan, MD
Assistant Professor of Pediatric Neurosurgery
Mount Sinai School of Medicine
New York, New York
83: *Dorsally Exophytic Brainstem Gliomas*

Tien T. Nguyen, MD
Division of Neurosurgery
Los Angeles Children's Hospital
Los Angeles, California
102: *Tumors of the Skull*

W. Jerry Oakes, MD
Professor of Neurosurgery
University of Alabama
Birmingham, Alabama
105: *Pediatric Intradural and Extramedullary*
    Spinal Cord Tumors

Cian J. O'Kelly, MD
Resident Physician
The Hospital for Sick Children;
Resident Physician
Division of Neurosurgery
The University of Toronto
Toronto, Ontario, Canada
76: *Optic Pathway Gliomas*

Nezih Oktar, MD
Professor
Department of Neurosurgery
Ege University School of Medicine
Izmir, Turkey
39: *Melanocytic Tumors*

Edward H. Oldfield, MD
Chief, Surgical Neurology Branch
National Institute of Neurological Disorders and
    Stroke
Bethesda, Maryland
68: *Spinal Cord Hemangioblastomas*

Alessandro Olivi, MD
Professor of Neurosurgery and Oncology
Johns Hopkins University School of Medicine;
Director of Neurosurgical Oncology
Johns Hopkins Hospital
Baltimore, Maryland
29: *Chordoid Glioma of the Third Ventricle*

Ian F. Parney, MD, PhD
Assistant Professor
Departments of Clinical Neurosciences and
    Oncology
University of Calgary
Calgary, Alberta
11: *Chemotherapy Principles*
19: *Glioblastoma Multiforme*
65: *Myxopapillary Ependymomas*

Andrew T. Parsa, MD, PhD
Assistant Professor
Department of Neurological Surgery
Principal Investigator, Brain Tumor Research
    Center
University of California, San Francisco,
    School of Medicine;
San Francisco, California
13: *Immunotherapy*
33: *Pineocytoma*
62: *Spinal Axis Tumors: Incidence, Classification,*
    and Diagnostic Imaging
65: *Myxopapillary Ependymomas*
66: *Intramedullary Ependymomas*
72: *Intrinsic Metastatic Spinal Cord Tumors*

James Pearlman, MD
Assistant Professor
University of South Florida;
Physician
H. Lee Moffitt Cancer Center;
Physician
VA-Hospital;
Physician
Tampa General Hospital
Tampa, Florida
18: *Anaplastic Astrocytoma*

Richard D. Pezner, MD
Clinical Professor, Department of Radiation
    Oncology
University of California Irvine
Orange, California;
Associate Chairman, Division of Radiation
    Oncology
City of Hope National Medical Center
Duarte, California
53: *Brain Metastasis from Non–Small Cell Lung
    Cancer*

Joseph H. Piatt, Jr., MD, FAAP
Professor of Neurological Surgery and Pediatrics
Drexel University College of Medicine;
Chief, Section of Neurosurgery
St. Christopher's Hospital for Children
Philadelphia, Pennsylvania
106: *Intramedullary Spinal Tumors*

Russell O. Pieper, PhD
Associate Professor of Neurological Surgery
University of California, San Francisco
San Francisco, California
2: *Molecular and Cell Biology*

Ian F. Pollack, MD
Walter Dandy Professor of Neurological Surgery
University of Pittsburgh School of Medicine;
Co-Director
University of Pittsburgh Cancer Institute Brain
    Tumor Center;
Professor of Neurosurgery
Children's Hospital of Pittsburgh;
Professor of Neurosurgery
University of Pittsburgh School of Medicine
Pittsburgh, Pennsylvania
79: *Supratentorial High-Grade Gliomas*

Martin G. Pomper, MD, PhD
Associate Professor
Departments of Radiology, Pharmacology and
    Molecular Sciences and Oncology
Johns Hopkins University
Baltimore, Maryland
29: *Chordoid Glioma of the Third Ventricle*

Michael D. Prados, MD
Professor of Neurological Surgery
Charles B. Wilson Endowed Chair in Neurological
    Surgery
Director, Clinical Neuro-Oncology Program
Brain Tumor Research Center
University of California, San Francisco,
    School of Medicine
San Francisco, California
11: *Chemotherapy Principles*
17: *Diffuse Astrocytoma*
19: *Glioblastoma Multiforme*
28: *Gliomatosis Cerebri*

Richard A. Prayson, MD
Professor of Pathology
Cleveland Clinic Lerner College of Medicine at
    Case Western Reserve University;
Section Head of Neuropathology
Department of Anatomic Pathology
The Cleveland Clinic
Cleveland, Ohio
30: *Mixed Neuronal and Glial Tumors*

James N. Provenzale, MD
Professor of Radiology;
Chief, Neuroradiology
Duke University Medical Center
Durham, North Carolina
25: *Ependymoma*

Alfredo Quinones-Hinojosa, MD
Neurosurgery Chief Resident
University of California, San Francisco,
    School of Medicine
San Francisco, California
26: *Choroid Plexus Tumors*

Ganesh Rao, MD
Resident, Neurosurgery
University of Utah School of Medicine
Salt Lake City, Utah
86: *Pleomorphic Xanthoastrocytoma*

Corey Raffel, MD, PhD
Professor of Neurosurgery
Mayo Clinic College of Medicine
Mayo Clinic
Rochester, Minnesota
89: *Medulloblastoma*

Vaneerat Ratanatharathorn, MD, MBA
Professor and Chairman of Radiation Oncology
University of Arkansas for Medical Sciences;
Head of Radiation Oncology
Arkansas Cancer Research Center;
Co-Director
University of Arkansas Gamma Knife Center
Little Rock, Arkansas
55: *Management of Central Nervous System
    Metastases from Breast Carcinoma*

Kevin P. Redmond, MD
Associate Clinical Professor, Department of
    Radiation Oncology
University of Cincinnati College of Medicine;
Associate Clinical Professor
Division of Radiation Oncology
Department of Radiology
Barrett Cancer Center
Cincinnati, Ohio
60: *Multidisciplinary Management of Patients with
    Brain Metastases from an Unknown Primary
    Tumor*

Amyn Rojiani, MD, PhD
Professor of Oncology and Pathology;
Director of Neuropathology
H. Lee Moffitt Cancer Center
University of South Florida
Tampa, Florida
18: *Anaplastic Astrocytoma*

Lucy B. Rorke, MD
Attending Neuropathologist
Department of Neuropathology
Childrens Hospital of Philadelphia
Philadelphia, Pennsylvania
99: *Atypical Teratoid/Rhabdoid Tumors*

James T. Rutka, MD, PhD, FRCSC
Professor and Chair of Neurosurgery
Dan Family Chair in Neurosurgery
Director, The Arthur and Sonia Labatt Brain
    Tumour Research Centre
The University of Toronto
Toronto, Ontario, Canada
76: *Optic Pathway Gliomas*
80: *Lhermitte-Duclos Disease*
84: *Cervicomedullary Astrocytomas*
92: *Pediatric Meningiomas*
94: *Pituitary Tumors in Children*
97: *Choroid Plexus Tumors*
108: *Neurocutaneous Syndromes*

Timothy Ryken, MD
Associate Professor
Departments of Neurosurgery and Radiation
    Oncology
University of Iowa College of Medicine;
University of Iowa Hospitals and Clinics
Iowa City, Iowa
58: *Intracerebral Metastatic Colon Carcinoma*

Madjid Samii, MD, PhD
Professor Emeritus
Hannover Medical School;
Director, International Neuroscience Institute
Hannover, Germany
43: *Acoustic Neuromas (Vestibular
    Schwannomas)*

John H. Sampson, MD, PhD
Associate Professor of Neurosurgery and
    Pathology
Duke University Medical Center
Durham, North Carolina
56: *Brain Metastases from Malignant Melanoma*

Robert A. Sanford, MD
Professor of Neurosurgery
Pediatric Neurosurgery, Semmes-Murphey Clinic
University of Tennessee College of Medicine
Semmes-Murphey Neurologic & Spine Institute
Memphis, Tennessee
88: *Ependymoma*

Michael Sargent, MD, MRCP, FRCR, FRCPC
Clinical Associate Professor
Department of Radiology
University of British Columbia;
Pediatric Neuroradiologist and Assistant
    Director
Department of Radiology
British Columbia Children's Hospital
Vancouver, British Columbia
103: *Epidural Spinal Tumors*

Raymond Sawaya, MD
Professor and Chair of Neurosurgery
Mery Beth Pawelek Chair in Neurosurgery
Director, Brain Tumor Center
University of Texas M.D. Anderson Cancer Center
Houston, Texas

S. Clifford Schold, Jr., MD
Professor and Chair
Department of Interdisciplinary Oncology
University of Southern Florida
Associate Center Director for Clinical Affairs
H. Lee Moffitt Cancer Center and Research
    Institute
Tampa, Florida
18: *Anaplastic Astrocytoma*

Ali Schwaiki, MD
Fellow, Hematology-Oncology
Department of Internal Medicine
University of Arkansas for Medical Sciences
Little Rock, Arkansas
55: *Management of Central Nervous System
    Metastases from Breast Carcinoma*

Theodore Schwartz, MD
Assistant Professor of Neurological Surgery
New York-Presbyterian Hospital
New York Weill Cornell Medical Center
Cornell Medical College
New York, New York
66: *Intramedullary Ependymomas*

Hilliard F. Seigler, MD
Professor of Surgery and Immunology
Duke University Medical Center School of
    Medicine
Durham, North Carolina
56: *Brain Metastases from Malignant Melanoma*

Timothy D. Shafman, MD
Department of Radiation Oncology
Duke University Medical Center
Durham, North Carolina
56: *Brain Metastases from Malignant Melanoma*

Patrick Shannon, MSc, FRCPC
Assistant Professor
Department of Pathobiology and Laboratory
    Medicine
The University of Toronto;
Staff Pathologist, Neuropathology
The Toronto Western Hospital;
Consulting Staff Pathologist, Fetal
    Neuropathology
The Mount Sinai Hospital
Toronto, Ontario, Canada
22: *Subependymal Giant Cell Astrocytoma and
    Tuberous Sclerosis Complex*

Dennis C. Shrieve, MD, PhD
Professor and Chair
Department of Radiation Oncology
University of Utah School of Medicine
Salt Lake City, Utah
45: *Meningiomas*

Sheila K. Singh, MD
Resident
Division of Neurosurgery
The University of Toronto
Toronto, Ontario, Canada
75: *Supratentorial Low-Grade Gliomas*

William H. Slattery III, MD
Clinical Professor
Department of Otolaryngology
University of Southern California;
Director of Clinical Research
House Ear Institute
Los Angeles, California
7: *Neurotology*

Andrew E. Sloan, MD
Assistant Professor
Wayne State University School of Medicine;
Chief of Neuro-Oncology
Karmanos Cancer Institute
Detroit, Michigan
35: *Medulloblastoma*

Jefferson C. Slimp, PhD
Associate Professor
Department of Rehabilitation Medicine;
Director, Neurophysiology Monitoring Program
University of Washington School of Medicine
Seattle, Washington
73: *Evaluation and Management of Benign
    Peripheral Nerve Tumors and Masses*

Edward R. Smith, MD
Instructor in Neurosurgery
Harvard Medical School;
Shillito Staff Associate in Pediatric Neurosurgery
Children's Hospital
Boston, Massachusetts
20: *Pilocytic Astrocytoma*

Justin S. Smith, MD, PhD
Resident
Department of Neurological Surgery
University of California, San Francisco,
    School of Medicine
San Francisco, California
28: *Gliomatosis Cerebri*

Susan Snodgrass, MD, RPh
Assistant Professor of Neuro-Oncology
H. Lee Moffitt Cancer Center and Research
    Institute
University of South Florida
Tampa, Florida
18: *Anaplastic Astrocytoma*

Mark M. Souweidane, MD, FACS
Associate Professor of Neurological Surgery
The Weill Medical College of Cornell University;
Vice Chairman and Director of Pediatric
    Neurosurgery
The Weill Medical College of Cornell University
Memorial Sloan-Kettering Cancer Center
New York, New York
77: *Thalamic Gliomas*

Paul Steinbok, MBBS, BSc, FRCSc
Professor
Department of Surgery
University of British Columbia;
Head, Division of Neurosurgery
British Columbia's Children's Hospital
Vancouver, British Columbia, Canada
103: *Epidural Spinal Tumors*

Caron Stralendorf, MB, BCh, FCP
Assistant Clinical Professor
University of British Columbia;
Pediatric Hematology, Oncology, Bone Marrow
    Transplantion
Children's and Women's Health Centre
Vancouver, British Columbia, Canada
103: *Epidural Spinal Tumors*

Mandeep S. Tamber, MD
Resident
Division of Neurosurgery
The University of Toronto
Toronto, Ontario, Canada
90: *Supratentorial Primitive Neuroectodermal
    Tumors*

Gianpiero Tamburrini, MD
Assistant Professor of Neurosurgery
Pediatric Neurosurgical Unit
Catholic University of Rome
Rome, Italy
85: *Desmoplastic Infantile Ganglioglioma*

Nancy J. Tarbell, MD
Professor of Radiation Oncology
Harvard Medical School;
Head, Pediatric Radiation Oncology
Massachusetts General Hospital
Boston, Massachusetts
20: *Pilocytic Astrocytoma*

Michael D. Taylor, MD, PhD
Neurosurgery Resident
Sonia and Arthur Labatt Brain Tumor Research
    Centre
The Hospital for Sick Children
Toronto, Ontario, Canada
91: *Dysembryoplastic Neuroepithelial Tumor*
99: *Atypical Teratoid/Rhabdoid Tumors*

Aramis Teixeira, MD
Department of Neurosurgery
University of Arkansas for Medical Sciences
Little Rock, Arkansas
49: *Paragangliomas of the Skull Base*

Tarik Tihan, MD, PhD
Associate Professor of Pathology
University of California San Francisco;
Attending Pathologist
University of California San Francisco School of
    Medicine
San Francisco, California
17: *Diffuse Astrocytoma*
21: *Pleomorphic Xanthoastrocytoma*
26: *Choroid Plexus Tumors*
34: *Pineoblastoma*
39: *Melanocytic Tumors*
62: *Spinal Axis Tumors: Incidence, Classification,
    and Diagnostic Imaging*

Tadanori Tomita, MD
Professor of Neurosurgery
Northwestern University Feinberg School of
    Medicine;
Chairman, Division of Pediatric Neurosurgery;
Director, Falk Brain Tumor Center
Children's Memorial Hospital
Chicago, Illinois
93: *Pineal Region Tumors in Children*

Ivo W. Tremont-Lukats, MD
Director of Neuro-Oncology and Brain Tumor
    Center
University of Texas M.D. Anderson Cancer Center
Houston, Texas
27: *Astroblastoma*

Eve C. Tsai, MD
Neurosurgery Resident
Toronto Western Hospital Research Institute
Toronto, Ontario
84: *Cervicomedullary Astrocytomas*

Martin J. van den Bent, MD, PhD
Neurologist, Neuro-Oncologist
Daniel den Hoed Cancer Center
Erasmus University Hospital
Rotterdam, The Netherlands
23: *Oligodendroglial Tumors*

Scott R. VandenBerg, MD, PhD
Professor of Pathology and Neurological Surgery;
University of California, San Francisco,
    School of Medicine
San Francisco, California
5: *Pathologic Classification*
31: *Neuronal Tumors*

G. Edward Vates, MD, PhD
Assistant Professor
University of Rochester School of Medicine;
Attending Neurosurgeon
Strong Memorial Hospital;
Director of Cerebrovascular and Skull Base
    Surgery
University of Rochester School of Medicine
Rochester, New York
28: *Gliomatosis Cerebri*
40: *Hemangioblastomas*

Corneila S. von Koch, MD, PhD
Clinical Instructor
Department of Neurosurgery
University of California San Francisco
San Francisco, California
81: *Cerebellar Astrocytomas*

Frank Vrionis, MD, PhD
Associate Professor of Neurosurgery, Oncology,
    and Neuro-Oncology Program
University of South Florida College of
    Medicine;
Associate Professor of Neurosurgery,
    Otolaryngology, and Oncology;
Director of Spinal and Skull Base Oncology
H. Lee Moffitt Cancer Center & Research
    Institute
Tampa, Florida
18: *Anaplastic Astrocytoma*

Toshihiko Wakabayashi, MD, PhD
Associate Professor
Center for Genetic and Regenerative Medicine
Nagoya University Hospital
Nagoya, Aichi, Japan
96: *Germ Cell Tumors in Children*

James Waldron, MD
Resident
Department of Neurosurgical Surgery
University of California, San Francisco,
    School of Medicine
San Francisco, California
13: *Immunotherapy*
63: *Nerve Sheath Tumors of the Spine*
69: *Benign Tumors of the Spine*

Sabrina M. Walski-Easton, MD
Neurosurgery Resident
University of Minnesota Medical School
Minneapolis, Minnesota
59: *Gynecologic Malignancies*

Jeremy Wang, MD
Chief Resident, Neurosurgery Service
Department of Surgery
The Weill Medical College of Cornell University
Memorial Sloan-Kettering Cancer Center
New York, New York
71: *Therapeutic Options for Treating Metastatic
    Spine Tumors*

Ronald E. Warnick, MD
Medical Director
The Jewish Hospital;
Director, Neuro-Oncology Division;
Professor, Department of Neurosurgery;
Director, Division of Surgical Neuro-Oncology
University of Cincinnati College of Medicine
Cincinnati, Ohio
60: *Multidisciplinary Management of Patients with
    Brain Metastases from an Unknown Primary
    Tumor*

Gordon A. Watson, MD, PhD
Department of Radiation Oncology
LDS Hospital
Salt Lake City, Utah
54: *Small Cell Lung Carcinoma*

K. Michael Webb, MD
Resident, Department of Neurosurgery
University of Virginia Health System
Charlottesville, Virginia
47: *Pituitary Adenomas*

Jason S. Weinstein, MD
Neurosurgery Resident
University of Oregon
Portland, Oregon
37: *Lipomatous Tumors*

Philip R. Weinstein, MD
Chief, Neurological Service
Veterans Administration Hospital;
Professor, Department of Neurological Surgery
Co-Director, Neurospinal Disorders Program;
Principal Investigator, Brain and Spinal Injury
    Center
University of California, San Francisco
San Francisco, California
63: *Nerve Sheath Tumors of the Spine*

John C. Wellons III, MD
Assistant Professor of Surgery and Pediatrics
Children's Hospital of Alabama
Birmingham, Alabama
105: *Pediatric Intradural and Extramedullary
    Spinal Cord Tumors*

Richard Wheeler, MD
Professor, Department of Internal Medicine;
Medical Director
Clinical Trials Office
Huntsman Cancer Institute
Salt Lake City, Utah
54: *Small Cell Lung Carcinoma*

John G. Wolbers, MD, PhD
Department of Neurosurgery
Erasmus University Medical Center
Rotterdam, The Netherlands
23: *Oligodendroglial Tumors*

Marguerite Wotoczek-Obadia, AHT
Coordinator of Neuro-Oncology Research
    Laboratory
H. Lee Moffitt Cancer Center and Research
    Institute
Tampa, Florida
18: *Anaplastic Astrocytoma*

Margaret Wrensch, PhD, MPH
Professor of Neurological Surgery
Co-Director, Division of Neuroepidemiology
University of California, San Francisco,
    School of Medicine
San Francisco, California
1: *Epidemiology of Brain Tumors*

Raafat Yahya, MD
Resident, Division of Neurosurgery
The University of Toronto
The Hospital for Sick Children
Toronto, Ontario, Canada
80: *Lhermitte-Duclos Disease*
97: *Choroid Plexus Tumors*

Jun Yoshida, MD, PhD
Professor and Chairman
Department of Neurosurgery
Nagoya University Graduate School of Medicine
Nagoya, Aichi, Japan
96: *Germ Cell Tumors in Children*

W.K. Alfred Yung, MD
Professor and Chairman
Department of Neuro-Oncology
University of Texas M.D. Anderson Cancer Center
Houston, Texas
24: *Mixed Gliomas*

Ping-pin Zheng, MD
Department of Pathology
Josephine Nefkens Institute
Erasmus Medical Center
Rotterdam, The Netherlands
23: *Oligodendroglial Tumors*

J. Chris Zacko, MD
Resident in Neurosurgery
Virginia Commonwealth University
Medical College of Virginia
Richmond, Virginia
38: *Fibrous Tumors*

Imad T. Zak, MD
Assistant Professor of Radiology
Director
Neuroradiology Fellowship Program
Harper University Hospital
Wayne State University
Detroit, Michigan
35: *Medulloblastoma*

Basic Essential Principles

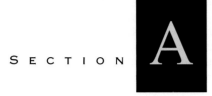

SECTION A **BASIC SCIENCE**

Section Editors

Mitchel S. Berger and Michael D. Prados

CHAPTER 1

EPIDEMIOLOGY OF BRAIN TUMORS

Margaret Wrensch, Terri Chew, Mitchel S. Berger, Yuriko Minn, Melissa L. Bondy

Epidemiology is concerned with measurements of health in human populations—quantifying the incidence and prevalence of a disorder, disability, or injury; its distribution; and the risk factors that may determine its occurrence and course. At times, epidemiologic evidence even suggests the root cause. Long restricted to evaluating mainly clinical, developmental, and environmental exposures, epidemiologists now have open to them molecular and genetic techniques that provide new areas for exploration and may lead to refinements in exposure measurements. In the study of brain tumors, molecular and genetic epidemiology may help define the disease.

Primary brain tumors are among the top 10 causes of cancer-related deaths in the United States, accounting for approximately 1.4% of all cancers and 2.4% of all cancer-related deaths.[1] About 14 per 100,000 people in the United States are diagnosed with a primary brain tumor each year, and 6 to 8 per 100,000 are diagnosed with a primary malignant brain tumor.[8] Approximately 35,000 people in the United States are newly diagnosed with a primary brain tumor each year. The prognosis for patients who develop these tumors is bleak, with average survival after diagnosis ranging from 6 to 8 years for those with low-grade astrocytoma or oligodendroglioma to 12 to 18 months for those with glioblastoma.[1] The only proven causes of brain tumors—inherited genetic syndromes,[6] therapeutic ionizing radiation,[30] and immunosuppression causing brain lymphoma[16,35]—account for a small number of the cases diagnosed each year.

Epidemiologic studies have an important role in research into the causes, progression, and outcome of primary brain tumors. Descriptive epidemiologic studies link histologic tumor type and demographic characteristics (such as age, sex, and race) of patients affected by primary brain tumors to associated incidence, prevalence, mortality, and survival rates. Analytic epidemiologic studies analyze suspected risk factors for

brain tumor, such as diet, smoking, alcohol consumption, occupational and industry hazards, exposure to radiation, and inherited genetic factors through either cohort studies (the risk of brain tumor in people with or without a specific characteristic) or case-control studies (comparative histories of people with and without brain tumors).

Recent dramatic progress in the molecular classification of brain malignancies and the identification of genes suspected to play a part in their progression have resulted in new approaches to delivering therapy to brain tumors and breaking down their resistance to drugs and radiation. These advancements lend renewed incentive in seeking means for prevention and cure of these devastating diseases.

DESCRIPTIVE EPIDEMIOLOGY: PATIENTS' CHARACTERISTICS AND THE ASSOCIATED RISK OF BRAIN TUMOR

Issues in Describing the Incidence of Brain Tumors

Among children younger than 14 and adults 70 years old and older, incidence rates for primary brain malignancies were significantly higher from 1991 to 1995 than from 1975 to 1979.[24] In the 15- to 44-year-old age group, there were no meaningful differences in overall rates between the two periods. For people in the 45- to 64-year-old age group, rates were somewhat lower for the more recent period. Increases in the incidence of primary malignant brain tumors, particularly among the elderly, have been attributed to several factors: improved diagnostic procedures, such as computed tomography and magnetic resonance imaging (MRI); a greater availability of neurosurgeons; changing patterns of access to medical care; and evolving medical approaches toward elderly patients.[11,19,24] Although environmental factors have been implicated in some analytic epidemiologic studies, no risk factors accounting for a large percentage of brain tumors have been identified. For this reason, researchers cannot yet hope to quantitatively explain temporal trends on the basis of changes in environmental factors. At present, any comparisons across time periods or across studies are complicated by a variety of factors. Incidence rates can differ among studies simply because of differences in definitions and methodologies in ascertaining and categorizing tumors.[29] Registry data can suffer from ascertainment biases as a result of reporting differences and variability in the availability of health care. The complexity of the anatomic, pathologic, and clinical classifications of brain tumors is problematic, and there is still dispute about how some tumor histologies, especially mixed tumor types, should be classified. This complexity is apparent when one considers that the Central Brain Tumor Registry of the United States categorizes 30 different histologic types of primary brain and central nervous system tumors resulting from 215 individual histology codes.[8] In the future, the use of genetic or other markers in conjunction with neuropathologic diagnosis may help to achieve a more precise system of tumor classification. Above all, a uniform, accurate, and unbiased method for the registration of both benign and malignant brain tumors in adults and children would help to clarify variations in the incidence of brain tumors.[11,18]

Age

Patients' median age at onset for all primary brain tumors is about 57 years.[8] Age distributions differ by site and by the histologic type of tumor, suggesting that different histologic types may have different etiologies. Some of this variation may be accounted for by differing diagnostic practices and access to diagnosis in different age groups. It seems probable that duration of exposure required for malignant transformation, the number of genetic alterations required to produce clinical disease, or poorer immune surveillance with advancing age accounts for those tumor types that increase in incidence with age. A peak in incidence of brain tumors among young children—some, but not all, of which can be attributed to medulloblastoma and other tumors of primitive neuroectodermal origin—remains an intriguing and incompletely explained feature of brain tumor epidemiology.

Sex

Overall, primary brain tumors are more common in males than females.[34] However, meningiomas are about twice as common in females as in males, and tumors of the cranial and spinal nerves and of the sellar region affect males and females almost equally.[8]

Geographic and Ethnic Variations

Both ascertainment bias and inconsistent reporting complicate the interpretation of geographic and ethnic variations in the incidence of brain tumors. Access to health care is an important geographic and ethnic factor because reported rates for primary malignant brain tumors tend to be higher in countries with more accessible and highly developed medical care.[20,30] However, an exception is in Japan, where access to medical care is similar to that in Northern Europe, but where the incidence rate for malignant brain tumors is less than half that in Northern Europe. Among other influences are cultural, ethnic, or geographic differences in risk factors. In the United States, glioma affects more whites than blacks, but the incidence of meningioma is nearly equal among blacks and whites. Thus the differences are not likely to be attributable only to differences between blacks and whites in their access to health care or in diagnostic practices.[34] The absolute variation in brain tumor incidence rates from high-risk to low-risk areas, in both the United States and the world, is about fourfold to fivefold.[20]

Survival and Prognostic Factors

The 5-year survival rate for all ages and all brain tumor types in the United States is 20% (95% confidence interval [CI], 18% to 22%).[12] Another measurement of patients' survival that is of interest is the conditional probability of survival to 5 years based on survival for the first 2 years after diagnosis.[14] In the United States between 1979 and 1993, the conditional probability of surviving another 3 years after survival to 2 years for all patients with primary malignant brain and other tumors of the central nervous system was 76.2% (95% CI, 74.8% to 77.6%); for glioblastoma, the conditional probability of survival for the same period was 36.4%; and the conditional probabilities of survival for patients with other tumor types were greater than 60%. Survival is known to be strongly related to the patient's age and tumor type.[8] Patients with glioblastoma multiforme consistently have the poorest survival rates in all age groups. Within any tumor type, older patients have poorer survival rates than younger patients. An exception is medulloblastoma or embryonal primitive tumors, which rarely occur in people older than 44 years. Children diagnosed before the age of 3 have poorer survival rates than children diagnosed at ages 3 to 14.[17] For all primary malignant brain tumors combined, the 5-year survival rate in children younger than 14 years is 72%.[17]

Overall survival for patients with primary malignant brain tumors has not improved much since the early 1970s,[24] but this factor, too, varies by age and histologic tumor type. Modest gains in survival time were achieved between 1975 and 1995 for people younger than 65, but there was little or no change for patients 65 years and older. Little progress has been made in survival from glioblastoma in the past 20 years, but 5-year survival rates for patients with medulloblastoma increased 20% from the 1970s to the 1980s. More recently, survival rates have leveled off.[12]

Age and tumor histology are still the strongest prognostic indicators for patients who have a brain tumor, although some other factors have been shown to influence survival to some extent. In all but 2 of 17 European countries, 5-year survival rates were somewhat better for women with primary malignant brain tumors than for men (20% versus 17%).[32] The location of a tumor and the extent of tumor resection are also factors predictive of overall or progression-free survival.[14]

Prevalence of Brain Tumors in the United States

The prevalence of brain tumors, which reflects their incidence and the duration of patients' survival, gives an idea of the extent

TABLE 1-1 **Potential Risk Factors for Primary Brain Tumors and Selected Epidemiologic Studies**

Authors	Potential Risk Factor	Outcome of Selected Epidemiologic Studies
Wrensch et al.[40]	Alcohol	Slight to no association.[40]
Schlehofer et al.[33] Wiemels et al.[39] Brenner et al.[7]	Allergies	An inverse association of allergic diseases with glioma.[7,33,39] Statistically significant inverse dose response of glioma with increasing numbers of allergens.[39]
Inskip et al.[21] Muscat et al.[28]	Cellular telephones	No association found in current studies.[21,28]
Caggana et al.[9] Chen et al.[10] Elexpuru-Camiruaga et al.[15] Kelsey et al.[22] Trizna [38]	Constitutive polymorphisms (in carcinogen metabolizing, DNA repair, and immune function genes)	Silent polymorphisms in DNA repair genes linked to oligoastrocytoma,[10] glioblastoma,[9] and astrocytoma.[9] Conflicting results for associations of cytochrome p4502D6 and glutathione transferase theta polymorphisms with increased risk.[15,22,38]
Blot et al.[2] Lubin et al.[27] Wrensch et al.[40]	Diet and vitamins	Mixed support for association of N-nitroso compounds, antioxidants, or specific nutrients with adult or childhood brain tumors.[2,28,40]
Preston-Martin & Mack[30]	Drugs and medications	Few statistically significant or consistent findings between brain tumor development and studied drugs.[30]
Lote et al.[26] Schlehofer et al.[33]	Epilepsy, seizures, or convulsions	Some association; causality is difficult to determine, because seizures are often a symptom of brain tumor.[26,33]
Wrensch et al.[41]	Family history of brain tumors	Reported relative risks range from almost 1 to 10.[41] Genetics or possible common exposure to environmental factors may contribute.
Bondy et al.[6]	Hereditary syndromes*	Convincing evidence that certain inherited genes may strongly influence the risk of primary brain tumor development.[6]
Inskip et al.[20] Gavin & Yogev[16] Taiwo[35]	Infectious agents or immunosuppression*	Some viruses cause brain tumors in experimental animals,[20] but except for studies of HIV-related brain lymphomas,[16,35] few epidemiologic studies have evaluated a potential role of viruses in human brain tumorigenesis.[20]
Loomis & Wolf[25] Preston-Martin & Mack[30] Wrensch et al.[40]	Ionizing radiation (therapeutic,* diagnostic, other)	Diagnostic radiation and nuclear material exposure may create elevated risk for some tumor types.[25,30] Therapeutic ionizing radiation is a strong risk factor for brain tumorigenesis.[30,40]
Bondy et al.[4] Bondy et al.[5]	Lymphocyte mutagen sensitivity (to gamma radiation)	Significantly associated with a risk of glioma.[4,5]
Thomas & Waxweiler[37]	Occupation and industry	Difficult to establish an association between exposure to specific occupational or industrial chemicals and human brain tumorigenesis.[37] Exposure to multiple chemicals and chemical interactions are two of the complicating factors.
Zahm[43]	Personal and residential chemical exposures	Some studies have shown a link between pesticide exposure and risk of childhood brain cancers.[43]
Wrensch et al.[42]	Power frequency electromagnetic field	No causal connection between EMF and risk of brain tumor has been established.[42] Measurement and unknown latency are complicating factors.
Teppo et al.[36]	Prior cancers	Increased risk among patients with small cell lung carcinoma and adenocarcinoma, but interpretation complicated by possibility of confusing metastatic and primary brain tumors.[36]
Boffetta et al.[3] Lee et al.[25]	Tobacco smoke exposure	No major contribution of maternal tobacco smoking to risk of childhood brain tumors,[3] small associations with paternal smoking. No important contribution of smoking filtered cigarettes to adult brain tumors.[23]
Raaschou-Nielsen et al.[31]	Traffic-related air pollution	No association between childhood brain tumor and exposure to traffic-related air pollution.[31]

*The only factors so far proved to cause primary brain tumors.
Cited references often have more detailed reviews of studies of these factors.

of the disease burden in an area, especially for brain tumor types associated with relatively long survival times, like meningioma. Davis and colleagues[13] recently published the first estimates of prevalence of primary brain tumors in the United States. They found that primary benign brain tumors had an estimated prevalence of 97.5 per 100,000 population for the year 2000 and emphasized the need for further studies of etiology and consideration of quality-of-life issues for this group of patients.

ANALYTIC EPIDEMIOLOGY OF BRAIN TUMORS: STUDIES OF RISK FACTORS

Within the brain tumor research community, there is little unanimity about the nature and magnitude of the risk factors for primary brain tumors. These tumors are highly heterogeneous histologically, and definitions and classifications of tumors often differ from one study to another. These factors, combined with retrospective assessments of exposure to risk factors and undefined latency periods, make for imprecise estimates of associations. Often, such limitations also make it difficult to compare studies. Differences in the eligibility criteria established for patients and control groups and the use of proxies further complicate the synthesis of results among studies. In addition, certain biologic and physiologic characteristics of the brain itself, such as the blood-brain barrier, add challenges to determining the risk factors for brain tumors.

Primary brain tumors are thought to develop through an accumulation of genetic alterations that permit cells to evade normal regulatory mechanisms and escape destruction by the immune system. In addition to inherited alterations in crucial genes that control the cell cycle, chemical, physical, and biologic agents that damage DNA are suspected potential neurocarcinogens. Unraveling the genetic, molecular, and cytogenetic errors in primary brain tumors is important to determining their pathogenesis. As work on elucidating patterns of molecular change continues, a more precise classification of brain tumors may evolve, making it possible to identify groups of tumors that are more homogeneous than current histologic groupings with respect to causal factors. Table 1-1, which summarizes only some of the vast number of epidemiologic studies of potential risk factors for brain tumor that have been performed, provides a sample of some of the major factors currently being analyzed.

CONCLUSION

There are very few proven causes for brain tumors, and they account for only a small proportion of cases. It is probable that primary brain tumors stem from multiple exogenous and endogenous events. Despite a persistently disheartening prognosis for patients who have a malignant brain tumor, the promise of molecular and genetic approaches has intensified efforts to define their biologic course and causes. Through these efforts, new concepts about neuro-oncogenesis are emerging to explicate the epidemiology of brain tumors and provide hope for a cure.

ACKNOWLEDGMENTS

This chapter was adapted with permission from Wrensch M, Minn Y, Chew T, Bondy M, Berger MS. Epidemiology of primary brain tumors: current concepts and review of the literature. Neuro-Oncol 4:278-99, 2002. The authors thank Sharon Reynolds for editorial collaboration and Susan Eastwood for helpful suggestions. Funding for this chapter was from National Institutes of Health grants R01CA52689 and 1P50CA97257.

References

1. ACS (American Cancer Society): Cancer Facts and Figures 2002. Atlanta, American Cancer Society, 2002.
2. Blot WJ, Henderson BE, Boice JD, Jr: Childhood cancer in relation to cured meat intake: review of the epidemiological evidence. Nutr Cancer 34:111–118, 1999.
3. Boffetta P, Tredaniel J, Greco A: Risk of childhood cancer and adult lung cancer after childhood exposure to passive smoke: a meta-analysis. Environ Health Perspect 108, 73–82, 2000.
4. Bondy ML, Kyritsis AP, Gu J, et al: Mutagen sensitivity and risk of gliomas: a case-control analysis. Cancer Res 56:1484–1486, 1996.
5. Bondy ML, Wang LE, El-Zein R, et al: Gamma radiation sensitivity and risk of glioma. J Natl Cancer Inst 93:1553–1557, 2001.
6. Bondy M, Wiencke J, Wrensch M, et al: Genetics of primary brain tumors: a review. J Neurooncol 18:69–81, 1994.
7. Brenner AV, Linet MS, Fine HA, et al: History of allergies and autoimmune diseases and risk of brain tumors in adults. Int J Cancer 99:252–259, 2002.
8. CBTRUS (Central Brain Tumor Registry of the United States): Primary Brain Tumors in the United States Statistical Report 1995–1999. Chicago, Central Brain Tumor Registry of the United States. 591–600, 2002–2003.
9. Caggana M, Kilgallen J, Conroy JM, et al: Associations between ERCC2 polymorphisms and gliomas. Cancer Epidemiol Biomarkers Prev 10:355–360, 2001.
10. Chen P, Wiencke J, Aldape K, et al: Association of an ERCC1 polymorphism with adult-onset glioma. Cancer Epidemiol Biomarkers Prev 9:843–847, 2000.
11. Davis FG, Bruner JM, Surawicz TS: The rationale for standardized registration and reporting of brain and central nervous system tumors in population-based cancer registries. Neuroepidemiology 16:308–316, 1997.
12. Davis FG, Freels S, Grutsch J, et al: Survival rates in patients with primary malignant brain tumors stratified by patient age and tumor histological type: an analysis based on Surveillance, Epidemiology, and End Results (SEER) data, 1973–1991. J Neurosurg 88:1–10, 1998.
13. Davis FG, Kupelian V, Freels S, et al: Prevalence estimates for primary brain tumors in the United States by behavior and major histology groups. Neuro-oncol 3:152–158, 2001.
14. Davis FG, McCarthy BJ, Freels S, et al: The conditional probability of survival of patients with primary malignant brain tumors: Surveillance, Epidemiology, and End Results (SEER) data. Cancer 85:485–491, 1999.

15. Elexpuru-Camiruaga J, Buxton N, Kandula V, et al: Susceptibility to astrocytoma and meningioma: influence of allelism at glutathione S-transferase (GSTT1 and GSTM1) and cytochrome P-450 (CYP2D6) loci. Cancer Res 55:4237–4239, 1995.

16. Gavin P, Yogev R: Central nervous system abnormalities in pediatric human immunodeficiency virus infection. Pediatr Neurosurg 31:115–123, 1999.

17. Grovas A, Fremgen A, Rauck A, et al: The National Cancer Data Base report on patterns of childhood cancers in the United States. Cancer 80:2321–2332, 1997.

18. Gurney JG, Wall DA, Jukich PJ, et al: The contribution of nonmalignant tumors to CNS tumor incidence rates among children in the United States. Cancer Causes Control 10:101–105, 1999.

19. Helseth A: The incidence of primary central nervous system neoplasms before and after computerized tomography availability. J Neurosurg 83:999–1003, 1995.

20. Inskip PD, Linet MS, Heineman EF: Etiology of brain tumors in adults. Epidemiol Rev 17:382–414, 1995.

21. Inskip PD, Tarone RE, Hatch EE, et al: Cellular telephone use and brain tumors. N Engl J Med 344:79–86, 2001.

22. Kelsey KT, Wrensch M, Zuo ZF, et al: A population-based case-control study of the CYP2D6 and GSTT1 polymorphisms and malignant brain tumors. Pharmacogenetics 7:463–468, 1997.

23. Lee M, Wrensch M, Miike R: Dietary and tobacco risk factors for adult onset glioma in the San Francisco Bay Area (California, USA). Cancer Causes Control 8:13–24, 1997.

24. Legler JM, Ries LA, Smith MA, et al: Cancer surveillance series [corrected]: Brain and other central nervous system cancers: recent trends in incidence and mortality. J Natl Cancer Inst 91:1382–1390, 1999.

25. Loomis DP, Wolf SH: Mortality of workers at a nuclear materials production plant at Oak Ridge, Tennessee, 1947–1990. Am J Ind Med 29:131–141, 1996.

26. Lote K, Stenwig AE, Skullerud K, et al: Prevalence and prognostic significance of epilepsy in patients with gliomas. Eur J Cancer 34:98–102, 1998.

27. Lubin F, Farbstein H, Chetrit A, et al: The role of nutritional habits during gestation and child life in pediatric brain tumor etiology. Int J Cancer 86:139–143, 2000.

28. Muscat JE, Malkin MG, Thompson S, et al: Handheld cellular telephone use and risk of brain cancer. JAMA 284:3001–3007, 2000.

29. Pobereskin LH, Chadduck JB: Incidence of brain tumours in two English counties: a population based study. J Neurol Neurosurg Psychiatry 69:464–471, 2000.

30. Preston-Martin S, Mack W: Neoplasms of the nervous system. In Schottenfeld D, Fraumeni JF, Jr (eds): Cancer Epidemiology and Prevention, ed 2. New York, Oxford University Press, 1996, pp 1231–1281.

31. Raaschou-Nielsen O, Hertel O, Thomsen BL, et al: Air pollution from traffic at the residence of children with cancer. Am J Epidemiol 153:433–443, 2001.

32. Sant M, van der Sanden G, Capocaccia R: Survival rates for primary malignant brain tumours in Europe. EUROCARE Working Group. Eur J Cancer 34:2241–2247, 1998.

33. Schlehofer B, Blettner M, Preston-Martin S, et al: Role of medical history in brain tumour development: results from the International Adult Brain Tumour Study. Int J Cancer 82:155–160, 1999.

34. Surawicz TS, McCarthy BJ, Kupelian V, et al: Descriptive epidemiology of primary brain and CNS tumors: results from the Central Brain Tumor Registry of the United States, 1990–1994. Neuro-oncol. [serial online], Doc. 98-13, January 19, 1999. URL neuro-oncology.mc.duke.edu. Neuro-oncol 1:14–25, 1999.

35. Taiwo BO: AIDS-related primary CNS lymphoma: a brief review. AIDS Read 10:486–491, 2000.

36. Teppo L, Salminen E, Pukkala E: Risk of a new primary cancer among patients with lung cancer of different histological types. Eur J Cancer 37:613–619, 2001.

37. Thomas TL, Waxweiler RJ: Brain tumors and occupational risk factors. Scand J Work Environ Health 12:1–15, 1986.

38. Trizna Z, de Andrade M, Kyritsis AP, et al: Genetic polymorphisms in glutathione S-transferase mu and theta, N-acetyltransferase, and CYP1A1 and risk of gliomas. Cancer Epidemiol Biomarkers Prev 7:553–555, 1998.

39. Wiemels JL, Wiencke JK, Sison JD, et al: History of allergies among adults with glioma and controls. Int J Cancer 98:609–615, 2002.

40. Wrensch M, Bondy ML, Wiencke J, et al: Environmental risk factors for primary malignant brain tumors: a review. J Neurooncol 17:47–64, 1993.

41. Wrensch M, Lee M, Miike R, et al: Familial and personal medical history of cancer and nervous system conditions among adults with glioma and controls. Am J Epidemiol 145:581–593, 1997.

42. Wrensch MR, Minn Y, Bondy ML: Epidemiology. In Bernstein M, Berger MS (eds): Neuro-Oncology: The Essentials. New York, Thieme Medical Publishers, 2000.

43. Zahm SH: Childhood leukemia and pesticides. Epidemiology 10:473–475, 1999.

CHAPTER 2

MOLECULAR AND CELL BIOLOGY

Russell O. Pieper and Joseph F. Costello

CELL BIOLOGY

Our understanding of human cell biology has been facilitated by our understanding of the structure of the cell. The human cell can be generally divided into two parts, the nucleus and the cytoplasm. The nucleus is the site of DNA and RNA synthesis and contains the genetic material of the cell arranged in 23 pairs of chromosomes, each of which varies by size and which, upon staining, can be distinguished one from another under a simple light microscope. The approximate 3 m of human chromosomal DNA is packaged to fit inside a human cell of approximately 20 μm in diameter by its association with histones, charged proteins around which the DNA is coiled and condensed. In addition to associating with histones, the chromosomal DNA is also attached in a transient manner to the nuclear matrix, a collection of scaffold proteins that further influences DNA packaging and accessibility of DNA to factors that influence gene expression. The nucleus is separated from the cytoplasm by the nuclear envelope, a double membrane breached by nuclear pores that allow import and export of factors critical in gene and protein expression. The cytoplasm itself is a viscous material filled with an interlaced pattern of protein filaments called the cytoskeleton. The cytoskeleton organizes the cytoplasm into compartments, which in turn contain the various intracellular organelles that carry out the intermediate metabolism of the cell. These organelles include the ribosome-studded endoplasmic reticulum, which carries out protein synthesis; the Golgi apparatus, which directs macromolecules to their appropriate intracellular locations; the mitochondria, which produce energy; lysozomes, which degrade molecules; and peroxisomes, which are involved in oxidative reactions. Surrounding the cytoplasm is the cell membrane, a lipid bilayer embedded with proteins critical for interactions between the cell interior and the extracellular environment. The proteins include transporters, growth-factor receptors, neurotransmitter receptors, and import and efflux proteins. Together, these components allow the cell to carry out all functions necessary for its contribution to the organism as a whole.

New cells are created by the process of cell division. Cell division is in turn intimately linked to the cell cycle. The human cell cycle is divided into four parts: G1, S, G2, and mitosis (M) (with a fifth phase, G0, reserved for cells not in the cell cycle).[14] Cells begin the process of cell division by preparing to replicate their DNA in the G1 phase. In this phase, nucleotides and all components necessary for duplication of DNA are created. The DNA is duplicated in the S phase. The movement from G1 to S phase is carefully regulated by the G1 checkpoint, which in turn is carefully controlled by the expression of cyclin and cyclin-associated proteins that monitor the process and allow or prohibit further cell-cycle progression. In S phase, the cell replicates its DNA and moves into the G2 phase, in which components necessary for physical division of the cell are synthesized. Movement of the cell out of G2 and into mitosis is also rigorously controlled by the G2 checkpoint, activation of which stalls entry into mitosis. Mitosis itself is divided into four parts—prophase, metaphase, anaphase, and telophase—during which the replicated chromosomes condense, align, are segregated into two daughter cells, and ultimately decondense to take their normal histone-associated conformation. Following completion of replication, the cells can divide again or move into the G0 phase of the cell cycle depending on the extracellular cues received.

The life of the cell following division consists of three primary functions: energy production, interaction with its environment, and interaction with neighboring cells. The process of energy production is accomplished in the cytoplasm by mitochondria and takes one of two paths depending on the availability of oxygen. In the presence of oxygen, cells rely on aerobic glycolysis to convert glucose to pyruvate, after which the pyruvate is converted via the citric acid cycle into CO_2 and H_2O with the concomitant production of adenosine 5′-triphosphate (ATP). In tumors, however, the growth rate of cells often exceeds the availability of oxygen, a problem compounded by the disordered growth and poor vascularization characteristic of tumors. In tumors (and in normal tissues in which oxygen is limited, such as exercising muscle), cells have the ability to produce energy in the absence of oxygen by converting pyruvate to lactate, a reaction that yields considerably less ATP than complete oxidative phosphorylation. Although anaerobic glycolysis remains a secondary, fallback means of energy production in most cells, tumors, even under well-oxygenated conditions, produce high levels of pyruvate and often rely on anaerobic metabolism more than aerobic energy generation.[7] This so-called "Warburg effect" in part explains why many tumor cells appear to have very high rates of glucose metabolism and further illustrates the idea that, although all cells need to produce energy, the multiple paths by which this can occur allow for differences between normal and tumor cells.

In addition to energy production, a second fundamental function of cells is interaction with the extracellular environment. As noted, the cell membrane is studded with a variety of proteins whose primary role is to sense signals in the extracellular environment and to relay these signals to the interior and to the nucleus. The sensing of the extracellular environment is mediated by four major types of molecules: transmembrane G–protein-linked receptors, receptor protein tyrosine kinases, ligand-gated ion channels, and intracellular receptors. Although the molecular details of how activation of these receptors is linked to cellular action vary, in each case ligand binding results in changes in the receptor or in receptor-associated proteins that lead either to alterations in ion movement in and out of the cells or in changes in gene expression. As an example, activation of the epidermal growth-factor receptor leads to activation of pathways that ultimately change gene expression in ways that stimulate cell-cycle progression and support cell survival. In addition, each signaling cascade has the potential to amplify the signal such that a small stimulus can lead to prolonged cellular effects. Most significantly, however, the overexpression of such receptors or the dysregulation of the intracellular pathways that link the receptors to cellular actions can lead to constitutive activation of these pathways. In the case of growth-factor pathways controlled primarily by receptor tyrosine kinases (such as the epidermal growth-factor receptor), this dysregulation can lead to unrestricted growth signaling and aberrant proliferation. Therefore, in cancers, and particularly in brain tumors, the pathways that cells use to sense their environment can serve as a driving force for the disease and potentially also as targets for therapeutic intervention.

Although energy production and interaction with the extracellular environment are key cellular functions, from a larger organism-based view the ability of cells to interact appropriately with neighboring cells is critical in keeping the organism functioning properly. The ability of cells to interact with their neighbors is controlled by membrane-bound receptors known as integrins. Integrin complexes exist as dimers of one of 16 alpha subunits and one of 8 beta subunits, each dimer interacting with a different extracellular component found in the extracellular matrix or in neighboring cell membranes.[4] The signaling pathways that emanate from ligated integrin complexes are complicated and involve both positive and negative signals regulating the cell cytoskeleton, cell adhesion, cell movement, protease expression and secretion, protein degradation, and cell division. Although appropriate balance of these signals leads to cells that function in a normal ordered environment, dysregulation of these signals can lead to degradation of extracellular proteins, movement of cells, growth of cells in the absence of cell contact, recruitment of blood vessels, and a variety of effects that are critical to the tumor phenotype. The disruption of normal cell-to-cell contact is therefore critical to the formation of tumors that must not only divide but also move through or displace existing cells in the environment. Cell-to-cell communication therefore represents an important control mechanism that is lost in tumorigenesis.

At the end of the life span of the cell, a variety of processes allow for cell removal and eventual replacement. The cell death process can be subdivided into necrotic cell death and apoptosis.[10] Necrotic cell death represents the most destructive form of cell elimination. In this process, cellular insults including but not limited to viruses, bacterial toxins, and complement lead to swelling of the cell, plasma membrane collapse, cell rupture, and release of cellular contents into the environment. This type of cell death, which is often considered to be nonprogrammed and not dependent on expression of new genes, initiates an immune response and can lead to the death of neighboring cells as well as the primary cell itself. In contrast, death by apoptosis results not in cell lysis but rather in cell shrinkage, disintegration of the cell into small, well-enclosed apoptotic bodies, and the display of unique lipids on the cell membrane that allow engulfment of the apoptotic bodies by professional macrophages or in many cases by neighboring cells. The apoptotic process, like necrosis, can be triggered by external toxic stimuli, but can also be activated by receptor-ligand binding or by other physiologic processes. A specialized form of apoptosis, referred to as *aniokis*, can be triggered by detachment of cells from components of the extracellular matrix. Because apoptosis is considered to be a form of programmed cell death, the process is rigorously controlled by both proapoptotic and antiapoptotic molecules that can swing the balance between cell survival and cell elimination. Furthermore, the process appears to be critically linked to energy metabolism, because apoptosis appears to be initiated in the mitochondria and can take place in the absence of a cell nucleus. Although the cell death process is critical for the remodeling of normal tissue, it has special importance in cancer states, in which cells outside their normal environment must suppress activation of programmed cell death pathways while at the same time maintaining activated growth pathways.

The normal life of the cell is a highly ordered process in which cell replication gives rise to cells that produce energy, interact with their environment and neighbors, and die in a highly ordered fashion. The initiation of the tumorigenic process alters many, if not all, of these pathways, such that the surviving tumor cell must not only activate growth pathways and divide but also produce energy and suppress cell death in sometimes hostile and foreign cellular environments. Certainly not all tumor cells can do so, and solid tumors such as gliomas often contain significant numbers of dead cells. Selection pressures, however, can allow the emergence of cells with the appropriate combination of alterations that allow survival and proliferation. Our understanding of normal cell biology has therefore provided significant clues about defects present in tumors, including brain tumors, and how to potentially use these defects for therapeutic advantage.

MOLECULAR BIOLOGY

All cellular functions depend on the coordinated activity of molecules. Molecules can be very small and detectable only through experimental molecular biology techniques, whereas others are macromolecules that are visible in the light microscope. It is the nature and activity of these molecules that together constitute the primary focus of molecular biology.

The flow of information between molecules is perhaps the most well-studied aspect of molecular biology. The central dogma of molecular biology is that information is encoded in DNA, transcribed to RNA, and then translated into protein. The proteins carry out the vast majority of molecular activities. Although this pattern is generally true, RNA itself can also provide important structural or catalytic activities. Proteins and RNA in turn regulate and maintain the information encoded in DNA, completing a continual and circular flow of information. Protein–protein interactions are essential to intrinsic cellular activities such as regulating the cell cycle. Proteins, lipids, and inorganic ions also mediate the cell's response to extracellular signals such as growth factors or cell–cell interactions through a multistep process called *signal transduction.* The cell's response to exogenous agents such as chemotherapy also involves transduction of information through proteins and the cell signaling machinery, as well as through the induced DNA damage itself. Regulation and fine tuning of the information flow also comes in the form of normal postsynthesis modifications of DNA, RNA, and proteins.

The starting point in the flow of information is the DNA molecule. DNA is the heritable material of genes and chromosomes that stores, or encodes, the information for creating proteins. The building blocks of DNA are nucleotides, which contain one of four bases, either adenine (A), guanine (G), cytosine (C), or thymine (T). A phosphodiester bond connects adjacent nucleotides asymmetrically, giving the DNA strand a 5' to 3' directionality. The two strands are then held together by specific base pairing along the strands, A with T and C with G. The combination of directionality and base pairing is the basis of the complementary, antiparallel nature of the two strands in a DNA double helix. This structure, seen in each chromosome, is essential for faithful DNA replication during mitosis, DNA repair, and heredity.

The human genome consists of 23 different chromosomes and is approximately 3×10^9 base pairs (bp) long.[6,15] In addition to this nuclear DNA, there are also 16,571 bp of DNA in each mitochondrion. More than 50% of the human genome is composed of repetitive elements, short sequences derived from formerly mobile genetic elements (transposons) that have been incorporated over millions of years, though their current function is unknown. In contrast to the repeat sequences, genes serve as the blueprint for RNA and proteins. The number of genes in the human genome is estimated at 30,000 to 40,000, only two times more than some worms and three times more than the fruit fly. The parts of genes that code for proteins, called exons, constitute less than 5% of the genome. Each gene has at least one promoter, which is a regulatory DNA sequence located at the start (5' end) of the gene, and an average of nine exons separated by contiguous noncoding DNA called *introns.* Fifty to sixty percent of all promoters are contained within DNA regions termed *CpG islands.*[3] CpG islands are typically 1000 bp and are unusual in their base content: They have a higher G and C content and approximately five times more CpG dinucleotides than the rest of the genome. A proportion of the promoters within CpG islands appears to function bidirectionally, regulating two genes that are in a head-to-head configuration.[1] Other gene regulatory elements in DNA include enhancers and repressors, which positively and negatively regulate transcription, respectively. These regulatory elements can be nearby or distant from the gene they influence, and their activity can be further influenced by intervening DNA sequences termed *insulators.*

Information flows from the DNA to the RNA by the process of transcription, the creation of an RNA copy of a gene. RNA polymerases and transcription factors initiate transcription within the promoter, and additional proteins such as positive transcription elongation factor b (P-TEFb) help elongate the RNA copy through the exons and introns to the 3' end of the gene to produce a relatively large heteronuclear RNA (hnRNA).[13] The elongation process can also be negatively regulated by molecules such as the Von Hippel Lindau (VHL) tumor suppressor gene. The introns are spliced out of the molecule to generate the mature messenger RNA (mRNA). Identical hnRNA molecules from a gene may be spliced differently to produce different mRNAs (i.e., differential splicing) and ultimately a greater diversity of proteins. Similarly to DNA, RNA also contains four bases, adenine, guanine, cytosine, and uracil (U) (rather than the thymine in DNA). RNA does not form a double helix like DNA but is composed of a single strand that adopts secondary structures, including regions of double-strand character. More than 95% of the RNA in a cell is ribosomal RNA (rRNA) and transfer RNA (tRNA), whereas only a few percent are mRNA. In addition to the protein-coding portions, mRNAs contain 5' and 3' regulatory elements. The protein-coding portion starts with the ATG codon, which encodes for a methionine in the corresponding protein. The protein-coding portion, also called the *open reading frame,* is preceded by a 5' untranslated region (5' UTR) and flanked on the 3' end with a 3' UTR and a poly(adenylic acid) (polyA) tail. The very abundant rRNA, in contrast, does not code for proteins but instead serves as a component of ribosomes, the protein and RNA complex where proteins are synthesized. tRNA also participates in protein synthesis by acting as an adapter to decode the mRNA through an anticodon and paired amino acid. Other noncoding RNAs serve unique functions in the cell. For example, the RNA produced from the X-inactivation-specific transcript (XIST) gene binds directly to one of the two X chromosomes in female cells to help initiate X inactivation.[8] RNA produced from an RNA-component-of-telomerase gene helps in the synthesis of telomeres, which are located at the ends of chromosomes.[12] There is also evidence that very short (21 to 23 bp) double-strand RNAs, termed *small inhibitory RNAs* (siRNAs), are produced in mammalian cells and appear to have a role in regulating gene expression. siRNAs are also a very useful experimental tool in molecular biology to selectively inhibit the expression of particular genes.[9] Thus DNA is transcribed into RNAs that either can be the guide for protein production or may feed back directly to maintain and regulate the DNA.

Following transcription, information flows from the mRNA to proteins through the process of translation. Translation is the production of proteins from amino acids, using the mRNA as a template and the tRNA as an amino acid donor. Translation follows the genetic code, a set of rules by which each specific set of three nucleotides (i.e., a codon) in the mRNA is translated into a particular amino acid in the protein being synthesized. The carboxyl terminus of one amino acid is then linked to the amino terminal of the next amino acid through a peptide bond. After translation, a protein may also be proteolytically processed to remove short pieces on either end, allowing the protein to adopt an active conformation. It is the precise sequence of amino acids in a protein that determines its final conformation. Many smaller, newly synthesized proteins undergo spontaneous folding into a three-dimensional structure (i.e., the tertiary structure), whereas larger proteins may require the assistance of additional proteins called *chaperones* (e.g., Hsp70) to fold correctly. The tertiary structure imparts the unique function to the protein. Proteins have one or more domains that perform specific functions, such as a helix-loop-helix domain that binds DNA, or a protein kinase domain that catalyzes the phosphorylation of other proteins. Some proteins function as a monomer, whereas others are assembled into multimers such as dimers (e.g., platelet-derived growth factor, or PDGF), trimers (e.g., collagen), or tetramers (e.g., p53 tumor suppressor). Proteins can be subdivided by their cellular location, being extracellular (e.g., soluble vascular endothelial growth factor, or VEGF), intracellular (e.g., p53 or cyclin-dependent kinases), or transmembrane (e.g., epidermal growth-factor receptor, or EGFR). Nuclear proteins such as transcription factors regulate transcription of specific genes by binding to the DNA, thereby completing the feedback loop of information from DNA to RNA to protein and back to DNA.

In addition to this central flow of information, the activity of DNA, RNA, and protein can be regulated and fine tuned through endogenous modifications. Nearly all nucleated cells in the human body contain exactly the same sequence of DNA, the same genes, and the same chromosomes. Clearly, additional mechanisms are required to determine which subset of genes is active in a given cell, although these are poorly understood. In humans, the only known covalent modification of DNA is methylation. DNA methylation involves the addition of a methyl group to cytosine within a CpG dinucleotide, catalyzed by proteins called DNA methyltransferases.[2,5] The pattern of methylation is critical for maintaining a properly functioning genome. Methylation stabilizes chromosomes particularly in the centromeres, constrains the activity of parasitic DNA elements such as transposons, and maintains patterns of gene expression. On a larger scale, proper methylation is necessary for normal brain development and function. In cancers, the pattern and level of DNA methylation is compromised, and this contributes to the overall instability of chromosomes and to aberrant loss of gene expression. Similar to DNA methylation, RNA can also be modified by methylation, typically on adenine residues. This modification may alter the properties of the RNA, although this is less well understood.

In contrast to DNA and RNA, the variety of posttranslational protein modifications is much more extensive. Protein activity can be modified by the addition of chemical groups in the processes of acetylation and methylation (e.g., on histones), phosphorylation or dephosphorylation (e.g., on retinoblastoma [RB], the cell-cycle regulator and tumor suppressor), hydroxylation (e.g., on collagen), and N-formylation (e.g., on melittin). In addition, many membrane and secreted proteins can be modified by the addition of sugar side chains (glycosylation). Lipids can also be added to proteins (acylation, on many membrane proteins, and myristolylation, on some protein kinases). Each modification occurs specifically on one or a few specific types of amino acids. One type of modification can have completely opposite effects on the activity of a protein depending on where in the protein the modification occurs. The function of histone proteins, the main protein component of chromosomes, is regulated by a variety of these modifications, including acetylation, methylation, and phosphorylation, the sum total of which is called the *histone code*. The histone code may participate with various transcription factors in the differential regulation of genes. The activity of proteins is also regulated by their cellular localization.[11] For example, in response to a steroid hormone entering the cell, the hormone binds its receptor in the cytoplasm, and the complex is actively transported into the nucleus to allow the receptor to bind to DNA and regulate gene expression. Finally, proteins can be targeted for degradation by the addition of ubiquitin. Ubiquitination represents an end stage

of the information flow and is essential for controlled molecular signaling and a finite molecular response to changing cellular conditions.

The coordinated modification of proteins and protein–protein interactions described previously is the primary driving force for the process of signal transduction. Unlike steroid hormones, many signals from outside the cell are not able to enter the cell and therefore require receptors on the cell surface to begin the signal transduction into the cytoplasm and beyond. These receptors are proteins that can be classified according to the manner in which they transduce the signal. G–protein-coupled receptors activate intracellular G-proteins, which then bind guanosine triphosphate (GTP) and control downstream biochemical reactions using the energy release as GTP is converted to guanosine diphosphate (GDP). Tryosine kinase receptors, such as EGFR, have intrinsic tyrosine kinase activity that can both autophosphorylate and add phospho groups to tyrosines on other intracellular proteins. Tryosine-kinase-associated receptors do not have intrinsic kinase activity but are associated with kinases (e.g., JAK, or Janus kinase) that then phosphorylate downstream proteins (e.g., JAK phosphorylates signal transducer and activator of transcription [STAT], which then moves into the nucleus to regulate genes). Other transmembrane receptors include serine-threonine-kinase receptors and ion channel receptors that control the movement of ions and small molecules through the cell membrane. Following the initiation of signal transduction, the signal can reach the nucleus and genes directly, as in the case of phosphorylated STAT, or may involve a signaling cascade such as occurs with the mitogen-activated protein kinases (MAPKs). The activation of Ras, an important intermediate molecule in signal transduction pathways, also leads to a cascade of phosphorylation and second messenger activation and ties into other pathways such as that of MAPK. Inappropriate activation of the Ras pathway underlies the excessive growth of many human cancers, including brain tumors.

In addition to proteins, signal transduction can be more indirect by using second messengers such as adenosine 3′,5′-cyclic monophosphate (cAMP), ions such as calcium, or lipid components of the intracellular membrane such as phosphatidylinositol-4,5-bisphosphate (PIP$_2$). Upon activation of a phospholipase, PIP$_2$ can be cleaved to inositol-1,4,5-trisphosphate (IP$_3$), a calcium channel opener, and another second messenger 1,2-diacylglycerol (DAG) that initiates additional signaling cascades. Signal transduction often involves both the protein and these nonprotein molecules.

Protein–protein signaling and phosphoregulation of protein activity also lie at the heart of the cell cycle.[14] As stated earlier, the cell cycle has distinct phases, including M, G1, S, and G2. Transition from one phase to the next is tightly controlled at cell-cycle checkpoints (G1 to S and G2 to M) that are regulated by the activity state of cell-cycle proteins. Center stage in regulation of the cell cycle is the RB protein. In the hypophosphorylated state, RB binds to the E2F family of transcription factors and prevents them from activating genes required for the next phase, S, thereby maintaining the cell in G1. Cell-cycle progression requires a cyclin (e.g., cyclin D) and a cyclin-dependent kinase (CDK) (e.g., CDK4 and CDK6) to form a complex and phosphorylate RB. Further regulation is provided by inhibitors of CDKs, such as CDK inhibitor 2A (CDKN2A, also called p16), which blocks the phosphorylation of RB by CDK-cyclin complexes. Similarly, the transition between the G2 and M phases is regulated by the cyclin B–CDC2 complex, which is in turn regulated by removal of a phosphate on CDC2 by a phosphatase, CDC25C. Exit from mitosis involves a ubiquitin-mediated degradation of cyclin B and inactivation of CDC2. The molecular guardians of the checkpoints restrain the cell cycle in response to stress to the cell and to the DNA. For example, in response to DNA damage, the ataxia telangiectasia mutated (ATM) and Rad3-related (ATR) proteins induce cell-cycle arrest in G2 by inhibiting CDC2. This inhibition is mediated in part by the tumor suppressor p53. The parallels between normal cell-cycle regulation and the dysregulation seen in most human cancers are remarkable. In brain tumors of glial origin, for example, the most common abnormalities are in the RB and p53 pathways, including overproduction of CDK4 or CDK6 by gene amplification, loss of the inhibitor p16 by homozygous deletion, or mutation and deletion of the p53 gene.

Understanding the exact molecular pathways of signal transduction and the elaborate molecular control of cellular processes such as the cell cycle are important goals of molecular biology. Because it is the imbalance of these mechanisms that underlie tumorigenesis, elucidation of the relevant molecules and mechanisms is essential to the development of targeted anticancer therapies.

References

1. Adachi N, Lieber MR: Bidirectional gene organization: a common architectural feature of the human genome. Cell 109:807–809, 2002.
2. Baylin S, Bestor TH: Altered methylation patterns in cancer cell genomes: cause or consequence? Cancer Cell 1:299–305, 2002.
3. Bird A, Taggart M, Frommer M, et al: A fraction of the mouse genome that is derived from islands of nonmethylated, CpG-rich DNA. Cell 40:91–99, 1985.
4. Hood JD, Cheresh DA: Role of integrins in cell invasion and migration. Nat Rev Cancer 2:91–100, 2002.
5. Jones PA, Baylin SB: The fundamental role of epigenetic events in cancer. Nature Reviews Genetics 3:415–428, 2002.
6. Lander ES, Linton LM, Birren B, et al: Initial sequencing and analysis of the human genome. Nature 409:860–921, 2001.
7. Lu H, Forbes RA, Verma A: Hypoxia-inducible factor 1 activation by aerobic glycolysis implicates the Warburg effect in carcinogenesis. J Biol Chem 277:23111–23115, 2002.
8. Ogawa Y, Lee JT: Xite, X-inactivation intergenic transcription elements that regulate the probability of choice. Mol Cell 11:731–743, 2003.
9. Paddison PJ, Hannon GJ: RNA interference: the new somatic cell genetics? Cancer Cell 2:17–23, 2002.
10. Proskuryakov SY, Gabai VL, Konoplyannikov AG: Necrosis is an active and controlled form of programmed cell death. Biochemistry (Mosc) 67:387–408, 2002.
11. Schwoebel ED, Moore MS: The control of gene expression by regulated nuclear transport. Essays Biochem 36:105–113, 2000.
12. Shay JW, Wright WE: Telomerase: a target for cancer therapeutics. Cancer Cell 2:257–265, 2002.
13. Shilatifard A, Conaway RC, Conaway JW: The RNA polymerase II elongation complex. Annu Rev Biochem 72:693–715, 2003.
14. Stewart ZA, Westfall MD, Pietenpol JA: Cell-cycle dysregulation and anticancer therapy. Trends Pharmacol Sci 24:139–145, 2003.
15. Venter JC, Adams MD, Myers EW, et al: The sequence of the human genome. Science 291:1289, 1304–1351, 2001.

CHAPTER 3

ANIMAL MODELS

Dominique B. Hoelzinger and Michael E. Berens

Animal models are tools used to study various aspects of cancer. The complexity of the disease leads to the adoption of a variety of models that, to varying degrees, embody oncogenic transformation events, tumor response to therapy, strategies for preventing cancer, testing mechanisms for novel agent delivery, and reporter systems of drug metabolism by tumors. Sporadic cancers in humans and in animals show substantial variation in histopathology, pace of progression, and associated molecular genetic events. Disparate genetic backgrounds, as well as likely multiplicity in etiologic paths for cancer induction, ensure great heterogeneity in cancer presentation. In the midst of this variability, development of reproducible animal models affords schemes for testing hypotheses that would be untenable in spontaneous tumors.

Animal models have utility in developing an understanding of the underlying genetic events of oncogenesis. Once tumors arise in controlled animal populations, they can be studied to learn how cancer progresses from local to disseminated disease, from low-grade to high-grade patterns of behavior. Such observations assist in the development of markers of tumor progression. Ideally, changes in tumor growth in animals consequent to therapy are indications of similar responses in human tumors. In this regard, animal models provide systems to test treatment response in the development of new interventions. The complexity of tumor physiology, which includes not only the self-renewing tumor stem cells but also neovascularization, stromal tissue encounters, drug metabolism and distribution, and immune cell interactions with the neoplastic mass, is also open to investigation using animal models.

Whereas there is no one ideal animal model of cancer that embodies all desired features, certain available methods work within critical research constraints. These restraints include a model that is highly reproducible, is affordable, shows fast tumor growth, shows features homologous to the human disease, and is amenable to scale-up so that nuances of research queries can be addressed. Different model systems manifest alignment with these constraints to varying degrees. Selection of the animal model to test a hypothesis should be determined by the degree to which features of the model best adhere to the research paradigm. In that sense, the abundance of different model systems represents a toolbox with which to advance the discovery, development, and delivery of new approaches to and treatments for cancer.

TRANSPLANTABLE TUMORS IN ANIMAL MODELS

The most demanding application for animal models of tumors is the testing and development of new therapies. Because these therapies will be applied in human treatments, the growth of human tumors in animal systems should approximate a testing environment close to the eventual clinical response of tumor cells. However, growing understanding of the role of the host environment on cancer cell behavior leads to the caveat that human tumors growing in nonhuman hosts may introduce artificial and uncontrollable changes in cell behavior and response.[8,21] Techniques for inducing such tumors might also engage molecular changes unrepresented by spontaneous tumors.

Brain Tumor Allografts in Mice

A variety of induced brain tumors in mice has been developed that can be serially transplanted into cohorts of test animals of the same strain of mice. Such tumors grow reproducibly and are nonimmunogenic. These models have been used as tools for exploring tumor-host relationships that include immune cell modulation for therapeutic application. These models are readily identified by searching the literature for the tumor names: GL261, CT-2A, VM/Dk, SR-B10.A, and EPEN. Some of these models have existed since the 1980s but have not enjoyed as widespread an application as have rat brain tumors.

Advantages

Mice are inexpensive. The breeding paradigms of mice have developed an exquisite immunologic perspective that is unrivaled in any other species of research animal. Tools for evaluating tumor-host relationships are likely to have the fastest maturation using the inventory of information on mice.

Disadvantages

The mouse models of brain tumors have gained only a limited amount of attention, largely because of the difficulties in orthotopic placement of tumors. In addition, these tumors have not yet received the degree of characterization that rat tumor models have.

Brain Tumor Allografts in Rats

Chemical treatment of pregnant rats with carcinogenic agents such as ethylnitrosourea leads to a heightened incidence of brain tumors in litters.[7] Consequently, induction of brain tumors in inbred rats has received considerable attention and effort. A panel of serially transplantable, syngeneic rat brain tumors exists. Their use is traceable through searching the literature for the names of the tumor models: C6, 9L, RG2, T9, BT4C, and CNS-1. Their popularity in the field has led to the assembly of a substantial body of literature characterizing these tumors for a wide variety of features such as growth properties, histology, angiogenesis, molecular genetics, and utility as markers of chemo- and radiation-responsiveness. The thousands of published articles on these tumors attest to their wide acceptance and utility.

Advantages

Rat brain tumors are widely accepted in the biomedical research community. Their wide use affords a common vocabulary.

Disadvantages

To varying degrees and with limited exceptions, syngeneic rat brain tumors show only modest invasiveness in the brain and do not always recapitulate the histopathology of human primary gliomas.

Xenografts

The central challenge facing researchers who propagate human cells in nonhuman hosts is that of immune rejection of the xenograft. Chemical or radiologic immunosuppression can establish a host that is unable to reject a transplanted tumor; these approaches have been employed in larger animals. Selective breeding of rodents has generated strains of mice and rats deficient in either T cells or additional major effectors of the immune system. These hosts necessitate husbandry in sterile environments, with extensive attention to preservation of barrier protection. By definition, studies of human xenografts in immune-deficient animals are unable to advance an understanding of the complex interactions between tumors and the host's immune system.

Propagation of a human tumor in immunocompromised animals has as its starting point the collection of a biopsy from a spontaneous growth. Not all resected masses demonstrate an ability to grow in an immune-deficient animal. Because tumor transplantation techniques are more successful when highly malignant cells are used as the innoculae, most xenograft studies of human tumors are uninformative for investigations of tumor progression; the transplanted cells are already highly malignant. Successful development of serially transplanted human xenografts may also bias the model in uncontrolled ways because of the in vivo selection of cells most capable of surviving in the xenogenic host.[17]

The range of species into which human tumors have been transplanted includes mice, rats, and cats. Rodent models are readily amenable to use in most research institutes' vivaria; cats necessitate a more sizable commitment to infrastructure. Cats adapt the xenograft model to a system closer in dimension to that of humans. Optimizing tumor response to novel delivery approaches, such as convection-based delivery systems, ideally would be conducted in models of anatomic scale much larger than a rodent.

Nude and Severe Combined Immunodeficient Mice

Selection of the host species in which to propagate a human tumor is a pragmatic decision driven by cost considerations. Their low cost is the reason that nude and severe combined immunodeficient (SCID) mice are the most used. Many commercial vendors provide well-characterized strains of immunodeficient and immunocompromised animals suitable for xenotransplantation of human tumors.

Nude and Severe Combined Immunodeficient Rats

In instances where a larger host is desirable, nude and SCID rats have been developed. These are models readily adopted by vivaria in most academic medical centers and in biotechnology and pharmaceutical companies. For reasons of scale, xenografts in rats are useful for stereotactic implants into the natural site of the tumor's origin (orthotopic), which in the case of brain cancers is of considerable value.

Subcutaneous Implants

Expanding masses of tumor cells grown in the subcutaneous space of mice have provided interpretations of response to treatments. Such tumors are typically well vascularized, highly proliferative, and amenable to caliper measurements of tumor volume. In this regard, subcutaneous tumors in mice operate as a fairly high throughput screening system in the preclinical assessment of tumor response to therapy. Implantable chip transponders for animal identification become tools that conveniently allow controlled, blinded studies that ensure optimal execution of the investigation.

A recent appreciation for differences in vascular endothelial cells by tissue or organ system has highlighted the need to approach transplantable xenografts using orthotopic sites of injection. Similarly, stromal cell responses to a neoplastic growth show variation by organ system, and a more keen appreciation for differences in the parenchymal cells residing in different tissues indicate a need for careful consideration of sites of implantation for xenografts into locations where the tumor would have naturally arisen.

Intracranial Implants, Stereotaxy in Small Dimensions

Intentionality for anatomic and tissue representation of the tumor's environment has fostered use of stereotactic deposition of tumors in the brains of experimental model hosts. A common deficiency of orthotopic xenograft models of brain tumors is the absence of glial tumor invasion, which is a central element to the behavior of such cancers in humans. It may be that species differences in the cell–cell interactions or the cell-matrix relationships that exist between rodents and humans are sufficiently large that the invasive phenotype of human xenografts is poorly supported in these hosts. Recent modifications in the preimplant handling of human tumors before intracranial implants, coupled with a protracted interval for the emergence of intracranial tumors in athymic rats, yields a model more complementary to the human disease that also affords glioma cell invasion.[2,13]

GENETICALLY ENGINEERED MOUSE MODELS OF ORTHOTOPIC TUMORIGENESIS

Conditional control of gene expression that leads to cellular transformation may more closely recapitulate the evolution of genetic changes found in cancers as they progress through the stages of malignancy. Genetically engineered mouse models of orthotopic tumorigenesis provide a platform for learning more about the early changes in a cell or the sequence of changes that lead to more malignant phenotypes.[10] A sizable variety of mouse models of human cancers has been generated, and the descriptive characterization of these tumors is maturing. The National Institutes of Health National Cancer Institute hosts a Web site for tracking the status of various iterations of these engineered models.[14]

Germline Manipulation

Models employing germline manipulations are those wherein the chromosomal DNA of every cell of the mouse carries an engineered construct. Transgenes are introduced into the genome by microinjection of fertilized eggs or embryonic stem cells. At its most basic it entails tissue-specific expression of an oncogene or mutated oncogene believed to be involved in tumor initiation. The expression of an oncogene (v-src) is driven through the astrocyte-specific glial fibrillary acidic protein (GFAP) promoter,[23] which results in the appearance of astrocytomas but also of tumors of different histologic lineage such as schwannomas. Verification of transgene expression is obtained by immunohistochemical staining for v-src and GFAP. Easy visualization of transgene expression and concomitant confirmation of appropriate histologic expression is achievable by using a bicistronic vector in which the reporter gene lacZ is expressed in tandem with V12Ha-ras but translated separately.[1] The addition of a reporter gene also allows the evaluation of the number of transgene integrations into the genome by measuring the relative level of reporter gene expression, illustrating the importance of gene dosage in tumor formation and progression.

Advantages

This system allows for a targeted re-creation of the activation of specific signaling pathways involved in the genesis of specific tumors.

Disadvantages

Introduction of genes into the germline affords no temporal regulation of expression; the engineered gene is turned on throughout the range of biologic activity of the promoter. This could potentially result in embryonal lethality. Multisite, multicopy integration of the DNA construct could generate secondary genetic modifications, making interpretation of results more difficult. Position effect variegation can cause varying degrees of penetrance, requiring the creation of various genetically engineered mice (GEM) to verify the levels of reporter gene or transgene expression. Finally, germline manipulation does not address the interplay between multiple genetic changes that results in true tumor biology.

Somatic Cell Manipulation In Situ

Intracranial delivery of a virus carrying platelet-derived growth factor B (PDGF-B), driven by a viral promoter,[18] induces formation of histologically varied brain tumors. The advantages of this technique are the localized effect of PDGF-B overexpression and the temporal control of the gene activation. Retroviral gene delivery through the replication-competent avian leukosis virus (ALV) splice (RCAS) system ensures specific gene activation in a timed and tissue-specific manner. It requires GEM expressing the RCAS receptor tv-a from a tissue-specific promoter (TSP) and the RCAS acceptor with the gene of interest. The viral vector is a retrovirus that infects only specific cell types at one time: those expressing the ALV receptor tv-a, which is not encoded in the mammalian genome. In gliomas two such mouse lines have been developed, one expressing tv-a from the GFAP promoter[4] and one expressing it from the nestin promoter.[3] The viral particles are delivered by local injection of avian producer cells. Only a few hundred cells are infected, which reduces the probability of the occurrence of secondary genetic alterations (through insertional mutagenesis).

Advantages

Somatic cell manipulation combines several conditionally expressed genes or specific mutations at the same time in the same tissue to more accurately reflect the tumor's genetic or genomic make-up or sequential genetic changes during tumor progression. The approach allows targeted-tissue delivery at anatomically determined sites at designated times. Titration of virus to low titers results in a limited number of tumors being formed, which allows monoclonality of the mass.

Disadvantages

The viruses have a small carrying capacity of 2.5 kb or less. To the extent that there may be leakiness of the ALV expression, this approach may lack cell-type specificity in the infection, and thus induction of gene expression may leak across different cell lineages.

Conditional Knock-Outs with the Cre-lox System

The Cre-lox approach enables timed, precise somatic inactivation of tumor suppressor genes. Two engineered mouse strains are required for conditional gene deletion: first, a conventional transgenic mouse line with Cre driven by a specific tissue or cell-type promoter, such as the whey acidic protein (WAP) employed in a breast cancer model,[24] and second, a mouse strain that embodies a target gene (BRCA1) flanked by two loxP sites in a direct orientation (floxed gene). Recombination (excision and consequent inactivation of the target gene) occurs only in those cells expressing Cre recombinase. Hence, the target gene remains active in all cells and tissues that do not express Cre. The same system can be used to create conditional activation (knock-in) of an oncogene. In a lung cancer model,[5] a mouse strain with an activated K-ras G12D mutation preceded by a stop codon in the 5′ untranslated region (UTR) flanked by two loxP sites has been created. The oncogene remains untranscribed until the tissue-specific removal of the lox-stop-lox sequences is activated. The Cre recombinase is delivered by adenoviral (AdenoCre) infection of the lung epithelium. This mimics the early events in the genesis of lung tumors. Other knock-in models require the crossing of the oncogene harboring GEM with a GEM carrying the Cre gene driven from a TSP.

Advantages

The utility of this approach has led to a growing palette of tissue-specific Cre GEM lines. This affords an inventory for manipulation of multiple genes in the same cell, including turning some on and others off. The timing of the viral activation circumvents embryonic lethality.

Disadvantages

Recombination is an irreversible genetic change; the targeted cell and all its potential progeny will manifest the same expression profile for the manipulated gene and the pathways it affects. There remains an inability to obtain exact temporal control over promoter activation.

Controlled Manipulation of Gene Expression

Fine-tuned temporal control over gene expression is the hallmark of inducible systems such as the tetracycline-dependent regulatory system. This binary transgenic approach requires a GEM with the TSP driving transcription of the tetracycline-controlled transactivator (tTA) of transcription, as well as carrying the tetracycline operon (tetO) fused to the open reading frame (ORF) of choice. tTA is produced in the specified cell type; systemic treatment with doxocyline (Dox) prevents tTA from binding to tetO sequences to induce transcription. The ORF is transcribed when the cell is depleted of Dox. Reverse tTA (rtTA) is another, related system in which the administration of Dox is needed for transcriptional activation.[6]

Advantages

Because of the chemical control afforded in this system, gene expression is temporally controlled. Thus it is possible to stop the transgene's expression and study factors needed not only for tumor induction but also for the maintenance of the tumor phenotype. Multiple genes can be turned on simultaneously, including reporter genes like luciferace.[22]

Disadvantages

This system requires both constructs to be stably integrated and expressed to be tissue specific. The model may manifest leakiness. Once administered, there is a time lag for the clearance of Dox from each tissue (1 to 7 days); this could result in slow activation of the rtTA system and slow inactivation of the tTA system.

Combination Approaches

Temporal fine tuning of Cre expression or activity results in the formation of one generation of tumors, which might more closely resemble individual cancerous lesions. Two approaches have been developed to control the transcription or the activity of Cre.[12] Transcriptional control of Cre is achieved by using the tet inducible system, such that Cre is produced only in the desired tissue during a timed administration of Dox. Functional control of Cre activity depends on a Cre variant that functions only in the presence of an exogenous inducer such as RU486 or tamoxifen. The Cre variant is continuously present in the desired tissue but can localize to the nucleus only in the presence of the inducer.

Advantages

The combined approach provides very sophisticated tissue and temporal control of the expression of genes of interest.

Disadvantages

The level of complexity within each approach is compounded.

VALIDATION OF THE TUMOR MODELS

With increasing characterization of human cancers using genomic and proteomic tools, the investigator has better platforms with which to defend the alignment of the model systems with the spontaneous disease. It should be anticipated that in the near future there will be extensive verification of the model tumor's histology, gene expression profile, and therapy response.

ASSESSMENT OF BRAIN TUMOR BEHAVIOR IN ANIMAL MODELS

The ultimate outcome for successful modeling of tumors in animals is an end point for illumination of tumor biology or response to therapy. These all require measurements, some of which necessitate the termination of the test subject. Where possible and appropriate, nonlethal end points allow serial studies of tumor growth, which allows a reduction in the number of animals needed for conclusive experiments. This is always a high priority. Statistical programs by which to evaluate the number of animals needed to generate results of sufficient power to draw statistical inference of the outcome of the study should be accessed. A free-ware program that has proved instructive can be accessed at http://calculators.stat.ucla.edu/powercalc/.

Invasive/Terminal Techniques

The growth and invasion behavior of brain tumors in animals can be assessed using histologic techniques. These require that the animal be euthanized; such end points necessitate pilot studies of the growth properties of the tumor to time the collection of the brain tissue. For xenograft studies, discrimination of the human cells from host cells can be readily accomplished by using immunostaining of HLA markers. Other reporter genes such as green fluorescent protein or one of its derivatives establish a method by which to readily detect the cells of interest under fluorescence microscopy. Linking reporter genes to the tumor cells allows technologies such as laser capture microdissection to be applied to tumors in animals for probing tumor-host interactions, tumor invasion mechanisms, or angiogenic responses to tumors.

Physiology of Transplantable Tumors

One novel recent application to tumor transplantation is the installation of physiologic windows over the tumor for intravital microscopy of the emerging tumor.[15,19] These studies afford exploration of tumor-host interactions, especially as related to the neoangiogenesis coincident to tumor expansion. The interspecies variations notwithstanding, such applications afford a research tool by which to assess unique but critical features of the tumor-host relationship as the neoplastic mass expands.

Noninvasive/Vital Techniques

When possible, maintenance of tumor-bearing animals during the end point analysis reduces the numbers of animals needed for the experiments. These end points, however, are only collected with technologically sophisticated instruments and may

be beyond the reach of many facilities. Some recent developments in photon imaging have introduced lower-cost options for animal studies.

Magnetic Resonance Imaging

Imaging technology for real-time assessment of tumor volume and invasion patterns in experimental animals has kept abreast of model development. These techniques are crucial allies in the support to fully utilize the applications of such model systems. Magnetic resonance imaging (MRI) has been successfully applied to brain tumor studies in mice[9,20] and in rats.[16]

Photon Imaging: Bioluminescence

Genetic engineering techniques allow the installation of reporter genes into tumor cells that afford novel detection strategies of biochemical events. One such application is the expression of a modified form of the luciferase gene that is only conditionally activated when cellular apoptosis is activated.[11] Use of luciferin as a substrate results in the elaboration of photons coincident to apoptosis (caspase-3-specific activation of luciferase) in the cells. This model has been used as an in situ reporter of the efficacy of cancer agents against brain tumors in rats. Matching of conditionally activated enzymes that become functional under specific biochemical signaling events will raise the utility of in vivo models for more accurate assessment of cancer interventions or tumor biology experiments.

References

1. Ding H, Roncari L, Shannon P, et al: Astrocyte-specific expression of activated p21-ras results in malignant astrocytoma formation in a transgenic mouse model of human gliomas. Cancer Res 61:3826–3836, 2001.
2. Guillamo JS, Lisovoski F, Christov C, et al: Migration pathways of human glioblastoma cells xenografted into the immunosuppressed rat brain. J Neurooncol 52:205–215, 2001.
3. Holland EC, Celestino J, Dai C, et al: Combined activation of Ras and Akt in neural progenitors induces glioblastoma formation in mice. Nat Genet 25:55–57, 2000.
4. Holland EC, Varmus HE: Basic fibroblast growth factor induces cell migration and proliferation after glia-specific gene transfer in mice. Proc Natl Acad Sci USA 95:1218–1223, 1998.
5. Jackson EL, Willis N, Mercer K, et al: Analysis of lung tumor initiation and progression using conditional expression of oncogenic K-ras. Genes Dev 15:3243–3248, 2001.
6. Jonkers J, Berns A: Conditional mouse models of sporadic cancer. Nat Rev Cancer 2:251–265, 2002.
7. Kindler-Rohrborn A, Koelsch BU, Buslei R, et al: Allele-specific losses of heterozygosity on chromosomes 1 and 17 revealed by whole genome scan of ethylnitrosourea-induced BDIX x BDIV hybrid rat gliomas. Mol Carcinog 26:163–171, 1999.
8. Kjaergaard J, Tanaka J, Kim JA, et al: Therapeutic efficacy of OX-40 receptor antibody depends on tumor immunogenicity and anatomic site of tumor growth. Cancer Res 60:5514–5521, 2000.
9. Koutcher JA, Hu X, Xu S, et al: MRI of mouse models for gliomas shows similarities to humans and can be used to identify mice for preclinical trials. Neoplasia 4:480–485, 2002.
10. Lampson LA: New animal models to probe brain tumor biology, therapy, and immunotherapy: advantages and remaining concerns. J Neurooncol 53:275–287, 2001.
11. Laxman B, Hall DE, Bhojani MS, et al: Noninvasive real-time imaging of apoptosis. Proc Natl Acad Sci USA 99:16551–16555, 2002.
12. Lewandoski M: Conditional control of gene expression in the mouse. Nat Rev Genet 2:743–755, 2001.
13. Mahesparan R, Read TA, Lund-Johansen M, et al: Expression of extracellular matrix components in a highly infiltrative in vivo glioma model. Acta Neuropathol (Berl) 105:49–57, 2003.
14. National Cancer Institute. MMHCC. The Mouse Models of Human Cancers Consortium. http://emice.nci.nih.gov/mouse_models (*last accessed* 9 June 2003).
15. Read TA, Farhadi M, Bjerkvig R, et al: Intravital microscopy reveals novel antivascular and antitumor effects of endostatin delivered locally by alginate-encapsulated cells. Cancer Res 61:6830–6837, 2001.
16. Ross BD, Chenevert TL, Rehemtulla A: Magnetic resonance imaging in cancer research. Eur J Cancer 38:2147–2156, 2002.
17. Schmidt EE, Ichimura K, Goike HM, et al: Mutational profile of the PTEN gene in primary human astrocytic tumors and cultivated xenografts. J Neuropathol Exp Neurol 58:1170–1183, 1999.
18. Uhrbom L, Hesselager G, Nister M, Westermark B: Induction of brain tumors in mice using a recombinant platelet-derived growth factor B-chain retrovirus. Cancer Res 58:5275–5279, 1998.
19. Vajkoczy P, Ullrich A, Menger MD: Intravital fluorescence videomicroscopy to study tumor angiogenesis and microcirculation. Neoplasia 2:53–61, 2000.

20. Verhoye M, van der Sanden BP, Rijken PF, et al: Assessment of the neovascular permeability in glioma xenografts by dynamic T(1)MRI with Gadomer-17. Magn Reson Med 47:305–313, 2002.

21. Visted T, Thorsen J, Thorsen F, et al: lacZ-neoR transfected glioma cells in syngeneic rats: growth pattern and characterization of the host immune response against cells transplanted inside and outside the CNS. Int J Cancer 85:228–235, 2000.

22. Vooijs M, Jonkers J, Lyons S, Berns A: Noninvasive imaging of spontaneous retinoblastoma pathway-dependent tumors in mice. Cancer Res 62:1862–1867, 2002.

23. Weissenberger J, Steinbach JP, Malin G, et al: Development and malignant progression of astrocytomas in GFAP-v-src transgenic mice. Oncogene 14:2005–2013, 1997.

24. Xu X, Wagner KU, Larson D, et al: Conditional mutation of Brca1 in mammary epithelial cells results in blunted ductal morphogenesis and tumour formation. Nat Genet 22:37–43, 1999.

CHAPTER **4**

DIAGNOSTIC IMAGING

Soonmee Cha

Brain tumors rank second as the cause of cancer-related deaths in children and young adults younger than the age of 34, and they affect adults of all ages. After cancer of the lung and pancreas, primary malignant brain tumors have the third-highest cancer-related mortality rate in the United States, and they take a disproportionate toll in disability and morbidity.[8] The Surveillance, Epidemiology, and End Results (SEER) program estimated that there were 17,400 new cases of brain tumors in the United States in 1998 and 13,300 deaths from brain and other central nervous system tumors.[11] There is now convincing evidence that the incidence of primary brain tumors is increasing.[5] Gliomas, the most common type of primary brain tumor, are extremely heterogeneous neoplasms that have defied many decades of therapeutic efforts, and they are one of the most difficult tumors to treat and cure. Glioblastoma multiforme (GBM), the most common and malignant type of glioma, has a poor prognosis, with fewer than 10% of patients remaining alive after 2 years, even with the most aggressive combination of therapies. Even the less common low-grade gliomas tend to dedifferentiate over time into more malignant varieties and eventually result in death.[2] Despite many years of research, technologic progress, and clinical trials, the diagnosis and therapy of brain tumors continue to challenge the medical and scientific community.

The current standard for diagnosis and classification of gliomas is histopathologic analysis of tissue specimens after imaging characterization and surgery. A histopathologic diagnosis of glioma relies on recognition of the tumor's presumed cell of origin, and grading is based on a qualitative histopathologic assessment of cellular proliferation, vascular hyperplasia, necrosis, and nuclear atypia or pleomorphism.[1,4] Preoperative imaging, however, plays several important roles in (1) characterizing the brain tumor and providing preliminary information on tumor type and grade; (2) establishing a differential diagnosis; (3) providing sufficient anatomic detail for surgical planning; and (4) identifying tumor-related complications such as hemorrhage, hydrocephalus, herniation, and mass effect.

BRAIN TUMOR IMAGING

Imaging plays a critical role in the diagnosis of a brain tumor and in patient management. Imaging provides a preliminary assessment of tumor type and grade, which is important in determining the patient's prognosis. Imaging also provides anatomic detail about the tumor, such as its location and size, and information about the surrounding brain, which directly influence surgical planning. Once the diagnosis of brain tumor is confirmed on histopathologic examination, imaging continues to play an important role in assessing residual or recurrent tumor and in monitoring the patient's response to treatment.

The timing of brain tumor imaging falls into five broad categories: (1) at initial presentation, (2) before surgery, (3) immediately after surgery, (4) before irradiation or chemotherapy, and (5) after adjuvant therapy.

Initial Presentation: Differential Diagnosis of Brain Tumors

Patients who have a brain tumor are usually initially seen in an acute setting, often an emergency room, because of an acute episode of seizure or the subacute development of focal neurologic deficit, personality changes, or headaches. In this acute environment, the first line of imaging is often a noncontrast computed tomography (CT) scan of the brain to exclude hemorrhage or a large area of infarction. It is important to note that less than 3% to 5% of all patients with acute stroke have seizure as their primary symptom. Therefore, when an adult patient has a seizure, brain tumor and not stroke should be considered the most likely diagnosis.

Once a mass lesion is suspected on noncontrast CT, contrast-enhanced CT or magnetic resonance imaging (MRI) should be performed to better characterize the mass. Its multiplanar capability and superior soft-tissue contrast make MRI, as opposed to CT, the preferred modality in evaluating patients with a brain tumor. The contrast agent gadolinium should be used routinely for MRI because it further enhances soft tissue contrast, improves delineation of the tumor, and provides information about the integrity of the blood-brain barrier, detecting areas of blood brain–barrier breakdown that allow leakage of contrast agent from the intravascular to the interstitial compartment.

When a brain tumor is suspected, the differential diagnosis can be narrowed by incorporating clinical information with imaging characteristics such as the tumor's location and contrast-enhancement pattern (Tables 4-1 and 4-2). The patient's age is an especially important clinical factor in narrowing the differential diagnosis of brain tumor because certain tumor types tend to occur more frequently in a particular age group. For instance, juvenile pilocytic astrocytoma (JPA) and GBM are common glial tumors distinctly associated with age. JPA is a grade I tumor with a relatively favorable prognosis that most often occurs in the pediatric age group.[7,13] In contrast, GBM is a grade IV tumor with aggressive biologic activity that tends to affect mostly adults, especially those older than 65 years. Imaging features further narrow the differential diagnosis. Tumor location is helpful in determining tumor type. Brain tumors can be classified by location into (1) intra-axial (within

TABLE 4-1	Differential Diagnosis of Brain Tumors Based on Tumor Location	
Intra-axial	**Extra-axial**	**Intraventricular Supratentorial**
Glial, Astrocytic	**Dural**	
Low-grade fibrillary astrocytoma	Meningioma	Choroid plexus tumor
Anaplastic astrocytoma	Hemangiopericytoma	Neurocytoma
Glioblastoma multiforme	Metastases	Meningioma
		Metastases
Glial, Nonastrocytic	**Pituitary**	
Oligodendroglioma	Adenoma	
Ganglioglioma		
Dysembryoblastic neuroepithelial tumor		
Nonglial	**Pineal**	
Primary cerebral lymphoma	Pineocytoma	
Metastases	Germ cell tumor	
	Pineoblastoma	
	Suprasellar	
	Craniopharyngioma	
	Germ cell tumor	
	Lymphoma	
	Metastases	
	Juvenile pilocytic astrocytoma	
	Skull Base	
	Chordoma	
	Plasmacytoma	
	Metastases	
	Chondroid tumor	
Infratentorial		
Glial, Astrocytic	**Dural**	
Juvenile pilocytic astrocytoma	Meningioma	Ependymoma/subependymoma
Astrocytoma (low-grade, anaplastic, glioblastoma)	Hemangiopericytoma	Choroid plexus tumor
	Metastases	
Nonglial	**Cerebellopontine Angle**	
Medulloblastoma	Meningioma	
Hemangioblastoma	Schwannoma	
Metastases	Epidermoid	

TABLE 4-2	Differential Diagnosis of Brain Tumors Based on Imaging Characteristics	
Imaging Characteristic	**Appearance**	**Tumor Type**
Contrast Enhancement Pattern	Homogeneous	Juvenile pilocytic astrocytoma Glioblastoma Metastases
	Heterogeneous, irregular	Glioblastoma Anaplastic astrocytoma Oligodendroglioma Metastases
	Focal nodular	Oligodendroglioma Ganglioglioma
	Absent	Low-grade fibrillary astrocytoma Gliomatosis cerebri
T2 Signal	Low to isointense to gray matter	Meningioma Primary cerebral lymphoma Ependymoma Medulloblastoma Pineoblastoma Metastases (mucinous variant)
	Hyperintense to gray matter	Glial tumor
Cyst		Juvenile pilocytic astrocytoma Ganglioglioma Oligodendroglioma Hemangioblastoma Pleomorphic xanthoastrocytoma
Hemorrhage		Glioblastoma Anaplastic astrocytoma Ependymoma Oligodendroglioma
Calcification		Oligodendroglioma Ependymoma
Necrosis		Glioblastoma Metastases

brain parenchyma) and extra-axial (outside brain parenchyma, including the intraventricular, pituitary, pineal, and meningeal locations); and (2) supratentorial and infratentorial tumors. Tumors within the cerebral white matter tend to be glial in origin, GBM being the most common. Tumors in the suprasellar location include pituitary adenoma and craniopharyngioma, whereas tumors in the pineal region include those originating from primitive neuroectodermal cells, such as pineoblastoma or pineocytoma. In the posterior fossa, medulloblastoma and JPA are the most common tumor types in children, and metastatic cancer and glial tumors are the most common in adults.

Imaging before Surgery

When a brain tumor is suspected based on initial imaging studies, most patients are then evaluated by a neurosurgeon for surgical resection and tissue diagnosis. Once surgery is planned, all patients should undergo preoperative MRI with intravenous gadolinium administration. The important goals of preoperative imaging are to (1) characterize tumor location, size, and imaging patterns to suggest a preliminary assessment of tumor type and grade; (2) provide sufficient anatomic detail for surgical planning; and (3) evaluate any tumor-related complications, such as hemorrhage, hydrocephalus, herniation, and mass effect.

Imaging after Surgery

The goals of immediate postoperative MRI are to assess the amount of any residual tumor and to evaluate postoperative complications, such as hemorrhage, infarction, contusion, or subdural collection of blood. The timing of immediate postoperative MRI is crucial to differentiate residual tumor and the reaction of brain tissue to surgery. Because postoperative granulation tissue, which can appear identical to residual tumor, is most conspicuous several days after surgery, immediate postoperative imaging should be done within 24 to 48 hours.

Most patients with high-grade brain tumors undergo radiation therapy, with or without adjuvant chemotherapy, within 6 weeks after their initial cytoreductive surgery. The primary aims of imaging before irradiation are to (1) assess residual or recurrent tumor; (2) determine the volume of tumor to be irradiated; and (3) plan the radiation isodose field.

Once irradiation is completed, postirradiation imaging should be performed to assess tumor response to radiation and any immediate radiation-related complications, such as edema, mass effect, or hemorrhage. Imaging at this time can also serve as a baseline scan before the patient starts adjuvant chemotherapy. For those patients enrolled in therapeutic clinical trials, a regular follow-up clinical and imaging evaluation is performed as part of the protocol—usually at intervals of 2 to 3 months, depending on the patient's clinical status. The goals of serial imaging studies during chemotherapy are to (1) assess response to treatment and (2) detect tumor recurrence and therapy-related complications.

After the completion of irradiation and chemotherapy, patients should undergo surveillance imaging to monitor them for tumor recurrence or emergence of a new tumor focus.

PRIMARY BRAIN TUMORS

Astrocytomas

Astrocytomas are the most common primary intra-axial brain tumor and the most common glial neoplasm, constituting approximately three quarters of all primary glial neoplasms. Astrocytomas are an extremely heterogeneous group of tumors, both histopathologically and prognostically. The grading of astrocytomas, which is important for prognosis and therapy, is based on histologic evaluation of a tissue specimen. There are several systems for the grading and classification of brain tumors, but a three-tiered grading system based on the World Health Organization (WHO) criteria is the most widely accepted and used. Regardless of the different grading systems and the degree of histopathologic differentiation, all infiltrating astrocytomas are considered malignant because, despite treatment, even the low-grade tumors tend to dedifferentiate into higher grade tumors.

Low-Grade Astrocytoma

Compared with their more malignant counterpart, low-grade astrocytomas are far less common, tend to affect a younger patient population, and have a more favorable prognosis. On imaging, low-grade astrocytomas tend to have a diffuse infiltrative tumor margin, but there are also those with a focal, well-circumscribed border. On angiography, they usually appear as an avascular mass with an absence of either arteriovenous shunting or early venous draining. On CT, low-grade astrocytomas tend to be isodense to hypodense to the adjacent brain, and intratumoral calcification may be seen, although it is not common. On contrast-enhanced CT, low-grade astrocytomas tend not to be enhanced. On MRI, they appear as fairly well-circumscribed lesions despite their infiltrative growth pattern, and they are homogeneously hyperintense on T2-weighted images. Contrast enhancement is usually minimal or absent and so is peritumoral edema (Figure 4-1). When there is robust and irregular contrast

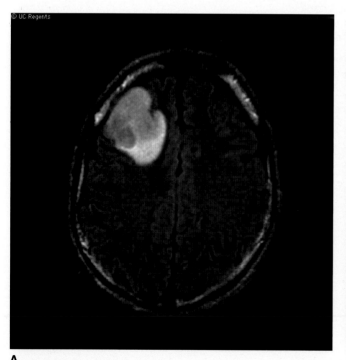

A

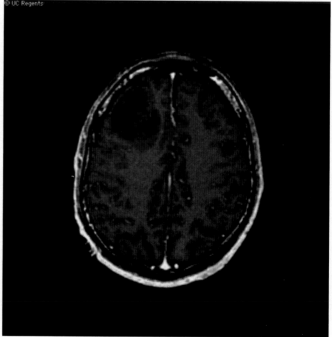

B

FIGURE 4-1   Low-grade glioma. *A,* Axial fluid-attenuated inversion recovery image demonstrates a hyperintense cortically based mass in the right frontal lobe. *B,* Axial postcontrast spoiled gradient recalled image shows no abnormal enhancement within the right frontal tumor.

enhancement of the lesion, the diagnosis of low-grade astrocytoma should not be considered the most likely choice.

Anaplastic Astrocytoma and Glioblastoma Multiforme

High-grade astrocytomas—anaplastic astrocytoma and GBM—are much more common than low-grade astrocytomas and tend to affect an older group of patients. GBM is not only the most common but also the most malignant of all primary glial neoplasms. The prognosis for patients with high-grade astrocytomas, especially a GBM, is usually poor, even with the most aggressive multimodality therapy. On imaging, high-grade astrocytomas tend to be vividly enhanced, albeit in a heterogeneous and irregular pattern. The tumor margins are often ill defined, and peritumoral edema tends to be moderate to severe. It is often difficult to differentiate anaplastic astrocytomas from glioblastomas, but the presence of tumor necrosis—as evidenced by a nonenhanced central region with a hyperintense T2 signal surrounded by a thick irregular enhanced rim (Figure 4-2)—is highly suggestive of glioblastoma. Some glioblastomas show no contrast enhancement or peritumoral edema, although such a case is very unusual.

As the name *multiforme* implies, GBMs are extremely heterogeneous and variegated tumors. Histologically, GBMs are characterized by increased cellularity, high proliferation indices, endothelial proliferation, and focal necrosis. Similarly, on imaging GBMs can appear markedly different from the more classic rim-enhanced necrotic mass, appearing to be a nonenhanced infiltrative lesion that at times can even be confused with an acute infarct.

Oligodendroglioma

Oligodendrogliomas, which constitute less than 10% of all primary glial neoplasms, are thought to have originated from oligodendrocytes of the brain. Histopathologically, oligodendrogliomas can be pure or mixed with astrocytic tumor cells. Variable contributions of the oligodendroglial and the astrocytic components make oligodendrogliomas appear different from one another on imaging. One of the commonly seen imaging hallmarks of oligodendroglioma is intratumoral calcification. The presence of a tumor-associated cyst and involvement of the cortical surface are also not unusual (Figure 4-3). The tumor can be quite large at initial presentation. There are no definitive imaging criteria to differentiate low-grade astrocytomas from anaplastic oligodendroglioma, although extensive edema and enhancement tend to be associated with the anaplastic variant.

Gliomatosis Cerebri

Gliomatosis cerebri is a rare neoplasm of the brain characterized by moderately pleomorphic glial cells that infiltrate along the preexisting structures without causing demonstrable destruction. One of the hallmarks of gliomatosis cerebri is increased cellularity without frank destruction of the infiltrated parenchyma or presence of neovascularity. Invasion of both the gray and white matter is seen, but it is distinctly unusual to find mitosis, necrosis, or angiogenesis.

On MRI, gliomatosis cerebri is seen as a focal or diffuse infiltrative signal abnormality involving white matter and expansion of cortex, usually without contrast enhancement.

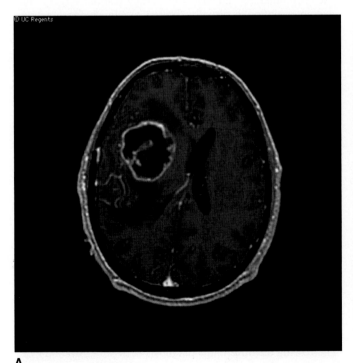

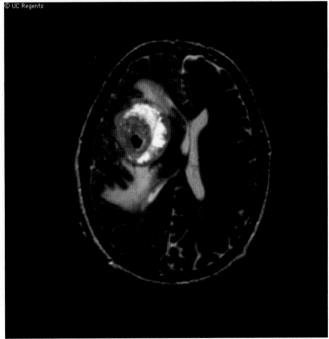

A   **B**

FIGURE 4-2   Glioblastoma multiforme. *A,* Axial postcontrast spoiled gradient recalled image demonstrates an irregularly rim enhancing, centrally necrotic mass in the right frontal lobe. *B,* Axial T2-weighted image shows edema surrounding and compression and displacement of the adjacent right lateral ventricle.

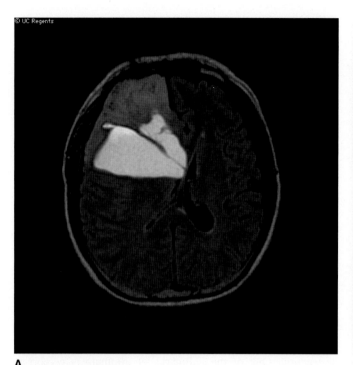

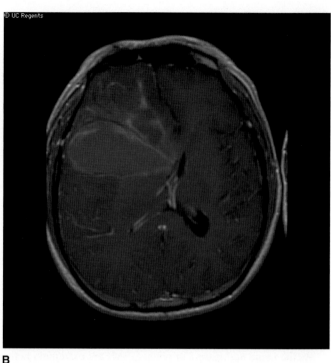

A   B

FIGURE 4-3 Low-grade oligodendroglioma. *A,* Axial fluid-attenuated inversion recovery image demonstrates a large hyperintense right frontal mass with complex architecture compressing the front of the right lateral ventricle. *B,* Axial postcontrast T1-weighted image shows rimlike linear enhancement along the peripheral margins of the tumor.

There is minimal, if any, mass effect or extensive vasogenic edema.[6,15,17,19,20] When there is new emergence of contrast enhancement, malignant degeneration into a higher grade tumor should be highly suspected.

Ganglioglioma

Gangliogliomas are most often seen in the pediatric patient population and are characterized by a biologically indolent growth pattern. The most common location is the temporal lobe, but they may be seen anywhere, including the posterior fossa.[10,14,] On imaging, they tend to have a well-circumscribed border, often composed of a solid enhanced nodule and a cystic component. Peritumoral edema is usually minimal, even in large lesions.

PRIMARY BRAIN TUMORS OF NONGLIAL ORIGIN

Primary Cerebral Lymphoma

Over the past 2 decades, the incidence of primary cerebral lymphoma (PCL) has substantially increased in both immunocompromised and immune-competent individuals—a phenomenon that cannot be entirely explained by changes in tumor classification, the increased prevalence of AIDS, or the growing number of organ transplantations. The incidence ratio of both PCL and GBM rose from 1 in 250 in 1974 to 1 in 6 in the period 1981 to 1990, with PCLs now accounting for 6.6% to 15.4% of all primary brain tumors.[5,18] Unlike other high-grade

intracranial neoplasms, PCLs are treated with combined high-dose chemotherapy and radiation therapy without surgery. Surgical intervention is usually limited to biopsy for obtaining tissue for a pathologic diagnosis.[9,12,16] It has been shown that surgical resection of PCL does not necessarily alter prognosis, and it can lead to profound functional deficit and increased postoperative morbidity. More important is that, when patients with PCL receive steroid therapy to reduce intracranial pressure before biopsy, the pathologic findings can be difficult to interpret, and a definitive diagnosis cannot be made. In addition, because PCLs tend to occur near eloquent areas of the brain and in a subependymal location, gross total resection may in fact be contraindicated, and performing a biopsy may be challenging. A minimally invasive and accurate diagnosis of PCL is therefore an important goal that could clearly alter patient management and reduce risk to the patient.

On imaging, PCLs are usually homogeneously enhanced. They can be multiple and tend to favor deep gray or subependymal locations, often involving the corpus callosum. At times they are indistinguishable from GBM. However, unlike GBM, which has a hyperintense signal on T2-weighted MR imaging, PCLs tend to show a hypointense T2 signal, presumably because of their dense cellularity and a high nuclear-to-cytoplasmic ratio that results in decreased extracellular fluid. Therefore the T2-signal intensity of the tumor can be helpful in narrowing the differential diagnosis between GBM and PCL. There are other brain tumors that are often hypointense in signal intensity on T2-weighted images, however, including primitive neuroectodermal tumors (e.g., medulloblastoma and pineoblastoma) and metastatic tumors, usually those metastatic from a mucinous adenocarcinoma primary.

Primary Nonglial Tumors of the Brain Coverings

Although a broad spectrum of neoplasms can originate from the coverings of the brain—the leptomeninges and dura—meningioma is by far the most common. Meningiomas are usually well-circumscribed lesions with a clearly demarcated tumor-brain interface. They tend to be biologically benign, although malignant variants occur.

On imaging, meningiomas show characteristics of an extra-axial tumor comprising a buckling or displacement of the gray-white matter junction and a cleaving of the subarachnoid space and vessels that surround the mass, separating it from the adjacent brain (Figure 4-4). Meningiomas are isointense to brain on unenhanced T1-weighted and T2-weighted images and tend to be vividly and homogeneously enhanced after the administration of contrast agent. The degree of peritumoral edema can be minimal to quite extensive (see Figure 4-4C).

SECONDARY BRAIN TUMORS (METASTASES)

Intracranial metastasis makes up almost 50% of all supratentorial brain tumors. Metastatic tumors spread into the central nervous system through a hematogenous route and induce neovascularization as they grow and expand. Intracranial metastatic tumors, especially those that cause neurologic symptoms, are associated with a variable degree of vasogenic edema. The capillaries within the area of vasogenic edema are consistently normal in appearance, and no tumor cells are found beyond the macroscopic boundaries of the tumor.[21] The radiologic diagnosis of intracranial metastases is usually straightforward and uncomplicated. Metastatic tumors tend to be multiple and well circumscribed and favor the gray-white matter junction. Patients generally have a known history of systemic malignancy. Solitary metastases, however—which can occur in 30% to 50% of cases—may pose a diagnostic challenge in differentiating them from a primary glioma, particularly when the patient has no known history of systemic cancer or when the medical evaluation does not identify a primary systemic malignancy. In general, metastatic tumors tend to have a more circumscribed border than do primary gliomas.

TUMOR-MIMICKING LESIONS

There are several non-neoplastic brain lesions that masquerade as intracranial neoplasms. These so-called tumor-mimicking lesions (TMLs) may present a considerable diagnostic challenge to both the clinician and the radiologist. Clinically, TMLs can present with symptoms suggestive of a mass lesion. The three most common TMLs in the brain are infarction, abscess, and large demyelinating plaques.

Infarction

A radiologic diagnosis of acute infarct is fairly straightforward since the introduction and wide clinical application of diffusion-weighted MRI. On diffusion-weighted imaging (DWI), acute infarcts are markedly hyperintense because of localized restriction of water within the area of infarcted tissue. In cases of subacute infarction or venous infarction, the imaging appearance can be quite confusing and misleading and hence may lead to an erroneous diagnosis of tumor. In this situation, the clinical history can be helpful in narrowing the differential diagnosis. It is important to recall that the most common presenting symptom of a brain tumor is seizure, whereas less than 3% of all patients with acute infarction have seizure as the primary initial symptom.

On CT, the early phase of acute infarction may not be discernible at all. There may be a subtle effacement of gray-white matter differentiation or a hyperdense artery suggestive of an occluded vessel. On MRI, the most important clue to the correct diagnosis of infarction is the abnormality seen on DWI. The degree of mass effect and gyral swelling is most prominent during the early phase of infarction, whereas contrast enhancement, usually of a gyral pattern, is most conspicuous several days after the onset of acute symptoms. In venous infarction, there may be a prominent hemorrhagic component as evidenced by marked hypointensity of signal on T2-weighted images or on gradient-echo images.

Brain Abscess

Brain abscess can simulate necrotic brain tumors. The use of antibiotics has substantially reduced the incidence of intracranial bacterial abscesses. With a growing number of AIDS and organ transplantation patients, however, the prevalence of opportunistic infections is on the rise, especially those caused by viral or protozoan organisms. Brain abscesses are usually the result of either a direct spread of infection from extracranial sites, such as the paranasal sinuses, or hematogenous dissemination from systemic bacteremia. The radiologic diagnosis of intracranial infections can be challenging because of the variable appearance of lesions as a result of different offending microbes and different stages of presentation.

On MRI, intracranial infection can present as a focal mass or a diffuse process, depending on the offending organism and the stage of infection. Bacterial infections can present as a nonspecific, diffuse signal abnormality with or without enhancement in the cerebritis stage, which precedes the formation of a well-defined abscess. Cerebral abscess, which is usually caused by pyogenic bacterial organisms, often presents as a ring-enhanced mass with marked surrounding edema. In imaging a well-formed abscess, there is a fairly uniform peripheral enhancement, a well-defined capsule that appears hypointense on T2-weighted images, and moderate to severe vasogenic edema.

Similarly to acute infarcts, brain abscesses have a characteristic abnormality on DWI, presumably because of a high viscosity of the pus that results in a restriction of water and hence a hyperintense signal on DWI. There are, however, brain tumors that have a diffusion abnormality similar to that seen with an abscess, such as epidermoid tumors, mucinous metastases, and primary cerebral lymphoma.

Tumefactive Demyelinating Lesions

Tumefactive demyelinating lesions (TDLs) are large demyelinating lesions that can mimic high-grade glial tumors. The literature contains many reports of large demyelinating lesions that masquerade as intracranial neoplasms.[3,22] These TDLs may

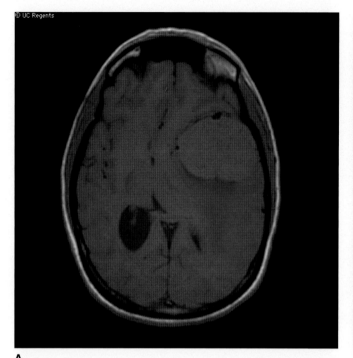

A

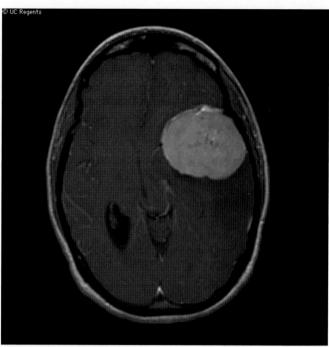

B

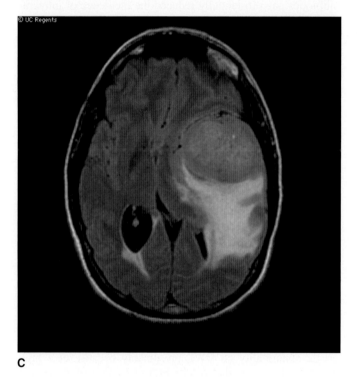

C

FIGURE 4-4   Meningioma. *A,* Axial unenhanced T1-weighted image shows a well-circumscribed left temporal extra-axial mass that has similar signal characteristics as the adjacent normal brain. *B,* Axial postcontrast T1-weighted image demonstrates avid and homogeneous enhancement of the mass. *C,* Axial fluid-attenuated inversion recovery image demonstrates extensive edema surrounding the mass.

pose a considerable diagnostic challenge to both the clinician and the radiologist. Clinically, TDLs may present with symptoms suggestive of a mass lesion. On MRI, TDLs are often indistinguishable from high-grade glial neoplasms, demonstrating ill-defined borders, mass effect, perilesional edema, central necrosis, contrast enhancement, and variable involvement of gray-matter structures. Even in the case of an established demyelinating disease such as multiple sclerosis, the

atypical appearance of a large lesion should cause concern about a concurrent neoplasm.

CONCLUSION

The differential diagnoses and imaging characteristics of brain tumors are quite variable, depending on tumor type and grade.

By using both clinical and imaging information, the differential diagnosis can be narrowed and an accurate diagnosis can be made. Imaging goals for patients who have a brain tumor depend on the clinical situation in which the imaging study is requested. The multiplanar capability and superior soft-tissue resolution of MRI with the intravenous administration of a contrast agent make MRI the preferred diagnostic modality for use with patients who have a brain tumor.

References

1. Burger P: Classification, grading, and patterns of spread of malignant gliomas. In Apuzzo ML (ed): Neurosurgical Topics: Malignant Cerebral Glioma. Park Ridge, Ill, American Association of Neurological Surgeons, 1990.
2. Burger PC, Vogel FS: The brain: tumors. In Burger PC, Vogel FS (eds): Surgical Pathology of the Central Nervous System and Its Coverings. New York, Wiley, 1982.
3. Dagher AP, Smirniotopoulos J: Tumefactive demyelinating lesions. Neuroradiology 38:560–565, 1996.
4. Daumas-Duport C, Scheithauer B, O'Fallon J, Kelly P: Grading of astrocytomas: a simple and reproducible method. Cancer 62:2152–2165, 1988.
5. Eby NL, Grufferman S, Flannelly CM, et al: Increasing incidence of primary brain lymphoma in the US. Cancer 62:2461–2465, 1988.
6. Essig M, Schlemmer HP, Tronnier V, et al: Fluid-attenuated inversion-recovery MR imaging of gliomatosis cerebri. Eur Radiol 11:303–308, 2001.
7. Garcia DM, Fulling KH: Juvenile pilocytic astrocytoma of the cerebrum in adults. A distinctive neoplasm with favorable prognosis. J Neurosurg 63:382–386, 1985.
8. Greenlee RT, Murray T, Bolden S, Wingo PA: Cancer statistics. CA Cancer J Clin 50:7–33, 2000.
9. Herrlinger U, Schabet M, Clemens M, et al: Clinical presentation and therapeutic outcome in 26 patients with primary CNS lymphoma. Acta Neurol Scand 97:257–264, 1998.
10. Lang FF, Epstein FJ, Ransohoff J, et al: Central nervous system gangliogliomas. Part 2: Clinical outcome. J Neurosurg 79:867–873, 1993.
11. Landis SH, Murray T, Bolden S, Wingo PA: Cancer statistics. CA Cancer J Clin 48:6–29, 1998.
12. Ling SM, Roach M, Larson DA, Wara WM: Radiotherapy of primary central nervous system lymphoma in patients with and without human immunodeficiency virus. Ten years of treatment experience at the University of California San Francisco. Cancer 73:2570–2582, 1994.
13. Mamelak AN, Prados MD, Obana WG, et al: Treatment options and prognosis for multicentric juvenile pilocytic astrocytoma. J Neurosurg 81:24–30, 1994.
14. Miller DC, Lang FF, Epstein FJ: Central nervous system gangliogliomas. Part 1: Pathology. J Neurosurg 79:859–866, 1993.
15. Porta-Etessam J, Berbel A, Martinez-Salio A, et al: Gliomatosis cerebri. MRI, SPECT and the study of pathology. Rev Neurol 29:287–288, 1999.
16. Reni M, Ferreri AJ, Garancini MP, Villa E: Therapeutic management of primary central nervous system lymphoma in immunocompetent patients: results of a critical review of the literature. Ann Oncol 8:227–234, 1997.
17. Rippe DJ, Boyko OB, Fuller GN, et al: Gadopentetate-dimeglumine-enhanced MR imaging of gliomatosis cerebri: appearance mimicking leptomeningeal tumor dissemination. AJNR Am J Neuroradiol 11:800–801, 1990.
18. Schabet M: Epidemiology of primary CNS lymphoma. J Neurooncol 43:199–201, 1999.
19. Schoenen J, De Leval L, Reznik M: Gliomatosis cerebri: clinical, radiological and pathological report of a case with a stroke-like onset. Acta Neurol Belg 96:294–300, 1996.
20. Spagnoli MV, Grossman RI, Packer RJ, et al: Magnetic resonance imaging determination of gliomatosis cerebri. Neuroradiology 29:15–18, 1987.
21. Strugar J, Rothbart D, Harrington W, Criscuolo GR: Vascular permeability factor in brain metastases: correlation with vasogenic brain edema and tumor angiogenesis. J Neurosurg 81:560–566, 1994.
22. Zagzag D, Miller DC, Kleinman GM, et al: Demyelinating disease versus tumor in surgical neuropathology. Clues to a correct pathological diagnosis. Am J Surg Pathol 17:537–545, 1993.

PATHOLOGIC CLASSIFICATION

Scott R. VandenBerg

The classification of tumors of the central nervous system (CNS) attempts to precisely define highly complex and dynamic biologic processes by a static, empirical framework. This is primarily based on histopathologic features that are defined by a combination of routine and immunohistochemical stains. Although these techniques have permitted useful characterization of a variety of neoplastic cellular phenotypes comprising the spectrum of CNS tumors,[57,58] the current classification scheme has limited utility for precisely predicting the invasive growth capacity, extent of recurrence, or the efficacy of specific adjuvant therapies for many tumor types.

The development of experimental molecular morphologic methods, including molecular cytogenetic techniques, promises to complement the current classification of CNS tumors. Laser capture microdissection of tissue sections now permits identifying specific gene amplification or expression, and the activation of signaling pathways regulating cell proliferation and invasion in selected tumor cell populations. Such genomic and proteomic approaches, when integrated into the current histopathologic framework, should provide the neuro-oncologist with a more accurate prediction of biologic activity and defined therapeutic targets. Molecular genetic assessment of brain tumors, especially with respect to astrocytic and oligodendroglial tumors, has already enhanced our understanding of oncogenesis and tumor progression in subtypes of tumors with similar or indistinguishable histopathology. Recent studies have suggested that gene-expression-based classification of malignant gliomas may have a stronger correlation with survival than only the histologic classification.[87]

Advances in neuroimaging and neurosurgical techniques for precise tumor localization, combined with the expanded use of stereotactic procedures, necessitate that pathologic diagnosis be rendered on minute tissue specimens from heterogeneous tumors. Thus for the most precise application of the current brain tumor classification, a clear and consistent definition of key pathologic features must be integrated with clinical and neuroimaging data for each tumor type. These histopathologic features will be enumerated in detail in Part II of this text, whereas the following discussion will be a selected overview of CNS tumor classification with specific emphasis on the advances in experimental neuro-oncology in which the molecular biology complements the World Health Organization (WHO) conceptual framework.

CENTRAL NERVOUS SYSTEM HISTOGENESIS AND TUMOR CLASSIFICATION

The complex histogenesis of the CNS from a primitive neuroepithelium must be considered when classifying the types and distribution of the neural neoplasms arising in both the developing and mature CNS. The development of the nervous system is an intricate and elaborate multistep process involving induction of the neuroepithelium, regional subdivision and morphogenesis, and cell-type specification with diverse neuronal and glial differentiation that culminates in an intricate arrangement of approximately 10^{11} neurons and 10^{12} glial cells.[50] These region-specific processes are associated with different constellations of regulated gene expression that are mediated by multiple homeobox genes, cell lineage–specific transcriptional activity, and gene methylation. Such differences in regulated gene expression may create cell targets for neoplastic transformation that are associated with specific developmental stages and regions.[43] The resultant transformed cells may likewise have different groups of activated regulatory pathways affecting cell migration, proliferation, senescence, and apoptosis. Such differences would affect the prognostic capability of a classification system.

The obvious differences in children's and adults' brains with respect to lineage and phenotypic differentiation are consistent with the existence of different cellular targets for neoplastic transformation. On the simplest level, this distinction is reflected by the different histogenetic potential and molecular biology of the most common malignant tumors, the medulloblastoma[25] and glioblastoma,[109] in children's and adults' brains, respectively. There are also differences in the genetic lesions and expression profiles between both the adult and pediatric low-grade astrocytomas[122,145] and the pediatric and adult glioblastomas.[16,105,129,130]

Although the adult CNS lacks the diverse constellation of stem cells and the differentiating neural cells that are present in the developing brain, recent studies unequivocally document the presence of neural progenitor cells that have specific regional distributions and variable potentials to generate glial and neuronal cellular lineages.[131] Experimental murine models suggest that primitive glial and neural progenitors and more differentiated glial cell lineages have different susceptibilities to neoplastic transformation and develop different constellations of gliomas after the introduction of the same genetic lesions, including activation of signaling pathways associated with platelet-derived growth factor B (PDGF-B), Ras, and Akt.[20,45,46,136] While the intriguing oncogenic roles of human adult neural progenitors, as compared with their counterparts in the developing brain, remain to be more completely defined, the concept that primitive progenitors and differentiated cell populations are targets with differing susceptibility for specific genetic and epigenetic events in the process of neoplastic transformation will have an impact on the future conceptual framework of tumor classification. Likewise, molecular biologic characterization of specific cell populations within tumors will also be defined within a developmental and brain region–specific context.

TUMORS ARISING FROM NEUROEPITHELIAL CELLS

Astrocytic Tumors

Diffuse Astrocytomas

The current WHO classification of CNS tumors[57,58] recognizes two different categories of astrocytic tumors. The first category, the *diffuse astrocytomas*, is so designated because these tumors invade the brain or spinal cord tissue by diffuse cellular infiltration at regional margins and cellular dispersion to distant sites. Aside from the capacity to diffusely invade the adjacent neuropil or white matter and to spread remotely, a diffuse-type astrocytoma has a significant potential to develop progressively more malignant biologic behavior with time. Therefore the grading of both anaplasia and the capacity for aggressive invasive growth is implicit in the histopathologic classification of the diffuse astrocytic tumors; and likewise, an increase in the WHO grade is accompanied by increased intratumoral heterogeneity. The classification defines three groups of diffuse astrocytic neoplasms: astrocytoma (WHO grade II); anaplastic astrocytoma (WHO grade III); and glioblastoma multiforme (GBM) and GBM variants, giant cell glioblastoma and gliosarcoma (astrocytoma, WHO grade IV).

According to the WHO scheme, tumors with nuclear atypia alone are considered grade II; those with mitotic activity in addition to nuclear atypia are grade III; and neoplasms showing atypia, mitoses, microvascular hyperplasia ("endothelial proliferation"), or necrosis are considered grade IV. The WHO classification recognizes three morphologic variants of cells comprising diffuse astrocytomas: *fibrillary*, *protoplasmic*, and *gemistocytic*. However, no cytoarchitectural variant appears to have any prognostic importance. The exception appears to be astrocytomas containing more than 20% gemistocytes.[66] Within these tumors, there is a highly variable population of small glial cells that appears to be the proliferative component, in contrast to the gemistocytic tumor cells that are not proliferative but are resistant to apoptosis. Although both the gemistocytic and small-cell components typically demonstrate nuclear p53 immunoreactivity, only the gemistocytes are immunoreactive for bcl-2,[139] suggesting a block in apoptosis. Gemistocytic astrocytomas tend to behave aggressively,[66] with approximately 80% of these tumors progressing to glioblastoma. Although these features

warrant communication to the neuro-oncologists, gemistocytic astrocytomas are currently considered grade II in the WHO classification, and a better definition of small glial cell lineages awaits further study.

Because the presence of mitotic cells is a key feature to distinguish WHO grade II from WHO grade III astrocytoma, immunohistochemical techniques have been used to more accurately enumerate proliferative cell populations. Immunostaining for the Ki-67 protein, as defined by monoclonal antibody MIB 1, is currently the most well-documented marker for "proliferative" cells. Although Ki-67 immunoreactivity alone is insufficient to definitively distinguish between anaplastic astrocytomas and glioblastomas, there is a good correlation between MIB-1 labeling indices and WHO grade in diffuse astrocytomas.[34]

The Ki-67 protein is a nuclear, nonhistone protein that is required for maintaining the cell cycle. It is expressed during G1, S, G2 and M phases but is absent in the G0 phase.[21,31–33] Ki-67 appears to be minimally expressed in mid to late G1 and significantly accumulates throughout S phase, with maximum levels attained in M phase. Levels rapidly drop in postmitotic cells with a half-life of less than 16% of G1 phase.[11] Therefore caution must be exercised when interpreting Ki-67 labeling indices in tumors that are treated with small molecular inhibitors with diverse effects on cell signaling, including disruption of the cell cycle in G1 phase or the G1-S transition, because these may result in a paradoxical increase in Ki-67 antigen indices despite a lower proliferative fraction.[19]

While the features of nuclear pleomorphism and mitotic activity are generally useful for broadly discriminating the WHO II tumors from either non-neoplastic, reactive lesions, or from WHO III neoplasms, the current histopathologic classification oversimplifies the biologic complexity of this neoplastic spectrum. Overlapping morphologic phenotypes thus preclude precise predictions as to the biologic behavior of individual tumors in the spectrum of the WHO II to III lesions. Molecular approaches, especially with respect to unique patterns and timing of genetic aberrations, may complement the current system to better define subtypes of low-grade astrocytomas and predict the biologic potential of individual tumors.[71,86] A comparative meta-analysis of genomic hybridization data demonstrated the correlation between the average number of copy alterations, the average number of affected GTG-bands, identified by Giemsa staining, for gains and losses, and the WHO grade in diffuse-type astrocytomas.[61] With respect to specific genetic loci, methylation of either p14^{ARF} or p16^{INK4a}, without deletions in either gene, occurs exclusively in low-grade astrocytomas. Such an epigenetic attenuation of gene function may be associated with blocking replicative senescence[7,48,72,90] to sustain mitogenic growth-factor stimulation. Although both TP53 gene mutations and the expression of PDGF and insulin-like growth factor 1 (IGF-1) appear to occur early in the tumorigenesis of the diffuse-type astrocytomas,[41,57,70] these molecular characteristics are not differential features for low-grade neoplasms.

GBM subtypes, with the same constellation of classic histopathologic features, have been identified on the basis of different sets of molecular genetic alterations in combination with the clinical features of age of onset and clinical duration of tumor growth.[56] The *primary* or *de novo* subtype of glioblastoma develops in older patients (mean age at onset is 56 years) with a short clinical interval (mean 1.7 months). The most common distinctive molecular biologic features of *primary* glioblastomas are a loss of PTEN (phosphatase and tensin homolog deleted on chromosome 10) (32%), epidermal growth-factor receptor (EGFR) amplification (40%), and MDM2 (human homolog of mouse double minute 2) amplification or overexpression (7% and 50%, respectively) in addition to loss of a number of growth-arrest pathways, more often by deletion (p14^ARF and p16^INK4a loss at 50% and 35%, respectively).

The *secondary* subtype of glioblastoma develops in younger patients (mean age at onset is 40 years) over a period of years from lower grade tumors. In this subtype, the most differential genetic lesion occurs in the TP53 gene. Retinoblastoma 1 (RB1) promoter hypermethylation (43%), loss of 14^ARF and p16^INK4a by methylation and deletion (75% and 31%, respectively), and cyclin-dependent kinase 4 (CDK4) amplification (13%) are also relatively common in *secondary* glioblastomas.

The rare *giant cell glioblastoma* subtype appears to have a distinctive "hybrid" molecular genetic profile between the *primary* and *secondary* glioblastomas with three notable features: (1) no genetic deletions of the CDK^4/6 inhibitors (CDKN2a gene); (2) no amplification of the EGFR or CDK4 genes;[77,92] and (3) a 30% frequency of PTEN mutations while yet having a higher frequency of TP53 mutations.[93] These differences from the other GBM subsets may account for a relatively more favorable clinical prognosis, including an apparently decreased capacity for brain invasion.

In contrast, the *gliosarcoma variant* of GBM[2] appears to be more closely related to the *primary* GBM subtype with a high incidence of PTEN mutations. However, there are important distinctions: (1) the incidence of TP53 mutations is approximately twice that in the primary GBM subtypes and lower than in the giant cell GBM or *secondary* GBM subset of tumors, whereas (2) MDM2 and EGFR gene amplifications are significantly lower than in the *primary* GBM subtype.

Localized Astrocytomas

The second category of astrocytic tumors in the WHO classification are the astrocytic tumors that share the feature of a relatively circumscribed pattern of growth and a limited capacity for infiltrative spread into the surrounding brain or spinal cord. Four distinct groups of astrocytic tumors compose this category, and all are more common in infants, children, and young adults.

Pilocytic astrocytoma (WHO I).   Pilocytic astrocytomas are typically composed of distinctive biphasic patterns of neoplastic astrocytes accompanied by Rosenthal fibers and eosinophilic granular bodies. Whereas pilocytic astrocytomas do not have a capacity for aggressive invasive growth and malignant progression within the brain or the spinal cord, compared with the *diffuse astrocytomas* the pilocytic tumor cells do appear to have selectively increased motility. Heterozygosity for the neurofibromatosis type 1 (NF1) tumor suppressor results in abnormalities in cell attachment spreading and motility in astrocytes,[36] with the resultant capacity to infiltrate the adjacent leptomeninges or white tracts, especially of the brain stem, optic nerves, and optic chiasm. Leptomeningeal infiltration may play a role in the rare disseminated forms that do not manifest anaplastic features. Pilocytic astrocytomas are slow-growing tumors that commonly arise in children and adolescents, with a peak incidence around 10 to 12 years of age. In

adults, these tumors tend to appear 1 decade earlier (mean of 22 years) than the diffuse astrocytomas.[30] Pilocytic astrocytomas are characteristically located in midline structures (e.g., cerebellum, third-ventricular region, optic chiasm or nerves, and brainstem) and may be cystic with a "mural nodule" of tumor. These tumors are not commonly located in the cerebral hemispheres but, when present, show a slight predilection for the temporal or temporoparietal regions and thalamus.[30] These tumors tend to occur in the spinal cord in older patients, more than at other sites, and may constitute a significant proportion (58%) of spinal astrocytic tumors in some series.[79]

In a large series of cerebellar pilocytic astrocytomas,[133] *de novo* anaplastic progression occurred in only 0.9%, and those, by flow cytometry, had higher S-phase fractions (5% to 11%) compared with 3.19 ($\pm$0.237 standard error of the mean). Although mitotic activity ($\leq$4 per 10 high-power field [HPF]) may be an unusual feature of otherwise typical tumors, brisk mitotic activity, in combination with increased cellularity, microvascular hyperplasia, or necrosis, may indicate anaplastic progression.

One histopathologic variant, the *monomorphous pilomyxoid pilocytic astrocytoma*, warrants particular notice.[132] This variant occurs in infants and young children in the region of the hypothalamus and optic chiasm. In comparison with typical pilocytic astrocytomas, these tumors have a more monomorphic histologic pattern, a prominent myxoid stroma, and inconspicuous or absent Rosenthal fibers and eosinophilic granular bodies. These tumors have a significantly higher recurrence rate and the progression-free survivals at 1 year appear to be only approximately 56% of those for typical pilocytic astrocytomas.

The molecular biologic profiles of pilocytic astrocytomas, like the histopathologic features, are clearly distinctive from the diffuse-type astrocytomas. While TP53 mutation and increased expression of PDGF-A and PDGF-Rα are common and probably early events in the formation of diffuse-type astrocytomas, there appears to be no role for either TP53 mutations or aberrant PDGF signaling in the development of pilocytic astrocytomas.[67,88] Comparative analyses of gene expression in sporadic astrocytomas demonstrates that these tumors are uniquely delineated from non-neoplastic white matter and other low-grade gliomas and have more similarity to fetal astrocytes.[37] However, pilocytic astrocytomas do also express a spectrum of genes associated with oligodendroglial lineages (natural killer cell restricted epitope PEN5, proteolipid protein PLP, peripheral myelin protein PMP-22, myelin basic protein MBP, and oligodendroglial myelin glycoprotein).[37,67]

Approximately 30% of pilocytic astrocytomas occur in patients with NF1 and, notably, these tumors typically develop in younger children (mean age of 4.5 years at diagnosis).[67] In this subset of tumors, the reduction or loss of NF1 gene expression appears to be a primary event in their development,[35] while in the sporadic tumors, the NF1 gene may even be overexpressed.[59,100,146] In addition to differences between NF1 and sporadic pilocytic astrocytomas with respect to NF1 gene expression, the elongation factor EF-1α2 gene appears to have increased expression only in the sporadic tumors. Thus the sporadic and NF1-associated pilocytic astrocytomas, despite the same histologic features, may develop and grow via different genetic alterations that culminate in similar histologic phenotypes.

Pleomorphic xanthoastrocytoma (WHO II, III).   Pleomorphic xanthoastrocytoma (PXA) occurs as a superficial cerebral

(95% supratentorial) tumor in children and young adults (average age younger than 20 years) who usually have an antecedent history of seizures. There is a predilection for involvement of the temporal lobe and the overlying leptomeninges, but growth into the dura is not common. These neoplasms are commonly cystic (approximately 50%) and may present as a mural nodule. Although there is usually a well-defined macroscopic border with the subjacent brain, there is always focal microscopic infiltration. The abundance of a reticulin-positive stroma is usually a conspicuous feature of this group of astrocytic tumors where it delineates fascicles of cells and is variably distributed between single tumor cells. However, a spectrum of PXA cases lacking this conspicuous stroma, but with otherwise typical features, have been described.[51] The prominence of this stroma may also vary between the initial and recurrent tumors, suggesting that this phenotypic feature of PXA results from interactions between tumor cells and specific types of brain extracellular matrices.

A small number of cases have demonstrated atypical ganglionic cells admixed with otherwise typical PXAs.[29,60,65,68,75] The proportion and pattern of the neuronal and glial components appear to vary from clusters of possibly entrapped neuronal elements to tumors in which the PXA appears to be the glial component of a ganglioglioma.[29,68] The histiogenic relationship between these rare cases and other desmoplastic glioneuronal neoplasms is currently unclear.

Although the initial clinical data of the PXA group suggested that these tumors should be considered a low-grade neoplasm,[53] the biologic behavior of PXA and its potential for anaplastic progression remain uncertain. A number of cases have recurred and exhibited anaplastic progression,[55,143] but this behavior appears to be significantly less common than for diffuse infiltrative astrocytomas. Nonetheless, when compared with the other more circumscribed, prognostically favorable variants of astrocytomas (i.e., pilocytic and subependymal giant-cell astrocytomas), PXA should be generally considered a tumor with a significant potential for aggressive biologic behavior. Accordingly, these tumors are designated as grade II or III (≥5 mitoses per HPF) by the WHO classification.[57,58] The histopathologic features at the infiltrating margin may be especially important for prospectively evaluating the potential for recurrence and anaplastic progression[55,143]; however, infiltration of Virchow-Robin spaces may occur without conferring a worse prognosis. PXA, in contrast to the diffuse-type astrocytomas, may recur after long intervals without anaplastic progression.[138]

The limited molecular analyses of PXA confirm its distinction from the diffuse-type astrocytomas, although there are no definitive data as to specific mechanisms of tumorigenesis and malignant progression from WHO II to WHO III. The genetic lesions that commonly present in the diffuse-type astrocytomas, the TP53 mutation and *EGFR* gene amplification, appear to be far less common in the pathogenesis of PXA, while genetic losses not common in diffuse-type astrocytomas (chromosome 8p) may play a more important role.[57,149]

Subependymal giant cell astrocytoma (WHO I). Subependymal giant-cell astrocytoma (SEGA) is a tumor that typically occurs in association with tuberous sclerosis in the first or second decades of life, but tumor development may be the primary manifestation of the disease. The tumors are conspicuously circumscribed, often nodular and multicystic with calcifications. They are most commonly located in the wall of the lateral ventricles at the level of the basal ganglia or, less commonly, adjacent to the third ventricle. Symptoms generally are related to the obstruction of the foramen of Monro.

The tumor cell populations in SEGAs exhibit a wide range of astroglial phenotypes but have the hallmark of giant pyramidal cells, with a "ganglioid" appearance. Most tumor cells demonstrate variable immunoreactivity for glial fibrillary acidic protein (GFAP) and S-100 protein, thus confirming the essentially astroglial nature of this tumor. A number of tumors, however, demonstrate both glial and neuronal-associated epitopes.[42,69] These tumors may also exhibit ultrastructural features suggestive of neuronal differentiation, including microtubules, occasional dense core granules, and rare synapse formation. These features recall those in tubers, the hamartomatous cortical lesions of tuberous sclerosis. Divergent glio-neuronal differentiation, a hallmark of tubers, may also be present in SEGAs.

In contrast to the diffuse-type astrocytomas, there is no correlation in the SEGAs between the anaplastic features of endothelial proliferation, necrosis, increased mitoses and marked cellular pleomorphism and any change in biologic behavior from typically indolent, noninvasive growth of these tumors. The rare examples of recurrent tumors have never undergone malignant transformation.[39]

Molecular genetics of SEGAs have demonstrated loss of heterozygosity in the TSC2 gene (16p13) and loss of the TSC2 gene product, tuberin, a Rap 1 homologue and putative tumor suppressor.[40,80] In a mouse model of TSC2 mutations, astroglial cells heterozygous for TSC2$^\pm$ had decreased expression of p27^{Kip1}, implicating a dysregulation of astrocyte proliferation (manifested by decreased contact inhibition in monolayer cell culture) in the development of these neoplastic lesions.[135] In addition, a functional loss of tuberin may stimulate vascular growth,[85] and SEGAs commonly have an abundance of abnormal blood vessels.

Oligodendroglial Tumors

The complex histogenesis of oligodendroglial tumors was recognized more than half a century ago and remains a current challenge to neuro-oncologists. Bailey and Bucy[5] highlighted glial heterogeneity as an intrinsic property of "oligodendrogliomas" with the variable presence of pleomorphic astrocytes and "all stages of transition" between "true" astrocytes, more primitive glia, and the predominant oligodendroglial tumor cells. Molecular genetic analyses combined with therapeutic response and survival data from clinical trials have significantly added more precision to the WHO histopathologic classification of oligodendrogliomas. There are distinct clinicogenotypic groups of tumors within the histologic continuum of gliomas that fall within the WHO oligodendroglioma classification. The first, which comprises the majority of oligodendrogliomas, has genetic losses on 1p (1p34-35; 1p36.2, 1p36.3-pter) (40% to 92%) and 19q (19q13.3) (50% to 80%). There is a tight association between 1p and 19q deletions and a mutual exclusion between this first group and the smaller numbers of histologic oligodendrogliomas that have TP53 mutation, EGFR amplification, or PTEN mutations.[26,44,107]

While multiple studies have shown that oligodendrogliomas, like low-grade astrocytomas, have hypermethylation of p14^{ARF}and CDKN2A (p16^{INK4a}) genetic loci, these loci are more commonly hypermethylated in oligodendrogliomas. Similarly, 5′-CpG island hypermethylation of multiple genetic loci may be an important epigenetic mechanism regulating gene expression at a number of sites in the tumors with 1p and 19q deletions.[147] Thus the 1p and 19q deletion appears to define a unique subset of oligodendrogliomas with a distinctive profile of gene expression.[82] This subset also has a significant responsiveness to specific chemotherapeutic agents and a best overall survival. In contrast, those oligodendrogliomas with genetic lesions other than 1p or 19q loss have poorer clinical responses and shorter overall survivals. Activation of both EGFR and PDGF receptor (PDGFR) pathways most likely play important roles in the biology of oligodendrogliomas,[142] but amplification of either EGFR or PDGFR genes is rare, even in anaplastic oligodendrogliomas with 1p or 19q loss. Wild-type EGFR may be overexpressed without the common mutation (EGFR vIII) detected in de novo glioblastomas.[76,108] Likewise, all components of the functional growth-regulated oncogene-1 (GRO1)-PDGF pathway (PDGFA, PDGFαR, the GRO1 chemokine and CXC chemokine receptor [CXCR2]) are expressed in the majority of oligodendrogliomas (WHO II and III), in contrast to diffuse-type astrocytomas (WHO II and III).[114]

Progression of oligodendrogliomas to anaplastic tumors may be accompanied by increasing alterations in cell-cycle regulatory genes, notably deletional mutations in addition to methylation at the 9p21 loci affecting CDKN2A/B/p14[ARF] and RB1 methylation.[44,107,140] Overexpression of the angiogenic growth factor vascular endothelial growth factor (VEGF) is also common with malignant progression. In addition, there are smaller subsets of anaplastic oligodendrogliomas that have a TP53 mutation,[139] 10q chromosomal loss of heterozygosity (LOH) (including PTEN) and EGFR amplification. Four subsets of histopathologic anaplastic oligodendrogliomas are defined on the basis of a hierarchy of molecular genetic alterations: (1) tumors with 1p and 19q loss without other detectable genetic lesions; (2) tumors with 1p loss without 19q loss or other detectable genetic lesions; (3) tumors with an intact 1p chromosome with TP53 mutations; and (4) tumors with an intact 1p chromosome without TP53 mutations. These neoplastic subsets have differences in the age of onset, common sites of involvement, clinical responses, and survival times.[107,141]

Oligodendroglioma (WHO II)

While approximately 5% to 15% of intracranial gliomas are classified as oligodendrogliomas, this tumor group, particularly among the low-grade gliomas, is most probably underdiagnosed as a result of its histogenetic complexity, as discussed above, and may account for a higher percentage of tumors, ranging from 19% to 25% of neoplasms. These tumors most often arise in adults, with an overall peak incidence in those in their fourth and fifth decade. In children, the peak incidence is between 6 and 12 years of age.[26] Any region of the neuroaxis may be involved, but the white matter of the frontotemporal region and the basal ganglia are common sites.

For oligodendrogliomas defined by using only the histopathologic features of the WHO classification, the criteria for grading oligodendroglial tumors as WHO II include (1) no or infrequent mitoses with overall low MIB-1 labeling indices (less than 5%); (2) no microvascular hyperplasia; and (3) no geographic necrosis. A study of Ki-67 in oligodendrogliomas showed that the mean MIB-1 labeling index (LI) in oligodendrogliomas (low-grade) is less than 2, and that tumors with MIB-1 LI greater than 5 were associated with shorter survival

time.[18,110] Correlation with neuroimaging data for clinical grading of oligodendrogliomas is strongly warranted. Magnetic resonance imaging of oligodendrogliomas (WHO II) commonly shows minimal peritumoral edema, sharply demarcated margins (60% to 70%), hypodensity on T1-weighted sequences, and hyperdensity on T2-weighted sequences. However, variable cystic degeneration and hemorrhage can result in more heterogeneous signal intensities of mixed hypodensities and isodensities on T1-weighted images.

Anaplastic Oligodendroglioma (WHO III)

Anaplastic oligodendrogliomas share the histopathologic features of oligodendrogliomas WHO II in addition to the features of necrosis, microvascular hyperplasia, and high cellularity with a high mitotic activity and increased nuclear pleomorphism. A definitive quantitative "grading" of these features as prognostic factors has been problematic. Although necrosis, increased mitotic rate, marked microvascular hyperplasia, and nuclear atypia may, in combination, be significant, extensive geographic necrosis may be a key prognostic feature. However, the molecular genetic analysis for 1p or 19q loss and other genetic aberrations, as described earlier, is an important prognostic complement to the tumor histopathology. Anaplastic tumors with brisk growth are marked by significant neovascularity and increased vascular enhancement with magnetic resonance imaging, although approximately two thirds of oligodendrogliomas (WHO II) may have a limited, patchy vascular enhancement.

Oligoastrocytoma (WHO II)

The majority of oligodendrogliomas contain variable numbers of reactive astrocytes that may be a conspicuous component of the non-neoplastic stroma. In contrast, the mixed oligoastrocytomas contain two populations of neoplastic cells that have variable astrocytic and oligodendroglial phenotypes. These different phenotypes may be focally or diffusely distributed. Smear preparations of the latter, in combination with GFAP and vimentin immunohistochemistry, highlight the distinct cytomorphologic features of the two cell populations.

Similarly to the oligodendrogliomas, molecular genetic studies have significantly complemented the histopathologic classification and have demonstrated that mixed oligoastrocytomas are a heterogeneous group of tumors with respect to molecular or genetic alterations.[8,9] One subset of these mixed tumors has the genetic lesions more typically associated with oligodendrogliomas, while another shares those molecular genetic profiles associated with the diffuse-type astrocytomas. Between 30% and 70% of oligoastrocytomas have allelic losses on chromosomes 1p and 19q in both oligodendroglial and astrocytic components,[63,74,106] while approximately 30% of tumors have genetic alterations often seen in diffuse astrocytomas, including TP53 gene mutations or 17p loss.[74,106] It appears that the subsets of oligoastrocytomas with 1p and 19q losses commonly have a predominance of oligodendroglial histologic features and more commonly occur outside the temporal lobes, while the mixed tumors with TP53 mutations or 17p loss are more often astrocytic predominant and more commonly arise in the temporal lobes.[74,81] Four subtypes of mixed oligoastrocytomas have been defined on the basis of chromosomal imbalances detected by comparative genomic hybridization: (1) tumors with losses on 1p or 19q, (2) tumors with gain on chromosome 7 (7q more than 7p) and losses on chromosome 10, (3) tumors with losses on 1p/19q, plus other chromosomal imbalances, and (4) tumors with imbalances other than in groups 1 to 3.[49] Unlike oligodendrogliomas, the mixed oligoastrocytomas do not have a well-characterized clinical behavior based on the profile of genetic aberrations. The apparent heterogeneity of mixed oligoastrocytomas suggests that glial progenitor cells with differing lineage plasticity[45] may develop tumors with similar histopathologic phenotypes but with dissimilar genotypes and gene expression profiles.

Anaplastic Oligoastrocytoma (WHO III)

The precise frequency of anaplastic progression from oligoastrocytomas is unknown. The histologic features of anaplasia are thus similar to those previously described for anaplastic astrocytomas.[83] Anaplastic progression in mixed oligoastrocytomas appears to be accompanied by more genetic aberrations than in anaplastic oligodendrogliomas, including EGFR and PDGF-R amplification, deletional loss of CDKN2A/B/p14^{ARF}, and PTEN mutation.

Ependymal Tumors

Ependymoma (WHO II)

Ependymomas represent approximately 10% of brain tumors and 6% of intracranial gliomas. Children and adolescents are affected most often, although the tumors may occur in adults. Ependymomas are most common in the second decade of life and preferentially arise in the fourth ventricle. In adults these tumors represent more than 60% of the spinal gliomas, with a peak incidence in the fourth decade. Multiple spinal cord ependymomas are typically associated with von Recklinghausen's disease.

The WHO classification recognizes four histopathologic variants of ependymomas: *cellular, papillary, clear cell,* and *tanycytic.* These tumors have essentially the same clinical behavior, but their recognition as ependymomas is important to eliminate confusion with anaplastic gliomas, meningiomas and choroid plexus tumors, oligodendrogliomas, and pilocytic astrocytomas, respectively.

Molecular genetic analyses demonstrate that the ependymomas are distinct from astrocytic and oligodendroglial tumors in that the common genetic alterations found in either of these gliomas are not common in the ependymomas. Loss of heterozygosity of chromosome 22 occurs in approximately 30% of cases in adult tumors but is uncommon in pediatric tumors,[61] and loss of the neurofibromatosis type 2 (NF2) gene on chromosome 22 may be a subset localized to the spinal cord.[24]

Anaplastic Ependymoma (WHO III)

Anaplastic progression of ependymomas can occur at most sites, but rarely in the spinal cord. For ependymal tumors, in comparison with astrocytomas, there are no features that appear to accurately grade anaplasia. Nevertheless, anaplastic ependymomas are recognized by the combination of increased cellularity and increased mitotic rate, microvascular proliferation, and variable degrees of cellular pleomorphism with nuclear atypia. Microscopic or geographic necrosis may be present, but necrosis alone is not a robust discriminating feature. A prognostic factor of particular significance in supratentorial lesions appears to be the mitotic index.[120] The importance of the proliferative component in predicting the biologic behavior has been confirmed by tumor growth-fraction measurements, either by bromodeoxyuridine (BUdR) uptake[4] or immunohistochemistry for MIB 1.[102,111,116,117,123] These studies showed that high labeling indices have a positive correlation with the histologic grade and early tumor recurrence. Alternatively, the presence of endothelial proliferation, as an independent feature, appears to be less relevant to prognosis.[115,121]

Myxopapillary Ependymoma (WHO I)

Myxopapillary ependymomas are a distinct variant of ependymoma, common in adults during their third or fourth decades, that are essentially restricted to the cauda equina. The neoplasms are usually discrete, elongate masses arising from the filum terminale or a spinal nerve root of the cauda equina. Rarely, extradural lesions in the sacral region occur, presumably from ependymal rests. Myxopapillary ependymomas contain an admixture of fibrillated and epithelioid cells with an exuberant connective tissue stroma, which may be mucin positive. Papillary arrangements of elongated fibrillary cells that extend delicate processes to hyalinized vessels are a histologic hallmark of these tumors. The unique histopathologic and biologic features of this ependymal neoplasm suggest that it may arise from cells derived from the distinctive caudal cell mass associated with the secondary caudal neural tube formation during development.

Subependymoma (WHO I)

Subependymomas are well-circumscribed, asymptomatic nodules in the walls of the fourth ventricle (66% to 70% of cases), lateral ventricles, septum pellucidum, foramen of Monro, or spinal cord. They may present with increased intracranial pressure caused by obstruction of cerebrospinal fluid (CSF) flow or with hemorrhage within the tumor, or they may be detected incidentally during autopsy. The cytoarchitectures of the tumor cells exhibit composite features of ependymal and astrocytic differentiation. Despite the occasional finding of increased atypia and mitotic activity, tumor location and successful resection are the most important prognostic factors. The histogenesis of these lesions remains to be determined, but discriminating them from ependymomas is important to avoid needless adjuvant therapy.

Choroid Plexus Tumors

Choroid plexus tumors arise from the specialized epithelium constituting the choroid plexus and therefore can arise in the lateral and fourth ventricles. However, they commonly arise in the lateral ventricles in children as *choroid plexus papillomas* (WHO I), although cases in adults and tumors arising in the fourth ventricle may also occur. Clinical symptoms are commonly caused by increased intracranial pressure, secondary to obstruction of the CSF pathways or an increased production of CSF. These clearly demarcated, often calcified tumors are distinctive for a conspicuously papillated surface that resembles the normal choroid plexus. The *choroid plexus carcinoma* (WHO III) shows anaplastic features and can be both locally invasive and diffusely disseminating in the CSF pathways.

These malignant tumors are rare (less than 20% of choroid plexus tumors) and typically occur in infants.

Neuroepithelial Tumors of Uncertain Origin

There are four neuroepithelial neoplastic lesions that have distinctive histopathologic features but for which the histogenesis is unclear. These are the *chordoid glioma of the third ventricle*, the *astroblastoma*, and *gliomatosis cerebri*. Although these tumors are considered by some authors to be individual entities, they may, in fact, represent only distinctive histopathologic variations of more well-defined ependymal, oligoastrocytoma, and astrocytic tumors.

Neuronal and Mixed Neuronal-Glial Tumors

Neuronal and mixed neuronal-glial tumors are a heterogeneous group of neoplasms that includes (1) tumors with only neuronal tumor cell phenotypes, comprising the *gangliocytoma* (WHO I) and the *dysplastic gangliocytoma of the cerebellum* (Lhermitte-Duclos disease) (WHO I); (2) tumors with a predominant neuronal cell phenotype and a minor, variable glial component, comprising *central neurocytoma* (WHO II) and *cerebellar liponeurocytoma* (WHO I to II); (3) tumors with mixed populations of neoplastic neuronal–glial populations, comprising *gangliogliomas* (WHO I to II), *desmoplastic infantile astrocytomas* and *gangliogliomas* (WHO I), and *dysembryoplastic neuroepithelial tumor (DNT)* (WHO I); and (4) tumors with neuroendocrine or neurosecretory phenotypes–neural crest derivation, comprising *paraganglioma* (WHO I). The biologic activity of DNTs especially reflects close interface between hamartomatous and neoplastic processes in tumor development.

With the exception of the dysplastic gangliocytoma of the cerebellum (see following discussion), the histogenesis and molecular genetic alterations of these tumors are not defined. Recent studies identified neural stem cells located within specific zones in the adult brain that are bipotential and unipotential progenitor cells, depending on both intrinsic and extrinsic cues.[43,131] Such cells, as targets for neoplastic transformation, could give rise to the neuronal and mixed neuronal-glial tumors. An important corollary to this hypothesis would be that the growth potential and cellular phenotypic composition of the tumors may vary according to both the temporal and spatial origin of the transformed progenitors and to the local extrinsic signals in the specific brain region. It is interesting to note that the glial component of gangliogliomas may undergo clonal evolution during tumor development.[6]

The *dysplastic gangliocytoma of the cerebellum* is a rare lesion of the CNS. The neoplasmic mass usually becomes clinically apparent between the third and fourth decades in patients with a reported mean age of 34 years; however, the lesions can clinically present from the neonatal period to 74 years. The multitude of diverse designations previously applied to this lesion, including granular cell hypertrophy, granomolecular hypertrophy of the cerebellum, diffuse hypertrophy of the cerebellar cortex, gangliomatosis of the cerebellum, and ganglioneuroma, pointedly reflect the lack of understanding about its histogenesis and disagreements as to its hamartomatous or neoplastic nature.

The majority of dysplastic gangliocytomas arise in association with the clinical manifestations of an autosomal dominant, systemic syndrome, Cowden's disease, leading to the development of multiple hamartomas and neoplasias.[114] The genetic lesion is a germline mutation of the PTEN gene. Cowden's disease has the hallmark mucocutaneous manifestations of trichilemmomas, related follicular malformations, and a distinctive type of hyalinizing, mucinous fibroma, in addition to acral keratoses and oral papillomas.[128] A significant number of patients also have thyroid adenoma or multinodular goiter, fibrocystic disease or adenocarcinoma of the breast, gastrointestinal polyps (colon, gastric, and esophageal), and ovarian cysts and polyps. The development of the cerebellar lesions in adolescents may herald the presence of Cowden's disease that usually does not more fully develop until the second to third decades.[144]

With the perspective of the germline PTEN mutation associated with this hypertrophic lesion, it is interesting to note that the tumor is composed of abnormal ganglion cells with abnormally myelinated parallel fibers, often with a reduction of the adjacent granular layer and demyelination of the cortical white matter. Thus the morphogenesis of this lesion may be an aberrant expansion of a specific neuroblastic population (possibly a block in apoptosis) in combination with altered, but limited, cellular migration. There is never any manifestation of invasiveness or evidence for a significant population of proliferating cells with dysfunctional cell-cycle regulation, as in the *de novo* GBMs that have PTEN mutations in combination with dysfunctional cell-cycle regulation and increased proliferative activity. Immunohistochemical studies suggest a histogenetic relationship to Purkinje cell lineages[27,124]; however, other data suggest an origin from granular cell progenitors.[112,148] Most likely, the neuronal proliferation arises from a more cytogenetically heterogeneous group of cells. Although most patients have a very favorable postoperative course, recurrences following subtotal resection do occur.

Pineal Parenchymal Tumors

Pineal parenchymal neoplasms account for less than 0.1% of all intracranial tumors and approximately 11% to 28% of the pineal-region tumors in children. Although these neoplasms have a wide spectrum of features, the current WHO classification designates three distinct groups. These range from the malignant *pineoblastomas* (WHO IV) to the well-differentiated *pineocytomas* (WHO I). The third group, the *pineal parenchymal tumors of intermediate differentiation*, are tumors composed of a more heterogeneous cell population encompassing the cytoarchitectural features, cellular patterns, and biologic behavior that are generally intermediate but without a predictable clinical behavior.

Embryonal Tumors

Embryonal tumors are primitive and clinically aggressive neoplasms that commonly arise during the first decade of life. They are histogenetically distinct from anaplastic variants of gliomas and glioneuronal tumors that more commonly arise in adults. All embryonal tumors, regardless of histogenesis, share the common features of high cellularity, numerous mitoses, and focal or more extensive necrosis. These features manifest a clinically aggressive behavior that corresponds to WHO IV tumors. In addition, there is a common propensity for leptomeningeal invasion and subsequent metastasis in the CSF pathways.

The classification of embryonal tumors over the past decade has been controversial with respect to the category of central primitive neuroectodermal tumors (PNETs). This category originally embraced the concept that such tumors arise from primitive neuroepithelial progenitor cells with equivalent developmental plasticity throughout the neuraxis. Although there is experimental evidence for a degree of autonomous developmental neural plasticity of stem cells,[134] this does not preclude the concept that embryonal tumors may arise from progenitor cell populations with a more limited, but different, histogenetic potential (multipotential or bipotential). Accordingly, this group of tumors would not necessarily represent a distinct clinicopathologic entity, but rather a category of tumors that could have a wide spectrum of histopathologic features and biologic behavior. Gene-expression profiling of supratentorial PNETs has demonstrated a lack of clustering and a molecular heterogeneity, possibly reflecting the diverse spectrum of tumors in this category.[101] Experimental immortalization of immature cells from the rodent cerebellum has demonstrated the existence of bipotential clonal stem cells that can differentiate into both neuronal or glial cell lineages, depending on extrinsic cues.[28] If analogous progenitor cells exist in selective regions of the immature human brain, their transformation would most likely result in the PNET histologic phenotypes with possibly distinctive epigenetic and genotypic alterations. It is most likely that the embryonal or primitive tumors of the CNS result from a combination of defects in signaling pathways that regulate the clonal expansion and differentiation of neural progenitor cell populations. The molecular biology of these tumors contrasts with the various combinations of attenuation or loss of replicative senescence, dysfunctional regulation of the cell cycle, and activation cell survival pathways that most often occur in tumors arising within the mature nervous system.

There are diverse cell populations in the immature nervous system that may be vulnerable targets for neoplastic transformation; however, special caution should be exercised in this context to avoid complete reliance on immunohistochemical techniques to establish the cell lineages of otherwise poorly differentiated tumors. Transient or heteroplastic expression of cell type–associated proteins, differential sensitivity of specific epitopes to routine tissue handling, and incomparable antibody reagents should always be carefully considered, and all results should be interpreted with these reservations. Despite this caveat, a small number of embryonal tumors may be characterized on the basis of distinctive features.

The current classification scheme recognizes a number of embryonal tumors with restricted and relatively limited neural histogenetic potentials along neuronal and glial or ependymal cell lineages: the supratentorial cerebral PNETs (*neuroblastoma* and *ganglioneuroblastoma*) and the *ependymoblastoma*, respectively. A rare embryonal neoplasm, the *medulloepithelioma*, merits separate mention. In contrast to the other tumors mentioned, this neoplasm has the hallmark of a mitotically active, pseudostratified columnar epithelium, often arranged in ribbons of tubules or papillary rosettes with variable interposition of delicate stromal elements, recapitulating the primitive epithelium of the neural tube. Approximately 50% of cases exhibit neuroblastic or neuronal, astroglial, or ependymal cell populations that are either intimately admixed with the tubules or present in more well-demarcated fields. Immunohistochemical studies demonstrate abundant IGF-1 and fibroblast growth factor (FGF)-2[125] in this primitive epithelium. In contrast, only rare sporadic expression of neuroblastic and glial cytoskeletal proteins (the neuron-specific class III β-tubulin isotype TUJI

and GFAP, respectively) is present in the epithelial structures, while these proteins can be readily demonstrated in the more differentiated cell populations surrounding the primitive neoplastic neuroepithelium.

Medulloblastoma (WHO IV)

Medulloblastoma is the most common and well characterized of embryonal tumors. In children it constitutes approximately one quarter of all intracranial tumors. The peak incidence for medulloblastomas is near the end of the first decade, and there is a slight male predilection. Most are situated in the cerebellar midline, although pediatric tumors may also appear in the cerebellar hemispheres. The latter tends to be a more common site in the rare adult cases. Rare variants of medulloblastoma include tumors showing striated muscle cell differentiation with populations of more primitive cells resembling rhabdomyosarcoma (medullomyoblastoma WHO IV) and pigmented papillary forms (melanotic medulloblastoma WHO IV) that are dissimilar to melanotic neuroectodermal tumors of infancy. The histogenetic relationships of these tumors to the more common forms of medulloblastoma are not understood.

Medulloblastomas exhibit various phenotypic manifestations of neuroblastic or neuronal differentiation as demonstrated by standard immunohistochemistry for neuronal cytoskeletal, membrane or vesicular, and neurosensory epitopes. Several histologic variants are recognized: (1) the *classic* subtype constituted by sheets of undifferentiated cells with variable numbers of neuroblastic rosettes and palisades, (2) the *desmoplastic* or *nodular* subtype with rows and nodules of neoplastic cells separated by an abundant collagen stroma, (3) the "*extensively nodular*" subtype, and (4) the *large-cell* or *anaplastic* subtype.

In the classic form, sporadic morphologic differentiation to ganglion cells within the primitive populations may occur without any apparent correlation with clinical behavior. In a large retrospective study,[23] moderate to severe grades of anaplasia occurred in approximately one quarter of the cases and were associated with aggressive clinical behavior. Anaplasia is defined by increased nuclear size, abundant mitoses, and the presence of a large-cell component resembling the large-cell or anaplastic subtype (see the following discussion).

The desmoplastic or nodular subtype has highly cellular sheets and trabeculae of typical tumor cells embedded in a conspicuous collagen stroma. Within the reticular-free zones, there is a variable decrease in cellularity that is accompanied by variably fibrillated processes and cells with morphologic evidence of increasing neuronal and ganglionic differentiation. In contrast, the desmoplastic areas are composed of highly cellular, proliferating cell populations. The designation of "extensive nodular subtype" is applied when this biphasic pattern becomes predominant with the formation of extensive, less cellular nodules of reticulin-free populations of prominently fibrillary, differentiated cells, as demonstrated by neuronal cytoskeleton and synaptophysin immunoreactivity. The characteristic nodular architectural pattern can be present in an initial specimen and may not be present in recurrent tumors.

Recent studies suggest that a combination of histopathologic taxonomy[23] and molecular analysis of medulloblastomas[25,101] may be the future basis for a more precise prognostic grading of these complex neoplasms. Gene-expression profiling shows that these desmoplastic or nodular subtypes are highly correlated with activation of the sonic hedgehog (SHH) pathway,[101] typically associated with disruption of the suppressive SSH receptor PATCHED (PTCH). This variant is also associated with germline mutations of PTCH (Gorlin syndrome). Downstream targets of SHH include regulation of the Gli zinc finger transcription factors and the N-MYC oncogene; both are up-regulated in experimental tumorigenesis associated with SHH activation,[25,38] and N-MYC up-regulation also promotes proliferation in granule neuron precursors.[52] Medulloblastomas with the best clinical prognosis appear to have down-regulation of N-MYC and up-regulation of tyrosin-kinase (Trk)-C (TrkC), a neurotrophin (NT) receptor subtype.[25] It is interesting to note that in experimental murine models, up-regulation of the SHH pathway results in tumors with the medulloblastoma phenotype. TP53 loss augments this experimental effect, and 17p deletions in association with Li-Fraumeni syndrome are associated with medulloblastomas. Likewise, LOH 17p may also occur in sporadic medulloblastomas (including classic subtypes), along with a variety of other cytogenetic aberrations, including deletions on 11p or 11q, 10q, 8, 16q, and 9q22 (PTCH) and amplifications on 7, 5p13, 11q22, and 8q24 (C-MYC). Mutations in the Wnt/APC pathway in association with type 2 Turcot syndrome (germline mutation in the APC gene) are also associated with the development of medulloblastomas; however, sporadic medulloblastomas rarely have mutations in the Wnt or APC pathway.

The most uncommon type of cytoarchitectural variant of medulloblastoma is the large-cell or anaplastic variant. This variant has an exceptionally aggressive biologic behavior[23] and is wholly populated by polygonal tumor cells with large round or lobated nuclei with prominent nucleoli and relatively more abundant cytoplasm than in the more common tumors. Abundant mitoses and nuclear molding are typical, as are conspicuous areas of necrosis.

Atypical Teratoid/Rhabdoid Tumor (WHO IV)

Atypical teratoid/rhabdoid tumor (AT/RT) refers to a group of rare childhood brain tumors that are distinctive for the presence of "rhabdoid cells." These tumors most commonly develop in the posterior fossa, although supratentorial tumors and tumors involving multiple sites are not uncommon.[89] Most patients are 3 years of age or younger, with a relative male predominance.

Tumor diagnosis is based on the combination of a distinctive histopathology, immunohistochemistry, and molecular genetic analysis. The histopathology is marked by large and polygonal rhabdoid cells with a conspicuous eosinophilic cytoplasm containing spherical fibrillary intracytoplasmic inclusions. In addition, there are often other tissue elements present, including primitive neuroepithelium, mesenchyme, and mature epithelium. The rhabdoid cells may be abundant or may be incorporated into these complex mixtures of primitive neuroepithelial cells. Although the hallmark cells are designated as "rhabdoid," they lack true muscle differentiation and are immunonegative with desmin. They may show variable immunopositivity with epithelial-membrane antigen (EMA), vimentin, and smooth muscle actin, and occasionally they react with GFAP, cytokeratin, and neurofilament protein. Germ cell markers are negative. Cytogenetic analysis of AT/RT reveals a loss of chromosome 22 or specific loss of 22q11 with aber-

rations in the chromatin remodeling/tumor suppressor gene hSNF5/INI1 ([human] sucrose nonfermentor/integrase interactor 1). These genetic alterations are restricted to malignant rhabdoid tumors or AT/RTs and are not present in medulloblastomas or other embryonal tumors arising in the CNS.[64,137] These embryonal tumors are extremely aggressive neoplasms associated with an overall median survival of 8.5 months, and gross total resection appears to increase this interval to 14 months.[89]

TUMORS OF THE MENINGES

Tumors of Meningothelial Cells

Meningioma (WHO I)

Meningiomas are tumors derived from the arachnoidal cells present in the arachnoidal villi and granulations and in the stroma of perivascular spaces and choroid plexus. They account for approximately 13% to 19% of intracranial tumors and one fourth of intraspinal tumors. Meningiomas usually become clinically evident in middle age and only rarely occur during childhood. There is a marked female predominance (3 to 1) in adults, especially with intradural tumors. Multiple meningiomas may occur in nearly 8% of the cases,[84] particularly in association with the neurofibromatosis type 2. Pediatric tumors are more likely to demonstrate malignant transformation[98] and have a higher proportion of the papillary variant. Loss of heterozygosity for loci on chromosome 22 has been demonstrated in 40% to 80% of sporadic tumors, and the genetic defect has been localized to the NF2 locus.

Meningiomas can occur anywhere in the meninges, but certain sites are favored. The intracranial examples are most common in the sagittal area along the superior longitudinal sinus, over the lateral cerebral convexities, at the tuberculum sellae and parasellar region, on the olfactory grooves, and over the sphenoidal ridge. Intraventricular meningiomas arise presumably from arachnoidal cells within the tela choroidea or stroma of the choroid plexus. They may also arise in the pineal region, in the orbit (3% of orbital expanding lesions), and in intraosseous locations at the cerebellopontine angle. In the spinal canal, meningiomas occur in the thoracic, cervical, and lumbar regions in order of decreasing frequency.

Numerous variants of meningiomas are described, reflecting the mesenchymal and epithelial histogenetic potential of arachnoidal cells (Table 5-1). Although the majority of these variants exhibit similar biologic behavior, some are associated with systemic diseases, such as Castleman's disease with the chordoid variant[54] and polyclonal gammopathies with lymphoplasmocyte-rich tumors.[47] The "epithelial" phenotype of meningiomas is expressed by the *microcystic, secretory, clear cell* (glycogen rich), *chordoid*, and *papillary* variants. Inclusions positive to periodic acid-Schiff (PAS) staining are commonly found in the secretory variant, the intracytoplasmic lumina within which they lie being lined by microvilli.[103] Both clear cell and chordoid variants behave in a more aggressive fashion, analogous to the atypical meningiomas. All three types of meningiomas are considered, accordingly, as WHO grade II neoplasms. Clear cell meningiomas are glycogen rich, often posterior fossa or spinal in location, and behave in an aggressive manner, which includes a very high recurrence rate and

TABLE 5-1

World Health Organization Grading of Meningiomas

Meningioma	WHO Grade
Low Risk of Recurrence and/or Aggressive Growth	
Meningothelial meningioma	I
Fibrous/fibroblastic meningioma	I
Transitional (mixed) meningioma	I
Psammomatous meningioma	I
Angiomatous meningioma	I
Microcystic meningioma	I
Secretory meningioma	I
Lymphoplasmocyte-rich meningioma	I
Metaplastic meningioma	I
Greater Risk of Recurrence and/or Aggressive Growth	
Atypical meningioma (with/without brain invasion)	II
Clear cell meningioma	II
Chordoid meningioma	II
Rhabdoid meningioma	III
Papillary meningioma	III
Anaplastic (malignant) meningioma	III

Source: Adapted from Kleihues P, Louis DN, Scheithauer BW, et al: The WHO classification of tumors of the nervous system. J Neuropathol Exp Neurol 61:215–225, 2002.

spinal seeding.[150] Chordoid meningiomas contain areas that recall the histologic pattern of chordomas with ribbons of eosinophilic, vacuolated cells in a myxoid matrix.

Atypical Meningioma (WHO II)

The WHO classification includes a variant of meningioma with biologic behavior intermediate between the typical meningioma (WHO grade I) and the anaplastic (malignant) meningioma (WHO grade III). Although these tumors lack histopathologic features clearly associated with malignancy, they show an increased tendency to recur and be locally aggressive. These tumors, along with the chordoid and clear cell variants, are designated as WHO grade II neoplasms. Important histopathologic features of such atypical tumors include hypercellularity, increased mitotic activity, diffuse or sheetlike growth, increased nuclear pleomorphism with nucleolar prominence, and the presence of micronecrosis. These features may be present in any histologic variant of meningioma and may be focal in a given tumor. Thus careful examination of multiple tissue sections is necessary in evaluating meningiomas. One of the most valuable parameters for predicting recurrence appears to be a quantitative assessment of mitotic activity, at least 4 or 5 mitotic figures per 10 HPFs being commonly accepted numbers.[73,95] Determination of tumor proliferative potential has been of value in identifying tumors that are likely to recur. Tumors with higher MIB-1 LI are known to exhibit a greater

chance for recurrence as compared with the usual meningioma.[15,97] Brain invasion with infiltration and integration of cerebral parenchyma is considered a strong indicator for recurrence.

Anaplastic Meningioma (WHO III)

The distinction between atypical and anaplastic meningiomas is a matter of degree, involving the same histopathologic features. Therefore anaplastic meningiomas display marked nuclear and cellular pleomorphism, high mitotic activity, and necrosis. A number of genomic alterations (in more than 30% of tumors) accumulate in the anaplastic progression from WHO I to WHO III meningiomas.[78,104] Meningiomas WHO I, in addition to a loss on 22q, may also have a loss on 18p, the location of the DAL-1 (Differentially expressed in Adenocarcinoma of the Lung) gene. Atypical meningiomas show gains on 1q, 9q, 12q, 15q, 17q, and 20q and losses on 1p, 6q10q, 14q, and 18q. Anaplastic tumors also show a loss on 17q and in the CDKN2A locus on 9p.[99]

Papillary Meningioma (WHO III)

Papillary meningioma, a rare malignant variant of meningioma, is more common in children and young adults, has a high tendency toward invasion and recurrence, and not uncommonly develops distant metastases. Accordingly, this variant is designated as WHO grade III. Histologically, this tumor is highly cellular, composed of epithelial-like cells with cuboidal or columnar shape and well-defined cytoplasmic borders. The tumor cells are often arranged in papillary structures around blood vessels or in "epithelial" ribbons that fuse into more patternless sheets, simulating metastatic adenocarcinoma. High cellularity and mitotic activity with evidence of brain invasion are common. Although the papillary pattern may be predominant, areas with the more classic meningothelial appearance are usually found after careful searching. Even the presence of a focal papillary pattern is associated with an increased likelihood of recurrence.[15]

Rhabdoid Meningioma (WHO III)

Meningiomas that contain a significant proportion of cells with a rhabdoid morphology are uncommon[96] but are notable for an aggressive biologic behavior similar to the anaplastic or malignant meningiomas. Therefore these neoplasms are designated, along with the anaplastic and papillary variants, as WHO grade III. The rhabdoid cells may be grouped in relatively large discohesive sheets or in a patchy pattern. The cytoarchitecture is similar to rhabdoid tumor cells described at other sites in that they are rounded and contain conspicuous eosinophilic cytoplasm filled with hyaline, paranuclear inclusions. Focal rhabdoid features without other evidence for malignancy may not necessarily signify an aggressive biologic behavior.

Mesenchymal, Nonmeningothelial Tumors

A number of mesenchymal neoplasms may occasionally arise in the meninges. Generally, these tumors have similar features to their counterparts outside the CNS. The more common benign tumors in this category include chondroma, osteochondroma, osteoma, lipoma, and fibrous histiocytoma. The most commonly encountered sarcomas include chondrosarcoma, malignant fibrous histiocytoma, and rhabdomyosarcoma.

Differential diagnosis of the rare solitary fibrous tumors (SFTs) from meningiomas is the most problematic. In contrast to fibroblastic meningiomas, SFTs do not show typical cellular patterns of meningothelial or syncytial whorling and psammomatous bodies, and the intercellular collagen tends to be more conspicuous and uniformly distributed. The collagenous matrix may be so abundant, focally, as to be the predominant feature, appearing as dense ropes of keloid-like bundles. Focal myxoid change may be present, but tumors in which this pattern predominates, as in tumors outside the CNS,[127] have not been described.

Regardless of cellular pattern, immunohistochemistry usually permits more precise recognition of these tumors.[94] CD34 (an antigen expressed on hematopoetic progenitor cells) immunoreactivity is typically strong and diffuse in contrast to the more focal, heterogeneously weaker staining of tumor cells in fibrous meningiomas and hemangiopericytomas. No immunoreactivity for S-100 protein or for epithelial cell phenotypes like the cytokeratins or EMA expression is detectable.

While the metastatic potential of the leptomeningeal solitary fibrous tumors appears to be low, tumor recurrence is common without total resection. Unlike tumors arising outside the CNS, the criteria for malignant SFTs in the CNS are not established and none have been reported. The combination of uniform, very high cellularity, higher mitotic indices, conspicuous cellular pleomorphism with prominent nucleoli, and nuclear atypia should most likely be considered suggestive for an increased malignant potential.

Hemangiopericytoma (WHO II,III)

Hemangiopericytomas of the meninges, accounting for approximately 1% to 7% of all meningeal tumors, are aggressive neoplasms with high rates of recurrence and direct metastatic spread. The majority of the tumors occur in adults, with a male predominance. The histogenesis of these tumors has been the subject of longstanding controversy among neuropathologists, but meningeal hemangiopericytomas are usually considered to be identical to their soft-tissue counterparts.

Melanocytic Lesions of the Meninges

Melanocytic tumors arising from leptomeningeal melanocytes are well circumscribed or diffuse and benign with aggressive potential or frankly malignant. This diverse group of neoplasms includes *diffuse melanocytosis, melanocytoma,* and *malignant melanoma.*

TUMORS OF UNCERTAIN HISTOGENESIS

Hemangioblastoma

CNS hemangioblastomas are relatively uncommon and are mostly found in adults, with a peak incidence in the fourth decade. Their classical location is the cerebellum, but they also occur in the brainstem and spinal cord. Supratentorial and multiple tumors are rare and more often associated with von Hippel-Lindau disease.[126]

PRIMARY LYMPHOMAS OF THE CENTRAL NERVOUS SYSTEM

Primary CNS lymphomas (PCNSLs) have remarkably increased in incidence over the past decade. Previously, these tumors were relatively rare, comprising 1% or fewer of all CNS tumors. In more recent series, PCNSLs have comprised nearly 7% of all primary CNS tumors. Although much of this increase may be attributed to an increase in immunocompromised patients, especially in association with AIDS, there is also an increase in CNS lymphomas among immunocompetent patients as well. Males in their sixth or seventh decade of life, with no apparent risk factors, appear to be most commonly affected by CNS lymphomas. In the immunocompromised population, the fifth, or in some series the fourth, decade is now the most common age threshold in large institutions.

PCNSLs usually arise in the supratentorium within the deep white matter of the cerebral hemispheres or in the basal ganglia, but periventricular locations are not uncommon. Unlike most primary CNS intra-axial tumors, these tumors are often multiple and multifocal, simulating metastatic tumors. PCNSLs are typically of the diffuse, large cell, or immunoblastic variety,[3,12] with more than 90% revealing a B-cell histogenesis, usually with immunoglobulin M (IgM) kappa production. T-cell PCNSLs are exceedingly rare but, when present, often involve the leptomeningeal space or posterior fossa of immunocompetent individuals. Much rarer is the Ki-1 anaplastic lymphoma subtype.[91] PCNSLs are generally high-grade tumors with very poor 5-year survival rates, particularly in patients with AIDS, and Epstein-Barr virus (EBV) appears to play a major role in the great majority of PCNSLs arising in immunocompromised individuals.[1] However, EBV genome has been identified in only a small population of PCNSLs arising in immunocompetent patients.[10] In contrast, human herpesvirus 8 DNA has recently been identified in PCNSLs in patients with and without AIDS.[14] A recent study of genetic alterations in immunocompetent individuals with PCNSLs (B-cell and T-cell lymphomas) has demonstrated frequent inactivation of the CDKN2A gene and only minor rare alterations of TP53 or BCL2 genes.[17]

The most common microscopic appearance of PCNSL reveals the cytologic features of large B-cell lymphomas: large cells with round or lobated nuclei with vesicular chromatin and prominent nucleoli that are typically admixed with variable numbers of reactive lymphocytes, histiocytes, microglia, and astrocytes. Most PCNSL infiltrates are poorly delineated and have a patchy distribution in an angiocentric pattern with both perivascular infiltrates and angioinvasion. Hypertrophic, reactive astrocytes are typically present and often conspicuous in the moderately cellular portions of the lesion.

GERM CELL TUMORS

Primary intracranial germ cell tumors are rare and occur primarily during childhood and adolescence. Like extragonadal germ cell tumors, they tend to arise almost exclusively in the midline structures, including the pineal and sellar regions, third ventricle, and hypothalamus, and only rarely in the spinal cord. The histogenesis and differentiation of germ cell tumors in the CNS are considered to be analogous to their gonadal and extragonadal counterparts. All types of germ cell tumors have been described in the CNS, including *germinomas, embryonal carcinomas, yolk sac tumors* (endodermal sinus tumors), *choriocarcinomas*, and *teratomas*. The *malignant variant* of teratoma shows malignant transformation of one or more of the three adult tissues, typically as encountered in other organs and tissues (e.g., sarcomas and carcinomas). Although the histologic picture of CNS teratomas is identical to that of those that arise in other regions, special mention will be made of the *immature variant*. In this type of teratoma, the immature component is not uncommonly composed of neuroepithelial elements, including patterns abundant in medulloepitheliomas, neuroblastomas, retinoblastomas, or ependymoblastomas. Unlike their neoplastic counterparts in embryonal-type tumors, their presence in infantile or young pediatric teratomas does not necessarily connote less favorable clinical behavior.

TUMORS OF THE SELLAR REGION

A spectrum of tumors may arise in the skull base in the region of the sella. The most common are *pituitary adenomas*, which comprise a variety of phenotypes that produce pituitary hormones (growth hormone [GH], prolactin [PRL], mixed GH-PRL, adrenocorticotropic hormone (ACTH), thyroid stimulating hormone [TSH]), the gonadotrophins (follicle-stimulating hormone (FSH), luteinizing hormone (LH), α-subunit), and nonfunctioning adenomas. Other neoplasms arising in this region include the *craniopharyngioma* and, in fewer patients, the *granular cell tumors* of the pituitary stalk.

Craniopharyngioma (WHO I)

Craniopharyngiomas are more common in children and adolescents, typically with a male predominance. Tumors in both neonates and adults may also occur. The majority of these tumors are in the intrasellar and suprasellar areas, where they may expand and compress the optic nerve and chiasma, and the third-ventricle region. In addition, craniopharyngiomas can arise as an "ectopic" tumor in surgical tracts. The current classification identifies two variants, the adamantinous and the papillary. Most commonly, the tumors contain variable proportions of these two histologic patterns. The papillary areas are composed of simple stratified squamous epithelium resting upon a connective stroma, usually forming pseudopapillary structures. Finger-like extensions of this epithelium commonly infiltrate the adjacent parenchyma. The adamantinous pattern is characterized by stratified epithelium with a palisading arrangement of the basal cells, keratin formation, and microcystic changes. The adjacent brain demonstrates exuberant astrogliosis with Rosenthal fiber formation.

Granular Cell Tumors of the Neurohypophysis (WHO I)

Granular cell tumors of the neurohypophysis are benign tumors arising from the neurohypophysis or infundibulum. The nests of large polygonal cells with eosinophilic cytoplasm contain abundant lysosomes and typically are immunoreactive for neuron-specific enolase (NSE), S-100, and a variety of lysosomal markers. Some tumors may also be immunoreactive for GFAP.

PERIPHERAL NEUROBLASTIC TUMORS

Neuroblastic tumors that arise outside the nervous system arise from histogenetically diverse cells. They range from *olfactory neuroblastomas*, with presumptive origins from the neurosensory portion of the nasal epithelium with both neuroblastic and neurosecretory or neuroendocrine phenotypes, to the primitive and differentiating neuroblastic tumors of the sympathetic nervous system and adrenal gland—*neuroblastomas, ganglioneuroblastomas*, and *ganglioneuromas*. The neural crest origin of the latter group confers a complex biology that presents both diagnostic and therapeutic challenges. Deletion of a presumptive tumor suppressor gene on chromosome 1p, N-MYC amplification, nerve growth-factor receptor (TrkA) expression, 17q23 gain amplification,[118] and ploidy are, in combination, molecular features important for prognostic tumor typing.

PERIPHERAL NERVE TUMORS

Most of the tumors that develop in relation to the peripheral nervous system are cells with lineages derived from neural crest progenitors or from mesenchymal cells that are intimately associated with the neural sheath. Putative targets for neoplastic transformation therefore include Schwann cells (*schwannoma*, WHO I), nerve sheath fibroblasts, which elaborate a specialized extracellular matrix, and with the microvascular elements form the endoneurial framework investing individual nerve fibers (*neurofibroma*, WHO I), and the perineurial cells, which play a specialized role in regulating diffusion into nerve fascicles (*perineuroma*, WHO I). Phenotypic features common to the neoplastic cells and these normal cellular constituents of the nerve sheath are the basis for classifying tumors as schwannomas, neurofibromas, or perineuromas. The schwannoma is a relatively homogeneous tumor, with cells restricted to Schwann cell phenotypes. In contrast, neurofibromas contain a more heterogeneous spectrum of both Schwann cell and neural sheath fibroblastic phenotypes. The perineuroma is a rare soft tissue tumor composed of cells with the morphologic and immunohistochemical features of perineurial cells.

Histologic variants of schwannoma include *cellular schwannomas, melanotic schwannomas*, and *schwannomas with a plexiform growth pattern* that arise in peripheral soft tissue (usually skin) in association with multiple schwannomas or NF2. Approximately 10% of schwannomas are a variant designated as cellular schwannoma. These tumors typically develop in a paravertebral or paraspinous location with or without a gross association with a nerve or autonomic ganglion. There is a distinctive combination of high cellularity, a predominance of Antoni A pattern with tightly interlacing fascicles of elongated tumor cells, sparse Antoni B zones, and nuclear hyperchromasia. Even with the feature of hypercellularity, the modest mitotic activity should not be considered as evidence of anaplastic change in this tumor. Nonetheless, it is notable that tumors in paravertebral, sacral, or intracranial locations may more likely recur as compared with peripherally situated tumors.[13]

Melanotic schwannomas (including psammomatous melanotic schwannoma) are a less common variant of schwannoma. The overall age at presentation is younger than other variants. Multiple tumors may arise in younger patients (third versus fourth decade for solitary tumors) in the setting of the Carney's complex, a distinctive autosomal dominant clinicopathologic complex of myxomas (heart, skin, and breast), spotty pigmentation, and pigmented nodular adrenocortical disease with endocrine overactivity (Cushing's syndrome), pituitary adenoma (acromegaly), and large cell calcifying Sertoli cell tumors. The melanotic tumor cells may be (1) spindled, dendritic forms, (2) fusiform cells, or (3) epithelioid forms. The vascular stroma is variable and ranges from regions with sparsely distributed thin-walled sinusoid microvessels to hyalinized, thick-walled forms typically present in schwannomas. Melanotic schwannomas may also develop as isolated lesions without evidence or familial history of Carney's complex. These tumors are typically more homogeneous and have a typical spectrum of Schwann cell phenotypes that express various stages of melanosomal differentiation. While most tumors have a benign biologic behavior, increased mitotic rate may be associated with a more aggressive behavior.

Solitary neurofibromas are the most abundant tumor of the peripheral nerve and most commonly arise as indolent tumors in the absence of NF1. Multiple neurofibromas occur as a hallmark manifestation of NF1. Neurofibromas may be classified into intraneural and diffusely infiltrative forms. Intraneural lesions are solitary, fusiform, or less often, multinodular with involvement of numerous branches. Such a "plexiform" growth pattern of a neurofibroma is pathognomonic of NF1. In contrast to schwannomas and solitary neurofibromas, neurofibromas in the context of NF1 show a distinct tendency to undergo malignant transformation, especially with plexiform neurofibromas.

Malignant Peripheral Nerve Sheath Tumors (WHO III-IV)

Malignant peripheral nerve sheath tumors (MPNSTs) refer to most spindle cell sarcomas arising from a nerve or a preexisting benign nerve sheath tumor and sarcomas showing nerve sheath differentiation. In the majority of the cases, MPNSTs represent malignant counterparts of neurofibromas, because malignant transformation of schwannomas is extremely rare. While MPNSTs may arise sporadically and *de novo*, most occur in the setting of NF1 in a preexisting lesion. Molecular studies of MPNST from patients with NF1 have demonstrated complete loss of heterozygosity of 17q loci, including loci within the NF1 gene. Some tumors also show deletions on 17p that may involve the TP53 gene and LOH of chromosome 22. Loss of p16 (chromosome 9p21) may accompany the malignant progression of neurofibromas to MPNST.[62]

MPNSTs show considerable cytologic and histologic variation. The majority of the tumors are composed of a densely cellular fascicle of spindle cells. Mitotic activity is quite high. Necrosis is often prominent and may exhibit a geographic aspect accompanied by peripheral cell palisading. Approximately 20% of the cases have heterologous differentiation, which is especially prominent in patients with NF1. This includes rhabdomyosarcomatous elements, composing the so-called malignant triton tumor, mature skeletal muscle, bone, cartilage, and epithelial and neuroendocrine elements.

References

1. Aboody-Guterman K, Hair L, Morgello S: Epstein-Barr virus and AIDS-related primary central nervous system lymphoma: viral detection by immunohistochemistry, RNA in situ hybridization, and polymerase chain reaction. Clin Neuropathol 15:79–86, 1996.
2. Actor B, Ludwig Cobbers JMJ, Büschges R, et al: Comprehensive analysis of genomic alterations in gliosarcoma and its two tissue components. Genes Chromosomes Cancer 34:416–427, 2002.
3. Altavilla G, Cssateill P, Salmaso R, Gardiman M: Primary central nervous system lymphomas: clinicopathology and immunohistochemical analysis of 30 cases. Tumors 85:19–27, 1999.
4. Asai A, Hoshino T, Edwards MS, Davis RL: Predicting the recurrence of ependymomas from the bromodeoxyuridine labeling index. Childs Nerv Syst 8:273–278, 1992.
5. Bailey P, Bucy PC: Oligodendrogliomas of the brain. J Pathol Bacteriol 32:735–751, 1929.
6. Becker AJ, Löbach M, Klein H, et al: Mutational analysis of TSC1 and TSC2 genes in gangliogliomas. Neuropathol Appl Neurobiol 27:105–114, 2001.
7. Besson A, Wee Yong V: Mitogenic signaling and the relationship to cell cycle regulation in astrocytomas. J Neurooncol 51:245–264, 2001.
8. Bigner SH, Matthews MR, Rasheed BKA, et al: Molecular genetic aspects of oligodendrogliomas including analysis by comparative genomic hybridization. Am J Pathol 155:375–386, 1999.
9. Bigner SH, Raheed A, Wiltshire R, McLendon RE: Morphologic and molecular genetic aspects of oligodendroglial neoplasms. J Neurooncol 1:52–60, 1999.
10. Bignon YJ, Clavelou P, Ramos F, et al: Detection of Epstein-Barr virus sequences in primary brain lymphoma without immunodeficiency. Neurology 41:1152–1153, 1991.
11. Bruno S, Darzynkiewicz Z: Cell cycle dependent expression and stability of the nuclear protein detected by Ki-67 antibody in HL-60 cells. Cell Prolif 25:31–40, 1992.
12. Camilleri-Broet S, Martin A, Moreau A, et al: Primary central nervous system lymphomas in 72 immunocopetent patients. Am J Clin Pathol 110:607–612, 1998.
13. Casadei GP, Scheithauer BW, Hirose T, et al: Cellular schwannoma. A clinicopathologic, DNA flow cytometric, and proliferation marker study of 70 patients. Cancer 75:1109–1119, 1995.
14. Cerboy JR, Garl PJ, Kleinschmidt-DeMasters BK: Human herpesvirus 8 DNA in CNS lymphomas from patients with and without AIDS. Neurology 50:335–340, 1998.
15. Chen WY, Liu HC: Atypical (anaplastic) meningioma: relationship between histologic features and recurrence. A clinicopathologic study. Clin Neuropathol 9:74–81, 1990.
16. Cheng Y, Ng HK, Zhang SF, et al: Genetic alterations in pediatric high-grade astrocytomas. Hum Pathol 30(11):1284–1290, 1999.
17. Cobbers JM, Wolter M, Reifenberger J, et al: Frequent inactivation of CDKN2A and rare mutation of TP53 in PCNSL. Brain Pathol 8:263–276, 1998.
18. Coons SW, Johnson PC, Pearl DK: The prognostic significance of Ki-67 labelling indices for oligodendrogliomas. Neurosurgery 41:878–884, 1997.
19. Couldwell WT, Weiss MH, Law RE, Hinton DR: Paradoxical elevation of Ki-67 labeling with protein kinase inhibition in malignant gliomas. J Neurosurg 82:461–468, 1995.

20. Dai C, Celestino JC, Okada Y, et al: PDGF autocrine stimulation dedifferentiates cultured astrocytes and induces oligodendrogliomas and oligoastrocytomas from neural progenitors and astrocytes in vivo. Genes Dev 15:1913–1925, 2001.
21. Duchrow M, Gerdes J, Schluter C: The proliferation-associated Ki-67 protein: definition in molecular terms. Cell Prolif 27:235–242, 1994.
22. Eberhart CG, Kepner JL, Goldthwaite PT, et al: Histopathologic grading of medulloblastomas: a pediatric oncology group study. Cancer 94(2):552–560, 2000.
23. Eberhart CG, Kratz JE, Schuster A, et al: Comparative genomic hybridization detects an increased number of chromosomal alterations in large cell/anaplastic medulloblastomas. Brain Pathol 12:36–44, 2002.
24. Ebert C, von Haken M, Meyer-Puttlitz B, et al: Molecular genetic analysis of ependymal tumors: NF2 mutations and chromosome 22q loss occur preferentially in intramedullary spinal ependymomas. Am J Pathol 155:627–632, 1999.
25. Ellison D: Classifying the medulloblastomas: insights from morphology and molecular genetics. Neuropathol Appl Neurobiol 28:257–282, 2002.
26. Engelhard HH, Stelea A, Cochran EJ: Oligodendroglioma: pathology and molecular biology. Surg Neurol 58:111–117, 2002.
27. Faillot T, Sichez JP, Brault JL, et al: Lhermitte-Duclos disease (dysplastic gangliocytoma of the cerebellum). Report of a case and review of the literature. Acta Neurochir (Wien) 105:44–49, 1990.
28. Frederiksen K, Jat PS, Valtz N, et al: Immortalization of precursor cells from the mammalian CNS. Neuron 1:439–448, 1988.
29. Furuta A, Takahashi H, Ikuta F, et al: Temporal lobe tumor demonstrating ganglioglioma and pleomorphic xanthoastrocytoma components. Case report. J Neurosurg 77:143–147, 1992.
30. Garcia DM, Fulling KH: Juvenile pilocytic astrocytoma of the cerebrum in adults. A distinctive neoplasm with favorable prognosis. J Neurosurg 63:382–386, 1985.
31. Gerdes J, Schwab U, Lemke H, Stein H: Production of a mouse monoclonal antibody reactive with a human nuclear antigen associated with cell proliferation. Int J Cancer 31:13–20, 1983.
32. Gerdes J, Lemke H, Baisch H, et al: Cell cycle analysis of a cell proliferation-associated human nuclear antigen defined by the monoclonal antibody Ki-67. J Immunol 133:1710–1715, 1984.
33. Gerdes J, Ki L, Schlüter C, et al: Cell cycle analysis of a cell proliferation-associated human nuclear antigen that is defined by monoclonal antibody Ki-67. Am J Pathol 138:867–873, 1991.
34. Giannini C, Scheithauer BW, Burger PC, et al: Cellular proliferation in pilocytic and diffuse astrocytomas. J Neuropathol Exp Neurol 58:46–53, 1999.
35. Gutmann DH, Donahor J, Brown T, et al: Loss of neurofibromatosis 1 (NF1) gene expression in NF1-associated pilocytic astrocytomas. Neuropathol Appl Neurobiol 26:(4)361–367, 2000.
36. Gutmann DH, Wu YL, Hedrick NM, et al: Heterozygosity for the neurofibromatosis 1 (NF1) tumor suppressor results in abnormalities in cell attachment, spreading and motility in astrocytes. Hum Mol Genet 10(26):3009–3016, 2001.
37. Gutmann DH, Medrick NM, Li J, et al: Comparative gene expression profile analysis of neurofibromatosis 1-associated and sporadic pilocytic astrocytomas. Cancer Res 62:2085–2091, 2002.
38. Hahn H, Wojnowski L, Specht K, et al: Patched target Igf2 is indispensable for the formation of medulloblastoma and rhabdomyosarcoma. J Biol Chem 275(37):28341–28344, 2000.
39. Halmagyi GM, Bignold LP, Allsop JL: Recurrent subependymal giant-cell astrocytoma in the absence of tuberous sclerosis. J Neurosurg 50:106–109, 1979.
40. Henske EP, Wessner LL, Golden J, et al: Loss of tuberin in both subependymal giant cell astrocytomas and angiomyolipomas supports a two-hit model for the pathogenesis of tuberous sclerosis tumors. Am J Pathol 151:1639–1647, 1997.
41. Hirano H, Lopes MBS, Carpenter J, et al: The IGF-I content and pattern of expression correlates with histopathologic grade in diffusely infiltrating astrocytomas. J Neurooncol 1:109–119, 1999.
42. Hirose T, Scheithauer BW, Lopes MB, et al: Tuber and subependymal giant cell astrocytoma associated with tuberous sclerosis: an immunohistochemical, ultrastructural, and immunoelectron and microscopic study. Acta Neuropathol 90:387–399, 1995.
43. Hitoshi S, Tropepe V, Ekker M, van der Kooy D: Neural stem cell lineages are regionally specified, but not committed, within distinct compartments of the developing brain. Development 129:233–244, 2002.
44. Hoang-Xuan K, He J, Huguet S, et al: Molecular heterogeneity of oligodendrogliomas suggests alternative pathways in tumor progression. Neurology 57:1278–1281, 2001.
45. Holland EC: Progenitor cells and glioma formation. Curr Opin Neurol 14:683–688, 2001.
46. Holland EC: Gliomagenesis: genetic alterations and mouse models. Nat Rev Genet 2:120–129, 2001.
47. Horten BC, Urich H, Stefoski D: Meningiomas with conspicuous plasma cell-lymphocytic components. Cancer 43:258–264, 1979.
48. Ivanchuk SM, Mondal S, Dirks PB, Rutka JT: The INK4A/ARF locus: Role in cell cycle control and apoptosis and implications for glioma growth. J Neurooncol 51:219–229, 2001.
49. Jeuken JW, Sprenger SHE, Boerman RH, et al: Subtyping of oligo-astrocytic tumours by comparative genomic hybridization. J Pathol 194:81–87, 2001.
50. Kandel ER, Schwartz JH, Jessel TM: Principles of Neuroscience. Norwalk, Conn, Appleton & Lange, 1991.
51. Kawano N: Pleomorphic xanthoastrocytoma (PXA) in Japan: its clinico-pathologic features and diagnostic clues. Brain Tumor Pathol 8:5–10, 1991.
52. Kenney AM, Cole MD, Rowitch DH: Nmyc upregulation by sonic hedgehog signaling promotes proliferation in developing cerebellar granule neuron precursors. Development 130:15–28, 2003.
53. Kepes JJ, Rubinstein LJ, Eng LF: Pleomorphic xanthoastrocytoma: a distinctive meningocerebral glioma of young subjects with relatively favorable prognosis. A study of 12 cases. Cancer 44:1839–1852, 1979.
54. Kepes JJ, Chen WYK, Connors MH, Vogel FS: "Chordoid" meningeal tumors in young individuals with peritumoral lymphoplasmacellular infiltrates causing systemic manifestation of Castleman Syndrome. A report of seven cases. Cancer 62:391–406, 1988.
55. Kepes JJ, Rubinstein LJ, Ansbacher L, Schreiber DJ: Histopathological features of recurrent pleomorphic xanthoastrocytomas: further corroboration of the glial nature of this neoplasm. Acta Neuropathol (Berl) 78:585–593, 1989.
56. Kleihues P, Ohgaki H: Primary and secondary glioblastoma: from concept to clinical diagnosis. Neurooncol 1:44–55, 1999.
57. Kleihues P, Cavenee WK: Tumours of the Nervous System: Pathology and Genetics. World Health Organization Classification of Tumours. IARC Press, Lyon, 2000.
58. Kleihues P, Louis DN, Scheithauer BW, et al: The WHO classification of tumors of the nervous system. J Neuropathol Exp Neurol 61:215–225, 2002.
59. Kluwe L, Hagel C, Tatagiba M, et al: Loss of NF1 alleles distinguish sporadic from NF1-associated pilocytic astrocytomas. J Neuropathol Exp Neurol 60:917–920, 2001.
60. Kordek R, Biernat W, Sapieja W, et al: Pleomorphic xanthoastrocytoma with a gangliomatous component: an immunohistochemical and ultrastructural study. Acta Neuropathol (Berl) 89:194–197, 1995.

61. Koschny R, Koschny T, Froster UG, et al: Comparative genomic hybridization in glioma: a meta-analysis of 509 cases. Cancer Genet Cytogenet 135:147–149, 2002.

62. Kourea HP, Orlow L, Scheithauer BW, et al: Deletions of the INK4A gene occur in malignant peripheral nerve sheath tumors but not in neurofibromas. Am J Pathol 155:1855–1860, 1999.

63. Kraus JA, Koopmann J, Kaskel P, et al: Shared allelic losses on chromosomes 1p and 19q suggest a common origin of oligodendroglioma and oligo-astrocytoma. J Neuropathol Exp Neurol 54:91–95, 1995.

64. Kraus JA, Oster C, Sorensen N, et al: Human medulloblastomas lack point mutations and homozygous deletions of the hSNF5/INI1 tumour suppressor gene. Neuropathol Appl Neurobiol 28:136–141, 2002.

65. Kros JM, Vecht CHJ, Stefanko SZ: The pleomorphic xanthoastrocytoma and its differential diagnosis: a study of five cases. Hum Pathol 22:1128–1135, 1991.

66. Krouwer HGJ, Davis RL, Silver R, Prados M: Gemistocytic astrocytomas: a reappraisal. J Neurosurg 74:399–406, 1991.

67. Li J, Perry A, James CD, Gutmann DH: Cancer-related gene expression profiles in NF1-associated pilocytic astrocytomas. Neurology 56:885–890, 2001.

68. Lindboe C, Cappelen J, Kepes J: Pleomorphic xanthoastrocytoma as a component of a cerebellar ganglioglioma. Case report. Neurosurgery 31:353–355, 1992.

69. Lopes MBS, Altermatt HJ, Scheithauer BW, et al: Immunohistochemical characterization of subependymal giant cell astrocytomas. Acta Neuropathol (Berl) 91:368–375, 1996.

70. Louis DN: A molecular genetic model of astrocytoma histopathology. Brain Pathol 7:755–764, 1997.

71. Louis ND, Holland EC, Cairncross JG: Glioma Classification. Am J Pathol 159:779–786, 2001.

72. Lundberg AS, Hahn WC, Gupta P, Weinberg RA: Genes involved in senescence and immortalization. Curr Opin Cell Biol 12:705–709, 2000.

73. Maier H, Ofner D, Hittmair A, et al: Classic, atypical, and anaplastic meningioma: three histopathological subtypes of clinical relevance. J Neurosurg 77:616–623, 1992.

74. Maintz D, Fiedler K, Koopmann J, et al: Molecular genetic evidence for subtypes of oligoastrocytomas. J Neuropathol Exp Neurol 56:1098–1104, 1997.

75. Maleki M, Robitaille Y, Bertrand G: Atypical xanthoastrocytoma presenting as a meningioma. Surg Neurol 20:235–238, 1983.

76. McLendon RE, Wikstrand CJ, Maatthews MR, et al: Glioma-associated antigen expression in oligodendroglial neoplasms: tenascin and epidermal growth factor receptor. J Histochem Cytochem 48:1103–1110, 2000.

77. Meyer-Puttlitz B, Haayashi Y, Whah A, et al: Molecular genetic analysis of giant cell glioblastomas. Am J Pathol 151:853–857, 1997.

78. Mimon M, Kokkino AJ, Warnick RE, et al: Role of genomic instability in meningioma progression. Genes, Chromosomes Cancer 16:265–269, 1998.

79. Minehan KJ, Shaw EG, Scheithauer BW, et al: Spinal cord astrocytoma: pathological and treatment considerations. J Neurosurg 83:590–595, 1995.

80. Mizuguchi M, Kato M, Yamanouchi H, et al: Loss of tuberin from cerebral tissues with tuberous sclerosis and astrocytomas. Ann Neurol 40:941–944, 1996.

81. Mueller W, Hartmann C, Hoffmann A, et al: Genetic signature of oligoastrocytomas correlates with tumor location and denotes distinct molecular subsets. Am J Pathol 161:313–319, 2002.

82. Mukasa A, Ueki K, Matsumoto S, et al: Distinction in gene expression profiles of oligodendrogliomas with and without allelic loss of 1p. Oncogene 21:3961–3968, 2002.

83. Muller W, Afra D, Schroder R: Supratentorial recurrences of gliomas: morphological studies in relation to time intervals with 544 astrocytomas. Acta Neurochir (Wien) 37:75–91, 1977.

84. Nakasu S, Hirano A, Shimura T, Llena JF: Incidental meningiomas in autopsy study. Surg Neurol 27:319–322, 1987.

85. Nguyen-Vu PA, Flackler I, Rust A, et al: Loss of tuberin, the turberous-sclerosis-complex-2 gene product is associated with angiogensis. J Cutan Pathol 28:470–475, 2001.

86. Nishizaki T, Ozaki S, Harada K, et al: Investigation of genetic alterations associated with the grade of astrocytic tumor by comparative genomic hybridization. Genes Chromosomes Cancer 21:340–346, 1998.

87. Nutt CL, Mani DR, Betensky RA, et al: Gene expression-based classification of malignant gliomas correlates better with survival than histological classification. Cancer Res 63:1602–1607, 2003.

88. Ohgaki H, Eibl RH, Schwab M, et al: Mutations of the p53 tumor suppressor gene in neoplasms of the human nervous system. Mol Carcinog 8:74–80, 1993.

89. Packer R, Biegel JA, Blaney S, et al: Atypical teratoid/rhabdoid tumor of the central nervous system: report on workshop. J Pediatr Hematol Oncol 24:337–342, 2002.

90. Parkinson EK, Munro J, Steeghs K, et al: Replicative senescence as a barrier to human cancer. Biochem Soc Trans 28:226–233, 2000.

91. Paulus W, Ott MM, Strik H, et al: Large cell anaplastic (Ki-1) brain lymphoma of T-cell genotype. Hum Pathol 25:1253–1256, 1994.

92. Peraud A, Watanabe K, Plate KH, et al: p53 mutations versus EGF receptor expression in giant cell glioblastomas. J Neuropathol Exp Neurol 56:1236–1241, 1997.

93. Peraud A, Watanabe K, Schwechheimer K, et al: Genetic profile of the giant cell glioblastoma. Lab Invest 79:123–129, 1999.

94. Perry A, Scheithauer BW, Nascimento AG: The immunophenotypic spectrum of meningeal hemangiopericytoma: a comparison with fibrous meningioma and solitary fibrous tumor of meninges. Am J Surg Pathol 21:1354–1360, 1997.

95. Perry A, Stafford SL, Scheithauer BW, et al: Meningioma grading: an analysis of histologic parameters. Am J Surg Pathol 21:1455–1465, 1997.

96. Perry A, Scheithauer BW, Stafford SL, et al: "Rhabdoid" meningioma: an aggressive variant. Am J Surg Pathol 22:1482–1490, 1998.

97. Perry A, Scheithauer BW, Stafford SL, et al: "Malignancy" in meningiomas: a clinicopathologic study of 116 patients, with grading implications. Cancer 85:2046–2056, 1999.

98. Perry A, Giannini C, Raghavan R, et al: Aggressive phenotypic and genotypic features in pediatric and NF2-associated meningiomas: a clinicopathologic study of 53 cases. J Neuropath Exp Neurol 60:994–1003, 2001.

99. Perry A, Banerjee R, Lohse CM, et al: A role for chromosome 9p21 deletions in the malignant progression of meningiomas and the prognosis of anaplastic meningiomas. Brain Pathol 12:183–190, 2002.

100. Platten M, Giordano MJ, Dirven CM, et al: Up-regulation of specific NF 1 gene transcripts in sporadic pilocytic astrocytomas. Am J Pathol 149:621–627, 1996.

101. Pomeroy SL, Tamayo P, Gaasenbeek M, et al: Prediction of central nervous system embryonal tumour outcome based on gene expression. Nature 415:436–442, 2002.

102. Prayson RA: Clinicopathologic study of 61 patients with ependymoma including MIB-1 immunohistochemistry. Ann Diagn Pathol 3:11–18, 1999.

103. Radley MG, Di Sant'Agnese PA, Eskin TA, Wilbur DC: Epithelial differentiation in meningiomas. An immunohistochemical, histochemical and ultrastructural study—with review of literature. Am J Clin Path 92:266–272, 1989.

104. Radner H, Katenkamp D, Reifenberger G, et al: New developments in the pathology of skull base tumors. Virchows Arch 438:321–335, 2001.

105. Raffel C, Fredrick L, O'Fallon JR, et al: Analysis of oncogene and tumor suppressor gene alterations in pediatric malignant

astrocytomas reveals reduced survival for patients with PTEN mutations. Clin Cancer Res 5:4085–4090, 1999.

106. Reifenberger G, Liu L, James CD, et al: Molecular genetic analysis of oligodendroglial tumors shows preferential allelic deletions on 19q and 1p. Am J Pathol 145:1175–1190, 1994.

107. Reifenberger G, Louis DN: Oligodendroglioma: toward molecular definitions in diagnostic neuro-oncology. J Neuropathol Exp Neurol 62:111–126, 2003.

108. Reifenberger J, Reifenberger G, Ichimura K, et al: Epidermal growth factor receptor expression in oligodendroglial tumors. Am J Pathol 149:29–35, 1996.

109. Reis RM, Könü-Leblblicioglu, Lopes JM, et al: Genetic profile of gliosarcomas. Am J Pathol 156:425–432, 2000.

110. Reis-Filho JS, Faoro LN, Carrilho C, et al: Evaluation of cell proliferation, epidermal growth factor receptor, and bcl-2 immunoexpression as prognostic factors for patients with World Health Organization grade 2 oligodendroglioma. Cancer 88:862–869, 2000.

111. Rezai AR, Woo HH, Lee M, et al: Disseminated ependymomas of the central nervous system. J Neurosurg 85:618–624, 1996.

112. Reznik M, Schoenen J: Lhermitte-Duclos disease. Acta Neuropathol (Berl) 59:88–94, 1983.

113. Robinson S, Cohen AR: Cowden disease and Lhermitte-Duclose disease: characterization of a new phakomatosis. J Neurosurg 46:371–383, 2000.

114. Robinson S, Cohen M, Prayson R, et al: Constitutive expression of growth-related oncogene and its receptor in oligodendrogliomas. Neurosurgery 48:864–873, 2001.

115. Ross GW, Rubinstein LJ: Lack of histopathological correlation of malignant ependymomas with postoperative survival. J Neurosurg 70:31–36, 1989.

116. Rushing EJ, Yashima K, Brown DF, et al: 1997 Expression of telomerase RNA component correlates with the MIB-1 proliferation index in ependymomas. J Neuropath Exp Neurol 56:1142–1146, 1997.

117. Rushing EJ, Brown DF, Hladik CL, et al: Correlation of bcl-2, p53, and MIB-1 expression with ependymoma grade and subtype. Mod Pathol 11:464–470, 1998.

118. Saito-Ohara F, Imoto I, Inoue J, et al: PPMID is a potential target for 17q gain in neuroblastoma1. Cancer Res 63:1876–1883, 2003.

119. Sawhney N, Hall, PA: Ki67: structure, function and new antibodies. J Pathol 168:161–162, 1992.

120. Schiffer D, Chib A, Giordana MT, et al: Histologic prognostic factors in ependymoma. Childs Nerv Syst 7:177–182, 1991.

121. Schiffer D, Chio A, Cravioto H, et al: Ependymoma: internal correlations among pathological signs: the anaplastic variant. Neurosurgery 29:206–210, 1991.

122. Schrock E, Blume C, Meffert MC, et al: Recurrent gain of chromosome arm 7q in low-grade astrocytic tumors studied by comparative genomic hybridization. Genes Chromosomes Cancer 15:199–205, 1996.

123. Schroder R, Ploner C, Ernestus RI: The growth potential of ependymomas with varying grades of malignancy measured by the Ki-67 labeling index and mitotic index. Neurosurg Rev 16:145–150, 1993.

124. Shiurba RA, Gessaga EC, Eng LF, et al: Lhermitte-Duclos disease. an immunohistochemical study of the cerebellar cortex. Review of reported cases. Acta Neuropathol (Berl) 75:474–480, 1988.

125. Shiurba RA, Buffinger NS, Spencer EM, et al: Basic fibroblastic growth factor and somatomedin C in human medulloepithelioma. Cancer 68:798–808, 1991.

126. Sims KB. Von Hippel-Lindau disease: gene to bedside. Curr Opin Neurol 14:695–703, 2001.

127. de Saint Aubain Somerhausen N, Rubin BP, Fletcher CDM: Myxoid solitary fibrous tumor: a study of seven cases with emphasis on differential diagnosis. Mod Pathol 12:463–471, 1999.

128. Starink TM: Cowden's disease: analysis of fourteen new cases. J Am Acad Dermatol 11:1127–1141, 1984.

129. Sung T, Miller DC, Hayes RL, et al: Preferential inactivation of the p53 tumor suppressor pathway and lack of EGFR amplification distinguish de novo high grade pediatric astrocytomas from de novo adult astrocytomas. Brain Pathol 10:249–259, 2000.

130. Sure U, Ruedi D, Tachibana O, et al: Determination of p53 mutations, EGFR over expression, and loss of p16 expression in pediatric glioblastomas. J Neuropathol Exp Neurol 56:782–789, 1997.

131. Temple S, Alvarez-Buylla A: Stem cells in the adult mammalian central nervous system. Curr Opin Neurobiol 9:135–141, 1999.

132. Tihan T, Fisher PG, Kepner JL, et al: Pediatric astrocytomas with monomorphous pilomyxoid features and a less favorable outcome. J Neuropathol Exp Neurol 58:1061–1068, 1999.

133. Tomlinson FH, Scheithauer BW, Hayostek CJ, et al: The significance of atypia and histologic malignancy in pilocytic astrocytoma of the cerebellum: a clinicopathologic and flow cytometric study. J Child Neurol 9:301–310, 1994.

134. Tropepe V, Hitoshi S, Sirard C, et al: Direct neuronal fate specification from embryonic stem cells: a primitive mammalian neural stem cell stage acquired through a default mechanism. Neuron 30:65–78, 2001.

135. Uhlmann EJ, Apicelli AJ, Baldwin RL, et al: Heterozygosity for the tuberous sclerosis complex (TSC) gene products results in increased astrocyte numbers and decreased p27-Kip1 expression in TSC2±cells. Oncogene 21:4050–4059, 2002.

136. Uhrbom L, Dai C, Celestino JC, et al: *Ink4a-Arf* loss cooperates with KRas activation in astrocytes and neural progenitors to generate glioblastomas of various morphologies depending on activated Akt[1]. Cancer Res 62:5551–5558, 2002.

137. Uno K, Takita J, Yokomori K, et al: Aberrations of the hSNF5/INI1 gene are restricted to malignant rhabdoid tumors of atypical teratoid/rhabdoid tumors in pediatric solid tumors. Genes Chromosomes Cancer 34:33–41, 2002.

138. VandenBerg SR: Current diagnostic concepts of astrocytic tumors. J Neuropath Exp Neurol 51:644–657, 1992.

139. Watanabe K, Peraud A, Gratas C, et al: p53 and PTEN gene mutations in gemistocytic astrocytomas. Acta Neuropathol (Berl) 95:559–564, 1998.

140. Watanabe T, Yokoo H, Yokoo M, et al: Concurrent inactivation of RB1 and TP 53 pathways in anaplastic oligodendrogliomas. J Neuropathol Exp Neurol 60:1181–1189, 2001.

141. Watanabe T, Nakamura M, Kros JM, et al: Phenotype versus genotype correlation in oligodendrogliomas and low-grade diffuse astrocytomas. Acta Neuropathol (Berl) 103:267–275, 2002.

142. Weiss WA, Burns MF, Hackett C, et al: Genetic determinants of malignancy in a mouse model for oligodendroglioma. Cancer Res 63:1589–1595, 2003.

143. Weldon-Linne GM, Victor TA, Groothuis DR, et al: Pleomorphic xanthoastrocytoma: ultrastructural and immunohistochemical study of a case with a rapidly fatal outcome following surgery. Cancer 52:2055–2063, 1983.

144. Wells GB, Lasner TM, Yousem DM, et al: Lhermitte-Duclos disease and Cowden's syndrome in an adolescent patient. J Neurosurg 81:133–136, 1994.

145. Wienecke R, Guha A, Maixe JC, Jr, et al: Reduced TSC2 RNA and protein in sporatic astrocytomas and ependymomas. Ann Neurol 42:230–235, 1997.

146. Wimmer K, Eckart M, Meyer-Puttlitz B, et al: Mutational and expression analysis of the NF1 gene argues against a role as tumor suppressor in sporadic pilocytic astrocytomas. J Neuropathol Exp Neurol 61:896–902, 2002.

147. Wolter M, Reifenberger J, Blaschke B, et al: Oligodendroglial tumors frequently demonstrate hypermethylation of the CDKN2A (MTS1, p16[INK4a], and 14[ARF], and CDKN2B (MTS2,

p15^{INK4b}) tumor suppressor genes. J Neuropathol Exp Neurol 60:1170–1180, 2001.

148. Yachnis AT, Trojanowski JQ, Memmo M, Schlaepfer WW: Expression of neurofilament proteins in the hypertrophic granule cells of Lhermitte-Duclos disease: an explanation for the mass effect and the myelination of parallel fibers in the disease state. J Neuropath Exp Neurol 47:206–216, 1988.

149. Yin XL, Hui AB, Liong EC, et al: Genetic imbalances in pleomorphic xanthoastrocytoma detected by comparative genomic hybridization and literature review. Cancer Genet Cytogenet 132:14–19, 2002.

150. Zorludemir S, Scheithauer BW, Hirose T, et al: Clear cell meningioma. A clinicopathologic study of a potentially aggressive variant of meningioma. Am J Surg Pathol 19:493–505, 1995.

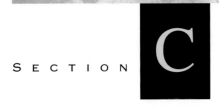

CHAPTER 6

NEUROENDOCRINOLOGY

Sandeep Kunwar

The pituitary gland is often considered the "master gland," regulating most of the body's hormonal balance. The gland itself is regulated by the hypothalamus through stimulatory and inhibitory hormones that travel through the infundibulum and pituitary stalk. The adult pituitary gland measures $12 \times 6 \times 9$ mm and weighs 0.6 g. It enlarges during pregnancy, when it may weigh 1 g or more. The gland is situated near the sella turcica ("Turkish saddle") formed by the sphenoid bone and is completely covered by dura and the sellar diaphragm above. The pituitary stalk enters the sella turcica through a hole in the sellar diaphragm. Laterally, the pituitary fossa is bounded by the cavernous sinuses containing the carotid artery and the third, fourth, fifth, and sixth cranial nerves. Superiorly, the optic nerves and chiasm traverse 4 to 6 mm above the sellar diaphragm. The human pituitary gland is divided into two parts: the adenohypophysis and the neurohypophysis.

The adenohypophysis is derived from the invagination of the hypophyseal-pharyngeal duct known as *Rathke's pouch*. The adenohypophysis constitutes approximately 80% of the entire pituitary and is divided into the pars distalis (anterior lobe), pars intermedia (intermediate lobe), and the pars tuberalis (pars infundibularis). The pars distalis is the largest and the functional part of the adenohypophysis. The pars intermedia in the human pituitary is a poorly developed, rudimentary structure lying between the anterior and posterior lobes. It often degenerates into a pars intermedia cyst (less than 5 mm) filled with colloid material. The pars tuberalis is an upward extension of the anterior lobe along the pituitary stalk and may be a source of suprasellar anterior-lobe pathology. The anterior lobe is the source of prolactin (PRL), growth hormone (GH), thyroid-stimulating hormone (TSH), gonadotropic hormones (follicle-stimulating hormone [FSH] and luteinizing hormone [LH]), and adrenocorticotropic hormone (ACTH).

The neurohypophysis is derived from the ventral outgrowth of the neuroectoderm. This is a funnel-shaped structure, with the base forming the tuber cinereum, median eminence, infundibulum, and infundibular process (pituitary stalk) and ending in the posterior lobe within the pituitary fossa. The posterior lobe is made up of axonal end bulbs containing neurosecretory vesicles (storing oxytocin and antidiuretic hormone) and pituicytes. These axons originate from the magnocellular neurons of the hypothalamus (in the supraoptic, paraventricular, and accessory nuclei), where the hormones are produced.

The pituitary receives its blood supply from the superior and inferior hypophysial arteries. Some data indicate that 70% to 80% of the anterior lobe blood comes from the large portal vessels that arise from the median eminence and traverse down the infundibulum, and the remainder of the pituitary blood supply comes from the short portal system. The communication between the hypothalamus and anterior lobe is through the blood via the portal circulation.

PITUITARY PHYSIOLOGY AND PATHOPHYSIOLOGY

Growth Hormone

Somatotrophs are GH-producing cells constituting approximately 50% of the anterior lobe, primarily located in the lateral wings. GH is a 191–amino acid polypeptide. GH-releasing hormone (GHRH) secreted by the hypothalamus induces transcription of the GH gene and stimulates secretion of GH. Somatostatin (somatotrophin release-inhibiting factor [SRIF]), also released by the hypothalamus, inhibits GH secretion, and is primarily responsible for the pulsatile secretion of GH.[12] As the name implies, GH's major function is growth promotion. Most of GH's effect occurs through stimulation of insulin-like growth factor 1 (IGF-1) or somatomedin C, primarily produced by the liver. IGF-1 causes growth of muscle, bone, and cartilage; protein synthesis and amino acid transportation; and DNA and

RNA synthesis and cell proliferation.[4] IGF-1 also suppresses the production of GH as part of a negative-feedback loop.

Hyposecretion of GH can occur as a result of a variety of pathologies, in isolation or as part of panhypopituitarism. Somatotrophic cells are very sensitive to trauma, radiation, and compression. Isolated GH deficiency has been reported after closed head injury,[6] and GH is one of the first hormones to be depressed by compression of the pituitary gland from a mass lesion. GH deficiency is most clinically relevant in children, resulting in short stature and delay in puberty, and is the most common presenting symptom in children with pituitary lesions.[7] Recently, GH-deficiency syndrome in adults has been recognized, although the diagnosis remains controversial. Symptoms include decreased energy and a feeling of social isolation. In addition, changes in body composition, with an increase in fat and decrease in lean body mass, are reported. Synthetic GH has improved treatment of GH deficiency. There is no orally bioavailable form, and replacement therapy currently requires daily injections. In children GH replacement is critical for growth and development; however, in adults replacement therapy has been controversial. For patients with normal IGF-1 levels, there may not be any benefit from GH therapy.[8] For patients with diminished IGF-1, GH can be titrated to normalize IGF-1 to determine if any benefit in energy or muscle mass is noted. Initial therapy can cause musculoskeletal pain that resolves with time or reductions in dose.

Hypersecretion of GH is related to a somatotroph adenoma in 98% of cases. Approximately 20% of GH-secreting adenomas also secrete PRL. Other causes include excess GHRH from a hypothalamic hamartoma or choristoma, or from ectopic production (i.e., bronchial carcinoid, pancreatic islet cell tumor, or small-cell lung cancer). Hypersecretion of GH leads to the clinical syndrome of acromegaly in adults and gigantism in children. Acromegaly is characterized by an enlarged protruding jaw (macrognathia) with associated overbite; enlarged tongue (macroglossia); enlarged, swollen hands and feet resulting in increased shoe and ring size; coarse facial features with enlargement of the nose and frontal bones; and spreading of the teeth (Table 6-1). Musculoskeletal symptoms are a leading cause of morbidity and include arthralgias leading to severe debilitating arthritic features. Skin tags; hyperhidrosis (in up to 50% of patients), often associated with body odor; hirsutism; deepening of the voice; neuropathies; and paresthesias (e.g., carpal tunnel syndrome) from nerve entrapment are common. Cardiovascular disease is accelerated with cardiomyopathy (left ventricular hypertrophy) and hypertension. GH is a potent antagonist of insulin action, and diabetes is a major determinant of mortality. The combination of macroglossia, mandible deformation, and mucosal hypertrophy can lead to airway obstruction, snoring, and sleep apnea in a majority of patients. Acromegaly is associated with a significant increased risk of colonic polyps and gastrointestinal cancer. The overall mortality rate in acromegaly is approximately two to four times that of the general population.[1,14]

The primary goal for treatment of acromegaly is normalization of GH levels; in particular, life-table analysis showed that GH levels less than 2.5 ng/mL were associated with survival rates equal to those of the general population.[1] The principal treatment for somatotroph adenomas is surgical resection of the tumor; however, because the symptoms of acromegaly are insidious in onset, tumors are often large at time of presentation and have invaded surrounding structures. In cases

TABLE 6-1

Clinical Manifestations of Acromegaly

Local Tumor Effects
Visual field defects
Cranial nerve palsy (diplopia)
Headache

Somatic
Acral enlargement
Thickening of soft tissue of the hands and feet (increased ring and shoe size)

Musculoskeletal
Prognathism
Malocclusion
Arthralgias
Carpal tunnel syndrome
Frontal bossing

Skin
Hyperhidrosis
Skin tags

Colon
Polyps

Cardiovascular
Left ventricular hypertrophy
Hypertension
Congestive heart failure

Sleep Disturbances
Sleep apnea
Narcolepsy

Visceral
Macroglossia
Hepatomegaly
Splenomegaly
Thyroid enlargement

Sexual Function
Menstrual abnormalities
Galactorrhea (hyperprolactinemia)
Decreased libido

Carbohydrate
Impaired glucose tolerance
Insulin resistance
Hyperinsulinemia
Diabetes mellitus

Lipids
Hypertriglyceridemia

where residual tumor remains, radiation therapy or medical management with somatostatin analogues may be necessary. Octreotide binds selectively to somatostatin receptor 2 (SSTR2) and inhibits GH release. Long-term treatment can result in normalized levels of GH and IGF-1 in more than 50% of patients, with amelioration of symptoms. Dopamine agonists have also been used, although GH normalization occurs in fewer than 15% of patients.

Prolactin

Lactotrophs are PRL-producing cells constituting 20% to 30% of the anterior lobe. They are scattered throughout the pars distalis with some accumulation within the posterolateral region. A sharp increase in the number of PRL cells (hyperplasia) occurs during pregnancy and lactation. PRL is a 198–amino acid peptide primarily known for its lactogenic properties. It is unique among pituitary hormones in that its secretion is spontaneous in the absence of any stimulation from the hypothalamus. The primary mechanism controlling PRL secretion is tonic inhibition by hypothalamic dopamine secretion. In addition, PRL secretion can be inhibited by somatostatin. PRL-releasing factors (PRFs), including thyrotropin-releasing hormone (TRH), estrogen, vasoactive intestinal peptide (VIP), and oxytocin, stimulate PRL. Serum levels range from 4 to 20 µg/L and are 20% to 30% lower in men. During the third trimester of pregnancy, the PRL levels increase up to 200 to 300 µg/L. PRL levels fall rapidly after delivery and return to resting levels within 2 to 3 weeks if breast-feeding does not occur. Surges in serum PRL levels are associated with suckling and can remain elevated 2 to 6 months after delivery if breast-feeding is continued.

PRL causes extensive proliferation of the lobuloalveolar epithelium, causing breast enlargement and breast milk production. PRL also inhibits gonadal activity by its influence on the hypothalamus, decreasing the release of gonadotropin-releasing hormone (GnRH) and subsequently LH. In women, this can result in infertility (lactational infertility is one consequence of high PRL values associated with breast-feeding), oligomenorrhea, and amenorrhea. In men hyperprolactinemia can result in loss of libido and impotence. PRL is also a brain-regulating hormone and is believed to be involved in maternal behavior patterns. The effects on the brain may also include stimulation of appetite, analgesia (through an opioid pathway), and increases in rapid-eye movement (REM) sleep activity.

Hypoprolactinemia occurs in the presence of panhypopituitarism. Rare cases of isolated PRL deficiency have been described and can be seen in patients on dopamine agonist therapy. Isolated PRL deficiency can result in lactational failure and reproductive difficulty, but no other obvious problems have been reported.[5]

Hyperprolactinemia is among the most common of pituitary disorders and may be seen in a variety of medical conditions and through different mechanisms (Table 6-2). Physiologic hyperprolactinemia is seen with both physical and emotional stress, pregnancy, nipple stimulation, and after sexual orgasm. Many medications can elevate PRL secretion, including certain antiemetics, antidepressants, antipsychotics, and narcotics, by antagonizing dopamine action. Medications that work primarily to diminish dopamine secretion (e.g., reserpine) or are dopamine receptor antagonists (e.g., phenothiazides, haldol) can often cause hyperprolactinemia. Pathologic hyper-

TABLE 6-2

Causes of Hyperprolactinemia

Hypothalamic
  Tumors
  Sarcoid
  Radiation therapy
Pituitary
  Hormonally active tumors
    Prolactinomas
    Somatotroph adenomas
    TSH adenomas
  Stalk effect
    Nonfunctioning adenomas
    Rathke's cleft cyst
    Parasellar tumors
  Stalk transection
Drugs
  Dopamine receptor antagonist
  Inhibitors of dopamine synthesis and release
  Estrogens
Neurogenic
  Chest wall/spinal cord lesions
  Breast stimulation
  Suckling
  Physical stress
Others
  Primary hypothyroidism
  Renal failure
  Pregnancy
  Idiopathic

prolactinemia can be seen with lesions in the sella and the parasellar region. PRL-secreting adenomas (prolactinomas) account for 40% to 60% of all pituitary adenomas. In prolactinomas PRL secretion is unregulated and directly proportional to tumor size. Hyperprolactinemia can also result from excessive glandular secretion as a result of distortion of the pituitary stalk or increased pressure within the gland causing disruption of the tonic dopamine inhibition of PRL secretion (stalk effect), resulting in PRL levels up to 150 µg/L. Thus large adenomas (macroadenomas) that do not secrete PRL, parasellar tumors that distort the pituitary stalk (i.e., tuberculum sellar meningioma), and pathology involving the hypothalamus (i.e., hypothalamic glioma, germinoma) can result in hyperprolactinemia from stalk effect. Moderate hyperprolactinemia can also be seen in approximately 20% of patients with hypothyroidism that results in elevated TRH secretion, which stimulates PRL release, or in thyrotropic hyperplasia of the gland and subsequent "stalk effect."

The clinical findings of hyperprolactinemia in women of reproductive age include amenorrhea, galactorrhea, and infertility. In most cases, changes in the menstrual cycle result in early evaluation and diagnosis of hyperprolactinemia, and thus most premenopausal women present with microprolactinomas (<1 cm). Hypoestrogenemia associated with hyperprolactinemia can result in dyspareunia and loss of libido, and long-lasting effects include osteopenia. Seborrhea and hirsutism may be present. In men the most common clinical manifestation of hyperprolactinemia is the progressive loss of libido and impotency. Oligospermia and other physical signs of hypogonadism (i.e., muscular hypotrophy, increased abdominal fat) are commonly reported. Galactorrhea or gynecomastia is present in 15% to 30% of male patients.[2] Prolactinomas among men and postmenopausal women are often macroadenomas (>1 cm), because changes in libido are not detected early. Hyperprolactinemia in both sexes can also be associated with anxiety, depression, fatigue, emotional instability, and hostility.[10,11]

Treatment of hyperprolactinemia depends on the cause. Normalization of PRL levels results in immediate restoration of menstrual function and fertility in women and libido and potency in men, assuming the residual normal gland remains functional. In cases of drug-induced hyperprolactinemia, cessation of the offending drug is often sufficient to return PRL levels to normal. In patients with psychosis, administration of antipsychotics that do not induce hyperprolactinemia should be instituted. For hypothyroid-related hyperprolactinemia, treatment of the hypothyroidism with thyroxine will result in normalization of PRL. In patients with a tumor or mass lesion, primary treatment should focus on the appropriate treatment for the tumor. For microprolactinomas, treatment options include surgical resection of the tumor or medical therapy with dopamine agonists. Surgical resection of microadenomas in experienced hands results in high cure rates with minimal morbidity.[13] Medical therapy (i.e., bromocriptine, cabergoline) is very effective in controlling the hyperprolactinemia and tumor growth for prolactinomas but requires life-long treatment. Dopamine agonists inhibit production and secretion of PRL from lactotroph adenomas and result in the shrinkage of the cell size with a decrease in secretory vesicles, which results in shrinkage of the overall tumor size. Dopamine agonists also prevent tumor cells from replicating, thus causing growth arrest. Discussion with both an endocrinologist and neurosurgeon with specialization in this therapy is required to determine the most appropriate treatment. For macroprolactinomas, because the local invasiveness results in lower surgical cure rates, surgery is reserved for patients desiring pregnancy (which requires cessation of medical therapy for at least the first trimester), those with visual deterioration, and those who are intolerant of or unresponsive to medical therapy. In idiopathic cases of hyperprolactinemia, correction of the PRL level with dopamine agonist or replacement of the sex hormones will correct the hypogonadal state.

Thyrotropin

Thyrotrophs, or TSH-producing cells, constitute approximately 5% of the anterior lobe. Thyrotrophs may undergo hyperplasia as a result of primary hypothyroidism that regresses after appropriate thyroxine therapy. TSH is composed of two subunits, α and β. The α-subunit is common to LH, FSH, and human chorionic gonadotrophin (HCG). The production and secretion of TSH is regulated by hypothalamic TRH. TRH is synthesized in the paraventricular nucleus of the hypothalamus and released into the portal capillary plexus. The main function of TRH is to stimulate TSH release, although TRH can also cause PRL secretion. TSH leads to increased formation and secretion of tetraiodothyronine (T_4) and to a lesser degree triiodothyronine (T_3). T_4 results in inhibition of both TRH and

TSH release as part of a negative-feedback loop. T_4 is the major hormone secreted by the thyroid gland. It is converted to T_3, the metabolically active hormone, by target tissues. Thyroid hormone is critical in the development of the brain in children and in regulating tissue metabolism in adults.

Hypothyroidism is considered primary when increased TSH levels accompany low T_3 and T_4 levels, suggesting thyroid pathology. In secondary or central hypothyroidism, low T_3 and T_4 are associated with low TSH and suggest pituitary insufficiency. Thyroid hormone deficiency causes mental retardation in infants, growth delay in children, and myxedema in adults. Symptoms of thyroid hormone insufficiency include cold intolerance, weight gain, memory loss, dry skin, hair loss, brittle nails, constipation, increased sleep demand, and fatigue. Severe, untreated hypothyroidism can lead to coma and even death. Hypothyroidism from TSH or TRH deficiency can result from hypothalamic or pituitary destruction (neoplastic, inflammatory, granulomatous, vascular, traumatic, autoimmune, or from radiation necrosis). In the presence of an expanding pituitary mass (i.e., pituitary adenoma), loss of TSH secretion is typically associated with other hormonal abnormalities because there is a step-wise loss of pituitary function starting with growth hormone, gonadotropins, and then thyrotropin (lastly ACTH). Treatment of most types of hypothyroidism is successful with replacement therapy using thyroxine, which is adjusted until normal serum hormone levels are achieved.

Hyperthyroidism, or thyrotoxicosis, is most commonly caused by thyroid gland pathology (Graves' disease, toxic multinodular goiter, and toxic adenoma), which is associated with low or undetectable TSH levels. TSH-secreting (thyrotroph) adenomas are rare and account for less than 1% of all pituitary adenomas. They are associated with long-standing hypothyroidism (characterized by high TSH and low T_4), or they can have high levels of TSH associated with high T_4 levels. In the former case, thyrotroph hyperplasia as a result of primary hypothyroidism must be ruled out. The symptoms of either primary or central cause of hyperthyroidism include tachycardia, heat intolerance, weight loss, diarrhea, tremor, osteoporosis, polyuria, and emotional lability. TSH-secreting adenomas can co-secrete other hormones, including GH, PRL, and gonadotropins, and tend to have more invasive features. Surgery is the primary treatment for thyrotroph adenomas. Successful resection depends on the extension and size of the tumor. Incompletely resected tumors will require radiation therapy or a trial of medical therapy with a dopamine agonist.

Adrenocorticotropic Hormone

Corticotroph cells produce ACTH and constitute 10% to 20% of the anterior lobe. Corticotrophs are concentrated in the central third of the gland but are also found in the lateral wings of the adenohypophysis and in the pars intermedia. Cortisol secretion is regulated by the hypothalamic-pituitary-adrenal axis. Corticotropin-releasing hormone (CRH) made by the paraventricular neurons in the hypothalamus stimulate the release of ACTH. ACTH is synthesized as part of the precursor proopiomelanocortin (POMC), which is cleaved into pro-ACTH and β-lipotropin (βLPH). Further processing of pro-ACTH yields ACTH, corticotrophin-like intermediate lobe peptide (CLIP), endorphin, lipotropin, and melanocyte-stimulating hormone (MSH). The major role of ACTH is to stimulate steroidogenesis in the adrenal cortex, which results in the synthesis and release of cortisol. Cortisol exerts negative feedback at the pituitary and the hypothalamus. Regulation of cortisol by the brain is through CRH release and involves a complex integration of neural inputs into the hypothalamus. Cholinergic and serotonergic input stimulate CRH secretion, whereas adrenergic pathways constitute an inhibitory pathway, all of which mediate stress-induced and circadian ACTH secretion. Peak levels of ACTH, and subsequently cortisol, are reached at 6 AM, decline during the day to 4 PM, and then further decline to a nadir between 11 PM and 3 AM.

The effects of ACTH pathology are primarily caused by cortisol dysregulation. Cortisol is a steroid hormone that does not bind to cellular receptors as in peptide hormones. Cortisol crosses the cell membrane and binds to cytosolic or nuclear receptors resulting in alteration of gene transcription and subsequent levels of protein synthesis of targeted genes. Cortisol is important in metabolic homeostasis and has a wide range of effects, including stimulation of protein breakdown for gluconeogenesis (catabolism) and anti-inflammatory effects.

Hypocortisolemia can be primary, in which there is a defect intrinsic to the adrenal gland, or secondary, when pituitary or hypothalamic dysfunction causes decreased secretion of CRH or ACTH. Primary adrenal insufficiency was described by Thomas Addison in 1855 and is most commonly associated with destruction of the adrenal glands, either by tuberculosis, acquired immunodeficiency syndrome (AIDS), autoimmune disorder, adrenal hemorrhage, or tumor. In such cases, ACTH levels are high in response to the low plasma levels of glucocorticoids. Secondary adrenal insufficiency is most often caused by suppression of the hypothalamic-pituitary axis by exogenous glucocorticoid therapy. Endogenous causes are a result of pituitary destruction by large tumors, apoplexy (hemorrhage into a pituitary adenoma), pituitary infarction (Sheehan's syndrome), inflammatory process (lymphocytic hypophysitis, Langerhans cell histiocytosis), or granulomatous disease (sarcoidosis). In almost all cases, loss of ACTH function is associated with panhypopituitarism. One exception is hypothalamic-pituitary suppression from long-standing Cushing's syndrome (described later), which results in impaired CRH and ACTH response up to 6 to 12 months after resolution of Cushing's syndrome. Clinically, hypocortisolism is associated with weakness, fatigue, anorexia, nausea and vomiting, diarrhea, and postural hypotension. The mineralocorticoid insufficiency that may accompany glucocorticoid insufficiency can lead to hyponatremia and hyperkalemia. In patients with primary adrenal insufficiency, hyperpigmentation can be detected (secondary to the elevated ACTH and associated MSH secretion). Adrenal insufficiency is typically diagnosed by detecting either a low early morning serum cortisol or an inadequate cortisol response (less than 18 μg/dL) to ACTH administration (Cortrosyn stimulation test). Treatment involves two to three doses throughout the day of cortisol replacement (e.g., 15 mg hydrocortisone at 8:00 AM and 10 mg at 3:00 PM). Patients with adrenal insufficiency should wear a medic alert indicator to avoid adrenal crisis at times of physical stress (severe illness, trauma, planned surgery), when stress dose steroids (e.g., hydrocortisone, 100 mg intravenously) should be initiated and maintained during the period of stress.

Hypercortisolemia leads to a syndrome first described by Harvey Cushing in 1912.[3] Cushing's syndrome is the eponym for the general clinical syndrome produced by chronic hypercortisolism. The most common cause of Cushing's syndrome is exogenous steroid use (e.g., in the treatment of arthritis, cerebral edema). Hypercortisolism resulting from excess ACTH secretion from the pituitary is termed *Cushing's disease*. Nearly all organ systems are affected by hypercortisolism (Table 6-3). Centripetal fat deposition is the most common manifestation of glucocorticoid excess and often the initial symptom. Fat accumulates in the face and the supraclavicular and dorsocervical fat pads, leading to the typical moon facies and buffalo-hump, often accompanied by facial plethora. The mechanisms that determine fat redistribution probably lie in the differential sensitivity of central and peripheral adipocytes to the opposite lipolytic and lipogenic actions of cortisol excess versus secondary hyperinsulinism. Other clinical features are related to the protein-wasting effect of cortisol, including skin thinning caused by the atrophy of the epidermis and connective tissue, purple to red striae, muscle wasting leading to fatigability, and large-muscle atrophy resulting in difficulty in getting up from

---

TABLE 6-3

Clinical Features of Cushing's Syndrome

Fat Distribution
Centripetal obesity
Generalized obesity
Moon facies
"Buffalo hump"
Supraclavicular fat pad

Skin Manifestations
Stria (red or purple)
Plethora
Hirsutism
Acne
Bruising
Pigmentation

Musculoskeletal
Osteopenia (pathological fractures)
Proximal muscle weakness

Sexual Function
Menstrual disorder
Decreased libido
Impotence

Metabolic/Cardiovascular
Glucose intolerance
Diabetes mellitus
Poor wound healing
Hypertension
Cardiac hypertrophy
Congestive heart failure

Mental Changes
Irritability
Psychosis
Emotional lability
Depression

a chair. Osteopenia with increased risk for pathologic fractures and compression fractures of the vertebral bodies may be presenting symptoms. Chronic hypercortisolism also results in impaired defense mechanisms against infections, hypertension-inducing cardiac hypertrophy and eventually congestive heart failure, and hirsutism caused by excess adrenocortical androgens. Psychic disturbances are extremely common and include anxiety, increased emotional lability and irritability, euphoria, and depression. Diagnosis involves a two-step process, first establishing that hypercortisolism or Cushing's syndrome exists and then identifying its cause. Plasma morning cortisol values can be easily measured; however, 50% of patients with Cushing's syndrome will have normal levels. Because patients with Cushing's syndrome usually lack a normal circadian rhythm, an evening serum or salivary cortisol level may be helpful. A 24-hour urine free-cortisol level is the most ideal measure of the cortisolic state. The most reliable means to confirm or rule out the diagnosis of Cushing's syndrome is the low-dose dexamethasone suppression test, which assesses the normal negative-feedback loop in the hypothalamic-pituitary-adrenal axis. Between 10 and 11 PM, 1 mg of dexamethasone is administered orally and plasma cortisol is measured the next morning at 8:00 AM. In normal patients, plasma cortisol values will be suppressed below a certain threshold depending on the assay used (typically less than 2 $\mu g/dL$). Although this test has very high sensitivity to Cushing's disease, the specificity is lower, with as many as 13% of obese patients lacking normal suppression.

When the diagnosis of Cushing's syndrome has been made, the cause is investigated. Plasma ACTH levels can be helpful in differentiating adrenocortical tumors (in which ACTH levels will be low), Cushing's disease (in which ACTH levels will be slightly above normal or normal), and ectopic ACTH tumors (in which ACTH levels are markedly elevated). The high-dose dexamethasone suppression test determines the pituitary dependency of the hypercortisolic state. The classic test requires 2 mg of dexamethasone given every 6 hours for 2 days. A 24-hour urine free-cortisol level is measured on the second day. Suppression of steroid levels of greater than 50% is seen in nearly all patients with Cushing's disease. No significant reduction of steroid levels is noted in patients with adrenal tumors. Similar results are seen with the use of a single 8-mg dose of dexamethasone at 11 PM and a plasma cortisol level at 8 AM. Patients with Cushing's disease have plasma cortisol decrease to 50% or less of the baseline value. An additional test is the metyrapone test, in which 750 mg of metyrapone are given every 4 hours for six doses, resulting in cortisol deprivation. Urine (24 hour) steroid levels are measured. In normal patients, the levels can rise twofold; however, in Cushing's disease (and in ectopic ACTH tumors) there is an explosive increase in urinary steroid levels after metyrapone in up to 98% of patients. If Cushing's disease is suspected, magnetic resonance imaging (MRI) is necessary to identify the corticotroph adenoma. If MRI is negative, suggesting a pituitary tumor too small to visualize or an ectopic ACTH tumor, bilateral inferior petrosal sinus (IPS) sampling (IPSS) is performed. ACTH measurements are made simultaneously from blood within the IPS from both sides and from a peripheral source. A central-to-peripheral ACTH gradient of greater than 2:1 is consistent with Cushing's disease. In patients with an ectopic ACTH tumor, this gradient is almost always lower than 1.7:1. Bilateral IPSS also can help to identify the location of a pituitary tumor. If the side-to-side gradient is greater than 1.5:1, and taking into account

anomalous venous drainage, the tumor is most likely located within the side of the gland with the higher ACTH level. The use of CRH stimulation increases the sensitivity of IPSS.[9] Treatment of Cushing's disease entails selective adenomectomy through a transsphenoidal operation. Because these tumors are often very small and invasive, surgical exploration should be performed by surgeons with significant experience with Cushing's disease. In certain cases, removal of half of the pituitary gland (hemihypophysectomy) guided by the IPSS can lead to cure in up to 80% of patients.[9]

Patients with long-standing hypercortisolemia have isolated hypothalamic-pituitary corticotropic suppression. Following successful treatment of Cushing's syndrome, patients will require replacement cortisol therapy for 6 to 12 months, until CRH and ACTH responses return to baseline. Total bilateral adrenalectomy is considered one of the last treatment options in patients with persistent or recurrent Cushing's disease not responding to other therapies. In such a case, the drastic cortisol deprivation induced by the hypocortisolism can trigger a boost in the growth and secretory activity of the corticotroph adenoma. This is associated with increased plasma ACTH levels and clinical hyperpigmentation with an expanding sellar mass, defining Nelson's syndrome.

Follicle-Stimulating Hormone and Luteinizing Hormone

Gonadotrophs produce both gonadotropic hormones (FSH and LH) and constitute 15% of the adenohypophysis. Both hormones share the same α-subunit, which is a 116–amino acid peptide that includes a 24–amino acid signal peptide. The β-subunit confers on each hormone its unique immunologic and biologic properties. The hypothalamus regulates gonadotrope release through GnRH. GnRH is a decapeptide released by neurons in the preoptic and arcuate nucleus within the hypothalamus. The relative amounts of LH and FSH secreted by gonadotroph cells in response to GnRH is a function of the frequency and concentration of administration of GnRH. The pulsatile release of LH and FSH is related to the pulsatile release of GnRH. In males, LH binds to receptors on Lyedig cells and stimulates testosterone production. The role of FSH remains uncertain in males but may work with testosterone for normal qualitative and quantitative spermatogenesis. In females, LH is a major regulator of ovarian steroid synthesis and oocyte maturation. FSH plays a critical role in follicle growth and in regulating estrogen production in the ovary.

Hypogonadism is separated into primary (dysfunction of the testis or ovary) or central (pituitary or hypothalamic). Clinical manifestations of hypogonadism in prepubertal children cause no symptoms, whereas in adolescents hypogonadism leads to delayed or absent pubertal development. In adult women, hypogonadism causes amenorrhea, infertility, loss of libido, vaginal dryness, and hot flashes. In men, hypogonadism leads to loss of libido, erectile dysfunction, and infertility. Causes of primary hypogonadism include genetic disposition, menopause, autoimmune reactions, viruses, radiation, and chemotherapeutic agents. Central hypogonadism is most often caused by pituitary adenomas. Through compression of the gland, these tumors can cause destruction of pituitary tissue or interference with GnRH input from the hypothalamus. Gonadotropin dysfunction is the second most common hormonal disorder from compression of the pituitary gland after GH suppression. Hypothalamic disorders, such as those associated with tumors or radiation therapy, and hypothalamic amenorrhea can lead to hypogonadism. Fasting, weight loss, anorexia nervosa, bulimia, excessive exercise, or stressful conditions result in defects in pulsatile GnRH secretion ("hypothalamic amenorrhea"). Elevated PRL levels can also suppress GnRH pulses and lead to hypothalamic hypogonadism. Diagnosis requires measurement of LH, FSH, and testosterone or estrogen with reference to age-adjusted normal values. Treatment of hypogonadism in men and premenopausal women is effectively accomplished by replacement hormonal therapy.

Overproduction of gonadotropins is a result of pituitary adenomas. Most of the previously classified "nonfunctioning" adenomas are in fact gonadotropin-producing. The abnormally high levels of α-subunit, FSH, or, rarely, LH does not produce any clinical syndrome, however. Furthermore, many of these tumors are inefficient in hormonal secretion or release improperly processed gonadotropins. Treatment of gonadotroph adenomas is surgical resection, most often through a transsphenoidal approach.

Antidiuretic Hormone

Antidiuretic hormone (ADH), or vasopressin, is a nonapeptide synthesized as a prohormone in the magnocellular neurons in the supraoptic and paraventricular nuclei of the hypothalamus. Neurosecretory granules are transported down axons that extend to the posterior pituitary, where the hormones are stored. Secretion of ADH is highly sensitive to osmotic regulation. Osmotic receptors located in the anterior aspect of the hypothalamus can be stimulated with as little as 1% change in plasma osmolality, causing release of ADH. Volume regulation of ADH secretion is less sensitive. These receptors are located in the aorta, carotid sinus, and left atrium and send their signal through the vagal and glossopharyngeal nerves to the brainstem. A 10% to 15% reduction in blood pressure is needed to stimulate release of ADH. Once secreted, ADH causes water retention in the kidneys. The hormone binds to receptors of the renal collecting ducts and stimulates free-water absorption from the distal convoluted tubules and collecting ducts.

Diabetes insipidus (DI) is the excretion of dilute urine related to hyposecretion of vasopressin (hypothalamic DI). Most patients with DI who are alert have a normal thirst mechanism and are able to drink sufficient water to maintain a relatively normal state of metabolic balance. These patients have secondary polydipsia and polyuria and nocturia. Because the posterior lobe is a storage depot for ADH, damage to the posterior lobe of the pituitary or the lower stalk seldom causes permanent DI. However, upper pituitary stalk and hypothalamic damage (e.g., germ cell tumors, craniopharyngioma, lymphocytic hypophysitis) is more likely to result in permanent DI, whereas pituitary adenomas are rarely associated with DI. Surgical pituitary stalk section can result in a triphasic response. An initial period of DI caused by shock to the posterior lobe is followed by excessive ADH secretion as the neurohypophyseal cells die off and release the stored ADH. Permanent DI eventually follows. Synthetic ADH (DDAVP, or desmopressin) can be used to treat patients who are unable to maintain adequate oral fluids (with resultant hypernatremia) or who display severe polyuria and nocturia. Transient DI may require therapy when urine specific gravity is below 1.005, urine output is greater

than 200 mL/hr for at least 2 hours, and the patient has hypernatremia, suggesting that the patient is unable to keep up oral intake with urinary output.

Hypersecretion of ADH represents the syndrome of inappropriate secretion of ADH (SIADH). SIADH is defined as continued secretion of ADH despite a low serum osmolality. The diagnosis of SIADH can be made only when there is a normal state of hydration; there is normal renal, thyroid, and adrenal function; and the patient is not taking diuretics. In all cases, the patient is hyponatremic and has urine that is less than maximally dilute. Possible causes of SIADH include ADH secretion from malignant systemic tumors (e.g., small-cell lung carcinoma, lymphoma, pancreatic tumors), chronic obstructive pulmonary disease (COPD), or drugs (e.g., induced by phenothiazine, tricyclic antidepressants, carbamazepine, lithium). Central nervous system disorders can be associated with SIADH, perhaps through loss of chronic inhibition of the brain on the magnacellular neurons. The clinical manifestations of hyponatremia are dependent on the onset and include confusion, stupor, coma, and seizures. Generally, symptoms do not develop in a normal individual until sodium levels fall below 125 mmol/L. The clinical manifestation probably represents brain edema caused by the osmotic water shifts into the brain because of the decreased plasma osmolality. Treatment of SIADH commonly involves restricting water intake to 600 to 800 mL per day, resulting in a gradual rise in sodium over 2 to 3 days. If patients are hyponatremic for a prolonged period, rapid sodium correction can lead to central pontine myelinolysis with quadriparesis and bulbar palsies. If patients rapidly develop hyponatremia and are very symptomatic, correction of the sodium level can occur with hypertonic (3%) saline in addition to fluid restriction.

Oxytocin

Oxytocin (OT) is the only other hormone stored within the posterior lobe. It is also a nonapeptide and is the most potent hormone to cause uterine contraction. Its effects have been utilized for the induction and augmentation of labor, as well as for prevention and treatment of postpartum hemorrhage. OT is also involved in lactation, causing milk ejection from the breast.

Panhypopituitarism

Pituitary dysfunction can involve selected hormones or complete loss of all pituitary function (panhypopituitarism). Loss of pituitary function from direct compression from a macroadenoma or from radiation therapy typically occurs in a stepwise fashion, with loss of GH secretion followed by loss of gonadotropin, thyrotropin, and finally corticotropic function. This graded loss of function relates to the sensitivity of pituitary cells to external trauma. Pituitary adenomas can cause symptoms related to hypersecretion of a hormone (hormonally active adenomas) or through progressive compression of the normal pituitary gland. In the latter case and in cases of Rathke's cleft cysts, the first hormonal symptoms typically include loss of libido in men and postmenopausal women and amenorrhea in premenopausal women. This can be caused by direct loss of gonadotropic function or because of hyperprolactinemia from stalk effect and subsequent GnRH suppression. Later, as the tumor or cyst enlarges, thyroid function and finally adrenal regulation can be affected, resulting in more pronounced symptoms. Often, signs and symptoms from local mass effect, causing headaches or pressure on the optic chiasm that result in a bitemporal hemianopsia, lead to the diagnosis. In patients who have diabetes insipidus or panhypopituitarism in the absence of symptoms of mass effect, nonadenoma sellar pathology should be considered. This pathology includes infection, sarcoidosis, lymphocytic hypophysitis, craniopharyngioma, glioma, germ cell tumor, lymphoma, Langerhans cell histiocytosis, or metastases. Acute pituitary failure can occur, with pituitary apoplexy caused by hemorrhage into a pituitary adenoma or infarction of the gland (Sheehan's syndrome). Radiation therapy involving the pituitary gland and, in particular, the pituitary stalk can result in pituitary failure in up to 50% of patients at 3 to 5 years. The clinical manifestations of hypopituitarism are detailed within the sections regarding individual hormones above.

References

1. Abosch A, Tyrrell JB, Lamborn KR, et al: Transsphenoidal microsurgery for growth hormone-secreting pituitary adenomas: initial outcome and long-term results. J Clin Endocrinol Metab 83:3411–3418, 1998.
2. Carter JN, Tyson JE, Tolis G, et al: Prolactin-screening tumors and hypogonadism in 22 men. N Engl J Med 299:847–852, 1978.
3. Cushing H: Medical Classic. The functions of the pituitary body: Harvey Cushing. Am J Med Sci 281:70–78, 1981.
4. Jones JI, Clemmons DR: Insulin-like growth factors and their binding proteins: biological actions. Endocr Rev 16:3–34, 1995.
5. Kauppila A: Isolated prolactin deficiency. Curr Ther Endocrinol Metab 5:29–31, 1994.
6. Kelly DF, Gonzalo IT, Cohan P, et al: Hypopituitarism following traumatic brain injury and aneurysmal subarachnoid hemorrhage: a preliminary report. J Neurosurg 93:743–752, 2000.
7. Kunwar S, Wilson CB: Pediatric pituitary adenomas. J Clin Endocrinol Metab 84:4385–4389, 1999.
8. Monson JP: Long-term experience with GH replacement therapy: efficacy and safety. Eur J Endocrinol 148 Suppl 2:S009–S014, 2003.
9. Oldfield EH, Doppman JL, Nieman LK, et al: Petrosal sinus sampling with and without corticotropin-releasing hormone for the differential diagnosis of Cushing's syndrome. N Engl J Med 325:897–905, 1991.
10. Reavley A, Fisher AD, Owen D, et al: Psychological distress in patients with hyperprolactinaemia. Clin Endocrinol (Oxf) 47:343–348, 1997.
11. Sobrinho LG: The psychogenic effects of prolactin. Acta Endocrinol (Copenh) 129(suppl 1):38–40, 1993.
12. Thorner MO, Vance ML: Growth hormone. J Clin Invest 82:745–747, 1988.
13. Tyrrell JB, Lamborn KR, Hannegan LT, et al: Transsphenoidal microsurgical therapy of prolactinomas: initial outcomes and long-term results. Neurosurgery 44:254–261; discussion 261–263, 1999.
14. Wright AD, Hill DM, Lowy C, et al: Mortality in acromegaly. Q J Med 39:1–16, 1970.

CHAPTER 7

NEUROTOLOGY

William H. Slattery III and Marlan R. Hansen

Benign lesions of the lateral skull base and cerebellopontine angle (CPA) often produce neurotologic symptoms such as hearing loss, dizziness, imbalance, facial weakness, and facial hypesthesia. Clinicians who manage patients with skull base lesions should have a working understanding of the clinical evaluation of these symptoms. This chapter focuses on the neurotologic evaluation of patients with benign lesions of the lateral skull base and CPA. We begin with a brief description of the more common surgical approaches to these regions from the neurotologic perspective. We then focus on key elements of the neurotologic examination and clinical testing that assist in establishing the diagnosis and selecting the most appropriate clinical management.

NEUROTOLOGIC SURGICAL APPROACHES

Surgical approaches to lesions of the lateral skull base and CPA often combine the expertise of a neurosurgeon and a neurotologist. We will provide a brief overview of four common approaches employed by this surgical team: translabyrinthine craniotomy, middle fossa craniotomy, petrosal approaches, and infratemporal fossa approaches. Lesions treated through these approaches include vestibular schwannomas, meningiomas, epidermoids, and paragangliomas of the infratemporal fossa and temporal bone.

Translabyrinthine Craniotomy

Translabyrinthine craniotomy accesses the internal auditory canal (IAC), CPA, and posterior fossa by removal of the mastoid, the semicircular canals, and the vestibule of the inner ear. It provides the most direct approach to the CPA, eliminating the need for cerebellar or temporal lobe retraction, and provides excellent exposure of the entire IAC.[3] Identification of the facial nerve as it exits the internal auditory canal facilitates nerve preservation. The main disadvantage of the translabyrinthine approach is that removal of the labyrinth results in hearing loss. This approach is best suited for medium to large lesions of the CPA that extend into the IAC, most commonly vestibular schwannomas or meningiomas. It is also appropriate for smaller lesions in patients with poor hearing in the affected ear. Removal of the cochlea with or without translocation of the facial nerve extends the translabyrinthine exposure to include the petrous segment of the internal carotid artery,

middle portion of the clivus, ventral pons, and the basilar artery.[1]

Middle Fossa Craniotomy

Middle fossa craniotomy involves a subtemporal craniotomy, extradural elevation of the temporal lobe from the middle fossa floor, and dissection of the IAC. This technically demanding approach provides exposure of the entire IAC without violation of the inner ear and offers the best chance of preserving hearing (up to 70%) in patients with small vestibular schwannomas.[10] It provides limited exposure of the posterior fossa and is generally restricted to lesions smaller than 2 cm. Most candidates for hearing-preservation approaches to the IAC have pure tone threshold averages above 50 dB hearing level and speech discrimination scores greater than 50%. Surgical approaches must be selected according to the individual situation; no strict audiometric criteria to exclude or demand attempts at hearing preservation exist. Anterior extension of the middle fossa approach involves bone removal between Meckel's cave (trigeminal nerve) and the IAC. This increases the exposure of the posterior fossa and petrous pyramid and is often useful for petroclival tumors, particularly meningiomas.[2]

Petrosal Approaches

Petrosal approaches combine posterior fossa and middle fossa exposure by transection of the superior petrosal sinus and tentorium cerebelli.[11] Posterior fossa exposure is gained via retrolabyrinthine or translabyrinthine craniotomy. In many circumstances a middle fossa craniotomy is also performed. Transection of the superior petrosal sinus and tentorium then provides excellent exposure of the lateral and ventral pons, lateral surface of the midbrain, clivus, and vertebrobasilar system.

Infratemporal Fossa Approaches

Fisch described three postauricular, lateral approaches to the infratemporal fossa.[7] Type A provides access to the jugular foramen, mandibular fossa, and posterior infratemporal fossa. Type B exposes the apical petrous bone, clivus, and petrous portion of the internal carotid artery, and type C is an anterior extension used for exposure of the infratemporal fossa, pterygopalatine fossa, parasellar regions, and nasopharynx. All variants typically involve removal of the external auditory canal and middle ear contents, resulting in maximum conductive hearing loss. Facial nerve translocation is often necessary, especially for type B and C variants, and may result in temporary paresis. Preauricular approaches to the infratemporal fossa, which do not require sacrifice of the external auditory canal and middle ear nor facial nerve translocation, are often appropriate for lesions that do not involve structures posterior to the intratemporal internal carotid artery.[5]

PHYSICAL EXAMINATION

Evaluation of the patient with lateral skull base, middle cranial fossa, or posterior fossa tumors requires a comprehensive neurologic and head and neck examination. Here we focus on those aspects of the examination most relevant to the neurotologist.

Otology Examination

Examination of the external ear focuses on swelling, skin lesions (viral eruptions or neoplasms), and evidence of prior surgery or trauma. The eardrum is examined for retraction, perforation, purulent drainage, cholesteatoma, middle ear effusion, and middle ear mass. Use of a microscope and pneumatic otoscopy greatly enhance the sensitivity of the examination, especially for assessing drum mobility and the detection of middle ear masses. Blanching of a middle ear mass with positive-pressure pneumatic otoscopy (Brown's sign) indicates a vascular lesion, such as glomus tumor or high jugular bulb.

Tuning forks help distinguish between sensorineural and conductive hearing loss. The Rinne test is performed by alternately placing a 512 Hz tuning fork on the mastoid (bone conduction) and directly in front of the external ear canal (air conduction). A positive result (air conduction louder than bone conduction) indicates normal hearing or a sensorineural hearing loss, whereas a negative result (bone conduction louder than air conduction) suggests a conductive hearing loss. The Weber test is performed by placing the 512 Hz tuning fork in the middle of the skull. In patients with unilateral hearing impairment, the sound will be localized in the affected ear if there is a conductive hearing loss, or it will be heard in the unaffected ear if the patient suffers from a sensorineural hearing loss.

The ability to understand words can be estimated by speaking phonetically balanced, single words at a conversational level into one ear while shielding the patient's eyes and providing masking noise in the opposite ear. Retrocochlear lesions (e.g., vestibular schwannomas) that affect the auditory nerve or its central projections typically result in significantly reduced word recognition, whereas cochlear and, especially, conductive forms of hearing loss generally maintain the ability to distinguish words.

Vestibular Examination

The vestibular system is highly integrated with the visual, propioceptive, cerebellar, and motor systems. Dysfunction of any one of these systems may result in dizziness or imbalance. The vestibular examination consists of two principal components: observation of eye movements to evaluate the vestibulocular reflex and examination of balance and coordination to evaluate the vestibulospinal, cerebellar, and proprioception function.

Vestibular nystagmus is characterized by a slower, physiologic eye movement in one direction, called the *slow phase,* followed by a rapid, compensatory movement of the eye in the opposite direction, called the *fast phase.* By contrast, ocular nystagmus is pendular with the speed of movement roughly equal in both directions. Vestibular nystagmus can have peripheral (labyrinthine) or central causes and is classified according to (1) direction and plane of movement, (2) inducing stimulus (spontaneous, gaze evoked, or induced), and (3) intensity. By convention, nystagmus is named for the direction of the fast phase. Nystagmus of labyrinthine origin is generally direction fixed and horizontal, although positional forms of labyrinthine nystagmus have a rotary component (Table 7-1). Central nystagmus resulting from central nervous system (CNS) disorders is often direction changing (as the eyes change direction of gaze, the fast phase of nystagmus changes to that direction) and may occur in vertical or oblique directions.

The sensitivity of testing for nystagmus can be increased by the use of Frenzel lenses. These are lighted, 20+ diopter lenses that provide the examiner a magnified view of ocular movements and prevent fixation suppression of the nystagmus by the patient.

Patients are first examined for spontaneous and gaze-evoked nystagmus by asking the patient to look at the examiner's finger in each direction of gaze. Examination for induced nystagmus also includes examination for head shaking and positional nystagmus. Head-shaking nystagmus is assessed by looking for nystagmus after the patient shakes his or her head vigorously 20 to 30 times in the horizontal plane. Head-shaking nystagmus indicates a peripheral vestibular lesion. Positional testing involves moving the patient from a sitting to supine position and then to a lying position on one side and then the other. Classic Hallpike positioning is also performed. Positional nystagmus indicates a vestibular disorder that may be caused by a peripheral or a central lesion.

TABLE 7-1

Differentiation of Labyrinthine from Central Nystagmus

Labyrinthine	Central
Usually horizontal or horizontorotary	Any direction including vertical and oblique
Direction fixed	Usually direction changing
Intensified by gaze in direction of fast phase and diminished by gaze in the direction of slow phase	Change of gaze generally does not affect intensity
Suppressed by visual fixation	Not suppressed by visual fixation and may be enhanced
Most intense at onset and diminishes with time	Continuous, may increase with time
Associated with intense nausea, anxiety, and cold sweats	Nonvertiginous symptoms less intense
Simultaneous and of equal intensity in both eyes	May affect only one eye or differ in intensity between eyes

Vestibular assessment also requires testing for balance and coordination. The Rhomberg and sharpened-Rhomberg tests assess stationary balance with the arms folded across the chest and the eyes closed. A positive test is characterized by obvious, uncontrollable falling, usually in the same direction, and indicates vestibular or cerebellar dysfunction. Gait is tested by observing the patient walk, make a quick turn, and walk back. Gait disturbances indicate imbalance but are nonlocalizing, although a wide-based gait is characteristic of cerebellar dysfunction. Tandem walking (heel to toe) is more sensitive than standard-gait testing and is often abnormal in patients with a balance disturbance. Finger-to-nose, finger-nose-finger, and rapid alternate-movement testing assess for asynergia, dysmetria, and adiadochokinesia, which are cerebellar findings.

Most lesions of the lateral skull base and CPA result in gradual loss of vestibular function. In such cases, gradual compensation for the unilateral vestibular loss occurs, and most patients do not exhibit spontaneous nystagmus; however, many exhibit unsteadiness with sudden movements. Patients with large tumors may demonstrate ataxia and cerebellar findings.

Cranial Nerve Assessment

A detailed assessment of all cranial nerves is an important part of the neurotologic evaluation. Here we limit our discussion to examination of the trigeminal and facial nerves. Together with the auditory-vestibular nerve complex, cranial nerves (CNs) V and VII are the most likely to be affected by lesions of the lateral skull base and CPA.

Trigeminal Nerve

Tumors of the middle fossa, CPA, cavernous sinus, infratemporal fossa, or paranasal sinuses may cause trigeminal disturbance. Usually the sensory function is affected first, and motor function is preserved. Facial sensation is assessed with a wisp of cotton (light touch), pin prick (pain), and warm and cold metal disks (temperature). All three divisions (V_1, V_2, and V_3) should be tested independently. Corneal reflex testing should be performed in all patients with CPA lesions. This reflex depends on V_1 sensory function and facial nerve motor function. The patient is asked to look away from the eye being tested and the examiner touches the sclera with a small wisp of cotton as a control. The cotton is then applied to the cornea, which should cause blinking in both eyes. If neither eye blinks, the patient has a V_1 deficit on the tested side. If only the opposite eye blinks, the patient has a facial nerve dysfunction. CPA lesions often disrupt the sensory function of the trigeminal nerve before they affect the motor function of the facial nerve.

Motor function of the trigeminal nerve is assessed by asking the patient to tightly clench the teeth. The examiner determines the strength of the masseter and temporalis muscles by direct palpation and by attempting to open the mouth with firm, downward pressure on the chin.

Facial Nerve

Motor function of the facial nerve is tested in all five peripheral branches of the facial nerve by asking the patient to raise the eyebrow, close the eye tightly, wrinkle the nose, smile, pucker the lips, and show the lower teeth while moving the skin on the front of the neck by drawing the lower lip and corner of the mouth downward and outward. Lesions involving the facial nucleus or main trunk of the facial nerve will affect all branches of the nerve, whereas distal lesions (e.g., parotid tumors) may affect only individual branches. Classically, supranuclear lesions (e.g., motor cortex) spare forehead function because of bilateral supranuclear innervation to the facial nucleus. Asking the patient to rapidly blink the eyes and observing for simultaneous movement of lower facial muscles assesses for synkinesis.

The extent of motor dysfunction should be estimated according to standardized grading systems. The modified House-Brackmann grading system consists of a six-point system (Table 7-2), and the American Academy of Otolaryngology—Head and Neck Surgery recommends that this system be used for reporting all facial nerve recoveries and treatment results.[9]

In addition to voluntary motor function, the facial nerve provides parasympathetic, taste, and general sensory innervation. Lesions of the facial nerve proximal to the geniculate ganglion often disrupt the parasympathetic innervation to the lacrimal gland and may exacerbate dry-eye symptoms caused by orbicular oculi weakness. The Schirmer II test can be used to quantitatively compare reflex tearing between the two eyes. Taste testing, although rarely clinically helpful, can be accomplished by placing sugar, salt, weak vinegar, and a bitter substance (quinine) on the anterior two thirds of the protruded tongue. Testing for loss of general sensory fibers can be accomplished by touching the posterior aspect of the ear canal and the conchal bowl with a sharp instrument. Decreased sensation of the posterior conchal bowl and ear canal, known as *Hitselberger's sign*, is often seen with vestibular schwannomas.

LABORATORY TESTS

Audiogram

Any patient known to have or suspected of having a lesion of the lateral skull base or CPA should undergo formal audiometric testing. Standard testing includes air and bone conduction pure tone thresholds, speech reception threshold, and speech discrimination scores. Lesions involving the middle ear typically result in a conductive hearing loss. Audiometrically conductive hearing losses manifest as elevated air conduction thresholds compared with bone conduction threshold (air-bone gap). Sensorineural hearing loss is caused by cochlear or auditory nerve dysfunction and demonstrates air and bone conduction thresholds elevated to the same degree. Lesions that involve the auditory nerve or auditory brainstem nuclei typically result in reduced speech discrimination scores out of proportion to their effect on pure tone thresholds. Any patient found to have an asymmetric sensorineural hearing loss or reporting unilateral tinnitus should be evaluated to exclude lesions of the IAC or CPA with magnetic resonance imaging (MRI) with gadolinium enhancement.

Auditory Brainstem Response Testing

Auditory brainstem response (ABR) testing uses surface electrodes and a computer to record and average auditory nerve and brainstem potentials in response to click stimuli delivered to the ear. It is useful to screen patients with asymmetric sensorineural hearing loss or unilateral tinnitus for retrocochlear lesions. Although ABR is less sensitive than MRI with gado-

TABLE 7-2	Modified House-Brackmann Facial Nerve Grading Scale	

Grade	Description	Characteristics
I	Normal	Normal facial function in all areas
II	Mild dysfunction	Gross: slight weakness noticeable on close inspection; may have very slight synkinesis
		At rest: normal symmetry and tone
		Motion:
		Forehead: moderate to good function
		Eye: complete closure with minimum effort
		Mouth: slight asymmetry
III	Moderate dysfunction	Gross: obvious but not disfiguring difference between two sides; noticeable but not severe synkinesis, contracture, or hemifacial spasm
		At rest: normal symmetry and tone
		Motion:
		Forehead: slight to moderate movement
		Eye: complete closure with effort
		Mouth: slightly weak with maximal effort
IV	Moderately severe dysfunction	Gross: obvious weakness or disfiguring asymmetry
		At rest: normal symmetry and tone
		Motion:
		Forehead: none
		Eye: incomplete closure
		Mouth: asymmetric with maximum effort
V	Severe dysfunction	Gross: only barely perceptible motion
		At rest: asymmetry
		Motion:
		Forehead: none
		Eye: incomplete closure
		Mouth: slight movement
VI	Total paralysis	No movement

linum for the detection of small vestibular schwannomas, it detects most schwannomas larger than 1 cm and is appropriate to screen patients unable or unwilling to undergo MRI or older patients who would be treated only for larger lesions.[6]

Preoperative ABR testing is useful for patients considered candidates for hearing-preservation approaches for removal of lesions in the IAC. Preoperative ABR testing confirms the presence of recordable responses that can be monitored intraoperatively. Poor or delayed ABR waveforms predict a lower likelihood of hearing preservation.[4]

Electronystagmogram

Although classically electronystagmogram (ENG) referred to the measurement of nystagmus using electro-oculography techniques, most modern ENG investigations use infrared videography to record eye movements during various vestibular and oculomotor tests. Typically, the ENG evaluates spontaneous, gaze-evoked, and positional nystagmus; optokinetic and saccadic eye movements; and caloric responses. Caloric testing offers quantitative evaluation of each labyrinth by measuring the nystagmus induced by placing cold and warm water in the external auditory canal. A 25% reduction in caloric response in one ear compared with the opposite ear suggests diminished vestibular function on the stimulated side.

When combined with a thorough history and neurotologic examination, ENG remains the most useful laboratory investigation of the vestibular system in the evaluation of patients with dizziness. ENG is sometimes useful in the evaluation of patients with lesions of the IAC (e.g., vestibular schwannoma) who are considered candidates for hearing-preservation procedures. Caloric stimulation primarily tests the lateral semicircular canal, which is innervated by the superior vestibular nerve. A reduced caloric response in a patient with a small vestibular schwannoma suggests that the tumor arises off the superior vestibular nerve. These patients have slightly better odds for hearing preservation than patients with inferior vestibular nerve tumors.[4] ENG is also helpful in elderly patients with vestibular schwannomas who have disabling dizziness. If an ENG demonstrates residual vestibular function in the affected ear, these patients often benefit from destruction of the labyrinthine function, even if the tumor does not require treatment. Other vestibular tests such as rotary chair and platform posturography offer little in the initial evaluation of patients with skull base lesions but occasionally help in monitoring vestibular compensation following destruction of the labyrinth or vestibular nerves.

Facial Nerve Electroneurography and Facial Electromyography

Facial nerve electroneurography (ENoG) uses surface or needle electrodes to quantify facial muscle action potentials in response to transcutaneous electrical stimulation of the facial nerve. Responses are evaluated by comparing the peak-to-peak amplitude of the maximum response obtained from the two sides of the face. The percentage reduction of amplitude on the affected side compared with the unaffected side is thought to represent the percentage of degenerated nerve fibers. ENoG is most commonly used to predict facial nerve recovery following acute palsy (Bell's palsy) and select patients most likely to benefit from facial nerve decompression.[8] It is also useful in the evaluation of lesions that intimately involve the facial nerve such as facial nerve schwannomas or hemangiomas. Any patient with a lesion in the IAC that appears as a vestibular schwannoma but demonstrates preoperative facial nerve weakness or reduced ENoG response should be counseled about the possibility of having a facial nerve schwannoma. Management of facial nerve schwannomas is significantly different from that for vestibular schwannomas.

Facial muscle electromyography (EMG) measures action potentials generated by spontaneous or voluntary activity, in contrast to ENoG, in which the facial nerve is electrically stimulated. Facial EMG is most valuable in the evaluation of patients who have suffered severe facial nerve injury and after 12 to 18 months demonstrate little or no recovery of facial movement. If an EMG demonstrates lack of polyphasic reinnervation potentials with or without fibrillation potentials, it is unlikely that further facial nerve regeneration will occur, and facial reanimation options should be considered (cross-facial to facial or hypoglossal to facial anastomosis). Likewise, facial EMG helps assess whether a nerve anastomosis (e.g., in the CPA) is unsuccessful in a patient with no recovery of motion at 18 months. Lack of polyphasic reinnervation potentials implies failed regeneration, and other reanimation options should be pursued.

CONCLUSION

Lateral skull base and CPA tumors often present with hearing loss, dizziness, imbalance, or facial weakness. Every member of the multispecialty team that evaluates and treats patients with skull base tumors should have a basic understanding of the examination and clinical tests necessary to evaluate these symptoms. As part of the skull base team, the neurotologist provides expertise in the clinical assessment of the auditory-vestibular system and facial nerve and on surgical approaches to the lateral skull base, especially those involving the temporal bone.

References

1. Angeli SI, De la Cruz A, Hitselberger W: The transcochlear approach revisited. Otol Neurotol 22:690–695, 2001.
2. Arriaga MA, Brackmann DE, Hitselberger WE: Extended middle fossa resection of petroclival and cavernous sinus neoplasms. Laryngoscope 103:693–698, 1993.
3. Brackmann DE, Green JD: Translabyrinthine approach for acoustic tumor removal. Otolaryngol Clin North Am 25:311–329, 1992.
4. Brackmann DE, Owens RM, Friedman RA, et al: Prognostic factors for hearing preservation in vestibular schwannoma surgery. Am J Otol 21:417–424, 2000.
5. Cass SP, Hirsch BE, Stechison MT: Evolution and advances of the lateral surgical approaches to cranial base neoplasms. J Neurooncol 20:337–361, 1994.
6. Chandrasekhar SS, Brackmann DE, Devgan KK: Utility of auditory brainstem response audiometry in diagnosis of acoustic neuromas. Am J Otol 16:63–67, 1995.
7. Fisch U, Fagan P, Valavanis A: The infratemporal fossa approach for the lateral skull base. Otolaryngol Clin North Am 17:513–552, 1984.
8. Gantz BJ, Rubinstein JT, Gidley P, et al: Surgical management of Bell's palsy. Laryngoscope 109:1177–1188, 1999.
9. House JW, Brackmann DE: Facial nerve grading system. Otolaryngol Head Neck Surg 93:146–147, 1985.
10. Slattery WH III, Brackmann DE, Hitselberger W: Middle fossa approach for hearing preservation with acoustic neuromas. Am J Otol 18:596–601, 1997.
11. Spetzler RF, Daspit CP, Pappas CT: The combined supra- and infratentorial approach for lesions of the petrous and clival regions: experience with 46 cases. J Neurosurg 76:588–599, 1992.

CHAPTER **8**

NEURO-OPHTHALMOLOGY

Creig S. Hoyt

Eye symptoms appear with significant frequency in patients with brain tumors. It has been estimated that some form of ocular sign can be observed in more than 50% of patients with brain tumors, and these are often the initial complaints. In more than 50% of patients with brain tumors, papilledema is found at some time during the course of the illness, and in 25% of patients ocular signs alone provide a fairly accurate localization of the tumor. There can be no doubt that the majority of eye signs in patients with brain tumors are of diagnostic or localizing significance.

A detailed history of visual symptoms is essential in examining these patients. Visual field defects are often not obvious to the patient, especially homonymous hemianopic defects, but history taking may document the consequence of visual-field defects on everyday life (e.g., frequent auto accidents). Loss of vision is an important symptom that may indicate tumors near the optic nerve, chiasm, or tract, but the patient often is not aware of the loss. Early signs of progressive visual loss are not always easy to detect, but a history of poor vision under poor lighting or disturbances of color sensation is suggestive of optic nerve dysfunction. Patients with papilledema may experience sudden visual loss lasting usually not more than 30 seconds and more often only a few seconds. These attacks may be preceded by photopsias—for example, a sensation of sparks or lightning—usually in both eyes and both visual fields.

Optic hallucinations may occur as the result of a lesion anywhere along the visual pathway. Unformed light sensations (e.g., luminous rings, stripes) are typical of occipital lesions, whereas formed and often complex sensations are more typical of a temporal lobe site. Micropsia and macropsia are sensations usually associated with retinal disease (macula) but may occur as the result of visual disturbances in the occipital or parietal cortex.

Paralysis of one or more extraocular muscles usually causes diplopia. This may be evident only in the field of gaze where the affected muscle acts or in primary gaze as well. The presence of a torsional component of the diplopia strongly suggests weakness of the superior oblique (fourth cranial nerve [CN] palsy). Vertical diplopia, especially when it is constant in all fields of gaze and not associated with torsional diplopia, may be the result of skew deviation, usually of a brainstem origin.

Headaches associated with elevated intracranial pressure may radiate into the eyes, but this is usually a minor complaint. If the eye ache is a primary complaint, localized ocular disease should be considered. In superior orbital fissure and cavernous sinus syndromes, there may be referred ocular pain associated with involvement of the first branch of the trigeminal nerve. A similar radiating pain into the eyes may be caused by tumors within the Gasserian ganglion or middle or posterior fossas.

Most important clinical findings on the neuro-ophthalmologic examination can be detected at the bedside with very little in the way of special instrumentation. Examination of the external aspect of the eyes may reveal important diagnostic findings. Unilateral widening of the palpebral fissure without proptosis of the globe is usually the result of an ipsilateral facial nerve paresis. Lagophthalmos, or the inability to fully close the eyes, usually accompanies a total facial paralysis and may lead to an exposure keratopathy requiring treatment. A unilateral narrowing of the lid fissure is usually caused by ptosis of the upper lid. This may be caused by paresis of the oculomotor nerve or sympathetic nerve. If the pupil is also affected, ptosis and a small pupil relative to the other eye indicate sympathetic damage, whereas ptosis and a large pupil is usually a sign of oculomotor nerve dysfunction.

Exophthalmos or proptosis may simulate widening of the lid fissure. Simple external examination of the two orbits and globes usually can differentiate the two, but objective measurements of proptosis can be obtained with a simple device known as an exophthalmometer. Exophthalmos is a primary sign of an orbital tumor or other orbital pathology such as thyroid ophthalmopathy. However, it may be a sign of sphenoid wing meningiomas. Exophthalmos associated with cavernous sinus thrombosis is usually easily distinguished because of the accompanying lid edema, severe chemosis, immobility of the globe, and corneal anesthesia.

Corneal sensitivity may be tested with a small paper strip or wisp of cotton. Unilateral anesthesia may be secondary to local corneal disease, especially herpetic infections that may also be a sign of dysfunction of the first branch of the trigeminal nerve. Unilateral absence or diminution of the corneal reflex may be an early sign of a cerebellopontine angle tumor.

Disturbances of pupil size, shape, and reactivity are common findings associated with brain tumors. During examination the size of the pupil should be noted first. Most important for diagnostic or localizing purpose are any differences in the size of the two pupils (anisocoria). Unilateral mydriasis may be caused either by stimulation of the sympathetic fibers or more commonly by paralysis of the pupillary sphincter resulting from injury to the oculomotor nerve. Pupillary dilation caused by oculomotor nerve dysfunction will be commonly associated with ipsilateral paresis of accommodation. Accommodation can be evaluated at the bedside by comparing visual acuities of the two eyes with a near-vision card. Pupillary mydriasis and accommodative paralysis without extraocular muscle dysfunction suggest a lesion of oculomotor subnucleus in the midbrain, whereas pupillary mydriasis, accommodative paralysis, and extraocular muscle dysfunction are seen in lesions affecting the oculomotor nerve itself. Unilateral mydriasis associated with oculomotor nerve dysfunction must be distinguished from drug-induced mydriasis, congenital anisocoria, Adie's syndrome, and local ocular pathology, including angle closure glaucoma and traumatic iris sphincter rupture.

Unilateral miosis is caused by stimulation of the iris sphincter or more commonly by paralysis of the dilator. Paralysis of the sympathetic fibers subserving the eye results in Horner's syndrome, which is characterized by mild ptosis of the upper lid, miosis, and mild enophthalmos. Hypopigmentation of the iris or heterochromia is usually seen in congenital Horner's syndrome but may be seen in young children with tumors of the chest or neck involving the sympathetic pathway. Confirmation of the diagnosis of Horner's syndrome may be established pharmacologically with topical 4% cocaine application. Cocaine blocks the normal reuptake of norepinephrine by the presynaptic nerve terminals. Therefore in a normal eye the pupil will dilate, but in Horner's syndrome the pupil will dilate poorly because little or no norepinephrine is being released into the synaptic cleft. An isolated Horner's syndrome is rarely caused by intrinsic brainstem disease but is much more commonly the result of involvement of the sympathetic pathway in the neck, cavernous sinus, or superior orbital fissure.

The Argyll Robertson pupil is miotic but is also associated with irregular pupillary shape and light-near dissociation. In light-near dissociation the affected pupil does not react to a bright light but does react to a near stimulus. This rare syndrome is usually associated with tertiary syphilis. Pupils with some of the features of the Argyll Robertson syndrome may be seen in patients with diabetes, alcoholism, encephalitis, or some degenerative syndromes of the central nervous system.

Assessment of pupillary function is a sensitive test for detecting optic nerve disease. This can be done with the so-called swinging flashlight test or Marcus Gunn pupil test. When a light is shone in an eye with normal optic nerve function, both pupils will quickly constrict and then slowly redilate. When the light is swung to the eye with optic nerve dysfunction, the normal initial pupillary constriction will be absent or diminished. The patient can also be asked to subjectively describe this phenomenon, because optic nerve disease causes the light to appear dimmer in the affected eye. A unilateral Marcus Gunn pupil is almost pathognomonic for optic nerve disease, although it may occur in amblyopia. A Marcus Gunn pupil may be seen in an optic tract lesion if there is more visual loss in one eye than the other. Occasionally, a Marcus Gunn pupil has been described in contralateral pretectal mesencephalic lesions despite the absence of visual field loss.

Although many ocular motor anomalies seen in patients with brain tumors are merely those seen as symptoms of elevated intracranial pressure, there are others that point to a specific diagnostic portion of the central nervous system (especially tumors located at the base of the skull). Extraocular muscle palsies indicate disturbed function of one or more extraocular muscles caused by a process in the muscle itself, the neuromuscular junction, or the CN or the nucleus innervating them. One first observes the position of the eyes in primary gaze. The most severe palsies result in a change in position of the eyes even in primary gaze. Then one tests the motility of the eyes by asking the patient to look to the right, left, up, and down. This should indicate the limitation of motility in a certain field of gaze that corresponds to the direction of the primary action of the paretic or paralyzed muscle. In some patients with only a partial muscle paresis, no limitation of motility may be seen. However, the speed of saccadic movements is slowed in the field of gaze in which the affected muscle is activated. In other patients the presence of so-called paretic nystagmus may be a valuable accompanying sign. In the terminal position of action of the paretic muscle there are some jerky, usually unsustained nystagmoid movements.

Documenting the presence of subjective diplopia can be essential in establishing the diagnosis of paretic strabismus. In many cases the patient will spontaneously report the presence of double vision during motility testing or normal activity. To make a latent diplopia obvious to the patient or to create a more distinct dissociation of the two images, it may be advisable to place a red lens over one eye. While the patient fixates on a bright light, the presence of red and white lights can be detected as well as the relative separation of the two images in the various fields of gaze. It has been reported that extraocular muscle palsies occur in approximately 10% to 15% of all patients with brain tumors. Sixth CN palsies are by far the most common, with those of the oculomotor nerve next most common. Isolated paresis of the fourth CN in patients with brain tumors is distinctly rare.

In contrast to isolated extraocular muscle palsies, with a disturbance of one or several individual muscles, gaze palsies are disturbances of the higher centers involving movements of both eyes. A gaze palsy is the inability to look in a given direction (right, left, up, or down). Horizontal gaze palsy is the inability to look to one side with both eyes. An isolated saccadic palsy with preservation of pursuit, vergence, and vestibular movements to one side is suggestive of a lesion in the contralateral frontal lobe or internal capsule. A focal motor seizure arising in this area will produce adversive eye movements. In contrast, when the paramedian pontine reticular formation is affected, a gaze palsy affecting saccades, pursuits, and vestibular eye movements results on the ipsilateral side. Convergence movements remain unaffected.

Vertical gaze palsies result in the patient's inability to look up or, very rarely, down. The rostral interstitial nucleus of the median longitudinal fasciculus in the mesencephalon acts as the immediate premotor pathway for upward eye movements. A lesion in this area results in paresis of upward gaze with retained upward movement of the eyes with forceful eyelid closure (Bell's phenomena). Paralysis of upward gaze is most commonly associated with compressive lesions at the level of the posterior commissure. Lesions in this area affecting the structures of the periaqueductal gray matter produce a typical disorder known as Parinaud's syndrome. The features of this syndrome include lid retraction, light-near dissociation of the pupils, convergence-retraction nystagmus, and papilledema. Downward gaze movements may be affected in Parinaud's syndrome, but isolated downward gaze palsies are distinctly rare.

Convergence palsy results in the inability to converge and fixate on a near object with preservation of accommodation and pupillary function. Isolated convergence palsy is quite rare but occurs commonly in combination with other symptoms, especially an upward gaze palsy. This is related to the location of the convergence center being in the midbrain. Divergence paralysis is poorly understood. Many experts believe that active divergence of the eyes does not occur and that so-called divergence palsies are merely bilateral sixth CN palsies.

Interconnecting the ocular motor nuclei in the pons in the midbrain is a fiber group known as the medial longitudinal fasciculus. It is located dorsally on either side of the brainstem midline. It connects the abducens nuclei to the trochlear and oculomotor nuclei. An intact median longitudinal fasciculus (MLF) is essential for the production of all conjugate eye movements. A unilateral lesion of the MLF produces a typical ocular motor disturbance characterized by slow adduction of the ipsilateral eye and nystagmus in the abducting eye. Convergence remains unaffected. This eye movement disorder is known as an internuclear ophthalmoplegia. Tumors affecting this area of the brainstem usually produce a bilateral internuclear ophthalmoplegia. Skew deviation is a nonlocalizing supranuclear vertical misalignment of the eyes often seen in conjunction with an ipsilateral internuclear ophthalmoplegia, in which case the hypertropic (higher) eye is usually ipsilateral to the medial rectus weakness.

Nystagmus is a rhythmic oscillation of the eyes in which each phase is of equal amplitude. Vestibular jerk nystagmus results from an altered input from nuclei to the horizontal or vertical gaze centers. The slow phase is initiated by the vestibular nuclei and the fast phase by the brainstem and frontomesencephalic pathway. Vestibular nystagmus can be horizontal, vertical, or rotary. Rotary nystagmus almost always is the result of a pathologic vestibular disorder. Gaze-evoked nystagmus is a jerk nystagmus of slow frequency that is similar to end-point nystagmus, except that it begins with the eyes in a less extreme field of gaze and is usually of a greater amplitude. It is often associated with cerebellar disease but may occur with cerebral hemispheric or brainstem lesions.

Acquired forms of vertical nystagmus are usually pathologic and localizing. Up-beating nystagmus that occurs in primary gaze is caused by impaired upward pursuit and results from lesions involving either the anterior vermis or lower brainstem. Sedatives, anticonvulsants, and many other drugs can produce an unsustained up-beating nystagmus, primarily in upward gaze, but they rarely affect primary gaze unless there is drug intoxication. Down-beating nystagmus that occurs in primary gaze is caused by impaired downward pursuit and is usually localized to the craniocervical junction. It is commonly associated with the Arnold-Chiari malformation but can also be seen in hydrocephalus, cerebellar atrophy, metabolic disorders, and drug intoxication. See-saw nystagmus is characterized by one eye rising and intorting while the other eye falls and extorts. If it is acquired, bitemporal field defects and third ventricular tumors are usually present. The etiology of this disorder is thought to be the result of interference with the connections to the interstitial nucleus of Cajal.

In children nystagmus may be a prominent feature of tumors affecting the intracranial portion of the optic nerve or chiasm. Bilateral sensory deprivation nystagmus occurs in young children when there is bilateral loss of central vision for any reason. When optic atrophy is also noted, then hydrocephalus, craniopharyngiomas, and optic nerve gliomas must be considered in the differential diagnosis. True monocular nystagmus is rare. In children, a benign self-limited disorder, spasmus nutans, can occur between 6 months and 2 years of age and is associated with binocular, often asymmetric, or even monocular nystagmus. The nystagmus is of small amplitude and very rapid and may be associated with head nodding or torticollis. Unfortunately, tumors of the hypothalamus, optic chiasm, or prechiasmal intracranial optic nerve may mimic this disorder, even in the absence of significant optic atrophy.

The external aspects of the eyes, corneal sensitivity, pupils, and ocular motility can easily be assessed by direct observation without special instruments. Examination of the ocular fundus, however, requires an ophthalmoscope, slit lamp with a special lens, or a fundus camera. By far the most important finding that can be identified in the ocular fundus of patients with brain tumors is papilledema. The term *papilledema* should be restricted to swelling of the optic disk produced by increased intracranial pressure. Early signs of papilledema include swelling of the peripapillary nerve fiber layer, hyperemia of the disk with dilated capillaries on the disk surface, dilated veins, loss of venous pulsations, and flame-shaped hemorrhages at the disk margin. The disk findings in early papilledema may be asymmetric, but unilateral papilledema is unusual. As papilledema evolves, hemorrhages and soft exudates on the disk become prominent. The disk becomes elevated, and the swelling of the nerve fiber layer may obscure the vessels at the disk margin. In the peripapillary retina, radial or concentric folds occur as the disk tissue exerts pressure on it. Venous dilation becomes prominent.

In its chronic form, the funduscopic appearance of papilledema changes. The disk elevation persists, but the hemorrhages and exudates disappear, and the venous dilation decreases or disappears. If chronic papilledema progresses, it may evolve to an atrophic form in which the disk elevation decreases, the hyperemia gives way to pallor, and the retinal vessels become narrow. Small calcific "pseudodrusen" may appear on the surface of the disk. Loss of vision occurs and blindness may result.

Damage to the anterior visual pathway results in degeneration of neurons of the optic nerve. Progressive visual loss associated with a central scotoma and a Marcus Gunn pupil is characteristic of compressive optic neuropathy. Occasionally, sudden expansion of a tumor by hemorrhage can cause a more acute visual loss. The optic nerve may appear swollen if there is an orbital mass, but with most intracranial compressive lesions the nerve appears normal and later becomes pale as atrophy becomes more apparent. Meningiomas of the optic nerve sheath and rarely optic gliomas may present a classic triad of visual loss, optic atrophy, and optociliary shunt veins. Proptosis is common.

Examination of the visual field is one of the most important procedures in the neuro-ophthalmologic evaluation of patients with brain tumors. Visual field changes occur commonly in patients with brain tumors. They occur in approximately 50% of all patients with brain tumors of any type and even more often with some specific tumors (e.g., in 70% to 80% of all patients with temporal lobe tumors). Moreover, the specific features of some visual field defects are definitive in locating the lesion. Many visual field defects can be detected at the bedside and do not require special instrumentation.

The arrangement of nerve fibers in the optic nerve corresponds generally to the distribution of fibers in the retina. The upper retinal fibers are representative in the upper portion of the nerve, the lower fibers are below, and the nasal and temporal fibers are on their respective sides. The fibers of the papillomacular bundle subserving central visual function enter on the temporal side of the disk. Visual field defects produced by optic nerve lesions can take several forms, including central, cecocentral, arcuate, and attitudinal scotomas. Only the central scotoma occurs often in compressive optic nerve lesions. Lesions affecting the optic chiasm may produce several different patterns of visual field loss. Lesions that involve the prechiasmal optic nerve produce a loss of vision and visual field loss in the ipsilateral eye and a superior temporal defect in the opposite eye. Damage to the chiasm itself produces bitemporal hemianopsias, usually without loss of central visual acuity but with impaired stereoacuity. Lesions that damage the posterior chiasm involve the posterior macular crossing fibers that result in bitemporal hemianopic scotomas. Sellar or supersellar lesions that expand posteriorly may compress fibers of the optic tract. This produces a homonymous hemianopia. Binasal hemianopias caused by lateral compression of the chiasm are very rare. Homonymous hemianopias produced by lesions in the temporal lobe tend to be slightly incongruous and denser in the superior quadrant. Homonymous hemianopias produced by lesions in the parietal lobe tend to involve the inferior quadrant. Abnormalities of optokinetic nystagmus may occur in deep parietal lobe lesions so that no normal optokinetic response is obtained as the targets are rotated away from the hemianopic field. Homonymous hemianopias resulting from occipital cortex lesions are extremely congruous. This is because the fibers subserving input from corresponding retinal elements of the two eyes lie extremely close together by the time the nerve fibers reach the occipital cortex. Field defects arising from the occipital cortex may spare fixation, although the cause remains controversial.

Evaluation of the patient with a brain tumor should include at least an abbreviated form of a neuro-ophthalmologic examination. Ocular findings occur commonly in these patients and are often of diagnostic and therapeutic significance.

CHAPTER 9

SURGICAL STRATEGIES IN THE MANAGEMENT OF BRAIN TUMORS

G. Evren Keles and Mitchel S. Berger

The incidence rate of all primary brain tumors, both benign and malignant, is 14 cases per 100,000 population per year.[16] The prevalence rate for all primary brain tumors is 130.8 per 100,000, with more than 359,000 persons living with a diagnosis of primary brain tumor in the United States in the year 2000.[19] Neuroepithelial tumors, tumors arising from glial or neuronal elements, account for 48% to 60% of primary intracranial neoplasms in adults, and the vast majority of these are glial tumors.[16,19,45] This chapter focuses on recent advances in the surgical management of intracerebral tumors.

PREOPERATIVE IMAGING

If clinical history, symptoms, and signs are suggestive of an intracranial tumor, the next step in diagnosis is to obtain an imaging study. In addition to magnetic resonance imaging (MRI), the gold standard for detecting intracranial tumors, recent advances in imaging techniques—such as functional MRI (fMRI), magnetic resonance spectroscopy (MRS), and magnetic source imaging (MSI)—provide valuable information in planning surgery.

An adjuvant technique to conventional neuroimaging techniques is proton MRS, which can be obtained simultaneously with the MRI examination in little additional time. This technique permits the detection of metabolite levels in specific brain voxels, thereby providing local physiologic data in addition to anatomic imaging. MRS has shown potential in differentiating neoplasms from inflammatory and demyelinating lesions,[20] as well as in detecting progression of neoplastic disease and providing for an evaluation of response to radiation therapy.[44,63]

The use of fMRI provides additional information helpful in planning tumor resection tailored to individual patients. The ability to detect the small changes in blood volume and in intrinsic T2-weighted signal that occur in eloquent cortex during physiologic activation[2] provides the potential for preoperative functional mapping of eloquent cortex. This information integrated with the anatomic information obtained from conventional MRI and intraoperative stimulation mapping data can allow for more precise and complete resection of tumor and enable the surgeon to avoid impinging on adjacent eloquent brain areas.[53]

Another functional imaging modality is MSI, which combines the temporal and spatial accuracy of magnetoencephalography (MEG) with the anatomic and pathologic specificity of MRI.[39] The resulting magnetic source image gives accurate information about cortical functional organization, such as the late neuromagnetic field elicited by simple speech sounds.[61] Like fMRI, this technique will be useful for preoperative mapping of rolandic cortex and determining hemispheric language dominance.[51,52]

SURGICAL MANAGEMENT

Principles guiding appropriate surgical treatment of gliomas include tumor biopsy for the purpose of histologic diagnosis, cytoreduction of tumor mass to the maximum extent consistent with optimal preservation of neurologic function, and judicious implementation of adjuvant therapies tailored to the specific clinical situation. The choice of operative procedure for resection of a neuroepithelial tumor depends on its location, size, gross characteristics, histologic characteristics, the sensitivity of the tumor to radiation, and the preoperative neurologic and medical condition of the patient. Contemporary neurosurgical methods, including frameless navigational systems, intraoperative imaging, ultrasonography, and functional mapping, enable the neurosurgeon to achieve optimal cytoreduction of the tumor with minimal postoperative neurologic morbidity.

Biopsy

Diagnostic biopsy is most often accomplished with a closed stereotactic procedure performed with local anesthesia. By using image-guided stereotactic biopsy techniques, optimal acquisition of diagnostic tissue material can be obtained with a low rate of morbidity and mortality. In a series from Toronto, Bernstein and colleagues[10] found that stereotactic brain biopsies are associated with a 6% overall complication rate, a 2% mortality rate, an 8% risk of failed biopsy because of inadequate material for diagnosis,[58] and a high rate of clinically silent hemorrhage postoperatively.[32] These data are similar to those in other series.[1,35,40] As modern neuroimaging techniques permit targeting the most representative portions of intracranial tumors, the diagnostic yield from stereotactic biopsies is likely to continue to improve. In current practice, stereotactic biopsy is limited to a subgroup of patients harboring suspected glial tumors, depending on the characteristics of the lesion; for example, depth, small size, multiplicity, diffuseness, or the clinical condition of the patient. An incorrect pathologic diagnosis is not unusual in cases of tumors of glial origin, and the misdiagnosis usually consists of misinterpreting a high-grade glial tumor as a low-grade glioma. Although the incidence of this problem varies in different series, it may be significantly reduced by serial sampling along the entire radius of the lesion and beyond. Close collaboration with an experienced neuropathologist is essential to the diagnostic efficiency of stereotactic biopsies. Despite imprints and smears having the advantage of being faster and leaving more tissue for paraffin sections, frozen sections, which are diagnostically accurate in 99% of cases, are more suitable for interpretation.[46] There are no randomized studies that examine the prognostic effect of stereotactic biopsy followed by radiation therapy for the initial management of patients with gliomas. Retrospective nonrandomized studies including selected patients do not show any substantial benefit in terms of overall survival for patients who receive a biopsy followed by radiation therapy when compared with those patients who undergo conventional surgical resection.[36,42,55,56]

Computer-Assisted Stereotactic Resection

Computer-assisted stereotactic resection is helpful for tumor resection in certain locations that are technically challenging and associated with high morbidity rates. This technique, by providing images of lesions in triplanar format and by accurately referencing the data to either a stereotactic frame or to the patient's surface anatomy, permits the neurosurgeon to plan precisely an approach that minimizes injury to critical neural structures. As an example, perioperative mortality for radical resection of gliomas in and around the thalamus now approaches zero with modern techniques.[59] Similarly, in resections involving the posteromedial temporal lobe, stereotaxy permits aggressive but safe resection, limiting the risk of injury to the lateral temporal lobe and cortical, optic, and vascular structures. Unnecessary brain resection and retraction are also minimized. In a series reported by Weiner and Kelly,[64] seven patients with posterior parahippocampal gyrus gliomas underwent gross total resection through a lateral occipitosubtemporal, computer-assisted stereotactic volumetric approach with no permanent morbidity or operative mortality.

Neuronavigation and Intraoperative Imaging

The development of neuronavigation systems was a major technical advance in neurosurgery. Neuronavigation methods help the neurosurgeon in planning surgery and approaching the tumor, as well as during resection and in evaluating the extent of resection. Although conventional neurosurgery training and subsequent experience enable the surgeon to navigate safely within the brain parenchyma, additional intraoperative anatomic information is still valuable, especially in situations where individual anatomic variations or prior treatment complicate the anatomy. Tumors, together with their surrounding edema, often distort normal anatomic relationships, thus posing significant

challenge to the neurosurgeon trying to navigate by using conventional landmarks. Intraoperative image guidance may also provide critical information during the resection of tumors with a consistency similar to normal brain tissue by delineating T2-weighted imaging margins. Registration of the surgical target with respect to surrounding structures and physical space, interacting with a localization device, integration of real-time data, and interfacing with a computer are the primary components of any contemporary navigational system.[67] Data from multiple images can be related to one another by using natural landmarks or external fiducial markers. Frameless stereotactic navigation systems include ultrasonic digitizer systems, magnetic field digitizers, multijointed encoder arms, infrared flash systems, and robotic systems. Multiple registration techniques are available to map images with respect to each other and to the surgical field. Regardless of the preferred registration method, frameless systems may provide an advantage over frame-based systems in defining precise localization because distortions of imagery are likely to be reflected in the landmarks as well in the anatomy of interest. In addition, because they do not require fixation to an immobile frame, they may be used for craniotomies and spine surgeries. Several frameless stereotactic systems are now available for use in procedures, together with ultrasound and light-emitting diode (LED)-based localization or with magnetic field-base tracking systems.[22,49]

Surgical retraction, the extent of the resection cavity, or cerebrospinal fluid leakage may cause intraoperative displacement of the brain tissue, which may result in alteration of the surgical field and the lesion itself.[26,31,47] The combination of the use of neuronavigation systems with data obtained from intraoperative ultrasound has provided the opportunity to partially overcome errors because of tissue movement.[23] Ultrasound has the unique distinction among other imaging modalities of producing real-time images. However, images are often difficult to interpret because echogenic structures cannot reliably discern normal from abnormal tissue. In addition, blood products in the surgical field may result in misinterpretation of ultrasound images. The greatest potential error results from intraoperative brain shift and not from registration of the target. The importance of brain shift has been demonstrated in detail, at both the cortical and subcortical levels, by using intraoperative imaging techniques.[37,38] To eliminate this problem, the use of a computational method based on data from intraoperative ultrasound or digital images that track cortical displacement and movements of known landmarks has been suggested.[48] More studies are needed to evaluate the efficiency of this and other mathematic models in the clinical setting. In our experience, intraoperative update by using ultrasound data appears to be an acceptable alternative when intraoperative imaging is not available.[6] Sononavigation provides real-time information during tumor removal in alignment with the preoperative magnetic resonance (MR) images, enabling the surgeon to detect intraoperative hemorrhage, cyst drainage, and tumor resection, and allows for calculation of brain shift during the use of standard navigation techniques.

Another new technology that provides valuable information to the surgeon is intraoperative MRI. Use of intraoperative MRI requires MR-compatible instruments—that is, titanium or ceramic instruments—to minimize artifact effects. Image distortion leading to inaccurate target registration may pose a significant problem with intraoperative MRI. Air-tissue interfaces may result in artifact effects and are currently being studied with respect to image distortion. Extravasation of contrast agent may occur as a result of surgical insult to the blood-brain barrier and may be interpreted as residual tumor. To reduce image inaccuracy, each system must be studied carefully and distortion measurements should be checked regularly with the use of phantoms. Moreover, correction programs should be used routinely to eliminate distortion.[13] Images obtained after the introduction of a higher contrast load before resection of a lesion can provide baseline films that distinguish extravasation from tumor.[11] Tronnier et al[62] reported their experience with intraoperative MRI, with special emphasis on technical details regarding MR-compatible monitoring equipment, anesthesia machines, and surgical instruments. They tested this new technology in 27 patients for updating data sets for navigational systems, extent of resection control for brain tumors, and MR-guided interventions, and they concluded that intraoperative MRI is beneficial in evaluating the extent of resection and in eliminating problems related to intraoperative brain shift encountered with conventional navigational systems. Similar conclusions were reached by Black et al[11] in a series of 140 patients including those with nontumor pathologies. They used an intraoperative MRI scanner with a vertical gap within its magnet, which provided the physical space for performing surgery. Despite potential misinterpretation regarding gadolinium enhancement around the resection margins caused by disruption of the blood-brain barrier, intraoperative MRI supplied valuable information in evaluating the resection, as well as being a reliable way of instrument tracking for biopsies. In another study, an "open" MRI scanner was used in an operating room adjacent to the main one, and patients were transferred from one room to the other.[60] Thirty-one of 55 cases included in this study were supratentorial brain tumors, and 18 patients had pituitary adenomas, where intraoperative MRI was used mainly to evaluate extent of resection. In 16% of the patients with a supratentorial tumor, an intraoperative postresection control MR image revealed significant residual tumor, which necessitated further resection. However, the authors concluded that intraoperative imaging did not facilitate "identification of the borders of low-grade gliomas, edema and normal brain tissue." Although the main operating room included conventional MR-incompatible instrumentation, the major disadvantage of this technique was the need to transport the patient to the scanner.

Stimulation Mapping Techniques

Intraoperative stimulation mapping of cortical and subcortical tissue in and around a tumor will identify functional tissue, and its preservation will minimize the risk of permanent postoperative deficit. It has been shown that resection of tumors located near or within functional brain areas may not be safe even if the surgeon remains within the boundaries of the macroscopically obvious tumor. In addition to its use to determine functional cortical sites, stimulation mapping is the only available method that provides reliable identification of descending subcortical motor, sensory, and language tracts.

Hemispheric gliomas located within or adjacent to functional areas, such as the rolandic cortex, supplementary motor area, corona radiata, internal capsule, and uncinate fasciculus, constitute the major indications for intraoperative motor mapping. Because of the tendency of infiltrative gliomas to invade underlying white matter tracts, it is important to identify both cortical motor sites and their descending pathways. Regardless of the gross appearance and consistency of the tumor, functional tissue may also reside within the mass itself and must be identified with stimulation mapping before definitive resection.[57]

Cortical language localization, through object naming and reading, is variable in each individual and does not follow any reproducible pattern across the population. The traditional concept regarding the cortical representation of language function involves an anterior language site, Broca's area (posterior part of the inferior frontal gyrus), and a posterior site, Wernicke's area (perisylvian in the temporoparietal cortex). This concept was challenged by some early studies in which electrical cortical stimulation was used. In addition, dominant temporal lobe resections guided by standard neurosurgical landmarks—that is, restricting the temporal lobe resections to within 4 cm of the temporal tip and limiting the removal of the superior temporal gyrus—have been associated with permanent postoperative language deficits.[24,25]

The patient is placed in the position appropriate for the area to be exposed. Special care is given to have all extremities well padded and protected. The core temperature is kept within 1°C of normal by using a heating blanket. Cortical stimulation mapping will be difficult if the patient's temperature drifts too low, especially with patients under general anesthesia. An intravenous propofol (Diprivan) or alfentanil drip maintains the sedative-hypnotic anesthesia. Oxygen is administered through a nasal cannula in case of a decrease in the arterial oxygen saturation. Regardless of the need for osmotic diuretics, a Foley catheter is inserted. Prophylactic antibiotics are used routinely and are given during the induction phase of anesthesia. The head is shaved and washed, and the incision is marked. In general, a wide exposure will be necessary to ensure that enough cortical sites are available for testing. The area of the scalp around the incision is infiltrated with a local anesthetic consisting of lidocaine (0.5%) and marcaine (0.25%) with sodium bicarbonate as a buffer. The craniotomy should be wide enough to expose the tumor and surrounding brain, including areas where language is likely to be located, to provide adequate cortical areas for language mapping. The tumor is localized with intraoperative ultrasound or surgical navigation systems. Because the dura is pain sensitive, the area around the middle meningeal artery should be infiltrated with the lidocaine-marcaine mixture to alleviate the patient's discomfort while awake.

Identification of the Motor Cortex and Subcortical Pathways

After the dura is opened, stimulation mapping should begin by first identifying the motor cortex. A bipolar electrode (5-mm spacing) on the surface for 2 to 3 seconds with a current amplitude between 2 and 16 mA is used. A constant-current generator is used to produce biphasic square-wave pulses at 60 Hz and a 1.25-msec single-peak (pulse) duration. The current necessary to evoke motor movement will vary depending on the anesthetic condition of the patient, with lower currents used when the patient is awake. The motor strip is stimulated with the patient asleep at a starting current of 4 mA, which is then reduced to 2 mA when stimulating with the patient awake. The amplitude of the current is adjusted, in 1- to 2-mA increments until motor movements are identified. The use of multichannel electromyographic recordings, in addition to visual observation of motor movements, results in greater sensitivity, permitting the use of lower stimulation levels to evoke motor activity[66]; it has never been necessary to use a current above 16 mA to evoke a sensory or motor response.[7] At this point in the operation, ice-cold Ringer's lactate solution should be immediately available for irrigation of the stimulated cortex in case a focal motor seizure develops. Rapid cortical irrigation at the stimulation site with ice-cold Ringer's solution is the best management of intraoperative stimulation-induced focal motor seizures,[50] and it will abruptly stop the seizure activity originating from the irritated cortex without using short-acting barbiturates.

First, the inferior aspect of the rolandic cortex is identified by eliciting responses in the face and hand. Because the leg motor cortex is out of view against the falx, a strip electrode may be inserted along the falx, and stimulation using the same current applied to the lateral cortical surface may be delivered through it to evoke leg motor movements. This maneuver is safe because of the lack of bridging veins between the falx and the leg motor cortex. Similarly, a subdural strip electrode may be inserted and stimulated to evoke the desired response if the craniotomy is near but not overlying the rolandic cortex.

After the motor cortex is identified, the descending tracts may be found by using similar stimulation parameters (Figure 9-1). Descending motor and sensory pathways may be followed into the internal capsule and inferiorly to the brainstem and spinal cord.[30a] This is especially important during resection of infiltrative glial tumors because functioning motor, sensory, or language tissue can be located within macroscopically obvious tumor or surrounding infiltrated brain.[57] A final postresection stimulation of cortical sites should be performed to confirm that the pathways are intact. This step will also ensure that the underlying functional tracts have been preserved if subcortical responses have not been obtained. Even if the patient's neurologic status is worse postoperatively, the presence of intact cor-

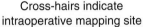

Cross-hairs indicate intraoperative mapping site

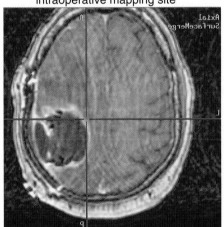

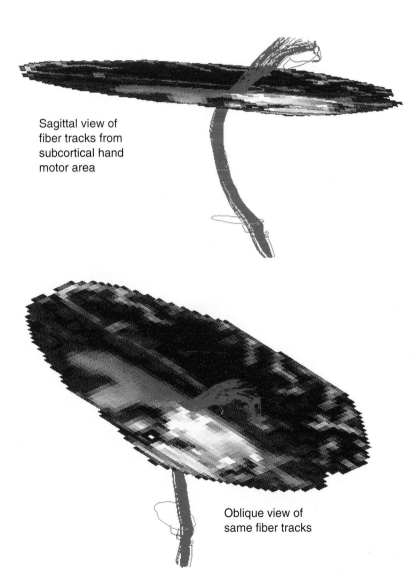

Sagittal view of fiber tracks from subcortical hand motor area

Oblique view of same fiber tracks

T2W EPI image at the same level with fiber track overlayed in red

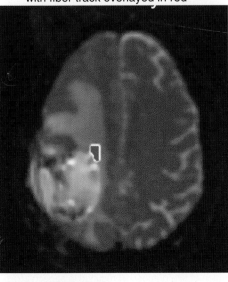

FIGURE 9-1   Visualization of the subcortical motor pathways that correspond to hand movement in a patient with a right parietal glioblastoma multiforme. EPI, Echo-planar imaging; T2W, T2-weighted.

tical and subcortical motor pathways implies that the deficit will be transient and will resolve within days to weeks.

Although somatosensory evoked potentials (SSEPs) may be helpful in identifying the central sulcus, they do not help to localize descending subcortical motor and sensory white matter tracts. Determination of the subcortical pathways is important when removing a tumor deeply located within or adjacent to the corona radiata, internal capsule, insula, supplementary motor area, or thalamus. Because the spread of current from the electrode contacts is minimal during bipolar stimulation, resection should be stopped when movement or paresthesia is evoked.

Identification of Language Sites

After bone removal under propofol anesthesia, the patient is kept awake during language mapping. The electrocorticography equipment is placed on the field and attached to the skull after the motor pathways have been identified. The recording electrode-cortex contact point is stimulated by using the bipolar electrode with electrocorticography in progress. This stimulation may result in after-discharge potentials that are seen on the monitor. The presence of such after-discharge potentials indicates that the stimulation current is too high and must be reduced by 1 to 2 mA until no after-discharge potential is seen following stimulation. At this point in the operation, the patient is asked to count from 1 to 50 while the bipolar stimulation probe is placed near the inferior aspect of the motor strip to identify Broca's area. Interruption of counting—that is, complete speech arrest without oropharyngeal movement—signifies the location of Broca's area (Figure 9-2). Speech arrest—the complete interruption of counting—is usually localized to the area directly anterior to the face motor cortex. As this ideal stimulation current is being applied, the patient is presented with object-naming slides that are changed every 4 seconds. The patient is asked to name the object during stimulation mapping, and the answers are carefully recorded. To ensure that there is no stimulation-induced error in the form of anomia and dysnomia, each cortical site is checked three times. All cortical sites essential for naming are marked on the surface of the brain with sterile numbered tickets. Throughout language mapping, the electrocorticogram is continuously monitored to signal multiple after-discharge spikes, both to reduce the chances of evoking a seizure by continued stimulation at that current and to reduce the chance that naming errors are caused by the propagated effects of the current.

A negative stimulation mapping may not provide the necessary security to proceed confidently with the resection. Therefore it is essential to document where language is located, as well as where it is not located, if feasible. This is also the reason for having a generous exposure, not only to maximize the extent of resection but also to minimize the possibility of obtaining negative data. It has been shown that the distance of the resection margin from the nearest language site is the most important factor in determining recovery from preoperative language deficits, the duration of postoperative language deficits, and whether the postoperative language deficits are permanent. Significantly fewer permanent language deficits occur if the distance of the resection margin from the nearest language site is more than 1 cm.

Surgical Options for Patients with Associated Epilepsy

The surgical management of patients with gliomas and seizures is controversial. Surgical options include focal excision of only the tumor, radical tumor resection without electrocorticography, and a radical resection with seizure foci mapping. In patients with low-grade gliomas who are under complete seizure control preoperatively and those who have an occasional seizure on medication, seizure control with or without

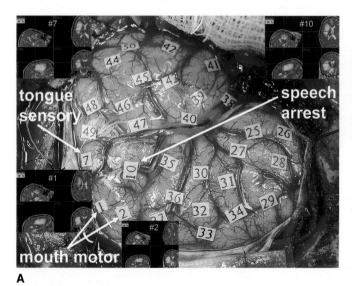

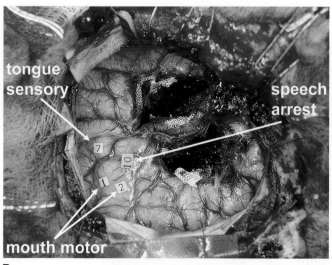

A   **B**

FIGURE 9-2   *A,* Preresection intraoperative image of an insular low-grade astrocytoma in the dominant hemisphere. Numbers 1 and 2 mark sites of mouth motor function, number 7 marks a site of tongue sensory function, and stimulation of site number 10 resulted in speech arrest. Inset images from the intraoperative navigation system depict the cortical sites that correspond to numbers 1, 2, 7, and 10 on a preoperatively obtained magnetic resonance data set. *B,* Postresection image from the same patient.

the need for postoperative anticonvulsants is often achieved with radical tumor resection alone. Management for patients with intractable epilepsy, however, differs from that for those patients whose seizures are well controlled with medication.

The literature suggests that acceptable seizure control may be achieved with lesionectomy alone in patients with tumor-associated epilepsy. It has been documented with serial electroencephalographic analysis that independent seizure foci may lose their epileptogenic activity following the excision of various lesions.[21,34] However, it should be noted that most patients in those earlier series had seizures that were not intractable according to contemporary criteria. Cascino et al[14,15] reported that computer-assisted stereotactic tumor resection, possibly the most precise form of focal tumor resection alone without removing adjacent, potentially epileptogenic brain, results in a reduced seizure frequency in the majority of patients who undergo this procedure. Although this proved to occur in 86% of their 30 patients with tumors, 97% remained on anticonvulsants to maintain that level of control. The proponents of this method conclude that tumor resection alone in a patient with medically refractory epilepsy is often inadequate, because removal of the seizure focus or foci adjacent to the lesion cannot be accomplished with that surgical technique, which does not use electrocorticography. Continued use of antiepileptic drugs is usually necessary, and in some patients an additional operation may be required to treat persistent seizure activity.

Authors of several published studies do not agree with the use of electrocorticography during tumor resection to maximize control of epilepsy associated with a tumor. However, in each of those studies, the resection strategy entailed removing the tumor and in addition removing brain adjacent to the lesion. Packer et al[41] reported their 10 years' experience with 60 patients with "cortical" low-grade gliomas. The patient population was not limited to patients with medically intractable seizures. Of those patients who had radical resection without the use of electrocorticography (78%), 75% were seizure free within the second postoperative year, although "relatively few patients who were seizure free at the 2-year point went on to develop seizures." Of those patients who were seizure free at the 2-year point, antiepileptic therapy was still needed for 47%. Recently, Burgeois et al[12] reported their experience with 200 epileptic patients with focal lesions. Although this series was histopathologically heterogeneous, 85% of the patients had medically intractable seizures. The authors defined their surgical approach as "lesionectomy including some of the surrounding cortex with no specific attempt to remove epileptogenic areas," and intraoperative electrocorticography was not used. For the group of patients whose seizures were medically refractory, a 71.3% seizure-free rate (Engel's class Ia status) was achieved over a mean follow-up period of 5.8 years.

With the use of intraoperative electrocorticography and excision of epileptogenic foci, a better seizure outcome may be achieved in children with hemispheric low-grade gliomas associated with intractable epilepsy, as compared with adults who have a similar pathology.[4,5] In both cases, patients have a greater chance of having a better quality of life, not dependent on antiepileptic medication, than do patients treated with other surgical methods that do not incorporate seizure-focus identification. In a study comparing lesionectomy with tumor resection combined with electrocorticographically identified epileptogenic-foci resection in patients with temporal lobe tumors, seizure-free status was achieved in 18.8% and 92.8%

of the patients, respectively.[27] Half of the patients undergoing only lesionectomy needed a second procedure, a temporal lobectomy, for seizure control, and 62.5% of that subgroup became seizure free. It is interesting that only 14% of the patients who underwent seizure-foci resection were taken off anticonvulsants at a mean follow-up time point of 52 months. The authors did not mention whether the seizures were intractable in the entire study population. In a well-documented retrospective analysis of a series of 146 patients with low-grade tumors and intractable epilepsy, Zentner et al[68] reported a 71% seizure-free rate, and 95% of their 124 patients with follow-up review showed significant (>75%) improvement regarding seizure frequency. Although various techniques, including extraoperative electrocorticography in 27% of the patients, were used in this large patient population, the authors stated that lesionectomy is successful in only a limited number of patients, and that in other patients excision of the epileptogenic zone, identified either intraoperatively or extraoperatively, is necessary to achieve satisfactory seizure control. Information regarding the need for antiepileptic drugs was not provided.

In our experience, the optimal control of epilepsy without postoperative anticonvulsants is provided when perioperative—that is, extraoperative or intraoperative—electrocorticographic mapping of separate seizure foci accompanies the tumor resection. When mapping is not used and a radical tumor resection is carried out with excision of adjacent brain, the occurrence of seizures will be lessened, but most patients will have to remain on antiepileptic drugs.[29]

PROGNOSTIC SIGNIFICANCE OF SURGERY

A recent review of the available studies of low-grade hemispheric gliomas in adults indicates there is growing evidence, though not of high quality, that favors more extensive surgical intervention at the time of the initial diagnosis as a positive prognostic indicator for longer survival.[30] Most of the published series have design-related limitations, including small study size and a small number of events (i.e., deaths for survival studies), and most include pediatric patients and various histologic tumor types (e.g., pilocytic, gemistocytic astrocytoma) with different natural histories. In addition, methods for determining extent of resection are subjective and qualitative in almost all studies. In two recent series, extent of resection that was not volumetrically determined was a statistically significant predictor of outcome in univariate analysis but did not show statistical significance in multivariate models.[43,54]

The prognostic effect of extensive surgery for low-grade gliomas is not well defined but there appears to be a positive effect on outcome.[3,8] The association between extent of resection and longer survival for patients with high-grade malignant gliomas is similarly controversial,[9] mainly because of a lack of randomized studies addressing the issue and the inconsistent and less-than-objective methodology used in determining extent of resection. The degree of cytoreduction achieved, as measured by extent of resection, appears to correlate with outcome. Patients with gross total resection live longer than those with partial resection, who in turn live longer than those who have biopsy only.[18,65] A further consideration is that partial resection is often accompanied by significant postoperative edema surrounding residual tumor tissue along with increased neurologic morbidity.[17] In a retrospective study of preoperative and postoperative tumor volumes in 92 patients with glioblastoma multiforme (GBM), extent of tumor removal and residual tumor volume were significantly correlated with median time to tumor progression and median survival.[28] In that study, a greater extent of resection did not compromise quality of life,

and patients who had no residual disease had a better postoperative performance status than did those patients who had less than total resection. In a recent study including 416 patients with glioblastoma multiforme, volumetrically assessed extent of resection had a statistically significant impact on survival in multivariate analysis.[33] In this study, a significant survival advantage was associated with resection of 98% or more of the tumor volume.

References

1. Apuzzo ML, Chandrasoma PT, Cohen D, et al: Computed imaging stereotaxy: experience and perspective related to 500 procedures applied to brain masses. Neurosurgery 20:930–937, 1987.
2. Belliveau JW, Kennedy DN, McKinstry RC, et al: Functional mapping of the human visual cortex by magnetic resonance imaging. Science 254:1224–1228, 1991.
3. Berger MS, Deliganis AV, Dobbins J, et al: The effect of extent of resection on recurrence in patients with low-grade cerebral hemisphere gliomas. Cancer 74:1784–1791, 1994.
4. Berger MS, Ghatan S, Geyer JR, et al: Seizure outcome in children with hemispheric tumors and associated intractable epilepsy: the role of tumor removal combined with seizure foci resection. Pediatr Neurosurg 17:185–191, 1991–1992.
5. Berger MS, Ghatan S, Haglund MM, et al: Low grade gliomas associated with intractable epilepsy: seizure outcome utilizing electrocorticography during tumor resection. J Neurosurg 79:62–69, 1993.
6. Berger MS, Keles GE: Intraoperative image update by interface with ultrasound. In Germano IM (ed): Advanced Techniques in Image-Guided Brain and Spine Surgery. New York, Thieme Medical Publishers, 2002.
7. Berger MS, Ojemann GA, Lettich E: Neurophysiological monitoring to facilitate resection during astrocytoma surgery. Neurosurg Clin N Am 1:65–80, 1990.
8. Berger MS, Rostomily RC: Low grade gliomas: functional mapping resection strategies, extent of resection, and outcome. J Neurooncol 34:85–101, 1997.
9. Berger MS, Wilson CB: Extent of resection and outcome for cerebral hemispheric gliomas. In Berger MS, Wilson CB (eds): The Gliomas. Philadelphia, WB Saunders, 1999.
10. Bernstein M, Parrent AG: Complications of CT-guided stereotactic biopsy of intra-axial brain lesions. J Neurosurg 81:165–168, 1994.
11. Black PM, Moriarty T, Alexander E III, et al: Development and implementation of intraoperative magnetic resonance imaging and its neurosurgical applications. Neurosurgery 41:831–845, 1997.
12. Bourgeois M, Sainte-Rose C, Lellouch-Tubiana A, et al: Surgery of epilepsy associated with focal lesions in childhood. J Neurosurg 90:833–842, 1999.
13. Burchiel K, Nguyen T, Coombs B, Szumoski J: MRI distortion and stereotactic neurosurgery using the Cosman-Roberts-Wells and Leksell frames. Stereotact Funct Neurosurg 66:123–136, 1996.
14. Cascino GD: Epilepsy and brain tumors: implications for treatment. Epilepsia 31(suppl 3):S37–S44, 1990.
15. Cascino GD, Kelly PJ, Hirschhorn KA, et al: Stereotactic resection of intra-axial cerebral lesions in partial epilepsy. Mayo Clinic Proceedings 65:1053–1060, 1990.
16. CBTRUS Statistical Report: Primary Brain Tumors in the United States, 1995–1999. Published by the Central Brain Tumor Registry of the United States, Hinsdale, Ill, 2002.
17. Ciric I, Ammirati M, Vick N, Mikhael M: Supratentorial gliomas, surgical considerations and immediate post-operative results. Neurosurgery 21:21–26, 1987.
18. Coffey RJ, Lunsford LD, Taylor FH: Survival after stereotactic biopsy of malignant gliomas. Neurosurgery 22:465–473, 1988.
19. Davis FG, Kupelian V, Freels S, et al: Prevalence estimates for primary brain tumors in the United States by behavior and major histology groups. J Neurooncol 3:152–158, 2001.
20. DeStefano N, Caramanos Z, Preul MC, et al: In vivo differentiation of astrocytic brain tumors and isolated demyelinating lesions of the type seen in multiple sclerosis using 1H magnetic resonance spectroscopic imaging. Ann Neurol 44:273–278, 1998.
21. Falconer MA, Driver MV, Serafetinides EA, et al: Temporal lobe epilepsy due to distant lesions: two cases relieved by operation. Brain 85:521–534, 1962.
22. Giorgi C, Casolino DS: Preliminary clinical experience with intraoperative stereotactic ultrasound imaging. Stereotact Funct Neurosurg 68:54–58, 1997.
23. Gronningsaeter A, Kleven A, Ommedal S, et al: SonoWand, an ultrasound-based neuronavigation system. Neurosurgery 47:1373–1379, 2000.
24. Heilman K, Wilder B, Malzone W: Anomic aphasia following anterior temporal lobectomy. Trans Am Neurol Assoc 97:291–293, 1972.
25. Hermann BP, Wyler AR, Somes G: Language function following anterior temporal lobectomy. J Neurosurg 74:560–566, 1991.
26. Hill DL, Maurer CR, Jr, Maciunas RJ, et al: Measurement of intraoperative brain surface deformation under a craniotomy. Neurosurgery 43:514–526, 1998.
27. Jooma R, Yeh HS, Privitera MD, et al: Lesionectomy versus electrophysiologically guided resection for temporal lobe tumors manifesting with complex partial seizures. J Neurosurg 83:231–236, 1995.
28. Keles GE, Anderson B, Berger MS: The effect of extent of resection on time to tumor progression and survival in patients with glioblastoma multiforme of the cerebral hemisphere. Surg Neurol 52:371–379, 1999.
29. Keles GE, Berger MS: Seizures associated with brain tumors. In Bernstein M, Berger MS (eds): Neuro-Oncology Essentials. New York, Thieme Medical Publishers, 2000.
30. Keles GE, Lamborn KR, Berger MS: Low-grade hemispheric gliomas in adults: a critical review of extent of resection as a factor influencing outcome. J Neurosurg 95:735–745, 2001.
30a. Keles GE, Lundin DA, Lamborn KR, et al: Intraoperative subcortical stimulation mapping for hemispherical perirolandic gliomas located within or adjacent to the descending motor pathways: evaluation of morbidity and assessment of functional outcome in 294 patients. JNS 100:369–375, 2004.
31. Kelly PJ: Measurement of intraoperative brain surface deformation under a craniotomy. Neurosurgery 43:527–528, 1998 (comment).
32. Kulkarni AV, Guha A, Lozano A, Bernstein M: Incidence of silent hemorrhage and delayed deterioration after stereotactic brain biopsy. J Neurosurg 89:31–35, 1998.
33. Lacroix M, Abi-Said D, Fourney DR, et al: A multivariate analysis of 416 patients with glioblastoma multiforme: prognosis, extent of resection, and survival. J Neurosurg 95:190–198, 2001.

34. Lourie H, Uemura K: Psychomotor seizures and mirror focus secondary to retained knife blade in temporal lobe. Resolution of mirror focus after extirpation of primary lesion. J Neurosurg 22:602–606, 1965.

35. Lunsford LD, Martinez AJ: Stereotactic exploration of the brain in the era of computed tomography. Surg Neurol 22:222–230, 1984.

36. Lunsford LD, Somaza S, Kondziolka D, Flickenger JC: Survival after stereotactic biopsy and radiation of cerebral non-neoplastic, non-pilocytic astrocytoma. J Neurosurg 82:523–529, 1995.

37. Nabavi A, Black PM, Gering DT, et al: Serial intraoperative MR imaging of brain shift. Neurosurgery 48:787–798, 2001.

38. Nimsky C, Ganslandt O, Cerny S, et al: Quantification of, visualization of, and compensation for brain shift using intraoperative magnetic resonance imaging. Neurosurgery 47:1070–1080, 2000.

39. Orrison WW: Magnetic source imaging in stereotactic and functional neurosurgery. Stereotact Funct Neurosurg 72:89–94, 1999.

40. Ostertag CB, Mennel HD, Kiessling M: Stereotactic biopsy of brain tumors. Surg Neurol 14:275–283, 1980.

41. Packer RJ, Sutton LN, Patel KM, et al: Seizure control following tumor surgery for childhood cortical low-grade gliomas. J Neurosurg 80:998–1003, 1994.

42. Piepmeier JM: Observations on the current treatment of low-grade astrocytic tumors of the cerebral hemispheres. J Neurosurg 67:177–181, 1987.

43. Pignatti F, van den Bent M, Curran D, et al: Prognostic factors for survival in adult patients with cerebral low-grade glioma. J Clin Oncol 20:2076–2084, 2002.

44. Pirzkall A, Nelson SJ, McKnight TR, et al: Metabolic imaging of low-grade gliomas with three-dimensional magnetic resonance spectroscopy. Int J Radiation Oncology Biol Phys 53:1254–1264, 2002.

45. Preston-Martin S: Epidemiology. In Berger MS, Wilson CB (eds): The Gliomas. Philadelphia, WB Saunders, 1999.

46. Reyes MG, Homsi MF, McDonald LW, Glick RP: Imprints, smears, and frozen sections of brain tumors, Neurosurgery 29:575–579, 1991.

47. Roberts DW, Hartov A, Kennedy FE, et al: Intraoperative brain shift and deformation: a quantitative analysis of cortical displacement in 28 cases. Neurosurgery 43:749–760, 1998.

48. Roberts DW, Miga MI, Hartov A, et al: Intraoperatively updated neuroimaging using brain modeling and sparse data. Neurosurgery 45:1199–1207, 1999.

49. Roessler K, Ungersboeck K, Czech T, et al: Contour-guided brain tumor surgery using a stereotactic navigating microscope. Stereotact Funct Neurosurg 1997, 68:33–38.

50. Sartorius CJ, Berger MS: Rapid termination of intraoperative stimulation-evoked seizures with application of cold Ringer's lactate to the cortex. J Neurosurg 88:349–351, 1998.

51. Schiffbauer H, Berger MS, Ferrari P, et al: Preoperative magnetic source imaging for brain tumor surgery: a quantitative comparison with intraoperative sensory and motor mapping. J Neurosurg 97:1333–1342, 2002.

52. Schiffbauer H, Ferrari P, Rowley HA, et al: Functional activity within brain tumors: a magnetic source imaging study. Neurosurgery 49:1313–1321, 2001.

53. Schulder M, Maldijian JA, Liu WC, et al: Functional image-guided surgery of intracranial tumors located in or near the sensorimotor cortex. J Neurosurg 89:412–418, 1998.

54. Shaw E, Arusell R, Scheithauer B, et al: Prospective randomized trial of low- versus high-dose radiation therapy in adults with supratentorial low-grade glioma: Initial report of a North Central Cancer Treatment Group/Radiation Therapy Oncology Group/Eastern Cooperative Oncology Group Study. J Clin Oncol 20:2267–2276, 2002.

55. Shaw EG, Scheithauer BW, O'Fallon JR, Davis DH: Mixed oligoastrocytomas: a survival and prognostic factor analysis. Neurosurgery 34:577–582, 1994.

56. Shibamoto Y, Kitakabu Y, Takahashi M, et al: Supratentorial low-grade astrocytoma. Correlation of computed tomography findings with effect of radiation therapy and prognostic variables. Cancer 72:190–195, 1993.

57. Skirboll SS, Ojemann GA, Berger MS, et al: Functional cortex and subcortical white matter located within gliomas. Neurosurgery 38:678–685, 1996.

58. Soo TM, Bernstein M, Provias J, et al: Failed stereotactic biopsy in a series of 518 cases. Stereotact Funct Neurosurg 64:183–196, 1995.

59. Souweidane NM, Hoffman HJ: Current treatment of thalamic gliomas in children. J Neurooncol 28:157–166, 1996.

60. Steinmaier R, Fahlbusch O, Ganslandt O, et al: Intraoperative magnetic resonance imaging with the Magnetom open scanner: concepts, neurosurgical indications, and procedures—a preliminary report. Neurosurgery 43:739–748, 1998.

61. Szymanski M, Rowley H, Roberts T: A hemispherically asymmetrical MEG response to vowels. NeuroReport 10:2481–2486, 1999.

62. Tronnier VM, Wirtz CR, Knauth M, et al: Intraoperative diagnostic and interventional magnetic resonance imaging in neurosurgery. Neurosurgery 40:891–902, 1997.

63. Vigneron DB, Nelson SJ: Magnetic resonance spectroscopy. In Bernstein M, Berger MS (eds): Neuro-Oncology: The Essentials. New York, Thieme Medical Publishers, 2000.

64. Weiner HL, Kelly PJ: A novel computer-assisted volumetric stereotactic approach for resecting tumors of the posterior parahippocampal gyrus. J Neurosurg 85:272–277, 1996.

65. Winger MJ, Macdonald DR, Cairncross JG: Supratentorial anaplastic gliomas in adults: the prognostic importance of extent of resection and prior low grade glioma. J Neurosurg 71:487–493, 1989.

66. Yingling CD, Ojemann S, Dodson B, et al: Identification of motor pathways during tumor surgery facilitated by multichannel electromyographic recording. J Neurosurg 91:922–927, 1999.

67. Zakhary R, Keles GE, Berger MS: Intraoperative imaging techniques in the treatment of brain tumors. Curr Opin Oncol 11(3):152–156, 1999.

68. Zentner J, Hufnagel A, Wolf HK, et al: Surgical treatment of neoplasms associated with medically intractable epilepsy. Neurosurgery 41:378–387, 1997.

CHAPTER 10

BASIC CONCEPTS UNDERLYING RADIATION THERAPY

Kristin Bradley and Minesh Mehta

Radiation is energy that is propagated in the form of waves or particles; it is categorized as electromagnetic or particulate. Particulate radiation is the propagation of energy by traveling particles characterized by mass, momentum, and position in time; examples include electrons, protons, and alpha particles. First described by Maxwell in the mid-nineteenth century, electromagnetic radiations are transverse waves consisting of oscillating electric and magnetic fields; examples include x-rays, gamma rays, radiowaves, visible light, ultraviolet light, and microwaves. The energy of electromagnetic radiation is often quantized as photons, or packets. The distinction between particulate and electromagnetic radiation is somewhat blurred. Sometimes photons behave more like waves and sometimes more like particles, whereas particles such as electrons and protons can exhibit wavelike properties. In general, low-energy photons, such as radiowaves, often act more like waves, and higher energy photons, such as x-rays, act more like particles.

In empty space, electromagnetic waves travel with the speed of light (c), equal to 3×10^8 m/second. Electromagnetic waves are characterized by their wavelength (λ) and frequency (v), related by the following equation: $c = \lambda v$. In addition, the energy (E) of electromagnetic radiation is expressed by the equation $E = hv$, where h is Planck's constant, with a value of 6.62×10^{-34} joule-second. The electromagnetic spectrum describes various types of radiations in terms of decreasing or increasing energy, wavelength, and frequency. Two types of electromagnetic radiation that are important in the field of radiation oncology, x-rays and gamma rays, are discussed in more detail later.

SOURCES FOR RADIATION THERAPY

Therapeutic radiation can be categorized by how it is produced—from high energy machines, such as linear accelerators, that generate electron beams or x-rays or through radioisotope decay. Most commonly, radiation therapy involves external-beam treatments using x-rays or electrons, but protons, neutrons, and gamma rays from cobalt-60 decay also may be used. The x-rays (photons) and electrons used in radiation oncology are of much higher energy than those used in diagnostic radiology. Most linear accelerators are capable of generating therapeutic x-rays and electrons of varying energies; this results in beams with different tissue-penetrating characteristics, making the treatment of malignancies in various anatomic locations possible. Unlike machine-generated x-rays, gamma rays are emitted when an unstable radioactive isotope decays. Cobalt-60, which emits gamma rays as it disintegrates, is commonly used as a source of external-beam radiation therapy; in the United States, high energy x-rays have largely replaced cobalt-60 as the choice for external-beam radiation therapy.

Heavy-particle beams, such as protons, neutrons, and alpha particles, are sometimes used for radiation therapy. Protons, the most common therapeutic heavy-particle beam, are generated in a cyclotron, which is a charged particle accelerator. Proton therapy can offer improved dose localization and distribution as compared with x-rays, but its use is limited to a few large institutions because of the enormous expense involved in the construction and operation of cyclotrons.

Although cobalt-60 has been eclipsed as the major source of external-beam radiation therapy, radioisotopes play a critical role in brachytherapy and systemic treatment of bone metastases, lymphoma, liver metastases, and hepatocellular carcinoma. Brachytherapy, commonly used to treat prostate cancer and gynecologic malignancies, is a method that places sealed radioactive sources close to the tumor. Radioisotopes can be gamma-, beta-, or alpha-emitters. Like gamma decay, alpha and beta decay result from disintegration of an unstable radioactive isotope, resulting in the production of energetic helium nuclei (alpha decay) or electrons (beta decay). Radium was the first radioisotope used clinically but has now been replaced by artificial radioisotopes, such as cesium-137, iodine-125, iridium-192, and palladium-103. Other isotopes such as samarium-153 and yttrium-90 are sometimes used for systemic radiation therapy, either singly or conjugated to monoclonal antibodies.

RADIATION PROCESSES

Direct versus Indirect Effect

Radiation can be either directly or indirectly ionizing. Directly ionizing radiation, such as protons and other charged particles, produce chemical and biologic damage by directly disrupting subcellular targets such as DNA. X-rays and gamma rays, however, are indirectly ionizing. When they are absorbed in a medium, usually rich in water content, they give up their energy to produce ultra-short-lived, fast-moving charged particles and radicals that cause chemical and biologic damage. There is strong circumstantial evidence that the primary target of this damage is DNA.[8]

DNA Damage

What happens when DNA is targeted by radiation? When cells are irradiated, many single-strand DNA breaks occur. Generally, single-strand breaks are easily repaired using the opposite strand of the DNA as a template, and therefore single-strand breaks have minimal biologic consequence. Double-strand DNA breaks, conversely, can be biologically significant. If both strands of the DNA break, and the breaks are directly opposite or very near to one another, then a double-strand break may occur. If the two breaks rejoin in their original configuration, then the next mitosis can proceed without difficulty. The two breaks may not reunite, leading to a deletion. Finally, the breaks in the two chromosomes may rejoin incorrectly, giving rise to distorted chromosomes at the next mitosis. Many types of chromosomal aberrations can occur—some are lethal to the cell, and some are nonlethal but are associated with carcinogenesis. Interestingly, aberrations can be scored in peripheral blood lymphocytes and used to estimate the total-body doses in radiation accidents.[5]

Cell Death

Cell death can be described as apoptotic or mitotic. Apoptosis, also called *programmed cell death*, is an active process of rapid cell death resulting from the triggering of a sequence of morphologic events that culminate with the fragmentation of DNA and phagocytosis of the apoptotic cell. Lymphoid and hemopoietic cells are particularly prone to radiation-induced apoptosis. Mitotic death occurs in the cell's attempt to divide and is caused by damaged chromosomes; this is the most common form of radiation-induced cell death and in some cells is the only mode of death.

Cellular radiosensitivity to mitotic death varies during the cell cycle. Cells are most sensitive at or close to mitosis and in the G2 phase, and most resistant in S phase. A family of genes, called *molecular checkpoint genes*, control progression through the cell cycle. These molecular checkpoint genes delay transition from G1 to S or G2 to M in cells that are exposed to radiation. This pause in cell-cycle progression allows the chromosomes to be checked for damage and the damage repaired before mitosis occurs. Certain syndromes associated with a predisposition to cancer or exquisite radiosensitivity have mutated genes that fail to induce arrest at molecular checkpoints.

MODIFYING THE EFFECT OF RADIATION THERAPY ON CELLS

Types of Radiation Damage

Damage to irradiated cells can be categorized as (1) lethal damage, which is irreversible and irreparable, leading to cell death; (2) sublethal damage, which normally can be repaired; or (3) potentially lethal damage, which is damage that is normally lethal but may be repaired if cells are held under proper postirradiation conditions. If an additional fraction of radiation is given and more sublethal damage is produced, this may result in lethal damage. Sublethal damage is also referred to as *split-dose recovery,* because when a dose of radiation is split into several fractions separated by a sufficient time interval, the cells

repair the sublethal damage, and more cells survive than if all the radiation had been delivered in a single fraction. This repair of sublethal damage may be seen as the "shoulder" of a cell survival curve when radiation dose is plotted against the surviving cell fraction. Some tumors, such as small-cell lung cancer, are very radiosensitive, have limited repair of sublethal damage, and exhibit a minimal shoulder on a cell survival curve. Other malignancies demonstrate a greater ability to repair sublethal damage and demonstrate a cell survival curve with a broader shoulder. Potentially lethal damage may be repaired if postirradiation conditions are suboptimal for growth. Its importance to clinical radiation oncology is uncertain. It has been postulated that some tumors that are radioresistant may be better able to repair potentially lethal damage than radiosensitive tumors.

The Four *R*'s of Radiobiology

There are three general categories of modifiers of radiation response: biologic, physical, and chemical. These modifiers of radiation response are intimately related to the four *R*'s of radiobiology: repair, reassortment, repopulation, and reoxygenation. The types of damage and repair have been discussed in the preceding paragraph. Reassortment is the redistribution of cells through the cell cycle between radiation fractions. After a dose of radiation selectively kills cells in sensitive phases of the cell cycle, the viable cells then reassort to a more even distribution of cell-cycle phases. Repopulation is the regrowth of a tumor resulting from cell division. Reoxygenation is the process by which surviving hypoxic clonogenic cells become better oxygenated during the period after irradiation of a tumor.

Effect of Dose Rate

Dose rate is crucial in determining the consequences of a given dose of radiation. Classically, the biologic effect of radiation is reduced as the dose rate is decreased and the exposure time is extended. This is caused by the repair of sublethal damage that occurs during a long radiation exposure time, generally when radiation dose rate is reduced from approximately 1 Gy/minute to 0.3 Gy/hour or less (or 100 cGy/minute to 30 cGy/hour). External-beam radiation therapy and high dose-rate brachytherapy generally deliver radiation at a dose rate greater than 12 Gy/hour and do not allow for repair of sublethal damage during the delivery of the given fraction of radiation.

The Rationale for Fractionation

Traditionally, external-beam radiation therapy is delivered in multiple daily fractions over several weeks. Dividing the total dose of radiation into multiple smaller fractions spares normal tissue because of its ability to repair sublethal damage and to repopulate between fractions. In addition, fractionation increases damage to the tumor, because reoxygenation and reassortment of cells into radiosensitive phases of the cell cycle occurs between fractions, increasing tumor killing when the next radiation fraction is delivered. If the total dose of radiation is divided into several small fractions that take several weeks to deliver, the excessive prolongation may allow surviving tumor cells to proliferate more rapidly, a phenomenon referred to as *accelerated repopulation,* which may be responsible for the ineffectiveness of very prolonged courses of radiation therapy.

Two common fractionation strategies used to modify radiation response are hyperfractionation and acceleration. *Hyperfractionation* refers to the concept of dividing a radiation dose into multiple smaller fractions given two or three times each day, with the total duration similar to that for conventional fractionation. By giving a smaller dose per fraction, the late effects of radiation are reduced, permitting the delivery of a higher total dose and thus possibly improving tumor control. Accelerated fractionation occurs when the overall treatment duration is shortened while the total numeric dose is kept approximately the same. This most commonly is achieved by giving more than one fraction per day at a reduced dose per fraction (accelerated hyperfractionation). Shortening the overall course of treatment could improve tumor control, especially where accelerated repopulation is common. Several studies have examined altered fractionation schedules with varying success in lung cancer, head and neck cancer, and brain tumors.[2,6,9]

Linear Energy Transfer

A process known as *linear energy transfer (LET)* can be a physical modifier of radiation response. LET is the average energy transferred to the medium by the ionizing particle per unit length of track. When radiation is absorbed in a medium, ionizations tend to occur along the tracks of individual charged particles. LET is important because it is a factor in the relative biologic effectiveness (RBE) of a particular type of radiation. RBE is used to compare the biologic effectiveness of different types of ionizing radiation. Radiation can be classified as high LET, such as protons, neutrons, and heavy charged particles, or low LET, such as x-rays and gamma rays. X-rays are an example of low LET radiation with low RBE because x-rays are more sparsely ionizing and have a lower probability of causing a double-strand break. Overall, high LET radiation has the advantages of (1) higher relative biologic effectiveness, (2) less resistance of hypoxic cells, (3) less resistance in resistant phases of the cell cycle, and (4) sometimes better dose distribution. The three main disadvantages of high LET radiation—lack of availability, high cost, and a loss of differential response between normal tissue and tumor—prohibit the use of high LET radiation at most radiation oncology centers.

Chemical Modifiers

Several chemical modifiers affect radiation response, either positively or negatively. The presence or absence of oxygen dramatically influences the biologic effect of x-rays. Oxygen "fixes" radiation-induced DNA damage, making it more difficult to repair. Only a very small amount of oxygen is needed for this effect; hypoxic tumor cells can escape cell death by repairing DNA damage more efficiently than do normoxic cells. In experimental tumors, approximately 10% to 15% of cells are hypoxic at any given time. The potential negative impact of tumor hypoxia is reduced by fractionation because tumor reoxygenation occurs between radiation fractions. There is clinical evidence that hypoxia may play an important role in radiation resistance in certain disease types, and this affords an opportunity to modulate hypoxia to improve radiation response. For example, in cervical cancer and head and neck carcinoma, pretreatment hemoglobin levels predict for outcome after radiation therapy, and transfusion improves radiation outcomes.[3,4]

FUNCTION OF RADIOSENSITIZERS AND RADIOPROTECTORS

A radiosensitizer is any agent that increases the sensitivity of cells to radiation damage. To be useful as a radiosensitizer, a chemical or pharmacologic compound must show a differential effect between tumor and normal tissue. Two types of radiosensitizers have commonly been used in clinical trials: hypoxic sensitizers and halogenated pyrimidines.

Hypoxic Sensitizers

Hypoxic sensitizers increase the radiosensitivity of hypoxic tumor cells by mimicking the action of oxygen in "fixing" free radical damage, but they have no effect on oxygenated cells. Because hypoxic sensitizers are metabolized more slowly than oxygen, they are able to penetrate farther and reach hypoxic cells beyond the diffusion range of oxygen. Misonidazole, etanidazole, and nimorazole are hypoxic sensitizers belonging to a class of compounds called *nitroimidazoles* that have been investigated in clinical trials. To date, the benefit of misonidazole has been minimal, and accompanying neurotoxicity has prevented the use of adequate levels of the drug throughout a course of radiation. Etanidazole has not proved beneficial. Nimorazole has shown some promise in a Danish head and neck cancer trial but has not been used elsewhere.[7]

Hypoxic Cytotoxins

Another class of drugs, bioreductive agents, selectively kills hypoxic cells rather than preferentially radiosensitizing hypoxic cells. These compounds are taken up by cells and are reduced preferentially in hypoxic cells to form cytotoxic compounds. Studies of bioreductive agents, such as tirapazamine, are ongoing.

Halogenated Pyrimidines

Halogenated pyrimidines, such as bromodeoxyuridine and iododeoxyuridine, are structurally similar to thymidine and are incorporated into DNA in place of thymidine, causing a "weakening" of the DNA, making cells more susceptible to damage by x-rays and ultraviolet light. Halogenated pyrimidines are ideally used to treat malignancies such as high-grade gliomas in which the tumor has a high growth fraction and the surrounding normal tissue has a low growth fraction. The rapidly proliferating tumor cells incorporate more drug and become preferentially radiosensitized. Although halogenated pyrimidines have worked well in laboratory experiments, they have not shown nearly as much promise in clinical practice.

Radioprotectors

Radioprotectors are chemicals that decrease the biologic effects of radiation, and often of chemotherapy as well. The best available radioprotectors are sulfhydryl compounds, which scavenge free radicals and reduce cellular damage. The radioprotector most commonly used in oncology clinics today is amifostine, a prodrug that requires conversion to its active moiety through the action of alkaline phosphatase, which is more abundant in normal cells than in tumors. Amifostine is taken up more rapidly by most normal tissues than by tumor cells. If radiation is delivered shortly after the drug is given, then normal cells will be protected preferentially. Amifostine has been demonstrated to protect salivary tissue, mucosa, and bone marrow.[1]

NEW TECHNOLOGIC INNOVATIONS IN RADIATION THERAPY

Three-Dimensional Conformal Radiation Therapy

Just a few years ago, most patients receiving radiation therapy were treated using conventional planning. In this process, a patient underwent simulation in which fluoroscopic x-ray studies were obtained, and then the physician outlined the treatment fields, blocking out normal tissue. Although this technique is still used, most commonly to palliate bone and brain metastases, the majority of treatments at major centers are now delivered using three-dimensional conformal radiation therapy (3-D CRT). The goal of 3-D CRT is to conform the delivered radiation to the tumor while decreasing the dose to the surrounding normal tissues. To accomplish this, a patient undergoes a planning computed tomography (CT) scan with the patient in the treatment position, and then the CT images are transferred to a computer equipped with three-dimensional visualization and planning software. The physician contours the tumor and critical normal structures on every slice and, by evaluating directional treatment factors, such as gantry, collimator, and couch angles, as well as blocking patterns, the optimal treatment plan is generated. Dose distributions can be evaluated by examining isodose curves and dose-volume histograms.

Intensity-Modulated Radiation Therapy

Intensity-modulated radiation therapy (IMRT) is an even more specialized 3-D CRT technique used to further minimize normal tissue dose. Like the 3-D CRT process described previously, a planning CT is performed, and the treatment plan is generated on a computer. It differs from the standard 3-D CRT approach in that the physician defines the target dose and dose constraints for normal structures, and then an optimal treatment plan is generated via computer algorithms that modulate the intensity of the radiation beams. This process creates a very large number of "sub-beams" with varying radiation intensity, resulting in very steep dose gradients between the tumor and adjacent structures. IMRT is implemented most often to treat head and neck cancer to spare the parotid glands and avoid xerostomia and to treat prostate cancer by conforming and

escalating dose to the prostate and minimizing the rectal dose. Motion by the patient and organs remain major constraints in the widespread implementation of IMRT for all body sites.

Radiosurgery and Fractionated Stereotactic Radiation Therapy

Stereotactic radiosurgery (SRS) and fractionated stereotactic radiation therapy (FSRT) rely on precise stereotactic localization of the target, substantial immobilization of the patient, and often cross-registration with other imaging studies, such as magnetic resonance imaging (MRI). Both techniques are most often used to treat intracranial tumors but are being investigated for extracranial disease as well. SRS is a single fraction treatment generally used for tumors up to 3 cm, and FSRT is used to deliver multiple treatments to larger tumors. The most common uses of SRS are to treat a limited number of brain metastases, vestibular schwannomas, meningiomas, trigeminal neuralgia, and other lesions. Generally, FSRT is used to treat some of the same tumors but is reserved for larger tumors and those close to critical structures, such as the brainstem and optic chiasm, where it is more prudent to give multiple smaller fractions than a single large fraction of radiation.

Brachytherapy

Brachytherapy, a mature and widely used radiation technique, is employed either alone or in conjunction with external-beam radiation therapy to treat a variety of cancers. It consists of placing radiation-active sources close to, or in contact with, the tumor. Treatments vary depending on the dose rate, mode of surgical implantation, and whether they are permanent or temporary. In the past, most brachytherapy treatments were low dose rate, but high dose rate (HDR) brachytherapy is increasing in popularity because the treatments are quick, lasting a few minutes, and delivered in the outpatient setting using a remote afterloading device that minimizes radiation exposure to others. These benefits come at the expense of the remote afterloading device and the construction of a shielded vault for brachytherapy.

Particle Beam Therapy

A last radiation therapy innovation that deserves to be mentioned is the use of particle beam therapy, such as with protons, neutrons, or heavy charged particles, which offers the advantages of high LET radiation with greater relative biologic effectiveness. Its use in radiation oncology has been hindered by the lack of widespread availability, high cost, and the paucity of clinical trials showing particle beams' superiority to conformal radiation therapy with photons.

References

1. Brizel DM, Wasserman TH, Henke M, et al: Phase III randomized trial of amifostine as a radioprotector in head and neck cancer. J Clin Oncology 18:3339–3345, 2000.
2. Fu KK, Pajak TF, Trotti A, et al: A Radiation Therapy Oncology Group (RTOG) phase III randomized study to compare hyperfractionation and two variants of accelerated fractionation to standard fractionation radiotherapy for head and neck squamous cell carcinomas: first report of RTOG 9003. Int J Radiat Oncol Biol Phys 48:7–16, 2000.
3. Grogan M, Thomas GM, Melamed I, et al: The importance of hemoglobin levels during radiotherapy for carcinoma of the cervix. Cancer 86:1528–1536, 1999.

4. Lee WR, Berkey B, Marcial V, et al: Anemia is associated with decreased survival and increased locoregional failure in patients with locally advanced head and neck carcinoma: a secondary analysis of RTOG 85–27. Int J Radiat Oncol Biol Phys 42:1069–1075, 1998.

5. Lindholm C, Salomaa S, Tekkel M, et al: Biodosimetry after accidental radiation exposure by conventional chromosome analysis and FISH. Int J Rad Biol 70:647–656, 1996.

6. Murray KJ, Scott C, Greenberg HM, et al: A randomized phase III study of accelerated hyperfractionation versus standard in patients with unresected brain metastases: a report of the Radiation Therapy Oncology Group (RTOG) 9104. Int J Radiat Oncol Biol Phys 39:571–574, 1997.

7. Overgaard J, Hansen HS, Overgaard M, et al: A randomized double-blind phase III study of nimorazole as a hypoxic radiosensitizer of primary radiotherapy in supraglottic larynx and pharynx carcinoma. Results of the Danish Head and Neck Cancer Study Protocol 5–85. Radiother Oncol 46:135–146, 1998.

8. Prise KM, Pinto M, Newman HC, Michael BD: A review of studies of ionizing radiation-induced double-strand break clustering. Radiation Res 156(5 Pt 2):572–576, 2001.

9. Saunders M, Dische S, Barrett A, et al: Continuous, hyperfractionated, accelerated radiotherapy (CHART) versus conventional radiotherapy in non-small cell lung cancer: mature data from the randomised multicentre trial. Radiother Oncol 52:137–148, 1999.

CHAPTER 11

CHEMOTHERAPY PRINCIPLES

Ian F. Parney and Michael D. Prados

Chemotherapy can be defined as administering pharmacologic agents that either destroy tumor cells directly or modify their biology such that tumor growth is impaired. Chemotherapy plays an important role in treating tumors affecting the nervous system. This role is expanding, and many options are now available to treat a wide variety of tumors. For example, whereas chemotherapy has been widely accepted in the management of highly malignant tumors such as glioblastoma multiforme, its use is now being considered in such nontraditional scenarios as lower grade astrocytomas and recurrent meningiomas. In addition, more cytostatic agents are being used that take advantage of insights into tumor biology. The way chemotherapeutic agents are administered is also being revised, with increasing emphasis on local delivery. In this chapter we review general chemotherapy principles with particular emphasis on how they may apply to nervous system tumors.

CLINICAL TRIALS AND TREATMENT RESPONSE

Chemotherapeutic agents generally undergo extensive preclinical and clinical studies before becoming widely available. The transition from experimental agent to standard treatment is based on progression through a series of clinical trials. Phase I clinical trials are generally conducted with few patients and are designed to determine toxicity and maximum tolerated dose. Once an appropriate starting dose has been determined, phase II trials are conducted to measure treatment response in a larger group of patients. Finally, if phase I and II trials have been promising, randomized phase III trials are performed to compare a new treatment with a standard treatment (or, less desirably for cancer trials, placebo or no treatment).

Many nervous system tumors present specific challenges to this chemotherapy evaluation schema. Antitumor response in clinical trials is usually measured by decreased tumor size shown on magnetic resonance imaging (MRI). Unfortunately, with diffuse central nervous system (CNS) tumors such as glioblastoma, exact tumor size is often difficult to determine on MRI. This can be particularly true when patients have previously undergone resection, irradiation, or chemotherapy. Furthermore, cytostatic chemotherapies may not have similar dose-limiting toxicities to standard cytotoxic agents. This can make it difficult to determine maximum tolerated dose in phase I trials. Despite these limitations, the traditional phase I through III clinical trials remain the mainstay for evaluating prospec-

tive chemotherapies for nervous system tumors. Surrogate biologic or pharmacologic end points have been developed in many cases to prevent these difficulties.

MULTIMODALITY TREATMENT, INTENT, AND TIMING

Patients with nervous system tumors usually receive chemotherapy as part of a multimodality treatment approach also involving surgery and radiation therapy. Chemotherapeutic agents may be given alone or in combination. Combining agents with different mechanisms of action and different toxicities is attractive and has been effective in many tumor types. Unfortunately, few chemotherapy combinations have proved more effective than single agents for nervous system tumors.

Chemotherapy can be administered with curative intent, to prevent disease recurrence, or as a palliative measure. Chemotherapeutic agents may be given at different times relative to diagnosis and other treatments. Adjuvant chemotherapy is delivered after diagnosis and initial therapy (e.g., surgery and irradiation for a glioblastoma) but before recurrence. In other words, adjuvant therapy is given in the setting of nonprogressive disease. Sometimes chemotherapy is administered concurrently with other initial therapies such as irradiation. Chemotherapy can also be given after diagnosis but before any other treatment (neoadjuvant). For malignant brain tumors, chemotherapy is often given at recurrence.

SYSTEMIC CHEMOTHERAPY: GENERAL PHARMACOLOGIC PRINCIPLES

For chemotherapy to be effective, it must be delivered to sensitive tumor cells in adequate concentrations. For nervous system tumors, as with all neoplasms, choosing appropriate chemotherapy administration routes and schedules is important in achieving adequate concentrations. In addition, CNS tumors have unique features, such as the blood-brain and blood-tumor barriers, that affect chemotherapeutic options.

Systemic chemotherapy may be given orally or intravenously. Oral bioavailability is important in deciding which route is more appropriate. This decision depends on several factors, including stability within gastric acid, absorption through the gastrointestinal tract, hepatic metabolism, biliary excretion, and treatment-related emesis. In addition, determining an appropriate treatment schedule can be critical. Some chemotherapeutic agents act primarily at specific time points within the cell cycle (cell-cycle specific). In brain tumors, the proportion of cells actively dividing at any given point in time can be quite small (<30%).[7] Therefore frequent dose administration may be desirable for cell-cycle specific agents to increase the number of actively dividing cells exposed to the agent. Theoretically, continuous intravenous infusion might be ideal for these agents. However, toxicities may also be increased, and logistic issues usually prohibit such rigorous administration schedules.

Physical characteristics unique to the CNS also affect drug concentration within CNS tumors. The blood-brain barrier (BBB) is an important limiting factor.[6] The BBB is made up of tight junctions between endothelial cells in CNS vasculature. Molecules larger than 40 kDa with poor lipid solubility or tight protein binding are unlikely to cross the BBB in significant amounts. Because the BBB is deficient in contrast-enhanced areas in CNS tumors, one might question its importance in choosing chemotherapy agents. However, agents that normally do not cross the BBB are still partially limited in their ability to enter contrast-enhanced areas. Their intratumoral concentration usually remains ineffective. Furthermore, tumor cells in nonenhanced areas adjacent to enhanced tumor are critical chemotherapy targets. These areas have an intact BBB. Finally, crossing the BBB does not ensure that a given agent will reach adequate numbers of tumor cells to be effective. It must also diffuse through the tumor and brain parenchyma. This depends on the physical properties of both the agent (size, lipophillicity) and the tissue (blood flow, cellularity, extracellular fluid composition).

Nonphysical factors can also affect chemotherapeutic efficacy in patients with brain tumor. Other common medications may interact with chemotherapeutic agents. For example, chemotherapeutic agents metabolized by the cytochrome p450 system may have to be given in larger doses in patients receiving antiepileptic medications that induce this enzyme system (e.g., phenytoin, carbamezepine, phenobarbital). Individual CNS tumors are also notoriously heterogeneous. Areas within a tumor may have marked resistance to a chemotherapeutic agent, even though the majority of the tumor is sensitive. These areas can quickly become the dominant population. Drug resistance can be either intrinsic or acquired and is mediated by several mechanisms. For example, P-glycoprotein, a 170-kDa membrane protein present on CNS endothelial cells and some CNS tumor cells, can act as a drug efflux pump that excludes xenobiotics, including a number of chemotherapeutic agents. O^6-alkylguanine-DNA alkyltransferase (O^6-AGAT) is a DNA repair enzyme that removes alkyl groups at the O^6 position of guanine, a location often alkylated by chemotherapeutic agents (see later discussion). This enzyme is up-regulated in many tumors and can mediate resistance to alkylating agents.

STRATEGIES TO INCREASE SYSTEMIC CHEMOTHERAPEUTIC EFFICACY

The most obvious choice to improve systemic chemotherapeutic efficacy is to find more effective agents. Considerable effort has gone into this, and a number of new small-molecule growth-factor pathway inhibitors are showing promise in early clinical

trials (see later discussion). Other strategies include administering high-dose chemotherapy and inhibiting drug resistance. High-dose chemotherapy has been proposed in the hope that higher serum drug levels will result in greater delivery across the BBB. This is typically accompanied by autologous bone marrow or stem cell transplant as a "rescue" from the marked myelosuppressive effects of high-dose cytotoxic chemotherapy. Although this strategy has shown some promise in children with medulloblastomas and germ cell tumors, the results have been much less favorable for adults with malignant gliomas. Several strategies have been proposed for inhibiting drug resistance. For example, the DNA repair enzyme O^6-AGAT can be inhibited using the agent O^6-benzyl guanine (O^6-BG). This is currently in clinical trials in combination with a number of alkylating agents. In addition to efforts to improve upon systemic chemotherapy, other strategies have been employed for local chemotherapeutic delivery. These will be discussed in detail.

CYTOTOXIC CHEMOTHERAPEUTIC AGENTS

Cytotoxic chemotherapeutic agents can be defined as those that inhibit tumor growth by killing tumor cells directly. These agents rely on tumor cells' dividing more rapidly than normal cells to achieve an acceptable therapeutic index. Still, their actions are necessarily nonspecific and many common cytotoxic chemotherapy side effects (e.g., myelosuppression, alopecia) reflect effects on normal dividing cells. General indications for cytotoxic chemotherapy include curing certain tumors, palliating symptoms, or prolonging progression-free survival. Most patients with a CNS tumor receive chemotherapy for this last reason. Relative contraindications include active infections, limited probability of prolonged survival even if tumor regression occurs, and severe debilitation.

Many cytotoxic agents mediate their effects by impairing DNA synthesis, a mandatory step in cell division. Cells that are not able to synthesize DNA cannot proceed through the cell cycle. They undergo apoptosis as a result. Alkylating agents such as temozolomide, carmustine (BCNU), lomustine (CCNU), procarbazine, carboplatin, and cisplatin cause alkyl groups to bind to DNA, producing DNA cross-links or single- or double-strand breaks. Antimetabolites such as methotrexate, 6-thioguanine, 5-fluorouracil, 6-mercaptopurine, and cytarabine impair such normal cellular metabolic activities as DNA synthesis. Camptothecin derivatives, such as irinotecan (CPT-11), and epipodophyllotoxins, such as etoposide (VP16), inhibit topoisomerases and lead to increased DNA strand breaks.

Other cytotoxic agents impair cell division by disrupting mitotic machinery. Vinca alkyloids such as vincristine and vinblastine act on tubulin to inhibit microtubule assembly by depolymerization. This leads to mitotic spindle dissolution. This effect can occur in G1 phase but is most effective in S phase. Taxanes such as paclitaxel and docetaxel bind to the microtubule β-subunit, producing polymerization. Like the vinca alkyloids, taxanes thus inhibit microtubule assembly by depolymerization, which leads to mitotic arrest and apoptosis. Antitumor antibiotics such as actinomycin, bleomycin, daunorubicin, doxorubicin, mithramycin, and mitomycin C are generally cell-cycle nonspecific agents. They act via several mechanisms, including intercalation into DNA (preventing

DNA replication and RNA transcription), DNA alkylation, and inducing DNA strand breaks.

Temozolomide, Procarbazine, and Dacarbazine

Temozolomide is an imidazotetrazine derivative of dacarbazine (DITC). It has excellent oral bioavailability. Temozolomide itself is inactive, but it is rapidly metabolized in vivo to an active derivative. This acts as an alkylating agent, methylating the O^6 position on guanine. Temozolomide has been shown to have activity against both malignant and low-grade gliomas as an adjuvant therapy and at recurrence.[14,17] Major toxicities include fatigue, headache, constipation, nausea and vomiting, and myelosuppression. However, temozolomide is relatively well tolerated as compared with many other cytotoxic chemotherapeutic agents. Its relative efficacy combined with a favorable side-effect profile have resulted in temozolomide's rapidly becoming the first line chemotherapeutic agent of choice for many patients with gliomas.

Procarbazine and DITC are methylating agents that produce single-strand DNA breaks. Procarbazine has good oral bioavailability. Its active metabolite acts as a cell cycle–nonspecific agent that inhibits DNA, RNA, and protein synthesis. Major toxicities include fatigue, nausea and vomiting, myelosuppression, and rash. It also acts as a monoamine oxidase inhibitor; therefore patients taking procarbazine need to avoid tyramine-containing foods such as red wine, sharp cheddar cheese, and flava beans. Procarbazine can be given as a single agent but is more commonly administered in combination with CCNU and vincristine (PCV chemotherapy). It has activity against malignant gliomas, low-grade gliomas, primitive neuroectodermal tumors (PNETs), and primary CNS lymphoma.[9,11]

Nitrosoureas

BCNU and CCNU are commonly used nitrosoureas that have formed the cornerstone of glioma chemotherapy for many years.[3,4,13] Both act as alkylating agents acting at multiple locations (primarily guanine but also adenine and cytosine). BCNU must be given intravenously. CCNU has better oral bioavailability and is administered as pills. Major toxicities for both BCNU and CCNU include fatigue, nausea and vomiting, myelosuppression, and dose-related pulmonary fibrosis. Nitrosoureas are active for the treatment of malignant gliomas, low-grade gliomas, PNETs, and (to a lesser degree) ependymomas.

Platinum Compounds

Carboplatin and cisplatin are cell-cycle nonspecific agents that alkylate the N^7 position on guanine.[16] Both are water-soluble, necessitating intravenous administration. Both are excluded by an intact BBB, but objective responses have been seen in CNS tumors, presumably because of partial intratumoral BBB disruption. Major toxicities related to carboplatin include fatigue, nausea and vomiting, and myelosuppression. Cisplatin causes very little myelosuppression but can lead to ototoxicity, nephrotoxicity, and peripheral neuropathy. Carboplatin and cisplatin can be used alone or in combination with other agents. They have activity against malignant gliomas, PNETs, ependymoma, and germ cell tumors.

Vinca Alkaloids and Epipodophyllotoxins

Vincristine and vinblastine are vinca alkaloids that act on tubulin to inhibit microtubule assembly. They result in S-phase–specific mitotic arrest. Resistance is mediated by the p170 membrane glycoprotein. These agents are water soluble, must be given intravenously, and have poor BBB penetration.[8] Toxicities are primarily neurologic, including peripheral neuropathy and (as a result) constipation. Vinblastine is seldom administered to patients with nervous system tumors. Vincristine is commonly used in combination with procarbazine and CCNU (PCV chemotherapy) and may have activity against malignant gliomas, PNETs, low-grade gliomas, ependymomas, and primary CNS lymphomas.

Epipodophyllotoxins such as VP16 (etoposide) inhibit the enzyme topoisomerase II and result in DNA strand breaks. This leads to G2-S cell-cycle arrest. VP16 can be given either by mouth or intravenously. Major toxicities include nausea and vomiting, peripheral neuropathy, and myelosuppression. VP16 can be given as a single agent, but is more commonly combined with other drugs. It has some activity as a single agent against malignant gliomas.[5] More commonly, it is used in pediatric patients to treat PNETs, malignant gliomas, low-grade gliomas, and ependymomas.

Camptothecins

Camptothecin derivatives such as topotecan and CPT-11 (irinotecan) are topoisomerase I inhibitors that result in DNA strand breaks (similar to etoposide). Both have poor oral bioavailability and must be administered intravenously. Major side effects include fatigue, nausea and vomiting, and myelosuppression. Diarrhea is a dose-limiting toxicity for CPT-11. Topotecan's effects in patients with nervous system tumors have been disappointing. However, CPT-11 has had some activity against malignant gliomas in early clinical trials.[2]

Taxanes

Taxanes such as paclitaxel and docetaxel impair microtubule assembly by stabilizing microtubule dynamics. They are water soluble and must be given intravenously. Major toxicities include myelosuppression, alopecia, neurotoxicity, cardiac arrhythmia, and hypersensitivity reactions. Taxanes have been used as single agents for malignant gliomas and as radiosensitizers. In both cases, results have been disappointing.

Nitrogen Mustards

Nitrogen mustards lead to reactive carbonium ion formation. These carbonium ions then react with electrophilic regions of DNA. They include cyclophosphamide, melphalan, ifosfamide, chlorambucil, and mechlorethamine. Toxicities include fatigue, myelosuppression, nausea and vomiting, pneumonitis, and pulmonary fibrosis. Cyclophosphamide is associated with hemorrhagic cystitis. Cyclophosphamide has shown some activity in recurrent malignant brain tumors, but the activity of other nitrogen mustards against nervous system tumors has been minimal.

Anthracyclines

Anthracyclines (antitumor antibiotics) are cell-cycle nonspecific DNA intercalating agents that impair DNA, RNA, and protein synthesis. They include doxorubicin, dactinomycin, bleomycin, and plicamycin. In general, they penetrate the BBB poorly and are often susceptible to multidrug-resistant phenotypes. Major toxicities include myelosuppression, mucositis, and cardiotoxicity. Their role in nervous system tumors is limited. However, doxorubicin combined with DITC may have some activity against malignant meningiomas. Bleomycin combined with vinblastine and carboplatin may have activity against intracranial germ cell tumors.

Antimetabolites

Methotrexate is an S-phase-specific folic acid analogue that blocks tetrahydrofolate production and decreases the intracellular reduced folate pool. It can be given orally or intravenously. Side effects include myelosuppression, nephrotoxicity, nausea and vomiting, diarrhea, mucositis, pneumonitis, and neurotoxicity. It has been used for primary CNS lymphoma, leptomeningeal metastases, and (in multiagent regimens) for pediatric PNETs.

Cytarabine is an S-phase-specific pyrimidine analogue. It can be given intravenously and does penetrate the BBB. Major toxicities include myelosuppression, nausea and vomiting, and neurotoxicity. Its indications are similar to methotrexate: primary CNS lymphoma and leptomeningeal metastases.

CYTOSTATIC AGENTS

Cytostatic agents can be defined as those that impair tumor growth without directly causing tumor cell death. Their mechanisms of action often affect specific facets of tumor biology. As such, they are often quite selective and have a favorable therapeutic index. As a result, these agents are assuming a larger role in chemotherapy.[10]

Cis-Retinoic Acid

Cis-retinoic acid (Acutane) is a vitamin A analogue that is commonly used in acne treatment. At higher doses, it has been shown to cause glioma cells to assume a less aggressive phenotype. It has excellent oral bioavailability. Toxicities are generally mild and include rash, photosensitivity, and dry mucous membranes. As a single agent, it has shown modest activity against malignant gliomas. More commonly, it is given in combination with other agents, including many standard cytotoxic agents.

Thalidomide

Thalidomide (α-phthalimidoglutarimide) was used extensively as a sedative and antiemetic in pregnant women in the 1960s and 1970s. It resulted in high rates of birth defects, particularly small deformed limbs. This effect was secondary to antiangiogenic properties that are now being exploited in cancer therapy. It has good oral bioavailability. Side effects include sedation, constipation, and peripheral neuropathy. Thalidomide has modest activity as a single agent against malignant gliomas but is more commonly given in combination with other agents.

Tamoxifen

Tamoxifen is an antiestrogen agent used extensively in breast carcinoma therapy. At higher doses, tamoxifen inhibits protein kinase C (PKC). This latter property gives it modest activity against malignant gliomas. It has excellent oral bioavailability. Major toxicities include increased risk of deep venous thrombus formation and pulmonary embolism.

Celecoxib

Celecoxib (Celebrex) is a cyclo-oxygenase-2 (COX-2) specific inhibitor used extensively in osteoarthritis treatment. COX-2 is overexpressed in many glioma cells and celecoxib has inhibited human glioma cell culture growth in vitro. Toxicities (when given for osteoarthritis) include gastritis and platelet function impairment despite its "selective" nature. Celecoxib is currently in clinical trial for malignant gliomas.

Small-Molecule Growth Factor Pathway Inhibitors

Currently, there is extensive clinical research interest in small molecules that block growth factor pathways overactive in many tumors. Although these agents are distinct from classic cytotoxic agents, it is not clear that they can be termed *cytostatic*, because objective responses to therapy with these agents, such as tumor shrinkage, have been noted. Compounds currently under investigation for malignant gliomas and several other nervous system tumors include OSI-774 and ZD1839 (epidermal growth factor receptor), R115-777 (Ras pathway or farnesyl transferase inhibitor), STI-571 (platelet-derived growth factor), SU5416 (vascular endothelial growth factor), and CCI-779 (mammalian target of rapamycin).

LOCAL OR INTRATUMORAL CHEMOTHERAPY

The preceding discussion has focused on systemic chemotherapy delivery. However, local delivery may be an attractive alternative for patients with CNS tumors.[12] These tumors are locally recurrent and rarely spread outside the CNS. Local high-dose chemotherapy without systemic administration may be efficacious but avoid systemic toxicities. Furthermore, local delivery may circumvent the BBB.

The simplest means to deliver chemotherapeutic agents locally to brain tumors has been direct injection, either intratumorally or intrathecally. Clinical studies have been performed that inject a number of chemotherapeutic agents (including BCNU, bleomycin, methotrexate, cisplatin, fluorouracil, and cyclophosphamide). Toxicities have been relatively mild, but clinical responses have been largely disappointing. This may relate to poor drug delivery after bolus injection. Slightly better results have been seen with primary CNS lymphoma (intrathecal methotrexate) and craniopharyngioma (intratumoral bleomycin). Ongoing studies may improve drug delivery with direct injection by preparing agents in such a way to promote diffusion. For example, BCNU dissolved in ethanol may have increased tissue penetration after bolus injection. This combination is currently in clinical trial (DTI-015).

Alternatively, chemotherapeutic agents may be delivered to brain tumors by intra-arterial infusion. This can lead to high intratumoral doses for a number of agents, including nitrosoureas, cisplatin, and methotrexate. This may have some benefit in primary CNS lymphomas but to date has not been associated with improved survival for patients with glioblastoma. Significant toxicities have occurred, including seizures, hearing loss, new focal neurologic deficits, and coma. Drug transfer can potentially be increased further by iatrogenic BBB disruption using intra-arterial mannitol or RMP-7 (a bradykinin analogue) infusion. However, this approach also continues to be associated with increased toxicities in the face of limited clinical success.

The pioneering work of Brem and colleagues[1] at Johns Hopkins has demonstrated the utility of another technique for intratumoral chemotherapy in malignant gliomas. Biodegradable wafers impregnated with chemotherapeutic agents can be used to line resection cavities after malignant gliomas are removed. This is associated with modestly prolonged survival.[1,15] As a result, these wafers have recently been approved by the Food and Drug Administration (FDA) for the treatment of both recurrent and newly diagnosed malignant gliomas.

Finally, convection-enhanced delivery (CED) utilizes catheters placed intraparenchymally around resection cavities at the time of surgery to deliver intratumoral chemotherapy infusions over several days. Rather than relying on diffusion to carry the agents into the brain, as occurs after direct injection, CED drives chemotherapeutic agents farther into brain and results in much larger volumes of distribution. This strategy has been evaluated in preclinical studies, and several clinical trials are ongoing. Agents being infused have included fusion proteins combining pseudomonas exotoxin with transferrin, interleukin-4, or interleukin-13.

CONCLUSION

Chemotherapy has an expanding role in nervous system tumors and is typically given as part of a multimodality treatment regimen. Many agents are available. In general, these can be subdivided into cytotoxic and cytostatic agents. Agents can be given either systemically (oral or intravenous) or locally (direct injection, intra-arterial, chemotherapy-impregnated wafers, or CED). Standard treatments have a significant impact on at least some patients with nervous system tumors. New agents and strategies are currently being evaluated that may improve on these results.

References

1. Brem H, Piantadosi S, Burger PC, et al: Placebo-controlled trial of safety and efficacy of intraoperative controlled delivery by biodegradable polymers of chemotherapy for recurrent gliomas. The Polymer-brain Tumor Treatment Group. Lancet 345:1008–1012, 1995.
2. Cloughesy TF, Filka E, Nelson G, et al: Irinotecan treatment for recurrent malignant glioma using an every-3-week regimen. Am J Clin Oncol 25:204–208, 2002.
3. Fewer D, Wilson CB, Boldrey EB, et al: The chemotherapy of brain tumors. Clinical experience with carmustine (BCNU) and vincristine. JAMA 222:549–552, 1972.
4. Fine HA, Dear KBG, Loeffler JS, et al: Meta-analysis of radiation therapy with and without adjuvant chemotherapy for malignant gliomas in adults. Cancer 71:2585–2597, 1993.
5. Fulton D, Urtasun R, Forsyth P: Phase II study of prolonged oral therapy with etoposide (VP16) for patients with recurrent malignant glioma. J Neurooncol 27:149–155, 1996.
6. Greig NH: Optimizing drug delivery to brain tumors. Cancer Treat Rev 14:1–28, 1987.
7. Hoshino T, Prados M, Wilson CB, et al: Prognostic implications of the bromodeoxyuridine labeling index of human gliomas. J Neurosurg 71:335–341, 1989.
8. Jackson DV, Jr., Sethi VS, Spurr CL, et al: Pharmacokinetics of vincristine in the cerebrospinal fluid of humans. Cancer Res 41:1466–1468, 1981.
9. Levin VA, Silver P, Hannigan J, et al: Superiority of postradiotherapy adjuvant chemotherapy with CCNU, procarbazine, and vincristine (PCV) over BCNU for anaplastic gliomas: NCOG 6G61 final report. Int J Radiat Oncol Biol Phys 18:321–324, 1990.
10. Parney IF, Chang S: Current chemotherapy for glioblastoma. Cancer J (in press), 2003.
11. Prados MD, Scott C, Curran WJ, Jr., et al: Procarbazine, lomustine, and vincristine (PCV) chemotherapy for anaplastic astrocytoma: a retrospective review of radiation therapy oncology group protocols comparing survival with carmustine or PCV adjuvant chemotherapy. J Clin Oncol 17:3389–3395, 1999.
12. Schmidt MH, Chang SM, Berger MS: An appraisal of chemotherapy: in the blood or in the brain? Clin Neurosurg 48:46–59, 2001.
13. Stewart LA: Chemotherapy in adult high-grade glioma: a systematic review and meta-analysis of individual patient data from 12 randomised trials. Lancet 359:1011–1018, 2002.
14. Stupp R, Dietrich PY, Ostermann Kraljevic S, et al: Promising survival for patients with newly diagnosed glioblastoma multiforme treated with concomitant radiation plus temozolomide followed by adjuvant temozolomide. J Clin Oncol 20:1375–1382, 2002.
15. Valtonen S, Timonen U, Toivanen P, et al: Interstitial chemotherapy with carmustine-loaded polymers for high-grade gliomas: a randomized double-blind study. Neurosurgery 41:44–48; discussion 48–49, 1997.
16. Warnick RE, Prados MD, Mack EE, et al: A phase II study of intravenous carboplatin for the treatment of recurrent gliomas. J Neurooncol 19:69–74, 1994.
17. Yung WK, Albright RE, Olson J, et al: A phase II study of temozolomide vs. procarbazine in patients with glioblastoma multiforme at first relapse. Br J Cancer 83:588–593, 2000.

CHAPTER 12

NEUROINTERVENTIONAL TECHNIQUES

Christopher F. Dowd, Van V. Halbach, and Randall T. Higashida

The past 2 decades have witnessed remarkable technical developments in the field of interventional neuroradiology. Nearly every subspecialty area within the clinical neurosciences has been enhanced by new endovascular applications, either as definitive therapies or as adjuvant treatments. The field of neuro-oncology has benefited most handsomely from its partnership with the field of interventional neuroradiology. This chapter outlines the basic principles involved in the application of neurointerventional techniques to brain tumors.

TECHNIQUES

Angiography

Angiography is the study of blood vessels using radiographic contrast agent. Most often, angiography means more specifically *arteriography,* or examination of arteries. One can also perform venography, or the examination of veins. Traditionally, angiography is performed by navigating an angiographic catheter through the access site (usually the femoral artery) under fluoroscopic guidance to the vessel under study. Once in position, radiographic contrast agent, or x-ray dye, is injected through the catheter, and a series of radiographs are obtained as the contrast agent moves with the circulation, allowing images of the arterial and venous systems to be captured. Angiography can be useful as a diagnostic tool in evaluating brain tumors by identifying tumor vascularity. This may assist in ascertaining the proper diagnosis (meningioma versus schwannoma, for example), identifying the arteries supplying the tumor and the pattern of venous drainage, the presence of arterial tumoral encasement or venous sinus occlusion, and feasibility of performing embolization.

Embolization

Embolization is the devascularization of a tumor by placing embolic material through a catheter in the feeding arteries to the tumor to block the internal architecture of the tumor's blood supply. This is usually a preoperative adjuvant in highly vascular extra-axial tumors (tumors arising outside the substance of the brain) to permit a more complete surgical resection with less operative time, less intraoperative blood loss, and less overall morbidity. The best candidate tumors are those with a rich blood supply from arteries accessible to microcatheter navigation, with limited risk of inadvertent embolization of important normal arteries. The classic example of such a tumor is the meningioma, a common vascular tumor of the covering of the brain that is usually supplied by accessible branches of the external carotid artery. Conversely, most intra-axial tumors (tumors arising within the substance of the brain such as gliomas and most metastases) are not candidates for preoperative embolization because the blood supply to these tumors also supplies normal brain parenchyma. An attempt to devascularize such a tumor would carry a likely risk of producing stroke from occlusion of normal brain arteries.

The development of the microcatheter in the mid-1980s revolutionized the process of embolization and permitted its widespread application. A diagnostic angiogram is performed to confirm tumor vascularity, to identify blood supply, and to determine feasibility and safety of embolization. A microcatheter (a flexible, small-lumen catheter placed coaxially through an angiographic catheter) is directed into the artery directly supplying the tumor using real-time digital subtraction fluoroscopy ("road-mapping" technology). Once in position, a superselective angiogram is obtained through the microcatheter. This allows confirmation of proper catheter position for embolization and identification of any normal arteries beyond the tip of the microcatheter, which might necessitate catheter repositioning or aborting the embolization procedure. Occasionally, provocative testing can also be used to identify blood supply to important structures such as cranial nerves.[23] This entails injection of a small dose of cardiac lidocaine through the microcatheter, a process that would cause temporary loss of function of a cranial nerve supplied by vessels beyond the microcatheter tip. Identification of a resulting new neurologic deficit during provocative testing may aid in evaluating the risk of embolization.

Once the microcatheter has been positioned safely, embolization is undertaken by injecting an embolic agent though the microcatheter into the tumor bed under digital-subtraction fluoroscopy. A wide variety of embolic materials exists from which to choose, including particulate agents (polyvinyl alcohol particles and acrylic microspheres[6]), liquid adhesives (cyanoacrylate "glue"), ethanol, and embolic microcoils. Generally, particulate agents are favored because of their relative ease of use; the permanence of glue or ethanol is unnecessary in the preoperative setting, and they may easily permeate small normal branches below the resolution capacity of even the best fluoroscopic units. After the tumor has been embolized, one can choose to place an occlusive microcoil in the feeding artery proximal to the tumor bed to allow easy transection of the artery facilitating surgical access to the tumor. The microcatheter is removed and a postembolization angiogram is performed to evaluate the angiographic efficacy of embolization. The risks of tumor embolization are generally small in properly selected cases and are inversely related to the experience of the interventional neuroradiologist.[23] Potential complications include transient cranial nerve palsies or inadvertent embolization of brain arteries through potential anastomoses of the external carotid branches to internal carotid or vertebral arteries.

Intra-Arterial Chemotherapy

Intra-arterial chemotherapy is the process by which chemotherapeutic agents are delivered directly into the arterial tumor supply (usually in gliomas) via a microcatheter. Most gliomas are treated by a combination of surgery, radiation therapy, and standard intravenous chemotherapy. However, selective intra-arterial chemotherapy was rendered possible by introduction of the microcatheter and has been undertaken in limited fashion in an effort to expose the tumor to the largest concentration of chemotherapeutic agent while limiting systemic effects. After determining the vascular territory encompassing the glioma, a microcatheter is navigated into the intracranial circulation to an optimal location depending on predicted tumor supply. Microcatheter positions beyond the ophthalmic artery origin were associated with diminished risk of visual impairment.[2] Infused chemotherapeutic agents have included carboplatin,[11] 5-fluorouracil, cisplatin, nitrosourea compounds,[9] and other agents that disrupt the blood-brain barrier.[17] Most practitioners now feel that intra-arterial chemotherapy may improve quality of life but may not improve survival time, and this technique has limited applications.

Balloon Test Occlusion

Many skull base tumors arise near or have the capacity to invade carotid or vertebral arteries. Before attempted surgical resection, a surgeon may wish to determine the patient's potential neurologic tolerance for sacrifice of the affected artery, in case this becomes necessary during surgery. This can be achieved by a preoperative balloon test occlusion of the internal carotid (or vertebral) artery. In an awake patient under anticoagulation, a double-lumen balloon catheter is directed to the artery in question. With the patient under constant neurologic surveillance to detect any change in neurologic function, the balloon is inflated to occlude the chosen artery and obstruct flow to the distal circulation for a limited time (usually 30 minutes). Tolerance is determined by lack of production of a new neurologic deficit. Adjunctive measures can include measurement of arterial back pressures, provocative tolerance test occlusion by artificially lowering the patient's blood pressure to identify the tolerance margin of safety, and measurement of cerebral blood flow (by positron emission tomography [PET], single photon emission computed tomography [SPECT], administration of xenon, or magnetic resonance [MR] perfusion).[18,35,41]

Venous Sampling

Venous sampling is a technique that assists in identifying the source of a hormone. It is especially applicable in the setting of adrenocorticotropic hormone (ACTH)-producing adenomas.[14,36] The primary goals of ACTH venous sampling are to differentiate a pituitary ACTH source (Cushing's disease) from a nonpituitary source and to lateralize the tumor if it is located in the pituitary gland.[33] Paired microcatheters are advanced through the venous system by femoral vein access and are placed in the inferior petrosal or cavernous sinuses, the direct recipients of ACTH hormone secreted from the pituitary gland. Venous samples are obtained, clearly marked by sample location, and sent to the laboratory for ACTH assay. The assay results are later compared with the sampling locations to identify the source of the abnormal ACTH production. Intravenous administration of corticotropin-releasing factor (CRF) has been used to stimulate release of ACTH from the anterior lobe of the pituitary gland during ACTH venous-sampling procedures to facilitate identification of the abnormal ACTH source. The pattern of petrosal sinus drainage can have direct bearing on interpretation of the assay results, because asymmetrical venous drainage can distort the lateralization process.[32]

DISEASE PROCESSES

Extra-Axial Tumors

Extra-axial tumors are brain tumors that arise on the surface of the brain or within the ventricles, and not within or among brain cells. The classic extra-axial tumor is the meningioma, and this is the tumor that most often requires preoperative embolization.

Meningiomas

Meningiomas are common benign extra-axial tumors that arise from arachnoid cells covering the brain. As such, these tumors are found in locations where the arachnoid cells are most plentiful: along the dural lining of the venous sinuses of the brain and skull base. They account for 20% of primary intracranial neoplasms.[34] Presenting signs and symptoms depend on the location and size of the tumor. Common locations include the lateral and parasagittal cerebral convexity, sphenoid wing, petrous ridge, cerebellopontine angle, tentorium, foramen magnum, and cavernous sinus. Common symptoms include headache, seizure, and neurologic deficit caused by local mass effect, although small meningiomas may be discovered incidentally when a patient undergoes brain imaging for unrelated symptoms. The diagnosis is usually straightforward on computed tomography (CT) or magnetic resonance imaging (MRI). The classic meningioma appearance is a well-circumscribed extra-axial mass with a distinct dural attachment and homogeneous contrast enhancement.

On angiography, a meningioma usually receives its blood supply primarily from *dural* arteries that supply the covering of the brain (as opposed to *pial* arteries that supply brain tissue directly.) Depending on tumor location, arterial supply is derived predominantly from middle meningeal, accessory meningeal, ascending pharyngeal, or occipital transmastoid perforating branches of the external carotid artery and may be bilateral, especially in a midline tumor. Dural arteries from the internal carotid (meningohypophyseal trunk, inferolateral trunk, ethmoidal branches of ophthalmic artery) and vertebral (posterior meningeal) arteries may also supply the tumor. As a meningioma grows, it may parasitize pial branches, which supply small twigs to the periphery of the tumor. Another characteristic feature of meningiomas is the angiographic staining pattern: a uniform radial arrangement of tiny tumor vessels in a well-defined tumor. Contrast opacification begins in the arterial phase, augments, and persists into the venous phase without washout.

The treatment goal for meningiomas is elimination of the tumor by complete surgical resection. Hindrances to this goal include tumor vascularity, invasion of an adjacent dural sinus, and encasement of major arteries or nerves. Because meningiomas are typically vascular tumors, preoperative devascularization by transcatheter embolization (Figure 12-1) can facilitate complete tumor resection by diminishing intraoperative blood loss and operative time.[21,25] Once the feeding arteries to a meningioma are identified and embolization is deemed safe and feasible, a microcatheter can be navigated into the feeding artery in preparation for embolization. Superselective angiography is carried out through the microcatheter to confirm proper microcatheter position and to identify any normal arteries beyond the catheter that might preclude safe embolization. Such arteries include the meningolacrimal branch of the middle meningeal artery (which can supply the retina directly), the odontoid branch of the ascending pharyngeal artery (which can anastomose with the vertebral artery), the neuromeningeal trunk of the ascending pharyngeal artery (which supplies cranial nerves IX, X, and XI), and the distal internal maxillary artery (which can communicate with cavernous branches of the internal carotid artery.) If adequate microcatheter position is confirmed, embolization can be carried out, usually with particulate agents,[7] to allow penetration of the embolic material into the vascular tumor bed to provide devascularization and subsequent tumor necrosis. Depending on the feeding artery, embolic microcoils can be placed to provide intraoperative arterial feeder occlusion after particulate devascularization of the tumor bed, which facilitates surgical transection of the feeding artery. Vigilance must be maintained to avoid reflux of embolic material into normal proximal branches by overly vigorous embolization. Secondary meningioma supply from pial arteries is generally not embolized preoperatively, because these branches provide only a small percentage of tumor vascularity, and the risk of embolization is greater than that of dural artery embolization. A postembolization control angiogram is performed to document adequate results. Some researchers advocate delaying surgery for several days to a week after embolization to permit necrosis to occur within the tumor, facilitating resection.[10,27]

Hemangiopericytomas

Hemangiopericytomas are soft tissue tumors that most often arise along the meningeal surface of the brain. There has been considerable debate as to the classification of this tumor, because it has been variously described as a variant of the meningioma or as an unrelated extra-axial tumor.[8] Although much less common than the meningioma, the hemangiopericy-toma is often extremely vascular and may exhibit more aggressive clinical and biologic behavior. Given its typical vascularity, preoperative embolization is helpful[8] to limit intraoperative blood loss and permit as complete a surgical resection as possible. The principles of embolization are the same as those covered in the section on meningiomas.

Choroid Plexus Papillomas

A choroid plexus papilloma is an unusual tumor that arises from choroid plexus cells within the cerebral ventricles. The normal function of the choroid plexus is to produce cerebrospinal fluid (CSF). These highly vascular tumors are usually identified in infants and children, are most often found within the lateral ventricles, and can produce hydrocephalus or ventriculomegaly from ventricular obstruction or overproduction of CSF.[22] Imaging studies show a contrast-enhanced mass with irregular borders within a cerebral ventricle.

Arterial supply to these tumors is derived from choroidal arteries, the same arteries that supply the normal choroid plexus. Thus the most common choroid plexus papilloma, which arises within the lateral ventricle, may be fed by the anterior choroidal artery (an important branch of the distal internal carotid artery) or by the lateral posterior choroidal artery (a branch of the posterior cerebral artery.) If the tumor is sufficiently large and vascular and the feeding artery is enlarged to permit microcatheter placement, preoperative embolization may be feasible.[38] An important caveat is that the anterior choroidal artery supplies vital neural structures (internal capsule, uncus, optic pathways) in addition to supplying the normal choroid plexus. Thus one must be extremely careful in undertaking embolization of this branch.[15]

Skull Base Tumors

Tumors of the skull base present a particular challenge because of the common involvement of crucial structures such as large arteries or cranial nerves and because of their relatively difficult surgical access. Endovascular techniques can improve operative outcomes by reducing intraoperative blood loss and operative time. The following represent the most common skull base tumors.

Paragangliomas

Paragangliomas (glomus tumors, chemodectomas) are benign, vascular, slow-growing tumors arising from paraganglionic glomic tissue of neuroectodermal origin. These tumors are found in adults and have a predilection for females.[3] The four most common sites are the jugular foramen (glomus jugulare), cochlear promontory of the middle ear (glomus tympanicum), carotid body, and vagus nerve (glomus vagale). Presenting clinical symptoms often include pulsatile tinnitus; other symptoms are caused by local mass effect and depend on tumor location.[26] On MRI, these tumors exhibit an internal "salt-and-pepper" appearance because of the abundant tumor vessels. Glomus jugulare tumors often erode the jugular foramen, a process best seen on CT scanning.[31]

Surgical resection of large paragangliomas may be complicated by intimate involvement of the temporal bone and posterior fossa structures. Given the extreme vascularity of

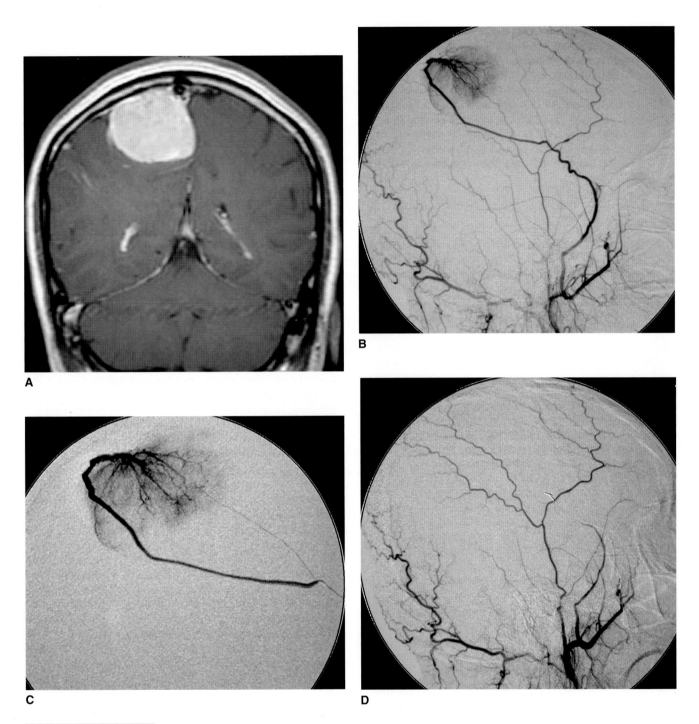

FIGURE 12-1 A 29-year-old man with a right parasagittal convexity meningioma. *A,* Coronal short repetition time (TR)/echo time (TE) magnetic resonance (MR) image with gadolinium contrast enhancement demonstrates a homogeneous mass consistent with this diagnosis. *B,* Pre-embolization right external carotid angiogram, lateral projection, shows tumor vascularity typical of a meningioma, supplied by an enlarged branch of the middle meningeal artery. *C,* Superselective right middle meningeal branch arteriogram, lateral projection, immediately before embolization. *D,* Postembolization right external carotid angiogram, lateral projection, after particulate embolization of the tumor bed and coil occlusion of the feeding artery. No residual tumor vascularity is seen. This patient is now prepared for surgical resection.

these tumors, preoperative embolization is warranted.[30] Angiographically, paragangliomas are highly vascular, are encapsulated, exhibit arteriovenous shunting, and are supplied primarily by branches of the external carotid artery. The ascending pharyngeal artery nearly always supplies glomus jugulare and glomus tympanicum tumors. Careful embolization, usually with particulate agents, is undertaken in the same fashion as for meningiomas. Particular care is necessary to preserve the neuromeningeal branch of the ascending pharyngeal artery (cranial nerves IX through XI) and the stylomastoid artery (facial nerve).[16]

Schwannomas

Schwannomas ("neuromas") are benign tumors arising from the cranial nerve sheaths, which are formed of Schwann cells. Ninety percent occur in the cerebellopontine angle,[24,39] and they are usually solitary. The so-called *acoustic schwannoma* is by far the most common tumor of this type; bilateral acoustic schwannomas are the hallmark of the central form of neurofibromatosis 2 (NF2).[5,28] The trigeminal nerve is the next most common site of origin.[24] Generally, schwannomas are firm, encapsulated tumors that may contain cysts. As the tumor grows, it may become lobulated, increase in vascularity,[29] or develop arachnoid adhesions that may result in arachnoid cysts. Clinical presentation depends on the size and site of origin of the tumor. Acoustic schwannomas initially present with tinnitus and progressive neurosensory hearing loss. Tumor enlargement into the cerebellopontine angle can produce ataxia or compression of the brainstem or exiting cranial nerves.

Cross-sectional imaging demonstrates that schwannomas are extra-axial, well-circumscribed tumors eroding the involved canal with variable contrast enhancement. Angiographically, schwannomas are generally less vascular than meningiomas, and the most suggestive angiographic finding is the presence of multiple small puddles of contrast agent that persist into the venous phase.[1] Most schwannomas are not sufficiently vascular to warrant preoperative embolization, but this has been shown to be efficacious in the more vascular schwannomas,[1,4] because it reduces tumor blood supply and eases surgical resection, as with meningiomas.

Juvenile Nasal Angiofibromas

Juvenile nasal angiofibromas are benign vascular tumors arising in the pterygopalatine fossa in adolescent males, usually presenting with epistaxis and nasal obstruction.[13] Large angiofibromas with posterior extension may invade the skull base, cavernous sinuses, or middle cranial fossa. On imaging, these markedly enhanced tumors are seen to arise in the pterygopalatine fossa and nasal cavity but may extend posteriorly to the skull base or to the adjacent paranasal sinuses. On angiography, these tumors appear dramatically vascular and are usually found to be supplied by the ascending pharyngeal artery and by multiple distal branches of the internal maxillary artery, often bilaterally. Transarterial particulate embolization has become the standard of care in preoperative devascularization.[12] Because of the high degree of correlation between the angiographic tumor blush and actual tumor boundary, this feature can be used to determine tumor extent before therapy and to assess efficacy of embolization.[30]

Malignant Skull Base Neoplasms

Malignant skull base tumors, such as squamous cell carcinomas arising in the head and neck region, have the capacity to encase or invade the carotid arteries. Internal carotid artery test occlusion with measurement of arterial pressures distal to the occlusion balloon enable the surgeon to determine whether the patient can tolerate carotid occlusion during skull base surgery. If permanent carotid occlusion is deemed mandatory for safe and successful skull base tumor resection, it can be carried out in the angiography suite following test occlusion.[20] One must adhere to the policy of vigorous volume expansion and strict limitation of activity following carotid occlusion to avoid hemispheric ischemia. The anesthesiology team should be apprised of the need to avoid episodes of hypotension during the subsequent operation for the same reason. Squamous cell carcinomas are not vascular tumors and generally do not require preoperative embolization.

INTRA-AXIAL TUMORS

Intra-axial tumors arise within glial or neural cells within the substance of the brain. Typical intra-axial tumors are gliomas and metastases. Although neurointerventional techniques are less applicable within this category than within the extra-axial group, there is an occasional role for endovascular therapy.

Hemangioblastoma

Hemangioblastomas are benign, highly vascular tumors that are found most often in the posterior fossa and spinal cord. The majority of these tumors consist of a vascular solid nodule associated with a cyst.[8] Hemangioblastomas can be sporadic or associated with von Hippel-Lindau disease, a condition of autosomal dominant inheritance that includes multiple hemangioblastomas, retinal angiomas, renal cell carcinoma, and pancreatic and hepatic cysts. Cerebellar hemangioblastomas are supplied primarily by pial arteries, such as branches of the posterior inferior cerebellar artery. Surgical resection can be aided by preoperative embolization[19,40,42] to produce tumor necrosis and reduce blood flow. Risk of embolization is greater than with many other types of tumor because of the apparent fragility of tumor arterioles that can lead to hemorrhage during embolization.

Glioma

Gliomas represent the largest group of primary brain tumors, accounting for two thirds of the tumors in this category. This heterogeneous group of intra-axial neoplasms includes astrocytomas, oligodendrogliomas, and ependymomas.[37] They demonstrate a wide spectrum of malignant potential, and survival rates depend on tissue type. Surgery, chemotherapy, and radiation therapy have been the mainstays of treatment for decades. Over the past decade, intra-arterial chemotherapy has been investigated to treat the more malignant gliomas, because of poor survival rates (see previous discussion of intra-arterial chemotherapy). Although the concept of direct arterial delivery of a chemotherapeutic agent to a malignant tumor that is otherwise difficult to treat holds promise, this technique has shown only limited efficacy and has not achieved a role as standard therapy.

CONCLUSION

The application of neurointerventional techniques has been of dramatic benefit in the treatment of patients with brain tumors. This chapter outlined the basic principles involved in the most common neurointerventional procedures. The interested reader is directed to a more detailed discussion of specific tumors in Part 2. Experience and new technical developments in microcatheters and embolic agents may permit safer and more efficacious therapy in the future.

References

1. Abramowitz J, Dion JE, Jensen ME, et al: Angiographic diagnosis and management of head and neck schwannomas. AJNR Am J Neuroradiol 12:977–984, 1991.
2. Ahuja A, Gibbons KJ, Hopkins LN: Endovascular techniques to treat brain tumors, Vol 4. In Youmans JR (ed): Neurological Surgery, 4th ed. Philadelphia, WB Saunders, 1996.
3. Alford BR, Guilford FR: A comprehensive study of tumors of the glomus jugulare. Laryngoscope 72:765–787, 1962.
4. Allcutt DA, Hoffman HJ, Isla A, et al: Acoustic schwannomas in children. Neurosurgery 29:14–18, 1991.
5. Aoki S, Barkovich AJ, Nishimura K, et al: Neurofibromatosis types 1 and 2: cranial MR findings. Radiology 172:527–534, 1989.
6. Beaujeux R, Laurent A, Wassef M, et al: Trisacryl gelatin microspheres for therapeutic embolization, II: Preliminary clinical evaluation in tumors and arteriovenous malformations. AJNR Am J Neuroradiol 17:541–548, 1996.
7. Bendszus M, Klein R, Burger R, et al: Efficacy of trisacryl gelatin microspheres versus polyvinyl alcohol particles in the preoperative embolization of meningiomas. AJNR Am J Neuroradiol 21:255–261, 2000.
8. Berger MS, Kros JM: Sarcomas and neoplasms of blood vessels, Vol 4. In Youmans JR (ed): Neurological Surgery, 4th ed. Philadelphia, WB Saunders, 1996.
9. Chiras J, Chedid G, DeBussche-Depriester C: Intraarterial chemotherapy of brain tumors. In Vinuela F, Halbach VV, Dion JE (eds): Interventional Neuroradiology: Endovascular Therapy of the Central Nervous System. New York, Raven Press, 1992.
10. Chun JY, McDermott MW, Lamborn KR, et al: Delayed surgical resection reduces intraoperative blood loss for embolized meningiomas. Neurosurgery 50:1231–1235; discussion 1235–1237, 2002.
11. Cloughesy TF, Gobin YP, Black KL, et al: Intra-arterial carboplatin chemotherapy for brain tumors: a dose escalation study based on cerebral blood flow. J Neurooncol 35:121–131, 1997.
12. Davis KR: Embolization of epistaxis and juvenile nasopharyngeal angiofibromas. AJR Am J Roentgenol 148:209–218, 1987.
13. Dillon WP, Mancuso AA: The oropharynx and nasopharynx, Vol 3. In Newton TH, Hasso AN, Dillon WP (eds): Modern Neuroradiology: Computed Tomography of the Head and Neck. New York, Raven Press, 1988.
14. Doppman JL, Miller DL, Patronas NJ, et al: The diagnosis of acromegaly: value of inferior petrosal sinus sampling. AJR Am J Roentgenol 154:1075–1077, 1990.
15. Dowd CF, Halbach VV, Barnwell SL, et al: Particulate embolization of the anterior choroidal artery in the treatment of cerebral arteriovenous malformations. AJNR Am J Neuroradiol 12:1055–1061, 1991.
16. Dowd CF, Halbach VV, Higashida RT, et al: Diagnostic and therapeutic angiography. In Jackler RK, Brackmann DE (eds): Neurotology. St. Louis, Mosby, 1994.
17. Elliott PJ, Hayward NJ, Huff MR, et al: Unlocking the blood-brain barrier: a role for RMP-7 in brain tumor therapy. Exp Neurol 141:214–224, 1996.
18. Erba SM, Horton JA, Latchaw RE, et al: Balloon test occlusion of the internal carotid artery with stable xenon/CT cerebral blood flow imaging. AJNR Am J Neuroradiol 9:533–538, 1988.
19. Eskridge JM, McAuliffe W, Harris B, et al: Preoperative endovascular embolization of craniospinal hemangioblastomas. AJNR Am J Neuroradiol 17:525–531, 1996.
20. Gonzalez CF, Moret J: Balloon occlusion of the carotid artery prior to surgery for neck tumors. AJNR Am J Neuroradiol 11:649–652, 1990.
21. Gruber A, Killer M, Mazal P, et al: Preoperative embolization of intracranial meningiomas: a 17-year single center experience. Minim Invasive Neurosurg 43:18–29, 2000.
22. Gupta N, Jay V, Blaser S, et al: Choroid plexus papillomas and carcinomas, Vol 4. In Youmans JR (ed): Neurological Surgery, 4th ed. Philadelphia, WB Saunders, 1996.
23. Halbach VV, Hieshima GB, Higashida RT, et al: Endovascular therapy of head and neck tumors. In Vinuela F, Halbach VV, Dion JE (eds): Interventional Neuroradiology: Endovascular Therapy of the Central Nervous System. New York, Raven Press, 1992.
24. Hasso AH, Vignaud J, Bird CR: Pathology of the temporal bone and mastoid, Vol 3. In Newton TH, Hasso AH, Dillon WP (eds): Modern Neuroradiology: Computed Tomography of the Head and Neck. New York, Raven Press, 1988.
25. Hieshima GB, Everhart FR, Mehringer CM, et al: Preoperative embolization of meningiomas. Surg Neurol 14:119–127, 1980.
26. Jackson CG, Glasscock ME III, Harris PF: Glomus tumors: diagnosis, classification, and management of large lesions. Arch Otolaryngol 108:401–410, 1982.
27. Kai Y, Hamada J, Morioka M, et al: Appropriate interval between embolization and surgery in patients with meningioma. AJNR Am J Neuroradiol 23:139–142, 2002.
28. Kanter WR, Eldridge R, Fabricant R, et al: Central neurofibromatosis with bilateral acoustic neuroma: genetic, clinical and biochemical distinctions from peripheral neurofibromatosis. Neurology 30:851–859, 1980.
29. Kasantikul V, Netsky MG, Glasscock ME III, et al: Acoustic neurilemmoma. Clinicoanatomical study of 103 patients. J Neurosurg 52:28–35, 1980.
30. Lasjaunias P, Berenstein A: Surgical Neuroangiography, Vol. 2: Endovascular Treatment of Craniofacial Lesions. Berlin, Springer-Verlag, 1987.
31. Lo WW, Solti-Bohman LG, Lambert PR: High-resolution CT in the evaluation of glomus tumors of the temporal bone. Radiology 150:737–742, 1984.
32. Mamelak AN, Dowd CF, Tyrrell JB, et al: Venous angiography is needed to interpret inferior petrosal sinus and cavernous sinus sampling data for lateralizing adrenocorticotropin-secreting adenomas. J Clin Endocrinol Metab 81:475–481, 1996.
33. Manni A, Latshaw RF, Page R, et al: Simultaneous bilateral venous sampling for adrenocorticotropin in pituitary-dependent Cushing's disease: evidence for lateralization of pituitary venous drainage. J Clin endocrinol Metab 57:1070–1073, 1983.
34. McDermott MW, Wilson CB: Meningiomas, Vol 4. In Youmans JR (ed): Neurological Surgery, 4th ed. Philadelphia, WB Saunders, 1996.
35. Monsein LH, Jeffery PJ, van Heerden BB, et al: Assessing adequacy of collateral circulation during balloon test occlusion of the internal carotid artery with 99mTc-HMPAO SPECT. AJNR Am J Neuroradiol 12:1045–1051, 1991.

36. Oldfield EH, Doppman JL, Nieman LK, et al: Petrosal sinus sampling with and without corticotropin-releasing hormone for the differential diagnosis of Cushing's syndrome. N Engl J Med 325:897–905, 1991.

37. Osborn AG: Astrocytomas and other glial neoplasms. In Osborn AG (ed): Diagnostic Neuroradiology. St. Louis, Mosby, 1994.

38. Pencalet P, Sainte-Rose C, Lellouch-Tubiana A, et al: Papillomas and carcinomas of the choroid plexus in children. J Neurosurg 88:521–528, 1998.

39. Russell DS, Rubenstein LJ: Pathology of tumors of the nervous system, 5th ed. Baltimore, Williams & Wilkins, 1989.

40. Standard SC, Ahuja A, Livingston K, et al: Endovascular embolization and surgical excision for the treatment of cerebellar and brain stem hemangioblastomas. Surg Neurol 41:405–410, 1994.

41. Steed DL, Webster MW, DeVries EJ, et al: Clinical observations on the effect of carotid artery occlusion on cerebral blood flow mapped by xenon computed tomography and its correlation with carotid artery back pressure. J Vasc Surg 11:38–43; discussion 43–34, 1990.

42. Tampieri D, Leblanc R, TerBrugge K: Preoperative embolization of brain and spinal hemangioblastomas. Neurosurgery 33:502–505; discussion 505, 1993.

13

IMMUNOTHERAPY

James Waldron and Andrew T. Parsa

The scientific advances of the past decade have led to an extraordinary increase in our understanding of how the human body protects itself from invading microbes, abnormal cell growth, and macromolecules that exist outside the context of a normal functional role. As our overall understanding of immunity has grown, so has our perspective on the interactions between cancer and the immune system. Several key concepts have become clear: (1) The immune system is able to recognize tumor. (2) Antitumor immunity is often suppressed. (3) The potential exists to manipulate the immune response as a tool in the treatment of cancer. Together these concepts have fueled the development of a large number of strategies that utilize intrinsic immune mechanisms as therapeutic modalities.

The potential for immunotherapy is strikingly evident in the field of neuro-oncology, where the traditional therapeutic modalities of chemotherapy, surgery, and irradiation fail to yield satisfactory outcomes from many types of central nervous system (CNS) cancer and are often associated with substantial morbidity. Gliomas continue to newly afflict approximately 17,000 people each year, with an average survival measured in months despite therapy.[8] This demonstrated need for improved outcomes, combined with the morbidity-limiting specificity that is implicit in most immunotherapeutic strategies, makes immunotherapy highly attractive. This chapter provides a brief overview of immunology, reviews the basic underpinnings of tumor immunobiology, and describes the current strategies being pursued in the development of effective immunotherapy.

OVERVIEW

Immunity is the means by which the body is able to resist potentially harmful microbes, macromolecules, and unregulated cell growth that threaten its integrity. The process of immunity can be viewed as a series of generalized defenses, known as *innate immunity*, that lead to an extremely potent and threat-specific reaction known as *adaptive immunity*. Although innate and adaptive immunity function through different mechanisms of action, the two responses are complementary and highly interconnected. Adaptive immunity depends on antigen presentation and activation signals from the innate system to generate a full response. In turn, innate system effector cells, such as macrophages, require stimulation by the adaptive system to become fully activated.

Innate immunity consists of first-line barrier defenses, such as the skin and mucosal membranes, and an immediate response that is generated within hours of the detection of a threat. The immediate response is mediated by nonspecific immune cells, inflammatory cytokines, and blood-borne proteins such as complement. Neutrophils and macrophages phagocytize microbes and other foreign substances. Natural killer (NK) cells destroy aberrant cells by recognizing characteristic changes in a cell's surface that signal potential infection or transformation. Common to these effector cells is the ability to recognize dangerous cells and substances through pattern recognition receptors that bind molecules that signal potential danger, such as unmethylated CpG, lipopolysaccharide (LPS), and double-strand RNA. This pattern recognition provides an immediate broad-based specificity to target innate effector activity without requiring the slow development of the unique specificity found in the adaptive response. In many cases the initial innate response is sufficient to deal with the identified threat.

The adaptive response is based on the premise of distinguishing self from nonself. Its defining characteristic is the extreme degree of specificity of its response. A large pool of B and T lymphocytes, each with a receptor specific to a unique nonself antigen, continually circulates through the body and lymph system in a naïve state awaiting exposure to the appropriate antigen. Activation of the adaptive immune response is primarily mediated through T cells (i.e., B-cell activation requires T-cell support) and requires two signals: T-cell receptor binding to antigen presented on major histocompatibility complex (MHC) molecules and a co-stimulatory second signal. Two classes of MHC molecules exist. MHC I molecules are expressed on the surface of all nucleated cells and present peptides derived from the products of degradation of intracellular proteins to CD8+ T cells. MHC II molecules are expressed on the surface of antigen presenting cells (APCs), which process and present antigen originating outside the APC to CD4+ cells. APCs represent a crucial cross-link with innate immunity. The classic APC is the dendritic cell, which phagocytizes peptides in the periphery and then travels to the lymph nodes, where it presents peptides in the context of both MHC I and MHC II to the concentrated T cells. In addition to presenting antigen in the context of MHC molecules, APCs also provide the co-stimulatory second signal necessary for activation. This signal is generated by the binding of T-cell surface proteins, such as CD28, to B7-1 or B7-2 molecules that are up-regulated on APCs activated during an innate immune response. In the absence of a co-stimulatory signal from the APC, T cells do not differentiate into their activated form and can become tolerant of the antigen. The two signal systems serve as an efficient mechanism to guard against potential autoimmunity in the

CD 8 T-CELL STAINING OF
INTRACRANIAL TUMOR

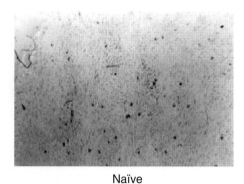

Naïve

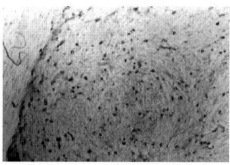

Immunized

FIGURE 13-1 CD8 T-cell infiltrate seen in Fischer rats with implanted 9L tumor after vaccination with a 9L tumor lysate. *Left*, Naïve animals; *right*, immunized animals.

instance that a T cell recognizes self antigen. After receiving the appropriate signals necessary for activation, T cells enter a phase of clonal proliferation that is further amplified by the autocrine and paracrine effects of cytokines such as interleukin 2 (IL-2) and interferon-gamma (IFN-gamma). During proliferation, T-cell effector forms emerge and mediate the effector response of adaptive immunity. The adaptive immunity effector response can be subdivided into two branches: humoral and cell-mediated immunity. One branch is favored over the other early in the response because of the local cytokine environment. The humoral response is mediated by Th2 helper cells with the support of IL-4, IL-5, and IL-10. Its primary mechanism of action is through antibodies that bind soluble and cell surface molecules and then induce phagocytosis or cell lysis through a number of pathways. These antigen-specific antibodies are secreted by plasma cells, a differentiated form of B cells. The cell-mediated response is mediated by Th1 helper cells, cytotoxic T cells (differentiated CD8+ cells), and macrophages with the support of IL2, IFN-gamma, and IL-12. Cytotoxic T cells induce cell lysis when they encounter nonself antigen in the context of MHC I on a cell's surface, effectively destroying cells expressing aberrant proteins. Simultaneously, the cell-mediated response activates the macrophages of the innate system through secretion of IFN-gamma, a potent macrophage stimulator. Once all nonself antigen has been cleared, the adaptive response self-limits with effector cells undergoing apoptosis, leaving only long-term memory cells to ensure the ability to rapidly react should the antigen be encountered again.

The CNS constitutes a unique immune environment. Historically the CNS has been viewed as an immunologically privileged environment as a result of early experiments in which allogeneic tissue transplanted into the CNS did not generate an immune response.[10] It was hypothesized that factors such as the presence of the blood-brain barrier and the absence of defined lymphatics led to this immunologically privileged environment. The current body of research supports a description of the CNS immune environment as one that is available to immunologic surveillance and the generation of an appropriate immune response to antigen, but with an overall climate that is biased against immune activity.[6] Basal levels of anti-inflammatory cytokines such as transforming growth factor (TGF)-β and low levels of leukocyte adhesion molecules on the blood-brain barrier mediate against the presence of a large immune cell population. However, activated T cells patrol through the CNS in their search for antigen, and when antigen is detected, mount an immune response in line with immune responses in the periphery. Although the brain lacks anatomic lymphatics, interstitial fluid has been shown to flow into the lymph system through the cribriform plate and trigger immune responses in the cervical lymph nodes.[7] Overall, despite a complex immunomodulatory environment, it is clear that immune response to antigen can occur in the CNS (Figure 13-1).

TUMOR IMMUNOBIOLOGY

The underlying principle of any immunotherapeutic strategy is the capability of the immune system to differentiate tumor from normal tissue and, once the tumor has been recognized as nonself, to mount an immune response. Several pieces of evidence support this capability. First, many tumors demonstrate the presence of an immune cell infiltrate (Figure 13-2). Although widely heterogeneous across tumor type, the presence of CD4+ T cells, CD8+ T cells, and other immune effector cells in the infiltrate has been documented by immunohistochemistry.[17] Isolation of tumor infiltrating lymphocytes (TILs) from a tumor specimen followed by stimulation in an in vitro system has demonstrated the ability of TILs to lyse tumor cells in a manner specific to the tumor cell population.[12] Together, the presence of an immune cell infiltrate and the demonstration of tumor-specific cell killing by cells isolated from the infiltrate strongly suggest the existence of an antigen-specific antitumor immune response. The existence of an antigen-specific antitumor immune response has been confirmed by the identification of a growing number of immunogenic tumor-associated antigens (TAAs) across a broad range of cancers. TAAs can arise from any protein expressed in the tumor cell and have their origin in the mutations and aberrant expression that accompany cell transformation. TAAs broadly fall into several groups: unique tumor antigens that are specific for a single tumor or tumor type (point mutations, Bcr and Abl translocations); shared tumor antigens that appear on a number of different tumor types but not in normal tissue (Ras mutations, p53 mutations, and melanoma-antigen [MAGE] genes);

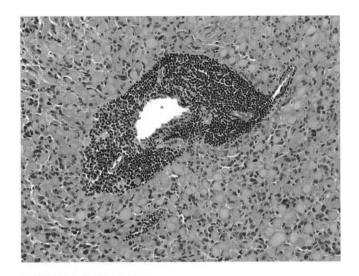

FIGURE 13-2 Inflammatory infiltrate seen in a gemistocytic glioma.

TABLE 13-1

Immune Escape Mechanisms

Failure of Antigen Presentation
Down regulation of MHC expression
Elimination of immunogenic antigens by tumor
Antigen expression level insufficient to generate a response
Heterogenicity of antigens across tumor cell population

Failure of the Immune Response
Lack of necessary costimulatory signals
T-cell tolerance/anergy toward tumor antigen
Active immunosupression via secreted or cell surface factors

MHC, Major histocompatibility complex.

and antigens that exist in normal tissues, but are overexpressed or inappropriately expressed in tumor populations.[1] TAAs identified to date for gliomas include matrix proteins such as tenascin and GP240 and a mutated form of the epidermal growth factor receptor (EGFR).

Within the context of antitumor immunity, the emergence of a tumor is a failure of the immune system on two fronts. As a first step, a tumor must avoid the initial mechanisms of immune surveillance. Immune surveillance is based on the hypothesis that circulating APCs and T cells will encounter, distinguish as nonself, and destroy cells expressing mutated proteins before the establishment of a tumor. A key step in this process is the ability of the APC to recognize the cell expressing mutant protein as a danger (Fuchs and Matzinger[4] have a detailed discussion of the danger hypothesis) and thereby become activated to present the antigen with the co-stimulatory signals that lead to T-cell activation. A failure by the APC to recognize the mutant protein as a danger leads to antigen presentation without the necessary co-stimulation. This has the potential to lead to T-cell tolerance and could form the basis for the establishment of a tumor. The second failure of the immune system is the generation of an ineffective response while the tumor is growing, continuing to produce antigenic mutations, and through its disruption of the local environment, creating an environment full of inflammatory signals. Mechanisms for tumor immune escape have been documented and are summarized in Table 13-1.

Gliomas are particularly well known for their immunosuppressive nature. Patients with gliomas often do not elicit delayed-type hypersensitivity reactions and demonstrate decreased responsiveness of peripherally derived T cells to nonspecific T-cell stimulants.[3] This response has been shown to normalize with tumor resection and then decline with tumor recurrence. TILs isolated from gliomas often exhibit aberrant phenotypes, and supernatants derived from glioma cell preparations have been shown to inhibit T-cell function in vitro.[3] This paints a picture of active immunosuppression via cell surface and secreted inhibitory molecules. The secretion of several inhibitory cytokines by gliomas has been documented, but none explains the observed widespread immunosuppression.[3] The immunosuppressive nature of gliomas represents a key hurdle that must be overcome in the development of effective immunotherapy.

APPROACHES

Current therapeutic modalities for brain tumors are able to achieve only modest improvements in long-term survival for many types of tumors. At the core of this is the fact that although surgery and irradiation are able to achieve significant cytoreduction in a cancer cell population, they are unable to effectively target cells that have migrated away from the primary tumor mass and are often associated with limiting side effects. The allure of immunotherapy lies in the ability of the immune system to address both of these issues by providing mechanisms that seek out tumor cells wherever they are located and generating a specific response with minimal side effects. Immunotherapeutic strategies include *active* and *passive* protocols.

Active immunotherapy attempts to up-regulate a potential immune response to a tumor. Examples include use of nonspecific immune stimulants such as inflammatory cytokines, immunization with tumor antigen, or more recently the use of dendritic cells. A key characteristic of active immunotherapy is that it can confer long-term immunity that mediates against a future recurrence. Passive immunotherapy involves the transfer of immune effectors to seek an immediate impact. Most passive strategies involve the use of tumor-specific antibodies or T cells that are activated against tumor. Unlike active strategies, passive immunotherapy is short lived and does not have the potential to generate long-term immunity.

Active Nonspecific Immunotherapy

The earliest attempts at immunotherapy were based on the concept that a generalized stimulation of the immune system might result in an increased immune response against tumor. To this end, nonspecific immune stimulants such as BCG (Bacille Calmette-Guérin) and toxoplasma were utilized with disappointing results.[2,9] The next evolution of nonspecific immunotherapy was the use of systemically and locally administered cytokines (IL-2, IFN-alpha, IFN-beta, IFN-gamma, tumor necrosis factor [TNF]-alpha, IL-4). IL-2 was found to be dose limited by cerebral edema, whereas the others failed to achieve a therapeutic response.[11]

Active Specific Immunotherapy: Tumor Vaccines

Tumor vaccine therapy is based on the premise that tumor antigen presented in the context of an adjuvant or other stimulatory immune signal may induce the immune system to generate an effective response against tumor. The main challenge of any active antitumor immunization strategy is to elicit an immune response against antigens to which the immune system is tolerant. A diverse set of vaccination strategies has been created in pursuit of this goal. The strategies fall into two main categories; those that immunize with an identified TAA and those that use either whole cells or components of whole cells. Tumor-specific antigen strategies include the use of purified antigenic peptide, whole proteins containing the antigenic peptide, and naked DNA that codes for the antigen, all administered in the context of a nonspecific adjuvant (e.g., Freund's incomplete adjuvant) or immunostimulatory cytokines such as GM-CSF (granulocyte-macrophage colony-stimulating factor). Whole-cell strategies seek to increase the innate immunogenicity of tumor cells through a variety of mechanisms (Figure 13-3). Examples include irradiation of tumor cells to increase expression of MHC I molecules, coadministration with adjuvant, and recent immunogene techniques in which cells are transfected with immunostimulatory cytokines or stimulatory cell-surface molecules (e.g., B7-1). Several very promising tumor vaccine strategies are in clinical trials for the treatment of melanoma (see Parmiani et al[14] for a review of cancer vaccines and a summary of trial results); however, to date, vaccine strategies for glioma have met with minimal success, although new immunogene techniques hold promise.[5]

Active Immunotherapy: Dendritic Cell Therapy

Dendritic cell therapy is a logical extension of the strategies developed for tumor vaccination. Whereas tumor vaccines seek to place tumor antigen in an immunostimulatory context designed to activate antigen uptake and presentation by APCs, dendritic cell therapy allows for the direct manipulation of the APC. Recent improvements in technique now allow for the isolation and in vitro expansion of dendritic cells in a manner practical for clinical application. One of the chief benefits of directly manipulating dendritic cells in vitro is that the cells can be activated and exposed to antigen in a precisely controlled environment that avoids any immunosuppressive influence that may exist in vivo. Once loaded with antigen and stimulated to an activated state, dendritic cells can then be readministered and mediate T-cell activation. Many different strategies are employed to deliver antigen and create an activated state. Dendritic cells have been loaded with antigenic peptide, tumor lysates, and apoptotic tumor cells; fused with tumor cells; transfected with the DNA or RNA of an antigenic peptide; and transfected with stimulatory cytokines in combination with peptide loading. As a group, these strategies generated preclinical

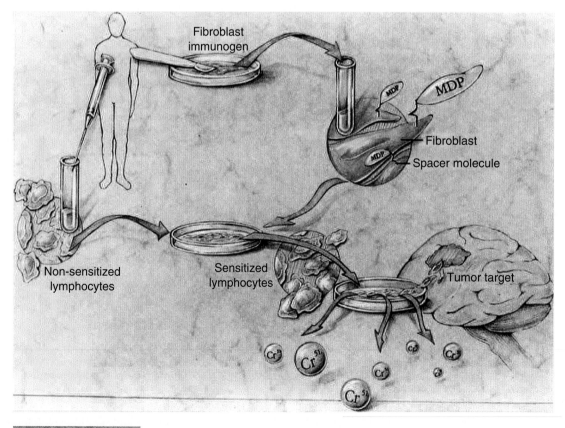

FIGURE 13-3 A model of adjuvant-linked autologous fibroblasts is shown for vaccination of patients against malignant glioma.

success in glioma and an assortment of other cancer models. Early clinical trials for melanoma have demonstrated encouraging results, but early glioma results have failed to demonstrate any benefit.[13,20]

Passive Immunotherapy: Antibody-Mediated Immunotherapy

Antibody-mediated immunotherapy is the use of monoclonal antibodies targeted against specific TAAs to mediate tumor cell destruction. Binding of antibody to a TAA can lead to cell death through the traditional pathways of phagocytosis or complement-mediated lysis or by serving as the delivery system for a tumoricidal compound conjugated to the antibody. A variety of tumoricidal compounds such as ricin and diphtheria toxin, radionuclides, and chemotherapeutic agents have been attempted. To date the most successful example of antibody-mediated immunotherapy is the monoclonal antibody against Her-2/Neu, a molecule that is highly expressed on some breast cancer tumors. The Her-2/Neu antibody has progressed from clinical trials and is now in widespread use. In patients with glioma, early clinical trials of ^{131}I-radiolabeled antibodies targeted against glioma-specific antigens such as tenascin have demonstrated minimal toxicity and improved survival. Recently reported phase II results by Reardon et al[16] of 33 patients with malignant glioma, who had ^{131}I-labeled antitenascin antibodies injected into the surgical resection cavity followed by external-beam radiation and a year of chemotherapy, yielded a mean survival of 86.7 weeks for all patients and 79.4 weeks for patients with glioblastoma multiforme (GBM).[16]

Passive Immunotherapy: Adoptive Transfer

Adoptive cellular transfer strategies are all derived from the concept that immune cells can be isolated from a patient with tumor, expanded in vitro, and then readministered to mediate a tumor-specific immune response. Early unsuccessful attempts at glioma therapy utilized autologous, nonactivated immune cells readministered at the tumor site.[19] Later strategies used lymphokine-activated killer (LAK) cells isolated from peripheral blood and nonspecifically activated with IL-2. LAK cell preparations are heterogeneous mixtures that contain a large proportion of NK cells that can lyse tumor cells in a non–antigen-specific manner. Clinical trials with LAK cells demonstrated mixed results with no clear clinical benefit.[18] The next generation of strategies has focused on inducing an antigen-specific immune response. To this end, two approaches have been explored. The first involves the harvest of tumor-infiltrating lymphocytes from surgically resected specimens and stimulating them in vitro with IL-2. Because of poor efficacy in animal models and technical difficulty, focus has switched to a second strategy in which the patient is immunized with irradiated tumor cells and adjuvant, and then lymphocytes are harvested from the draining lymph nodes, stimulated, and readministered. The most successful application of this strategy to date is a phase I trial conducted by Plautz et al.[15] In this trial, irradiated tumor cells were coadministered with GM-CSF and T cells harvested from the draining lymph nodes; activated and expanded in vitro with a bacterial superantigen, anti-CD3, and IL-2; and readministered peripherally to 10 patients with recurrent malignant gliomas. Of 10 patients, 3 demonstrated a partial response radiographically that lasted approximately 6 months in two patients and 13 months in the third. Given this evidence of response and lack of side effects, phase II trials with newly diagnosed patients with glioma are currently under way.

CONCLUSION

Immunotherapy holds a great deal of potential for the treatment of brain tumors and cancers of all types because of its ability to target tumor cells regardless of their location and the side-effect-limiting specificity of its response. In particular, immunotherapy seems a logical adjuvant to therapies such as surgery and chemotherapy that result in bulk cytoreduction but are unable to eliminate the last cell populations that lead to recurrence. The development of effective immunotherapy for brain tumors must overcome several hurdles, the most daunting of which is the active immunosuppression associated with gliomas. The immune strategies that have yielded the most success to date in patients with glioma have avoided this immunosuppression by utilizing effectors such as antibodies that are unresponsive to cytokines or by priming and activating immune cells in a controlled in vitro environment removed from in vivo immune suppression. Future strategies will benefit from an improved understanding of glioma-mediated immunosuppression.

References

1. Borrello IM, Sotomayor EM: Cancer vaccines for hematologic malignancies. Cancer Control 9:138–151, 2002.
2. Conley FK: Influence of chronic Toxoplasma infection on ethylnitrosourea-induced central nervous system tumors in rats. Cancer Res 40:1240–1244, 1980.
3. Dix AR, Brooks WH, Roszman TL, Morford LA: Immune defects observed in patients with primary malignant brain tumors. J Neuroimmunol 100:216–232, 1999.
4. Fuchs EJ, Matzinger P: Is cancer dangerous to the immune system? Semin Immunol 8:271–280, 1996.
5. Herrlinger U, Kramm CM, Johnston KM, et al: Vaccination for experimental gliomas using GM-CSF-transduced glioma cells. Cancer Gene Ther 4:345–352, 1997.
6. Hickey WF: Basic principles of immunological surveillance of the normal central nervous system. Glia 36:118–124, 2001.
7. Kida S, Weller RO, Zhang ET, et al: Anatomical pathways for lymphatic drainage of the brain and their pathological significance. Neuropathol Appl Neurobiol 21:181–184, 1995.
8. Landis SH, Murray T, Bolden S, Wingo PA: Cancer statistics, 1999. CA Cancer J Clin 49:8–31, 31, 1999.
9. Mahaley MS, Jr., Aronin PA, Michael AJ, Bigner D: Prevention of glioma induction in rats by simultaneous intracerebral inoculation of avian sarcoma virus plus bacillus Calmette-Guerin cell-wall preparation. Surg Neurol 19:453–455, 1983.
10. Medawar P: Immunity to homologous grafted skin: III. The fate of skin homografts transplanted to the brain, to subcutaneous

tissue, and to the anterior chamber of the eye. Br J Exp Pathol. 29:58–69, 1948.

11. Merchant RE, Ellison MD, Young HF: Immunotherapy for malignant glioma using human recombinant interleukin-2 and activated autologous lymphocytes. A review of pre-clinical and clinical investigations. J Neurooncol 8:173–188, 1990.

12. Miescher S, Whiteside TL, de Tribolet N, von Fliedner V: In situ characterization, clonogenic potential, and antitumor cytolytic activity of T lymphocytes infiltrating human brain cancers. J Neurosurg 68:438–448, 1988.

13. Nestle FO, Alijagic S, Gilliet M, et al: Vaccination of melanoma patients with peptide- or tumor lysate-pulsed dendritic cells. Nat Med 4:328–332, 1998.

14. Parmiani G, Castelli C, Dalerba P, et al: Cancer immunotherapy with peptide-based vaccines: what have we achieved? where are we going? J Natl Cancer Inst 94:805–818, 2002.

15. Plautz GE, Miller DW, Barnett GH, et al: T cell adoptive immunotherapy of newly diagnosed gliomas. Clin Cancer Res 6:2209–2218, 2000.

16. Reardon DA, Akabani G, Coleman RE, et al: Phase II trial of murine (131)I-labeled antitenascin monoclonal antibody 81C6 administered into surgically created resection cavities of patients with newly diagnosed malignant gliomas. J Clin Oncol 20:1389–1397, 2002.

17. Saito T, Tanaka R, Yoshida S, et al: Immunohistochemical analysis of tumor-infiltrating lymphocytes and major histocompatibility antigens in human gliomas and metastatic brain tumors. Surg Neurol 29:435–442, 1988.

18. Sankhla SK, Nadkarni JS, Bhagwati SN: Adoptive immunotherapy using lymphokine-activated killer (LAK) cells and interleukin-2 for recurrent malignant primary brain tumors. J Neurooncol 27:133–140, 1996.

19. Young H, Kaplan A, Regelson W: Immunotherapy with autologous white cell infusions ("lymphocytes") in the treatment of recurrrent glioblastoma multiforme: a preliminary report. Cancer 40:1037–1044, 1977.

20. Yu JS, Wheeler CJ, Zeltzer PM, et al: Vaccination of malignant glioma patients with peptide-pulsed dendritic cells elicits systemic cytotoxicity and intracranial T-cell infiltration. Cancer Res 61:842–847, 2001.

CHAPTER 14

GENE THERAPY FOR MALIGNANT GLIOMAS

Devin K. Binder

High-grade glial tumors, in particular anaplastic astrocytoma and glioblastoma multiforme (GBM), are the most common primary brain tumors in adults. Despite optimal current therapy, high-grade gliomas are associated with a poor prognosis. There is increasing hope that understanding the molecular derangements that give rise to these aggressive glial neoplasms may lead to targeted therapies. In particular, the identification of overlapping but recurring genetic alterations within gliomas[13,44,91] has led to the idea of gene therapy to reverse or "treat" these alterations. In this regard, a variety of promising preclinical findings in animal models have encouraged the development of gene therapy for gliomas in early clinical trials in humans.[1,11,76]

The term *gene therapy* comprises techniques aimed at delivering and expressing selected genetic material in cells and tissues of interest for therapeutic application.[9] There are three basic components of this therapeutic strategy: (1) expression of the gene or genetic material in the desired cell population (*vector strategy*); (2) selection of the gene or genetic material to be expressed (*transgene strategy*); and (3) delivery of the transgene-containing vector to the therapeutic target (*delivery strategy*). In this review, I discuss these three components and summarize current strategies in preclinical and clinical development for gene therapy of human gliomas.

VECTOR STRATEGIES

Viral vector gene therapy has been divided into two general strategies.[11] The first uses *replication-defective* viruses in which the viral genome has been altered to delete key viral genes involved in viral replication. In this approach, the virus cannot grow in cells but is used to deliver an anticancer transgene to effect tumor toxicity. Examples of this approach include retrovirus, adenovirus, adeno-associated virus (AAV), and herpes simplex virus type 1 (HSV-1). Advantages of this strategy include low toxicity and versatility of genetic construction. The primary potential disadvantage is a low volume of distribution in the tumor because of the viral inability to replicate.

An alternative strategy is the use of replication-competent viruses that are designed to selectively replicate in tumor cells but not in normal cells; these are also called *replication-selective* or *oncolytic* viruses. Examples include adenovirus, HSV-1, and reovirus.[11] The primary advantage is improved

volume of distribution in tumor. Disadvantages include potential toxicity, which may result from loss of selective replication, and higher immunogenicity.

Retroviral Vectors

Retroviruses are enveloped RNA viruses that possess the ability to integrate into the host cell genome by transcribing DNA from their RNA template via viral reverse transcriptase.[19] The transcribed viral DNA is then integrated into the host cell genome nonspecifically. There is relative specificity for tumors because, except for lentiviruses,[8] retroviral DNA preferentially integrates into the genome of dividing cells. Retroviral vectors have been derived from the Moloney murine leukemia virus (M-MuLV) established by Baltimore and colleagues.[51] The replication-defective retroviral vector is constructed as follows. DNA plasmid constructs containing long-terminal repeats (LTRs) and the packaging signal ψ together with the transgene of interest are transfected into modified cultured cells termed *vector-producer cells (VPCs)*. These VPCs, which are usually derived from the murine fibroblast 3T3 cell line, have been stably transfected with a plasmid with the entire retroviral genome, save the packaging signal ψ. Thus the VPCs are able to transcribe and translate viral RNA but are unable to package viral genomic RNA into virions. Nevertheless, they efficiently complement the plasmid construct (containing the packaging signal ψ), leading to packaging of the transgene of interest into virions, which can then be harvested from the medium of VPCs.

Advantages of retroviral vectors include (1) integration into dividing cells, which is particularly advantageous for tumor therapy, and (2) low toxicity because of replication deficiency. Disadvantages include (1) low transgene capacity, (2) the necessity of implanting transfected VPCs, which may not survive long in the host, and (3) a risk of insertional mutagenesis in host cells (e.g., by insertion at a proto-oncogene locus).

In the attempt to improve transduction efficiency, replication-competent retroviruses (RCRs) have recently been developed. RCRs are able to transduce human and rat glioma cell lines in vitro much more effectively than replication-defective retroviral vectors at the same dose.[90] In addition, RCRs capably and selectively transduce established U-87 gliomas in vivo.[90] To date, RCRs have not been used in clinical trials.

Adenoviral Vectors

Adenoviruses are nonenveloped DNA viruses associated with upper respiratory tract infections.[89] Subgroup C adenovirus is used for the construction of adenoviral vectors and usually causes a mild upper respiratory infection in immunocompetent hosts. Generation of adenoviral vectors is accomplished as follows. The transgene of interest is cloned into a plasmid and flanked by DNA homologous to adenoviral DNA sequences. Adenoviral DNA with E1 deleted—a gene needed for adenoviral growth in cells—is co-transfected with the transgene-containing plasmid into a cell line (e.g., 293 cells) engineered to express the E1 gene. Homologous recombination between the E1-deleted adenoviral DNA and the transgene-containing plasmid DNA creates a new replication-defective (because E1 has been deleted) adenoviral vector which is complemented by (i.e., can grow in) 293 cells expressing E1. The E1-deleted vector can then be harvested from cells and used to infect tumor cells in which it will express the transgene of interest but be unable to replicate.

Whereas some adenoviral vectors are replication-defective, others are replication-selective or "oncolytic." A potential advantage of replicative oncolytic viruses is that viral replication within infected tumor cells produces new viral progeny to infect additional cells within the tumor mass.[64] For example, one strategy is to produce an adenoviral vector with a deletion in the E1B region; because E1B inactivation of the tumor-suppressor gene p53 is necessary for viral replication, this restricts replication in this mutant to cells lacking p53.[5] This provides some tumor selectivity to viral replication, and could be useful in the subset of gliomas with p53 mutations.[26,44] Another strategy involves oncolytic adenoviruses that replicate selectively in cells with mutations in the p16 tumor-suppressor gene pathway.[25,33]

An important trend in the development of adenoviral vectors has been deletion of a portion of wild-type viral DNA (total 36 kb) to accommodate large amounts of foreign DNA (up to 10 kb).[21,43] Other than this high cloning capacity, important advantages to adenoviral vectors include (1) high viral titers, (2) high virion stability, unlike retroviruses, (3) broad host cell range, and (4) ability to infect both proliferating and quiescent cells.[43]

Disadvantages of adenoviral vectors include (1) virulence of wild-type virus and (2) immunogenicity.[2,50] "First-generation" adenoviral vectors have induced strong immune responses in the host as well as acute and chronic toxicity from the vector itself.[38,50] Aside from toxicity, one deleterious result of a robust host adaptive response is loss of vector genomes locally in the inflamed tissue. Progressive attenuation of the vectors and deletion of specific viral coding sequences will presumably mitigate these responses in future trials.[2,50]

Adeno-Associated Virus Vectors

AAV is a parvovirus that is nonpathogenic to human cells and incapable of autonomous replication without the presence of helper virus, usually adenovirus.[57,68] Recombinant adeno-associated virus (rAAV) vectors are replication-defective and can infect a broad host range of cells and tissues.

Advantages of rAAV vectors include (1) infection of both quiescent and proliferating cells, which is particularly impor-

tant for gene therapy directed at postmitotic neurons,[37] (2) lack of pathogenicity and immunogenicity,[55] and (3) site-specific integration.[21,43] Site-specific integration on human chromosome 19q is a unique feature of rAAV vectors and confers the ability of rAAV vectors to mediate long-term transgene expression in a variety of tissues.[21] Disadvantages of rAAV vectors include (1) low transgene capacity (4.7 kb) and (2) low titers.

Herpes Simplex Virus Type 1 Vectors

HSV-1 is an enveloped double-stranded DNA virus with a large genome (152 kb). Wild-type HSV-1 is neurotropic and can invade and replicate in both neurons and glial cells, resulting in a hemorrhagic necrotizing encephalitis (HSV-1 encephalitis).

As a gene therapy vector, advantages of HSV-1 include (1) high transgene capacity (30 kb, compared with approximately 8 kb in retroviral vectors, 10 kb in adenovirus vectors, and 4.7 kb in AAV vectors); (2) high titer; (3) high virion stability; (4) neurotropism; and (5) availability of a specific antiviral agent (ganciclovir).[11,53] In addition, unlike retroviral vectors, there is no risk of insertional mutagenesis, because the HSV-1 genome does not integrate but instead persists as an episome in the host cell cytoplasm. Disadvantages include (1) difficulty of genetic manipulation given a large viral genome, (2) preexisting immunity in the majority of humans (60% to 90%), which could stimulate host-immune response and limit transgene delivery, and (3) potential toxicity caused by virulence of wild-type virus.[11,53]

For glioma therapy, replication-selective (oncolytic) HSV-1 viruses have been constructed by deletion of various viral genes.[10,53] These include viral thymidine kinase, DNA polymerase, uracil DNA glycosylase, ribonucleotide reductase, and γ34.5. For example, the G207 virus carries deletions in both copies of γ34.5 (encoding a protein essential for viral replication in neurons) and a lacZ insertion in the U_L39 gene (viral ribonucleotide reductase).[53] This virus has been tested in a phase I clinical trial[54] (see later discussion).

Advances in Vector Design

Developments in vector design offer new avenues for exploration. For example, reovirus, a nonenveloped DNA virus that replicates selectively in cells with an activated Ras pathway,[12] has shown promise in preclinical animal models[60,93] and is being developed for human clinical trials.[11] In addition, advances in vector targeting include capsid modification for individual cell type targeting[7,30] and differential transduction by use of serotypes.[43]

TRANSGENE STRATEGIES

Transgene strategies have included (1) prodrug activation, (2) correction of genetic defects, and (3) provision of immune response-modifying genes.[1,11]

Prodrug Activation

The most common transgene strategy to date used in clinical trials of gene therapy for malignant gliomas is the herpes simplex virus–thymidine kinase (HSV-TK)/ganciclovir system.[11,42,52] Ganciclovir is an acyclic nucleoside analog that is clinically useful as an antiherpetic drug, because it has specificity for viral TK over human nucleoside kinase. Thus viral TK monophosphorylates ganciclovir, which is then dually phosphorylated to ganciclovir triphosphate by cellular kinases. Ganciclovir triphosphate binds viral better than human DNA polymerase and serves as a false substrate, leading to DNA chain termination and cellular toxicity.

For gene therapy, the most important observation is that transduction of glioma cells with HSV-TK increases their ganciclovir sensitivity 5000-fold.[82] Because it targets DNA, ganciclovir affects rapidly dividing cells such as tumor cells. In vivo efficacy in animal models was initially demonstrated by a dramatic increase in length of survival following intratumoral implantation of HSV-TK retroviral vectors and intraperitoneal ganciclovir in a rat gliosarcoma model.[14,15] This was subsequently confirmed by other investigators.[74]

The bystander effect of HSV-TK/ganciclovir has been crucial to its widespread application in cancer gene therapy. The bystander effect refers to the ability of ganciclovir to eradicate an entire population of tumor cells despite the expression of HSV-TK in only a fraction, often a minority, of cells.[24] This effect has been shown to require cell–cell contact. Because HSV-TK$^+$ cells contain mostly ganciclovir monophosphate and "bystander" HSV-TK$^-$ cells contain mostly ganciclovir triphosphate,[34] the bystander effect presumably involves transfer of ganciclovir triphosphate from HSV-TK$^+$ cells to HSV-TK$^-$ cells. The transfer is thought to occur across astrocyte–astrocyte gap junctions in gliomas,[3,22] and indeed the magnitude of the bystander effect correlates with the extent of gap junctional coupling.[23]

Other prodrug activation models are now in development, such as the cytosine deaminase/5-fluorocytosine (5-FC) system. 5-FC is a prodrug that is converted in vivo into 5-fluorouracil (5-FU) by cytosine deaminase (CD). 5-FU is a toxic chemotherapeutic agent that works primarily via chain termination and perturbation of DNA synthesis.[11] Adenovirus-mediated transfer of CD followed by systemic administration of 5-FC has led to improved survival in rodent glioma models.[18,56]

Correction of Genetic Defects

A distinct transgene approach has involved replacement of genes mutated in gliomas. P53 gene mutations are associated with a subset of glioblastomas, so-called secondary glioblastomas.[40,91] In preclinical studies, reintroduction of wild-type p53 has been associated with glioma growth inhibition in vitro and in vivo.[26,31,41,46,48] This result led to a phase I trial of adenovirus-mediated p53 gene therapy[45] (see later discussion).

Immune Response Modification

Another approach has involved transducing tumor cells with genes that will increase immunogenicity. This has commonly been accomplished with cytokine genes. Cytokines used for this purpose have included interleukin (IL)-2,[28] IL-4,[94] IL-12,[63] and interferon (IFN)-β,[58,66,84] and IFN-γ.[27] A significant potential problem with this approach is that significant toxicity as a consequence of cerebral edema has been associated with IL-2 and IFN-γ secretion.[85]

CLINICAL TRIALS OF GENE THERAPY FOR MALIGNANT GLIOMA

Based on the strategies and preclinical work just outlined, several clinical trials of gene therapy for malignant gliomas are under way or completed.

Retroviral HSV-TK Trials

The first study of gene therapy for brain tumors involved implantation of murine cells modified to produce a retroviral vector with an HSV-TK transgene into recurrent brain tumors.[78] Fifteen patients with brain tumors (12 with malignant gliomas, 3 with metastases) were studied. The results demonstrated survival of vector-producing cells (VPCs) at 7 days, but limited gene transfer into tumors; TK transcripts were identified in surviving VPCs but in less than 0.2% of neighboring tumor cells by in situ hybridization. Antitumor activity was observed in only five of the smaller tumors (1.4 ± 0.5 mL).[78]

In France a phase I and II study of gene therapy for recurrent glioblastoma was performed.[39] This trial involved 12 patients in whom HSV-TK VPCs were injected into the cavity margins following tumor resection. Seven days postoperatively, ganciclovir was administered for 14 days. An important result was that no treatment-related adverse events were reported. Median survival was 206 days, and 25% of the patients survived longer than 12 months. One patient survived for 3 years after gene therapy and ultimately died of disseminated breast cancer with no evidence of glioblastoma recurrence on postmortem analysis.[87]

Another phase I trial involved 12 children (ages 2 to 15) with recurrent tumors treated with VPCs carrying HSV-TK retroviral vectors, followed by ganciclovir treatment.[61] Again, no treatment-related adverse events were reported. Median time to disease progression was 3 months, with the three longest times to progression being 5, 10, and 24 months.

An international phase II trial conducted between 1997 and 1998 involved 48 patients with recurrent glioblastoma.[81] In this trial, retroviral VPCs were administered intracerebrally following tumor resection, and ganciclovir was infused intravenously 14 to 27 days after surgery. Median survival was 8.6 months, and the 12-month survival rate was 13/48 (27%). There was no evidence of tumor recurrence on magnetic resonance imaging (MRI) in seven of the patients for at least 6 months and in two patients for at least 12 months.

To further evaluate the rate of tumor cell transduction, immune response, and degree of antitumor effect, another study combined gene marking and a therapeutic trial in five patients.[32] In this study, two trials of intratumoral VPC implantation were separated by intermediate tumor harvest to assay TK protein, enzymatic activity, and immune response. Stereotactic biopsy sampling and intratumoral implantation with VPCs was performed; after 5 days, the tumor was resected, the cavity was reimplanted with VPCs, and ganciclovir was given. Four patients tolerated the treatment well but had tumor progression. One patient developed a lethal brain abscess after the second operation. Increased HSV-TK enzymatic activity was demonstrated in one tumor specimen, but immunohistochemical evidence of TK gene expression was limited to VPCs with no obvious tumor cell transduction. In addition, minimal immune response was seen.[32]

These uncontrolled trials indicated that HSV-TK gene therapy with retroviral VPCs was largely safe but was quite likely limited by poor viral transduction to tumor cells. Of course, efficacy could be established only by a phase III randomized clinical trial, which occurred between 1996 and 1998. In that study—the only phase III study of gene therapy for brain tumors published to date—patients with newly diagnosed and previously untreated GBM were divided into two groups of 124 patients each.[69] The control group received standard therapy (surgery and radiation therapy), and the gene therapy group received standard therapy plus adjuvant gene therapy during surgery. Following tumor resection, HSV-TK VPCs were manually implanted into the tumor bed via multiple injections, and ganciclovir was given intravenously from days 14 to 27. In the gene therapy group versus the control group, progression-free median survival was 180 days versus 183 days; median survival was 365 versus 354 days; and 12-month survival was 50% versus 55%. This trial demonstrated feasibility and safety, but lack of efficacy—again presumably because of poor tumor transduction. A separate immunophenotyping study of a subset of 13 patients from this study demonstrated a mild systemic immune response but no difference in numbers of tumor-infiltrating lymphocytes.[75]

A distinct retroviral vector in development is the pLIL-2-TK, which co-expresses the suicide gene HSV-TK and the immunomodulatory gene IL-2 in an attempt to amplify the antitumor effect. A pilot study has been reported of four patients with recurrent GBM who received stereotactic injection of retroviral VPCs. No treatment-related adverse effects were reported, and evidence of transgene expression in treated tumors is promising.[62]

Adenoviral HSV-TK Trials

Adenoviral HSV-TK vectors have also been studied in early clinical trials. Between 1996 and 1998, 13 patients with recurrent malignant brain tumors (nine with GBM, one with gliosarcoma, and three with anaplastic astrocytoma) were treated with intratumoral injection of between 2×10^9 and 2×10^{12} vector particles (VP) of a replication-defective adenoviral vector carrying HSV-TK followed by ganciclovir treatment.[86] At the highest dose (2×10^{12} VP), central nervous system (CNS) toxicity was manifested by confusion, hyponatremia, and seizures. Within 10 months after treatment, 10 of 13 patients died: 9 from tumor progression and 1 from sepsis. Two patients survived more than 25 months, and one was alive 29.2 months after treatment. Postmortem neuropathologic examination demonstrated variable inflammation within the residual tumors.[86]

In a similar trial from the Netherlands, performed between 1998 and 2001, 14 patients with recurrent high-grade gliomas were treated with a replication-defective adenoviral vector carrying HSV-TK followed by ganciclovir treatment.[83] The vector was injected intraoperatively into the tumor bed following resection. Although there were no treatment-related adverse effects in this study, all patients had recurrence or progression, with an overall median survival of 4 months following treatment.

A phase I and II trial conducted in Finland between 1998 and 1999 directly compared retroviral with adenoviral vector-mediated delivery of the HSV-TK transgene.[80] This study involved two experimental groups—retroviral vector treatment in seven patients and adenoviral vector treatment in seven patients—and a control group of seven patients receiving *Escherichia coli* β-galactosidase marker vector treatment.[65] Adverse effects included fever in two patients with adenoviral vector therapy and an increase in seizure frequency in two patients. In the group treated with retroviral vector, all patients showed progression on MRI by 3 months, whereas three of the seven patients treated with adenoviral vectors did not. Mean survival times for retroviral, adenoviral, and control groups were 7.4, 15, and 8.3 months, respectively. On the basis of this comparison, the authors speculated that adenoviral vectors may be therapeutically advantageous, considering their greater titer and ability to infect nonreplicating cells.

Oncolytic HSV-1 Trials

The third virus used in clinical trials for glioma is oncolytic (replication-selective) HSV-1. Two phase I trials have been reported.[54,79] In a Scottish study,[79] nine patients with recurrent high-grade gliomas (eight with GBM, one with anaplastic astrocytoma) were treated with intratumoral inoculation of 1716, a γ34.5 mutant oncolytic HSV-1. No treatment-related adverse effects were documented. Of the nine patients, four were alive and well 14 to 24 months after 1716 administration.

In a trial performed in the United States,[54] 21 patients with recurrent malignant glioma were treated with intratumoral inoculation of G207, an HSV-1 double mutant for γ 34.5 and ribonucleotide reductase (see previous discussion).[53] No toxicity or serious adverse effects could be unequivocally ascribed to viral inoculation, and no patient developed HSV encephalitis. Four of twenty-one patients were alive at the time the results were published. The most encouraging result was that examination of tissue from re-resections demonstrated expression of HSV-1 and the *lacZ* reporter gene in two patients at 56 and 157 days after inoculation.

Other Trials

Many new clinical trials of novel vectors and transgenes for glioma therapy are open and in various stages of development.[9,11] For example, two new transgene strategies focus on the introduction of immunomodulatory genes or genetic correction with p53. A phase I trial using a recombinant adenovirus that expresses human IFN-b is under way at the University of Pennsylvania.[20] The primary goal of that study is to examine toxicity of intratumoral injection of the vector in patients with recurrent or progressive malignant glioma; other goals include obtaining evidence of gene transfer in resected tissue specimens and clinical or biologic response.

A phase I trial of adenovirus-mediated p53 gene therapy has recently been reported.[45] In this multicenter study, 15 patients with recurrent malignant glioma were enrolled for a two-stage treatment. In the first stage, a replication-defective E1-deleted adenoviral vector carrying p53 (Ad-p53) was stereotactically injected as a single bolus into the tumor by using an implanted catheter. In the second stage, the tumor and catheter were resected en bloc 3 days later, and the resection cavity treated again with Ad-p53. The intratumoral injection of Ad-p53 led to minimal toxicity and resulted in p53 gene transfer and p53 protein expression. However, this study also demonstrated that Ad-p53 did not penetrate far from the injection site.[45]

DELIVERY STRATEGIES

One point made clear by preclinical and early clinical trials of gene therapy for gliomas is the importance of delivery strategy,[73] the goal being optimal delivery of the transgene-containing vector to as many tumor cells as possible. So far, as described above, clinical studies of gene therapy for glioma have used direct injection of the vector into the tumor or tumor bed.[1,11]

One possibility is to optimize infusion into the tumor or tumor bed. Freehand injection of VPCs is inaccurate and offers little control of injection parameters. Other problems include tissue disruption from forceful injection and injectate reflux along the needle tract.[67] Novel strategies involving stereotactic needle guidance and mechanical control over VPC infusion and needle withdrawal may improve tumor saturation.[67]

Convection-enhanced drug delivery (CEDD) may optimize the delivery of infusate into a defined tissue volume. Developed by Oldfield and colleagues,[6,49] CEDD overcomes the limitations of simple diffusion by adjusting the infusion parameters to induce bulk flow in the interstitial space, thereby distributing macromolecules into brain interstitium centimeters instead of millimeters from the infusion site. Drug distribution can be controlled by varying infusion volume or rate. In recent important work, Bankiewicz and colleagues[4,16,59] have demonstrated the efficacy of CEDD to deliver rAAV vectors to CNS parenchyma in rats and monkeys.

Two clinical trials using CEDD have been reported. First, Oldfield and colleagues[47] used CEDD to administer transferrin-CRM107, a conjugate of transferrin and a mutant diphtheria toxin, to 15 patients with malignant glioma. At least 50% reduction in tumor volume occurred in 9 of 15 patients.[47] Second, a clinical trial using CEDD for intratumoral administration of IL-4 *Pseudomonas* exotoxin (NBI-3001) for patients with recurrent malignant glioma has recently been reported.[92] In that study, 31 patients received various doses of NBI-3001 administered via CEDD; safety and toxicity evaluations were performed, but the volume of drug distribution is unclear.

Another delivery approach is intra-arterial vector infusion combined with blood brain–barrier disruption. One study in a 9L gliosarcoma rat model used intra-arterial delivery of HSV-1 vector and bradykinin-induced blood brain–barrier disruption.[77] Delivery of HSV-1 into 9L gliosarcoma cells was enhanced by intracarotid bradykinin. A follow-up study demonstrated that intra-arterial infusion of an attenuated HSV-1 vector followed by blood brain–barrier disruption and systemic ganciclovir administration led to regression of established tumors.[70] Adenoviruses have also demonstrated promise when administered using this approach.[72]

A distinct delivery strategy is nonviral DNA delivery via liposome-gene complexes. Potential advantages of cationic liposomes include (1) uncomplicated preparation, (2) minimal safety requirements, (3) ability to complex a large amount of DNA, (4) lack of immunogenicity, and (5) greater stability.[29,88] Liposome systems deliver DNA to the cytoplasm of cells by plasma membrane fusion and endocytosis. Liposome-mediated HSV-TK gene transfer led to decrease in tumor volume and tumor regression in an experimental F98 glioma model.[95] In another study, cationic liposome-plasmid DNA complexes showed increased efficacy but reduced specificity of gene transfer following intra-arterial delivery compared with adenovirus vectors.[72] A phase I and II trial of cationic liposome-HSV-TK treatment in patients with recurrent malignant gliomas is under way.[88]

Yet another possibility is the use of lipophilic prodrugs. Prodrugs, such as ganciclovir or 5-FC, must be efficient and selective substrates for the activating enzyme and must be metabolized to potent cytotoxins. Lipophilicity of the prodrug determines blood brain–barrier penetration, and furthermore the lipophilicity of the activated prodrug is pivotal in determining bystander effects.[17] For example, ganciclovir triphosphate is highly polar, cannot diffuse across cell membranes, and therefore requires intercellular gap junctions for its bystander toxicity (see previous discussion). In principle, lipophilic prodrugs could better penetrate the blood-brain barrier and in their activated forms could cause a tumor-killing bystander effect without requiring cell–cell contact.[71]

Whereas a full discussion of the advantages and disadvantages of these macroscopic delivery methods is beyond the scope of this chapter, refinement of vector delivery is clearly critical to optimizing vector-target interaction.

THE FUTURE

Despite a great deal of development, gene therapy for brain tumors is still at an early stage.[11,76] Completed clinical trials demonstrate the overall safety of the approach, but also show limited efficacy due largely to poor tumor transduction. A combination of advances in vector design and creative transgene approaches, together with optimized macroscopic delivery systems, should improve therapeutic efficacy and minimize toxicity. Molecular imaging techniques using marker substrates will also be important to track transgene expression in tissue noninvasively.[35,36] Combination therapies may help to target the many distinct genetic alterations known to exist within glial tumors, and could in principle be tailored to the molecular signature of individual lesions. Significant parallel progress in all of these areas should foster ongoing interest in further translational clinical trials of novel gene therapy for gliomas.

References

1. Alavi JB, Eck SL: Gene therapy for high grade gliomas. Expert Opin Biol Ther 1:239–252, 2001.
2. Amalfitano A, Parks RJ: Separating fact from fiction: assessing the potential of modified adenovirus vectors for use in human gene therapy. Curr Gene Ther 2:111–133, 2002.
3. Asklund T, Appelskog IB, Ammerpohl O, et al: Gap junction-mediated bystander effect in primary cultures of human malignant gliomas with recombinant expression of the HSVtk gene. Exp Cell Res 284:185–195, 2003.
4. Bankiewicz KS, Eberling JL, Kohutnicka M, et al: Convection-enhanced delivery of AAV vector in parkinsonian monkeys: in vivo detection of gene expression and restoration of dopaminergic function using pro-drug approach. Exp Neurol 164:2–14, 2000.

5. Bischoff JR, Kirn DH, Williams A, et al: An adenovirus mutant that replicates selectively in p53-deficient human tumor cells. Science 274:373–376, 1996.
6. Bobo RH, Laske DW, Akbasak A, et al: Convection-enhanced delivery of macromolecules in the brain. Proc Natl Acad Sci USA 91:2076–2080, 1994.
7. Buning H, Ried MU, Perabo L, et al: Receptor targeting of adeno-associated virus vectors. Gene Ther 10:1142–1151, 2003.
8. Chang LJ, Gay EE: The molecular genetics of lentiviral vectors: current and future perspectives. Curr Gene Ther 1:237–251, 2001.
9. Chiocca EA: Gene therapy: a primer for neurosurgeons. Neurosurgery 53:364–373, 2003.
10. Chiocca EA: Oncolytic viruses. Nat Rev Cancer 2:938–950, 2002.
11. Chiocca EA, Aghi M, Fulci G: Viral therapy for glioblastoma. Cancer J 9:167–179, 2003.
12. Coffey MC, Strong JE, Forsyth PA, et al: Reovirus therapy of tumors with activated Ras pathway. Science 282:1332–1334, 1998.
13. Collins VP: Genetic alterations in gliomas. J Neurooncol 24:37–38, 1995.
14. Culver KW, Ram Z, Wallbridge S, et al: In vivo gene transfer with retroviral vector-producer cells for treatment of experimental brain tumors. Science 256:1550–1552, 1992.
15. Culver KW, Van Gilder J, Link CJ, et al: Gene therapy for the treatment of malignant brain tumors with in vivo tumor transduction with the herpes simplex thymidine kinase gene/ganciclovir system. Hum Gene Ther 5:343–379, 1994.
16. Cunningham J, Oiwa Y, Nagy D, et al: Distribution of AAV-TK following intracranial convection-enhanced delivery into rats. Cell Transplant 9:585–594, 2000.
17. Denny WA: Prodrugs for gene-directed enzyme-prodrug therapy (suicide gene therapy). J Biomed Biotechnol 2003:48–70, 2003.
18. Dong Y, Wen P, Manome Y, et al: In vivo replication-deficient adenovirus vector-mediated transduction of the cytosine deaminase gene sensitizes glioma cells to 5-fluorocytosine. Hum Gene Ther 7:713–720, 1996.
19. Dornburg R: The history and principles of retroviral vectors. Front Biosci 8:818–835, 2003.
20. Eck SL, Alavi JB, Judy K, et al: Treatment of recurrent or progressive malignant glioma with a recombinant adenovirus expressing human interferon-beta (H5.010CMVhIFN-beta): a phase I trial. Hum Gene Ther 12:97–113, 2001.
21. Einfeld DA, Roelvink PW: Advances towards targetable adenovirus vectors for gene therapy. Curr Opin Mol Ther 4:444–451, 2002.
22. Estin D, Li M, Spray D, et al: Connexins are expressed in primary brain tumors and enhance the bystander effect in gene therapy. Neurosurgery 44:361–368; discussion 368–369, 1999.
23. Fick J, Barker FG, Dazin P, et al: The extent of heterocellular communication mediated by gap junctions is predictive of bystander tumor cytotoxicity in vitro. Proc Natl Acad Sci USA 92:11071–11075, 1995.
24. Freeman SM, Abboud CN, Whartenby KA: The "bystander effect": tumor regression when a fraction of the tumor mass is genetically modified. Cancer Res 53:5274–5283, 1993.
25. Fueyo J, Alemany R, Gomez-Manzano C, et al: Preclinical characterization of the antiglioma activity of a tropism-enhanced adenovirus targeted to the retinoblastoma pathway. J Natl Cancer Inst 95:652–660, 2003.
26. Fulci G, Ishii N, Van Meir EG: p53 and brain tumors: from gene mutations to gene therapy. Brain Pathol 8:599–613, 1998.
27. Gansbacher B, Bannerji R, Daniels B, et al: Retroviral vector-mediated gamma-interferon gene transfer into tumor cells generates potent and long lasting antitumor immunity. Cancer Res 50:7820–7825, 1990.
28. Gansbacher B, Zier K, Daniels B, et al: Interleukin 2 gene transfer into tumor cells abrogates tumorigenicity and induces protective immunity. J Exp Med 172:1217–1224, 1990.
29. Gao X, Huang L: Cationic liposome-mediated gene transfer. Gene Ther 2:710–722, 1995.
30. Girod A, Ried M, Wobus C, et al: Genetic capsid modifications allow efficient re-targeting of adeno-associated virus type 2. Nat Med 5:1052–1056, 1999.
31. Gomez-Manzano C, Fueyo J, Kyritsis AP, et al: Adenovirus-mediated transfer of the p53 gene produces rapid and generalized death of human glioma cells via apoptosis. Cancer Res 56:694–699, 1996.
32. Harsh GR, Deisboeck TS, Louis DN, et al: Thymidine kinase activation of ganciclovir in recurrent malignant gliomas: a gene-marking and neuropathological study. J Neurosurg 92:804–811, 2000.
33. Heise C, Hermiston T, Johnson L, et al: An adenovirus E1A mutant that demonstrates potent and selective systemic antitumoral efficacy. Nat Med 6:1134–1139, 2000.
34. Ishii-Morita H, Agbaria R, Mullen CA, et al: Mechanism of 'bystander effect' killing in the herpes simplex thymidine kinase gene therapy model of cancer treatment. Gene Ther 4:244–251, 1997.
35. Jacobs A, Voges J, Reszka R, et al: Positron-emission tomography of vector-mediated gene expression in gene therapy for gliomas. Lancet 358:727–729, 2001.
36. Jacobs AH, Winkeler A, Hartung M, et al: Improved herpes simplex virus type 1 amplicon vectors for proportional coexpression of positron emission tomography marker and therapeutic genes. Hum Gene Ther 14:277–297, 2003.
37. Janson CG, McPhee SW, Leone P, et al: Viral-based gene transfer to the mammalian CNS for functional genomic studies. Trends Neurosci 24:706–712, 2001.
38. Kielian T, Hickey WF: Inflammatory thoughts about glioma gene therapy. Nat Med 5:1237–1238, 1999.
39. Klatzmann D, Valéry CA, Bensimon G, et al: A phase I/II study of herpes simplex virus type 1 thymidine kinase "suicide" gene therapy for recurrent glioblastoma. Hum Gene Ther 9:2595–2604, 1998.
40. Kleihues P, Ohgaki H: Primary and secondary glioblastomas: from concept to clinical diagnosis. Neurooncol 1:44–51, 1999.
41. Kock H, Harris MP, Anderson SC, et al: Adenovirus-mediated p53 gene transfer suppresses growth of human glioblastoma cells in vitro and in vivo. Int J Cancer 67:808–815, 1996.
42. Kramm CM, Sena-Esteves M, Barnett FH, et al: Gene therapy for brain tumors. Brain Pathol 5:345–381, 1995.
43. Lai CM, Lai YK, Rakoczy PE: Adenovirus and adeno-associated virus vectors. DNA Cell Biol 21:895–913, 2002.
44. Lang F, Miller D, Koslow M, et al: Pathways leading to glioblastoma multiforme: a molecular analysis of genetic alterations in 65 astrocytic tumors. J Neurosurg 81:427–435, 1994.
45. Lang FF, Bruner JM, Fuller GN, et al: Phase I trial of adenovirus-mediated p53 gene therapy for recurrent glioma: biological and clinical results. J Clin Oncol 21:2508–2518, 2003.
46. Lang FF, Yung WK, Sawaya R, et al: Adenovirus-mediated p53 gene therapy for human gliomas. Neurosurgery 45:1093–1104, 1999.
47. Laske DW, Youle RJ, Oldfield EH: Tumor regression with regional distribution of the targeted toxin TF-CRM107 in patients with malignant brain tumors. Nat Med 3:1362–1368, 1997.
48. Li H, Alonso-Vanegas M, Colicos MA, et al: Intracerebral adenovirus-mediated p53 tumor suppressor gene therapy for experimental human glioma. Clin Cancer Res 5:637–642, 1999.
49. Lieberman DM, Laske DW, Morrison PF, et al: Convection-enhanced distribution of large molecules in gray matter during interstitial drug infusion. J Neurosurg 82:1021–1029, 1995.
50. Liu Q, Muruve DA: Molecular basis of the inflammatory response to adenovirus vectors. Gene Ther 10:935–940, 2003.
51. Mann R, Mulligan RC, Baltimore D: Construction of a retrovirus packaging mutant and its use to produce helper-free defective retrovirus. Cell 33:153–159, 1983.

52. Maria BL, Friedman T: Gene therapy for pediatric brain tumors. Semin Pediatr Neurol 4:333–339, 1997.

53. Markert JM, Gillespie GY, Weichselbaum RR, et al: Genetically engineered HSV in the treatment of glioma: a review. Rev Med Virol 10:17–30, 2000.

54. Markert JM, Medlock MD, Rabkin SD, et al: Conditionally replicating herpes simplex virus mutant, G207 for the treatment of malignant glioma: results of a phase I trial. Gene Ther 7:867–874, 2000.

55. Mastakov MY, Baer K, Symes CW, et al: Immunological aspects of recombinant adeno-associated virus delivery to the mammalian brain. J Virol 76:8446–8454, 2002.

56. Miller CR, Williams CR, Buchsbaum DJ, et al: Intratumoral 5-fluorouracil produced by cytosine deaminase/5-fluorocytosine gene therapy is effective for experimental human glioblastomas. Cancer Res 62:773–780, 2002.

57. Monahan PE, Samulski RJ: Adeno-associated virus vectors for gene therapy: more pros than cons? Mol Med Today 6:443–440, 2000.

58. Natsume A, Tsujimura K, Mizuno M, et al: IFN-beta gene therapy induces systemic antitumor immunity against malignant glioma. J Neurooncol 47:117–124, 2000.

59. Nguyen JB, Sanchez-Pernaute R, Cunningham J, et al: Convection-enhanced delivery of AAV-2 combined with heparin increases TK gene transfer in the rat brain. Neuroreport 12:1961–1964, 2001.

60. Norman KL, Coffey MC, Hirasawa K, et al: Reovirus oncolysis of human breast cancer. Hum Gene Ther 13:641–652, 2002.

61. Packer RJ, Raffel C, Villablanca JG, et al: Treatment of progressive or recurrent pediatric malignant supratentorial brain tumors with herpes simplex virus thymidine kinase gene vector-producer cells followed by intravenous ganciclovir administration. J Neurosurg 92:249–254, 2000.

62. Palù G, Cavaggioni A, Calvi P, et al: Gene therapy of glioblastoma multiforme via combined expression of suicide and cytokine genes: a pilot study in humans. Gene Ther 6:330–337, 1999.

63. Parker JN, Gillespie GY, Love CE, et al: Engineered herpes simplex virus expressing IL-12 in the treatment of experimental murine brain tumors. Proc Natl Acad Sci USA 97:2208–2213, 2000.

64. Post DE, Khuri FR, Simons JW, et al: Replicative oncolytic adenoviruses in multimodal cancer regimens. Hum Gene Ther 14:933–946, 2003.

65. Puumalainen A-M, Vapalahti M, Agrawal RS, et al: ß-galactosidase gene transfer to human malignant glioma in vivo using replication-deficient retroviruses and adenoviruses. Hum Gene Ther 9:1769–1774, 1998.

66. Qin XQ, Tao N, Dergay A, et al: Interferon-beta gene therapy inhibits tumor formation and causes regression of established tumors in immune-deficient mice. Proc Natl Acad Sci USA 95:14411–14416, 1998.

67. Qureshi NH, Bankiewicz KS, Louis DN, et al: Multicolumn infusion of gene therapy cells into human brain tumors: technical report. Neurosurgery 46:663–668, 2000.

68. Rabinowitz JE, Samulski RJ: Building a better vector: the manipulation of AAV virions. Virology 278:301–308, 2000.

69. Rainov NG: A phase III clinical evaluation of herpes simplex virus type 1 thymidine kinase and ganciclovir gene therapy as an adjuvant to surgical resection and radiation in adults with previously untreated glioblastoma multiforme. Hum Gene Ther 11:2389–2401, 2000.

70. Rainov NG, Dobberstein KU, Heidecke V, et al: Long-term survival in a rodent brain tumor model by bradykinin-enhanced intra-arterial delivery of a therapeutic herpes simplex virus vector. Cancer Gene Ther 5:158–162, 1998.

71. Rainov NG, Dobberstein KU, Sena-Esteves M, et al: New prodrug activation gene therapy for cancer using cytochrome P450 4B1 and 2-aminoanthracene/4-ipomeanol. Hum Gene Ther 9:1261–1273, 1998.

72. Rainov NG, Ikeda K, Qureshi NH, et al: Intraarterial delivery of adenovirus vectors and liposome-DNA complexes to experimental brain neoplasms. Hum Gene Ther 10:311–318, 1999.

73. Rainov NG, Kramm CM: Vector delivery methods and targeting strategies for gene therapy of brain tumors. Curr Gene Ther 1:367–383, 2001.

74. Rainov NG, Kramm CM, Aboody-Guterman K, et al: Retrovirus-mediated gene therapy of experimental brain neoplasms using the herpes simplex virus-thymidine kinase/ganciclovir paradigm. Cancer Gene Ther 3:99–106, 1996.

75. Rainov NG, Kramm CM, Banning U, et al: Immune response induced by retrovirus-mediated HSV-tk/GCV pharmacogene therapy in patients with glioblastoma multiforme. Gene Ther 7:1853–1858, 2000.

76. Rainov NG, Ren H: Gene therapy for human malignant brain tumors. Cancer J 9:180–188, 2003.

77. Rainov NG, Zimmer C, Chase M, et al: Selective uptake of viral and monocrystalline particles delivered intra-arterially to experimental brain neoplasms. Hum Gene Ther 6:1543–1552, 1995.

78. Ram Z, Culver KW, Oshiro EM, et al: Therapy of malignant brain tumors by intratumoral implantation of retroviral vector-producing cells. Nat Med 3:1354–1361, 1997.

79. Rampling R, Cruickshank G, Papanastassiou V, et al: Toxicity evaluation of replication-competent herpes simplex virus (ICP 34.5 null mutant 1716) in patients with recurrent malignant glioma. Gene Ther 7:859–866, 2000.

80. Sandmair AM, Loimas S, Puranen P, et al: Thymidine kinase gene therapy for human malignant glioma, using replication-deficient retroviruses or adenoviruses. Hum Gene Ther 11:2197–2205, 2000.

81. Shand N, Weber F, Mariani L, et al: A phase 1–2 clinical trial of gene therapy for recurrent glioblastoma multiforme by tumor transduction with the herpes simplex thymidine kinase gene followed by ganciclovir. Hum Gene Ther 10:2325–2335, 1999.

82. Shewach DS, Zerbe LK, Hughes TL, et al: Enhanced cytotoxicity of antiviral drugs mediated by adenovirus directed transfer of the herpes simplex virus thymidine kinase gene in rat glioma cells. Cancer Gene Ther 1:107–112, 1994.

83. Smitt PS, Driesse M, Wolbers J, et al: Treatment of relapsed malignant glioma with an adenoviral vector containing the herpes simplex thymidine kinase gene followed by ganciclovir. Mol Ther 7:851–858, 2003.

84. Tada H, Maron DJ, Choi EA, et al: Systemic IFN-beta gene therapy results in long-term survival in mice with established colorectal liver metastases. J Clin Invest 108:83–95, 2001.

85. Tjuvajev J, Gansbacher B, Desai R, et al: RG-2 glioma growth attenuation and severe brain edema caused by local production of interleukin-2 and interferon-gamma. Cancer Res 55:1902–1910, 1995.

86. Trask TW, Trask RP, Aguilar-Cordova E, et al: Phase I study of adenoviral delivery of the HSV-tk gene and ganciclovir administration in patients with recurrent malignant brain tumors. Mol Ther 1:195–203, 2000.

87. Valéry CA, Seilhean D, Boyer O, et al: Long-term survival after gene therapy for a recurrent glioblastoma. Neurology 58:1109–1112, 2002.

88. Voges J, Weber F, Reszka R, et al: Liposomal gene therapy with the herpes simplex thymidine kinase gene/ganciclovir system for the treatment of glioblastoma multiforme. Hum Gene Ther 13:675–685, 2002.

89. Wadell G: Molecular epidemiology of human adenoviruses. Curr Top Microbiol Immunol 110:191–220, 1984.

90. Wang WJ, Tai CK, Kasahara N, et al: Highly efficient and tumor-restricted gene transfer to malignant gliomas by replication-competent retroviral vectors. Hum Gene Ther 14:117–127, 2003.

91. Ware ML, Berger MS, Binder DK: Molecular biology of glioma tumorigenesis. Histol Histopathol 18:207–216, 2003.

92. Weber F, Asher A, Bucholz R, et al: Safety, tolerability, and tumor response of IL4-Pseudomonas exotoxin (NBI-3001) in patients with recurrent malignant glioma. J Neurooncol 64:125–137, 2003.

93. Wilcox ME, Yang W, Senger D, et al: Reovirus as an oncolytic agent against experimental human malignant gliomas. J Natl Cancer Inst 93:903–912, 2001.

94. Yu JS, Wei MX, Chiocca EA, et al: Treatment of glioma by engineered interleukin 4-secreting cells. Cancer Res 53:3125–3128, 1993.

95. Zhu J, Zhang L, Hanisch UK, et al: A continuous intracerebral gene delivery system for in vivo liposome-mediated gene therapy. Gene Ther 3:472–476, 1996.

CHAPTER 15

FUNCTIONAL OUTCOMES

Christina A. Meyers

SYMPTOM CLUSTERS THAT AFFECT QUALITY OF FUNCTIONAL OUTCOMES

Patients with brain tumors experience a number of adverse symptoms that negatively affect their ability to function in usual work, leisure, and social roles. These include cognitive impairment, neurologic signs and symptoms, fatigue, mood disturbance, sleep disturbance, and sexual dysfunction. These symptoms occur in a majority of patients on active therapy, and occasionally are the first symptoms that herald the initial diagnosis. In addition, these symptoms often persist after treatment is discontinued. Most patients who have a brain tumor experience cognitive impairment, including restricted working memory capacity (e.g., how much information the person can process "on-line"), distractibility, and problems multitasking. They often experience generalized slowing and must exert increased effort when performing even routine activities. In addition, many patients experience fatigue related to their disease and treatment that compounds cognitive impairment. This fatigue is an unusual, persistent tiredness that is not relieved by rest, and thus has pervasive effects on the person's ability to function. A recent study at The University of Texas M. D. Anderson Cancer Center indicated that more than 40% of outpatients receiving chemotherapy for non–brain cancer experienced severe fatigue, resulting in significant impairment of their daily function.[2] Fatigue can be so distressing for patients during and after cancer therapy that it is a principal reason they stop treatment. The cluster of cognitive dysfunction, fatigue, and mood disturbance is extremely common.

More than half of long-term survivors of glioma develop significant cognitive impairments and severe short-term memory deficits. There are a number of pathophysiologic mechanisms by which brain tumor treatments injure the brain, including vascular and immunologic mechanisms. There are in addition neurochemical and neurotransmitter changes that underlie the development of neurocognitive deficits. Neurochemical changes in the brains of glioma patients distant from treatment-induced white matter changes have been demonstrated by magnetic resonance spectroscopic (MRS) imaging.[19] This study showed a loss of choline in areas with normal-appearing white matter, reflecting membrane damage at sites remote from the tumor and radiation. The degree to which the changes in the neurochemical makeup of the brain distant from the original site of the tumor affect brain function is poorly understood.

Cognitive function and fatigue may also be caused by other factors. For instance, both are associated with anemia and are improved by normalization of hemoglobin. Preliminary evidence indicates that cognitive dysfunction and fatigue may also be associated with fluctuations in inflammatory cytokines,[6] the production of which is either promoted or inhibited by various agents used to treat cancer (see Treatment-Specific Factors below).

Cognitive impairment and other symptoms also cause significant distress in non–brain cancer patients. Cognitive function studies performed with untreated cancer patients suggest that memory, motor dexterity, and executive functions (frontal subcortical components) tend to be impaired concurrently, whereas attention, reasoning, and psychomotor speed are not. Working memory (the ability to process information and do multiple tasks) is often impaired, whereas hippocampal components of memory (retention and consolidation) are not. Cognitive impairment that develops in chronic myelogenous leukemia patients receiving IFN-α appears not to correlate with depression, suggesting that immunotherapy-induced depression and cognitive dysfunction could be mediated by different mechanisms.[14]

There are numerous sources that contribute to the manifestation of distressing symptoms in brain tumor patients, including tumor effects, treatment effects, host factors, and factors unrelated to the diagnosis of brain tumor.[13] Brain tumor treatment is truly successful only if these adverse symptoms are managed, and symptom assessment guidelines are now being introduced as part of routine patient care. However, successful management of these symptoms is often hampered by a lack of knowledge about the mechanisms, and thus improved knowledge may lead to targeted, more successful intervention strategies.

Disease-Specific Factors

The site of the brain tumor will be a major determinant of the type of cognitive symptoms patients experience, following well-established brain–behavior relationships. However, because many brain tumors grow insidiously and are infiltrative rather than destructive, many patients experience milder and more variable cognitive deficits than what would be predicted by site alone. Now that functional neuroimaging is becoming more commonly used for presurgical planning, it is apparent that a significant proportion of patients have some alterations in the usual pattern of cerebral localization of function, suggesting that cerebral plasticity and reorganization of function, to some degree, is more prevalent than previously thought. Lesion momentum, the speed at which tumors grow, is a significant factor in the presentation of cognitive deficits. For instance, a patient with a secondary glioblastoma that developed from a lower grade tumor over time may have fewer cognitive problems than a person with a primary glioblastoma that became rapidly symptomatic.

Patient-Specific Factors

Age of the patient is a long-known determinant of functional outcome, with older individuals being more at risk regardless of the histopathology of the tumor. There is very little known about the effect of other demographic characteristics, such as race and sex of the patient. However, there is evidence that some individuals are more vulnerable to the neurotoxic effects of treatment regardless of age and other demographic variables. Thus patients with similar characteristics and treatment factors may have very different outcomes (e.g., the development of rampant radiation necrosis). Assessment of possible risk factors, including potentially vulnerable genotypes, is currently under way, but none has been identified as of yet.

Medical complications also contribute to functional outcome. In addition to the effects of primary brain tumor treatment, adjuvant medications may also cause cognitive and mood disturbance. Steroid therapy, which is ubiquitous in this population of patients, can independently contribute to memory loss and psychiatric symptoms. Such medications as antiemetics and pain medications may also contribute to the patient's overall functional status. Patients with brain tumor often have medical complications, such as seizures, that further compromise brain function and have a negative impact on the person's social function, ability to drive, and so on. Brain tumor patients may also have co-existing neurologic or psychiatric illness, such as learning disabilities, cerebrovascular disease, or bipolar illness. Reactive mood and adjustment disorders may also contribute to cognitive impairment; a patient who is depressed and preoccupied with his or her situation may exhibit attentional problems.

Treatment-Specific Factors

Radiation therapy to the brain is widely known to cause injury to white matter and cognitive impairments related to frontal-subcortical dysfunction. It also causes significant fatigue; in fact, cancer patients receiving radiation therapy to non-CNS sites (e.g., prostate or breast cancer) also experience fatigue during treatment that is centrally mediated. Induction of inflammatory cytokines, disruption of the hypothalamic-pituitary-adrenal axis, and alterations of neurotransmitters have been implicated in radiation-induced fatigue and cognitive impairment.

Chemotherapy can also cause additional functional impairments; patients often refer to their experience as "chemobrain." The effects appear to vary somewhat depending on the agent administered, but little is known about the actual side-effect profile of most agents other than through self-report and quality of life questionnaires, neither of which capture all significant symptoms. Although most cognitive effects tend to be diffuse and reversible off treatment, some agents may cause specific cognitive effects related to their mechanism of action.

Immunotherapy is increasingly being utilized in brain tumor treatment. Interferon-alpha (IFN-α), in particular, can cause significant cognitive impairments and organic mood disturbance. Several physiologic mechanisms have been proposed for the neurotoxic effects of IFN-α, including actions mediated through neuroendocrine, neurotransmitter, and cytokine pathways.[14] Inductions of other inflammatory cytokines, such as interleukin-1β (IL-1β), tumor necrosis factor-α (TNF-α), and IL-6, are major mechanisms of immunotherapy neurotoxicity. IL-1 and its receptors are found in many areas of the brain. IL-1 mRNA is found in abundance in the hippocampus, a critical structure for memory processes. IL-1 depresses the influx of calcium into hippocampal neurons, which may explain the preponderance of memory impairment in patients with immunotherapy toxicity. TNF is also neurotoxic and is associated with demyelination in the brain. TNF and IL-1 are synergistically toxic and are associated with the development of multiple sclerosis plaques and gliosis.[3] Patients with Alzheimer's disease have elevated levels of IL-6. In addition to their direct effects on brain function, these cytokines also provoke a stress hormone cascade that can affect mood and cognition, as well as having discrete effects on brain neurotransmitter systems.[6] Patients with IFN-α neurotoxicity have been reported to exhibit mild to moderate symptoms of frontal-subcortical brain dysfunction, including cognitive and behavioral slowing, apathy, impaired executive functions, and decreased memory. The cognitive and behavioral symptoms of chronic IFN-α administration have been compared with those of Parkinson's disease.

The use of hormonal agents, such as Tamoxifen, can also cause cognitive impairment. Estrogen receptors have been found in many brain regions, including the hypothalamus and hippocampus. Animal studies have indicated several mechanisms by which estrogen affects memory, including increasing cholinergic activity, maintaining dendritic spine density in certain cells of the hippocampus, and facilitating long-term potentiation in the hippocampus, which is crucial to memory encoding. Tamoxifen also stimulates the induction of inflammatory cytokines, including IL-1 and IL-6, which have profound effects on brain function, as mentioned earlier.

FUNCTIONAL IMPAIRMENTS

The cognitive and functional impairments that patients with brain tumor experience have a profound effect on their daily life. They often have difficulty multitasking and become easily overwhelmed when more than one thing is happening at a time. They may be easily distracted and lose track of their train of thought. Because of generalized slowing, they may miss points in conversation and have difficulty keeping deadlines at work. In general, all tasks require increased effort, including tasks that were previously performed automatically. The lack of any "auto pilot" contributes to fatigue, as well.

The impact of these symptoms on a patient's function is related to a number of individual factors, including the patient's developmental stage in life and the type and pace of his or her normal work and leisure activities. The impact of neurocognitive and neurologic symptoms will vary; patients who are working parents will have many more functional problems than patients who are retired and can take activities at their own pace. Thus a specific impairment of brain function, which may cause similar disabilities in terms of cognitive performance, will cause vastly different degrees of handicap. Interventions for these impairments will by necessity be highly individualized; there is no "one size fits all" treatment of distressing cancer-related symptoms.

ENHANCING FUNCTIONAL OUTCOMES

Medical Interventions

Correction of underlying medical conditions may be overlooked when the focus is on cancer treatment. Yet many medical conditions that are relatively easy to handle may contribute to impaired function. Correction of borderline anemia, for instance, can greatly enhance quality of life even though the situation may not be medically serious. In addition, many brain tumor patients have deficient endocrine function following treatment. Correction of thyroid and other hormonal abnormalities can improve cognitive function, libido, mood, and overall quality of life.

Pharmacologic Interventions

Pharmacologic interventions may be extremely helpful in improving a patient's function and general well-being. Clinicians often use psychostimulants to treat the declines in cognitive and emotional functioning that are so ubiquitous among brain tumor patients. Psychostimulants are effective, in part, because they counter the effects that tumor and treatment produce on the monoamine pathways of the frontal-brainstem reticular system. Methylphenidate, dextroamphetamine, and pemoline have each been reported to ameliorate depression and fatigue in cancer patients. In the brain tumor population, only methylphenidate, in immediate release form, has been investigated as a possible treatment for declines in neurocognitive functioning (i.e., neurobehavioral slowing and impairments in attention and working memory). For example, in children with acute lymphoblastic leukemia and malignant brain tumors, treatment with methylphenidate was shown to improve sustained attention.[17] In adult patients with brain tumors, methylphenidate treatment was successful in treating the concentration difficulties related to the side effects of irradiation or chemotherapy.[20] Recently, a phase I trial (single treatment group, open label, dose-escalating design) demonstrated that treatment with methylphenidate improved cognition, mood, and some areas of functioning in 30 patients with malignant glioma.[8] The treatment effect was observed at a relatively low dose of 10 mg twice daily. Improvements in cognitive functioning and mood occurred despite progressive disease (23%) and worsening radiation injury (27%). In addition, no patient experienced increased seizure activity. Further, the dose and schedule can easily be titrated for a paticular individual.

Although methylphenidate has relatively transient and minimal side effects, the drug may be contraindicated for some and, in such cases, clinicians may defer to alternative pharmacologic treatments. Modafinil, a novel vigilance-promoting drug, has also been used by clinicians to treat cancer-related impairments in cognitive functioning but has not been formally investigated for this purpose in this population. Modafinil is used to treat the excessive daytime sleepiness (EDS) that is associated with narcolepsy and idiopathic hypersomnia.[9]

Agents used to treat other neurologic illnesses, such as Alzheimer's disease, are also being investigated. For instance, donepezil inhibits centrally active acetylcholinesterase, which is responsible for hydrolysis of acetylcholine (Ach). This may result in increased concentrations of Ach available for synaptic transmission and has been found useful in the treatment of patients with Alzheimer's disease, in whom choliner-gic deficiency contributes to memory loss and other cognitive deficits. Ach deficiency may play more of a role than is appreciated in brain tumor patients who have neurocognitive impairments, and it may serve as a target for attempts to improve cognitive function.

Targeted pharmacologic therapy against specific mechanisms of toxicity is currently being piloted. For instance, radiation therapy may induce release of inflammatory cytokines that cause more widespread brain injury. Cytokine antagonists such as the recombinant soluble human TNF receptor (p75)-Fc fusion protein (etanercept) have been used successfully to treat TNF-α-mediated diseases, including rheumatoid arthritis, Crohn's disease, and psoriasis. One study found a significant improvement in symptoms related to myelofibrosis with myeloid metaplasia (MMM), another TNF-α-mediated disease that causes night sweats, severe fatigue, fever, and weight loss. Although objective responses (e.g., increased hemoglobin, transfusion independence) occurred in only 20% of patients treated with etanercept, 60% percent of the patients had improved constitutional symptoms, including cessation of night sweats, weight gain, and improved energy.[16]

Anti-inflammatory agents may also be helpful in treating symptoms. The most common pharmacologic agents used to antagonize sickness behaviors in animals are the nonsteroidal anti-inflammatory drugs (NSAIDs), which include aspirin, acetaminophen, ibuprofen, and selective COX inhibitors. These agents are being investigated for their antineoplastic properties;[12] close monitoring of cognitive function and symptoms during these trials may also shed light on their ability to attenuate symptoms.

Neuroprotective agents, although still awaited in the future, represent an exciting area of potential intervention. Agents such as erythropoietin (EPO) may reduce the generalized brain injury caused by brain tumor treatment. In animal studies, it has been shown that EPO crosses the blood-brain barrier and is neuroprotective if given before 24 hours and up to 6 hours after experimental brain injury resulting from induced focal brain ischemia/hypoxia and stroke, trauma, excessive neuronal excitation, and immune mediated inflammation.[1] No data on clinical applicability of EPO as a neuroprotective agent in humans are yet available. There are, however, many studies in humans of the beneficial effect of EPO on functional outcomes relative to its role in treating anemia. The specific components of quality of life that showed improvements included energy level, activity level, and daily activities.[5] In addition, a number of psychophysiologic studies have reported improvements in evoked potentials in patients following EPO treatment. Specifically, increases in amplitude and decreases in latency of the P300 component were noted. The reported changes in electrophysiologic parameters on late components of the evoked potential indicate an effect on the central components of neurobehavioral functioning and may be reflected in improvements in working memory and processing speed.[11]

Behavioral Interventions

Formal rehabilitation, including physical therapy, occupational therapy, cognitive rehabilitation, and vocational rehabilitation are underutilized in the population of patients with brain tumor. Health care providers and families may believe that such strategies lack benefit for patients who have a poor prognosis. However, formal rehabilitation has the potential to allow patients with brain tumor to function at the highest level possible for the longest time possible and has been shown to be cost effective.[15]

There are a number of behavioral strategies that can also enhance functional outcome in brain tumor patients. There is a growing literature about the positive effects of exercise on cancer-related symptoms.[4] Behavioral interventions such as relaxation therapy and self-hypnosis may be very useful as well. Such strategies can alleviate symptoms such as pain, nausea, and fatigue and help patients relax and focus when they feel overwhelmed. Life-style alterations may also be useful. For instance a person with increased distractibility may be able to maintain employment given reasonable accommodations, such as flexibility of deadlines and a quieter work environment. Students may be able to continue in school if allowed to tape lectures and to take tests without time constraints.

CONCLUSION

The assessment and treatment of symptoms experienced by patients with brain tumor adds an important dimension to overall patient care. Furthermore, the objective assessment and documentation of cognitive deficits could lead to the implementation of measures to protect patients from the adverse effects of disease or treatment on cognitive functioning. Such general measures have included (e.g., in the case of interferon-associated neurotoxicity) stimulant therapy for fatigue and neurobehavioral slowing, opiate antagonist therapy for cognitive deficits, and antidepressant therapy for mood disturbance.[18] If specific relationships can be established between cognitive deficits and increased cytokine levels or decreased activity in specific neuronal circuits, anti-cytokine therapy (e.g., the recently available TNF antagonists) or pharmacologic agents (e.g., dopamine agonists) to improve functional outcome can be implemented. In addition, antineoplastic therapies that improve cognitive function or slow expected cognitive deterioration would add a great deal to the benefits versus the risks of new treatments. For example, a recent study found delayed time to neurocognitive progression in patients with brain metastases from non–small-cell lung cancer treated with a radiosensitizer in addition to whole brain irradiation, as compared with those receiving whole brain radiation therapy alone,[7] and it is likely that more such studies will be performed to supplement survival as an outcome. The development of interventions to improve functional outcome has been deemed a research priority in the report of the Brain Tumor Progress Review Group co-sponsored by the National Cancer Institute and the National Institute of Neurological Disorders and Stroke.[10]

References

1. Cerami A, Brines ML, Ghezzi P, Cerami CJ: Effects of epoetin alfa on the central nervous system. Semin Oncol 28:66–70, 2001.
2. Cleeland CS, Mendoza TR, Wang XS, et al: Assessing symptom distress in cancer: the M. D. Anderson symptom inventory. Cancer 89:1634–1646, 2000.
3. Dantzer R, Wollman EE, Yirmiya R: Cytokines and depression: an update. Brain Behav Immun 16:501–502, 2002.
4. Dimeo F: Radiotherapy-related fatigue and exercise for cancer patients: a review of the literature and suggestions for future research. Front Radiat Ther Oncol 37:49–56, 2002.
5. Gabrilove JL, Cleeland CS, Livingston RB, et al: Clinical evaluation of once-weekly dosing of epoetin alfa in chemotherapy patients: improvements in hemoglobin and quality of life are similar to three-times-weekly dosing. J Clin Oncol 19:2875–2882, 2001.
6. Larson S, Dunn AJ: Behavioral effects of cytokines. Brain Behav Immun 15:371–387, 2001.
7. Meyers CA, Smith JA, Bezjak A, et al: Neurocognitive function and progression in patients with brain metastases treated with whole-brain radiation and motexafin gadolinium: results of a randomized phase III trial. J Clin Oncol 22:157–165, 2004.
8. Meyers CA, Weitzner MA, Valentine AD, Levin VA: Methylphenidate therapy improves cognition, mood, and function of brain tumor patients. J Clin Oncol 16:2522–2527, 1998.
9. Mitler MM, Harsh J, Hirshkowitz M, Guilleminault C: Long-term efficacy and safety of modafinil (Provigil®) for the treatment of excessive daytime sleepiness associated with narcolepsy. Sleep Medicine 1:231–243, 2000.
10. National Cancer Institute, National Institute of Neurological Disorders and Stroke (November, 2000): Report of the Brain Tumor Progress Review Group. Available at http://osp.nci.nih.gov/Prg_assess/PRG/BTPRG.
11. Nissenson AR: Epoetin and cognitive function. Am J Kidney Dis 20:21–24, 1992.
12. Raz A: Is inhibition of cyclooxygenase required for the antitumorigenic effects of nonsteroidal, anti-inflammatory drugs (NSAIDs)? In vitro versus in vivo results and the relevance for the prevention and treatment of cancer. Biochem Pharmacol 63:343–347, 2002.
13. Scheibel RS, Meyers CA, Levin VA: Cognitive dysfunction following surgery for intracerebral glioma: influence of histopathology, lesion location, and treatment. J Neurooncol 30:61–69, 1996.
14. Scheibel, RS, Valentine AD, O'Brien S, Meyers CA: Cognitive dysfunction and depression during treatment with interferon-alpha and chemotherapy. J Neuropsychiatry Clin Neurosci 16:1–7, 2004.
15. Sherer M, Meyers CA, Bergloff P: Efficacy of post acute brain injury rehabilitation for patients with primary malignant brain tumors. Cancer 80:250–257, 1997.
16. Steensma DP, Mesa RA, Li CY, Gray L, Tefferi A. Etanercept, a soluble tumor necrosis factor receptor, palliates constitutional symptoms in patients with myelofibrosis with myeloid metaplasia: results of a pilot study. Blood 99:2252–2254, 2002.
17. Thompson SJ, Leigh L, Christensen R, et al: Immediate neurocognitive effects of methylphenidate on learning-impaired survivors of childhood cancer. J Clin Oncol 19: 1802–1808, 2001.
18. Valentine AD, Meyers CA, Kling MA, et al: Mood and cognitive side effects of interferon-alpha therapy. Sem Oncol 25(suppl 1):39–47, 1998.
19. Virta A, Patronas N, Raman R, et al: Spectroscopic imaging of radiation-induced effects in the white matter of glioma patients. Magn Reson Imaging 18:851–857, 2000.
20. Weitzner MA, Meyers CA, Valentine AD: Methylphenidate in the treatment of neurobehavioral slowing associated with cancer and cancer treatment. J Neuropsychiatry Clin Neurosci 7:347–350, 1995.

CHAPTER 16

CLINICAL TRIALS

Susan M. Chang and Kathleen R. Lamborn

The clinical outcome for patients with primary brain tumors, especially high-grade glioma, remains poor. As more understanding of the complex processes of oncogenesis, growth, and invasion of central nervous system (CNS) tumors is acquired, the hope is that this will translate into the development of novel therapeutic strategies that will improve outcome. Before a new therapy is used in patients, much work is done preclinically to try to determine the mechanism of activity and the relevance of the therapy in the treatment of malignancy and to establish the toxicity in animal studies.

Once the preclinical work has been completed, clinical trials—experiments in human subjects—are conducted. The design and conduct of these clinical trials are the critical component for evaluating these new therapies. Clinical trials are used to evaluate the safety, effectiveness, and benefit of new therapies. These new therapies could be novel single agents or treatment combinations. The systematic evaluation of new treatments prevents widespread use of ineffective, potentially toxic therapies. The overall goal of clinical trials is to identify effective new therapies, to avoid the inappropriate use of scarce resources, and to protect future patients from unnecessary morbidity by the determination of appropriate expectations of therapies.

Clinical trials are scientific experiments. They require the formal structure of an experiment, including a well-defined question in a specified patient population, prospective planning, and controlled conditions. This planning is all the more important because those included in the experiments are patients, and it is critical to assure that the information provided will directly address the therapeutic question being posed. The results of these experiments are used to reach conclusions about the therapy. In general, the types of clinical therapeutic trials can be described as phase I, II, or III. In all these phases, a specific question is posed, clear objectives are defined, outcome measures are determined, and statistical rigor is incorporated.

Regardless of protocol phase, important components of any clinical trial need to be addressed[7] (Table 16-1). The scientific rationale and background for the study should be outlined in the introduction to the protocol. Information on the mechanism of action, preclinical data to support the study, as well as any clinical data that may be relevant should be outlined. The objectives of the study, including the primary and secondary end points, should be listed. Patients' eligibility criteria should be described. Relevant information includes age range, tumor type, tumor stage, prior allowed therapies, organ function parameters, performance status, medical status, and informed consent. The treatment plan and design, including follow-up evaluations, both clinical and laboratory based, also

need to be specified. Drug information that includes the chemical formulation and mode of administration, as well as toxicity information, should be provided. How toxicities will be assessed and addressed also needs to be incorporated. The criteria for evaluation of the appropriate endpoints and statistical considerations have to be defined. A justification of the sample size and methodology of the analysis of the data should be provided. Reasons for study discontinuation and any early stopping rules should be clear. A data safety monitoring plan should be outlined, and the regulatory documents and consent form must be included. Overall, the clinical trial should be feasible, important, novel, ethical, and relevant. In the following sections, we review the basic principles of different types of cancer clinical trials (Table 16-2).

PHASE I CANCER TRIALS

Phase I studies have the primary objective of establishing a phase II dose.[15] For cytotoxic agents, the phase II dose is assumed to be the maximally tolerated dose (MTD) based on dose-limiting toxicities (DLTs). For some phase I cancer studies, the selection of patients may be important. Although patients with refractory disease are often included, the important factor is normal organ function. In some instances, patients who have previously been heavily pretreated with other agents may be excluded for fear of underestimating the MTD. The design of the phase I trial depends on the nature of the therapy.[1] The most common is a phase I study of a new cytotoxic agent where, as noted previously, the goal is to find an MTD. The classic design for such a study starts with a low dose that is not expected to cause any serious adverse side effects. Usually this dose is determined as one tenth of the median lethal dose, expressed as milligrams per meter squared of body surface area, in the most sensitive species tested in preclinical work. The dose is then escalated among cohorts of patients according to prespecified increments with the assumption that "more drug will equal more effect" and that the mechanisms of action of the toxic and therapeutic effects are the same. Patients are assessed for toxicities, usually based on the National Cancer Institute Common Toxicity Criteria, and the decision to escalate depends on the tolerance at the dose levels. A common escalation plan is to treat three patients at a certain level. If there are no DLTs in these three patients, the dose is escalated for the next cohort. If the incidence of DLT is one third, the cohort is expanded to a maximum of six patients. If no further DLTs are seen, the dose is escalated. Otherwise, dose escalation stops. If the incidence of DLT is greater than one third at a given level, dose escalation also stops. The phase II dose is taken as the highest dose for which the incidence is less than 33%. Usually, at least six patients are treated at the recommended dose. The dose levels are commonly based on the modified Fibonacci series[11] (Table 16-3). Although there is no scientific rationale for choosing this scheme, experience has shown that it is safe and reasonably effective. Other escalation designs have been proposed with the goal of more quickly and accurately defining the MTD and decreasing the number of patients treated at less than the MTD. These include the accelerated titration design and the continual reassessment method. A summary of these alternative techniques is presented by O'Quigley et al.[8]

Most phase I studies have corollary pharmacokinetic and pharmacodynamic studies associated with them. For the brain tumor patient population, it has been important to characterize the pharmacologic interaction of the experimental agent with known agents that alter the hepatic metabolism of drugs. These agents include some anticonvulsants and corticosteroids. Because of hepatic enzyme induction by these agents, some chemotherapeutic agents may have accelerated metabolism, and thereby decreased concentrations may be achieved in the serum, resulting in lower efficacy. A different toxicity profile may also be noted at higher doses. It is important therefore that for new agents metabolized through the hepatic enzyme systems, patients be stratified in phase I studies based on whether they are receiving enzyme-inducing agents.

More novel, cytostatic agents are now being evaluated in clinical trials.[4] These targeted therapies include growth-factor inhibitors such as epidermal growth factor inhibitors, antiangiogenic agents, and anti-invasive agents. Because these have specific biologic activity, classic phase I designs for cytotoxic agents may not be appropriate.[2] These agents are expected to have a lower toxicity profile than standard cytotoxics, and the toxic effects may be produced through different mechanisms than the therapeutic effect. Instead of determining the MTD, the more relevant end point for these agents is the optimal biologically effective dose of the agent. Indeed, sometimes the MTD may not be the most effective dose. This has been seen in immune modulatory agents where there may be a narrow window of therapeutic efficacy below and above which the agent may not exhibit its desired effect on tumor growth. The difficulty is determining an appropriate measure of biologic effectiveness. Because these agents are targeted to specific abnormalities within the tumor, selection of patients based on the presence of these abnormalities is of relevance. Ideally, measurement of the target and the subsequent effects of the agent following administration would best define the optimal biologically effective dose. Determining the effect on the tumor is best done by repeated samples of the tumor both before and following therapy. This is particularly difficult for patients with brain tumors.

There are definite limitations to what is known about toxicity of a therapy at the end of phase I studies. Relatively few patients will have received treatment, leaving the possibility for substantial undetected toxicities. Also, because phase I studies normally utilize a dose-escalation scheme based on immediate toxicity, they do not adequately address long-term toxicities. This is particularly problematic for cytostatic therapies. These therapies tend to be administered in chronic dosing and may be given in conjunction with radiation or other cytotoxic agents. It is unlikely that studies in the future will enroll larger numbers of patients or follow patients for longer periods before starting clinical trials for efficacy (phase II). Therefore careful monitoring for safety and early-stopping rules for unexpected toxicity need to be incorporated in these trials, as discussed later.

PHASE II CANCER TRIALS

Once a therapeutic dose has been determined, the next step in evaluation of a treatment is to determine if there is evidence of efficacy. Although response to therapy can be described in a phase I study, this is not the primary objective. Also, phase I trials tend to be performed in patients with refractory cancers of various types, so the determination of benefit among a specific tumor type is limited by small numbers and multiple dose levels. In phase II studies, a specified tumor type is studied because the main biologic response of interest is the tumor

---

TABLE 16-1

Important Components of Clinical Trials

Scientific background and rationale for the study
Objectives and end points
Patients' eligibility criteria
Treatment plan and design, including follow-up evaluations
Drug information
Toxicity assessment and modifications
Treatment-effect evaluation and statistical considerations
Regulatory considerations, including consent and data safety monitoring plan

---

TABLE 16-2   Summary of Typical Conditions for the Different Types of Cancer Clinical Trials

	Phase I	Phase II	Phase III
Patient population	All refractory tumors	Tumor specific	Tumor specific
Dose of drug	Escalating	Specified	Specified
Primary objective	Establish phase II dose	Antitumor activity	Effectiveness compared with standard
Study design	Single arm	Usually single arm	Randomized
Number of patients	<30	20–40	>200
Typical end point	Toxicity	Response	Survival
Statistical design	Escalating cohorts	Two-stage design	Randomized, controlled

TABLE 16-3

Modified Fibonacci Series for Phase I Cytotoxic Dose Escalation

Starting dose	A
Level 1	2A = B
Level 2	$\frac{2}{3}$ B = C
Level 3	$\frac{1}{2}$ C = D
Level 4	$\frac{2}{5}$ D = E
Level 5	$\frac{1}{3}$ E = F
Level 6	$\frac{1}{3}$ F = G
Level 7	$\frac{1}{3}$ G = H

itself.[17] The main objective of phase II studies is the determination of efficacy for an agent administered at the dose and schedule identified in phase I trials. The preferred design includes patients most likely to show a favorable effect but for whom no effective therapy is available. Most patients have a good "performance status" and limited prior exposure to chemotherapeutic agents. A phase II study serves to evaluate whether a therapy has sufficient antitumor activity to warrant further investigation in larger groups of patients or as an alternative to a currently accepted therapy.

These efficacy trials typically accrue 40 to 50 patients, and a common end point may be determination of whether the tumor shrinks in response to therapy. For tumor types where spontaneous regression is infrequent, the identification of a therapy that has at least a 20% response rate might signify that the agent is worthy of further clinical evaluation. To minimize the number of patients receiving an inactive medication, a two-stage design is often used.[13] For example, following accrual of 10 to 14 patients, the study is expanded to a further 10 to 14 patients if enough responses are seen in the first group of patients to justify the expansion. The exact number of patients and number of responses required depend on the therapeutic goal and willingness to accept specified probabilities of false-positive and false-negative results.

Most cancer phase II studies are open labeled and single arm in design. If multiple agents are concurrently available for testing or alternative regimens of the same agent are under consideration, a "randomized phase II study" may be conducted. In such a study patients are randomized among multiple phase II regimens with the goal not to directly test which regimen is best but to prevent bias in assigning the "best" or "worst" cases to a particular treatment. Because a single-arm trial uses historical data to determine if the therapy is active, such a bias would make it difficult to assess the new treatment. Occasionally, as with some of the autologous vaccines, there is no way to provide an appropriate historical comparison. In these cases, a concurrent control group is required. However, with the variability among patients, it is unrealistic to expect to prove a hypothesis of treatment difference with sample sizes appropriate for initial efficacy evaluation. Thus these trials emphasize estimation of potential differences in determining the likely usefulness of the therapy.

The interpretation of the results of phase II studies can be difficult because of the use of different outcome measures and nonrandomized studies. In the majority of phase II studies, response rate has been accepted as a measure of efficacy, as it is believed to indicate activity of the agent, even if not long-term clinical benefit.[3] However, for studies in some patient groups—for example, those with complete tumor resection—tumor regression is not a useful end point. For these studies, the median time to tumor progression may be a study outcome. In these instances, the frequency of evaluating disease status needs to be stated, as the end point depends on the time intervals at which progression will be assessed. The use of a set time at which the status of disease is assessed has also been used—for example, 6-month progression-free survival. This has the advantage of not requiring a specific event to take place and can allow for more timely completion of studies. The use of these alternative end points is made more difficult because of the nonrandomized nature of the studies. Historical data are less likely to provide an adequate control group, and bias in both patient selection and follow-up, a problem for any single-arm study, is even more likely to confound results when these alternative end points are used.

Cytostatic agents may prevent further growth without shrinkage of the existing tumor, another example of where response rate may not be an appropriate endpoint for evaluation of efficacy. Possible end points include changes in tumor markers, measures of target inhibition, noninvasive functional imaging changes, time to progression, or proportion of patients with evidence of progression at a defined time point after the start of therapy.

Recently, more attention has been given to the important outcome of quality-of-life assessments using validated patient questionnaires.[16] Although this is an appropriate end point from the standpoint of medical care, it is a difficult one to evaluate, because as patients' tumors progress, their quality of life tends to decrease. What may be of most importance is the time during which the patient's quality of life was maintained above a certain level.[6]

To date we have focused on the design of the studies. Although it is beyond the scope of this chapter to discuss analysis plans in detail, a few general comments can be made. In phase II trials, there has been a history of reporting on "evaluable" patients, where these were the patients who received a certain minimum duration of treatment. The logic for this approach was that, unless the patients received a certain minimum treatment, the treatment could not be expected to be of help. The problem with this approach was that it resulted in overestimates of the success rate, because patients who failed early or who could not tolerate the therapy were not included in the report. More recently the concept of intent-to-treat has become the accepted analysis. This method describes the number of successes—by whatever definition provided in the study design—in terms of the number of patients entered in the study. Thus the study estimates the proportion of those who agree to the treatment who will be labeled a treatment success.

In the discussion of the phase I trials, it was noted that the numbers of patients studied are too small to provide assurance as to the nature of the toxicities that would be seen when a larger group of patients is studied. Thus toxicity assessment is an important secondary goal for phase II studies. However, phase II studies still enroll relatively few patients, leaving considerable imprecision in estimates of both efficacy and safety. When analyzing the results of these studies, it is important to acknowledge the limitations of the information. This is most easily done by providing confidence intervals for the estimates.

Thus instead of saying that 20% of the patients responded, the report would note that the 95% confidence interval for the response rate is, for example, 10% to 30%. The width of the confidence interval depends on the sample size, and the need for precise estimates is one of the items that should be considered in planning the size of the clinical trial.

PHASE III CANCER TRIALS

Phase III studies are generally designed to corroborate previous positive findings in phase II trials or to evaluate modifications in an established regimen. They are designed to assess clinical benefit—as distinct from measuring activity of the therapy, which is often the end point for phase II studies. Clinical outcome in a group of patients receiving the new treatment is compared with the outcome in a group of similar patients treated with a control, or standard, therapy. Because phase III trials are designed as the definitive study, two issues related to patient heterogeneity are of particular concern when designing these trials—the effect of chance and the effect of bias. These issues are addressed by including adequate numbers of patients and using randomization for treatment assignment. Randomizing the patients separately within different risk groups (strata) based on known prognostic factors can help to assure balance between the groups. Including strata in the statistical analysis can explain apparently variable results and so increase the power to detect treatment differences.[10,12,14] Primary and secondary outcome measures should be predefined with a description of the statistical analyses that will be used to determine the significance of the findings. A large number of patients is usually needed for these studies. This can be difficult to achieve for diseases such as primary brain tumors, which occur with relatively low incidence. This means that the time for accrual can be very long and these studies may be possible only through the cooperative effort of several institutions.

In noncancer clinical trials, phase III studies almost always are double blind; that is, neither the patient nor the physician is aware of which therapy the patient is receiving. Single blinding—where the patient is unaware of the treatment assignment—is important if the treatment of one of the arms is commercially available and the patient could access a supply during their time on the study. It may also be important if the standard therapy is thought to be of low efficacy. In this case, patients may choose to drop out of the study if they find they are receiving this treatment. In either case, the results of the study can become meaningless if blinding is not used. A double-blind placebo-controlled trial is preferred when important end points are subjective. Although studies may be randomized, some cannot be double blind, for example, if the active treatment is highly effective with respect to one of the outcomes, like a laboratory measure, or if it has a distinctive side effect. In cancer clinical trials the problem is more often that the comparison treatment is another active treatment that has a different schedule or route of administration, making blinding impractical.

For some end points, such as progression-free survival, investigator bias cannot be eliminated, but the obvious advantage of phase III studies, given their randomized design, is the minimization of bias in assessment and the ability to balance for the effect of unrecognized prognostic factors on outcome. An intent-to-treat analysis of outcome is important to maintain the comparability in expectations across treatment groups that is gained by randomization.[9]

CONCLUSION

We reviewed the basic principles of cancer clinical trial design. Not only rigorous design but also high standards of conduct and reporting,[5] as well as ethical considerations, are important to ensure good-quality studies that can truly evaluate the value of new therapies.

References

1. Eisenhauer EA, O'Dwyer PJ, Christian M, et al: Phase I clinical trial design in cancer drug development. J Clin Oncol 18:684–692, 2000.
2. Fox E, Curt GA, Balis FM: Clinical trial design for target-based therapy. Oncologist 7:401–409, 2002.
3. Harrington DP, Anderson JW: Common methods of analyzing response data in clinical trials (with discussion by Simon R.). Oncology 4:95, 1990.
4. Korn EL, Arbuck SG, Pluda JM, et al: Clinical trial designs for cytostatic agents: are new approaches needed? J Clin Oncol 19:265–272, 2001.
5. Moher D, Schulz KF, Altman DG for the CONSORT Group: The CONSORT statement: revised recommendations for improving the quality of reports of parallel-group randomised trials. Lancet 357:1191–1194, 2001; comment in Lancet 358:585, 2001.
6. Moinpour CM, Feigl P, Metch B, et al: Quality of life end points in cancer clinical trials: review and recommendations. J Natl Cancer Inst 81:485–495, 1989.
7. Nottage M, Siu LL: Principles of clinical trial design. J Clin Oncol 20:42S–46S, 2002.
8. O'Quigley J, Pepe M, Fisher L: Continual reassessment method: a practical design for phase 1 clinical trials in cancer. Biometrics 46:33–48, 1990.
9. Peto R, Pike MC, Armitage P, et al: Design and analysis of randomized clinical trials requiring prolonged observation of each patient. II. Analysis and examples. Br J Cancer 35:1–39, 1977.
10. Pocock SJ: Randomised clinical trials. Br Med J 1:1661, 1977.
11. Schneiderman M: Mouse to man: statistical problems in bringing a drug to clinical trial, in Proceedings of the Fifth Berkeley Symposium on Mathematical Statistical Probability. University of California at Berkeley, 1967, Vol 4.
12. Simon R: Importance of prognostic factors in cancer clinical trials. Cancer Treat Rep 68:185–192, 1984.
13. Simon R: Optimal two-stage designs for phase II clinical trials. Control Clin Trials 10:1–10, 1989.
14. Simon R: Randomized clinical trials in oncology. Principles and obstacles. Cancer 74:2614–2619, 1994.
15. Storer BE: Design and analysis of phase I clinical trials. Biometrics 45:925–937, 1989.
16. Testa MA, Simonson DC: Assessment of quality-of-life outcomes. N Engl J Med 334:835–840, 1996.
17. Wittes RE, Marsoni S, Simon R, et al: The phase II trial. Cancer Treat Rep 69:1235–1239, 1985.

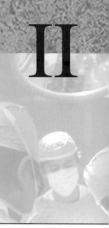

Tumor-Specific Principles

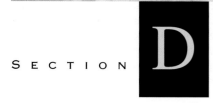

CHAPTER 17

DIFFUSE ASTROCYTOMA

G. Evren Keles, Tarik Tihan, Eric C. Burton, Michael D. Prados, and Mitchel S. Berger

Diffuse astrocytomas reviewed in this chapter are grade II tumors according to the World Health Organization (WHO) classification.[42] WHO grade II tumors correspond to the Kernohan grading system[41] grades I and II tumors and the St. Anne–Mayo classification[17] grade II tumors. They include fibrillary, protoplasmic, and gemistocytic astrocytomas.[42] In the literature these histologic entities are usually grouped and referred to as *low-grade gliomas*. Although this terminology is helpful in differentiating these tumors from higher grade gliomas that have a significantly different prognosis, grouping all histologic subtypes results in a heterogeneous mix of tumors with different natural histories and therefore provides limited prognostic information. Various grading systems further complicate the overall picture.

Approximately 50% of newly diagnosed brain tumors are primary brain tumors of glial origin. Astrocytomas represent 26.6% of all newly diagnosed glial primary brain tumors.[53] This corresponds to 1500 to 1800 new cases of low-grade gliomas diagnosed in North America each year.[18,53] Age-specific data show that low-grade astrocytomas constitute 15% of brain tumors in adults and 25% of brain tumors in children.[26] Pediatric low-grade gliomas, which include cerebellar astrocytomas, optic pathway and hypothalamic gliomas, brainstem gliomas, and hemispheric low-grade gliomas, are discussed in detail in Chapters 75 to 88.

The etiology of low-grade gliomas is unknown. Except for patients with one of the phakomatoses, it has not been documented that genetic predisposition plays a role in the development of these tumors. There is no indication in the literature that low-grade gliomas are more prevalent in a specific ethnic or national group.

The only molecular genetic alteration consistently observed in otherwise healthy patients with low-grade astrocytomas is mutation of p53.[30] The p53 gene is located at chromosomal location 17p13.1, and this site is often deleted in astrocytomas. The remaining copy of p53 is usually inactivated through a subtle mutation. The end product of this gene is a nuclear DNA-binding phosphoprotein that has transcriptional activity that is essential in the regulation of apoptosis and cell cycle progression. It has been shown that loss of normal p53 function promotes the accelerated growth and malignant differentiation of astrocytes.[8,103] Astrocytomas are the only type of brain tumor to have significant p53 mutation rates. That 50% to 60% of grade II and grade III astrocytomas exhibit p53 mutations suggests that this tumor suppressor gene inactivation is an early lesion among gene alterations associated with the development of malignant gliomas.[98] Although some glioblastomas exhibit p53 mutations, a significant subset of them do not and instead have amplification of the epidermal growth factor receptor (EGFR) gene, suggesting that they arise from different genetic pathways. Other recurrent alterations observed in adult low-grade astrocytomas are gain of chromosome 7 and double-minute chromosomes. Losses of chromosomes 10, 13, 15, 20, and 22 and structural rearrangements involving chromosomes 4, 11, 12, 13, 16, 18, and 21 are observed in isolated patients.[76]

PATHOLOGY

In recent years the critical progress in our understanding of gliomas has led to the distinction between circumscribed and infiltrating types of astrocytoma. Circumscribed and infiltrating astrocytomas display distinct characteristics in their morphologic, clinical, radiologic, and genetic features.[20] The current nosology of brain tumors considers infiltrating astrocytomas as diffuse and progressive gliomas that gradually accumulate more aggressive histologic and molecular features.[43] The term *infiltrating astrocytoma* without additional qualifiers is a WHO grade II neoplasm, even though the term can be used to identify all astrocytomas from grade II to IV.[42] WHO grade II astrocytoma is synonymous with low-grade infiltrating astrocytoma (LGIA). *Astrocytoma, NOS* (not otherwise specified) is a highly vague and confusing term that should not be considered as a specific diagnostic entity. *Well-differentiated astrocytoma* is another vague term that should be avoided as a final diagnostic category.

Intraoperative Evaluation

The fundamental purpose of the intraoperative evaluation, or the frozen section, is to provide necessary information to the surgeon to complete the surgical procedure. As in all cases submitted for intraoperative evaluation, a few critical steps facilitate proper interpretation of infiltrating astrocytomas. The first step is the issue of sample adequacy and the studies needed for adequate interpretation of cytologic and architectural detail. We believe the standard hematoxylin-eosin (H&E) stain is sufficient for such an evaluation and should be adhered to until better and more detailed alternatives are discovered. Second, it is imperative to obtain intraoperative smears that provide the best venue for accurate interpretation of the cytologic detail. Finally, intraoperative evaluation should never be considered as a substitute for final diagnosis, and adequate sample should always be saved for permanent sections. The pathologist should clearly communicate to the neurosurgeon that frozen sections always have the potential to require additional tissue. Requests for frozen section after the completion of the surgical procedure or when additional tissue will not be available are superfluous.

Frozen sections are particularly challenging for LGIA because there is a great tendency for tissue to exhibit marked freezing artifact, often in the form of clear spaces and vacuoles. In addition, frozen section greatly distorts the nuclear size and shape. It is also difficult to estimate the degree of cellularity and the relation of cells to each other. Vacuolar artifacts may be difficult to distinguish from microcysts that are often filled with a faintly basophilic material. In most of these problems, the intraoperative smear proves to be an invaluable aid to interpretation.

Grading of infiltrating astrocytomas during intraoperative evaluation is a nagging problem in surgical neuropathology. Particularly with the advent of more sophisticated treatment options that require intraoperative decisions, there is increasing pressure for a tentative grading of the pathology material. The problem is often resolved if the surgical pathologist can unequivocally identify the highest grade, but in the case of LGIA it is best to evaluate histologic features in relation to clinical and radiologic evidence. For a more effective and appropriate evaluation of the intraoperative samples from LGIA, a visit to the operating room and a discussion with the neurosurgeon are invaluable.

Interpretation of tissue previously used for a frozen section should also be done with great caution and with the understanding that artifacts in nuclear size and shape can cause misinterpretations. Postfrozen samples can mislead the interpreter to diagnose gliosis as glioma and cause misinterpretations on the grade and type of the tumors.

Macroscopic Features

The external appearance of LGIA largely depends on the extent of cortical involvement, in other words, the involvement of superficial structures. There may be little or no external abnormality in tumors that are deep seated within the cerebral hemisphere. In tumors involving the cortex, the gyri appear edematous, expanded, and slightly discolored. Infiltrative astrocytomas almost imperceptibly blend with the brain parenchyma, and boundaries are often difficult to define. In surgical and autopsy material, LGIAs cause gray-dusky discoloration of the white matter with focal cystic appearance and soft to gelatinous consistency. The cysts may be large enough to be noticed during surgery, but they are often small and can be seen after examination of the cut surface of the pathology specimen. The outlines of anatomic structures are typically effaced, and the boundary between white matter and cortex becomes indistinct. In the brainstem LGIA can expand the pons and medulla and fill the cerebellopontine angle or interpeduncular fossa. These tumors can also distort the fourth ventricle and encase the basilar artery.

Microscopic Features

An astrocytoma is traditionally described as a tumor resembling normal astrocytic cells.[12] However, the microscopic attributes of astrocytes vary—hence an astrocytoma's microscopic appearance. Nevertheless, the morphologic features of cells recognized as fibrillary or protoplasmic astrocytes constitute the standards for defining an astrocytoma.

Typically, LGIA is hypercellular by a factor of two or more when compared with normal white matter. Recognizing the hypercellularity and the disruption of the architecture are the first clues to the diagnosis. Occasionally, the cell density may only minimally exceed that of normal white matter. In such cases correct diagnosis depends on accurate interpretation of the cytologic features.

The microscopic nature of infiltrating astrocytomas is evident in their ability to penetrate the brain parenchyma and permeate among glia, neuronal cells, and axonal segments.

The infiltrating astrocytomas have substantial nuclear hyperchromasia and pleomorphism. The nuclei often display striking irregularities with invaginations, sharp edges, and irregular contours. The chromatin is much coarser than those of normal astrocytes. Most astrocytic nuclei do not exhibit prominent nucleoli, or the nucleoli are rather indistinct within a markedly condensed chromatin. The size and shape of tumor nucleoli are quite variable among tumors as well as within a single specimen. Tumor cells occasionally display a fibrillary, eosinophilic cytoplasm. In paucicellular areas the cytoplasm appears even more indistinct, and it may not be easy to associate the nuclei with the background fibrillarity.

Perinuclear haloes, or the so-called "fried-egg" appearance of the cytoplasm, can be seen in astrocytomas and do not necessarily imply an oligodendroglial component. Nevertheless, prominence of such cells always raises the differential issue of oligodendroglioma or the dubious category of oligoastrocytoma.

The most common pattern for infiltrating astrocytoma is the microcystic pattern, which is a reliable indicator of an infiltrating low-grade glioma, because it rarely occurs in reactive conditions. However, microcystic pattern is not specific to LGIA and can also be observed in oligodendrogliomas and glioneuronal tumors.

A rare pediatric type of infiltrating astrocytoma with a unique histologic pattern has been termed *bipolar angiocentric astrocytoma*.[96] It is still not clear whether this pattern represents a unique entity or a morphologic variant of LGIA.

LGIAs display secondary structures such as perineuronal satellitosis and subpial or leptomeningeal spread. Although these features are helpful in defining a low-grade glial neoplasm, they are neither specific nor common in LGIA. Mineralizations either as amorphous or concentric forms can be seen in association with LGIA. These mineralizations often occur within the gray matter and are more typical of an oligodendroglioma than astrocytoma.

Chondroid metaplasia or chondroid pattern is an extremely rare but striking finding in LGIA. The production of cartilage by neoplastic astrocytes may be related to their ability to secrete basement membrane material and other forms of mucopolysaccharides, which may become condensed to form a chondroid ground substance.[40] The chondroid cells in these metaplastic regions are also glial fibrillary acidic protein (GFAP) positive.[40]

The histologic definition of LGIA practically excludes the presence of mitoses.[43] The significance of a solitary mitosis in a fairly well-sampled tumor is still controversial. A recent study found a trend for better prognosis for infiltrating astrocytomas with a single mitotic figure when compared with frankly anaplastic astrocytomas. However, this trend could not be substantiated in multivariate analyses.[67] Nevertheless, it has been suggested that a single mitotic figure in a resection specimen may not impact prognosis significantly, and some authors accept the presence of a solitary mitosis in a well-sampled grade II astrocytoma.[12] In such cases it is even more critical to be aware of the radiologic, surgical, and clinical findings to better interpret the biopsy. In our opinion it is not appropriate to view the microscopic features in isolation from the clinical and radiologic data.

Neither the presence of necrosis nor vascular proliferation is acceptable in LGIA. Nevertheless, it is rarely possible that LGIA might show focal necrosis due to vascular compression and ischemia. A rare LGIA that was inadvertently or deliberately subjected to radiation treatment can also present with necrosis. Accurate clinical information and knowledge of biopsy site are often helpful to avoid overgrading such lesions.

Granular Cell Astrocytoma

Granular cell astrocytoma is a unique and rare form of infiltrating astrocytoma that has been recently described.[9,14] This neoplasm is described as an infiltrating glioma that contains individual or sheets of large, round cells packed with eosinophilic, PAS-positive granules. Most granular cell astrocytomas contain lymphocytic infiltrates, either perivascular or admixed with neoplastic cells, and often there is a transition to typical infiltrating astrocytoma. Granular cell astrocytomas can be grade II, but most reported cases are higher grade neoplasms.[9]

Gemistocytic Astrocytoma

Some LGIAs primarily consist of plump cells with abundant eosinophilic, hyaline cytoplasm and an asymmetric array of short processes. These tumors are designated as *gemistocytic astrocytomas*. Gemistocytic astrocytomas rarely occur in pure form and often coexist with the classic infiltrating astrocytoma pattern. Perivascular lymphocytic infiltrates, occasionally creating germinal centers, are common and typical for these neoplasms. Gemistocytic astrocytomas possess brightly eosinophilic bodies resembling Rosenthal fibers in their highly fibrillary cytoplasm. However, typical Rosenthal fibers are not seen in these tumors. Gemistocytic astrocytomas also contain a second population of small astrocytic cells with hyperchromatic nuclei, mitoses, and a higher MIB-1 labeling index compared with the gemistocytic cell population. They are believed to represent the main proliferating element of this variant of astrocytoma.[99] Krouwer et al[46] suggest that the presence of at least 20% gemistocytes in a glial neoplasm is a poor prognostic sign, irrespective of the pathologic background. These authors also propose that gemistocytic astrocytomas be classified with anaplastic astrocytomas and treated accordingly.[46] Current WHO classification does not provide an automatic designation of grade III for gemistocytic astrocytomas.[43] Currently, there is little doubt that gemistocytic cells in infiltrating astrocytomas are neoplastic rather than reactive. The frequency of p53 mutations is significantly higher (approximately twofold) in gemistocytic astrocytomas as compared with other astrocytoma subtypes.[44] Further studies on the cytogenetics of gemistocytes confirm that the gemistocytic cells in most infiltrating astrocytomas are neoplastic.[45]

A critical issue for gemistocytic astrocytomas is their distinction from oligodendrogliomas that typically contain plump cells known as *minigemistocytes*. The minigemistocyte has an eccentric, spherical GFAP-positive cytoplasm, and GFAP staining can be even more pronounced than for typical astrocytic cells. True gemistocytes seen in astrocytomas are larger, more eosinophilic, and have less distinct cytoplasm with short processes. In contrast to the minigemistocyte, GFAP positivity is confined to the periphery of the gemistocyte, and the central portion of the perikarya is weakly positive. There is considerable overlap in the appearances of gemistocytes and minigemistocytes, and neither is absolutely diagnostic of any specific entity.

Immunohistochemical Features

In essence, the diagnosis of LGIA is primarily done on routine H&E stains, and immunohistochemical stains can hardly make up for a poorly sampled specimen. Nevertheless, a number of immunohistochemical stains are useful adjuncts in the interpretation of LGIA. The commonly used antibodies for neurofilament (NF) protein aid in defining axons within the specimen and confirm the infiltrative nature of the tumor. Even though astrocytomas and astrocytes are strongly positive for GFAP, this antibody is often unhelpful in determining the type and the grade of the neoplasm, because the cells of many astrocytomas have little cytoplasm. In addition, the strongest GFAP positivity is seen in reactive rather than neoplastic astrocytes. The gemistocytic cells are often weakly positive for GFAP, and the staining is usually in the periphery of the cytoplasm. In contrast, minigemistocytes of oligodendroglioma are strongly GFAP positive. Staining for MIB-1 (Ki-67 antibody) is usually less than 2%, and a neoplasm with higher than 5% MIB-1 labeling suggests a higher grade neoplasm. Despite extensive studies on the Ki-67 labeling index and its relation to grade and survival, changing the grade of the lesion based on the MIB-1 labeling index is not justified in the current WHO classification.[51,91] A significant percentage of LGIAs are immunoreactive for p53.[16] This is particularly predominant in gemistocytic astrocytomas.[97,99]

Ultrastructural Features

The ultrastructural examination of an LGIA is rarely undertaken for diagnostic purposes, except to explain an unusual histologic feature. The fine structure of the astrocytic cell bodies and the processes are fundamentally similar to those of normal or developing astrocytes. The nuclei often display marked chromatin condensation and irregularities. The astrocytomas differ in their less developed cell junctions and poorly formed peripheral processes. The processes often consist of small microvilli or pseudopod-like protrusions. The cytoplasm of astrocytoma cells often contains few or no intermediate filaments, except in areas with increased cellularity.[27] The cytoplasm of gemistocytes is typically loaded with organelles and is sparse in intermediate filaments. The granular cell astrocytomas contain partially membrane-bound, dense bodies compatible with secondary lysosomes. The granular cells also contain intermediate filaments corresponding to GFAP,[59] supporting their glial origin.

CLINICAL CHARACTERISTICS

It is important to obtain a history and perform a physical examination, together with a thorough neurologic examination preoperatively, to obtain relevant details and information regarding the patient's general medical condition. Currently, with the help of better health-care systems and advanced diagnostic technology, patients are diagnosed at an earlier stage of the disease. In modern series, approximately half of the patients have a seizure disorder, and half of the patients with a low-grade glioma appear neurologically intact.[80]

The median age of patients with low-grade astrocytomas is approximately 35 years, which is considerably lower than that of patients with higher grade gliomas. There is a biphasic age distribution with two peak incidences at 6 to 12 years and 26 to 46 years. Most studies have shown that males constitute between 55% and 65% of patients with low-grade astrocytomas.[26] This corresponds to a sex ratio of male-to-female incidence rates of approximately 1.5.[93] The frontal lobe is the most common location, followed by the temporal and parietal lobes.[105] Low-grade astrocytomas may be lobar and relatively well circumscribed or deep and diffusely infiltrating.

The most common feature for patients with low-grade astrocytomas is seizures. One half to two thirds of patients with low-grade gliomas have seizures. Approximately 50% of the patients have headaches. In larger series and community-based studies, the presence of a brain tumor was detected in 8% to 30% of patients who had partial seizures, with age increasing the risk of epilepsy being caused by a tumor.[37,54,102] Together with gangliogliomas, tumors reviewed in this chapter constitute the gliomas that are most commonly associated with intractable epilepsy.[37] This fact is attributed to the characteristics of the tumor's growth pattern, with a higher seizure incidence being associated with relatively slow-growing tumors. In Penfield's series, including 230 astrocytomas, low-grade gliomas were associated with epilepsy twice as often as glioblastomas.[65] The clinical course of 48% of 209 patients with hemispheric astrocytomas presented by Gonzales and Elvidge[24] was complicated by seizures.

Headache, lethargy, and personality change may be caused by the general increase in intracranial pressure. Papilledema may be present. Focal neurologic deficits due to direct tumor infiltration or by local pressure depend on the location of the lesion. Depending on the location of the low-grade glioma, disinhibition, irritability, impaired judgment, abulia, apathy, motor and sensory loss, dysphasia, aphasia, and anosognosia may be present. Tumors involving the parietooccipital area may cause visual agnosias.

Magnetic resonance imaging (MRI) and computed tomography (CT) are the two neuroradiologic tools that provide valuable diagnostic information. The diagnostic procedure of choice, however, is MRI because of its higher sensitivity in differentiating tumor tissue from normal brain. Although low-grade astrocytomas are often not associated with significant mass effect, a mass effect upon surrounding ventricular structures and cortical sulci is common, and in some cases considerable mass effect may be seen in patients without neurologic deficit due to the slow-growth characteristics of these tumors. The typical CT image is a nonenhanced isodense or hypodense mass. Calcification may be detected in 15% to 20% of cases, and mild to moderate inhomogeneous contrast enhancement can be seen in up to 40% of all cases.[78] Cystic changes are not rare. On MRI, T1-weighted images reveal an isointense to hypointense nonenhanced mass that is hyperintense on T2-weighted images. Enhancement, when it occurs, is generally faint. In an earlier study, contrast enhancement was found to have no prognostic effect for patients with low-grade gliomas.[87] In contrast, more recent studies showed that enhancement has a negative prognostic effect on time to progression and overall outcome.[55,69]

An adjunct to conventional neuroimaging techniques is magnetic resonance spectroscopy (MRS), which can be obtained during the MRI examination with little additional time. This technique allows detection of metabolite levels in and around tumors, therefore providing metabolic data in addition to morphologic imaging. Additional functional information may be obtained preoperatively with functional MRI and magnetic source imaging (MSI). This information, integrated with the anatomic information obtained from conventional MRI and intraoperative stimulation mapping data, can allow for more precise and complete resection of tumor and enable the surgeon to minimize morbidity when operating in functionally eloquent brain areas.[4]

TREATMENT AND OUTCOME

Treatment options for diffuse astrocytomas at the time of initial diagnosis include observation, surgery in the form of biopsy or resection, and radiation therapy. The efficiency of chemotherapy is also being studied, mostly for recurrent tumors.

Surgery

The extent and timing of surgical resection are still controversial in the management of diffuse astrocytomas, mainly because of lack of conclusive studies addressing these issues. In the literature, reports question the value of immediate treatment when an imaging study suggests a low-grade glioma.[75] Although there is no class 1 evidence in favor of early intervention, there is also no study showing an outcome benefit for patients when treatment is deferred. Furthermore, there are several potential risks that the patients would be exposed to by delaying surgery, including the risk of malignant degeneration, probability of developing irreversible neurologic deficit, and a more persistent seizure disorder refractory to medical treatment.

Dedifferentiation, or malignant transformation, is a well-described phenomenon observed in low-grade gliomas. In the literature, 13% to 86% of tumors initially diagnosed as low grade recur at a higher histologic grade.[5,47,55,58,61,69,89,94,100] Similar to its broad range of incidence, the time to malignant differentiation is also variable, ranging from 28 to 60 months.[5,55,75,81,94] However, the factors resulting in the change to a malignant phenotype remain unclear. In a recent study investigating the relationship between anaplastic transformation and patient's age, a strong inverse relationship was found between age at initial diagnosis and time to progression to a higher grade glioma.[81] The effect of treatment on malignant transformation is controversial. In a series by Recht et al.,[75] 58% of patients who did not initially undergo biopsy and treatment of a suspected low-grade glioma after diagnostic imaging studies eventually required surgery at a median interval of 29 months, and 50% of the tumors then showed anaplastic features. Although a higher incidence of malignant transformation at the time of operation and shorter time to tumor progression was observed compared with that in patients who initially were operated upon, the authors stated that no difference was observed in terms of survival.[75] The opposite was found in a series of 53 hemispheric low-grade gliomas volumetrically analyzed regarding recurrence patterns.[5] The risk of recurrence, either as low-grade or at a higher histologic grade, was minimized when less residual tumor volume was present postoperatively. Residual tumor volume was found to be more important than the percentage of resection in predicting the histologic phenotype of recurrence. In addition, time to tumor progression was longer with more extensive resections associated with a smaller volume of residual tumor.[5] Additional studies evaluating the role of residual tumor volume on survival provided inconclusive results.[48,57]

Surgical treatment of diffuse astrocytomas consists of several different approaches depending on the patient's clinical condition and the surgeon's preferences. Surgical intervention may range from a simple stereotactic biopsy to obtain tissue diagnosis to an extensive resection coupled with seizure surgery in patients with diffuse astrocytomas associated with intractable epilepsy. Surgical intervention is the essential treatment modality in management of low-grade gliomas, and the main goals are histologic diagnosis and reducing the tumor bulk to decrease intracranial pressure, improve neurologic deficit, prevent malignant dedifferentiation, and obtain seizure control.

Stereotactic techniques or frameless methods (i.e., neuronavigation) have a lower morbidity and mortality (i.e., 1.2% to 6.4%)[1,7] than open surgical approaches. However, with the exception of computer-assisted stereotactic resections, they serve the aim of only obtaining tissue diagnosis. Therefore the use of stereotactic biopsy is limited to a subgroup of patients with suspected low-grade glial tumors and depends on the characteristics of the lesion (e.g., depth, small size, multiplicity,

diffuseness, or the clinical condition of the patient). Incorrect pathologic diagnosis is not uncommon for tumors of glial origin, and the misdiagnosis usually consists of misinterpreting a high-grade tumor as a low-grade glioma. Although the incidence of this problem varies in different series, it may be significantly reduced by serial sampling along the entire radius of the lesion and beyond. Close collaboration with an experienced neuropathologist is essential to the diagnostic efficiency of stereotactic biopsies. There are no randomized studies examining the prognostic effect of stereotactic biopsy followed by radiation therapy for the initial management of patients with diffuse astrocytomas. Retrospective nonrandomized studies do not show any substantial benefit in terms of overall survival for patients who receive a biopsy followed by radiation therapy when compared with those patients who receive conventional surgical resections.[52,69,85,86]

Computer-assisted stereotactic resections are helpful for tumor resection in certain locations that are technically challenging and associated with high morbidity rates. This technique, by providing images of lesions in triplanar format and by accurately referencing the data to either a stereotactic frame or to the patient's surface anatomy, permits the neurosurgeon to plan precisely an approach that minimizes injury to critical neural structures. As an example, perioperative mortality for radical resection of gliomas in and around the thalamus now approaches zero with modern techniques.[90] Unnecessary brain resection and retraction are also minimized.

Open surgical interventions for the treatment of diffuse astrocytomas are conducted using general neurosurgical principles of tumor surgery as detailed in Chapter 9, Surgical Strategies in the Management of Brain Tumors. Contemporary neurosurgical methods, including ultrasonography,[6,39] functional mapping,[36] frameless navigational resection devices, and intraoperative imaging techniques,[104] enable the neurosurgeon to achieve more extensive resections with less morbidity.

Reviewing the four prospective randomized studies currently available for diffuse astrocytomas in adult patients, age, histology, and tumor size appear to be generally accepted prognostic factors influencing outcome.[19,34,71,83] The prognostic effect of surgical intervention, however, is controversial.[38] The majority of low-grade gliomas seen in adults are located in the cerebral hemispheres, and their natural history is significantly different from their pediatric counterparts. The trend in the literature, unfortunately, has been inclusion of all low-grade gliomas in the series regardless of the age group and location, making the data difficult to interpret. A review of the literature from 1970 to 2000 shows that in the 1990s there was a noticeable increase in the number of studies that support more extensive resections, along with a decrease in the number of reports showing no difference in terms of outcome.* All of these studies are nonrandomized except for two,[19,35] and in all studies extent of resection is determined by nonvolumetric methods, mostly depending on the surgeon's intraoperative estimate.

Studies with a distinct subgroup of patients who had a macroscopically gross total resection of their tumor† found a statistically significant effect of the extent of surgery on

---

*See references 2, 3, 19, 29, 31, 33, 35, 47, 48, 50, 56, 57, 60, 61, 66, 68–70, 74, 77, 79, 82, 84–86, 88, 89, 92, 101.
†See references 2, 29, 47, 56, 57, 60, 61, 66, 68–70, 74, 79, 85, 89, 101.

survival. Results of studies in which gross total resections were combined with less than total resections* were also consistent with an improved survival observed in patients with a higher degree of resection. Although longer 5-year survival rates were observed for patients who received a more extensive resection, the difference of survival benefit was less pronounced when compared with those patients who received a gross total resection. However, there was no indication that more extensive resections were associated with a less favorable outcome.

There are few studies that simultaneously excluded pediatric patients and pilocytic and gemistocytic histologies, which have significantly different prognosis, and included more than 75 patients.[48,68,74,89,92] Despite these five studies being all retrospective and nonmatched, they are the most homogeneous series that are available in the literature regarding patient population and histologic characteristics. The prognostic effect of extent of resection was found to be statistically significant in univariate analysis in all studies. In multivariate analysis, however, extent of resection was a significant independent factor in four of these five series.[48,68,89,92]

Since 2001 there have been five studies that addressed the issue of extent of resection for diffuse astrocytomas as it relates to outcome. Two of these studies[71,83] are prospective and randomized and, although they were not designed to evaluate extent of resection specifically, both had this parameter as a variable in their statistical analysis. The volume assessments, however, were not volumetric. In both studies extent of resection was found to be a statistically significant predictor of outcome in univariate analysis, but not in multivariate statistics.[71,83] In the remaining three retrospective studies extent of resection had a significant prognostic impact for low-grade tumors.[28,32,49]

The surgical management of patients with low-grade gliomas and seizures is controversial. Surgical options include focal excision of the tumor alone, radical tumor resection without electrocorticography, and a radical resection with seizure foci mapping. In patients with low-grade gliomas who are under complete seizure control preoperatively or those who have an occasional seizure on medication, seizure control with or without the need for postoperative anticonvulsants is often achieved with radical tumor resection alone. Management of patients with intractable epilepsy, however, is different from that of those individuals whose seizures are well controlled with medication. Various surgical approaches used for the treatment of patients with diffuse astrocytomas associated with epilepsy are discussed in Chapter 9, Surgical Strategies in the Management of Brain Tumors.

Radiation Therapy

Radiation therapy is one option for treatment of patients with low-grade glioma. Other options include postoperative observation or chemotherapy. The role of radiation has been controversial for many decades, with physician and patient bias supporting the decision to treat once the diagnosis is made or to defer therapy until further tumor progression or symptoms

occur, prompting intervention. Retrospective, single-institution reviews seemed to suggest a benefit for the use of radiation therapy at the time of initial diagnosis. Fortunately, over the past several years, a number of prospective clinical trials have been reported that should be helpful as guidelines for treatment decision.

In general, treatment is reserved for patients with symptomatic residual disease despite optimal surgical resection or for patients who are felt to have high-risk features. Further studies are needed to fully define high-risk features, but the current hypothesis is that patients older than the age of 40 with residual disease represent a subset of cases in which earlier intervention may be warranted. The basis for these recommendations is three prospective studies done over the past 10 years.[34,35,83] The studies were designed to address two specific questions: Is there a radiation dose that might improve survival, and does early intervention with radiation improve outcome compared with observation? A fourth study sought to evaluate the survival impact of chemotherapy in addition to radiation.[19]

The European Organization for Research and Treatment of Cancer (EORTC) conducted two prospective studies in adults with low-grade glioma, which included astrocytoma, oligodendroglioma, and mixed oligoastrocytoma.[34,35] EORTC protocol 22845 randomized 311 patients to postoperative observation versus postoperative radiation (54 Gy), whereas EORTC 22844 randomized 379 patients to high-dose (59.4 Gy) versus low-dose (45 Gy) radiation. The two studies were conducted simultaneously, with similar eligibility and stratification factors. No survival benefit was seen with high-dose radiation compared with low-dose radiation, and perhaps more importantly, no survival benefit was seen when radiation was used postoperatively compared with patients who were followed with observation alone. The 5-year overall survival rate for observation was 66% compared with 63% with radiation of 54 Gy, 58% for low-dose radiation of 45 Gy, and 59% for radiation of 59.4 Gy. There was no difference in the 5-year progression-free survival rate comparing the low dose (47%) versus higher dose radiation (50%). However, there was an improvement in the 5-year progression-free survival in patients randomized to radiation (44%) compared with patients who were observed (37%). The conclusions from these two large prospective studies support the notion that a survival benefit does not exist when radiation is used in the initial treatment of adults with low-grade glioma, although there does appear to be a difference in progression-free survival.

The Southwest Oncology Group (SWOG) conducted a small prospective randomized study of radiation alone (55 Gy) versus radiation plus adjuvant chemotherapy using single-agent lomustine (CCNU).[19] This study included adult patients with subtotal resections or biopsies of astrocytoma, oligodendroglioma, or mixed oligoastrocytoma. Only 60 patients were randomized. There appeared to be a trend toward better median survival with chemotherapy (7.4 years) compared with radiation alone (4.45 years), but the 10-year survival rate was 40% for radiation alone compared with radiation plus CCNU (20%). Thus this study also suggests that more therapy is not necessarily better.

Finally, the North Central Cancer Treatment Group (NCCTG), the Radiation Therapy Oncology Group (RTOG), and the Eastern Cooperative Group conducted a large phase III study in adult patients with newly diagnosed low-grade glioma

---

*See references 3, 19, 31, 33, 35, 48, 50, 77, 82, 86, 88, 92.

(astrocytoma, oligodendroglioma, and oligoastrocytoma), randomizing patients to high-dose (64.8 Gy) versus low-dose (50.4 Gy) radiation.[83] As with the EORTC 22844 trial, no survival benefit was seen with the higher dose radiation. There appeared to be a higher incidence of neurotoxicity at 5 years with the higher dose strategy (10% rate) compared with lower dose radiation (2% rate). The 5-year overall survival rate was 72% and 65% with low-dose radiation compared with higher dose radiation, respectively. Important negative prognostic factors included age younger than 40, tumor size larger than 5 cm, and astrocytoma histology. Extent of resection was an important prognostic factor in the EORTC 22844 study.

The RTOG recently completed accrual to a large randomized phase III study comparing radiation alone versus radiation plus adjuvant chemotherapy using procarbazine, CCNU, and vincristine (PCV) chemotherapy in patients with high-risk features, which they defined as age older than 40 or any age with less than a gross-total resection. Patients younger than 40 with a gross-total resection were followed with observation. The results of this study have not been analyzed but will be of interest and are hoped to add further information about prognostic subgroups and the impact of combination radiation and chemotherapy. Other randomized studies are ongoing in the EORTC as well. These new studies will be of great interest not only for the outcomes data but also for the results of tissue correlation studies that will compare biologic factors in the outcomes analysis. We hope molecular pathology and genetic characterization of tumors will become as important as age, histology, and extent of resection as prognostic factors. The goal of these studies is to ultimately allow specific stratification of patients toward treatment more likely to improve survival with minimal risk.

Radiation frequently will be necessary in patients with low-grade glioma. Older, newly diagnosed patients with larger tumors or any patient with symptomatic lesions should be considered for radiation. The alternative approach is to use chemotherapy in an attempt to defer the need for radiation (see later discussion). In general, radiation is given to a dose of 50 Gy to 54 Gy, in 1.8 Gy to 2.0 Gy fractions, to a focal field with 2-cm margins. Whole-brain radiation is rarely indicated and can cause significant neurocognitive deficits over time. This is especially relevant in older patients who appear to have less tolerance to radiation-associated injury. Younger patients, who may live for decades, are also at greater risk for late radiation effects. The volume of brain irradiated, total dose given, and tumor location may play a role in the development of late radiation effects. Unfortunately, there is limited prospective data concerning the scope and degree of neurotoxicity in long-term survivors treated with radiation. Improved techniques now exist for radiation-treatment planning that make it possible to limit normal brain exposure to higher dose radiation, and we hope these advances will minimize the potential negative impact of radiation-associated injury.

With the results thus far presented in the literature, a practical approach to treating the patient with low-grade glioma would be to consider prognostic factors and make specific recommendations based on age, extent of resection, tumor location, and presence of symptoms related to the residual disease. One could strongly consider the option of observation, particularly for a younger patient with a gross-total resection of disease. Observation of the older patient with gross-total resection is also an option, although the risk of earlier progression may be higher compared with younger patients. More frequent scanning may be indicated in this setting. Younger patients (older than 40 years) with partially resected disease, who are without significant symptoms, could also be given the option of observation as well, given the fact that a survival benefit has not been demonstrated with early intervention using radiation. This is not to state categorically that radiation is not indicated, because there may appear to be some benefit in progression-free survival. Some patients and physicians may believe that the potential to defer growth is an appropriate reason to choose radiation early. In this circumstance, the risks of radiation need to be weighed against this nonsurvival benefit. Smaller lesions in noneloquent areas of the brain would seem to offer less long-term risk and thus may be a situation where radiation would be a reasonable approach. Younger patients with symptomatic disease, despite optimal surgery, could be given the option of radiation, or perhaps chemotherapy, and, as noted previously, should consider enrollment in clinical trials. Older patients with residual disease, with or without symptoms, appear to represent the highest risk group for early progression and should be considered for radiation treatment. Whenever possible, enrollment in clinical studies should be encouraged, given the uncertainty of specific therapies on survival outcomes within patient subgroups.

Chemotherapy

Management options for adults with low-grade astrocytomas (LGAs) include observation, surgery, radiation, or chemotherapy, but there is no well-established standard approach. Patients who have undergone a complete radiographic resection of their tumor are often followed with surveillance MRI scans and treated at progression. In the past, patients who have undergone subtotal resections have been treated with radiation therapy. However, there is now a trend to avoid up-front radiation based on an EORTC study that suggests there is no survival benefit.[34] Adjuvant chemotherapy after radiation has not typically been given. However, the RTOG is conducting a study that addresses the question of a possible benefit with this approach. In this trial patients older than 40 or those with incompletely resected low-grade tumors will receive radiation with or without PCV.

The role of chemotherapy in adult patients with LGA has not been extensively investigated. This section will focus on the use of chemotherapy in the treatment of adults with LGA and the relevant clinical studies that have been completed or are being conducted.

In the available literature describing the use of chemotherapy for low-grade gliomas in adults there are differences in trial methodology that can confound an interpretation of the results. Most studies are retrospective and have a mixture of low-grade histologies included. Patients may also have had different therapies before receiving chemotherapy, such as radiation. Chemotherapy in adults with LGA has most commonly been used as salvage treatment for post–radiation therapy progression.[10,13,22] However, in many instances it is not clear that the tumor has remained low grade at progression, because tissue confirmation has not been obtained. Up-front chemotherapy has been used primarily to treat children to prevent the potential long-term deleterious effects of radiation.[21,72]

To date there has only been a single published randomized trial to assess the role of chemotherapy in patients with LGAs. SWOG conducted a prospectively randomized study to evaluate the addition of CCNU to radiation therapy for the treatment of low-grade gliomas. This study included grade I or II astrocytomas that were pilocytic astrocytomas, gemistocytic astrocytomas, mildly anaplastic astrocytomas, mixed gliomas, oligodendrogliomas, and gangliogliomas.[19] Fifty-four patients were randomized after incomplete resection to receive radiation or radiation in combination with CCNU. There was no statistically significant difference in survival time between the two groups. The median survival for patients who received radiation alone was 4.5 years, and for patients who received radiation plus CCNU median survival was 7.4 years; P was .7. Other clinical factors that impacted survival in this study were age, functional status, and extent of resection.

Temozolomide (Temodar), an oral alkylating agent, is now being investigated in several trials for patients with progressive low-grade gliomas. In a study published by Quinn et al, temozolomide was administered at 200 mg/m^2/day for 5 consecutive days to 46 patients with progressive low-grade gliomas.[73] Histologic types included in this cohort were astrocytoma, oligodendroglioma, mixed glioma, and pilocytic astrocytoma. Thirty-five percent of the patients had astrocytomas. The median period of follow-up was 11.2 months. Fifteen percent of patients had prior radiation, and 22% had prior chemotherapy. The objective response rate for all histologic types was 61%, with an additional 35% having stable disease. Median progression-free survival was 22 months. In the 16 patients with astrocytomas, the overall objective response rate was 69% (31%, 5/16 complete response, and 38%, 6/16 partial response).

Pace et al have also looked at temozolomide in 43 patients with progressive low-grade gliomas.[62] Tumor types included grade II astrocytomas, oligodendrogliomas, and mixed gliomas. Patients began therapy at the time of documented radiographic progression. Thirty patients had previously received radiation. Sixteen patients had already been treated with PCV chemotherapy. Temodar was administered at 200 mg/m^2/day for 5 consecutive days. They observed 4 complete responses and 16 partial responses for an objective response rate of 47%. Seventeen patients had stable disease, making the overall response rate 86%. Median length of response was 10 months. Progression-free survival at 12 months was 39.6%.

Viviers et al assessed the efficacy of temozolomide in patients with stable or progressive low-grade gliomas.[95] Patients in this study had no antitumor therapy other than resection. Twenty-five patients were enrolled (18 grade II astrocytoma and 7 oligodendroglioma). All patients had radiographic residual disease at study entry. Of the 12 patients who received a minimum of six cycles, an overall objective response rate of 67% was seen.

Based on these studies it is apparent that temozolomide is an effective therapy for patients with recurrent or progressive low-grade gliomas. This raises the question of a role for this agent in patients with newly diagnosed low-grade gliomas. Currently, a single-institution phase II investigation is being conducted at the University of California at San Francisco (UCSF) that will address this question. In this study newly diagnosed patients will be treated with temozolomide as the primary therapy after an incomplete resection. The goals are to determine efficacy by radiographic response criteria and time until disease progression.

Other chemotherapy regimens that have been investigated in adults are carboplatin and PCV. Christina et al treated 22 patients with progressive low-grade gliomas using carboplatin.[15] Carboplatin was given at 560 mg/m^2 every 4 weeks. Maximum response was stable disease in 12 patients (55%). The 3-year progression-free survival was 20%. Median follow-up was 28 months. Carboplatin in combination with vincristine has been used often to treat children with low-grade gliomas.[63,64]

The reported data using the PCV regimen has been predominantly for patients with low-grade oligodendroglioma and oligoastrocytoma, which is outside the focus of this review.[11]

The best management for adult patients with low-grade gliomas has not been defined. And the only clear role for chemotherapy in adults with LGA is in the setting of postradiation progression. In those patients with gross totally resected tumors follow-up alone after surgery is a treatment option, reserving further therapy until tumor progression. At the time of progression both radiation and chemotherapy may be considered. Investigations also show that chemotherapy can be used effectively in some patients with progressive tumors that have not been previously treated. Postoperative high-risk patients (those older than 40 years and those with significant residual disease) with stable tumors may also receive radiation or chemotherapy. There is an emerging trend to forgo or delay radiation and use chemotherapy in this setting. The efficacy of this approach is currently being evaluated in a single-institution phase II trial using temozolomide.

CONCLUSION

Despite a better prognosis when compared with higher grade glial tumors, low-grade glioma patients have a median survival of 5 to 10 years and a 10-year survival rate that ranges from 5% to 50%.* Between 50% and 75% of the patients will eventually die of their disease. Within the past 10 years, several studies analyzing the prognostic impact of tumor resection on outcome reveal lower recurrence rates and improved overall survival with radical resection. Moreover, aggressive resection minimizes the chances of misdiagnosis as a result of sampling error and also relieves symptomatic mass effect, obstructive hydrocephalus, and neurologic deficit. Our standard practice is radical resection whenever feasible. This approach requires precise delineation of both the tumor margins and functional regions of involved and adjacent brain. A combination of methods, including intraoperative navigation techniques, intraoperative ultrasonography, and cortical and subcortical functional mapping, may be used to minimize the incidence of morbidity. Adjuvant postoperative therapy is usually not required in the treatment of localized, low-grade gliomas resected with minimal or no residual tumor volume. The tumor is followed with sequential imaging, and recurrence is treated with another operation and radiation, chemotherapy, or both. Overall, the management of low-grade gliomas is still controversial, and practice parameters are ill defined. This is caused by our limited knowledge regarding the natural history of this entity and lack of high-quality evidence supporting various treatment options.

---

*See references 19, 23, 25, 31, 48, 55, 68, 69, 86, 94.

References

1. Apuzzo MLJ, Chandrasoma PT, Cohen D, et al: Computed imaging stereotaxy: experience and perspective related to 500 procedures applied to brain masses. Neurosurgery 20:930–937, 1987.

2. Bahary JP, Villemure JG, Choi S, et al: Low-grade pure and mixed cerebral astrocytomas treated in the CT scan era. J Neuro-oncol 27:173–177, 1996.

3. Bauman G, Lote K, Larson D, et al: Pretreatment factors predict overall survival for patients with low-grade glioma: a recursive partitioning analysis. Int J Radiat Oncol Biol Phys 45:923–929, 1999.

4. Berger MS, Ghatan S, Haglund MM, et al: Low grade gliomas associated with intractable epilepsy: seizure outcome utilizing electrocorticography during tumor resection. J Neurosurg 79:62–69, 1993.

5. Berger MS, Deliganis AV, Dobbins J, Keles GE: The effect of extent of resection on recurrence in patients with low grade cerebral hemisphere gliomas. Cancer 74:1784–1791, 1994.

6. Berger MS, Keles GE: Intraoperative image update by interface with ultrasound. In Germano IM (ed): Advanced Techniques in Image-Guided Brain and Spine Surgery. New York, Thieme Medical Publishers, 2002.

7. Bernstein M, Parrent AG: Complications of CT-guided stereotactic biopsy of intra-axial brain lesions. J Neurosurg 81:165–168, 1994.

8. Bogler O, Huang HJ, Cavenee WK: Loss of wild-type p53 bestows a growth advantage on primary cortical astrocytes and facilitates their in vitro transformation. Cancer Res 55:2746–2751, 1995.

9. Brat DJ, Scheithauer BW, Medina-Flores R, et al: Infiltrative astrocytomas with granular cell features (granular cell astrocytomas): a study of histopathologic features, grading, and outcome. Am J Surg Pathol 26:750–757, 2002.

10. Buckner JC, Brown LD, Kugler JW, et al: Phase II evaluation of recombinant interferon alpha and BCNU in recurrent glioma. J Neurosurg 82:430–435, 1995.

11. Buckner JC, Gesme D, Jr, O'Fallon JR: Phase II trial of procarbazine, lomustine, and vincristine as initial therapy for patients with low-grade oligodendroglioma or oligoastrocytoma: efficacy and associations with chromosomal abnormalities. J Clin Oncol 21:251–255, 2003.

12. Burger PC, Scheithauer BW, Armed Forces Institute of Pathology (U.S.), Pathology: UAfRaEi. Tumors of the Central Nervous System. Washington, DC, Armed Forces Institute of Pathology, 1994.

13. Cairncross G, Macdonald D, Ludwin S, et al: Chemotherapy for anaplastic oligodendroglioma. National Cancer Institute of Canada Clinical Trials Group. J Clin Oncol 12:2013–2021, 1994.

14. Castellano-Sanchez AA, Ohgaki H, Yokoo H, et al: Granular cell astrocytomas show a high frequency of allelic loss but are not a genetically defined subset. Brain Pathol 13:185–194, 2003.

15. Christina M, Cavazos SG, Herndon J II et al: A phase II study of low-dose carboplatin (CBDCA) chemotherapy in adults with progressive low-grade gliomas. Proc Am Soc Clin Oncol, 2001.

16. Cunningham JM, Kimmel DW, Scheithauer BW, et al: Analysis of proliferation markers and p53 expression in gliomas of astrocytic origin: relationships and prognostic value. J Neurosurg 86:121–130, 1997.

17. Daumas-Duport C, Scheithauer BW, O'Fallon J, Kelly P: Grading of astrocytomas: a simple and reproducible method. Cancer 62:2152–2165, 1988.

18. Davis FG, Malinski N, Haenszel W, et al: Primary brain tumor incidence rates in four United States regions, 1985–1989: a pilot study. Neuroepidemiology 15:103–112, 1996.

19. Eyre HJ, Crowley JJ, Townsend JJ, et al: A randomized trial of radiotherapy plus CCNU for incompletely resected low-grade gliomas: a Southwest Oncology Group study. J Neurosurg 78:909–914, 1993.

20. Fisher PG, Breiter SN, Carson BS, et al: A clinicopathologic reappraisal of brain stem tumor classification. Identification of pilocystic astrocytoma and fibrillary astrocytoma as distinct entities. Cancer 89:1569–1576, 2000.

21. Gajjar A, Heideman RL, Kovnar EH, et al: Response of pediatric low grade gliomas to chemotherapy. Pediatr Neurosurg 19:113–118; discussion 119–120, 1993.

22. Galanis E, Buckner JC, Burch PA, et al: Phase II trial of nitrogen mustard, vincristine, and procarbazine in patients with recurrent glioma: North Central Cancer Treatment Group results. J Clin Oncol 16:2953–2958, 1998.

23. Gannett DE, Wisbeck WM, Silbergeld DL, Berger MS: The role of postoperative irradiation in the treatment of oligodendroglioma. Int J Radiat Oncol Biol Phys 30:567–573, 1994.

24. Gonzales D, Elvidge AR: On the occurrence of epilepsy caused by astrocytoma of the cerebral hemispheres. J Neurosurg 19:470–482, 1962.

25. Guidelines and Outcomes Committee of the AANS: Practice parameters in adults with suspected or known supratentorial nonoptic pathway low-grade glioma. Neurosurg Focus 4:Article 10, 1998.

26. Guthrie BL, Laws ER: Supratentorial low-grade gliomas. Neurosurg Clin North Am 1:37–48, 1990.

27. Hang Z, Wei Y, Liao W: [A comparison between astrocytoma cells and the developing astrocytes in human embryo brain by electron microscopy]. Zhonghua Bing Li Xue Za Zhi 24:65–68, 1995.

28. Hanzely Z, Polgar C, Fodor J, et al: Role of early radiotherapy in the treatment of supratentorial WHO Grade II astrocytomas: long-term results of 97 patients. J Neurooncol 63:305–312, 2003.

29. Ito S, Chandler KL, Prados MD, et al: Proliferative potential and prognostic evaluation of low-grade astrocytomas. J Neurooncol 19:1–9, 1994.

30. James CD, Carlbom E, Nordenskjold M, et al: Mitotic recombination of chromosome 17 in astrocytomas. Proc Natl Acad Sci USA 86:2858–2862, 1989.

31. Janny P, Cure H, Mohr M, et al: Low grade supratentorial astrocytomas. Management and prognostic factors. Cancer 73:1937–1945, 1994.

32. Jeremic B, Milicic B, Grujicic D, et al: Hyperfractionated radiation therapy for incompletely resected supratentorial low-grade glioma: a 10-year update of a phase II study. Int J Radiat Oncol Biol Phys 57(2):465–471, 2003.

33. Jeremic B, Shibamoto Y, Grujicic D, et al: Hyperfractionated radiation therapy for incompletely resected supratentorial low-grade glioma. A phase II study. Radiother Oncol 49:49–54, 1998.

34. Karim ABMF, Afra D, Cornu P, et al: Randomized trial on the efficacy of radiotherapy for cerebral low-grade glioma in the adult: European Organization for Research and Treatment of Cancer Study 22845 with the Medical Research Council Study BR04: an interim analysis. Int J Radiat Oncol Biol Phys 52:316–324, 2002.

35. Karim ABMF, Maat B, Hatlevoll R, et al: A randomized trial on dose-response in radiation therapy of low-grade cerebral glioma: European Organization for Research and Treatment of Cancer (EORTC) Study 22844. Int J Radiat Oncol Biol Phys 36:549–556, 1996.

36. Keles GE, Berger MS: Functional mapping. In Bernstein M, Berger MS (eds): Neuro-Oncology Essentials. New York, Thieme Medical Publishers, 2000.

37. Keles GE, Berger MS: Epilepsy associated with brain tumors. In Kaye AH and Laws ER (eds): Brain Tumors: An Encyclopedic Approach, 2nd ed. London, Churchill Livingstone (Harcourt Publishers), 2001.

38. Keles GE, Lamborn KR, Berger MS: Low-grade hemispheric gliomas in adults: a critical review of extent of resection as a factor influencing outcome. J Neurosurg 95:735–745, 2001.

39. Keles GE, Lamborn KR, Berger MS: Coregistration accuracy and detection of brain shift using intraoperative sononavigation during resection of hemispheric tumors. Neurosurgery 53:556–562, 2003.

40. Kepes JJ, Rubinstein LJ, Chiang H: The role of astrocytes in the formation of cartilage in gliomas. An immunohistochemical study of four cases. Am J Pathol 117:471–483, 1984.

41. Kernohan JW, Mabon RF, Svien HJ, Adson AW: A simplified classification of the gliomas. Proc Staff Meet Mayo Clin 24:71–75, 1949.

42. Kleihues P, Burger PC, Scheithauer, BW: The new WHO classification of brain tumours, Brain Pathol 3:255–268, 1993.

43. Kleihues P, Cavenee WK: Pathology and Genetics of Tumours of the Nervous System. World Health Organization Classification of Tumours. Lyon, France, IARC Press, 2000.

44. Kosel S, Scheithauer BW, Graeber MB: Genotype-phenotype correlation in gemistocytic astrocytomas. Neurosurgery 48:187–193, 2001.

45. Kros JM, Waarsenburg N, Hayes DP, et al: Cytogenetic analysis of gemistocytic cells in gliomas. J Neuropathol Exp Neurol 59:679–686, 2000.

46. Krouwer HG, Davis RL, Silver P, Prados M: Gemistocytic astrocytomas: a reappraisal. J Neurosurg 74:399–406, 1991.

47. Laws ER, Taylor WF, Clifton MB, Okazaki H: Neurosurgical management of low-grade astrocytoma of the cerebral hemispheres. J Neurosurg 61:665–673, 1984.

48. Leighton C, Fisher B, Bauman G, et al: Supratentorial low-grade glioma in adults: an analysis of prognostic factors and timing of radiation. J Clin Oncol 15:1294–1301, 1997.

49. Lo SS, Hall WA, Cho KH, et al: Radiation dose response for supratentorial low-grade glioma—institutional experience and literature review. J Neurol Sci 214:43–48, 2003.

50. Lote K, Egeland T, Hager B, et al: Survival, prognostic factors, and therapeutic efficacy in low-grade glioma: a retrospective study in 379 patients. J Clin Oncol 15:3129–3140, 1997.

51. Louis DN: The p53 gene and protein in human brain tumors. J Neuropathol Exp Neurol 53:11–21, 1994.

52. Lunsford LD, Somaza S, Kondziolka D, Flickenger JC: Survival after stereotactic biopsy and radiation of cerebral non-neoplastic, non-pilocytic astrocytoma. J Neurosurg 82:523–529, 1995.

53. Mahaley MS, Mettlin C, Narajan N: National survey of patterns of care for brain-tumor patients. J Neurosurg 28:659–665, 1989.

54. Manford M, Hart YM, Sander JWAS, et al: National General Practice Study of Epilepsy (NGPSE): partial seizure patterns in a general population. Neurology 42:1911–1917, 1992.

55. McCormack BM, Miller DC, Budzilovich GN, et al: Treatment and survival of low-grade astrocytoma in adults 1977–1988. Neurosurgery 31:636–642, 1992.

56. Medberry III CA, Straus KL, Steinberg SM, et al: Low-grade astrocytomas: treatment results and prognostic variables. Int J Radiat Oncol Biol Phys 15:837–841, 1988.

57. Miralbell R, Balart J, Matias-Guiu X, et al: Radiotherapy for supratentorial low-grade gliomas: results and prognostic factors with special focus on tumour volume parameters. Radiotherapy and Oncology 27:112–116, 1993.

58. Muller W, Afra D, Schroder R: Supratentorial recurrences of gliomas: morphological studies in relation to time intervals with astrocytomas. Acta Neurochir 37:75–91, 1977.

59. Nakamura T, Hirato J, Hotchi M, et al: Astrocytoma with granular cell tumor-like changes. Report of a case with histochemical and ultrastructural characterization of granular cells. Acta Pathol Jpn 40:206–211, 1990.

60. Nicolato A, Gerosa MA, Fina P, et al: Prognostic factors in low-grade supratentorial astrocytomas: a uni-multivariate statistical analysis in 76 surgically treated adult patients. Surg Neurol 44:208–223, 1995.

61. North CA, North RB, Epstein JA, et al: Low-grade cerebral astrocytomas. Survival and quality of life after radiation therapy. Cancer 66:6–14, 1990.

62. Pace A, Maschio M, Carosi MA, et al: Temozolomide chemotherapy for progressive low grade glioma. Proc Am Soc Clin Oncol 22:107, 2003.

63. Packer RJ, Lange B, Ater J, et al: Carboplatin and vincristine for recurrent and newly diagnosed low-grade gliomas of childhood. J Clin Oncol 11:850–856, 1993.

64. Packer RJ, Ater J, Allen J, et al: Carboplatin and vincristine chemotherapy for children with newly diagnosed progressive low-grade gliomas. J Neurosurg 86:747–754, 1997.

65. Penfield W, Erickson TC, Tarlov IM: Relation of intracranial tumors and symptomatic epilepsy. Arch Neurol Psychiatr 44:300–315, 1940.

66. Peraud A, Ansari H, Bise K, Reulen HJ: Clinical outcome of supratentorial astrocytoma WHO Grade II. Acta Neurochir 140:1213–1222, 1998.

67. Perry A, Jenkins RB, O'Fallon JR, et al: Clinicopathologic study of 85 similarly treated patients with anaplastic astrocytic tumors. An analysis of DNA content (ploidy), cellular proliferation, and p53 expression. Cancer 86:672–683, 1999.

68. Philippon JH, Clemenceau SH, Fauchon FH, Foncin JF: Supratentorial low-grade astrocytomas in adults. Neurosurgery 32:554–559, 1993.

69. Piepmeier JM: Observations on the current treatment of low-grade astrocytic tumors of the cerebral hemispheres. J Neurosurg 67:177–181, 1987.

70. Piepmeier J, Christopher S, Spencer D, et al: Variations in the natural history and survival of patients with supratentorial low-grade astrocytomas. Neurosurgery 38:872–879, 1996.

71. Pignatti F, van den Bent M, Curran D, et al: Prognostic factors for survival in adult patients with cerebral low-grade glioma. J Clin Oncol 20:2076–2084, 2002.

72. Prados MD, Edwards MS, Rabbitt J, et al: Treatment of pediatric low-grade gliomas with a nitrosourea-based multiagent chemotherapy regimen. J Neurooncol 32(3):235–241, 1997.

73. Quinn JA, Reardon DA, Friedman AH, et al: Phase II trial of temozolomide in patients with progressive low-grade glioma. J Clin Oncol 21:646–651, 2003.

74. Rajan B, Pickuth D, Ashley S, et al: The management of histologically unverified presumed cerebral gliomas with radiotherapy. Int J Radiat Oncol Biol Phys 28:405–413, 1993.

75. Recht LD, Lew R, Smith TW: Suspected low-grade glioma: is deferring therapy safe? Ann Neurol 31:431–436, 1992.

76. Rey JA, Bello MJ: Cytogenetics. In Berger MS, Wilson CB (eds): The Gliomas. Philadelphia, WB Saunders, 1999.

77. Rudoler S, Corn BW, Werner-Wasik M, et al: Patterns of tumor progression after radiotherapy for low-grade gliomas. Am J Clin Oncol 21:23–27, 1998.

78. Salcman M: The natural history of low grade gliomas. In Apuzzo MLJ (ed): Benign Cerebral Gliomas. Park Ridge, Ill, AANS Publications, 1995.

79. Scerrati M, Roselli R, Iacoangeli M, et al: Prognostic factors in low grade (WHO grade II) gliomas of the cerebral hemispheres: the role of surgery. J Neurol Neurosurg Psychiatry 61:291–296, 1996.

80. Schuurman PR, Troost D, Verbeeten B Jr, Bosch DA: 5-year survival and clinical prognostic factors in progressive supratentorial diffuse "low grade" astrocytoma: a retrospective analysis of 46 cases. Acta Neurochir 139:2–7, 1997.

81. Shafqat S, Hedley-White ET, Henson JW: Age-dependent rate of anaplastic transformation in low-grade astrocytoma. Neurology 52:867–869, 1999.

82. Shaw EG, Daumas-Duport C, Scheithauer BW, et al: Radiation therapy in the management of low-grade supratentorial astrocytomas. J Neurosurg 70:853–861, 1989.

83. Shaw E, Arusell R, Scheithauer B, et al: Prospective randomized trial of low-versus high-dose radiation therapy in adults with supratentorial low-grade glioma: initial report of a North Central Cancer Treatment Group/Radiation Therapy Oncology Group/Eastern Cooperative Oncology Group study. J Clin Oncol 20: 2267–2276, 2002.

84. Shaw EG, Scheithauer BW, Gilbertson DT, et al: Postoperative radiotherapy of supratentorial low-grade gliomas. Int J Radiat Oncol Biol Phys 16:663–668, 1989.

85. Shaw EG, Scheithauer BW, O'Fallon JR, Davis DH: Mixed oligoastrocytomas: a survival and prognostic factor analysis. Neurosurgery 34:577–582, 1994.

86. Shibamoto Y, Kitakabu Y, Takahashi M, et al: Supratentorial low-grade astrocytoma. Correlation of computed tomography findings with effect of radiation therapy and prognostic variables. Cancer 72:190–195, 1993.

87. Silverman C, Marks JE: Prognostic significance of contrast enhancement in low-grade astrocytomas of the adult cerebrum. Radiology 139:211–213, 1981.

88. Singer JM: Supratentorial low grade gliomas in adults. A retrospective analysis of 43 cases treated with surgery and radiotherapy. Eur J Surg Oncol 21:198–200, 1995.

89. Soffietti R, Chio A, Giordana MT, at al: Prognostic factors in well-differentiated cerebral astrocytomas in the adult. Neurosurgery 24:686–692, 1989.

90. Souweidane NM, Hoffman HJ: Current treatment of thalamic gliomas in children. J Neurooncol 28:157–166, 1996.

91. Tihan T, Davis R, Elowitz E, et al: Practical value of Ki-67 and p53 labeling indexes in stereotactic biopsies of diffuse and pilocytic astrocytomas. Arch Pathol Lab Med 124:108–113, 2000.

92. van Veelen MLC, Avezaat CJJ, Kros JM, et al: Supratentorial low grade astrocytoma: prognostic factors, dedifferentiation, and the issue of early versus late surgery. J Neurol Neurosurg Psychiatry 64:581–587, 1998.

93. Velema JP, Walker AM: The age curve of nervous system tumor incidence in adults: common shape but changing levels by sex, race and geographical location. Int J Epidemiol 16:177–183, 1987.

94. Vertosick FT, Selker RG, Arena VC: Survival of patients with well-differentiated astrocytomas diagnosed in the era of computed tomography. Neurosurgery 28:496–501, 1991.

95. Viviers L, Hines F, Britton J, et al: A phase II trial of primary chemotherapy with temozolomide in patients with low-grade cerebral gliomas. Proc Am Soc Clin Oncol, 2000.

96. Wang M, Tihan T, Rojiani AM, et al: Angiocentric bipolar astrocytoma: a distinctive infiltrating astrocytoma of children. J Neuropathol Exp Neurol 61:475, 2002.

97. Watanabe K, Peraud A, Gratas C, et al: p53 and PTEN gene mutations in gemistocytic astrocytomas. Acta Neuropathol (Berl) 95:559–564, 1998.

98. Watanabe K, Sato K, Biernat W, et al: Incidence and timing of p53 mutations during astrocytoma progression in patients with multiple biopsies. Clin Cancer Res 3:523–530, 1997.

99. Watanabe K, Tachibana O, Yonekawa Y, et al: Role of gemistocytes in astrocytoma progression. Lab Invest 76:277–284, 1997.

100. Weingart J, Olivi A, Brem H: Supratentorial low-grade astrocytomas in adults. Neurosurg Q 1:141–159, 1991.

101. Whitton AC, Bloom HJG: Low grade glioma of the cerebral hemispheres in adults: a retrospective analysis of 88 cases. Int J Radiat Oncol Biol Phys 18:783–786, 1990.

102. Wyke BD: The cortical control of movement: a contribution to the surgical physiology of seizures. Epilepsia 1:4–35, 1959.

103. Yahamada AM, Bruner JM, Donehower LA, et al: Astrocytes derived from p53-deficient mice provide a multistep in vitro model for development of malignant gliomas. Mol Cell Biol 15:4249–4259, 1995.

104. Zakhary R, Keles GE, Berger MS: Intraoperative imaging techniques in the treatment of brain tumors. Curr Opin Oncol 11:152–156, 1999.

105. Zulch KJ: Brain Tumors: Their Biology and Pathology, 3rd ed. Berlin, Springer-Verlag, 1986.

CHAPTER 18

ANAPLASTIC ASTROCYTOMA

Steven Brem, Susan Snodgrass, Margaret Booth-Jones, James Pearlman, Reed Murtagh, Frank Vrionis, S. Clifford Schold, Jr., Marguerite Wotoczek-Obadia, and Amyn Rojiani

Anaplastic astrocytomas (AAs) command increasing interest in neuro-oncology. Optimal outcomes can be expected when the tumor is recognized, histologically confirmed, and treated in a robust, interdisciplinary manner, because patients will benefit from the application and integration of current advances in surgery, oncology, radiation therapy, and rehabilitation. The starting point for the diagnosis is the World Health Organization (WHO) classification.[60] AAs are located at the crossroads between the slow-growing, low-grade gliomas (WHO grade II) and highly malignant glioblastoma (WHO grade IV). Once the diagnosis is clearly established, adherence to the clinical guidelines developed for malignant gliomas by the National Cooperative Cancer Network (NCCN)[43] provides a valuable treatment paradigm—what we term at our institution *total cancer care*. In earlier literature, AA was generally grouped with glioblastoma, but new FDA-approved treatments for AA highlight the reality that these tumors are distinctive from glioblastoma in their biology and therapy.

There has been little change in the survival of patients with glioblastoma during the past 3 decades,[22] but the prognosis for a patient with AA is significantly better. At the molecular level, these gliomas provide specific targets for potential control of malignancy to avert progression to glioblastoma. Confusion abounds in the literature, because these tumors have been commonly grouped with glioblastomas. However, it is clear that AAs are more than a precursor of glioblastoma and respond to therapy with improvements in the time and quality of survival.

DEFINITION AND LOCATION

AAs are diffusely infiltrating astrocytomas with focal or dispersed *anaplasia* and a marked proliferative potential.[60] Localization of AAs generally corresponds to that of other diffusely infiltrating astrocytomas, with a preference for the cerebral hemispheres.[60] In the Moffitt series (*n* = 43 patients), the resected tumors were located throughout the cerebrum, but predominantly in the frontal lobe (64%) followed by the temporal lobe (29%). AAs can arise from low-grade astrocytomas (WHO grade II) but also can be diagnosed *de novo* at first biopsy without signs of a less malignant precursor.[60] AAs have an innate tendency toward malignant progression to glioblastoma. Like glioblastoma, these tumors tend to

recur locally, often at the margin of the surgical operation, even when the initial operation has been a macroscopic total removal.[121]

CLINICAL FEATURES

Patients' initial symptoms and signs are similar to those of other types of gliomas[60] and include seizures, increasing neurologic deficit, and symptoms of raised intracranial pressure (headache, nausea, blurred vision, lethargy, personality change). Headaches and seizures are the most common presentation (Figure 18-1).

Diagnosis is made by tissue histopathology, either using a stereotactic needle biopsy or by resection of the tumor guided by magnetic resonance imaging (MRI). Because of the clinical overlap in symptoms and signs with low-grade astrocytomas (WHO grade II) and glioblastoma (WHO grade IV), the specific diagnosis can be made only by an accurate histologic diagnosis. Confusion until recently with the WHO classification system has abounded, resulting in large, multicenter studies using central review, reclassifying as many as 20% to 30% of patients with the initial diagnosis of AA.[1]

In our experience the use of stereotactic, magnetic resonance (MR)-guided craniotomy provides a more accurate diagnosis, because it can avoid the sampling error of a needle biopsy; selective biopsies of areas of greatest gadolinium enhancement, or "hot spots" (Figure 18-2), can be made. What appears to be an AA by needle biopsy can be upgraded to glioblastoma multiforme (GBM) at the time of craniotomy.[80]

EPIDEMIOLOGY, INCIDENCE, PROGNOSTIC FACTORS

The age distribution of AAs is consistent with their place as an intermediate in malignant progression from the most benign (WHO grade II) to the highly malignant glioblastoma (WHO grade IV). The average age at diagnosis is approximately 40,[60,94] higher than that of patients with WHO grade II tumors (age 34) and younger than the age of patients with glioblastoma (mean age 53).[60] In the Moffitt series, the median age of presentation was also 40. AAs are more common in

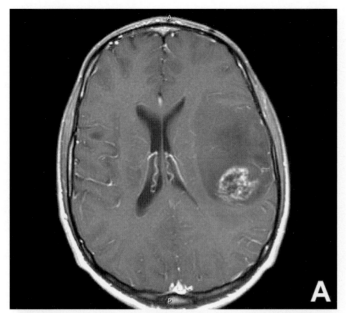

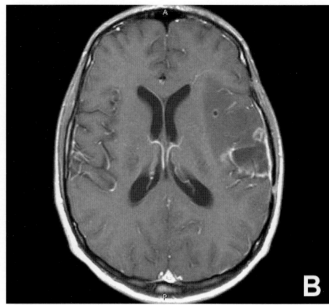

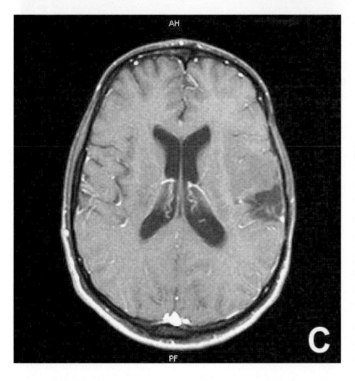

FIGURE 18-1 Magnetic resonance imaging (MRI) scans of a 19-year-old man who underwent a biopsy showing a low-grade glioma in the left temporal lobe. Three years later, he presented with a headaches and seizures. An MRI *(A)* showed a temporal-parietal tumor with associated vasogenic edema and irregular enhancement. A craniotomy with motor mapping was performed and the tumor removed was an anaplastic astrocytoma (AA). The patient was placed on temozolomide and given radiation. At 4 months *(B)* the mass effect was significantly improved. The patient received a New Approaches to Brain Tumor Therapy (NABTT) protocol of procarbazine and then had 5 cycles of carmustine, vincristine, and etopside. After 31 months, the patient was radiographically and clinically stable *(C)*. The patient continued to do well at 4-year follow-up.

males,[94] with a male-to-female ratio in one series of 1.8 : 1,[60] consistent with our experience at H. Lee Moffitt Cancer Center of 30 men and 13 females, a male-to-female ratio of 2.3:1.

The median survival for AA ranges between 2.5[117] to 3 years.[94] Favorable prognostic features[94,117] include (1) age younger than 50 years; (2) high Karnofsky performance scale (KPS) score; (3) a proliferative rate (Ki-67 index) of 5%; (4) absence of ring enhancement on CT scan, which reflects the degree of tumor angiogenesis[129]; and (5) presence of an oligodendroglial component.[117] Intensive salvage therapy of radiation and chemotherapy adds 1 year of survival.[94]

NEUROIMAGING

The well-established MRI features of intra-axial glial neoplasms provide clues to the tumor grade based on characteristics that define the extremes of the neoplastic spectrum, between benignity and malignancy.[2,24,31,86] Low-grade, benign astrocytic tumors tend to be well circumscribed anatomically, often with little mass effect, and devoid of enhancement following contrast administration (Figure 18-3A). These features reflect the biology of GBM in minimal invasiveness and angiogenesis, but not necrosis. Glioblastomas on MRI show extensive mass effect, extreme contrast enhance-

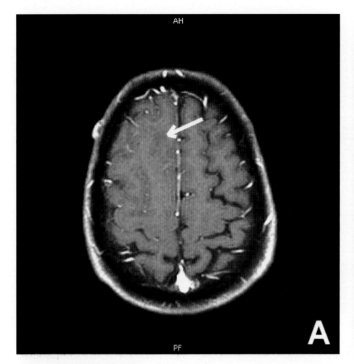

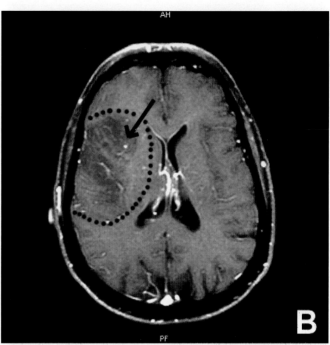

FIGURE 18-2   A 56-year-old man who presented with headaches and cognitive changes. A magnetic resonance imaging (MRI) scan showed two nonenhancing lesions in the right cerebral frontal lobe. *A,* Superior frontal gyrus *(arrow). B,* Inferior frontal gyrus near the operculum and Sylvian fissure *(dotted outline).* These lesions, before admission to Moffitt Cancer Center, were initially diagnosed as "strokes." Note the subtle mass effect with obliteration of the sulci in *A* and compression of the lateral ventricle in *B.* Progression of symptoms led to resection of the lesions, showing anaplastic astrocytoma. A small, gadolinium-enhancing "hot spot" *(black arrow)* in *B,* however, revealed a focal area of glioblastoma.

ment, necrosis, and occasional hemorrhage (see Figure 18-3C).

Between these two ends of the glial spectrum lies the AA.[2,31] The problem in identifying these tumors accurately preoperatively relates to their broad spectrum and the overlap between the benign and malignant forms. Specifically, AAs can appear as totally devoid of enhancement, mimicking a low-grade astrocytoma. This subpopulation can show histologically a relatively low proliferative rate and fewer mitotic figures, just sufficient to qualify as an AA. Sometimes, tumors with sufficient mitotic figures to qualify histologically as an AA will not enhance on MRI. These tumors could be in an early stage of neoplastic development (Figure 18-4A) and not stimulate sufficient angiogenesis to result in breakdown of the blood-brain barrier and contrast enhancement.

In the spectrum of malignancy, tumors that are less malignant will not demonstrate the elevated choline over creatinine (Cho/Cr) levels that are the hallmark of malignant activity on MR spectroscopy (MRS), and these tumors will not destroy sufficient neurons to result in decreased *N*-acetyl aspartate (NAA) levels.[77,86] On MRI perfusion studies, the rate of tissue capillary filling as represented by increased regional cerebral blood flow (rCBF) parameters may not be any more elevated than in a more benign tumor. Diffusion-tensor MRI[84] may not have increased directional flow caused by excessive vasogenic edema, and of course, diffusion-weighted image sequences will not be positive for the same reasons in these AAs that are barely over the threshold of anaplasia on the path toward increased malignancy.[5]

Higher grade tumors within the spectrum of AAs that are more aggressive will display increased membrane turnover and angiogenesis but may not meet all the main histologic criteria to be termed GBM (i.e., absence of necrosis). These tumors, by MRS, show increased Cho/Cr ratios and decreased NAA. Increased vascular permeability and disruption of the blood brain barrier result in (1) marked contrast enhancement on MRI, (2) increased rCBF on perfusion MRI, and (3) increased vasogenic edema on diffusion tensor MRI. These tumors closely resemble glioblastoma by MR criteria, and only a histologic diagnosis can distinguish the grade III AAs from the grade IV glioblastoma.

Positron-emission tomography (PET) uses ^{18}F-fluorodeoxyglucose (^{18}F-FDG) as an indicator of relative metabolism. AA tumors that are on the benign side of the spectrum relative to GBM would therefore be expected to not have much higher uptake of ^{18}F-FDG than normal brain, whereas the more malignant varieties can have the intense uptake of a GBM.[56,77] This may not be any more helpful than any of the other characteristics described previously in the preoperative diagnosis of AA.[23] In summary, MRI can delineate the clear-cut cases of benign (see Figure 18-3A) and highly malignant astrocytomas (glioblastoma, see Figure 18-3C). When findings are not pathognomonic for either one, AA should be in the preoperative differential diagnosis.

MRS may be a useful technique to predict survival and response after radiation therapy. In a study of 51 malignant gliomas, including 33 patients with AAs, survival correlated strongly with tumor grade and patient age, but the strongest

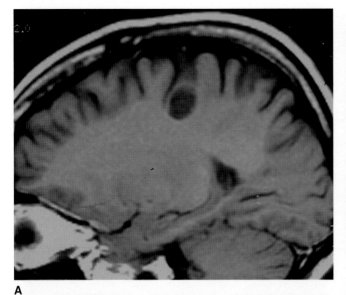

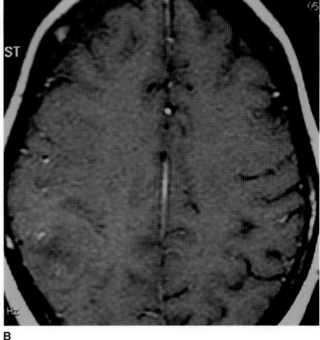

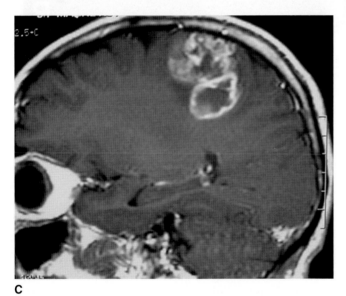

FIGURE 18-3 Magnetic resonance brain images of three main tumor types. *A,* Low-grade intra-axial astrocytoma. *B,* Anaplastic astrocytoma. *C,* Glioblastoma multiforme.

prognostic factor was the lactate to NAA ratio.[115] There was a significant difference in those patients whose tumors had a high lactate to NAA ratio (>2) compared with those patients with a good prognosis when the ratio of lactate to NAA was low (<2). For those patients with high lactate, the 1-year survival rate was 20%, and for those with low lactate to NAA values, the 1-year survival rate was 85%. Because lactate levels can be a surrogate marker of necrosis, another interpretation of the data is that the lactate to NAA ratio separates the glioblastomas from the AAs and the higher grade AAs that are close to becoming a glioblastoma from the patients with less aggressive AAs. Occasionally, the same patient will develop both AA and glioblastoma from different topographic areas (see Figure 18-2). These studies confirm that MRS can be useful: an elevated Cho/Cr ratio is a reliable indicator of malignancy for gliomas and correlates better for AAs compared with glioblastomas because of the confounding variable of tumor necrosis, which is more prevalent in glioblastoma.[52] Quantification of lipids and

macromolecules at short echo time (TE) provided a good marker for tumor grade, and a scatter plot of the sum of alanine, lactate, and delta 1.3 lipid signals versus myo-Inositol (mI)/Cho provided a simple way to separate most tumors by type and grade.[52]

Because of the role of angiogenesis in malignant progression of gliomas,[9,10,13] perfusion MRI also complements the histologic diagnosis.[71,72] Cerebral blood volume is significantly higher in glioblastoma compared with AA ($P < .05$) and much higher in both forms of malignant gliomas than low-grade gliomas (WHO grade II) ($P < .01$).[71]

TUMOR HISTOLOGY

The validity of distinguishing AAs from glioblastomas was confirmed by a large study of approximately 1500 malignant gliomas.[15] In both groups, advancing age was associated with

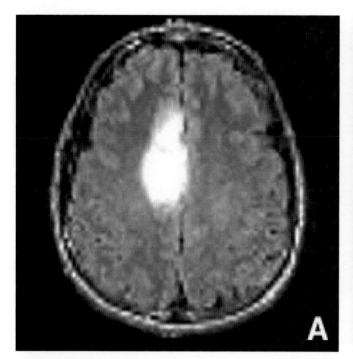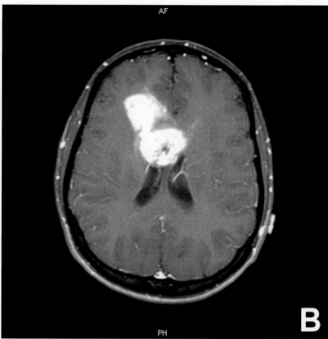

FIGURE 18-4 Magnetic resonance imaging (MRI) scans of a 44-year-old woman who initially presented with a grand-mal seizure and had a 5 × 3 × 3.5 cm noncontrast-enhancing mass in the right superior frontal gyrus detected on fluid attenuated inversion recovery (FLAIR) image *(A)*. The patient had a gross total removal of the tumor; the pathology report showed an anaplastic oligoastrocytoma. She was treated with 5940 cGy and 8 cycles of temozolomide. Her Karnofsky Performance Scale (KPS) score was 100. Fourteen months later, she presented with a large contrast-enhancing mass showing intense angiogenesis and recurrent tumor *(B)*. The pathology confirmed an anaplastic astrocytoma.

shorter survival. As with all glial tumors, glial fibrillary acidic protein (GFAP) positivity distinguishes AA from epithelial tumors such as cerebral metastases.[37] For AAs, the appearance of gemistocytes or lymphocytes does not affect survival, but advancing age is correlated with decreased time of survival.[15,97] Gemistocytic cells, although themselves of low proliferative potential, indicate a variant of low-grade glioma (WHO grade II) more prone to progression to AA (WHO grade III) than the standard fibrillary type of low-grade glioma.[101]

Histopathologic Diagnosis, Classification, and Grading

The generic reference to astrocytomas is that of the diffuse infiltrating, predominantly supratentorial tumor derived from fibrillary astrocytes. In their normal state, astrocytes are readily found in the neuropil, with many stellate processes, often reaching out to extend foot-processes that rest on nearby blood vessels. The neoplastic transformation of these cells is responsible for the widest range of clinical presentations, an array of histologic features and wide-ranging prognostic implications. Histopathologic diagnostic criteria developed by broad consensus and standardized nomenclature is perhaps the most important element needed to decipher the results of multicenter therapeutic trials or progress in neuro-oncology. There is no dearth of classification systems, particularly as they attempt to

define prognostic features for gliomas. The most widely accepted of these remains the WHO system that was recently modified (2000). Within this system, the anaplastic astrocytoma is assigned the WHO grade III, with the well-differentiated, low-grade astrocytoma as grade II and the highly malignant glioblastoma multiforme as grade IV. The validity of distinguishing AA from glioblastomas was confirmed by a large study of approximately 1500 malignant gliomas.[15] In both groups, advancing age was associated with shorter survival.

It behooves the pathologist to inquire into the clinical and neuroimaging features of the patient from whose neoplasm an often very limited specimen is presented for final diagnosis. Thus knowledge of advanced age of the patient or presence of contrast enhancement may be critical in suggesting inadequate sampling and the need for additional tissue for accurate diagnosis. Histologic criteria that determine grade within the spectrum of astrocytic neoplasms are cellular pleomorphism, mitotic activity, vascular proliferation, and necrosis (Figure 18-5). Although exceptions abound, cells of the low-grade tumor display some variability in nuclear shape and size, hyperchromasia, and altered nuclear-cytoplasmic ratio. The identification of mitotic figures in the specimen typically places the tumor in the next grade (i.e., AA; WHO grade III). There still remains some debate with regard to the number of mitoses required to make this diagnosis. Although some may argue for even a single mitosis being sufficient, others demand multiple mitotic figures. In the situation of a limited needle biopsy specimen, it

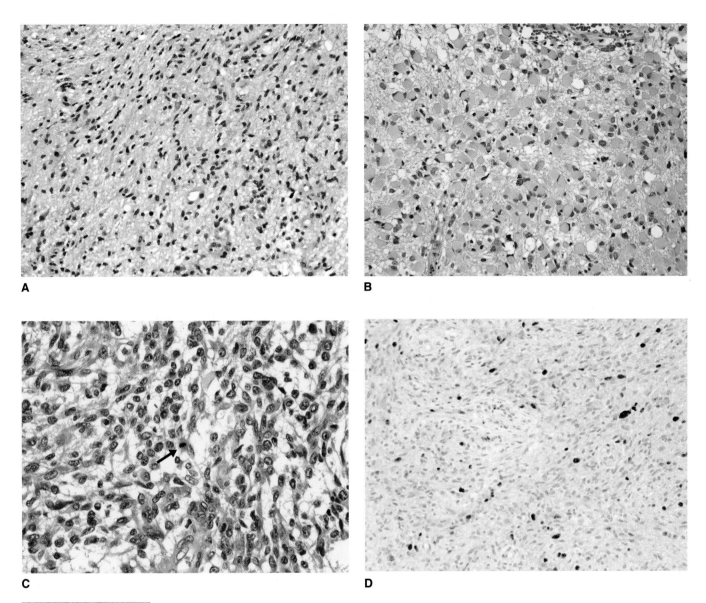

A

B

C

D

FIGURE 18-5 Anaplastic astrocytomas manifest a wide morphologic spectrum, extending from fibrillary tumors *(A)* to the predominantly gemistocytic neoplasm *(B)*. The histologic features defining the grade are pleomorphism and mitosis *(arrow in C)*. The latter is supplemented by immunohistochemical markers such as MIB-1 labeling, which identifies cell proliferation *(D)*.

is our practice to lend greater credence to the presence of a single mitosis. In the context of a specimen spanning multiple histologic slides, a single mitosis resulting from a concerted search is unlikely to warrant a diagnosis of AA. In contrast, tumors, which in addition to the above-described pleomorphism and mitosis also have foci of necrosis or multilayered (glomeruloid) vascular proliferation, are readily classified as glioblastoma multiforme. Many previous classification systems and investigative studies required the identification of necrosis for a designation of GBM. Tumors with vascular proliferation were thus relegated to the anaplastic category, although recent studies have clearly shown that they behave in a manner identical to glioblastomas. It is often tempting for the pathologist to flirt with the idea of calling the tumor something "in between" histologic grades II and III or III and IV. This is a reflection of the spectrum that may exist even within the category of AA: the presence of significant pleomorphism but lack of mitosis (having excluded the diagnosis of pleomorphic xanthoastrocytoma), a well-differentiated tumor with mild atypia and rare mitoses, or a tumor with marked pleomorphism and mitotic activity but lacking the vascular proliferation or necrosis requisite for a diagnosis of GBM. In cases such as this the histologic diagnosis must be reviewed in the context of the total clinical picture. Another variant within the category of astrocytic neoplasms, the gemistocytic astrocytoma, is distinctive in its appearance, with generous eosinophilic cytoplasm with a "stuffed" stellate appearance. These tumors may be low-grade astrocytomas in their own right; however, they commonly house a population of small, often proliferative astrocytes that would demand a diagnosis of a higher (anaplastic) grade.

The histologic diagnosis and grading of astrocytomas is most commonly accomplished on frozen sections and on routinely processed paraffin-embedded sections with the standard hematoxylin and eosin stain. There is no role for electron microscopy in the diagnostic process, and immunohistochemistry for glial fibrillary acidic protein (GFAP), as with all astrocytic tumors, distinguishes AA from epithelial tumors such as cerebral metastases and lymphoma. Determination of proliferation index using antibodies raised against MIB-1 protein is a useful although not incontrovertible tool in the process of defining grade. There still remain significant variables in technical aspects of performing this immunoreaction such as its correct interpretation, counting and sampling procedures, and the use of means versus "hot spots." Cut-off values range from 5% to 8%, and therefore no specific values have been set, particularly within the WHO classification system.

Genomic and molecular classification can identify subsets of patients with AA, whose symptoms resemble changes in GBM and correlate directly with age and inversely with survival.[66] Genetic subgroups are thought to determine the outcome of AAs. In a study of 80 AAs by comparative genomic hybridization, specific chromosomal aberrations (+7p/q, −9p, −10q, −13q, +19q) were related to aberrations that are common in grade IV astrocytoma, whereas others (+10p, −11q, +11p, −Xq) were more common in grade III astrocytoma. More common in tumors from older patients were +7p, +19, and −4q, whereas −11p was more common in tumors from younger patients. Finally, gains of 7p and 7q were associated with shorter patient survival, independent of age. These findings indicate that genetic events underlie the well-known effects of age on survival in AAs and underscore the importance of molecular classification of astrocytic tumors.[66]

Patients with AA and mutations of PTEN, an immunohistochemical, prognostic marker linked to astrocytoma progression and malignancy in preclinical models[124] and in human tissues,[36] have significantly shorter survival.[63,110] PTEN mutation can, in turn, activate signaling pathways that promote angiogenesis, including vascular endothelial growth factor (VEGF).[93]

The absence of necrosis is a key histologic hallmark, characteristic of AA. The molecular mechanisms that lead to necrosis, such as a postulated overexpression of tumor necrosis factor, may provide molecular targets to halt malignant progression and prevent the conversion of AA to glioblastoma.[98]

Gene expression profiling using cDNA microarray technology promises to be as accurate an alternative as histologic diagnosis and a more objective molecular approach than standard histologic criteria, with the prospect of identifying subsets of patients with better prognosis.[35] The molecular approach to tumor classification can generate clinically meaningful patient stratification, and more importantly, is an efficient discovery tool for human gliomas, permitting the identification of previously unrecognized, clinically relevant tumor subsets that predict response to chemotherapy or radiation therapy.[98] Identification of sets of genes will supplement standard histologic examination in the future as molecular classification of gliomas, using microarrays, elucidates the genetic signature of AAs.[59] Two-gene and three-gene combinations thus provide robust classifiers possessing the potential to translate expression microarray results into diagnostic histopathologic assays for clinical use. Some of the identified genes, such as insulin-like growth factor–binding protein 2, have been confirmed to be associated with one of the tumor types.[59]

Genetic instability caused by the impaired ability of p53 to mediate DNA damage repair further facilitates the acquisition of new genetic abnormalities, leading to malignant progression of an astrocytoma to AA. This is reflected by a high rate of p53 mutation (60% to 70%) in AAs.[87] There are two types of glioblastoma. One arises de novo, is associated with epidermal growth factor receptor (EGFR) amplification, and is radioresistant. The other has an early mutation in p53 and passes through a stage of being an AA. A large percentage of AA tumors can be distinguished by the genetic change of a p53 abnormality.[87] Loss of function of the p53 tumor-suppressor gene because of mutation occurs early in astrocytoma tumorigenesis in approximately 30% to 40% of cases. This is believed to confer a growth advantage to the cells, allowing them to clonally expand because of loss of the p53-controlled G1 checkpoint and apoptosis. The cell cycle control is further compromised in astrocytoma by alterations in one of the G1-S transition control genes, either loss of the p16 and CDKN2 or RB genes or amplification of the cyclin D gene. The final progression process leading to GBM appears to require additional genetic abnormalities in the long arm of chromosome 10, one of which is deletion or functional loss of the PTEN-MMAC1 gene.

For malignant progression to glioblastoma, there are two major molecular pathways. One arises de novo, the other from patients who have an AA or low-grade glioma.[9,61,87] There are two lineage pathways of glioblastoma: one that derives de novo (primary glioblastoma, often in older patients) and another (secondary glioblastoma in younger patients), characterized by p53 mutation as the earliest detectable change.[61] The secondary glioblastomas may have passed through an intermediate stage as an AA. The primary glioblastomas show amplification of the EGFR gene, CDKN2A (p16) deletions, and less commonly, MDM2 amplification. In contrast to the secondary glioblastomas that evolve from astrocytoma cells with p53 mutations in younger patients, primary glioblastomas seem to be resistant to radiation therapy and thus show a poorer prognosis.

Recurrence and progression to higher grade lesions are characteristic of the clinical course of astrocytic tumors. P53 expression is linked to tumor progression from low-grade to AA.[107] Though p53 gene mutation is an important initiating event in astrocytic tumorigenesis, its role in malignant progression remains controversial. Sarkar et al. analyzed p53 protein expression in paired histologic samples from 48 cases of astrocytic tumors and their recurrences—29 diffuse (low-grade) astrocytomas, 10 AAs, and 14 GBM.[107] Malignant progression at recurrence was noted in 93% of diffuse astrocytomas and 64% of AAs. We observed an association between p53 protein immunopositivity and malignant progression at recurrence. Thus 27 of 48 (56%) primary tumors were initially p53 positive, whereas in recurrent tumors associated with malignant progression this frequency increased to 71% (34/48 cases). This was because 7 of the 13 cases (4/8 diffuse and 3/5 AA) that were initially p53 negative acquired immunopositivity on malignant progression at recurrence. In contrast, none of the 19 tumors that recurred to the same grade showed any change of p53 status at recurrence. Furthermore, recurrence was associated with increase in the percentage of p53 immunopositive cells (p53 labeling index, LI), which was also higher in tumors with progression. Thus this study conclusively indicates the role of p53 in malignant progression of astrocytic tumors. Also, it suggests a potential role of p53 LI in predicting malignant progression at recurrence because the highest initial LI was noted in tumors that progressed to GBM compared with those that recurred to the same grade or progressed to AA. No correlation could, however, be demonstrated between p53 immunoreactivity and time to recurrence.[107]

More subtypes of glioblastomas may exist with intermediate clinical and genetic profiles, a factor exemplified by the giant cell glioblastoma that clinically and genetically occupies a hybrid position between primary (de novo) and secondary glioblastomas.[61] The evaluation and design of therapeutic modalities aimed at preventing malignant progression of astrocytomas and glioblastomas should now be based on stratifying patients with astrocytic tumors according to their genetic diagnosis.[61,87]

In the progression of AA to GBM, angiogenesis is a molecular checkpoint that could be a target for future therapy.[9] Angiogenesis, as measured by microvascular density, is significantly higher in GBM compared with AA.[11,13,85] Detailed molecular studies of astrocytoma progression point to a number of pathways that could be therapeutically modulated.[9] Despite the wide range of genetic events that ultimately lead to GBM, the vascular changes that evolve are remarkably similar.[85] Microvascular hyperplasia is spatially and temporally associated with pseudopalisading necrosis in GBM and is believed to be driven by hypoxia-induced expression of pro-angiogenic cytokines such as VEGF.[9] Understanding genetic events and their relation to angiogenic regulation in astrocytic neoplasms may eventually lead to therapies that are specifically directed at molecularly defined subsets of these diseases.[9]

For example, *endostatin*, an endogenous inhibitor of angiogenesis, is also significantly higher in blood vessels of GBM compared with AA, suggesting the host response counteracts pathologic angiogenesis.[85] During the angiogenic process, an isoform of fibronectin accumulates specifically around growing blood vessels. The "angiogenic index" based on the domain B sequence of *fibronectin (B-FN)* is a precise diagnostic tool, with a higher correlation to the histologic grade of astrocytoma than the microvascular density (based on factor VIII) staining or the endothelial proliferative rate (based on Ki-67 labeling).[17] Fibroblast growth factor (FGF) expression increases as the tumor malignancy progresses[13,125]; a specific *FGF receptor, FGFR-4*, can distinguish two subtypes of AA: one FGFR-negative that behaves like a low-grade glioma with a long survival time, and the other FGFR-positive that behaves similar to a glioblastoma with a poor survival time.[125] *Thymidine phosphorylase (TP)*, a proangiogenic molecule associated with macrophage infiltration, highly correlates with prognosis and astrocytoma progression, possibly better than classic histologic criteria.[126] Regardless of glioma grading, patients with TP-positive tumors had a significantly shorter mean survival time than those with TP-negative tumors. TP could play a crucial role in angiogenesis during astrocytoma progression; immunodetection of TP is useful for clinical prediction, as well as a molecular target for antiangiogenesis therapy.[126] Other molecular markers that could complement or surpass classic histologic criteria of astrocytoma progression include the guanosine triphosphate (GTP) binding proteins *Rho A and Rho B*. The expression of these proteins is inversely correlated with the

WHO histologic grades of astrocytoma II, III (AA), and IV (glioblastoma).[34] Ultimately, microarray analysis offers great promise to identify specific genes and groups of genes linked to malignant progression of astrocytomas.[32]

THERAPY

Treatment Overview

The basic principles of the treatment of AAs are outlined in the National Cooperative Cancer Network (NCCN) guidelines[43] (Figure 18-6). The diagnosis of a primary brain tumor is made on MRI. Next, the clinical impression determines whether "maximal safe resection" is feasible. For the treatment of AAs, and nearly all other histologies, neurosurgeons generally provide the best outcome for their patients if as much tumor as possible is removed.[16,43] Because these tumors are heterogeneous, maximal resection often provides the most accurate histologic diagnosis. Modern, MR-guided, stereotactic biopsies or craniotomies enable the resection of "hot spots," areas of contrast enhancement with gadolinium, that likely contain the focus of anaplastic, angiogenic tissue. Selective biopsies can provide accurate tissue diagnosis and minimize sampling error. The general objective is to remove more than 90% of the tumor volume with surgical debulking. The actual extent and percentage of "gross total removal" will be determined by the location of the tumor, quality of the computer-assisted image guidance; experience of the surgeon and the surgical team; and pattern of tumor growth. For example, a well-circumscribed tumor in the frontal lobe can be easily resected, whereas a deep, or multifocal, temporal lobe tumor invading the ventricular system and extending into the diencephalon or the brainstem cannot. Because the pathologic diagnosis is pivotal for patient management, the importance of obtaining adequate amounts of tissue to be reviewed by an experienced neuropathologist cannot be overemphasized.

The most important prognostic factors in patients with AA (and glioblastoma) are the histologic diagnosis, the performance status, age, type and duration of symptoms, and extent of surgical resection.[20]

An objective of surgery, in addition to tissue diagnosis, is improvement in quality and duration of life. First, patients with AAs often have symptoms of raised intracranial pressure, seizures, or focal neurologic findings related to tumor size and location and associated peritumoral edema (Table 18-1). AAs generally do not have associated hemorrhage or calcifications but produce considerable edema and mass effect (Figure 18-4B). Because tumor cells are commonly found in the peritumoral zone of edema, which corresponds to the T2-weighted MRI, the tumor and zone of edema is often used to define the radiation portals for external-beam radiation therapy (EBRT).

Once a patient's tumor has a clinical and radiologic picture consistent with an AA, the first step is a neurosurgical consultation to determine the maximal feasible resection of tumor.[43] Because numerous studies support the concept that the time to tumor progression (TTP) and the survival is improved with maximal tumor debulking, a major tumor removal should be performed. One exception to this rule is if the initial MRI appearance suggests a lymphoma and a frozen section establishes the diagnosis of a lymphoma, then extensive tumor resec-

Anaplastic Astrocytoma

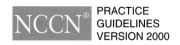

PRACTICE
GUIDELINES
VERSION 2000

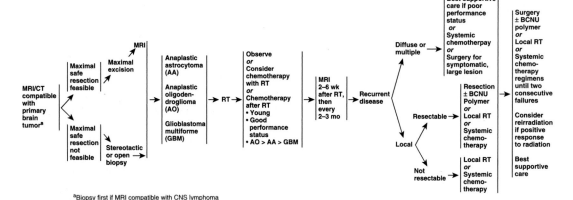

aBiopsy first if MRI compatible with CNS lymphoma

FIGURE 18-6 NCCN Guidelines, version 2000, for Treatment of Anaplastic Astrocytomas. These guidelines are also recommended for treatment of anaplastic oligodendrogliomas and glioblastomas. NCCN, National Comprehensive Cancer Network. (Courtesy of Dr. Rodger Winn/NCCN.)

TABLE 18-1

Indications and Objectives of Surgery for Anaplastic Astrocytoma

1. Establish histological diagnosis
2. Improve survival and time to tumor progression using maximal safe resection
3. Improve symptoms by decreasing local mass effect and raised ICP
4. Reduce steroid dependence
5. Remove cell populations with potential for malignant progression to GBM
6. Enhance adjuvant therapy by target reduction and removal of necrotic, cystic, and hypoxic areas that are chemoresistant and radioresistant
7. Implant biodegradable wafers for local drug delivery of BCNU chemotherapy
8. Enable experimental focal therapy (e.g., immunotoxins, convection therapy, radiation therapy balloon devices, alginate beads, monoclonal antibodies, stem cells)

GBM, Glioblastoma multiforme; ICP, intracranial pressure.

---

tion is reserved for only alleviating mass effect and not as part of an algorithm for disease management. The extent of tumor resection can best be gauged with a baseline, contrast-enhanced MRI obtained within 72 hours after surgery, before reparative angiogenesis (i.e., surgical scar) confounds measurements of residual tumor volume and the physiologic host response. Other factors that can mimic tumor progression by altering vascular permeability and affecting extravasation of gadolinium include radiation therapy, corticosteroid tapering, and implantation of BCNU-impregnated wafers.

Following tumor surgery, radiation therapy is the next step. Chemotherapy is of marginal benefit for glioblastomas but is important in the treatment of AAs, because these tumors are more chemoresponsive (see Figures 18-1 and 18-7). Recently, the FDA has approved BCNU-wafers in the initial treatment of AAs and temozolomide (TMZ) for the recurrence.[123,128] There has been a tendency to give patients with AA chemotherapy with procarbazine, CCNU, and vincristine (PCV) and to use systemic BCNU for patients with glioblastoma, but the data favoring PCV over BCNU for AA are meager.[43] As with surgery, those most likely to benefit from chemotherapy are young patients with good performance status and lower grades of malignant tumors in contrast to patients with poor prognosis.[43]

Follow-up care during or after adjuvant treatment consists of monitoring (i.e., surveillance therapy) with an initial baseline MRI 2 to 4 weeks after completion of radiation therapy, then every 2 or 3 months. MRI scans performed in the first few months after radiation therapy allow for appropriate titration of corticosteroids, guided by the degree of mass effect and peritumoral brain edema. Later scans are useful to identify tumor recurrence.

At the time of tumor recurrence, if the tumor is diffuse or multifocal, options for salvage treatment include (1) surgery, for reduction of mass effect; (2) systemic chemotherapy; or (3) best supportive care if performance status is poor. By contrast, if the tumor recurs locally and is resectable, therapeutic options

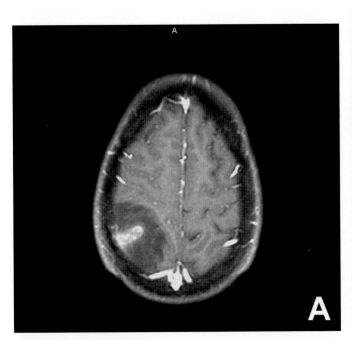

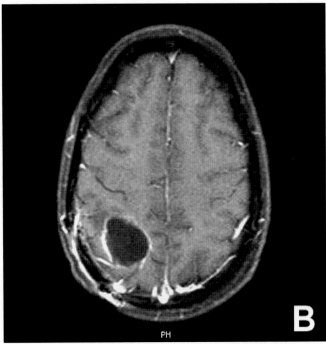

FIGURE 18-7 Magnetic resonance imaging (MRI) scans of a 31-year-old woman who presented with numbness and paresthesias in the left arm. A stereotactic biopsy revealed an anaplastic astrocytoma. The MRI showed a 5 × 4.4 × 4 cm mass, with patchy enhancement, in the right parietal lobe, including the primary sensory cortex (A). The patient had motor mapping, and a gross total resection was obtained. B, Postoperative MRI after external-beam radiation therapy. The patient was started on temozolomide and remained progression free after 2-year follow-up.

include (1) surgical resection with the possibility of placing a BCNU polymer, (2) local radiation ("boost") therapy, or (3) systemic chemotherapy.

The benefit of a multimodality interdisciplinary approach using maximal safe resection, radiation therapy, and intensive chemotherapy has been validated in numerous studies, using multivariate and univariate analysis, by correlating response to treatment methods.[96,103] These studies show a benefit in survival with combined multimodality therapy. However, these studies are retrospective, uncontrolled, and have an inherent selection bias (i.e., the patients who survive the longest and have the most favorable tumors receive cycles of chemotherapy, boost radiation therapy, and repeat surgery for recurrent disease).

Surgery

The indications for surgery are listed in Table 18-1. The advent of computer-assisted, three-dimensional, interactive, real-time neuronavigation devices has greatly increased the indications for, efficacy of, safety of, and efficiency of glioma surgery in general, and the surgery for AAs in particular.[30,105,130] At the H. Lee Moffitt Cancer Center, the median length of stay for patients undergoing a craniotomy for supratentorial AA was 1 day. Of 43 patients, 15 had tumors in "eloquent" areas of the brain, 13 had intraoperative motor mapping, and 3 had awake speech mapping. One patient had both. The benefits of MR-guided surgery are listed in Table 18-2. The use of MR guid-

ance has become the gold standard for glioma surgery. As with the introduction of the surgical microscope, neuronavigation has proved to be revolutionary for optimizing results of brain tumor surgery and is under continual refinement as faster, more precise techniques are being developed with fusion of images and other technologies that enable anatomic, functional, and metabolic mapping to be performed by the tumor surgeon. By delineating tumor margins and preserving surrounding eloquent brain[81,104] and vascular structures,[67] computer-assisted, MR-guided surgery enables the neurosurgical oncologist to focus on *tumor surgery*, not brain surgery.

Frameless stereotactic biopsy has been shown in both laboratory and clinical studies to achieve a level of accuracy equal to frame-based (Cosman-Roberts-Wells, CRW) stereotactic biopsy.[29] In clinical use, frameless stereotactic biopsies led to significant reduction of (1) time of anesthesia and surgery, (2) surgical complications, (3) hospital stay, and (4) overall cost, despite the additional cost of MR scanning. The superior imaging, target visualization, and flexibility of the technique of frameless stereotactic biopsy translate into tangible advantages for safety, time, and cost.

The extent of surgical debulking is a key preoperative and intraoperative concern. Use of image guidance has made many tumors previously thought to be inoperable amenable to a near-total resection, particularly those tumors near eloquent brain, such as the speech, motor, and visual cortex. In patients referred to a major cancer center who previously had only a stereotactic needle biopsy, the majority could safely undergo gross-total

Magnetic Resonance–guided, Stereotactic Volumetric Surgery for Anaplastic Astrocytoma: Advantages

1. Preoperative planning of entry points and target sets; definition of "safe corridors"
2. Delineation of tumor margins from surrounding brain
3. Enables use of CSF-containing cisterns, sulci, and fissures rather than transcortical approaches
4. Identifies regional vascular anatomy, including tumor arterial feeders and draining veins
5. Enables "minimally invasive" linear and sigmoid incisions versus traditional large flaps
6. Enables segmentation of tumor and fusion with CT scan, fMRI, MRA, etc. for superior visualization
7. Defines tumor margins, enabling more complete en bloc resections, maximally effective cytoreduction
8. Complication avoidance (e.g., avoidance of ventricular entry if tumor is periventricular or trapped ventricular horn)
9. Avoid "brain shift" through judicious use of mannitol, positioning of patient
10. Avoid need and morbidity of brain retraction to gain "exposure"
11. Shortened length of hospital stay
12. Selective biopsy of "hot spots" for heterogeneous gliomas (e.g., anaplastic astrocytoma)
13. Customization of skin, bone, and dural flaps for second-stage surgery for recurrent gliomas

CSF, Cerebral spinal fluid; CT, computed tomography; fMRI, functional magnetic resonance imaging; MRA, magnetic resonance angiography.

(>95%) resection.[54] Furthermore, stereotactic volumetric resection yielded a different diagnosis in 40 of 82 cases (49%); this discrepancy was reduced to 38% when the biopsy slides from an outside institution were reviewed preoperatively by neuropathologists at the cancer center.[54]

Volumetric frameless stereotaxy can be combined with awake anesthesia for maximal, safe resection of AAs in the language area, such as the dominant Broca's area, operculum, posterior superior temporal lobe, or angular gyrus.[81] The goal of surgery is to resect the maximum neurologically permissible tumor volume defined on preoperative T2 imaging, with tumor resection stopped at the onset of speech dysfunction.[81] The majority of patients (52%) had achieved greater than 90% volumetric reduction. Of interest, in 26 patients considered to have low-grade astrocytomas (WHO grade II) based on preoperative imaging, nearly one half (n = 12) had AAs (WHO grade III) based on histology. Intraoperative deficits were present in 74%, but the majority (71%) recovered postoperatively within 3 months.[81]

The basic limitation of surgery for AAs and other malignant gliomas is the spatial distribution. There are two basic forms of glioma growth: infiltrative, where cells replace surrounding brain, and expansive, where tumor displaces surrounding brain.[84] Stereotactic volumetric resection is most useful for tumors that present as discrete masses on MR imaging.[21] For diffuse AAs, multifocal tumors, tumors spread-

ing into the corpus callosum, ventricular subependymal lining, the diencephalon, hypothalamus, or brainstem or those that are predominantly infiltrative with minimal mass effect, stereotactic biopsy may still provide the best result, comparable to surgical debulking.[27] Whether performing a stereotactic biopsy[58] or a craniotomy, care must be taken to avoid seeding tumor cells, because AA has the capacity for iatrogenic spread, a rare complication that can be readily avoided.[58] These tumors often arise or extend near the subependymal surface of the ventricle. It is important to avoid, using image guidance, entering the ventricle, because entry into the ventricle carries a higher risk of postoperative hydrocephalus,[78] which can occur in these patients merely because of the higher protein levels in CSF associated with a brain tumor. If recognized, hydrocephalus can be treated by an appropriate shunting procedure.[78]

The advisability of a second operation for recurrent GBM or AA depends on the expected duration and quality of subsequent survival.[49]

In one large series, both operative morbidity and mortality were close to 5%, for a combined rate of 10%. The median duration of survival after reoperation was 88 weeks in those with AA. The median duration of high-quality survival (KPS > 70) after reoperation was 83 weeks for patients with AA. Often, patients can expect to spend a greater portion of life at a higher level of function than they would have without reoperation. As adjunctive forms of therapy improve, reoperation plays an increasingly prominent role in the management of recurrent AAs.[49]

The postoperative control of seizures in patients with astrocytic tumors is correlated with preoperative incidence of seizures, tumor recurrence, or postoperative hemorrhage. Meticulous regulation of anticonvulsant medication significantly reduces the risk of postoperative seizures.[53]

Radiation Therapy

Radiation therapy is an integral part of the standard treatment for AAs. The overall treatment with regard to radiation dose and field planning is similar for all high-grade gliomas. The initial fields encompass the T2-weighted target with a margin of 1 to 3 cm. The dose to this region is approximately 4500 to 4680 cGy in 180-cGy fractions. A "cone down" follows this to treat the T1-weighted postcontrast target with a 1- to 3-cm margin. Treatment is continued to bring the total dose to this target to approximately 5940 cGy in 180 cGy per fraction. All margins are in three dimensions. *The side effects of treatment are similar to other partial brain treatments and are described in Part 1 of this book.* Because survival is significantly longer with AAs than GBM, the potential for developing a late radiation complication is greater. In covering the margin one may treat the optical structures, which have a tolerance to radiation lower than the total prescribed dose. The risk and benefit of including or avoiding these structures needs to be discussed with the patient. The most significant concern, however, is the inevitable progression of the tumor after radiation.

To improve the outcome of patients with AA, several different strategies have been tried over the years with limited success. One strategy was to increase the dose to the tumor either by adding more daily treatments or by alternating the fractionation schema. The latter included delivery twice a day and even three times a day. The results were no better than the historical controls, and in fact, as the effective doses increased, the outcomes were worse. Another strategy was similar, but with additional radiation added by particles such as neutrons or with brachytherapy. However, the Radiation Therapy Oncology Group (RTOG) found again that the "median survival decreased as the aggressiveness of the treatment increased."[69] Others found no significant difference when brachytherapy was added to standard radiation for the initial treatment of AA.[68] Although it did not lengthen survival when used in initial therapy, interstitial brachytherapy used at the time of tumor progression was associated with increased survival.[94] The addition of chemotherapy has been evaluated in several trials. In some series, a small benefit was detected with the addition of BCNU to radiation.[121] Subsequently, numerous other chemotherapy regimens or radiation sensitizers failed to make a significant impact on survival time.[18,96]

Ongoing trials (e.g., RTOG-98-13) are looking at newer agents such as TMZ (Temodar). The future of radiation therapy for treating AAs and high-grade brain tumors, in general, will be in functional planning, where the target is based on tumor activity or density and not a geometric distance from the contrast-enhanced edge of the tumor. We believe that such tumor-specific targeting, in addition to novel radiation sensitizers, will improve outcome over current treatments.

Chemotherapy

General Considerations

AAs represent approximately 25% of malignant gliomas. Because they are less common, they typically compose a small part of the study group in clinical trials for malignant gliomas. Misclassification has been problematic as well. In a large phase III trial of PCV chemotherapy with or without BUdR as a radiation sensitizer, 78 of 268 patients enrolled were ineligible primarily on the basis of central pathology review findings, the most common scenario being that tumors classified as anaplastic at the local institutions were upgraded to GBM after central review.[96a] Patients with AA have a median survival of about 4 years,[75] as opposed to approximately 1 year for patients with GBM.[89a] In general, AAs are more responsive to chemotherapy than are the more malignant forms of gliomas (i.e., the glioblastoma).[51] Furthermore, whereas glioblastomas show a 12% to 13% biologic response by imaging criteria,[41,123a] AAs show a complete or partial response in 55% of cases in a small series.[51] The time of survival is the key end point to evaluate chemotherapy. Objective responses, in the traditional sense of tumor shrinkage (partial response) or disappearance on radiographic studies (complete response), are rare. Studies that appear at first to have a high response rate (RR) typically include stable disease as part of the response. The durability of response—progression-free survival (PFS)—and TTP are used as end points in most recent studies, as is the overall survival (OS).

Initial Studies

An early study by the Brain Tumor Study Group (BTSG) randomized 303 patients with anaplastic glioma to one of four treatments: best supportive care, radiation therapy (50 to 60 Gy to the whole brain), BCNU, or a combination of radiation therapy and BCNU. Survival was increased in both of the radiation therapy arms, but no advantage was seen in the combination arm. There was an increase in the surviving fraction of patients at 18 months that was statistically significant.[120] Only 9% of the valid study group was confirmed to have AA, and they were equally distributed among the treatment groups.

Up-Front Therapy for Anaplastic Astrocytoma

The Northern California Oncology Group (NCOG) stratified a chemotherapy trial based on tumor type. The investigators first compared single-agent BCNU with PCV in patients with malignant glioma. PCV was found to be superior to BCNU but only in the patients with AA.[76] This difference was observed in a retrospective analysis of the data. The number of patients with AA was relatively small: 37 in the BCNU arm and 36 in the PCV arm. This advantage was not observed for patients with GBM. Retrospective subset analysis of the RTOG brain tumor database failed to show a treatment advantage of PCV over that of carmustine (BCNU).[95]

A second NCOG study suggested that the use of the radiation sensitizer bromodeoxyuridine (BUdR) with radiation therapy and PCV increased the median survival of patients with AA to 4 years.[75] The additional benefit of BUdR was not confirmed in a follow-up study done by RTOG. This study was closed after accruing 281 of a planned 293 patients, because of stochastic analysis suggesting that the addition of BUdR would not statistically improve survival.[96] The use of halogenated pyrimidines, with an agent such as 5-iododeoxyuridine (IUdR), as a chemical modifier of the radiation response continues to be advocated by some.[119]

A recently published, nonrandomized study of 31 patients with AA focused on predictors of long-term survivorship.[103] This study found that significant predictors of survival were preoperative and postoperative KPS score, age under 40, number of chemotherapy cycles, and radiation dose.[103] Though virtually every known approved chemotherapy agent has been tested in malignant glioma at recurrence, few new agents were tested for AA in the newly diagnosed up-front setting (Table 18-3), possibly because of the perception that no single or combination therapy was superior to PCV.

There are some data that the combination of chemotherapy plus radiation therapy could be more effective than radiation therapy alone for patients with AA.[109] Forty-one AA patients received 4 to 5 cycles of chemotherapy (BCNU + cisplatin), subsequent radiation therapy (median dose 56.5 Gy), and PCV at recurrence. The group of AA patients was compared with a homogeneous group of 39 AA patients treated only with radiation therapy after surgery. The median TTP of patients on the protocol was 24.5 months. The median survival time for AA patients treated with the chemotherapy plus radiation therapy was 38.8 months, compared with 21 months for patients treated with radiation therapy but without chemotherapy.[109]

Recently, Levin et al[73] reported that survival of patients with anaplastic gliomas was significantly increased by using PCV as a postirradiation adjuvant therapy in combination with an inhibitor of ornithine decarboxylase, DFMO (alpha-difluoromethyl ornithine; eflornithine). Survival analysis from registration found a DFMO-PCV median survival of 6.3 years, whereas that for PCV alone was 5.1 years.

TABLE 18-3	Up-front Trials of PCV for Patients with Anaplastic Astrocytoma			
Radiation Therapy	Chemotherapy During XRT	Postradiation Chemotherapy	Median Survival, (wk)	No. of Patients with AA Histology
60 Gy WB (Levin et al, 1990 NCOG 6G61)[76]	Hydroxyurea	PCV	157	36
60 Gy LF (Levin et al, 1995)[75]	BUdR	PCV	208	116
Varies (Ron et al, 2002)[103]	None	PCV	80	31

AA, Anaplastic astrocytoma; LF, limited-field irradiation; PCV, procarbazine, lomustine (CCNU), and vincristine; WB, whole-brain; XRT, radiation therapy.

Response to PCV is much better when there is an oligodendroglial component, in contrast to a "pure" AA.[64] The TTP and the time of survival in a group of patients with "pure" AA ($n = 24$) was compared with 24 patients with an oligodendroglial component, including anaplastic oligodendroglioma (AO, $n = 20$) and anaplastic oligoastrocytoma (AOA, $n = 4$). The groups were evenly matched for gender, performance score, tumor localization, extent of tumor resection, and dose of radiation therapy, but the mean age of the patients with AA was 10 years older at entry (48.5 years), compared with the patients with an oligodendroglial component. The median TTP (26.8 months) and survival time (27.9 months) in the AA group was significantly less than the AO and the AOA group. A new neurologic deficit, following surgery, occurred in 14.5% of the patients. The most significant toxicity of PCV chemotherapy was hematologic, becoming grades 3 and 4 toxicities in 30% of the patients. In a retrospective review of RTOG studies, Prados et al found that PCV is not superior to classic chemotherapy, such as BCNU.[95]

TMZ is a novel second-generation oral alkylating agent with demonstrated efficacy and safety in patients with recurrent AA.[40] It is a prodrug that undergoes spontaneous chemical degradation at physiologic pH to form the highly reactive alkylating agent 5-(3-methyltriazeno)-imidazole-4-carboxamide (MTIC). In clinical trials, TMZ has activity in gliomas and is approved for treatment of recurrent AA.[89] Pharmacokinetic studies show that it easily crosses the blood-brain barrier with significant levels in the cerebrospinal fluid.[89]

A multicenter, open-label, phase II study of TMZ in AA at first recurrence enrolled 162 patient in 32 centers worldwide. Most of the patients had a KPS score of 70 or greater. Most patients had AA or anaplastic oligoastrocytoma (AOA) (69%), and 60% had prior chemotherapy. For patients with AA, the progression-free survival was 5.5 months the overall survival was 14.2 months.[128] Gilbert et al published a multicenter trial of preirradiation TMZ in patients with glioblastoma and AA. Of the 57 patients, 21 had AA; 18 were adults. Up to four cycles of TMZ (200 mg/m^2/day for 5 consecutive days every 28 days) were given to patients before external beam radiation therapy. TMZ was safe and well tolerated in adult and pediatric patients. Common toxicity criteria grade 3 adverse events occurred in 16 (28%) patients, and grade 4 toxicities occurred in 7 (12%) patients.[40] Of 21 patients (18 adult, 3 pediatric) with AA, two (10%) achieved complete response, five (24%) achieved partial response, and eight (38%) had stable disease. These results were similar to the subgroup of patients with glioblastoma.

Among adult patients with AA, the median PFS and OS rates were 7.6 and 23.5 months, respectively, less than those observed in earlier studies. Because the diagnosis of AA in some patients was made by needle biopsy alone, there may have been a sampling error. Therefore the preirradiation treatment approach appears promising but requires additional evaluation in comparative studies.[40]

There are numerous problems associated with brain tumor trials. One of the most important is the inherent difficulty in grading malignant gliomas. This problem is compounded by the sampling error seen in patients who have only biopsies rather than resections. Greater than 20% of AA were upgraded after a central pathology review in the course of two AA trials.[1,5] Older studies are limited by variability in response criteria and by the lack of or limited availability of MRI.

Given the distinct improvement in survival and despite the small numbers and study flaws, adjuvant chemotherapy has become part of the treatment guideline for newly diagnosed AA.[43] Because of the marked survival benefit of adjuvant PCV in patients with AA, there has been a trend to study new agents in the up-front setting only in GBM or in AA patients randomized to PCV or BCNU as the standard arm. One of these studies, RTOG 98-13, randomizes patients to TMZ, BCNU, or a combination of the two.

Side Effects and Drug Interactions

PCV is not, however, an innocuous therapy, and for a disease in which cure is desired by all but not expected except by the patient, less toxic therapies are necessary. Lomustine (CCNU) is a potent marrow toxin with a delayed nadir. Effects on marrow worsened with repeat dosing. One must avoid cumulative doses of more than 1100 mg/m^2 because of possible pulmonary fibrosis and secondary leukemias.[91] Procarbazine is a mild monoamine oxidase inhibitor. There are potential interactions with medications and tyramine-containing foods.[94] Vincristine causes a neuropathy, with numbness in the extremities and constipation. This effect may be compounded in patients with preexisting neuropathies.[94]

In addition, the concomitant use of antiepileptic drugs (AEDs) and chemotherapy may increase clearance of the chemotherapy and therefore decrease response, especially with the taxanes irinotecan[65,79] and 9-aminocamptothecan.[42] Conversely, chemotherapy can cause fluctuations in the serum concentrations of phenytoin, allowing for breakthrough seizure activity and mandating frequent serum monitoring.[38,44] Elevated serum phenytoin levels and clinical toxicity have been reported during treatment with fluorouracil.[39] Heightened hematologic toxicity has been reported in patients treated with cisplatin-nitrosourea-based chemotherapy and valproic acid.[8] Studies are now commonly stratified as to the use of cytochrome p450-inducing AEDs. Patients taking these enzyme-inducing agents (phenytoin, carbamazepine, etc.) are typically entered into companion dose-finding phase I studies of new agents, whereas patients on no AED or non–enzyme inducing AEDs (gabapentin, valproic acid, etc.) are entered into phase II studies.

Treatment at Recurrence

Studies for recurrence often enroll patients under the broad label of "malignant glioma," which can include a heterogeneous group of four distinct pathologies—AA, AO, mixed oligoastrocytoma (MOA), and GBM—in the study group.

The most important new drug for the treatment of recurrent AA is TMZ. It is a second-generation alkylating agent. TMZ is rapidly absorbed after oral administration and undergoes spontaneous hydrolysis at physiologic pH to its active metabolite, MTIC.[89] A further breakdown leads to an intermediary in the purine biosynthesis pathway,[26,128] methyldiazonium, which forms DNA adducts. The methylation at the O^6 position on guanine is cytotoxic.[89] It is lipophilic with good penetration of the CSF. It penetrates the central nervous system and passes through the blood-brain barrier with a 30% to 40% CSF-to-plasma ratio.[62,116,128]

An open-label, multicenter phase II trial (Table 18-4) enrolled 162 patients, 111 of whom had AA or malignant oligoastrocytoma. The primary study end point of a PFS of 6 months was achieved by 46%, and the median PFS was 5.4 months. The median OS was 13.6 months. The objective response rate (RR) was 35% (8% complete response [CR] and 27% partial response [PR]). If stable disease was included, the RR rose to 61%. Hematologic toxicities occurred in less than 10% of patients and were not cumulative.[127] Yung et al concluded that TMZ demonstrated good single-agent activity, an acceptable safety profile, and documented health-related quality of life (HQL) benefits in patients with recurrent AA.[128]

A review of the effectiveness of TMZ in the treatment of recurrent AA and glioblastoma was commissioned by the National Health Service and based on a randomized controlled trial and four uncontrolled studies.[28] The key conclusion was that TMZ increases PFS but does not significantly affect OS. TMZ appears to produce few serious adverse effects and may also have a positive impact on HQL. Large, well-designed randomized controlled trials conducted in a wider patient population are needed.[28]

To try to improve the RR with monotherapy, TMZ has been paired with other chemotherapy agents or given in alternative treatment schedules. One such pairing is that of TMZ and irinotecan. Heightened activity of irinotecan is observed following the administration of TMZ and is attributed to the placement of an adduct at the O^6 position of methylguanine. Preclinical studies are promising. A phase I trial and additional studies are ongoing.[47,99] Other combinations using TMZ are being evaluated for use in patients with recurrent malignant glioma. These include cisplatin[14] and BCNU. Investigators combined BCNU-impregnated polymer wafers (Gliadel) implanted at the time of surgery with TMZ.[19,102]

There has not yet been a large-scale up-front phase III trial comparing TMZ with the gold standard of PCV in patients with newly diagnosed AA. RTOG has opened a three-armed study comparing radiation plus BCNU, radiation plus TMZ, and radiation therapy plus a combination of TMZ and BCNU. The rationale of the combination is that TMZ might help overcome BCNU resistance by depleting the repair enzyme alkyl guanine alkyltransferase (AGT).[92] Similarly, O^6-benzyl guanine (O-6 BG) has been used to reduce AGT-associated nitrosourea resistance.[113]

Biologic Response Modifiers

TMZ is easily tolerated, and attempts have been made to increase response without substantially increasing toxicity. Although TMZ is active against recurrent malignant glioma, responses in many patients are modest and short-lived. TMZ may prove more effective in combination with other agents; therefore combination oral chemotherapy for these patients is a particularly attractive approach.[62] Investigators paired TMZ with such biologic response modifiers as cis-retinoic acid, a proapoptotic and cellular differentiating agent,[55] and interferon-α-2a.[127] TMZ has been paired with the matrix-metalloproteinase inhibitors marimastat[45] and Prinomastat with varying results.[74] The results of these trials have been compared with TMZ as a single agent (see Table 18-4).

More recently, TMZ has been paired with the cyclooxygenase-2 (COX-2) inhibitor celecoxib. COX-2 is expressed in the majority of brain tumors and is shown to inhibit growth in human glioma cell lines. The TMZ dose was given on a twice daily schedule, and the dose of celecoxib ranged from 60 mg/m^2 twice daily to 240 mg/m^2 twice daily. The result in a subset of patients (7) after two cycles was 85% (two partial responses [29%] + four SD [57%]). There was hematologic toxicity grades 3 and 4 of 14%.[88] The retinoids suppressed epidermal growth factor (EGF)-induced COX-2 expression in head and neck tumors and may be one mechanism of action of this class of drug. There is an ongoing trial of the combination

TABLE 18-4

Trial of Temozolomide for Recurrent Anaplastic Astrocytoma

PFS-6	46%
PFS-6 Median	5.4 mo
RR (CR + PR)	35% (8% + 27%)
Overall RR % (CR + PR + SD)	61% (8% + 27% + 26%)
Median Overall Survival from Time of Recurrence	13.6 mo

CR, Complete response; PFS-6, progression-free survival at 6 mos; PR, partial response; RR, response rate; SD, stable disease.
Source: Hildebrand J, De Witte O, Sahmoud T: Response of recurrent glioblastoma and anaplastic astrocytoma to dibromodulcitol, BCNU and procarbazine—A phase-II study. J Neurooncol 37:155–160, 1998.

of celecoxib and isotretinoin (c-RA) for recurrent malignant glioma.[118]

TMZ has been paired with the antiangiogenesis agent thalidomide. The activity of thalidomide as a monotherapy in malignant glioma was minimal.[33] However, the combination was found to have a 35% RR in AA and a 21% RR in the larger glioblastoma subset of patients. The dose used in this study was relatively low, 200 to 400 mg/day.[90] The North American Brain Tumor Consortium (NABTC) study 99-04 paired thalidomide with TMZ for recurrent GBM. The dose of thalidomide was higher (400 mg twice daily). The PFS was 13 weeks and not believed to be a significant increase from historical control.[46] Studies of the triple therapy of TMZ, thalidomide, and celecoxib are ongoing.

EGFR is overexpressed in a large percentage of malignant gliomas, especially in older patients. These patients may have more radiation-resistant tumors.[6] ZD1839 (Iressa) is an oral EGFR inhibitor. Diarrhea and rash are side effects. It is being tested as a radiation sensitizer for up-front treatment for GBM and is being tested alone and in combination with TMZ for recurrent GMB. Similarly, OSI-774 (Tarceva), another EGFR inhibitor, is being tested alone and in combination with TMZ to treat recurrent malignant glioma.

Summary

The treatment of AA consists of maximal safe resection, followed by chemotherapy and radiation therapy. Studies are ongoing to determine whether TMZ is as effective as nitrosourea in the initial-treatment setting or whether a combination of the two is superior. In the setting of recurrent disease, TMZ is FDA approved and may be more effective if paired with certain biologic response modifiers. It is common for patients to receive chemoradiation with TMZ in the initial-treatment setting because of results of a European Organization for Research and Treatment of Cancer (EORTC) trial.[114] In that case, CCNU can be considered in the recurrent setting. Participation in a clinical trial is suggested. One of the unanswered questions with TMZ therapy is when a patient with an AA whose disease is stable should discontinue treatment. Some neuro-oncologists will arbitrarily stop at 1 year, but there are no data as yet to determine the best course of action.

Targeted Therapy for Anaplastic Astrocytomas: Experimental Molecular Approaches

Angiogenesis

The onset of the "angiogenic switch" is central to the development of malignancy.[7,12] VEGF promotes tumor growth and angiogenesis. A key molecular difference between AA and glioblastoma is the expression of vascular endothelial isoforms. Whereas VEGF is up-regulated in only a portion of AAs, it is overexpressed in most GBMs, and the level of expression is correlated with grade of glioma.[111] Sonoda et al developed an experimental model of AA using genetically modified mutant H-ras–transformed cells that form AA-like tumors when implanted intracranially.[111] The tumors formed by the cells

expressing exogenous VEGF(121) or VEGF(165) retained the phenotype of AA, lacking areas of necrosis that are the hallmark of the glioblastoma phenotype. These results suggest that, whereas the VEGF(121) and VEGF(165) isoforms can contribute to glioma vascularization, oxygenation, and growth, they do not in and of themselves drive the formation of the GBM phenotype.[111]

This group also showed that activation of the Akt pathway was sufficient to transform AA to glioblastoma.[112] Human malignant gliomas are thought to develop as the result of stepwise accumulations of multiple genetic alterations. Human astrocytes that expressed a constitutive activated form of Akt tended to mimic the Akt activation noted in grade IV GBM, had large areas of necrosis surrounded by neovascularization and were consistent in appearance with grade IV human glioblastoma, in contrast to the poorly vascularized, necrosis-free, genetically engineered cells that mimic AA. These results show that activation of the Akt pathway is sufficient to allow the "switch" of human AA to human GBM.[112]

Because of the central role of angiogenesis in the diagnosis and formation of AA from low-grade glioma, it is possible that AAs would be highly susceptible to treatment with antiangiogenesis agents. Thus identifying and targeting specific pathways that promote malignant astrocytoma-induced angiogenesis could have substantial therapeutic benefit.[57] Khatua et al, using gene expression profiling of childhood astrocytomas, found that only the 133 angiogenesis-related genes distinguished high-grade astrocytoma (HGA) from low-grade astrocytoma in 100% of the samples analyzed, as did unsupervised analyses using the entire set of 9198 expressed genes represented on the array, indicating that the angiogenesis-related genes were reliable markers of pathologic grade between high-grade astrocytomas and benign low-grade astrocytomas. In par-ticular, there was significant overexpression of hypoxia-inducible transcription factor (HIF)-2α, as well as high level expression of FK506-binding protein (FKBP) 12 by high-grade astrocytomas. The EGFR–FKBP12–HIF-2α pathway was recently discovered to be of particular importance in glioma-genesis and angiogenesis and represents a novel therapeutic target.[57]

There is epigenetic expression of specific forms of VEGF-D and specific antigens on glioma cells as they undergo malignant progression from benign to malignant. It is proposed that these findings provide molecular targets during this switch for antiangiogenesis therapy or specific vaccines.[25] Debinski et al identified a new ubiquitous angiogenic factor in high-grade astrocytomas, a VEGF-D, and showed that the activating protein-1 (AP-1) family of transcription factors plays a potentially critical role in the progression of gliomas by eliciting uncontrolled up-regulation of VEGF-D and other compounds essential for cancer cell proliferation, tumorigenesis, and infiltration. The possibility exists that an unopposed constitutive increase in AP-1 activity in high-grade astrocytomas is related to epigenetic silencing of the inhibitors of AP-1 activity. Drugs or vaccines with anti-AP-1 activity could be effective in preventing the formation or progression of high-grade astrocytomas from more benign forms.[25]

Phenylbutyrate

The possibility of controlling the growth of malignant glioma cells using a biologic response modifier such as phenylbutyrate has been found ineffective as monotherapy to increase survival of patients with malignant glioma. However, we observed one patient with a recurrent, multicentric AA, treated with oral phenylbutyrate, who experienced a durable remission lasting more than 4 years.[4] Sodium phenylbutyrate acts as a dose-dependent inhibitor of glioma cell proliferation, migration, and invasiveness in vitro, possibly by inhibition of urokinase and c-myc pathways. Further studies should be considered to identify a subset of patients with tumors sensitive to phenylbutyrate, either as a single agent or in combination with radiation therapy or other chemotherapeutic agents.[4]

Recent molecular analysis[50] of human AA taken from biopsy specimens identifies signaling pathways that contribute to cell proliferation. These molecular targets include the src kinase, focal adhesion kinase (FAK), cyclin A and D pathways, and Ras. All of these regulators of cell growth show elevated activity in biopsy specimens of AA patients.[50] FAK is a nonreceptor tyrosine kinase that on activation promotes cell proliferation by signaling through the Ras-mitogen-activated protein kinase cascade. Overexpression of exogenous FAK lacking alternative splicing in malignant astrocytoma clones injected intracerebrally into severe combined immunodeficiency (SCID) mouse brains promotes tumor cell proliferation.[50]

Inhibitors of Ras prenylation, including farnesyl transferase inhibitors (FTIs), offer promise as radiosensitizers and are undergoing evaluation in the clinic.[70,108] Lovastatin inhibits the prenylation of several key regulatory proteins including Ras and the small guanosine triphosphate binding proteins. Eighteen patients with either anaplastic glioma or GBM were entered in a trial testing the safety of high-dose lovastatin with or without radiation, showing safety and tolerance of concurrent radiation with high doses of lovastatin, as more selective FTIs are brought into the clinic as radiation sensitizers.[70]

An overview of biologic approaches showing promise for the treatment of malignant gliomas,[3] including AAs, highlights multiple potential strategies, including gene therapy, immunotherapy, antiangiogenesis, antagonists of protein kinase C, metalloproteases, and modulation of drug resistance (e.g., by P-glycoprotein antagonists or 06-alkyl-guanine-DNA-transferase inhibitors).[3]

QUALITY OF LIFE AND REHABILITATION

Primary brain tumors can be a devastating condition to patients and their families. Unlike other forms of cancer, primary brain tumors can lead to marked changes in all aspects of functioning, including cognition, personality, and mood. AA presents a unique situation for QOL and rehabilitation because, unlike more malignant tumors, with aggressive treatment survival can be many years, allowing for return to premorbid roles in many cases. There is recent evidence that more aggressive medical treatment is associated with better QOL and increased independence.[100] There is additional evidence that neuropsychologic evaluation followed by appropriate pharmacologic interventions and cognitive rehabilitation can maintain higher quality of life and reduce dependence on others.[83]

Quality of Life

Assessing QOL in the population of patients with AA needs to be multidimensional at the time of diagnosis as well as throughout treatment. Assessment of physical status with the KPS and the Eastern Cooperative Oncology Group (ECOG) Performance Status Rating is relatively routine but does not adequately assess other aspects of functioning such as cognition and emotional well-being, nor does it assess the effect on the spouse and family.

As with all brain tumors, cognitive changes observed with AA at the time of diagnosis are usually a direct consequence of tumor location and size. Many patients with AA experience a significant improvement in cognitive function following surgery secondary to the reduction of tumor burden. Tumors in the left hemisphere are generally associated with impairment in verbal memory, language, and right-side physical function. Tumors in the right hemisphere are associated with nonverbal impairment, such as face recognition, and left-side physical function. Changes in emotional function also lateralize, with an increase in depression with left hemisphere tumors and poorer mood modulation with right hemisphere tumors. Cognitive effects of brain tumor therapy, specifically radiation therapy and chemotherapy, are generally observed weeks or months into treatment and are generally characterized by psychomotor slowing and executive dysfunction caused by white matter changes.[48,82] Decline in cognitive function often precedes MRI evidence of tumor recurrence and change in activities of daily living by 6 weeks.[82]

Regardless of tumor location, many AA patients experience increased emotional reactivity, lowered frustration tolerance, and distress in their family and occupational life. It has been shown that patients with tumors involving the right hemisphere or the frontal regions have lower QOL scores than patients with left-side tumors.[106] Though some of these changes can be attributed to the site of the tumor, others are caused by the treatment. Increased fatigue is a common complaint of patients undergoing radiation therapy and some forms of chemotherapy. Steroid therapy, for example, can directly cause reduced frustration tolerance, increased irritability, alterations in sleep and appetite, and delirium in some cases. Some patients develop seizures secondary to their tumors and others are treated with antiseizure medications prophylactically. Neurobehavioral slowing and problems with attention and concentration have been attributed to seizures and antiseizure medication.

Clinical interview and administration of the Mini-Mental Status Examination are not comprehensive or sensitive enough to fully determine the extent of cognitive, behavioral, and emotional disruption caused by AA and its treatment. Some patients are acutely aware of their deficits and may be overly distraught, whereas others may have limited insight into their deficits and their effect on family and friends. Clinical interview of the patient and a family member usually provides a more thorough and realistic picture of the true extent of the impact of the tumor on the patient and his or her family. Neuropsychological assessment using standard measures of attention, memory, executive function, and psychomotor speed is a valuable tool for identifying cognitive dysfunction and designing rehabilitative strategies. A comprehensive neuropsychological evaluation at or near the time of diagnosis is essential to determine the patient's neurobehavioral status and to design an individualized psychosocial plan of care to maximize and maintain independent functioning for the longest period possible.

Rehabilitation

Most cognitive rehabilitation is designed for the stroke or head trauma patient. Brain tumor patients have often had more time to develop their symptoms, rather than experiencing a sudden onset. Many patients with AA will have only subtle cognitive changes and may not require rehabilitation or other intervention. For those with cognitive and behavioral changes, cognitive rehabilitation is designed to address the loss or impairment of a cognitive function including, but not limited to, attention and concentration, memory, reasoning and problem solving, neurobehavioral modulation, visuospatial processing, and verbal expression. Strategies can be designed to address any or all of these specific functions or their application. Cognitive rehabilitation usually takes one of three forms: (1) restoration of a function that has been compromised, (2) substitution of a lost function through compensatory strategies and assistive devices, and (3) restructuring of the environment by changing the demands and responsibilities on the patient. Neuropsychologists, occupational therapists, and speech or language pathologists can provide cognitive rehabilitation services. Physical dysfunction can be treated with physical therapists.

Pharmacotherapy is another important aspect of treating cognitive and emotional changes associated with AA and treatment. Whether caused by the tumor or an emotional reaction to the tumor, timely diagnosis and treatment of symptoms of depression or anxiety are essential to minimize the emotional suffering of the patient and maintain a higher QOL. Some patients may require medication to assist with sleep or appetite. Stimulant medications, such as methylphenidate (Ritalin), have been shown to be effective in improving psychomotor slowing, attention, and short-term memory and reducing fatigue, elevating mood, and maintaining QOL.[83] Though there is limited evidence, potential exists for improvement in memory function with medications typically used in neurodegenerative diseases such as Alzheimer's disease, including donepezil (Aricept) and galantamine hydrobromide (Reminyl).

The QOL of patients with AA and their family members may be improved with support groups designed to provide psychoeducation as well as peer support. National and local organizations provide such services. These include the American Brain Tumor Association (ABTA), the Brain Tumor Society (BTS), the Florida Brain Tumor Association (FBTA), and the National Brain Tumor Foundation (NBTF). Most have their own Web sites with frequent updates of meetings, latebreaking news, research developments, and information on clinical trials. The Internet also provides information on current clinical trials. The following organizations have Web sites for patients with AAs: National Cancer Institute (NCI), Al Musella's Virtual Trials, the New Approaches to Brain Tumor Therapy (NABTT), and the NABTC.

References

1. Afra D, Kerpel-Fronius S, Szinai I, et al: Combined treatment of anaplastic astrocytoma (grade 3–4) with diacetyl-dianhydrogalactitol (DADAG). J Neurooncol 8:85–91, 1990.
2. Aldape K, Simmons ML, Davis RL, et al: Discrepancies in diagnoses of neuroepithelial neoplasms: The San Francisco Bay Area Adult Glioma Study. Cancer 88:2342–2349, 2000.
3. Andratschke N, Grosu AL, Molls M, Nieder C: Perspectives in the treatment of malignant gliomas in adults. Anticancer Res 21:3541–50, 2001.
4. Baker MJ, Brem S, Daniels S, et al: Complete response of a recurrent, multicentric malignant glioma in a patient treated with phenylbutyrate. J Neurooncol 59:239–242, 2002.
5. Barker FG II, Chang SM, Huhn SL, et al: Age and the risk of anaplasia in magnetic resonance-nonenhancing supratentorial cerebral tumors. Cancer 80:936–941, 1997.
6. Barker FG, Simmons ML, Chang SM: EGFR overexpression and radiation response in glioblastoma multiforme. Int J Radiat Oncol Biol Phys 51:410–418, 2001.
7. Bergers G, Benjamin LE: Angiogenesis: tumorigenesis and the angiogenic switch. Nat Rev Cancer 3:401–410, 2003.
8. Bourg V, Lebrun C, Chichmanian RM, et al: Nitroso-urea-cisplatin-based chemotherapy associated with valproate: increase of haematologic toxicity. Ann Oncol 12:217–219, 2001.
9. Brat DJ, Castellano-Sanchez A, Kaur B, Van Meir EG: Genetic and biologic progression in astrocytomas and their relation to angiogenic dysregulation. Adv Anat Pathol 9:24–36, 2002.
10. Brem S: The role of vascular proliferation in the growth of brain tumors. Clin Neurosurg 23:440–453, 1976.
11. Brem S, Cotran R, Folkman J: Tumor angiogenesis: a quantitative method for histological grading. J Natl Cancer Inst 48:347–356, 1972.
12. Brem S, Medina D, Gullino PM: Angiogenesis: a marker for experimental neoplastic transformation of mammary hyperplasia. Science 195:880–882, 1977.
13. Brem S, Tsanaclis AMC, Gross JL, Herblin WF: Immunolocalization of basic fibroblast growth factor to the microvasculature of human brain tumors. Cancer 70:2673–2680, 1992.
14. Britten CD, Rowinsky EK, Baker SD, et al: A Phase I and pharmacokinetic study of temozolomide and cisplatin in patients with advanced solid malignancies. Clin Cancer Res 5:1629–1637, 1999.
15. Burger PC, Vogel FS, Green SB, Strike TA: Glioblastoma multiforme and anaplastic astrocytoma. Pathologic criteria and prognostic implications. Cancer 56:1106–1111, 1985.
16. Burton EC, Prados MD: Malignant gliomas. Curr Treat Options Oncol 1:459–68, 2000.
17. Castellani P, Borsi L, Carnemolla B, et al: Differentiation between high- and low-grade astrocytoma using a human recombinant antibody to the extra domain-B of fibronectin. Am J Pathol 161:1695–1700, 2002.
18. Chamberlain MC, Jaeckle KA: Medical Research Council adjuvant trial in high-grade gliomas. J Clin Oncol 19:3997–3999, 2001.
19. Colvin OM, Cokger I, Edwards S, et al: Phase I trials of Gliadel plus CPT-11 or Temodar. 36th Ann. Mtg of ACSO, May 22–23, 2000. (Abstr 668).
20. Curran WJ, Jr, Scott CB, Horton J, et al: Recursive partitioning analysis of prognostic factors in three radiation therapy

oncology group malignant glioma trials. J Natl Cancer Inst 85:704–710, 1993.

21. Daumas-Duport C, Scheithauer BW, Kelly PJ: A histologic and cytologic method for the spatial definition of gliomas. Mayo Clin Proc 62:435–449, 1987.

22. Davis FG, Freels S, Grutsch J, et al: Survival rates in patients with primary malignant brain tumors stratified by patient age and tumor histological type: an analysis based on Surveillance, Epidemiology, and End Results (SEER) data, 1973–1991. J Neurosurg 88:1–10, 1998.

23. De Witte O, Lefranc F, Levivier M, et al: FDG-PET as a prognostic factor in high-grade astrocytoma. J Neurooncol 49:157–163, 2000.

24. Dean BL, Drayer BP, Bird CR, et al: Gliomas: classification with MR imaging. Radiology 174:411–415, 1990.

25. Debinski W, Gibo D, Mintz A: Epigenetics in high-grade astrocytomas: opportunities for prevention and detection of brain tumors. Ann NY Acad Sci 983:232–242, 2003.

26. Denny BJ, Wheelhouse RT, Steven MRG, et al: NMR and molecular modeling investigation of the mechanism and activation of the antitumor drug temozolomide and its interaction with DNA. Biochemistry 33:9045–9051, 1994.

27. Devaux BC, O'Fallon JR, Kelly PJ: Resection, biopsy, and survival in malignant glial neoplasms. A retrospective study of clinical parameters, therapy, and outcome. J Neurosurg 78:767–775, 1993.

28. Dinnes J, Cave C, Huang S, Milne R: A rapid and systematic review of the effectiveness of temozolomide for the treatment of recurrent malignant glioma. Br J Cancer 86:501–5, 2002. Comment in Br J Cancer 86:499–500, 2002.

29. Dorward NL, Paleologos TS, Alberti O, Thomas DG: The advantages of frameless stereotactic biopsy over frame-based biopsy. Br J Neurosurg 16:110–118, 2002.

30. Dunn IF, Black PM: The neurosurgeon as local oncologist: cellular and molecular neurosurgery in malignant glioma therapy. Neurosurgery 52:1411–1424, 2003.

31. Earnest F, 4th, Kelly PJ, Scheithauer BW, et al: Cerebral astrocytomas: histopathological correlation of MR and CT contrast enhancement with stereotactic biopsy. Radiology 166:823–827, 1988.

32. Fathallah-Shaykh HM, Rigen M, Zhao LJ, et al: Mathematical modeling of noise and discovery of genetic expression classes in gliomas. Oncogene 21:7164–7174, 2002.

33. Fine HA, Figg WD, Jaeckle K, et al: Phase II trial of the antiangiogenic agent thalidomide in patients with recurrent high-grade gliomas. J Clin Oncol 18:708–715, 2000.

34. Forget MA, Desrosiers RR, Del M, et al: The expression of rho proteins decreases with human brain tumor progression: potential tumor markers. Clin Exp Metastasis 19:9–15, 2002.

35. Fuller GN, Hess KR, Rhee CH, et al: Molecular classification of human diffuse gliomas by multidimensional scaling analysis of gene expression profiles parallels morphology-based classification, correlates with survival, and reveals clinically-relevant novel glioma subsets. Brain Pathol 12:108–116, 2002.

36. Fults D, Pedone C: Immunocytochemical mapping of the phosphatase and tensin homolog (PTEN/MMAC1) tumor suppressor protein in human gliomas. Neuro-oncol 2:71–79, 2000.

37. Galloway PG, Roessmann U: Anaplastic astrocytoma mimicking metastatic carcinoma. Am J Surg Pathol 10:728–732, 1986.

38. Ghosh C, Lazarus HM, Hewlett JS, Creger RJ: Fluctuation of serum phenytoin concentrations during autologous bone marrow transplant for primary and secondary central nervous system tumors. J Neuro-Oncol 12:25, 1992.

39. Gilbar RJ, Brodribb TR: Phenytoin and fluorouracil interaction. Ann Pharmacother 35:1367–1370, 2001.

40. Gilbert MR, Friedman HS, Kuttesch JF, et al: A phase II study of temozolomide in patients with newly diagnosed supratento-

rial malignant glioma before radiation therapy. Neuro-oncol 4:261–267, 2002.

41. Grossman SA, Burch PA: Quantitation of tumor response to anti-neoplastic therapy. Semin Oncol 15:441–454, 1988.

42. Grossman SA, Hochberg F, Fisher J, et al: Increased 9-aminocamptothecin dose requirements in patients on anticonvulsants. NABTT CNS Consortium. The New Approaches to Brain Tumor Therapy. Cancer Chemother Pharmacol 42:118–126, 1998.

43. Grossman SA and the NCCN Brain Tumor Panel: NCCN adult brain tumor practice guidelines. Oncology 11:237–277, 1997. Update v.1.2002, CNS cancers, http://www.nccn.org/physician_gls/f_guidelines.html.

44. Grossman SA, Sheidler VR, Gilbert MF: Decreased phenytoin levels in patients receiving chemotherapy. Am J Med 87:505, 1989.

45. Groves MD, Jaeckle KA, Puduvalli VK, et al: A phase II study of temozolomide (Temodar®) plus marimastat for recurrent glioblastoma multiforme (GBM). Neuro-Oncology 2:266, 2000. Abstract 86.

46. Groves MD, Tremont-Lukats IW, Conrad C, et al: A phase II trial of temozolomide plus thalidomide (NABTC 99-04) for recurrent glioblastoma multiforme. Neuro-Oncol 4:s41, 2002.

47. Gruber M, Gruber D: Phase II treatment of recurrent malignant astrocytoma with temozolomide and irinotecan. 37th Annual Meeting of the American Society of Clinical Oncology, San Francisco, May 12–15, 2001.

48. Hahn CA, Dunn RH, Logue PE, et al: Prospective study of neuropsychologic testing and quality-of-life assessment of adults with primary malignant brain tumors. Int J Radiat Oncol Biol Phys 55:992–999, 2003.

49. Harsh GR, IV, Levin VA, Gutin PH, et al: Reoperation for recurrent glioblastoma and anaplastic astrocytoma. Neurosurgery 21:615–621, 1987.

50. Hecker TP, Grammer JR, Gillespie GY, et al: Focal adhesion kinase enhances signaling through the Shc/extracellular signal-regulated kinase pathway in anaplastic astrocytoma tumor biopsy samples. Cancer Res 62:2699–2707, 2002.

51. Hildebrand J, De Witte O, Sahmoud T: Response of recurrent glioblastoma and anaplastic astrocytoma to dibromodulcitol, BCNU and procarbazine—A phase-II study. J Neurooncol 37:155–160, 1998.

52. Howe FA, Barton SJ, Cudlip SA, et al: Metabolic profiles of human brain tumors using quantitative in vivo 1H magnetic resonance spectroscopy. Magn Reson Med 49:223–232, 2003.

53. Hwang SL, Lieu AS, Kuo TH, et al: Preoperative and postoperative seizures in patients with astrocytic tumours: analysis of incidence and influencing factors. J Clin Neurosci 8:426–429, 2001.

54. Jackson RJ, Fuller GN, Abi-Said D, et al: Limitations of stereotactic biopsy in the initial management of gliomas. Neuro-oncol 3:193–200, 2001.

55. Jaeckle KA, Yung WKA, Prados M, et al: NABTC 98-03: Phase II evaluation of temozolomide and 13-cis retinoic acid (isotretinoin; cRA) for the treatment of recurrent and progressive malignant gliomas. 5th Annual Meeting of the Society of Neuro-Oncology, Nov 9–12. Abstract 103.

56. Janus TJ, Kim EE, Tilbury R, et al: Use of [18F] fluorodeoxyglucose positron emission tomography in patients with primary malignant brain tumors. Ann Neurol 33:540–548, 1993.

57. Khatua S, Peterson KM, Brown KM, et al: Overexpression of the EGFR/FKBP12/HIF-2alpha pathway identified in childhood astrocytomas by angiogenesis gene profiling. Cancer Res 63:1865–1870, 2003.

58. Kim JE, Kim CY, Kim DG, Jung HW: Implantation metastasis along the stereotactic biopsy tract in anaplastic astrocytoma: a case report. J Neurooncol 61:215–218, 2003.

59. Kim S, Dougherty ER, Shmulevich L, et al: Identification of combination gene sets for glioma classification. Mol Cancer Ther 1:1229–1236, 2002.

60. Kleihues P, Davis RL, Coons SW, Burger PC: Anaplastic astrocytoma. In Kleihues P, Cavenee WK (eds): Pathology and Genetics of Tumours of the Nervous System, World Health Organization Classification of Tumours, Lyon, IARC Press, 2000.

61. Kleihues P, Ohgaki H: Primary and secondary glioblastomas: from concept to clinical diagnosis. Neuro-oncol 1(1):44–51, 1999.

62. Korones DN, Benita-Weiss M, Coyle TE, et al: Phase I study of temozolomide and escalating doses of oral etoposide for adults with recurrent malignant glioma. Cancer 97:1963–1968, 2003.

63. Korshunov A, Golanov A, Sycheva R: Immunohistochemical markers for prognosis of anaplastic astrocytomas. J Neurooncol 58:203–215, 2002.

64. Kristof RA, Neuloh G, Hans V, et al: Combined surgery, radiation, and PCV chemotherapy for astrocytomas compared to oligodendrogliomas and oligoastrocytomas WHO grade III. J Neurooncol 59:231–237, 2002.

65. Kuhn JG: Influence of anticonvulsants on the metabolism and elimination of irinotecan. A North American Brain Tumor Consortium preliminary report. Oncology (Hunting) 16(8 Suppl 7):33–40, 2002.

66. Kunwar S, Mohapatra G, Bollen A, et al: Genetic subgroups of anaplastic astrocytomas correlate with patient age and survival. Cancer Res 61:7683–7688, 2001.

67. Lang FF, Olansen NE, DeMonte F, et al: Surgical resection of intrinsic insular tumors: complication avoidance. J Neurosurg 95:638–650, 2001.

68. Laperriere NJ, Leung PM, McKenzie S, et al: Randomized study of brachytherapy in the initial management of patients with malignant astrocytoma. Int J Radiat Oncol Biol Phys 41:1005–11, 1998.

69. Laramore GE, Martz KL, Nelson JS, et al: Radiation Therapy Oncology Group (RTOG) survival data on anaplastic astrocytomas of the brain: does a more aggressive form of treatment adversely impact survival? Int J Radiat Oncol Biol Phys 17:1351–1356, 1989.

70. Larner J, Jane J, Laws E, et al: A phase I-II trial of lovastatin for anaplastic astrocytoma and glioblastoma multiforme. Am J Clin Oncol 21:579–583, 1998.

71. Lee SJ, Kim JH, Kim YM, et al: Perfusion MR imaging in gliomas: comparison with histologic tumor grade. Korean J Radiol 2:1–7, 2001.

72. Lev MH, Hochberg F: Perfusion magnetic resonance imaging to assess brain tumor responses to new therapies. Cancer Control 5:115–123, 1998.

73. Levin VA, Hess KR, Choucair A, et al: Phase III randomized study of postradiotherapy chemotherapy with combination alpha-difluoromethylornithine-PCV versus PCV for anaplastic gliomas. Clin Cancer Res 9:981–990, 2003.

74. Levin VA, Phuphanich S, Glantz MJ, et al: Randomized phase II study of temozolomide (TMZ) with and without the matrix metalloprotease (MMP) inhibitor Prinomastat in patients (pts) with glioblastoma multiforme (GBM) following best surgery and radiation therapy. Proceedings of ASCO 21:99, 2002, abstract 100.

75. Levin VA, Prados MR, Wara WM, et al: Radiation therapy with bromodeoxyuridine followed by CCNU, procarbazine, and vincristine (PCV) chemotherapy for the treatment of anaplastic gliomas. Int J Radiat Oncol Biol Phys 32:75, 1995.

76. Levin VA, Silver R, Hannigan J, et al: Superiority of post radiotherapy adjuvant chemotherapy with CCNU, procarbazine and vincristine (PCV) over BCNU for anaplastic gliomas:

NCOG 6G61 final report. Int J Radiat Oncol Biol Phys 18:321, 1990.

77. Luyten PR, Marien AJ, Heindel W, et al: Metabolic imaging of patients with intracranial tumors: H-1 MR spectroscopic imaging and PET. Radiology 176:791–799, 1990.

78. Marquardt G, Setzer M, Lang J, Seifert V: Delayed hydrocephalus after resection of supratentorial malignant gliomas. Acta Neurochir (Wien) 144:227–231; discussion 231, 2002.

79. Mathijssen RH, Spaerboom A, Dumez H, et al: Altered irinotecan metabolism in a patient receiving phenytoin. Anticancer Drugs 13:139–140, 2002.

80. McGirt MJ, Villavicencio AT, Bulsara KR, et al: MRI-guided stereotactic biopsy in the diagnosis of glioma: comparison of biopsy and surgical resection specimen. Surg Neurol 59:279–283, 2003.

81. Meyer FB, Bates LM, Goerss SJ, et al: Awake craniotomy for aggressive resection of primary gliomas located in eloquent brain. Mayo Clin Proc 76:677–687, 2001. Comment in Mayo Clin Proc 76:670–672, 2001.

82. Meyers CA, Hess KR: Multifaceted end points in brain tumor clinical trials: cognitive deterioration precedes MRI progression. Neuro-oncol, 5:89–95, 2003.

83. Meyers CA, Weitzner MA, Valentine AD, et al: Methylphenidate therapy improves cognition, mood, and function of brain tumor patients. J Clin Oncol 16:2522–2527, 1998.

84. Mori S, Frederiksen K, van Zijl PC, et al: Brain white matter anatomy of tumor patients evaluated with diffusion tensor imaging. Ann Neurol 51:377–380, 2002.

85. Morimoto T, Aoyagi M, Tamaki M, et al: Increased levels of tissue endostatin in human malignant gliomas. Clin Cancer Res 8:2933–2938, 2002.

86. Nelson SJ, McKnight TR, Henry RG: Characterization of untreated gliomas by magnetic resonance spectroscopic imaging. Neuroimaging Clin N Am 12:599–613, 2002.

87. Nozaki M, Tada M, Kobayashi H, et al: Roles of the functional loss of p53 and other genes in astrocytoma tumorigenesis and progression. Neuro-oncol 1:124–137, 1999.

88. Panullo S, Serventi J, Balmaceda C, Burton J: Temozolomide plus celecoxib for treatment of malignant gliomas. Proc Am Soc Clin Oncol 22:114, 2003 (abstr 455).

89. Patel M, McCully C, Godwin K, Balis FM: Plasma and cerebrospinal fluid pharmacokinetics of intravenous temozolomide in non-human primates. J Neurooncol 61:203–207, 2003.

89a. Phillips TL, Levin VA, Ahn DK, et al: Evaluation of bromodeoxyuridine in glioblastoma multiforme: a Northern California Cancer Center Phase II study. Int J Radiat Oncol Biol Phys 21:709, 1991.

90. Phuphanich S, Selph J, Snodgrass S: Low dose thalidomide and Temodar as salvage therapy for recurrent malignant gliomas. Neuro-oncol 4:374, 2002. Abstract 240.

91. Physicians Desk Reference, 55th ed. Montvale NJ, Medical Economics Company, 2001.

92. Plowman J, Waud WR, Koutsoukos AD: Preclinical antitumor activity of temozolomide in mice: efficacy against human brain tumor xenografts and synergism with 1,3-bis(2-chloroethyl)-1-nitrosourea. Cancer Res 54:3793–3799, 1994.

93. Pore N, Liu S, Haas-Kogan DA, et al: PTEN mutation and epidermal growth factor receptor activation regulate vascular endothelial growth factor (VEGF) mRNA expression in human glioblastoma cells by transactivating the proximal VEGF promoter. Cancer Res 63:236–241, 2003.

94. Prados MD, Gutin PH, Phillips TL, et al: Highly anaplastic astrocytoma: a review of 357 patients treated between 1977 and 1989. Int J Radiat Oncol Biol Phys 23:3–8, 1992.

95. Prados MD, Scott C, Curran WJ Jr, et al: Procarbazine, lomustine, and vincristine (PCV) chemotherapy for anaplastic astrocytoma: a retrospective review of radiation therapy oncology

group protocols comparing survival with carmustine or PCV adjuvant chemotherapy. J Clin Oncol 17:3389–3395, 1999. Comment in J Clin Oncol 19:3997–3999, 2001.

96. Prados MD, Scott C, Sandler H, et al: A phase 3 randomized study of radiotherapy plus procarbazine, CCNU, and vincristine (PCV) with or without BUdR for the treatment of anaplastic astrocytoma: a preliminary report of RTOG 9404. Int J Radiat Oncol Biol Phys 45:1109–1115, 1999. Comment in Int J Radiat Oncol Biol Phys 45:1105–1106, 1999.

96a. Prados MD, Sieferheld W, Sandler, et al: Phase III randomized study of radiotherapy plus procarbazine, lomustine, and vincristine with or without BUdR for treatment of anaplastic astrocytoma: final report of RTOG 9404. Int J Radiat Oncol Biol Phys 58:1147–1152, 2004.

97. Rasheed A, Herndon JE, Stenzel TT, et al: Molecular markers of prognosis in astrocytic tumors. Cancer 94:2688–97, 2002.

98. Raza SM, Lang FF, Aggarwal BB, et al: Necrosis and glioblastoma: a friend or a foe? A review and a hypothesis. Neurosurgery 51:2–12; discussion 12–13, 2002.

99. Reardon DA, Friedman HS, Gilbert M, et al: Promising activity in the treatment of malignant glioma. Oncology 17(suppl 5):9–14, 2003.

100. Recht L, Glantz M, Chamberlain M, et al: Quantitative measurement of quality outcome in malignant glioma patients using an independent living score (ILS). Assessment of a retrospective cohort. J Neurooncol 61:127–136, 2003.

101. Reis RM, Hara A, Kleihues P, Ohgaki H: Genetic evidence of the neoplastic nature of gemistocytes in astrocytomas. Acta Neuropathol (Berl) 102:422–425, 2001.

102. Rich J et al: Phase I/II trial of Gliadel® plus Temodar for adult patients with recurrent high-grade glioma. 37th Annual Meeting of the American Society of Clinical Oncology, San Francisco, May 12–15, 2001.

103. Ron IG, Gal O, Vishne TH, Kovner F: Long-term follow-up in managing anaplastic astrocytoma by multimodality approach with surgery followed by postoperative radiotherapy and PCV-chemotherapy: phase II trial. Am J Clin Oncol 25:296–302, 2002.

104. Russell SM, Kelly PJ: Incidence and clinical evolution of postoperative deficits after volumetric stereotactic resection of glial neoplasms involving the supplementary motor area. Neurosurgery 52:506–516; discussion 515–516, 2003.

105. Russell SM, Kelly PJ: Volumetric stereotaxy and the supratentorial occipitosubtemporal approach in the resection of posterior hippocampus and parahippocampal gyrus lesions. Neurosurgery 50:978–988, 2002.

106. Salo J, Niemela M, Joukamaa M, et al: Effects of brain tumour laterality on patients' perceived quality of life. J Neurol, Neurosurg Psychiat 72:373–377, 2002.

107. Sarkar C, Ralte AM, Sharma MC, Mehta VS: Recurrent astrocytic tumours—A study of p53 immunoreactivity and malignant progression. Br J Neurosurg 16:335–342, 2002.

108. Saxman S, Dancey J: Overview of specific molecular targeted agents for combined modality therapy. In Choy H (ed): Chemoradiation in Cancer Therapy. Totawa, NJ, Human Press, 2003.

109. Silvani A, Salmaggi A, Pozzi A, et al: Effectiveness of early chemotherapy treatment in anaplastic astrocytoma patients. Tumori 81:424–428, 1995.

110. Smith JS, Tachibana I, Passe SM, et al: PTEN mutation, EGFR amplification, and outcome in patients with anaplastic astrocytoma and glioblastoma multiforme. J Natl Cancer Inst.

111. Sonoda Y, Kanamori M, Deen DF, et al: Overexpression of vascular endothelial growth factor isoforms drives oxygenation and growth but not progression to glioblastoma multiforme in a human model of gliomagenesis. Cancer Res 63:1962–1968, 2003.

112. Sonoda Y, Ozawa T, Aldape KD, et al: Akt pathway activation converts anaplastic astrocytoma to glioblastoma multiforme in a human astrocyte model of glioma. Cancer Res 61:6674–6678, 2001.

113. Spiro TP, Gerson SL, Liu L: O6-benzylguanine: a clinical trial establishing the biochemical modulatory dose in tumor tissue for alkyltransferase-directed DNA repair. Cancer Res 59:2402–2410, 1999.

114. Stupp R, Dietrich PY, Ostermann Kraljevic S, et al: Promising survival for patients with newly diagnosed glioblastoma multiforme treated with concomitant radiation plus temozolomide followed by adjuvant temozolomide. J Clin Oncol 20:1375–1382, 2002.

115. Tarnawski R, Sokol M, Pieniazek P, et al: 1H-MRS in vivo predicts the early treatment outcome of postoperative radiotherapy for malignant gliomas. Int J Radiat Oncol Biol Phys 52:1271–1276, 2002. (See comment in Int J Radiat Oncol Biol Phys 54:1576, 2002.

116. Temozolomide (Temodar™) Prescribing Information. Kenilworth, NJ, Schering-Plough Corp, 1999.

117. Tortosa A, Vinolas N, Villa S, et al: Prognostic implication of clinical, radiologic, and pathologic features in patients with anaplastic gliomas. Cancer 97:1063–1071, 2003.

118. Tremont-Lukats IW, Gilbert MR: Advances in molecular therapies in patients with brain tumors. Cancer Control 10:125–137, 2003.

119. Urtasun RC, Kinsella TJ, Farnan N, et al: Survival improvement in anaplastic astrocytoma, combining external radiation with halogenated pyrimidines: final report of RTOG 86–12, Phase I-II study. Int J Radiat Oncol Biol Phys 36:1163–1167, 1996. Comment in: Int J Radiat Oncol Biol Phys 36:1281–1282, 1996.

120. Walker MD, Alexander E, Jr, Hunt WE, et al: Evaluation of BCNU and/or radiation in the treatment of anaplastic gliomas, a cooperative clinical trial. J Neurosurg 49:333–343, 1978.

121. Walker MD, Green SB, Byar DP, et al: Randomized comparisons of radiotherapy and nitrosoureas for the treatment of malignant glioma after surgery. N Engl J Med 303:1323–1329, 1980.

122. Wallner KE, Galicich JH, Krol G, et al: Patterns of failure following treatment for glioblastoma multiforme and anaplastic astrocytoma. Int J Radiat Oncol Biol Phys 16:1405–1409, 1989.

123. Westphal M, Hilt DC, Bortey E, et al: A phase 3 trial of local chemotherapy with biodegradable carmustine (BCNU) wafers (Gliadel wafers) in patients with primary malignant glioma. Neuro-oncol 5:79–88, 2003.

123a. Wong ET, Hess KR, Gleason MJ, et al: Outcomes and prognostic factors in recurrent glioma patients enrolled onto phase II clinical trials. J Clin Oncol 17:2572, 1999.

124. Xiao A, Wu H, Pandolfi PP, et al: Astrocyte inactivation of the pRb pathway predisposes mice to malignant astrocytoma development that is accelerated by PTEN mutation. Cancer Cell 1:157–168, 2002.

125. Yamada SM, Yamada S, Hayashi Y, et al: Fibroblast growth factor receptor (FGFR) 4 correlated with the malignancy of human astrocytomas. Neurol Res 24:244–248, 2002.

126. Yao Y, Kubota T, Sato K, Kitai R: Macrophage infiltration-associated thymidine phosphorylase expression correlates with increased microvessel density and poor prognosis in astrocytic tumors Clin Cancer Res 7:4021–4026, 2001.

127. Yung WKA, Jaeckle K, Kyritsis A, et al: A combination of temozolomide and interferon-α in recurrent malignant gliomas, a phase II study. 4th Annual Meeting of the Society of Neuro-Oncology, Nov 17–21, 347, 1999. Abstract 217.

128. Yung WK, Prados MD, Yaya-Tur R, et al: Multicenter phase II trial of temozolomide in patients with anaplastic astrocytoma

or anaplastic oligoastrocytoma at first relapse. Temodal Brain Tumor Group. J Clin Oncol 17:2762–2771, 1999. Erratum in: J Clin Oncol 17:3693, 1999.

129. Zagzag D, Goldenberg M, Brem S: Angiogenesis and blood-brain barrier breakdown modulate CT contrast enhancement: an experimental study in a rabbit brain tumor model. Am J Roentgenol 153:141–146; 1989.

130. Zakhary R, Keles GE, Berger MS: Intraoperative imaging techniques in the treatment of brain tumors. Curr Opin Oncol 11:152–156, 1999.

CHAPTER 19

GLIOBLASTOMA MULTIFORME

Ian F. Parney and Michael D. Prados

Glioblastoma multiforme (GBM) is a cancerous brain tumor thought to develop from astrocytes. It is both the most common and the most malignant primary central nervous system (CNS) tumor. In this chapter, we review clinical principles for GBM.

EPIDEMIOLOGY

Glioblastomas develop in approximately 5 per 100,000 individuals per year in North America, making them the most common primary CNS tumor.[24] Furthermore, GBMs result in 2% of adult cancer deaths even though they only account for 1% of adult cancers. They may occur at any age, but the peak incidence is between ages 65 and 74. They occur in men approximately 40% more often than women. Recently, there has been concern that the incidence of glioblastoma multiforme is increasing. This appears to be unfounded when rigorous population-based studies are performed.[19] Rather, there has been an increase in glioblastoma diagnosis that correlates with improved access to imaging such as computed tomography (CT) and magnetic resonance imaging (MRI). Geographic factors may play a role in gliomagenesis, because it appears that GBMs occur less frequently in some locales (e.g., Japan). GBM incidence is higher in North American Caucasians than in other ethnic groups, suggesting ethnic background may also contribute to risk.

In most GBM patients, no specific risk factors can be identified. Glioblastomas can occur in association with specific genetic disorders such as Li-Fraumeni syndrome or neurofibromatosis or as part of nonspecific familial aggregations, but this accounts for a minority of patients. Other factors, such as presence of allergies, asthma, or autoimmune diseases, may be somewhat protective.[24] Numerous environmental exposures have been loosely associated with GBMs, including nitrates, pesticides, synthetic rubber, petrochemicals, polyvinyl chloride, and formaldehyde. However, the strengths of these associations are not compelling. Ionizing radiation can definitely predispose to GBM development, but this also accounts only for a small minority of GBM patients. Electromagnetic fields generated by power lines or cell phones have not been associated with GBMs to date.[7]

MOLECULAR PATHOGENESIS

Molecular derangements in GBMs can be divided into two broad categories: (1) proto-oncogene up-regulation by mutation or overexpression or (2) tumor suppressor gene down-regulation by mutation or deletion.[6] Many overactive oncogenes in GBMs form part of the receptor tyrosine kinase (RTK)–Ras–Akt pathway. These include the epidermal growth factor receptor (EGFR), platelet-derived growth factor (PDGF), platelet-derived growth factor receptor (PDGFR), and Ras. Many tumor suppressor genes lost in GBMs are involved in cell-cycle regulation (p16^{INK4a}, p14^{ARF}, p53, Rb, cyclin D, cyclin E, cyclin-dependent kinase (CDK) 4/6). Some tumor suppressor genes normally inhibit the RTK–Akt pathway (PTEN).

Glioblastomas can be subdivided based on molecular and clinical factors into primary and secondary GBMs.[25] Primary GBMs occur *de novo* without preceding lower grade astrocytomas. They tend to occur in older individuals and are strongly associated with increased EGFR and MDM2 activity and decreased PTEN and p16^{INK4a}. Secondary GBMs arise as malignant degeneration of lower grade tumors. They occur in younger individuals and are associated with early p53 loss and PDGF overexpression followed by Rb and CDK4/6 loss with progression. In addition to these molecular abnormalities, both primary and secondary GBMs have other derangements that promote angiogenesis, apoptosis-resistance, and escape from immune surveillance. Common molecular abnormalities in GBMs are summarized in Figure 19-1.

PATHOLOGY

Glioblastomas are diffuse intra-axial brain tumors largely made up of neoplastic cells resembling primitive astrocytes. Grossly, they are poorly delineated diffuse masses. Areas of hemorrhage of varying ages are common. Central necrotic areas occur frequently and may occupy a large part of the total tumor mass. They occur throughout the CNS but are most common in the cerebral hemispheres and deep gray matter. Brainstem GBMs are infrequent and typically affect children or young adults (malignant brainstem gliomas). GBMs in the cerebellum and spinal cord are rare.

Microscopically, GBMs show evidence for nuclear pleomorphism, mitotic activity, endothelial hyperplasia, and necrosis.[9] Presence of any three of these four characteristics is enough to result in the diagnosis of a grade IV astrocytoma (glioblastoma multiforme) in most classification schemes. In practice, all four are often present if tissue sampling is adequate. In smaller samples, it may be more difficult to be definitive regarding tumor grade because of the marked histopathologic variability that can be seen within a given

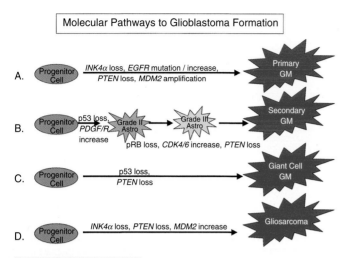

Molecular Pathways to Glioblastoma Formation

A. Progenitor Cell → *INK4α* loss, *EGFR* mutation / increase, *PTEN* loss, *MDM2* amplification → Primary GM

B. Progenitor Cell → p53 loss, *PDGF/R* increase → Grade II Astro → pRB loss, *CDK4/6* increase, *PTEN* loss → Grade III Astro → Secondary GM

C. Progenitor Cell → p53 loss, *PTEN* loss → Giant Cell GM

D. Progenitor Cell → *INK4α* loss, *PTEN* loss, *MDM2* increase → Gliosarcoma

FIGURE 19-1 Schematic diagram showing molecular pathways to formation of *(A)* primary glioblastoma multiforme, *(B)* secondary glioblastoma multiforme, *(C)* giant cell glioblastoma multiforme, and *(D)* gliosarcoma.

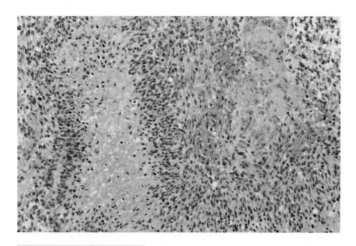

FIGURE 19-2 Typical microscopic features of glioblastoma. Note the nuclear pleomorphism, endothelial hyperplasia, and areas of pallisading necrosis.

tumor. Figure 19-2 shows the typical microscopic appearance of a GBM. As discussed previously, glioblastomas can be subdivided into primary and secondary categories based on their clinical and molecular phenotype. These categories are indistinguishable by light microscopy. However, at least two distinct histopathologic GBM subtypes are recognized.

Giant cell glioblastomas are characterized by numerous large multinucleated giant cells, small fusiform syncytial cells, and a reticulin network. These findings are seen in addition to the classic characteristics of a glioblastoma. They arise *de novo* (like primary GBMs) but tend to occur in younger individuals (like secondary GBMs). Their molecular phenotype is similarly mixed, with relatively common p53 mutations (like secondary GBMs) and PTEN loss (like primary GBMs). They are often located in subcortical temporal and parietal lobes and appear relatively circumscribed on imaging. Although their overall prognosis is poor, it may be slightly better than other glioblastomas.

Gliosarcomas display a mixed pattern of gliomatous and sarcomatous tissue on light microscopy. The gliomatous portion has the typical features of a GBM including glial fibrillary acidic protein (GFAP) reactivity. The sarcomatous portions often have densely packed spindle-shaped cells in herring bone patterns suggestive of fibrosarcoma. These areas form a prominent reticulin network and are negative with GFAP immunostaining. They have a genetic phenotype similar to primary GBMs, except that EGFR amplification appears rare. The sarcomatous and gliomatous portions of the tumor have similar clonal genetic abnormalities, suggesting a common cell of origin. The prognosis for patients with gliosarcomas does not appear to be significantly different from other GBMs.

DIAGNOSIS

Clinical Presentation

Symptoms and signs in GBM patients are relatively uniform but nonspecific. Raised intracranial pressure phenomena (headache, nausea and vomiting, blurred or double vision, drowsiness) are common. These may be associated with objective papilledema, extraocular motor palsies, pupil abnormalities, or decreased level of consciousness. Typically, these symptoms and signs are most prominent in the morning and improve over the course of the day. Seizures occur frequently. Up to one third of glioblastoma patients will have seizures. Neurologic deficits are also common. These may be global (personality change, altered cognition) or focal, depending on the tumor's location. Although many patients will have neurologic deficits, they are often relatively subtle and may go unrecognized until after a brain tumor is identified.

Laboratory Evaluation

Currently, there are no specific serum markers for GBM. Standard laboratory investigations (complete blood count, serum electrolytes, urea, creatinine, glucose, liver enzymes, partial thromboplastin time, international normalized ratio [PTT–INR]) are often obtained in the course of initial evaluation and preparation for therapy but do not provide specific diagnostic information.

IMAGING

Like most aspects of neuro-oncology, imaging GBMs revolves around CT and MRI. On noncontrast CT, glioblastomas are most commonly (but not exclusively) low density. They tend to be enhanced nonuniformly in a ring pattern around a central hypodense area and have a further surrounding hypodense area. From inside out, these regions are thought to represent necrosis, active tumor, and edema. However, viable tumor cells may be seen in all of these regions. Enhancement on CT is generally associated with aggressiveness, but this is not an absolute correlation. Some GBMs may have minimal or no enhancement on CT.

MRI has largely replaced CT as the imaging modality of choice for GBM patients. The improved anatomic detail and multiplanar imaging provided by MRI are invaluable for modern surgical and radiation therapy planning. On MRI,

GBMs tend to be isointense or hypointense on noncontrast T1 and hyperintense on T2 and fluid-attenuated inversion recovery (FLAIR) sequences. The MRI enhancement pattern is similar to CT. Again, there is a rough but not absolute correlation with MRI enhancement and tumor grade. The T2 and FLAIR signal abnormality usually extends farther on MRI than the corresponding hypodensity on CT. Neither modality can clearly distinguish the margin of these infiltrating tumors. A typical MRI appearance for a GBM is shown in Figure 19-3.

Many GBM patients get a CT scan during their initial work-up. This is usually followed quickly by an MRI scan once a mass lesion is identified. MRI is often the primary determinant of treatment response. However, interpretation after treatment can be difficult and must be made in light of other factors. For example, surgery itself can result in inflammation that leads to enhancement indistinguishable from tumor. This is maximal between 48 hours and 4 weeks after surgery. Corticosteroid use can also alter the degree of enhancement, without altering the underlying tumor burden. MRI scans must be interpreted in light of a patient's current corticosteroid dose and any recent changes in that dose. Finally, an effective treatment response (particularly to radiation therapy) may result in tissue changes and necrosis that enhance on MRI in a manner that cannot be reliably distinguished from tumor on anatomic studies alone.

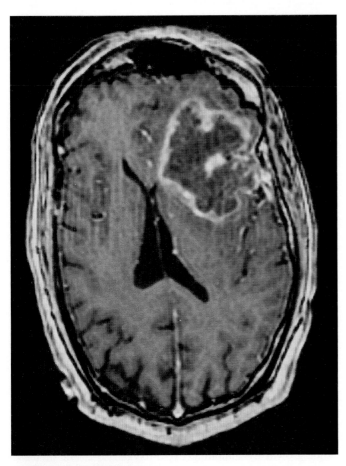

FIGURE 19-3 Axial T1 postcontrast magnetic resonance image showing a typical ring-enhanced left frontal glioblastoma multiforme. Note that, although this appearance is typical for glioblastoma, it is not pathognomonic.

With this in mind, biologic imaging studies are taking an increasing role in GBM patient management. In particular, they can be a useful adjunct when evaluating new enhanced areas of uncertain significance in previously treated patients. Fluorodeoxyglucose positron emission tomography (FDG-PET) scans can be useful to distinguish metabolically active areas such as tumor from inactive areas such as necrosis. However, PET scans require a cyclotron to generate appropriate isotopes, and access to these scans can be limited in some areas. Increasingly, MRI techniques that are potentially more universally available are being used to provide similar biologic information. Proton magnetic resonance spectroscopy (MRS) can be used to detect metabolites in normal and abnormal brain tissue.[22] Common metabolite peaks generated include choline (Cho), creatine (Cr), N-acetyl aspartate (NAA), lactate (Lac), and lipid (Lip). Active tumor will often show increased choline and decreased NAA compared with normal brain. Necrotic material typically shows a global decrease in metabolites except for lipid. Similarly, magnetic resonance perfusion studies can indicate blood volume and vascularity. Aggressive tumors typically exhibit increased blood volume compared with normal brain, whereas necrotic areas usually have decreased vascularity.

Other imaging modalities have a more limited role in GBM patient management. Functional MRI can be used to identify eloquent cortical areas, but this is largely experimental. Digital subtraction angiograms have been largely superseded by MR angiography and are rarely necessary. When performed, they may be normal, may show mass effect, or may show a tumor "blush." Skull x-ray studies are often normal. Any findings that may be seen (e.g., calcifications) are nonspecific.

TREATMENT

General Management

The initial management of GBM patients is necessarily nonspecific, because they have typically only recently sought treatment for neurologic signs and symptoms and had some form of neuroimaging whose results were compatible with a malignant brain tumor. The diagnosis has not yet been confirmed pathologically. Management is aimed at symptom control and preparing patients for surgery (biopsy or resection). Dexamethasone is helpful to reduce vasogenic edema surrounding the tumor, reducing symptoms and making surgery safer. A typical dose regimen would be 10 mg intravenous load followed by 4 mg four times a day. Similarly, an antiepileptic medication such as phenytoin is often advisable to reduce risk of perioperative seizures for patients with supratentorial tumors. Mild analgesics such as acetaminophen with or without codeine may be necessary to control headache. Typically, these interventions may be performed on an outpatient basis. Occasionally, sicker patients may require admission for stabilization.

Once surgery has been performed and the diagnosis is established, specific adjunctive therapies may be instituted (see later discussion). Patients who are still taking corticosteroids should be weaned from them to the lowest dose possible to minimize the side effects of prolonged high-dose corticosteroid therapy. In patients who have had seizures, most authorities recommend continuing antiepileptic medications. Patients who have not had seizures should have antiepileptic medication discontinued. If antiepileptic medications are prescribed, consideration must be given to potential interactions with other therapies, particularly chemotherapy. Some antiepileptic medications such as carbamazepine are inherently myelosuppressive and should be avoided when possible in this patient population. Some (e.g., phenytoin, carbamazepine, phenobarbital) induce the cytochrome p450 enzyme system in the liver. This alters the metabolization of some chemotherapy agents, and doses may need to be adjusted accordingly.

Surgery

Surgery plays a key role in GBM patient management. Indications may include confirming histopathologic diagnosis, reducing tumor burden, relieving mass effect, introducing local antineoplastic agents, and performing cerebrospinal fluid (CSF) diversionary procedures. Relative contraindications include medical frailty, poor performance status, and eloquent or inaccessible location. Options for surgery include frame-based and frameless stereotactic biopsy, open biopsy, debulking, and gross-total resection. Numerous studies have shown that gross-total resection is associated with improved prognosis.[5,10] However, these studies have been largely retrospective, and no randomized controlled trials have been performed comparing aggressive surgical resection with more conservative approaches. This area remains controversial as a result. Still, most authorities advocate gross-total resection whenever possible if this can be accomplished without unacceptable risk of neurologic deficit.

Increasingly, tumors that have traditionally been thought to be unresectable can be safely removed using intraoperative image guidance, awake craniotomy, and intraoperative electrophysiologic mapping.[8,14] In addition to resection, surgery's role in GBM therapy is being expanded. Increasingly, craniotomy is used as an opportunity to introduce other antineoplastic agents, including low-dose permanent brachytherapy seeds and various chemotherapeutic agents.[20]

Surgery, whether it is a limited biopsy or an attempt at more aggressive resection, is associated with some risk. In a recent prospective multi-institutional series, the total morbidity rate (neurologic, regional, or systemic complications) among 408 patients undergoing craniotomy for resection of a previously untreated malignant glioma was 24%.[4] Mortality was 1.5%. Of note, 53% of patients improved neurologically after craniotomy and resection, whereas only 8% were worse. There is no opportunity for a corresponding improvement in neurologic function after biopsy. However, the overall morbidity risk appears to be lower for stereotactic biopsy. The University of Toronto group has reported that total symptomatic morbidity was 6% in a prospective series of 300 patients undergoing stereotactic biopsy for an intra-axial lesion.[1] Mortality was still 1.7%.

Radiation Therapy

Conventional fractionated radiation therapy has a role in virtually all GBM patients unless they refuse active treatment in favor of supportive care.[11] This is typically given as an adjuvant in the early postoperative phase. Multiple randomized controlled trials have demonstrated a survival benefit for patients receiving radiation in addition to resection versus patients undergoing surgery alone. Outcome is improved (i.e., less toxicity) when radiation is given focally to the tumor and to a margin of several centimeters compared with giving whole-brain radiation. Typically, total doses of 60 Gy are administered in 1.8 to 2.0 Gy fractions given 5 days per week for 6 to 6.5 weeks. Alternate fractionation schemes and radiosensitizers have not proved beneficial to date.

Stereotactic radiosurgery (SRS), delivering a single very high-dose radiation fraction to a carefully defined treatment volume with the aid of stereotactic localization, has an evolving role in GBM management. This can be delivered using either linear accelerators or a Gamma Knife®. SRS boost in addition to standard fractionated radiation therapy has appeared to be beneficial in single-arm studies, and results from a randomized controlled trial are pending.[13] SRS may also have a role in treating small recurrent GBMs.[3]

Other means to deliver radiation to GBMs continue to be investigated. Temporary high dose brachytherapy was shown to be ineffective in randomized controlled trials.[12,21] However, low-dose permanent brachytherapy may have a role in select patients and is being tested at some centers. Similarly, studies with particle beam therapy and with intraoperative radiotherapy are ongoing.

Chemotherapy

Chemotherapy also plays a role in GBM management.[17] Although results to date have been somewhat disappointing on a population basis, some individuals have had dramatic responses. Timing can vary. Some protocols give agents concurrent with radiation therapy, after radiation as further adjuvant treatment, or at recurrence. Cytotoxic agents (agents that result in tumor cell death) remain the mainstay of GBM chemotherapy. First-line cytotoxic agents include temozolomide, carmustine (BCNU), and PCV (a combination of procarbazine, CCNU, and vincristine). All of these agents work by disrupting DNA synthesis except vincristine, which disrupts the mitotic spindle apparatus in dividing cells. Temozolomide is often the first choice because it has similar efficacy to BCNU and PCV but is associated with a better side-effect profile. Second-line cytotoxic chemotherapy options include carboplatin, VP16 (etopiside), and CPT-11 (irinotecan). These agents have some activity against GBM but are, in general, less effective than first-line options. New cytotoxic agents continue to be developed and tested.

In addition, agents designed to overcome chemotherapy resistance mechanisms are currently undergoing clinical trial. For example, O^6-alkylguanine-DNA alkyltransferase (O^6-AGAT) is a DNA repair enzyme that mediates resistance to several alkylating agents. O^6-benzyl guanine (O^6-BG) blocks this enzyme and is now being studied in combination with standard agents such as BCNU and temozolomide.

In addition to cytotoxic agents, increasing numbers of cytostatic agents are available that have activity against GBM. For example, cis-retinoic acid has been shown to promote neoplastic astrocyte differentiation to less malignant phenotypes and inhibit tumor growth as a result. Thalidomide can inhibit GBM growth by impairing angiogenesis. Celecoxib can slow tumor growth by inhibiting cyclo-oxygenase-2. All of these agents are FDA approved for other indications and may be used off-label for GBM treatment. Several small molecule growth factor inhibitors affecting EGFR (ZD1839, OSI774), PDGFR (STI571), and Ras (R115777) are currently in clinical trial for GBM treatment.

In addition to options for systemic chemotherapy outlined previously, strategies to increase chemotherapeutic agent concentration within the tumor are increasingly important in GBM management.[20] Biodegradable wafers impregnated with BCNU can be used to line resection cavities to deliver BCNU to the tumor bed. Moderately improved survival has been reported for recurrent GBM patients treated with these wafers.[2] Several ongoing clinical trials postoperatively administer chemotherapeutic agents or immunologically targeted toxins by convection-enhanced delivery via intraparenchymal catheters placed around the resection cavity at surgery. The results are pending. Finally, considerable experimental effort is being made to evaluate the role of intra-arterial chemotherapy with and without blood-brain barrier modification.

Experimental Therapy

Numerous experimental strategies for treating glioblastomas are currently in clinical trial. Many of these involve variations on standard therapy (surgery, radiation, chemotherapy) and have been discussed previously. However, several novel biologically based strategies are currently in clinical trials and will be briefly reviewed here.

Gene therapy can be defined as transferring genetic material to human cells to treat human disease. Many different vectors are available for gene transfer, and many diseases and genes are potential targets.[26] Target genes may be selected to kill transfected cells (suicide gene therapy), replace mutated or deleted tumor suppressor genes, or stimulate antitumor immune responses (immunogene therapy). For example, glioma cells may be transduced in situ with the herpes simplex virus–thymidine kinase (HSV-TK) gene, making them susceptible to ganciclovir-mediated killing. This strategy was very impressive in preclinical studies but has been less so in early clinical trials. This may in part reflect difficulties in gene transfer in situ. This is a common problem for gene therapy, and overcoming it will require both improved vector systems and mechanical delivery strategies.

Immunotherapy has long held promise for glioma treatment because of its potential to be a "silver bullet" that specifically kills tumor cells while leaving normal cells unharmed. Unfortunately, early clinical efforts were unrewarding and led to declining interest in this treatment modality. However, recent advances in immunology, tumor biology, and molecular biology have led to renewed interest in glioma immunotherapy.[18] Active specific immunotherapies via immunogene therapy and dendritic cell vaccines have received particular attention, as have passive but specific monoclonal antibody therapies.

Cytotoxic viral therapy is another novel therapeutic approach that is beginning to attract more interest. For example, glioblastoma patients may be exposed to replication-competent (but attenuated) herpes simplex virus strains that are followed by ganciclovir treatment. This is similar to HSV-TK and ganciclovir gene therapy. Reovirus, a common virus that causes mild upper respiratory tract infections in healthy individuals, appears to be tumoricidal in glioma models in vivo,[23] possibly by targeting tumors with Ras-pathway overactivity.

RECURRENT GLIOBLASTOMAS

At present, it is an unfortunate truism to state that all GBMs will recur. The only variant is timing. Median time to recurrence after treating a newly diagnosed GBM is 7 months. Clinical presentation at recurrence is often similar to that at initial diagnosis. In addition, asymptomatic progression on routine follow-up imaging is not uncommon, particularly if follow-up scans are obtained frequently. As noted previously, interpreting MRI scans of previously treated GBM patients can be challenging and must be done in light of factors such as timing relative to surgery, corticosteroid dose, and previous therapy.

Once progression has been recognized, appropriate management is necessary. Dexamethasone may be helpful once again in controlling symptoms related to cerebral edema. Antiepileptic medication may be appropriate if seizures have occurred. Surgery may be a viable option. There is an increased risk of neurologic worsening with repeat craniotomy and resection compared with first craniotomy (18% versus 8%). However, significantly more patients are neurologically improved following second surgery than are worsened (40% versus 18%). Generally, surgery for recurrent GBMs is considered if the diagnosis is in question and for symptomatic relief for large tumors. Repeating standard fractionated external-beam therapy beyond a total cumulative dose of 6000 cGy is not an option because of intolerably high toxicity risk. However, radiosurgery (either Gamma Knife or linear-accelerator (LINAC) based) can be helpful for small (<2 cm) recurrences. Chemotherapy options also can be reviewed at recurrence. If progression occurred while receiving systemic chemotherapy, this regimen should be discontinued and a new regimen instituted. If progression occurred while off therapy, it may be possible to return to some agents used previously (e.g., temozolomide) if the patient had not progressed while on treatment with these agents. For others, such as BCNU and CCNU, cumulative toxicity precludes return.

It may be appropriate at recurrence to consider supportive care without further active intervention. This decision is best made on a case-by-case basis by the patient in consultation with family, friends, and physician. This decision should reflect both patients' physical health and performance status and their underlying values and desires. Although the overall prognosis for patients with recurrent glioblastoma is poor, it should be remembered that some of these patients do respond to treatment. Therapeutic nihilism at recurrence should be avoided.

REHABILITATION

Patients with glioblastomas frequently develop substantial neurologic deficits at some point in the course of their disease. In many cases, particularly after surgery, formal rehabilitation efforts may be helpful in minimizing the impact of these deficits. Deficits in cognition, strength, and visual perception have been among the most common reasons for referring brain tumor patients to a comprehensive interdisciplinary rehabilitation program. Programs such as these have had documented success in improving functional status in brain tumor patients.[15]

OUTCOME AND QUALITY OF LIFE

Despite advances in diagnosis, surgery, radiation, and chemotherapy, median survival for patients diagnosed with a glioblastoma multiforme remains approximately 1 year. Median survival for patients with recurrent glioblastomas is approximately 4 months. However, some patients have relatively prolonged survival (>5 years). It is difficult to predict which patients will fall into this category when they are newly diagnosed, but some factors are associated with a slightly better prognosis. Age younger than 45 years, better functional status (often measured by preoperative Karnofsky performance score), and gross-total resection have all been associated with improved survival. In addition to these clinical factors, molecular and cytogenetic factors may help predict outcome. EGFR overexpression (as opposed to mutation) has been associated with prolonged survival, particularly when combined with normal p53 status. Prolonged survival is also associated with 1p through 19q chromosome deletions.

Given the overall prognosis for patients with glioblastomas despite aggressive therapy, quality of life during treatment is an important concern. If quality of life becomes very poor at any point, it argues against further aggressive treatment that is unlikely to result in cure or even remission. Measuring quality of life can be elusive, however. Common functional rating systems such as the Karnofsky scale may not correlate well with patients' perceived quality of life. Quality of life is mul-

tifaceted and is influenced by both physical and psychosocial factors. Broad-based tools that reflect these factors have been developed, including the European Organization for Research and Treatment of Cancer Quality of Life (EORTC-QOL) and the Brain Cancer Module (BCM) questionnaires. These tools are beginning to yield more objective information concerning quality of life in brain tumor patients.[16]

CONCLUSION

GBM remains a difficult clinical problem. However, advances in conventional diagnosis and therapy are beginning to have an impact on survival. Increased knowledge about the biology of these tumors is beginning to pay dividends in terms of novel biologically based therapies. There are more viable treatment options available for patients with glioblastomas than ever before. Physicians treating patients diagnosed with a glioblastoma still face a daunting prognosis, but options available now can help many patients, and the prospects for the future are exciting.

References

1. Bernstein M, Parrent AG: Complications of CT-guided stereotactic biopsy of intra-axial brain lesions. J Neurosurg 81:165–168, 1994.
2. Brem H, Piantadosi S, Burger PC, et al: Placebo-controlled trial of safety and efficacy of intraoperative controlled delivery by biodegradable polymers of chemotherapy for recurrent gliomas. The Polymer-brain Tumor Treatment Group. Lancet 345:1008–1012, 1995.
3. Chamberlain MC, Barba D, Kormanik P, et al: Stereotactic radiosurgery for recurrent gliomas. Cancer 74:1342–1347, 1994.
4. Chang S, Parney IF, McDermott M, et al: Perioperative complications and neurological outcome of first versus second craniotomy among patients enrolled in the Glioma Outcomes (GO) Project. J Neurosurg 98:1175–1181, 2003.
5. Devaux BC, O'Fallon JR, Kelly PJ: Resection, biopsy, and survival in malignant glial neoplasms. A retrospective study of clinical parameters, therapy, and outcome. J Neurosurg 78:767–775, 1993.
6. Holland EC: Brain tumor animal models: importance and progress. Curr Opin Oncol 13:143–147, 2001.
7. Inskip PD, Tarone RE, Hatch EE, et al: Cellular-telephone use and brain tumors. N Engl J Med 344:79–86, 2001.
8. Kaibara T, Saunders JK, Sutherland GR: Advances in mobile intraoperative magnetic resonance imaging. Neurosurgery 47:131–137; discussion 137–138, 2000.
9. Kleihues P, Burger PC, Collins VP, et al: Glioblastoma. In Kleihues P, Cavanee WK (eds): Tumours of the Nervous System. Lyon, France, IARC Press (WHO), 2000.
10. Lacroix M, Abi-Said D, Fourney DR, et al: A multivariate analysis of 416 patients with glioblastoma multiforme: prognosis, extent of resection, and survival. J Neurosurg 95:190–198, 2001.
11. Laperriere N, Zuraw L, Cairncross G: Radiotherapy for newly diagnosed malignant glioma in adults: a systematic review. Radiother Oncol 64:259, 2002.
12. Laperriere NJ, Leung PM, McKenzie S, et al: Randomized study of brachytherapy in the initial management of patients with malignant astrocytoma. Int J Radiat Oncol Biol Phys 41:1005–1011, 1998.
13. Loeffler JS, Alexander E III, Shea WM, et al: Radiosurgery as part of the initial management of patients with malignant gliomas. J Clin Oncol 10:1379–1385, 1992.
14. Matz PG, Cobbs C, Berger MS: Intraoperative cortical mapping as a guide to the surgical resection of gliomas. J Neurooncol 42:233–245, 1999.
15. Mukand JA, Blackinton DD, Crincoli MG, et al: Incidence of neurologic deficits and rehabilitation of patients with brain tumors. Am J Phys Med Rehabil 80:346–350, 2001.
16. Osoba D, Brada M, Prados MD, et al: Effect of disease burden on health-related quality of life in patients with malignant gliomas. Neuro-oncol 2:221–228, 2000.
17. Parney IF, Chang S: Current chemotherapy for glioblastoma. Cancer J 9:149–156, 2003.
18. Parney IF, Hao C, Petruk KC: Glioma immunology and immunotherapy: a review. Neurosurgery 46:778–792, 2000.
19. Radhakrishnan K, Modir B, Parisi JE, et al: The trends in incidence of primary brain tumors in the population of Rochester, Minnesota. Ann Neurol 37:67–73, 1995.
20. Schmidt MH, Chang SM, Berger MS: An appraisal of chemotherapy: In the blood or in the brain? Clin Neurosurg 48:46–59, 2001.
21. Selker RG, Shapiro WR, Burger P, et al: The Brain Tumor Cooperative Group NIH Trial 87-01: a randomized comparison of surgery, external radiotherapy, and carmustine versus surgery, interstitial radiotherapy boost, external radiation therapy, and carmustine. Neurosurgery 51:343–355; discussion 355–347, 2002.
22. Vigneron D, Bollen A, McDermott M, et al: Three-dimensional magnetic resonance spectroscopic imaging of histologically confirmed brain tumors. Magn Reson Imaging 19:89–101, 2001.
23. Wilcox ME, Yang W, Senger D, et al: Reovirus as an oncolytic agent against experimental human malignant gliomas. J Natl Cancer Inst 93:903–912, 2001.
24. Wrensch M, Minn Y, Chew T, et al: Epidemiology of primary brain tumors: current concepts and review of the literature. Neuro-oncol 4:278–299, 2002.
25. Zhu Y, Parada LF: The molecular and genetic basis of neurological tumours. Natl Rev Cancer 2:616–626, 2002.
26. Zlokovic BV, Apuzzo MLJ: Cellular and molecular neurosurgery: pathways from concept to reality. Part I—target disorders and concept approaches to gene therapy of the central nervous system. Neurosurgery 40:789–803, 1997.

CHAPTER 20

PILOCYTIC ASTROCYTOMA

Edward R. Smith, David H. Ebb, Nancy J. Tarbell, and Fred G. Barker II

Pilocytic astrocytomas (PAs) are defined as a unique entity under the World Health Organization (WHO) Classification of Tumors of the Nervous System. They are a common variant of low-grade astrocytomas, which are primary tumors of the central nervous system. These histologically benign lesions (WHO grade I) have little tendency toward malignant degeneration. They typically arise in children and young adults and in patients with neurofibromatosis type I (NF1). These low-grade glial tumors are distinguished from other astrocytomas by their radiographic characteristics, histology, and unusually favorable prognosis.

LOCATION

PAs have been reported in all regions of the brain, although they tend to present in several characteristic locations. Most of these favored locations are in or near the midline, including the optic pathways, region of the third ventricle, tectum of the midbrain, pons, cervicomedullary junction, and cerebellum. They can also occur in the cerebral hemispheres. Case reports have documented rare presentations of PAs within the lateral ventricular system and as disseminated subarachnoid tumor.

Cerebellum

PAs are most commonly found in the cerebellum, both as midline lesions in the roof of the fourth ventricle and also in the cerebellar hemispheres. In one study, 62 of 78 cerebellar astrocytomas in children were pilocytic.[43] Many cerebellar PAs are well circumscribed, although some may also extend through the cerebellar peduncle into the brainstem.

Brainstem

PAs can generally be identified in three regions of the brainstem: the tectum of the midbrain, the pons, and the cervicomedullary junction.

At the most rostral aspect of the brainstem is the relatively common tectal glioma. These lesions, involving the tectum and periaqueductal region, often present with hydrocephalus. In one study, four out of four biopsies of tectal lesions were PAs.[6]

Pontine gliomas can be divided into two groups, based on location. The diffuse astrocytomas of the ventral pons typically occur in young children, presenting with cranial nerve palsies and long tract signs. These tumors pursue a malignant course and are much more common than pontine PAs. Astrocytomas

occurring in the dorsal pons, typically with an exophytic component, are almost always the pilocytic subtype. In one study of 76 patients, the findings of a lesion outside the ventral pons and dorsal exophytic growth were associated with a statistically significant likelihood ($P = .001$ and $P = .013$, respectively) of histology and behavior consistent with PA.[11] In another study, 11 of 12 patients with dorsally exophytic lesions of the pons had pilocytic histology.[23]

Cervicomedullary gliomas are less homogeneous. In one series of 39 cervicomedullary tumors, only 3 were PAs.[50] In contrast, a second series of 11 cervicomedullary astrocytomas found the majority to be PAs.[51] Though cervicomedullary gliomas appear to be more variable in their histology, the majority of exophytic lesions arising in the cervicomedullary region are PAs.

Supratentorial

PAs are commonly found in the midline, with many reports of these tumors involving the optic nerves and chiasm. Unlike PAs in other areas of the brain, the tumors involving the optic nerves or chiasm can often grow along the nerve, demonstrating a multilobed appearance. Tumors in this region can also involve the borders of the third ventricle, including the hypothalamus and thalamus. Supratentorial hemispheric lesions often occur in the medial aspects of the temporal and parietal lobes. Cerebral hemispheric cases of PA are relatively uncommon. In one study of 20 cases of PA, only 3 were found in the cerebral hemispheres.[5] A study of these lesions found them to be indistinguishable from PAs in other parts of the brain.

DIAGNOSIS

The diagnosis of PA is often made based on symptoms or signs referable to three distinct mechanisms common to many intrinsic brain tumors: (1) focal invasion or destruction of neural tissue, (2) local mass effect, or (3) a general increase in intracranial pressure. The salient findings on presentation will relate to the location of the tumor.

Cerebellum

PAs of the cerebellum often present with findings of elevated intracranial pressure, including headache, lethargy, and emesis, especially when the lesion causes obstructive hydrocephalus. In addition, tumors arising in the lateral aspect of the cerebellum often present with ipsilateral dysmetria and appendicular ataxia. Truncal ataxia is common in midline lesions. This deficit may be noticeable only by examining gait. In a group of 102 cerebellar astrocytomas in children, the average duration of symptoms was 5.8 months, with presenting findings most commonly attributed to intracranial hypertension.[7] This may include chronic emesis (especially after waking), weight loss, and papilledema. Rarely, there is evidence that these tumors can present acutely with spontaneous intratumoral hemorrhage.

Brainstem

Although most intrinsic brainstem tumors present with long tract signs (such as spastic quadriparesis or sensory changes), cranial nerve dysfunction, and cerebellar deficits, these findings are unusual for PAs and are more characteristic of diffuse fibrillary pontine gliomas. Tectal pilocytic lesions most often present with hydrocephalus due to obstruction of the cerebral aqueduct. Diffuse fibrillary astrocytomas of the ventral pons often present with a sixth nerve palsy, whereas dorsal PAs usually do not. In addition, pontine PAs often have a longer clinical prodrome than other, more aggressive pontine lesions. A series of 12 patients, of whom 11 had pontine PAs, reported a 7-month prodrome of symptoms that were referable to elevated intracranial pressure. These patients demonstrated minimal cranial nerve abnormalities (including near normal brainstem auditory-evoked potentials) and a striking absence of pyramidal tract findings.[23]

Cervicomedullary lesions have similar presentations to those in the pons. In a study of 17 cervicomedullary tumors in children, the mean duration of symptoms before diagnosis was 2.1 years and at least 1 year in 80% of the patients.[39]

Supratentorial

PAs in the optic apparatus often present with visual-field defects, decreased acuity, or proptosis. Tumors that involve the chiasm, third ventricle, or hypothalamus can cause endocrine deficiencies, such as diabetes insipidus (DI), the syndrome of inappropriate antidiuretic hormone release (SIADH), or precocious puberty. Obstructive hydrocephalus can be caused by a large midline tumor in this region. Multicentric intraventricular PAs have also been reported, which presumably arise from the subependymal glia. Patients with tumors involving the area of the optic apparatus or third ventricle should be considered for formal ophthalmologic and endocrinologic evaluations.

Supratentorial hemispheric PAs can present with seizure, headache, or focal deficits. These symptoms may persist for a prolonged period of time before a diagnosis is made, reflecting the indolent character of these tumors. In a review of cases of supratentorial PA, the duration of symptoms before diagnosis has been reported to be more than a year.

Leptomeningeal (LM) presentation is rare, but has significant prognostic implications. Approximately 3% of PAs present in this fashion, often with signs or symptoms such as paraparesis, sphincter dysfunction, hydrocephalus, ataxia, seizures, or cognitive dysfunction.[20] Because of the association between LM disease and diencephalic tumors, care should be taken to look for LM spread when patients have PAs in this location.

EPIDEMIOLOGY, INCIDENCE, PREVALENCE

The Central Brain Tumor Registry of the United States (CBTRUS, available at www.cbtrus.org) has pooled and analyzed the data from 61.5 million people, approximately 23% of the U.S. population. From 1992 to 1997, 719 cases of PA were reported. Thus PAs represent 1.9% of all brain tumors, with a mean age at diagnosis of 17 years. Adjusted to the U.S. population, the incidence of PAs is 0.23 cases per 100,000 person years, or roughly 700 new cases per year in the United States. PAs are more common in children (younger than 20 years of age), with an incidence of 0.57 cases per 100,000 person years. Cerebellar PAs are diagnosed at a younger age (9 to 10 years) than cerebral PAs, which are diagnosed at an average age of 22 years.[22]

A recent review of 340 primary central nervous system tumors in children identified PA as the most common tumor, at 23.5%.[38] PAs (as do most gliomas) appear to be more common in males, with a prevalence of 62%, although the CBTRUS data suggest an incidence rate that is approximately equal between males and females.

Although the majority of PAs are sporadic, there is a notable association with NF1. In particular, optic gliomas (nearly all pilocytic) have been reported in 5% to 19% of NF1 cases, although higher estimates have come from retrospective analyses of referral clinics.[3,42,48] Conversely, approximately 20% of patients who have optic glioma will have NF1, supporting the policy of screening patients with optic glioma for NF1.[22]

IMAGING

PAs demonstrate characteristic features on imaging studies. They are often well-demarcated, circumscribed lesions, with the exception of tumors involving the optic apparatus, that commonly enlarge the nerves or grow in a multilobed fashion. They are usually isodense or hypodense relative to surrounding brain on computed tomography (CT). On magnetic resonance imaging (MRI), they are hyperintense on T2 and hypointense on T1. PAs enhance brightly with contrast on both CT and MRI studies. The tumors characteristically have a cystic component with an enhancing mural nodule. When investigated with angiography, only 30% were "hypervascular," with the other 70% reported as avascular or normal.[12] PAs can demonstrate increased glucose metabolism on positron-emission tomography (PET), corresponding to the enhanced regions on MRI.[13] The current diagnostic procedure of choice for a patient suspected of having a PA is an MRI with and without contrast.

Of interest is a study of three tumors in which the wall of the tumor cyst did not demonstrate any tumor cells.[2] However, if the cyst wall enhances, there is an increased likelihood of tumor cells being present in the cyst lining.[22]

Unlike other enhanced astrocytomas, the enhancement associated with PAs does not portend a poor prognosis. Evidence suggests that the enhancement is due to chronic glomeruloid degenerative hyalinization of blood vessels (in contrast to endothelial proliferation, believed to be the cause of enhancement in more aggressive gliomas).[27] PAs often cause minimal edema and may exert surprisingly little mass effect. Despite sharp radiographic margins, these tumors may infiltrate the surrounding parenchyma.

The tumors are often single, but disseminated lesions, including LM spread, have been reported. In the brainstem, tectal PAs are often isodense on CT, hyperintense on T2-weighted MRI, and inconsistently enhancing. The dorsally exophytic pontine PAs have similar radiographic features. Cervicomedullary tumors are also T1 hypointense and T2 bright, commonly expanding the medulla and proximal cervical spinal cord. The clear superiority of MRI in detecting these lesions supports employing this modality to assess patients with a clinical history and examination suggestive of a mass lesion in the brain.

TUMOR HISTOLOGY

The histology and molecular genetic characteristics of PAs have been studied extensively. Much of this interest is derived from the discordance between the benign clinical course typical of this disease and the radiographic and histologic features that suggest a far more aggressive biology. Moreover, the relationship of PA with NF1 has been a source of multiple insights regarding tumor biology.

Gross Pathology

PAs are usually gray-pink lesions, often with a large cyst (or cysts). In the setting of a single cyst, a mural nodule that may be calcified is commonly present. Hemorrhage within these lesions has also been reported.[30]

Histology

PAs exist in two histologic subtypes: juvenile and adult. The juvenile subtype is more common and is identified by bipolar-appearing tumor cells with elongated nuclei. The cells have characteristic fine hairlike (hence *pilo*) cytoplasmic processes and often form tight clusters around blood vessels. These compact areas commonly have characteristic eosinophilic Rosenthal fibers. In addition, the juvenile subtype can also have components of the tumor composed of cystic cells, filled with eosinophilic material. The adult subtype does not often exhibit cystic areas but shares the cellular morphology characteristic of the juvenile variant. These tumors usually have some calcification and may exhibit gemistocytic cells.

Interpreting the pathology of PAs can be difficult, because features commonly indicative of malignancy may be present. Though features such as vascular proliferation or necrosis are typically associated with aggressive neoplasms, they may not be associated with a poor prognosis when identified in the context of a PA.

Molecular and Genetic Analysis

In view of the difficulty in reconciling some of the histologic characteristics of these tumors, multiple attempts have been made to elucidate their unique biology.

One avenue of investigation has focused on the association between NF1 and PAs, including chromosomal analysis. A study of both sporadic and NF1-associated PAs found that 4 out of 20 tumors had allelic losses on chromosome 17q, in the region of the known NF1 tumor suppressor gene.[49] Another report documented that eight of eight PAs in patients with NF1 had a loss of NF1 gene expression.[15] Although it is tempting to hypothesize that loss of function of the NF1 gene may contribute to the formation of PAs, this potential relationship is difficult to reconcile with the finding that sporadic astrocytomas overexpress the NF1 gene product at levels up to fourfold higher than normal brain.[35] Moreover, a series comparing sporadic PAs to those found in patients with NF1 found that 92% of the NF1-associated tumors had loss of the NF1 gene, in marked contrast to only 4% of the sporadic PAs exhibiting loss of the NF1 locus.[24]

Other genetic analyses of these tumors have been described, including an increased incidence of abnormalities on chromosomes 7, 8, 9, and 11.[40,52] Gene expression profiles of NF1-associated and sporadic PAs, compared with multiple cell lines of various lineages, demonstrated that PAs are genetically unique gliomas with gene expression profiles that resemble those of fetal astrocytes, and, to a lesser extent, oligodendroglial precursors.[16]

A variety of markers of cellular proliferation and apoptosis have been evaluated as indicators of tumor behavior in both sporadic and NF1-associated PAs. The proliferative index of these tumors is often low, commonly less than 5%, with a concomitant high apoptotic ratio.[8,31] Many of the markers commonly associated with proliferation, such as Ki-67 or MIB-1, have not been consistently reliable as prognostic indicators for these tumors. Other markers that have been investigated in PAs include mouse double minute 2 (MDM2), p21, p16, p53, and PTEN. Despite this extensive research, no clear genetic markers or prognostic indicators have emerged for PAs.

Evidence suggests that the impressive vascularity of these tumors is associated with increased expression of vascular endothelial growth factor (VEGF), with a concomitant increase in the activity of VEGF-associated receptors.[28] It has been suggested that increased perivascular cellularity may be associated with anaplastic change, although this finding was only reported in a single case series.[26] However, further support for this hypothesis is present in a study demonstrating increased presence of von Willenbrand factor (vWF) in association with more aggressive tumors.[41]

THERAPY

Surgery

If the tumor is surgically accessible, the definitive therapy for PA is surgical extirpation. One series with a median follow-up of 14.9 years reported a 100% 10-year survival rate for patients who had undergone a gross-total (or radical subtotal) resection, versus 74% for those patients undergoing subtotal removal or biopsy.[12] This finding has been corroborated by other studies, including 100% 5-year survival with complete resection in a series of patients reported by Haapasalo.[17] Because the rate of recurrence following a gross-total resection is extremely low, adjuvant postoperative radiation treatment is not indicated unless clear recurrence is documented.

After subtotal resection, close observation is warranted with serial imaging. PAs are notable for their tendency to remain stable for long periods. Some tumors may undergo spontaneous regression. There are multiple reports of tumors becoming undetectable on imaging after subtotal resection. If there is a recurrence, the preferred treatment is a second resection if the tumor is surgically accessible. In one series of 20 cases of recurrent PA, 10 patients had a gross-total resection at second surgery.[5] Reoperation should be considered particularly for tumors located in the cerebral hemispheres or in the cerebellum.

The role of surgery is more controversial in tumors located in sensitive midline structures, such as the optic apparatus or brainstem. Operation on lesions of the optic apparatus can be technically challenging, and tumor may be intimately associated with the optic nerves. Although conservative surgery, such as decompression of the optic canal or tumor debulking, may be useful, there is also evidence supporting the use of radiation therapy (discussed later).[45] Tectal lesions can often be followed and treated with radiation if they progress. If a brainstem tumor is dorsally exophytic, then a subtotal resection followed by observation or radiation therapy may be indicated. Of note, patients with NF1 and brainstem lesions suspected of being PAs may manifest a more benign biologic behavior that differs significantly from sporadic lesions.[36] In this group of patients, observation may be a safe course of action, because these tumors may spontaneously involute or remain stable for prolonged periods.

In addition to the considerations of surgical resection, biopsy, or observation, patients with brainstem lesions (in particular, tectal and pontine lesions) may need to be evaluated for cerebrospinal fluid (CSF) diversion. Traditionally, this has involved the use of a ventriculoperitoneal shunt, although endoscopic third ventriculocisternostomy is gaining favor as an alternative approach.

Cervicomedullary tumors require careful consideration before surgery. There are varying reports of efficacy and safety of surgery. One group reported a gross-total resection in 12 out of 39 patients, with 1 death. In a second series there was no postoperative mortality, although 5% of patients developed a new postoperative neurologic deficit.[9,50] There may be an association between preoperative radiation therapy and postoperative complications. In a series of 17 cervicomedullary gliomas, it was noted that out of five patients with postoperative complications, four had received preoperative radiation.[39] The decision to treat cervicomedullary tumors surgically should balance the experience of the individual surgeon with the expected natural history of the lesion.

The goal of surgery for any PA is maximal resection of the lesion with minimal effects to the patient. Complete removal is the ideal objective, if safe. Cystic lesions should have intraoperative biopsies of the cyst wall to determine if resection of the wall is necessary. If the tumor is in a difficult location, stereotactic guidance or intraoperative MRI may assist in resection or biopsy. Patients should receive a postoperative MRI scan within 48 hours (to avoid postoperative artifactual enhancement) to assess the extent of resection, as well as to serve as a baseline study against which future studies can be compared. It has been demonstrated that postoperative imaging is more reliable than the surgeon's subjective assessment of the degree of tumor removal, a potentially important consideration in determining the need for future treatments.

Radiation

The role of radiation therapy in PA is limited, given the excellent outcomes achievable with surgery. Use of radiation therapy has been proposed primarily for surgically inaccessible lesions such as optic system or hypothalamic tumors or when there is a significant volume of residual postoperative tumor.

As previously discussed, PA is notable for the propensity for residual tumor to remain stable in size or even to involute after surgery. As noted previously, recurrence after subtotal resection can be often be treated successfully with reoperation. However, in the setting of a recurrent, symptomatic PA in a surgically inaccessible region, radiation is a useful treatment. In a group of 37 recurrent or unresectable PAs, stereotactic radiosurgery (SRS) was used in conjunction with other treatment modalities. The median radiosurgical dose to the tumor margin was 15 Gy (in a range of 9.6 to 22.5 Gy). In this group, 10 of 37 patients had complete disappearance of the tumor, 15 had stable or decreased tumor volume, and 12 had delayed tumor progression. At 28 months after radiation, 89% were alive.[18] There is often a long delay between treatment and a demonstrable response on MRI, particularly in fractionated radiation therapy.[1]

Interstitial radiation has been used, including iodine-125 implants with low dose rates (≤10 cGy/hour) and a reference dose of 60 to 100 Gy calculated to the outer rim of the tumor. The 5- and 10-year survival rates in patients with PAs (97 patients) were 84.9% and 83%, respectively.[25]

The use of fractionated radiation therapy is supported in patients with unresectable optic gliomas. A series of 24 patients evaluated the use of fractionated radiation therapy in the setting of decreasing vision or clinical or radiographic evidence of progressive disease. Radiation doses ranged from 4500 to 5660 cGy (median 5400 cGy). At a median of 6 years of follow-up, 88% of patients had freedom from disease progression and 100% were alive. Although 91% had symptomatic improvement or stabilization of vision, 15 of 18 patients had postradiation endocrine abnormalities (predominately growth hormone deficiency).[34,48] Fractionated radiation therapy has also been used as an adjunct in the treatment of LM disease.[46]

In general, radiation arrests tumor growth, although there are reports of irradiated tumors shrinking or completely disappearing. Following radiation therapy, these tumors may initially grow and then reduce their volume. Such early changes in tumor volume and MRI signal characteristics are often difficult to interpret, although new radiographic modalities, such as magnetic resonance spectroscopy and PET, may prove to be helpful adjuncts in discriminating between tumor progression and radiation-induced tissue injury. In rare cases, fulminant, symptomatic radionecrosis can occur, particularly after radiosurgery.[47]

Chemotherapy

The primary role of chemotherapy for PAs resides in the treatment of young children who have surgically inaccessible lesions or progressive recurrences. Although radiation therapy is typically administered to older patients with unresectable progressive disease, the potential neurocognitive and neuroendocrine morbidity of cranial radiation make this modality far less appealing for young children. The availability of several active chemotherapeutic regimens has permitted postponement or avoidance of radiation therapy in this vulnerable subset of patients. The use of chemotherapy has also been reported as salvage therapy for patients with multiple recurrences or LM disease. A variety of regimens have demonstrated clinical benefit, most notably the combination of vincristine with low dose carboplatin (Packer) and the combination of procarbazine, CCNU, vincristine, and 6-thioguanine (Prados).[21,29,32,33,37] Both of these regimens have permitted deferral of radiation therapy for 2 to 3 years in children with tumors in the first 5 to 10 years of life. In a multi-institutional study, Packer and colleagues treated 78 children with progressive low-grade astrocytomas with a regimen that employed vincristine and low-dose carboplatin, given 4 weeks out of 6 for a total of 18 months. This schedule produced an objective response rate of 56%, with 2- and 3-year progression-free survival rates of 75% and 68%, respectively. Prados and colleagues have reported similar success in controlling progressive disease in young children using a regimen that consists of 6-thioguanine, procarbazine, CCNU, and vincristine given over 12 months. This treatment program achieved stabilization or tumor shrinkage in all but 3 of the 41 patients followed (92.7%), with a median progression-free survival of 30 months. These two regimens are now being compared in a randomized study sponsored by COG (Children's Oncology Group), the North American pediatric oncology cooperative group.[21,32,33,37] Side effects include hematologic toxicity, with bone marrow suppression, as well as otologic and renal damage.

Of note, there appears to be no difference in response to chemotherapy between NF1-associated and sporadic PAs.[32] However, it appears that children younger than 5 have longer progression-free survival in response to chemotherapy than older children.[32] Packer's study demonstrated a 3-year progression-free survival rate of 74% for children younger than 5 years old, versus a progression-free survival of only 39% over the same interval in children older than 5 years at diagnosis. The efficacy of these chemotherapeutic regimens in producing temporary and, less frequently, durable disease stabilization supports deferral of radiation therapy in children younger than 7 to 10 years who have progressive disease.

RECURRENCE

In general, the long-term prognosis for PA is excellent, with a very low rate of recurrence, dependent primarily on the degree of surgical resection. Moreover, patients with cerebellar or cerebral hemispheric lesions have a longer progression-free survival than patients with lesions in other locations.[14] As previously discussed, many tumors can remain stable for long periods or spontaneously involute. Recurrence can occur in a delayed fashion, however, with one recurrence documented after a 45-year interval.[4]

The volume of postoperative tumor is one of the factors that is most closely linked to disease progression. In one study, 3 of 23 patients with gross-total resections had recurrences of

their tumors within 2 to 5 years, and all had re-excision with no disease detectable at 4 to 10 years of follow-up. Of those who had a subtotal resection, 9 of 13 required reoperation within an average of 12 months. In 4 of these 9, the recurrent tumor was reclassified as anaplastic astrocytoma (11% of the total series).[26] Another study of 103 patients with subtotally resected PAs found that 33 patients had progression requiring retreatment at a mean of 39 months after operation.[10]

Most recurrence is local, although LM disease has been reported, particularly with hypothalamic tumors. LM recurrence rates as high as 11% have been reported in patients with hypothalamic PAs.[20] Rarely, LM disease can spontaneously regress, although it most commonly requires treatment with radiation or chemotherapy, as previously discussed.

OUTCOME

Outcomes for patients with PAs are generally excellent, particularly for those who undergo a gross-total resection. In general, most patients can anticipate a normal or near-normal neurologic status after treatment, with the notable exception of NF1 patients, who may have significant comorbidity related to their genetic disorder. In a study of 51 patients with PA, 82% were alive at 10 and 20 years (with a median follow-up of 15 years). Among those long-term survivors, 89% were fully active.[12] A 100% 10-year survival has been reported for gross-total resection (or radical subtotal resection) and 74% 10-year survival with only a subtotal resection.[12]

By location, brainstem PAs have an overall reported 5-year survival of 95%.[11] Cerebellar PAs have a 100% 5-year survival with a gross-total resection and a 93% 5-year survival overall.[17] Optic gliomas treated with radiation had a 100% survival with 6 years of follow-up, and 88% of these were disease free.[34] Patients with tectal lesions have been reported to have a 100% survival at 4 years of follow-up. A study looking at all midline gliomas reported high survival rates over long periods (96% survival at 1 year, 91% survival at 5 years, and 80% survival at 10 years).[19,44] In one series of 427 patients with low-grade astrocytomas, LM disease was documented in 13 of the 177 patients (7%) whose tumors progressed or recurred. Despite a 5-year progression-free survival of only 18%, the majority of these patients (68%) were still alive 10 years after their LM recurrence. This is further testimony to the remarkably indolent behavior of these tumors.[20]

Patients younger than 5 years seem to have slightly worse outcomes than older children, regardless of histology or location.[14] Younger children with PAs seem to respond better to chemotherapy than their older counterparts and have longer progression-free survival.[32] Patients with PAs associated with NF1 are more difficult to assess, because they may have considerable additional morbidity associated with their neurogenetic disorder.

In summary, PA is a tumor notable for slow growth and a good long-term prognosis. Despite useful advances in chemotherapeutics and radiation treatments, surgery remains the primary treatment modality, with patient outcome heavily influenced by the degree of resection.

References

1. Bakardjiev AI, Barnes PD, Goumnerova LC, et al: Magnetic resonance imaging changes after stereotactic radiation therapy for childhood low grade astrocytoma. Cancer 78:864, 1996.

2. Beni-Adani L, Gomori M, Spektor S, Constantini S: Cyst wall enhancement in pilocytic astrocytoma: neoplastic or reactive phenomena. Pediatr Neurosurg 32:234, 2000.

3. Blatt J, Jaffe R, Deutsch M, Adkins JC: Neurofibromatosis and childhood tumors. Cancer 57:1225, 1986.

4. Boch AL, Cacciola F, Mokhtari K, et al: Benign recurrence of a cerebellar pilocytic astrocytoma 45 years after gross total resection. Acta Neurochir (Wien) 142:341, 2000.

5. Bowers DC, Krause TP, Aronson LJ, et al: Second surgery for recurrent pilocytic astrocytoma in children. Pediatr Neurosurg 34:229, 2001.

6. Boydston WR, Sanford RA, Muhlbauer MS, et al: Gliomas of the tectum and periaqueductal region of the mesencephalon. Pediatr Neurosurg 17:234, 1991.

7. Desai KI, Nadkarni TD, Muzumdar DP, Goel A: Prognostic factors for cerebellar astrocytomas in children: a study of 102 cases. Pediatr Neurosurg 35:311, 2001.

8. Dirven CM, Koudstaal J, Mooij JJ, Molenaar WM: The proliferative potential of the pilocytic astrocytoma: the relation between MIB-1 labeling and clinical and neuro-radiological follow-up. J Neurooncol 37:9, 1998.

9. Epstein F, Wisoff J: Intra-axial tumors of the cervicomedullary junction. J Neurosurg 67:483, 1987.

10. Fisher BJ, Leighton CC, Vujovic O, et al: Results of a policy of surveillance alone after surgical management of pediatric low grade gliomas. Int J Radiat Oncol Biol Phys 51:704, 2001.

11. Fisher PG, Breiter SN, Carson BS, et al: A clinicopathologic reappraisal of brain stem tumor classification. Identification of pilocytic astrocytoma and fibrillary astrocytoma as distinct entities. Cancer 89:1569, 2000.

12. Forsyth PA, Shaw EG, Scheithauer BW, et al: Supratentorial pilocytic astrocytomas. A clinicopathologic, prognostic, and flow cytometric study of 51 patients. Cancer 72:1335, 1993.

13. Fulham MJ, Melisi JW, Nishimiya J, et al: Neuroimaging of juvenile pilocytic astrocytomas: an enigma. Radiology 189:221, 1993.

14. Gajjar A, Sanford RA, Heideman R, et al: Low-grade astrocytoma: a decade of experience at St. Jude Children's Research Hospital. J Clin Oncol 15:2792, 1997.

15. Gutmann DH, Donahoe J, Brown T, et al: Loss of neurofibromatosis 1 (NF1) gene expression in NF1-associated pilocytic astrocytomas. Neuropathol Appl Neurobiol 26:361, 2000.

16. Gutmann DH, Hedrick NM, Li J, et al: Comparative gene expression profile analysis of neurofibromatosis 1-associated and sporadic pilocytic astrocytomas. Cancer Res 62:2085, 2002.

17. Haapasalo H, Sallinen S, Sallinen P, et al: Clinicopathological correlation of cell proliferation, apoptosis and p53 in cerebellar pilocytic astrocytomas. Neuropathol Appl Neurobiol 25:134, 1999.

18. Hadjipanayis CG, Kondziolka D, Gardner P, et al: Stereotactic radiosurgery for pilocytic astrocytomas when multimodal therapy is necessary. J Neurosurg 97:56, 2002.

19. Hoffman HJ, Soloniuk DS, Humphreys RP, et al: Management and outcome of low-grade astrocytomas of the midline in children: a retrospective review. Neurosurgery 33:964, 1993.

20. Hukin J, Siffert J, Velasquez L, et al: Leptomeningeal dissemination in children with progressive low-grade neuroepithelial tumors. Neuro-oncol 4:253, 2002.

21. Kato T, Sawamura Y, Tada M, et al: Cisplatin/vincristine chemotherapy for hypothalamic/visual pathway astrocytomas in young children. J Neurooncol 37:263, 1998.

22. Kaye AH, Laws ER: Brain Tumors: An Encyclopedic Approach, 2nd ed. London, Churchill Livingstone, 2001.

23. Khatib ZA, Heideman RL, Kovnar EH, et al: Predominance of pilocytic histology in dorsally exophytic brain stem tumors. Pediatr Neurosurg 20:2, 1994.

24. Kluwe L, Hagel C, Tatagiba M, et al: Loss of NF1 alleles distinguish sporadic from NF1-associated pilocytic astrocytomas. J Neuropathol Exp Neurol 60:917, 2001.

25. Kreth FW, Faist M, Warnke PC, et al: Interstitial radiosurgery of low-grade gliomas. J Neurosurg 82:418, 1995.

26. Krieger MD, Gonzalez-Gomez I, Levy ML, McComb JG: Recurrence patterns and anaplastic change in a long-term study of pilocytic astrocytomas. Pediatr Neurosurg 27:1, 1997.

27. Lee YY, Van Tassel P, Bruner JM, et al: Juvenile pilocytic astrocytomas: CT and MR characteristics. AJR Am J Roentgenol 152:1263, 1989.

28. Leung SY, Chan AS, Wong MP, et al: Expression of vascular endothelial growth factor and its receptors in pilocytic astrocytoma. Am J Surg Pathol 21:941, 1997.

29. McCowage G, Tien R, McLendon R, et al: Successful treatment of childhood pilocytic astrocytomas metastatic to the leptomeninges with high-dose cyclophosphamide. Med Pediatr Oncol 27:32, 1996.

30. Mesiwala AH, Avellino AM, Roberts TS, Ellenbogen RG: Spontaneous cerebellar hemorrhage due to a juvenile pilocytic astrocytoma: case report and review of the literature. Pediatr Neurosurg 34:235, 2001.

31. Nakamizo A, Inamura T, Ikezaki K, et al: Enhanced apoptosis in pilocytic astrocytoma: a comparative study of apoptosis and proliferation in astrocytic tumors. J Neurooncol 57:105, 2002.

32. Packer RJ, Ater J, Allen J, et al: Carboplatin and vincristine chemotherapy for children with newly diagnosed progressive low-grade gliomas. J Neurosurg 86:747, 1997.

33. Packer RJ, Lange B, Ater J, et al: Carboplatin and vincristine for recurrent and newly diagnosed low-grade gliomas of childhood. J Clin Oncol 11:850, 1993.

34. Pierce SM, Barnes PD, Loeffler JS, et al: Definitive radiation therapy in the management of symptomatic patients with optic glioma. Survival and long-term effects. Cancer 65:45, 1990.

35. Platten M, Giordano MJ, Dirven CM, et al: Up-regulation of specific NF 1 gene transcripts in sporadic pilocytic astrocytomas. Am J Pathol 149:621, 1996.

36. Pollack IF, Shultz B, Mulvihill JJ: The management of brainstem gliomas in patients with neurofibromatosis 1. Neurology 46:1652, 1996.

37. Prados MD, Edwards MS, Rabbitt J, et al: Treatment of pediatric low-grade gliomas with a nitrosourea-based multiagent chemotherapy regimen. J Neurooncol 32:235, 1997.

38. Rickert CH, Paulus W: Epidemiology of central nervous system tumors in childhood and adolescence based on the new WHO classification. Childs Nerv Syst 17:503, 2001.

39. Robertson PL, Allen JC, Abbott IR, et al: Cervicomedullary tumors in children: a distinct subset of brainstem gliomas. Neurology 44:1798, 1994.

40. Sanoudou D, Tingby O, Ferguson-Smith MA, et al: Analysis of pilocytic astrocytoma by comparative genomic hybridization. Br J Cancer 82:1218, 2000.

41. Selby DM, Woodard CA, Henry ML, Bernstein JJ: Are endothelial cell patterns of astrocytomas indicative of grade? In Vivo 11:371, 1997.

42. Singhal S, Birch JM, Kerr B, et al: Neurofibromatosis type 1 and sporadic optic gliomas. Arch Dis Child 87:65, 2002.

43. Smoots DW, Geyer JR, Lieberman DM, Berger MS: Predicting disease progression in childhood cerebellar astrocytoma. Childs Nerv Syst 14:636, 1998.

44. Squires LA, Allen JC, Abbott R, Epstein FJ: Focal tectal tumors: management and prognosis. Neurology 44:953, 1994.

45. Sutton LN, Molloy PT, Sernyak H, et al: Long-term outcome of hypothalamic/chiasmatic astrocytomas in children treated with conservative surgery. J Neurosurg 83:583, 1995.

46. Tamura M, Zama A, Kurihara H, et al: Management of recurrent pilocytic astrocytoma with leptomeningeal dissemination in childhood. Childs Nerv Syst 14:617, 1998.

47. Tandon N, Vollmer DG, New PZ, et al: Fulminant radiation-induced necrosis after stereotactic radiation therapy to the posterior fossa. Case report and review of the literature. J Neurosurg 95:507, 2001.

48. Tao ML, Barnes PD, Billett AL, et al: Childhood optic chiasm gliomas: radiographic response following radiotherapy and long-term clinical outcome. Int J Radiat Oncol Biol Phys 39:579, 1997.

49. von Deimling A, Louis DN, Menon AG, et al: Deletions on the long arm of chromosome 17 in pilocytic astrocytoma. Acta Neuropathol (Berl) 86:81, 1993.

50. Weiner HL, Freed D, Woo HH, et al: Intra-axial tumors of the cervicomedullary junction: surgical results and long-term outcome. Pediatr Neurosurg 27:12, 1997.

51. Young Poussaint T, Yousuf N, Barnes PD, et al: Cervicomedullary astrocytomas of childhood: clinical and imaging follow-up. Pediatr Radiol 29:662, 1999.

52. Zattara-Cannoni H, Gambarelli D, Lena G, et al: Are juvenile pilocytic astrocytomas benign tumors? A cytogenetic study in 24 cases. Cancer Genet Cytogenet 104:157, 1998.

CHAPTER 21

PLEOMORPHIC XANTHOASTROCYTOMA

Ziya Gökaslan and Tarik Tihan

Pleomorphic xanthoastrocytoma (PXA) is a circumscribed astrocytic neoplasm often associated with leptomeninges. The neoplasm was first described by Kepes et al[8] as a distinctive form of supratentorial astrocytoma in young individuals and with a more favorable prognosis than infiltrating astrocytomas. The authors of the original study as well as others have suggested the subpial astrocyte as the cell of origin.[2]

LOCATION

The typical location of PXA is the cerebral hemispheres and particularly the temporal lobe. In a recent large series with 71 patients, the most common single location was the temporal lobe followed by other supratentorial loci.[1] Examples of this unusual neoplasm have also been reported in the cerebellum,[19] spinal cord,[9] and even the retina.[21] There has been one case report of an intrasellar PXA with a quite unusual clinical and histologic appearance.[1]

PXA is typically a solitary superficial mass associated with leptomeninges, and displays, at least in part, a distinct interface with the underlying brain. Rare examples are located deep within the parenchyma without obvious leptomeningeal attachment.[14] PXA can be multicentric either at presentation or after recurrence.

DIAGNOSIS

Due to its superficial location, most patients with PXA have seizures of long duration, and the history of seizures may occasionally be traced back a few decades. Focal or generalized seizures are observed in more than two thirds of patients with PXA. The supratentorial PXAs can also cause headaches and visual disturbance and may be associated with focal weakness and sensory impairment.

The clinical course of the disease is often without acute exacerbations, and the symptoms often develop gradually. In rare instances, the tumor is discovered incidentally. Sometimes the patients carry diagnoses such as fibrous xanthoma, monstrocellular sarcoma, or even glioblastoma multiforme at initial presentation.

Even though radiologic studies may suggest the diagnosis in the differential based on location and solid-cystic appearance, the definitive diagnosis of PXA is made after histopathologic examination. Before the use of immunohistochemistry, most PXAs were classified as mesenchymal neoplasms such as fibrous xanthoma or monstrocellular sarcoma.

EPIDEMIOLOGY

PXA is an uncommon glial neoplasm and accounts for less than 1% of all astrocytic neoplasms. However, true incidence is difficult to establish because of lack of accurate epidemiologic statistics specifically for PXA.

PXA is most commonly seen during the first 3 decades of life. In their original report Kepes et al have reported patients between the ages of 7 and 25.[8] Recent reviews also reported a median age of 22 years.[1] However, there have been occasional reports of older individuals with PXA.[15] The male to female ratio has been equal in most studies.

Little is known about the epidemiologic characteristics of PXAs. Because of their rarity, it has not been possible to associate the neoplasm with any particular region, profession, or risk factor.

NEUROIMAGING

PXA typically appears as a solid-cystic mass in most imaging modalities. Even though PXA can be suggested within the differential diagnosis, the neoplasm does not have specific characteristics on computed tomography (CT) or magnetic resonance imaging (MRI). PXAs can be partially solid (i.e., solid-cystic) or, less commonly, entirely solid masses.[7]

Computed Tomography

PXA appears as a discrete, mixed high and low attenuation mass with at least partially well-defined margins. Some examples of PXA may not be well visualized by noncontrast CT or appear as ill-defined low attenuation lesions. Calcification is not a prominent feature of PXA. After contrast administration, the solid components are homogeneously enhanced, and the solid-cystic tumors appear as cysts with an enhanced mural nodule. Rarely, contrast enhancement is in a gyral form. Some PXAs remodel the inner table of the skull, causing bony erosions.

Magnetic Resonance Imaging

The tumor is typically a cortical-based lesion isointense to gray matter on nonenhanced T1-weighted images. On T2, the tumor is often hyperintense, but the T2 appearance is often more variable. The solid cystic tumors can be readily recognized on MRI, particularly after gadolinium administration (Figure 21-1). Most tumors demonstrate a homogeneous and strong enhancement in their solid components on postgadolinium images. Occasionally, one can also identify surrounding leptomeningeal enhancement as well as gyriform enhancement, similar to that seen with CT. Entirely solid PXAs can easily be confused with meningiomas, and rare cases have been reported as having dural tail.[17]

There have been a few recent reports on the positron-emission tomography (PET) findings in patients with PXA. This modality has been found useful in determining the presence or absence of recurrence after initial surgery and in assessing the aggressiveness of the neoplasm and the effect of treatment.[2]

PATHOLOGIC FEATURES

The definitive diagnosis of PXA rests on accurate and appropriate interpretation of pathologic findings. Pathologic evalua-

tion can distinguish these lesions from other gliomas or nonglial tumors.

Macroscopic Features

Intraoperatively, consistency of the neoplasm is often rubbery. The xanthomatous component may give the tumor a yellow-tan appearance.

Microscopic Features

The most consistent feature of PXA is compact and largely noninfiltrating architecture that is common to the circumscribed astrocytomas such as pilocytic astrocytoma. Overall, most slides containing tumor tissue have only a small amount of incorporated brain parenchyma, but this feature is often lost in recurrences.

The tumor is characterized by the components that can be inferred from its name, and the histologic appearance is often very ominous to the untrained eye (Figure 21-2A). The amount of pleomorphism is often at the degree that is seen in glioblastomas or high-grade sarcomas; hence the previous designation, *monstrocellular sarcoma*. The pleomorphic astrocytes are often admixed with spindled forms as well as those that resemble ganglion cells with bizarre nuclei and large cytoplasm (see Figure 20-2B). Pleomorphic cells are always present but vary in number, size, and shape from case to case. In addition, among the pleomorphic cells are the xanthomatous or lipidized cells that resemble lipoblasts with highly vacuolated cytoplasm (see Figure 20-2C). Through special histochemical stains, these cells have been shown to contain lipid material but

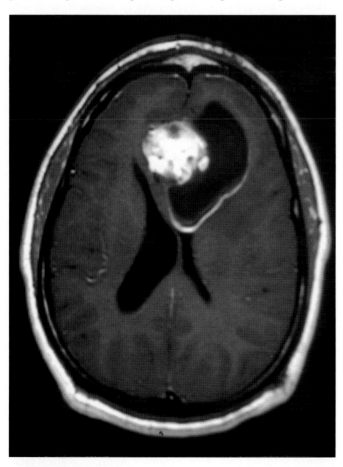

FIGURE 21-1 Axial, contrast-enhanced T1-weighted image of a typical pleomorphic xanthoastrocytoma. The tumor is considered one of a group of tumors that commonly present as cystic masses with an enhancing mural nodule. Note the smooth contours of the focal rim enhancement.

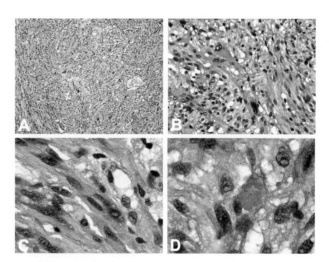

FIGURE 21-2 Typical histological appearance of pleomorphic xanthoastrocytoma. *A,* On low power magnifications the tumor appears rather cellular and compact. In most part, the tumor is noninfiltrating. *B,* The tumor cells are predominantly spindle shaped with frequent bizarre nuclei, giving the pleomorphic appearance. *C,* Occasional cells have multiple cytoplasmic vacuoles resembling adipocytes (i.e., xanthomatous cells). *D,* High-power magnification of an eosinophilic granular body (EGB). EGBs are frequently observed in compact portions of the neoplasm.

also clearly show astrocytic differentiation, hence the term *xanthoastrocytoma*.

Most PXAs demonstrate a fascicular pattern that on occasion appears storiform and mesenchymal so as to mimic that of a fibrohistiocytic neoplasm. The tumor associated with the brain surface can spread along the subarachnoid space, and into perivascular (Virchow-Robin) spaces. In that case, the tumor may appear even more mesenchymal or sarcomatoid.

The astrocytic quality of the PXA is often conspicuous in the variably fibrillary cytoplasm, glial fibrillary acidic protein (GFAP) positivity, and in some cases, in a focal and peripheral infiltrating component resembling classical infiltrating astrocytoma. The astrocytic quality is also more pronounced in the smaller, spindled cells that accompany the bizarre giant cells.

Large ganglion-like cells are present in some PXAs. To distinguish trapped nonneoplastic ganglion cells from a true neoplastic component is not always simple and may require the identification of features such as binucleation or bizarre cytologic forms. Immunohistochemistry may be necessary when ganglion-like cells occur as isolated cells or as a minor component. In some cases, ganglion-like cells are seen in the recurrent but not original specimen. Although PXAs with a neuronal component are, in effect, a form of ganglioglioma, they are considered PXAs with ganglionic differentiation, rather than grade I gangliogliomas. PXAs have also been reported as a component of a composite tumor that exhibits a distinct ganglioglioma. There have been a number of elaborate reports that describe tumors with clearly distinctive components of PXA and ganglioglioma.[16] Currently, it is not clear whether these neoplasms are a distinct group or more pronounced examples of the former PXA category.

Lymphocytes are typically seen around the vessels and within the substance of the tumor. Most inflammatory cells are of T-cell phenotype and are often accompanied by plasmacytes. PXAs are rarely calcified, but calcospherites are sometimes found in the adjacent cortex.

The presence of eosinophilic granular bodies (EGBs) is a critical but not specific feature of PXA. EGBs are small clusters of eosinophilic, hyaline spheroids that aggregate similar to bundles of grapes among tumor cells (see Figure 20-2*D*). EGBs characteristically occur in low-grade lesions that should be principally treated by surgical resection. Even though the presence of EGBs was not emphasized in the original reports of PXAs, further studies point to the value of these protein clusters for diagnosis. EGBs are found in most PXAs and are strong evidence against the alternative diagnosis of giant cell glioblastoma. Special stains help in the detection of these proteinaceous structures.

Reticulin fibers are generally present in the solid regions of the tumor and around individual or clusters of cells. Reticulin staining is not always diffuse within the tumor, but the diagnosis should be suspected in the absence of reticulin.

Immunohistochemistry

There have been a number of studies to understand the immunophenotypical characteristics of PXAs.[8] Typically, almost 100% of tumors exhibit positivity with antibodies against GFAP and S-100 protein. The immunohistochemical staining for GFAP is often positive in most tumor cells, but one should not expect to see positivity in every tumor cell. In addition, a significant number of tumors exhibit positivity with

neuronal markers such as synaptophysin and neurofilament proteins. In almost all cases that exhibit positivity with neuronal markers, the positive staining identifies individual cells and often the large bizarre cells within the tumor. An elaborate study has also determined that these large cells exhibit glial as well as neuronal markers, suggesting that PXAs are closer to glioneuronal tumors such as gangliogliomas.[18]

In summary, the findings originally described by Kepes et al, and further substantiated in close to 100 publications, provide a set of pathologic features for the diagnosis of PXA. These features can be summarized as follows: (1) pleomorphic astrocytic cells with bizarre cytologic features; (2) lipidization of astrocytes, otherwise known as xanthomatous astrocytes; (3) perivascular lymphocytes; (4) reticulin staining about single or grouped tumor cells; (5) EGBs; and (6) a compact, predominantly noninfiltrating architecture.

PXA with anaplastic elements has been recently described in carefully conducted clinicopathologic studies. These neoplasms have the characteristic features of PXA in addition to increased mitotic figures and necrosis. Even though some may prefer to call such lesions *anaplastic* or *malignant* PXA, the current WHO classification recommends referring to these lesions as *PXA with anaplastic elements*. Typically, such lesions are interpreted as WHO grade III lesions as compared with the classical PXA, which is a grade II neoplasm.

Molecular Genetics

Molecular genetics of PXA has recently become a topic of interest because of early recognition of such cases and collection of tissue suitable for such analyses. Previous studies failed to identify genetic alterations that are typical of infiltrating gliomas such as PTEN mutations.[5] A recent study of three PXAs revealed multiple genetic alterations in one tumor with a poor prognosis, and gain on chromosome 7 and loss on 8p were demonstrated in two cases. The authors of this study suggest that the candidate genes located on these regions may play a role in the development of PXA.[20] A more recent study indicates that the chromosomal and genetic aberrations in PXAs are different from those typically associated with the diffusely infiltrating astrocytic and oligodendroglial gliomas.[10] Further studies are needed to identify the residing candidate genes that are involved in the tumorigenesis of PXA.

Pathologic Differential Diagnosis

A pathologic differential diagnosis includes the giant cell glioblastoma, fibrous xanthoma, fibrous histiocytoma, an occasional pleomorphic sarcoma, and finally a ganglioglioma.

THERAPY

The primary goal in surgical treatment of PXA is the complete removal of tumor with clean margins.[7,6] Although cortical location of the tumor makes it easily accessible, proximity to eloquent cortex may prove challenging in achieving a clean resection. However, the most recent advances in functional MRI, cortical mapping techniques, and awake craniotomy now allow most neurosurgeons to radically remove these locally invasive tumors. Because most patients have seizures[7] caused by cortical irritation, intraoperative recording of seizure foci may be necessary to ensure the complete removal of epileptogenic foci. Additionally, it is critical to determine the mitotic index of a surgically resected neoplasm, to determine whether the patient will require any adjuvant treatment.[7]

Because high mitotic rate has been correlated with higher local recurrence rate, its presence may necessitate local radiation therapy (RT) or chemotherapy. The experience with chemotherapy specifically in PXA is very limited. Usually, regimens such as procarbazine, CCNU, and vincristine (PCV), temozolomide, or other glioma protocols can be tried, and the treatment is modified depending on the clinical or radiographic stability of the tumor or response to the therapy. Specifically, vincristine and carboplatin have been shown to result in decreased tumor vascularity, allowing complete resection.[3]

Radiosurgery can also be used following conventional RT or instead of it if the lesion volume is appropriate (i.e., tumor diameter <3.0 cm in a spherical lesion), although experience in this particular tumor is lacking.

RECURRENCE

PXAs are often known as neoplasms with favorable prognosis, yet this statement requires clarification. Recurrent PXAs can be identical to typical glioblastomas, and some may have the appearance of a small cell glioblastoma.[12] The interval between initial surgery and recurrence can be extremely variable, and there are limited studies that analyze sufficient numbers of tumors long enough to determine predictors of recurrence. Currently, the most important prognostic indicators appear to be the extent of resection and mitotic index of the original tumor.[7] On pathologic examination, recurrent PXAs can demonstrate an infiltrative element that may closely resemble a typical infiltrating astrocytoma.

OUTCOME

Overall, PXA is an astrocytic tumor with a relatively favorable prognosis. Mitotic index and extent of resection have been found to be the main predictors of outcome. In the study by Giannini et al from Mayo Clinic, the reported overall survival rate was 72% at 5 years and 70% at 10 years, and recurrence-free survival rates were 72% at 5 years and 61% at 10 years. Seizures were present in 71% of the patients. Extent of tumor resection was gross total in 68% of cases and subtotal in 32% of the cases. Postoperative radiation therapy was administered with or without chemotherapy in 29% and 12.5% of the cases, respectively.[7]

Malignant transformation of PXA, although rare, has been reported.[4] Thus these patients require lifelong follow-up with serial imaging studies.

References

1. Arita K, Kurisu K, Tominaga A, et al: Intrasellar pleomorphic xanthoastrocytoma: case report. Neurosurgery 51:1079–1082; discussion 1082, 2002.
2. Bicik I, Raman R, Knightly JJ, et al: PET-FDG of pleomorphic xanthoastrocytoma. J Nucl Med 36:97–99, 1995.
3. Cartmill M, Hewitt M, Walker D, et al: The use of chemotherapy to facilitate surgical resection in pleomorphic xanthoastrocytoma: experience in a single case. Childs Nerv Syst 17:563–566, 2001.
4. Chakrabarty A, Mitchell P, Bridges LR, Franks AJ: Malignant transformation in pleomorphic xanthoastrocytoma—A report of two cases. Br J Neurosurg 13:516–519, 1999.
5. Duerr EM, Rollbrocker B, Hayashi Y, et al: PTEN mutations in gliomas and glioneuronal tumors. Oncogene 16:2259–2264, 1998.
6. Fouladi M, Jenkins J, Burger P, et al: Pleomorphic xanthoastrocytoma: favorable outcome after complete surgical resection. Neuro-oncol 3:184–192, 2001.
7. Giannini C, Scheithauer BW, Burger PC, et al: Pleomorphic xanthoastrocytoma: what do we really know about it? Cancer 85:2033–2045, 1999.
8. Giannini C, Scheithauer BW, Lopes MB, et al: Immunophenotype of pleomorphic xanthoastrocytoma. Am J Surg Pathol 26:479–485, 2002.
9. Herpers MJ, Freling G, Beuls EA: Pleomorphic xanthoastrocytoma in the spinal cord. Case report. J Neurosurg 80:564–569, 1994.
10. Kaulich K, Blaschke B, Numann A, et al: Genetic alterations commonly found in diffusely infiltrating cerebral gliomas are rare or absent in pleomorphic xanthoastrocytomas. J Neuropathol Exp Neurol 61:1092–1099, 2002.
11. Kepes JJ: Pleomorphic xanthoastrocytoma: the birth of a diagnosis and a concept. Brain Pathol 3:269–274, 1993.
12. Kepes JJ, Rubinstein LJ, Ansbacher L, Schreiber DJ: Histopathological features of recurrent pleomorphic xanthoastrocytomas: further corroboration of the glial nature of this neoplasm. A study of 3 cases. Acta Neuropathol (Berl) 78:585–593, 1989.
13. Kepes JJ, Rubinstein LJ, Eng LF: Pleomorphic xanthoastrocytoma: a distinctive meningocerebral glioma of young subjects with relatively favorable prognosis. A study of 12 cases. Cancer 44:1839–1852, 1979.
14. Kros JM, Vecht CJ, Stefanko SZ: The pleomorphic xanthoastrocytoma and its differential diagnosis: a study of five cases. Hum Pathol 22:1128–1135, 1991.
15. MacKenzie JM: Pleomorphic xanthoastrocytoma in a 62-year-old male. Neuropathol Appl Neurobiol 13:481–487, 1987.
16. Perry A, Giannini C, Scheithauer BW, et al: Composite pleomorphic xanthoastrocytoma and ganglioglioma: report of four cases and review of the literature. Am J Surg Pathol 21:763–771, 1997.
17. Pierallini A, Bonamini M, Di Stefano D, et al: Pleomorphic xanthoastrocytoma with CT and MRI appearance of meningioma. Neuroradiology 41:30–34, 1999.
18. Powell SZ, Yachnis AT, Rorke LB, et al: Divergent differentiation in pleomorphic xanthoastrocytoma. Evidence for a neuronal element and possible relationship to ganglion cell tumors. Am J Surg Pathol 20:80–85, 1996.
19. Wasdahl DA, Scheithauer BW, Andrews BT, Jeffrey RA Jr: Cerebellar pleomorphic xanthoastrocytoma: case report. Neurosurgery 35:947–950; discussion 950–951, 1994.
20. Yin XL, Hui AB, Liong EC, et al: Genetic imbalances in pleomorphic xanthoastrocytoma detected by comparative genomic hybridization and literature review. Cancer Genet Cytogenet 132:14–19, 2002.
21. Zarate JO, Sampaolesi R: Pleomorphic xanthoastrocytoma of the retina. Am J Surg Pathol 23:79–81, 1999.

CHAPTER 22

SUBEPENDYMAL GIANT CELL ASTROCYTOMA AND TUBEROUS SCLEROSIS COMPLEX

Asis Kumar Bhattacharyya, Patrick Shannon, and Mark Bernstein

Subependymal giant cell astrocytoma (SGCA) is one of the fascinating manifestations of tuberous sclerosis complex (TSC), a heredofamilial multisystem disease. Though SGCA is the only condition of neurosurgical interest, a myriad of clinicopathologic abnormalities affect the brain in TSC. For clarity of understanding, the whole spectrum should be reviewed as a single entity.

The concept of TSC has evolved over the past 2 centuries. In 1835 Pierre Francois Olive Rayer[45] published an atlas of skin disease, and in one of the pictures in that book he produced a color drawing of a man's face dotted with erythematous papules that resembled facial angiofibroma. In 1862 Friedrich Daniel Recklinghausen[59] presented the autopsy finding of cardiac myomata and cerebral sclerosis of a newborn who died almost immediately after birth. In 1880 Deisire-Magloire Bourneville[10] described a girl with mental retardation, seizures, and facial angiofibroma. The girl died at the age of 15. At autopsy he discovered opaque whitish sclerotic areas on the cerebral convolutions and a nodular tumor of the corpus striatum projecting into the lateral ventricle. To denote these lesions of potato-like consistency in cortical gyri he coined the term *tuberous sclerosis*. He concluded that the tuber was the cause of the seizures. In fact, it is Bourneville who established tuberous sclerosis as a distinct disease entity, so TSC is also known as *Bourneville's disease*. In 1890 Pringle[44] reported that adenoma sebaceum was often found in mentally retarded patients and subsequently was found to be associated with tuberous sclerosis. In 1905 Perusini[42] presented the microscopic description of a cortical tuber and its association with cardiac, renal, and dermal lesions in patients with TSC.

Heinrich Vogt[58] in 1908 made a great contribution by describing the classic clinical triad of adenoma sebaceum, seizures, and mental retardation for the diagnosis of TSC. But in 1914 Schuster[48] described a patient with TSC without mental retardation. This patient was categorized as having a "forme fruste of Tuberous Sclerosis." In 1920 van der Hoeve[56] described a retinal astrocytic tumor as a part of the disease complex and introduced the term *phakomatosis*. Subsequently, with increasing clinical awareness and availability of newer imaging modalities, the whole spectrum of TSC unfolded. In 1992 the Diagnostic Criteria Committee of the National Tuberous Sclerosis Association[46] classified the gamut of clinical manifestations according to their relative significance. In 1993 the European Chromosome 16 Consortium[18] defined and characterized the TSC2 gene. The TSC1 gene, though identified in 1987, was fully evaluated in more recent times.[54]

EPIDEMIOLOGY

Clinical presentation of TSC may be subtle, and hence it can go unrecognized or misdiagnosed for many years. The reported prevalence varies widely. Initially it was reported to be 1 in 1000 to 1 in 170,000 live births.[19] However, a Swedish study in 1994 found the prevalence to be 1 in 6800 children.[1] Both sexes are equally affected and no racial predilection is observed.

It is a genetic disease with autosomal dominant inheritance and 80% penetrance. In most patients, however, *de novo* mutation is the cause.[28] Both of the genes (TSC1 and TSC2) are equally responsible in familial cases.[43] The majority of sporadic cases are due to TSC2 gene mutation.[4] Mental retardation is also found to be more frequent in TSC2 sporadic cases than TSC1 sporadic cases.[30] Recent genetic linkage analysis demonstrates that germline mosaicism without an overt clinical manifestation in parents of TSC patients is not uncommon.[18,19] Approximately 6% to 15% of TSC patients develop SGCA, and the majority of them seek treatment in the first 2 decades of life.[11,32,50,51] Only 20% are diagnosed in adulthood.[27,38] Very rarely, SGCA arises without TSC,[21,31] usually in older patients. Simultaneous occurrence in siblings without TSC is also reported.[15]

GENETICS IN TUBEROUS SCLEROSIS COMPLEX

Recent identification of mutation of two genes (TSC1 and TSC2) has led to rapid progress in the understanding of the molecular and cellular pathogenesis of TSC. How these genetic mutations manifest in such a wide variety of clinical presentations is under intense research.

The TSC2 gene is located on chromosome 16p13. This gene contains 41 coding exons and spans 43 kb of DNA.[18] Its organization is evolutionarily conserved from pufferfish,[35] through rodents,[33] to humans. A wide variety of mutations of this gene have been reported; these are deletion, rearrangement, or missense mutation and mutations leading to premature truncation of proteins. The TSC2 gene is located very close to PKD1 (polycystic kidney disease) gene. In a few patients with TSC associated with infantile polycystic kidney disease, a contiguous genetic deletion affecting both TSC2 and PKD1 genes has been demonstrated.[13] The TSC2 gene has a 5.5 kb transcript that encodes a protein, called *tuberin*, that contains 1807 amino acids and has a molecular weight of 200 kDa.[18] Fifty-eight amino acids near its C terminal show homology to part of guanosine 5'-triphosphate (GTP)-ase activating protein (GAP).[18]

The TSC1 gene is located in chromosome 9q34. This gene contains 23 exons.[54] It has no homology to any known vertebrate genes. Many causative mutations of it have been reported, and like the TSC2 gene, they are deletion, rearrangement, or missense mutation and mutations leading to premature truncation of proteins. The TSC1 gene has an 8.6 kb transcript that encodes a protein, called *hamartin*, which contains 1164 amino acids and has a molecular weight of 130 kDa.

Tuberin and hamartin are distributed in fetal and adult brain, liver, cardiac muscle, kidney, and adrenal cortex.[61] Several pieces of evidence suggest that both TSC genes are tumor-suppressor genes and their protein products act in a single cellular pathway; hence they lead to the same clinical manifestations.

Tuberin appears to be located in the Golgi apparatus.[62] It has GAP activity of Rap1 and Rab5. Both Rap1[61] and Rab5[65] are small GTP-ase signaling molecules in the Ras superfamily. Activation of the Rap1 pathway leads to enhancement of cell proliferation[53] and incomplete cellular differentiation.[52] Activation of the Rab5 pathway leads to increased rate of endocytosis.[65] Tuberin can also modulate transcription mediated by members of the steroid receptor superfamily of genes.[22] Restoration of normal tuberin function in the cells cultured from the Eker rat suppresses tumorigenicity.[29] Loss of heterozygosity (LOH) of both TSC genes has been demonstrated in renal angiolipoma, cardiac rhabdomyoma, renal cell carcinoma, subungual fibroma, and SGCA.[14,23,49] This implies that TSC is recessive at the cellular level and requires a "second hit" in a single cell that forms the lesion.[24]

CLINICAL PRESENTATIONS OF TUBEROUS SCLEROSIS COMPLEX

Vogt's classic triad of seizures, mental retardation, and adenoma sebaceum is present in less than 50% of all cases of TSC. Moreover, a wide variety of clinical manifestations and their variable expressions make the diagnosis more difficult. So in 1992 the National Tuberous Sclerosis Association formulated the diagnostic criteria for TSC.[46] For a definitive diagnosis the presence of one primary criterion, two secondary criteria, or one secondary and three tertiary criteria are required (Table 22-1). When one secondary and one tertiary or three tertiary criteria are present, the disease is a possibility. If only one secondary or two tertiary criteria are detected, the disease is suspected.

Seizures and mental retardation are the most common symptoms, but they are not included in the diagnostic criteria because of lack of specificity. Seizures are initially flexion

TABLE 22-1

Diagnostic Criteria of Tuberous Sclerosis Complex

Primary Criteria
Facial angiofibroma
Multiple subungual fibroma
Multiple retinal astroblastoma
Cortical tuber (histologically confirmed)
Subependymal giant cell astrocytoma (SGCA)
Multiple calcified subependymal nodules protruding into the ventricles

Secondary Criteria
Cortical tuber (radiologically confirmed)
Noncalcified subependymal nodule (radiologically confirmed)
Forehead plaque
Shagreen patch
Other retinal hamartoma or achromic patch
Cardiac rhabdomyoma
Pulmonary lymphangiomyomatosis (histologically confirmed)
Renal angiolipoma
Renal cyst (histologically confirmed)
Affected first-degree relative

Tertiary Criteria
Hypomelanotic macules
Confetti skin lesions
Gingival fibroma
Enamel pits in deciduous or permanent teeth
Cerebral white matter migration tracts or heterotopias
Pulmonary lymphangiomyomatosis (radiologic evidence)
Renal cysts (radiologic evidence)
Hamartomatous rectal polyps (histologically confirmed)
Bone cyst (radiologically confirmed)
Hamartoma of other organs (histologically confirmed)
Infantile spasm

myoclonus with hypsarrhythmia but may gradually evolve into grand mal or psychomotor epilepsy. Many of these patients have features of autism; rarely, there may be chorea and athetosis. With time higher mental function deteriorates. Approximately two thirds of patients with normal mental function have seizures. On the other hand, all patients with mental retardation suffer seizure disorders.[19] A loose correlation exists between a large number of cortical lesions, developmental delay, and poor seizure control.

In TSC the brain is the most common organ to be affected. Spinal cord and peripheral nerves are always spared. The cerebral manifestations include cortical tubers, cerebral white matter migration tracts, subependymal nodules, and SGCA. Ophthalmic manifestations include retinal astrocytomas, retinal hamartomas, and achromic patches. Retinal astrocytomas are detected in approximately 50% of patients with TSC. They are usually bilateral and multiple. In children they must be differentiated from retinoblastomas.

Adenoma sebaceum (facial angiofibroma) is the most distinctive dermal manifestation (Figure 22-1). These reddish

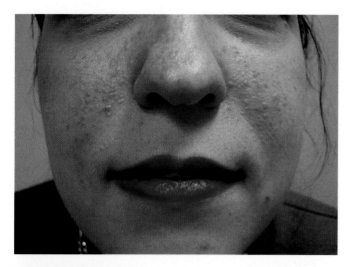

FIGURE 22-1 Facial rash of a 32-year-old woman with tuberous sclerosis complex (TSC) who underwent resection of a subependymal giant cell astrocytoma (SGCA) 9 years previously and remains well in follow-up. Her 10-year-old daughter also has TSC. (Photo used by permission of patient.)

papules appear on the nose, cheeks, and chin in 70% of the affected population. They usually develop between 5 years of age and puberty. Polygonal or ash-leaf shaped hypomelanotic macules are better seen by Wood's lamp (ultraviolet light) and may have been present since birth. Pitting in the teeth is found in 90% of adults with TSC as opposed to 9% of the general population.

Renal cysts occur in children. These may occasionally lead to hypertension and end-stage renal disease. Renal angiolipoma is more often seen in adults. This may give rise to retroperitoneal hemorrhage[19] or renal cell carcinoma.[2] Multiple cardiac rhabdomyomas are present at birth and usually regress over time. They may even be diagnosed antenatally by ultrasonography. Rarely, they cause ventricular outflow obstruction leading to heart failure. Pulmonary lymphangiomyomatosis is a very rare manifestation characterized by the patient's slow decline to end-stage lung disease. There are several case reports of TSC associated with cerebral aneurysm,[8,12] fibrillary astrocytoma,[17] and glioblastoma multiforme.[16] It is not yet established whether these are incidental findings or there is any causal relationship with TSC.

CORTICAL TUBERS

Cortical tubers are the most common cerebral manifestation in TSC. They are most often seen in the supratentorial compartment, and the frontoparietal region is the most common location. They are multiple, a few millimeters to several centimeters, and asymmetrically involve the hemispheres. On macroscopic examination they are firm, pale, flat, dimpled or wart-like protrusions on the cortical surfaces causing expansion of gyri and blurring of gray and white matter junction.[28] Microscopically atypical giant astrocytes, dysmorphic neurons with disrupted radial orientation and abnormal arbors, many intermediate cells, numerous glial processes, gliosis, and abnormal myelination characterize them. The typical hexalaminar archi-

tecture of the cerebral gray matter is lost. Rarely the cerebellum may be affected.

Magnetic resonance imaging (MRI) is the best diagnostic investigation. It can detect cortical tubers in 95% of patients with TSC. The inner core is usually hypointense to isointense to gray matter on T1-weighted images and hyperintense on T2-weighted images. The peripheral part is isointense to mildly hyperintense on both T1- and T2-weighted images.[11] Less than 5% of tubers are enhanced with gadolinium (Gd-diethyl triamine penta-acetic acid [DTPA]).[28] Associated expansion and thickening of cortical gyri and blurring of gray-white matter junctions are important findings. In neonates and in small children normal white matter contains more water and less myelination, so the inner core appears hyperintense in T1-weighted and hypointense in T2-weighted images.[16] Small cortical tubers may be obscured by the partial-volume effect caused by cerebrospinal fluid in hemispheric cisterns. In that situation fluid attenuation inversion recovery (FLAIR) image or magnetic transfer imaging is a better alternative.

Computed tomography (CT) is less sensitive in detecting these lesions. They appear hypodense on CT; calcification may be detected in 54% of cases,[3] and occasionally calcification may be gyriform mimicking Sturge-Weber syndrome.[63]

WHITE MATTER LESIONS

White matter lesions are clusters of bizarre and gigantic heterotopic cells with characteristics of both neurons and glia. Many of them are microscopic lesions only. They are distributed along the most direct line between the ependymal wall and the cortex, and this might represent the normal migratory pathway of spongioblasts during embryogenesis.

On CT scan they appear hypodense and nonenhanced. Calcification may be present. On MRI they may be of two varieties. The majority are hypointense on T1-weighted and hyperintense on T2-weighted images. Less commonly they are hyperintense on both T1- and T2-weighted images. The first variety may occur in three subtypes: straight or curvilinear bands, wedge-shaped lesions, and cerebellar radial bands.[28] Enhancement on contrast administration (Gd DTPA) is seen in only 12% of such cases.[11] In neonates they may be hyperintense on T1-weighted and hypointense on T2-weighted images, similar to cortical tubers.

SUBEPENDYMAL NODULE

Subependymal nodules are well-circumscribed periventricular hamartomas most commonly found in the lateral ventricular wall, with their deeper part abutting the head of the caudate nucleus or thalamus. They are covered by an intact layer of ependyma. On pneumoencephalography performed before the modern positive-imaging era, multiple adjacent nodules resembled drippings of wax, hence the description *candle-dripping appearance*. Rarely, subependymal nodules are seen along the walls of the third ventricle, aqueduct of Sylvius, or fourth ventricle.

Histologically, they contain giant cells that are similar to those found in cortical tubers. With increasing age they undergo progressive calcification. On CT scan calcification may be globular or ringlike, and these lesions usually do not become enhanced on contrast CT scan. On MRI they appear isointense

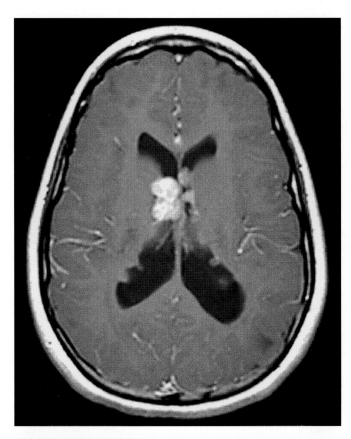

FIGURE 22-2 Axial T1-weighted magnetic resonance image with gadolinium enhancement of a 12-year-old girl with tuberous sclerosis complex (TSC) and severe seizures. The tumor is presumed to be a subependymal giant cell astrocytoma (SGCA). Subependymal nodules are also present. (Photo courtesy of Dr. Susan Blaser, Hospital for Sick Children, Toronto.)

to hyperintense on T1-weighted images and isointense to hypointense on T2-weighted images (Figure 22-2). A gradient echo T2-weighted image (T2* image) may be useful for detection of calcification. Administration of Gd-DTPA enhances 30% to 80% of nodules. Enhancement does not necessarily denote neoplastic transformation.[64] Most subependymal nodules remain static, but a few may enlarge and lead to SGCA. Those nodules near the foramen of Monro are particularly prone to this transformation and hence should be followed up carefully. In addition, partially calcified nodules of more than 5 mm diameter in patients with family history of TSC are at higher risk for transformation.[37]

SUBEPENDYMAL GIANT CELL ASTROCYTOMA

Clinical Presentation

The fascinating entity SGCA is of considerable neurosurgical interest. It occurs in 6% to 15% of cases of TSC.[11,32,50,51] Progressive enlargement of a subependymal nodule leads to SGCA.[36] It commonly presents in adolescents and young adults,

although a few cases have been described in neonates,[40,41] in which case they are more commonly associated with sporadic TSC.[40] With enlargement, SGCA may obstruct the foramen of Monro, leading to obstructive hydrocephalus and features of raised intracranial pressure. Rarely, they may lead to intraventricular hemorrhage.[60] Though most of them are intraventricular, they may arise in the brain parenchyma as well.

Pathology

On gross examination SGCAs appear as well-circumscribed, pinkish-white, firm, gritty, well-vascularized lesions. Areas of dilated vessels may give rise to angiomatous appearance. Some of these tumors are coarsely nodular with cysts of varying sizes. Focal calcification is frequent (Figure 22-3).

Histologically, they are characterized by large pyramidal or fusiform-shaped cells with short stubby processes, containing bulky homogeneous eosinophilic cytoplasm and large nuclei with eccentrically located vesicular nucleoli. Some of the cells resemble gemistocytes and some others mimic astroblasts. Foci of calcification and pseudo-rosette formation are fairly common. Mitotic figures and necrotic areas are rare. When present, they have little prognostic significance and should not prompt misclassification of the tumor as a glioblastoma multiforme (see Figure 22-3).

Immunohistochemically, some of the cells have features of glial origin and others have features of neuronal origin. The features of glial lineage[30,57] are reactivity for glial fibrillary acidic protein (GFAP), vimentin, and S-100 protein and CD44. The features of neuronal lineage[26,30,34,57] are reactivity to neuron specific enolase (NSE), tubulin, microtubule-associated proteins (MAPs), neuropeptide Y, met-enkephalin, and beta-endorphin. Ultrastructurally, microtubules, dense-core granules, and synapses may be seen.[39] This signifies that SGCA may be a neoplasm of developmental origin in which multipotential progenitor cells within the germinal mantle of the developing brain fail to migrate and fail to commit to one line of differentiation.[9,20] Some dysembryonic cells completely migrate to the cerebral cortex, producing cortical tubers; some may incompletely migrate, producing white matter lesions; and some may not migrate at all, producing subependymal nodules and SGCA.[5,7]

Imaging

On CT scan, SGCAs are partially calcified, solid, intraventricular tumors with varying degree of enhancement and associated with unilateral or bilateral ventriculomegaly. On MRI, they are isointense to slightly hypointense on T1-weighted images, hyperintense on T2-weighted images, and show marked enhancement with gadolinium (see Figure 22-2).[11] Perilesional edema is usually minimal. Occasional serpentine signal voids represent dilated vessels.[11] Cerebral angiography may reveal a tumor blush in late arterial phase.[25] These imaging features help to differentiate SGCA from other tumors of the same location, namely central neurocytoma, meningioma, oligodendroglioma, pilocytic astrocytoma, and choroid plexus papilloma.

Treatment

The main indication for neurosurgical intervention is obstructive hydrocephalus leading to increased intracranial pressure. Less commonly, surgery may be required for patients with

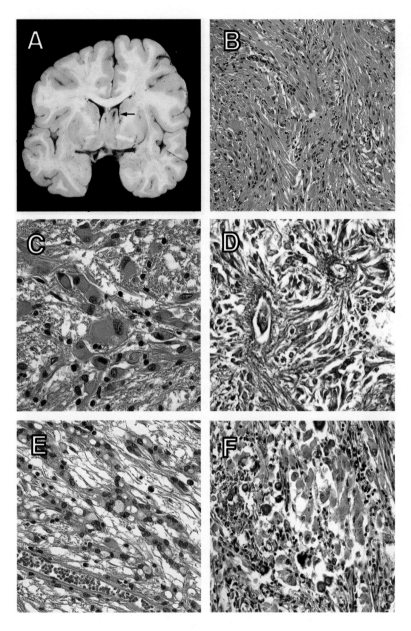

FIGURE 22-3 *A,* Gross photograph of a paraseptal subependymal giant cell astrocytoma (SGCA) with cystic degeneration *(arrow).* The histopathology is highly variable between tumors. *B,* At low power, there is frequently a fascicular architecture (hematoxylin and eosin [H&E], ×200). *C,* Aggregates of large bizarre glial-like cells, often with densely hyperchromatic nuclei, are characteristic. *D,* A papillary astroblastic pattern may be prominent (Martius Scarlet Blue, ×400). *E,* Clusters and strands of vacuolated cells with a "chordoid" appearance can sometimes be seen (H&E, ×400). *F,* Often the tumor cells are a mixture of giant and spindled cells in a densely calcified stroma (phosphotungstic acid-hematoxylin [PTAH], ×400).

seizures that do not respond to medical treatment. The aim of surgery is to achieve gross-total removal.[55] Cerebrospinal fluid (CSF) diversion techniques should be reserved for patients who are poor surgical candidates because they have medical comorbidities, unresectable tumors, or hydrocephalus that persists even after removal of tumor.[55]

The operative approach depends on the location and size of the tumor. A transcortical transventricular approach or interhemispheric transcallosal approach is used in most cases. Recently, endoscopic removal of such tumors has been described.[6] Surgical outcome is generally satisfactory, but the result is considerably worse in neonates because in many of them associated cardiac rhabdomyomas lead to cardiac arrhythmia, heart failure, and death.[40,41] Hence, in view of the multisystem involvement of the TSC, preoperative evaluations of the cardiac, pulmonary, and renal functions are of utmost importance.

These lesions are histologically benign, and the recurrence rate is very low, but they may recur a long time after surgery.[21] Clear benefit of radiation therapy has never been established,

and this modality is reserved only for recurrences. To defer radiation in very young children, chemotherapy with nitrosourea-based cytotoxic regimens has been tried with some success.[47]

Follow-Up

After a successful surgery a reasonably good quality of life is expected. But patients should be followed up clinically and with MRI for other manifestations of TSC. Asymptomatic relatives should be screened for possible TSC.

THE FUTURE

The future lies in genetic research. Genetic mutation as a useful diagnostic tool and as a method of genetic counseling is a realistic possibility. However, gene therapy appears to be a distant goal. Until then, skilled microsurgical techniques remain the mainstay of SGCA management.

References

1. Ahlsen G, Gillberg IC, Lindblom R, et al: Tuberous sclerosis in Western Sweden. A population study of cases with early childhood onset. Arch Neurol 51:76–81, 1994.
2. Al-Saleem T, Wessner LL, Scheithauer BW, et al: Malignant tumors of the kidney, brain and soft tissues in children and young adults with tuberous sclerosis. Cancer 83:208–216, 1998.
3. Altman NR, Purser RK, Post MJ: Tuberous sclerosis: characteristics at CT and MR imaging. Radiology 167:525–532, 1988.
4. Au K, Rodriquez J, Finch J, et al: Germline mutational analysis of the TSC2 gene in 90 tuberous sclerosis patients. Am J Hum Genet 62:286–294, 1998.
5. Barkovich AJ, Kjos ES, Jackson DE, Jr, et al: Normal maturation of the neonatal and infant brain. MR imaging at 1.5T. Radiology 166:173–180, 1988.
6. Beems T, Grotenhuis JA: Subependymal giant cell astrocytoma in tuberous sclerosis: endoscopic images and the implications for therapy. Minim Invasive Neurosurg 44:58–60, 2001.
7. Benders BL, Yunis ES: Cerebral nervous system pathology of tuberous sclerosis in children. Ultrastruct Pathol 1:287–299, 1980.
8. Blumenkopf B, Huggins MJ: Tuebrous sclerosis and multiple intracranial aneurysms: case report. Neurosurgery 17:797–800, 1985.
9. Bonnin JM, Rubinstein LJ, Papasozomenos SC, et al: Subependymal giant cell astrocytoma: significance and possible cytogenic implications of a immunohistochemical study. Acta Neuropathol (Berlin) 62:185–193, 1984.
10. Bourneville DM: Sclerose tubereuse des circonvolutions cerebrales: idiotie et epilepsie hemiplegique. Arch Neurol (Paris) 1:81–91, 1880.
11. Braffiman BH, Bilaniuk LT, Naidich TP, et al: MR imaging of tuberous sclerosis: Pathogenesis of this phakomatosis, use of gadopentetate dimeglumine, and literature review. Radiology 183:227–238, 1992.
12. Brill CB, Peyster RG, Hoover ED, et al: Giant intracranial aneurysm in a child with tuberous sclerosis: CT demonstration. J Comput Assist Tomogr 9:377–380, 1985.
13. Brook-Carter PT, Peral B, Ward CJ, et al: Deletion of the TSC2 and PKD1 genes associated with severe infantile polycystic kidney disease—a contiguous gene syndrome. Nat Genet 8:328–332, 1994.
14. Carbonara C, Longa L, Grosso E, et al: 9q34 loss of heterozygosity in a tuberous sclerosis astrocytoma suggests a growth suppressor like activity also for TSC1 gene. Hum Mol Genet 3:1829–1832, 1994.
15. Cheng TM, Coffey RJ, Gelber BR, et al: Simultaneous presentation of symptomatic subependymomas in siblings: case report and review. Neurosurgery 33:145–150, 1993.
16. Christopher C, Bartholome J, Blum D, et al: Neonatal tuberous sclerosis. US, CT and MR diagnosis of brain and cardiac lesions. Pediatric Radiol 19:446–448, 1989.
17. Eren S, Polat Z: An unusual tuberous sclerosis case presenting with fibrillary astrocytoma. Pediatr Neurosurg 37:118–121, 2002.
18. The European Chromosome 16 Consortium: Identification and characterization of the tuberous sclerosis gene on chromosome 16. Cell 75:1305–1315, 1993.
19. Gomez MR: Tuberous Sclerosis, 2nd ed. New York, Raven Press, 1988.
20. Gyure AK, Prayson RA: Subependymal giant cell astrocytoma: a clinico-pathological study with HMB45 and MIB-1 immunohistochemical analysis. Mod Pathol 104:313–317, 1997.
21. Halmagyi GM, Bignold LP, Allsop JL: Recurrent subependymal giant cell astrocytoma in the absence of tuberous sclerosis: case report. J Neurosurg 50:106–109, 1979.
22. Henry KW, Yuan X, Koszewski NJ, et al: Tuberous sclerosis gene 2 product modulates transcription mediated by steroid hormone receptor family members. J Biol Chem 273:20535–20539, 1998.
23. Henske EP, Neumann H, Scheithauer B, et al: Loss of heterozygosity in the tuberous sclerosis (TSC2) region of chromosome band 16p13 occurs in sporadic as well as TSC-associated renal angiomyolipomas. Gene Chrom Cancer 13:295–298, 1995.
24. Henske EP, Wessner LL, Golden J, et al: Loss of tuberin in both subependymal giant cell astrocytomas and angiolipomas supports a two-hit model for the pathogenesis of tuberous sclerosis tumors. Am J Pathol 151:1639–1647, 1997.
25. Herz DA, Liebeskind A, Rosenthal A, et al: Cerebral angiographic changes associated with tuberous sclerosis. Radiology 115:647–649, 1975.
26. Hirose Y, Scheithauer BW, Lopes MBS, et al: Tuber and subependymal giant cell astrocytoma associated with tuberous sclerosis: an immunohistochemical, ultrastructural and immuno-electronmicroscopic study. Acta Neuropathol 90:387–399, 1995.
27. Holanda FJ, Holanda GM: Tuberous sclerosis: neurosurgical indications in intraventricular tumors. Neurosurg Rev 3:139–150, 1980.
28. Inoue Y, Nemato Y, Ryuusuke M, et al: CT and MR imaging of cerebral tuberous sclerosis. Brain Dev 20:209–221, 1998.
29. Jin F, Wienecke R, Xiao G, et al: Suppression of tumorigenicity by the wild type of tuberous sclerosis 2 (TSC2) gene and its C-terminal region. Proc Natl Acad Sci USA 93:9154–9159, 1996.
30. Jones AC, Shyamsundar MM, Thomas MW, et al: Comprehensive mutation analysis of TSC1 and TSC2 and phenotypic correlation in 150 families with tuberous sclerosis. Am J Hum Genet 64:1305–1315, 1999.
31. Kashiwagi N, Yoshihara W, Shimada N, et al: Solitary subependymal giant cell astrocytoma: case report. Eur J Radiol 33:55–58, 2000.
32. Kingsley DP, Kendall BE, Fits CR: Tuberous sclerosis: a clinicopathological evaluation of 110 cases with particular reference to atypical presentation. Neuroradiology 28:38–46, 1986.
33. Kobayashi T, Urakami S, Cheadle JP, et al: Identification of a leader exon and a core promoter for the rat tuberous sclerosis (TSC2) gene and structural comparison with the human homolog. Mamm Genome 8:554–558, 1997.
34. Lopes MBS, Altermatt HJ, Scheithauer BW, et al: Immunohistochemical characterization of subependymal giant cell astrocytoma. Acta Neuropathol 91:368–375, 1996.
35. Maheshwar MM, Sandford R, Nellist M, et al: Comparative analysis and genomic structure of the tuberous sclerosis 2 (TSC 2) gene in human and pufferfish. Hum Mol Genet 5:562, 1996.
36. Morimoto K, Mogami H: Sequential CT study of subependymal giant cell astrocytoma associated with tuberous sclerosis. J Neurosurg 65:874–877, 1986.
37. Nabbout R, Santos M, Rolland Y, et al: Early diagnosis of subependymal giant cell astrocytoma in children with tuberous sclerosis. J Neurol Neurosurg Psychiatry 66:370–375, 1999.
38. Naguib MG, Haines SJ, Erickson DL et al: Tuberous sclerosis: a review for the neurosurgeon. Neurosurgery 14:93–98, 1984.
39. Nakamura Y, Becker LE: Subependymal giant-cell tumor: astrocytic or neuronal? Acta Neuropathol (Berlin) 60:271–277, 1983.
40. Oikawa S, Sakamoto K, Kobayashi N: A neonatal huge subependymal giant cell astrocytoma: case report. Neurosurgery 35:748–750, 1994.
41. Painter MJ, Pang D, Ahdab-Barmada M, et al: Connatal brain tumors in patients with tuberous sclerosis. Neurosurgery 14:570–573, 1984.
42. Perusini G: Uber einen Fall von Sclerosis tuberosa hypertrophica. Monatsschr Psychiatr Neurol 17:69–255, 1905.

43. Povey S, Burley M, Attwood J, et al: Two loci of tuberous sclerosis: one on 9q34 and one on 16p13. Ann Hum Genet 58:107–127, 1994.

44. Pringle JJ: A case of congenital adenoma sebaceum. Br J Dermatol 2:1–14, 1890.

45. Rayer PFQ: Traite theorique et pratique des maladies de la peau, 2nd ed. Paris, JB Bailliere, 1835.

46. Roach ES, Smith M, Huttenlocher P, et al: Diagnostic criteria: tuberous sclerosis complex. Report of the Diagnostic Criteria Committee of the National Tuberous Sclerosis Association. J Child Neurol 7:221–224, 1992.

47. Rock JP: Pilocytic astrocytoma and other indolent tumors. In Bernstein M, Berger MS (eds): Neuro-oncology: The Essentials, New York, Thieme Medical Publishers, 2001.

48. Schuster P: Beitrage zur Klinic der tuberosen Sklerose desGehirns. Dtsch Z Nervenheilk 50:96–133, 1914.

49. Sepp T, Yates J, Green A: Loss of heterozygosity in tuberous sclerosis hamartomas. J Med Genet 33:962–964, 1996.

50. Shepherd CW, Scheithauer BW, Gomez MR, et al: Subependymal giant cell astrocytoma: a clinical, pathological, and cytometric study. Neurosurgery 28:864–868, 1991.

51. Smirniotopoulos JG, Murphy FM: The phakomatoses. Am J Neuroradiol 13:725–746, 1992.

52. Soucek T, Holzl G, Bernaschek G, et al: A role of the tuberous sclerosis gene 2 product during neonatal differentiation. Oncogene 16:2197–2204, 1998.

53. Soucek T, Pusch O, Wienecke R, et al: Role of the tuberous sclerosis gene 2 product in cell cycle control. J Biol Chem 272:29301–29308, 1997.

54. The TSC1 Consortium (1997): Identification of the tuberous sclerosis gene TSC1 on chromosome 9q34. Science 277:805–808, 1997.

55. Turgut M, Akalan N, Ozgen T, et al: Subependymal giant cell astrocytoma associated with tuberous sclerosis: diagnosis and surgical characteristics of five cases with unusual features. Clin Neurol Neurosurg 98:217–221, 1996.

56. van der Hoeve J: Eye symptoms in tuberous sclerosis of the brain. Trans Ophthamol Soc UK 20:329–324, 1920.

57. Verhoef S, Bakker L, Tempelaar S, et al: High rate of mosaicism in tuberous sclerosis complex. Am J Hum Genet 64:1632–1637, 1999.

58. Vogt H: Zur Pathologie und pathologischen Anatomie der verschiedenen Idiotieform. Monatsschr Psychiatr Neurol 24:106–150, 1908.

59. von Recklinghausen FD: Ein Herz von einem Neugeborene welches mehrere theils nach aussen, theils nach den Hohlen prominirende Tumoren (Myomen) trug. Monatsschr Geburtsheilk 20:1–2, 1862.

60. Waga S, Yamamoto Y, Kojima T, et al: Massive hemorrhage in tumor of tuberous sclerosis. Surg Neurol 8:99–101, 1977.

61. Wienecke R, Maize J, Reed J, et al: Expression of the TSC2 product tuberin, its target Rap1 in normal human tissues. Am J Pathol 150:43–50, 1997.

62. Wienecke R, Maize J, Shoarinejad F, et al: Co-localization of the TSC2 product tuberin with its target Rap1 in the Golgi apparatus. Oncogene 13:913–923, 1996.

63. Wilms G, van Wijek E, Demaerel P, et al: Gyriform calcification in tuberous sclerosis simulating the appearance of Sturge-Weber disease. Am J Neuroradiol 13:295–297, 1992.

64. Wippold FJ, Baber WW, Gado M, et al: Pre- and post contrast MR studies in tuberous sclerosis. J Comput Assist Tomogr 16:69–72, 1992.

65. Xiao G, Shoarinejad F, Jin F, et al: The tuberous sclerosis 2 gene product, tuberin, functions as a Rab5 GAP in modeling endocytosis. J Biol Chem 272:6097–6100, 1997.

66. Yates JR, van Bakel I, Sepp T, et al: Female germline mosaicism in tuberous sclerosis confirmed by molecular genetic analysis. Hum Mol Genet 6:2265–2269, 1997.

CHAPTER 23

OLIGODENDROGLIAL TUMORS

Johan M. Kros, Ping-pin Zheng, John G. Wolbers, and
Martin J. van den Bent

The diagnosis and treatment of oligodendrogliomas has become a major topic in current neuro-oncology. There are basically two reasons for this development. One is the clinical observation that oligodendrogliomas respond to treatment with chemotherapy. The other reason is the laboratory finding of specific genotypical aberrations in these tumors. These genotypical characteristics are losses on the short arm of chromosome 1 and the long arm of chromosome 19. Because the histopathologic diagnosis of oligodendroglioma and delineation of this glioma subtype from other gliomas suffers from a great deal of subjectivity, genotypical characteristics offer objective criteria for making the diagnosis. Moreover, the genotypical hallmarks of this tumor may be traced in gliomas that lack the classic histology and therefore must be identified by other means than the gold standard of histopathology. Current investigations aiming at the correlation between histology, genomic aberrations, and response to therapy will redefine the oligodendroglioma, delineate it from gliomas of astrocytic lineage, and possibly split the entity into subtypes.

DEFINITION AND CLINICAL PRESENTATION

Definition

The current World Health Organization (WHO) definition of oligodendroglioma is "a well-differentiated, diffusely infiltrating tumor of adults, typically located in the cerebral hemispheres and composed predominantly of cells morphologically resembling oligodendroglia." Oligodendrogliomas certainly diffusely infiltrate brain tissue, but areas of remarkably sharp borders with surrounding brain tissue are, in contrast to astrocytomas, characteristic of this glioma subtype. Most oligodendrogliomas arise in the cerebral hemispheres, but this location is by no means exclusively involved. Oligodendrogliomas are encountered throughout the central nervous system (CNS), including infratentorial sites and the spinal cord. Certainly most oligodendrogliomas present in adults, who show two age peaks around 35 and 55 years, but children are not exempt from being affected by this glioma. Within the variable group of gliomas that may be encountered in children, not all tumors with oligodendroglioma-like features represent genuine oligodendrogliomas. Round nuclei and perinuclear halos are not specific for neoplastic oligodendroglial cells. Many pediatric gliomas consist of cells that may somewhat resemble oligodendroglial cells simply because they lack signs of astrocytic, ependymal, or ganglion cell differentiation.

The definition given by the WHO for anaplastic oligodendroglioma is "An oligodendroglioma with focal or diffuse histological features of malignancy and a less favorable prognosis." Oligodendrogliomas gradually become more anaplastic (i.e., lose the hallmarks of tissues of their putative origin, also indicated with the term *dedifferentiation*) and evolve from low-grade, well-differentiated gliomas into high grade gliomas with anaplastic features and high indices of cellular proliferation. This process, however, will take more time in oligodendrogliomas than in gliomas of astrocytic lineage. Diffuse gliomas are histologically graded, for which procedure various features should be scored. Because the morphologic changes that are characteristic of high-grade glioma, like high cell density or microvascular proliferation, appear gradually within a glioma, the exact delineation of low- and high-grade (or anaplastic) oligodendroglioma is somewhat unclear.

The diagnosis of oligodendroglioma is based on histologic verification of tumor tissue. Apart from tumors with classic histology there is large histologic variation within individual tumors and between different tumors. In addition to histologic analysis, fluorescent in situ hybridization (FISH) or loss of heterozygosity (LOH) analysis to detect losses on 1p or 19q may be added to make the diagnosis. Tracing these genotypical characteristics may be especially helpful to make the diagnosis of oligodendroglioma in cases of disputable histology or in situations of sampling errors. It should be admitted at this point, however, that the diagnosis of oligodendroglioma as defined by the WHO does not yet include these molecular properties. It may very well be that genotypical changes soon will be mandatory for the diagnosis. None of the many immunohistochemical markers proposed as specific for oligodendroglioma have been sustained so far, but immunohistochemistry certainly may be helpful in narrowing down the differential diagnosis. Also, immunohistochemistry for glial fibrillary acidic protein enables delineating oligodendrogliomas from gliomas harboring neoplastic astrocytic cells.

Clinical Presentation

The symptomatology encountered in patients with oligodendroglial tumors is well within the spectrum of diffuse gliomas in general. Compared with patients with other diffuse gliomas, a relatively large proportion of patients with oligodendrogliomas suffer from generalized or focal seizures for many years. A minority of patients present with signs of increased intracranial pressure, focal deficits, or mental changes. The prognosis of patients with symptoms of increased intracranial pressure or focal deficits is generally worse than for patients suffering from seizures.

Location

The majority of oligodendrogliomas are located in the cerebral hemispheres, preferentially affecting the cerebral cortex. More than 50% of oligodendrogliomas are found in the frontal lobes. Larger tumors may involve more than one lobe. Some tumors may be present in deeper structures of the brain like the basal ganglia. Incidentally, oligodendrogliomas are encountered in the cerebellum, pons, brainstem, or spinal cord. Rare cases of pure leptomeningeal localization (oligodendrogliomatosis) have been reported and must be distinguished from intracerebral tumors with arachnoidal invasion. In these cases clear cell ependymomas, chromophobic adenomas of the pituitary, or metastatic cancers should be eliminated from the differential diagnosis. The development of leptomeningeal involvement during the course of the disease is a relatively frequent event, but metastases outside the CNS are very rare. The lung seems to be the organ mainly targeted for oligodendroglioma metastases.

Neuroradiologic Imaging

Neuroradiologic imaging is often nonspecific and in most cases the presentation on computed tomography (CT) or magnetic resonance imaging (MRI) does not differ from that of any other diffuse glioma. On MRI, calcifications are not unequivocally appreciated, but in approximately 40% of cases calcifications are visualized on CT. Calcifications are indicative of, though not specific for, oligodendroglioma. Infiltration in or spread along the arachnoidal space is characteristically seen in oligodendroglioma but is nonspecific by itself. On CT, low-grade oligodendrogliomas appear as less dense masses that are not enhanced. Cysts may be present. Tumor borders may appear rather well defined at neuroimaging and may match with focal areas of sharp delineation from surrounding brain tissue found in pathology specimens. Intratumoral hemorrhage may be present in up to 20% of patients. MRI of low-grade oligodendrogliomas shows an increased signal intensity on T2-weighted images without enhancement. Anaplastic oligodendrogliomas will be enhanced because of disruption of the blood-brain barrier.

Incidence

In the literature, the incidence of oligodendrogliomas ranges from 5% to 18% of all primary CNS tumors. In a Norwegian population-based survey dated from 1986, 4% of primary tumors of the CNS appeared to be oligodendrogliomas. The Central Brain Tumor Registry of the United States registered 3.5% in the admissions between 1992 and 1997. However, in recent studies incidence percentages as high as 25% of all primary brain tumors are reported. There are various reasons to explain this large variation in incidence. First, most data are derived from investigations made on materials from local centers and there exist relatively few original data based on population-based surveys. Second, the notorious difficulties

regarding the histopathologic criteria and definition of oligodendroglioma cause large interobserver variability. The delineation of pure oligodendroglioma from mixed oligoastrocytomas and pure astrocytomas is subject to dispute. Criteria as to what percentage of tumor cells with oligodendroglial phenotype would define the threshold of either pure oligodendroglioma or, alternatively, mixed oligoastrocytoma, has been variably used by authors. Percentages range from 10% to 50%, although 25% seems accepted by the majority.

Prognosis

Oligodendrogliomas may arise in childhood, but most patients are older than 30. The distribution curves show a typical biphasic pattern with one age peak around 35 years and a second age peak around 55 years. Age has been invariably found to be the most important prognosticator in oligodendrogliomas. Low-grade tumors are typically seen in patients younger than 40, whereas most patients suffering from high-grade (anaplastic) oligodendrogliomas are older. Several publications from single institutions addressed the effects of various patient characteristics and treatment-related factors on the prognosis. It should be kept in mind that these series often span many decades. Effects of changing therapeutic approaches and variability in patient care over time certainly had their influence on the survival data shown in these studies. Favorable prognostic factors include younger age at presentation, absence of focal deficits or increased intracranial pressure at presentation, tumor localization in the frontal lobe, no contrast enhancement on preoperative neuroimaging, and good postoperative performance status. Ring enhancement of the tumor at CT or MRI, in contrast to diffuse (nonring) enhancement, is related to a worse prognosis. In recent studies some specific genetic aberrations have been linked to survival statistics. Loss of the short arm of chromosome 1 is related to a longer progression-free survival after radiation therapy (RT). Patients with 1p loss had a median progression-free survival of 49.8 months, in contrast to the 5.7 months for patients lacking 1p loss. In a series of anaplastic oligodendrogliomas treated with chemotherapy, the 1p status was a significant predictor of chemosensitivity, and loss of both 1p and 19q was associated with prolonged recurrence-free survival after chemotherapy. Another genetic aberration associated with prognosis appeared to be the CDKN2A gene; deletion of this locus was related to poor survival.

The histologic delineation between oligodendroglioma and mixed oligoastrocytoma is subject to large interobserver variability (see later discussion). The survival statistics of patients diagnosed with mixed oligoastrocytomas are reportedly better than those of patients with pure astrocytomas but worse than those of pure oligodendrogliomas of similar malignancy grade. Patients with mixed oligoastrocytomas have 5- and 10-year survival rates of 63% and 33%, respectively, whereas patients with pure oligodendrogliomas have rates of 75% and 46%, respectively. It may be concluded that mixed oligoastrocytomas represent an intermediate group with respect to biologic aggressiveness. An explanation for the differences in survival statistics may also be that the mixed oligoastrocytomas actually consist of tumors that behave as either pure oligodendroglioma or pure astrocytoma. Arguments for this hypothesis depend on recent data of genotyping of mixed oligoastrocytomas. The finding of TP53 mutations (considered an astrocytoma feature) was mutually exclusive with the finding of losses on the chromosome arms 1p and 19q (considered a feature of oligodendroglioma). Among 50 patients diagnosed with anaplastic oligodendroglioma, 23 patients with tumors with 1p or 19q deletions had a higher response rate (100%) to chemotherapy and a longer median survival (123 months) compared with 8 patients with TP53 mutations (33% response rate; 71-month median survival).

PATHOLOGY

Histology

In 1926 Harvey Cushing and Hamilton Bailey classified intracerebral tumors by matching the phenotypes of tumor cells with those of cells they knew were from normal embryologic development. Since the end of the 19th century it had been generally believed that neoplasms would arise from cells that had arrested somewhere between the stage of stem cell and end-differentiated cell. Hence the terms used in the various tumor classifications of cancers of various organs referred to embryonic morphology. Glial tumors consisting of cells resembling mature oligodendrocytes were called oligodendrogliomas. Some authors coined the term *oligodendroblastomas* for more primitive variants of oligodendroglial tumors, and they reserved the term *oligodendrocytomas* for tumors consisting of cells with a more mature phenotype. In the first report on a series of oligodendrogliomas by Percival Bailey and Paul Bucy in 1929, the similarity of the tumor cells with normal mature oligodendrocytes was recapitulated.[1]

Although normal oligodendrocytes produce myelin in the CNS, no trace of myelin has ever been observed in an oligodendroglioma. The resemblance with oligodendrocytes is merely based on the monotonous phenotypes of the cells. The nuclei are fairly round. In most specimens the nuclei are positioned in the center of a so-called perinuclear halo, which basically is a shrinkage artifact of the cytoplasm of these cells, especially induced when the specimen has not been placed in formalin within minutes after removal. The cytoplasm of the classic neoplastic oligodendrocyte does not contain glial fibrillary acidic protein (GFAP)-positive filaments as encountered in astrocytic tumors. In a fair number of cases there is mucoid degeneration of the tumor tissue. Incidentally, eosinophilic granular cells or signet-ring cells are present—probably representing degenerating tumor cells—and the former are encountered in astrocytomas as well. Ultrastructural findings in oligodendrogliomas are nonspecific; the classic tumor cells lack intermediate filaments as characteristically seen in astrocytic cells. The presence of crystalline structures, concentric laminar structures, autophagic vacuoles, perikaryal microtubules, and a variable number of mitochondria have been reported by different authors. Except for the crystalline structures, whose nature and origin remain obscure, none of these structures may be considered specific for the neoplastic oligodendrocyte.

The oligodendroglial tumor cells may grow in queues and mimic the alignment of normal oligodendrocytes along axons. The most characteristic picture of oligodendroglioma is that of honeycomb-like structures, caused by the tumor cells lying close together, displaying their round nuclei in small empty boxes that represent the shrunken cytoplasm (Figure 23-1A). The tumor cells in readily fixed specimens will show some

cytoplasm instead of the perinuclear empty space (halo) (see Figure 23-1B). Tumor borders with surrounding brain tissue may be surprisingly well defined (see Figure 23-1C). Invasion of the subarachnoidal space is a feature often encountered in oligodendroglioma (see Figure 23-1D). In rare instances dissemination along the routes of CSF is seen. Tumor calcification is basically a nonspecific feature but is characteristically present in classic cases of oligodendroglioma and is a diagnostic clue for many pathologists. The presence of calcifications may be in the form of minuscule particles or large clumps. In more extensive resection specimens one may occasionally see the typical bands of calcium deposits parallel to the pial surface. The mechanism of calcification is unknown. It may be considered as a dystrophic event, occurring as sequel of circulatory disturbances in the prolonged initial course of this neoplasm.

Etiology and Cell of Origin

The etiology is unknown. Oligodendrogliomas are not known to arise following irradiation or treatment with particular drugs or toxins. Despite scarce reports of tumors in which sequences of SV-40 virus are documented, there is no proof of viral genesis. By now, there is a worldwide reappraisal of the so-called stem cell as source of the development of tissues and also neoplastic derivatives of tissues. The concept of a glial precursor cell for gliomas, possibly arrested somewhere in its development and giving rise to various tumors depending on the phase of development at which the arrest took place, was basically proposed in the very first classifications of gliomas. In well-known experiments by Raff et al published in 1983, aiming to isolate glial precursor cells, antibodies to differentiated glial cells (galactocerebroside for oligodendroglial lineage and GFAP for astrocytic lineage) were used in addition to antibodies for precursor cells. These antibodies have been used on tissue slides of oligodendroglioma and mixed oligoastrocytoma to determine the lineage of the neoplasms. The A2B5 antibody, which stains the precursor cells of oligodendrocytes and a subset of astrocytes, appeared to be immunoreactive with oligodendrogliomas and part of mixed oligoastrocytomas, whereas the astrocytomas remained negative.[7] The results of these immunohistochemical investigations pointed to the theory that oligodendroglial tumors would be derived from A2B5-positive precursor cells. The results were, however, never reproduced by others.

Glial Fibrillary Acidic Protein–Positive Cells in Oligodendroglioma

In approximately half of oligodendrogliomas, GFAP-positive tumor cells are found. These GFAP-positive tumor cells should be carefully distinguished from interspersed reactive astrocytes that merge with the diffusely infiltrating tumor tissue (Figure 23-2A). The GFAP-positive cells may be gliofibrillary oligodendrocytes (GFOCs), miniature gemistocytes (minigemistocytes), or larger gemistocytic cells (see Figure 23-2B). Any of these cells may be found scattered throughout the tumor or incidentally aligned in clusters. Few tumors are almost entirely composed of transitional cells, and especially in these cases the designation of the glioma as either a pure oligodendroglioma or a mixed oligoastrocytoma is controversial. The GFOCs are

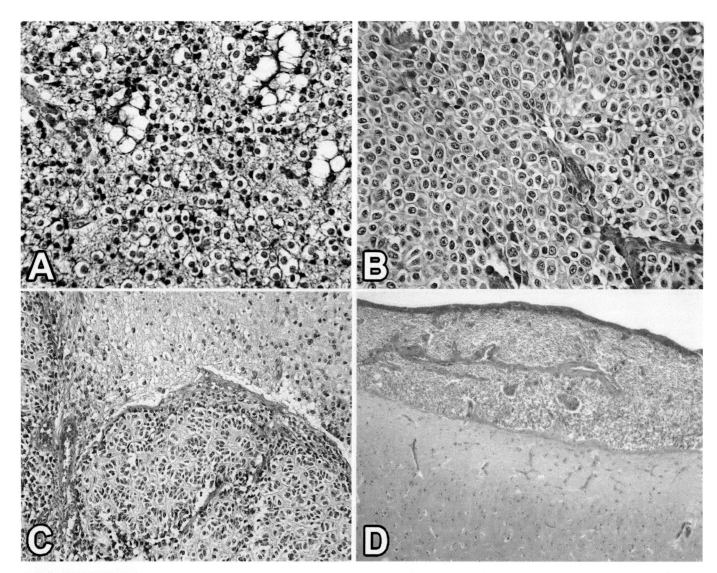

FIGURE 23-1   Histology of oligodendroglioma. *A,* Classic histology of oligodendroglioma. There is monotonous histology, and the tumor cells have perinuclear shrinkage artifacts (halos) that give the impression of a honeycomb (hematoxylin and eosin [H&E], ×400). *B,* Oligodendroglioma in which the tumor cells still have some cytoplasm. The absence of the shrinkage artifact is due to rapid fixation after removal of the specimen (H&E, ×400). *C,* The oligodendroglial tumor tissue may be sharply delineated from surrounding brain tissue (H&E, ×250). *D,* The arachnoidal space is filled with oligodendroglial tumor tissue, indicative of arachnoidal spread. At this point the cortex is not infiltrated (H&E, ×100).

morphologically similar to the GFAP-negative oligodendroglial tumor cells and are otherwise not distinguishable from surrounding GFAP-negative oligodendroglial tumor cells. The GFAP colocalizes with the intermediate filaments that are present in the GFOCs and miniature gemistocytes. The origin of these cells, or the trigger for the appearance of GFAP in oligodendroglial tumor cells, is not known. Oligodendroglial tumors harboring transitional (GFAP-positive) cells are generally considered to be pure oligodendroglioma and not mixed oligoastrocytoma.

Immunohistochemical Tumor Markers

Various immunohistochemical markers have been introduced as lineage specific for oligodendrogliomas. Unfortunately, virtually none have been sustained as practical tumor markers.

Some antibodies react only with part of the tumors or tumor cells, whereas others seem not specific for tumors histologically matching the diagnosis of oligodendroglioma. The intermediate filament-related GFAP is a reliable and specific marker for astrocytic lineage and thus its use may be helpful in the distinction of oligodendroglioma from astrocytoma. However, the interpretation of the staining results for GFAP may be problematic. The immunomorphologic identification of neoplastic astrocytes from reactive astrocytes may be difficult if not impossible. Myelin basic protein, Leu-7, and myelin-associated glycoprotein specifically are found in oligodendroglial cells and sometimes also in oligodendroglial tumors, but these proteins have not been established as markers for oligodendroglioma. Recently, the expression of particular glycolipids was found to correlate with either oligodendroglioma, mixed oligoastrocytoma, or astrocytoma.[23] For instance, the presence

The expression of markers mirroring neuronal differentiation and the recently described immunopositivity for neuronal markers in oligodendroglioma is somewhat confusing. In 1982 the term central neurocytoma was introduced for a glioma subtype found in the subependymal areas around the ventricles. These neoplasms showed remarkable morphologic similarity to oligodendrogliomas, although classic cases displayed an even more monotonous histology than oligodendrogliomas. Proof of the neuronal lineage of the central neurocytoma was obtained by positive immunohistochemistry for synaptophysin and electron microscopically by visualization of the synaptic vesicles in the tumor cells. Only incidental cases of oligodendrogliomas have been described in which neuronal differentiation is substantiated by positivity of the tumor cells for synaptophysin or rosette-like structures. The precise relation between these oligodendrogliomas with neuronal differentiation and their delineation from the central neurocytomas remains to be established.

Delineation of Oligodendrogliomas from Astrocytomas and Mixed Oligoastrocytomas

The delineation of mixed oligoastrocytomas from pure oligodendrogliomas is troublesome.[3] Moreover, the existence of true mixed gliomas is an unsettled matter. Mixed oligoastrocytomas are defined as a mixture of neoplastic oligodendroglial and neoplastic astrocytic cells. There is ongoing debate about the percentage of neoplastic oligodendrocytes necessary to make the diagnosis of pure astrocytoma, pure oligodendroglioma, or mixed oligoastrocytoma. As mentioned previously, there are no definite criteria to identify a neoplastic oligodendrocyte in the first place. In Radiation Therapy Oncology Group (RTOG) and European Organization for Research and Treatment of Cancer (EORTC) trials on (neo)adjuvant procarbazine, CCNU, and vincristine (PCV) chemotherapy, tumors are considered "oligodendroglial," that is, true oligodendroglioma or mixed oligoastrocytoma, if they have at least 25% oligodendroglial tumor cells. Obviously, this criterion is prone to large subjectivity: There may be regional variation in cellular composition of the tumor, and there is substantial interobserver variation in the appreciation of the lineage characteristics. The results of some genetic investigations support the idea that gliomas are either oligodendroglial or astrocytic in nature, leaving the mixed oligoastrocytomas a nonexisting entity (see previous discussion). Others found genetic characteristics of oligodendroglioma (losses on 1p and 19q) and astrocytoma (mutations of TP53) within the same tumors, supporting the idea of the existence of a genetically mixed glioma. Attempts to divide the mixed oligoastrocytomas in tumors consisting of diffusely interspersed tumor cells of either oligodendroglial or astrocytic lineage, or alternatively, tumors with distinct areas consisting purely of one tumor cell type, have never gained practical application. Morphologically, most cases consist of a diffuse mixture of either astrocytic or oligodendroglial tumor cells. In larger resection specimens of brain tissue infiltrated by oligodendroglioma, it is apparent that the classical oligodendroglioma tumor center is often flanked by areas of astrocytic proliferation similar to fibrillary astrocytoma. Some authors have taken this to the extreme by supposing that fibrillary astrocytomas simply do not exist and all gliomas basically represent oligodendroglioma.[6] Oligodendrogliomas with transitional cells are

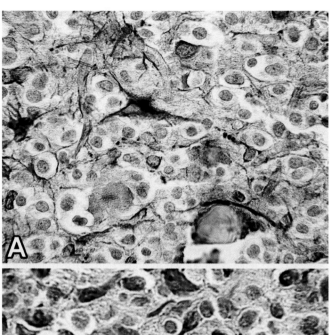

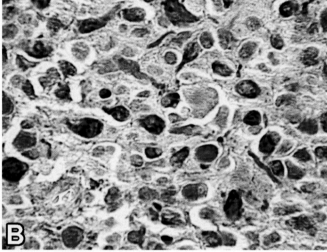

FIGURE 23-2   Glial fibrillary acidic protein (GFAP)-positive cells in oligodendrogliomas. *A,* Oligodendroglial tumor cells are immunonegative for GFAP. Interspersed astrocytes (recognized by their cell processes) are strongly immunostained (anti-GFAP immunohistochemistry, ×400). *B,* Transitional cells in oligodendroglioma. Depending on the cytoplasmic volume, the GFAP-positive oligodendroglial tumor cells are called *gliofibrillary oligodendrocytes* (GFOC) or *miniature gemistocytes*—the latter identified by more voluminous cytoplasm (anti-GFAP immunohistochemistry, ×400).

of asialoGM1 and the absence of paragloboside correlates with an oligodendroglial phenotype. The glycolipids are synthesized by glycosyltransferases that are variably expressed by gliomas. Overexpression, deletion, or mutations in these genes are expected to correlate with glioma histology and lineage, and future studies will reveal if the glycolipids will be sustained as markers and used in pathology practice. Olig 1 and olig 2 are recently discovered oligodendrocytic lineage-specific transcription factors, and these proteins also have yet to prove their practical value as oligodendroglial tumor markers.[12] Another recently reported lineage marker, the microtubule-associated protein 2 (MAP2), though expressed in oligodendrogliomas, seems to be of limited specificity.

considered pure oligodendrogliomas by some, mixed oligoastrocytomas by others. The genetic background of such tumors has not been determined.

Grading and Proliferation Indices

The obsolete terms *oligodendrocytoma* and *oligodendroblastoma*, which were soon coined following Bailey and Cushing's initial tumor typing, reflected the earliest attempt to grade oligodendrogliomas. Following the example provided by Broders, who had initiated the grading of colon cancers, James W. Kernohan from the Mayo Clinic began to grade gliomas to provide information as to the expected clinical behavior of the tumors. Certain histologic parameters were estimated and weighed for the attribution of a malignancy grade. Initially, four grades of malignancy were distinguished, the lowest corresponding to the most indolent biologic behavior of the tumor and longest survival curves, the highest to the most aggressive tumor behavior paired with short survival. The grading procedure yielded sensible information as to the biologic behavior to be expected of gliomas of the astrocytic group. However, with respect to oligodendrogliomas it was reported that grading did not result in useful prognostic information. For the astrocytic tumor group, four malignancy grades had been distinguished, but the oligodendrogliomas were divided into only two categories (oligodendrogliomas, or "oligodendrocytomas," and "oligodendroblastomas"). The disappointing results of grading oligodendrogliomas may have been due to the relatively small series involved. A long list of histologic parameters was used for grading according to Kernohan's system for the astrocytomas, but neither the way of scoring of these parameters nor the respective tumor grades were clearly defined. The value of the mitotic index for tumor grade has been particularly troublesome in oligodendroglioma. In otherwise low-grade oligodendrogliomas there may be an abundance of mitoses. Soon other grading schemes for oligodendrogliomas, variably composed of two, three, or four tiers, were launched. Grading schemes like those of Davis (1950), Ringertz (1950), Horrax (1951), and Afra (1978) had limited acclaim, mainly because they were not accurate in the definition of the respective grades.

In 1983 Smith developed a four-tiered grading scheme that attracted attention because of the relative limited number of features used and the simple way of scoring.[19] This scheme certainly succeeded in providing easily recognizable features that could be comprehensively scored. Important practical issues concerning interobserver variability in grading oligodendrogliomas have been the subject of recent investigations. Not only the interobserver variability in scoring histologic features but also the individual prognostic value of each variable has been evaluated by multivariate analyses. One recent study on grading oligodendrogliomas assessed hyperchromasia, coarse chromatin and pleomorphism of nuclei, nuclear-cytoplasmic ratio, cytologic malignancy (anaplasia), mitoses, subpial infiltration, invasion of the leptomeninges, microcysts, calcifications, endothelial hypertrophy and proliferation, increased vascularization, necrosis, and the presence of transitional cells.[8] In this analysis, in which 13 experienced observers were involved, only age of the patient and the presence of endothelial proliferation were found to be independently associated with survival. In earlier studies, tumor necrosis has almost invariably been identified as a feature with independent prognostic value. The WHO distinguishes oligodendroglioma and anaplastic oligodendroglioma. The histologic features of malignancy include cellularity, cytologic atypia, and mitotic activity. These histopathologic features may, when present or sufficiently high, be enough to diagnose anaplastic oligodendroglioma. The presence of microvascular proliferation or necrosis alone would be sufficient for that diagnosis. Because no exact definition of the two grades is provided, many pathologists use either the grading scheme of Smith or apply the St. Anne–Mayo grading scheme, which has been developed for astrocytomas, to oligodendroglial tumors.

Various techniques to measure cell proliferation in tumors have been developed in recent decades. Immunohistochemistry for Ki-67, a protein that is present in the cell nucleus in all phases of the cell cycle except G0, is widely used because of its reproducible and reliable results. The anti-Ki-67 antibody MIB-1 has terminated the use of immunohistochemistry for proliferating cell nuclear antigen (PCNA). MIB-1 labeling indices (LIs) have been shown to correlate well with biologic behavior in oligodendroglioma. A labeling of 5% is usually taken as the cutoff point between low and high proliferation. The MIB-1 LI has not yet been included in any of the grading schemes. A measure of cell loss may also be a factor in tumor progression. Various methods for labeling apoptotic cells have been developed, and although the value of some of these has been estimated in oligodendrogliomas, none was implemented in a grading scheme.[18]

Differential Diagnosis

There are various glial neoplasms with histopathology mimicking oligodendroglioma. The histology of the central neurocytomas may be indistinguishable from classic oligodendroglioma; ventricle-related tumor sites and expression of neuronal markers like synaptophysin or neurofilament may be helpful in making the distinction. Classical oligodendrogliomas should be distinguished from other tumors with clear cell morphology, like clear cell ependymomas and chromophobic adenomas of the pituitary. Also in these cases tumor site and immunophenotype will assist in making the right diagnosis. It is well known that pilocytic astrocytomas, in older literature referred to as *cerebellar astrocytomas*, especially the examples found in the cerebellum, may harbor clear cell tumor parts mimicking oligodendroglioma. Dysembryoplastic neuroepithelial tumors (DNTs) partly consist of oligodendrocytes and may cause confusion in small biopsies. In case of DNTs the typical radiologic presentation will aid in the differential diagnosis.

GENETICS: GENOTYPICAL CHARACTERISTICS

In the early 1990s it was discovered that oligodendrogliomas lose parts of the short arm of chromosome 1 and the long arm of chromosome 19.[17] This finding holds true today, and the alteration is particularly associated with the classic histology of oligodendroglioma. The coincidence of the two aberrations is unique for oligodendroglioma. Deletion mapping studies have narrowed regions on 1p, but tumor-suppressor genes have not yet been identified. The cyclin-dependent-kinase inhibitor gene CDKN2C (p18^{INK4c}) on 1p32, RAD54 on 1p32, and TP73 on 1p36.3 have all been mentioned as putative tumor-suppressor genes in this respect, but no mutations have been found in any of these genes. The promotor of TP73 was found to be hypermethylated, and a transcriptional silencing of the TP73 gene has been found in the minority of anaplastic oligodendrogliomas. TP73 may serve a function as an oncogene because one of its transcripts is frequently up-regulated in tumors. Loss of 19q is, in contrast to loss of 1p, also frequently found in astrocytomas and glioblastomas. Four candidate genes on 19q13.3 have been proposed, but no mutations have been found so far.

Whereas losses on chromosome arms 1p and 19q are characteristic of oligodendroglial lineage, mutations of TP53 are rare in oligodendrogliomas and are more specific for gliomas of astrocytic descent. Mutations of the tumor-suppressor PTEN are incidentally found in anaplastic oligodendrogliomas and are not associated with losses on 1p or 19q. Losses on chromosome 10q (the PTEN tumor-suppressor locus) are less often found in oligodendroglioma than in glioblastomas and astrocytomas. There are indications of yet another tumor suppressor gene located at 10q that possibly plays a role in glial tumor progression. The epidermal growth factor receptor (EGFR) gene is rarely amplified in oligodendroglioma, but the protein is frequently found to be overexpressed in low- and high-grade oligodendroglioma. Another proto-oncogene implicated in at least some gliomas with oligodendroglial phenotype is plateletderived growth factor R (PDGF-R). Other genetic alterations frequently encountered in oligodendroglioma include losses on chromosomes 4, 6, and 14 and the chromosome arms 11p and 22q. Deletions on 9p and 10q are associated with oligodendroglial tumor progression and are more often found in anaplastic oligodendrogliomas. In a significant number of cases the CDKN2A gene at 9p21 was found to be deleted. In a number of cases, also, the tumor-suppressor genes p14^{ARF} and CDKN2B, also located on 9p, are lost. The proteins p16^{INK4a} and p15^{INK4b}, encoded by CDKN2A and CDKN2B, respectively, regulate the cell cycle by inhibiting the activity of cyclin-dependent kinases CDK4 and CDK6. The latter phosphorylate the retinoblastoma protein pRB, which serves a function in controlling the G1-S phase of the cell. Other chromosomes involved in oligodendroglial tumor progression are 4, 6, 7, 11, 13q, 15, 18, and 22q.

Whatever the relation between losses on 1p alone or in combination with loss on 19q and tumor responsiveness to chemotherapy may be, tracing these aberrations obviously became clinically important for making decisions as to best treatment. Genotyping for 1p and 19q is currently being done by several centers and will yield interesting correlations with the phenotypes of the tumors. Loss of 19q seems to be predictive of sensitivity to treatment with PCV only when 1p has been lost as well. The correlation has been revealed in low- as well as high-grade tumors. Not only phenotype and sensitivity to PCV, but also clinical presentation of the oligodendroglial tumor has been shown to correlate with genotype.[22] In a recent publication a relation between tumor localization and specific genotype was found, possibly reflecting different precursor cells of these subsets.[14]

The testing for loss of 1p and 19q is mainly done by LOH analysis and FISH. The advantage of LOH analysis is that results are quickly scored. Once optimized, the technique is relatively easy to carry out. Its disadvantage is that for reliable results, normal DNA (mostly derived from blood) is needed. In contrast, FISH (Figure 23-3) does not need a source of normal DNA. A disadvantage of FISH is that results may vary consid-

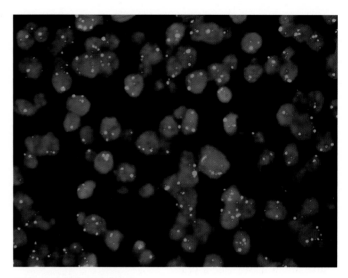

FIGURE 23-3 Fluorescent in situ hybridization for 1p36 in an oligodendroglioma. The *green spots* represent the hybridization product of the probe for the centromeric region of chromosome 1, whereas the locus-specific *red spots* show hybridization with 1p36. Nuclei of normal cells would have two homologous chromosomes and thus two green and two red spots each. However, counting results are statistically corrected for a truncation artifact: Because the slide thickness is 4 µm, parts of nuclei are chopped off. Therefore a correction of the counting is necessary to avoid the erroneous interpretation of loss. In this specimen under-representation of red spots (i.e., 1p36), may be appreciated, indicative of loss of this representing the chromosomal part. The *green spots* representing the centromeric region of chromosome 1 demonstrate that this part of the chromosome is retained (DAPI counterstained, ×400).

erably between tumor sections. Particularly, results on material taken from different laboratories may show variations, mainly due to differences in fixation. Furthermore, scoring the spots is laborious. However, the technique yields interesting correlations with tumor morphology. Good correlations between both techniques' results have been reported.

THERAPY

So far, there are no data from results of randomized studies regarding the effects of treatment applied to patients with oligodendrogliomas. Generally, for patients with primary brain tumors, including oligodendrogliomas, one should base the treatment decision on clinical condition and the expected behavior of the tumor. To some extent, tumor progression correlates with the clinical presentation, the age and condition of the patient, and neuroimaging characteristics (namely, mass effect and enhancement).

Wait and See

In cases of young patients who have only seizures and neuroimaging abnormalities compatible with low-grade primary brain tumor (no enhancement, no mass effect), a wait-and-see policy may be applied. This approach is, however, controversial in the field of neuro-oncology. The key argument in favor of the wait-and-see approach is that the low-grade lesions may remain stable over a prolonged period, whereas treatment (in particular, surgery and radiation therapy) may cause clinical symptoms, particularly cognitive deficits. In a series of 106 patients with low-grade oligodendroglioma and mixed oligoastrocytoma, the median overall survival time was 16.7 years.[15] Of the patients treated with RT, 15% suffered radiation necrosis and 21% developed delayed cognitive deterioration. Patients with focal neurologic deficits with tumors showing enhancement or mass effect unquestionably require treatment. In older patients with low-grade oligodendrogliomas a more aggressive approach may be considered, but there may still be reasons to withhold treatment. In all cases in which a wait-and-see strategy is applied, strict follow-up is necessary, requiring neuroimaging at least twice a year.

Surgery

Surgical resection is the primary treatment modality for patients with resectable tumors and provides tissue for the classification, grading, and genetic analysis of the tumor. Tumor typing, distinguishing oligodendroglioma from astrocytoma in particular, is essential for guiding therapeutic intervention. Further, histologic grading cannot be replaced by estimating tumor grade by neuroimaging. Basically, in any case in which treatment is considered, histologic typing and grading is necessary. In many instances direct surgical intervention will be necessary to relieve symptoms due to mass effects of the tumor and may also help control seizures. The results of some studies concerning both low- and high-grade gliomas pointed to beneficial effect of the extent of surgery on outcome. There are data supporting the notion that gross-total resection is associated with a longer disease-free interval,[11] but studies specifically addressing oligodendroglioma are scarce, and prospective data are not available. In the studies claiming that gross-total tumor resections relate to better survival curves, confounding factors like age, tumor grade, and type of presentation were not always eliminated.[2,16] The beneficial effects of extent of surgery were not demonstrated in other studies, although these were invariably performed retrospectively and uncontrolled.[10] From prospective trials it is clear that low-grade glioma patients with smaller tumors have a better prognosis, and also that smaller tumors are more often completely removed. This may at least in part explain the better outcome of patients who underwent complete tumor resections—and therefore the effects of complete tumor resection remain unknown. So far, the conclusion is justified that once a resection is planned, the tumor should be resected as extensively as safely possible without impairing the neurologic state of the patient.

Adjuvant Treatment

Adjuvant therapy following surgery, particularly radiation therapy and chemotherapy, is indicated in a variety of situations. Patients who undergo partial tumor resections may also need additional treatment. Furthermore, patients with enhancing or progressive lesions, lesions with mass effect, or anaplastic tumors, should also be eligible for additional treatment

following surgery. Adjuvant therapy should be applied to those patients who suffer from neurologic deficits and to elderly patients.

Radiation Therapy

The results of randomized trials comparing adjuvant RT and best standard of care following surgery have confirmed that adjuvant RT provides significant yet modest improvements in survival for patients with high-grade gliomas. The role of RT in low-grade glioma is less clear. Despite the observation made in an EORTC study of early RT leading to increased time to progression, no effect on overall survival was noticed.[9] Studies in which the effects of postoperative RT in oligodendroglial tumors was investigated are contradictory, mainly due to the lack of prospective, randomized trials. The results of several retrospective studies suggest beneficial effects of postoperative RT in patients with oligodendroglioma. This would particularly be true for the subgroup of patients with neurologic deficits and the group of patients who had undergone limited surgery or only a biopsy. In patients with low-grade oligodendrogliomas who underwent an extensive resection, RT can be deferred until tumor progression becomes apparent. Postsurgical RT is indicated in patients with focal or cognitive deficits, tumor enhancement, or mass effect of the tumor. EORTC and RTOG phase III trials in low-grade glioma have shown that there is no improvement of survival following RT with a dose of more than 55 Gy compared with 45 to 50 Gy. An important rationale for deferral of RT is provided by compelling data demonstrating pronounced cognitive deficits and late side effects of RT in patients with low-grade gliomas who have undergone early RT.

Chemotherapy

An observation of paramount importance to all involved in neuro-oncology is the sensitivity of oligodendroglial tumors to chemotherapy. In three studies on relatively large, homogeneous populations, two thirds of patients with anaplastic oligodendrogliomas were responding to chemotherapy treatment with PCV[4,20,21] (Figure 23-4). In these studies, comparable median times to progression were recorded: 12 to 16 months for the partial responders, 25 to 46 months for the complete responders, and 7 to 9 months for the 19% to 27% of patients with stable disease. Similar response rates were reported in studies on preirradiation PCV chemotherapy. The best timing of chemotherapy in oligodendroglioma has not been determined. It is unclear if chemotherapy should be given immediately before or following RT, or at the time of recurrence. The results of RTOG and EORTC randomized, controlled trials answering this question are expected to be out in 2004.

Until recently, there were few data on the effectiveness of PCV chemotherapy in low-grade oligodendroglioma.[13] Although monitoring the response is difficult in the usually nonenhancing low-grade tumors, there are strong indications that a significant percentage of low-grade oligodendrogliomas may respond favorably to PCV chemotherapy. Small series have found improvement of cognitive functions and better seizure control following chemotherapy. The application of other chemotherapeutic agents, such as carboplatin, cisplatin, etoposide, paclitaxel, and temozolomide, has been investigated.

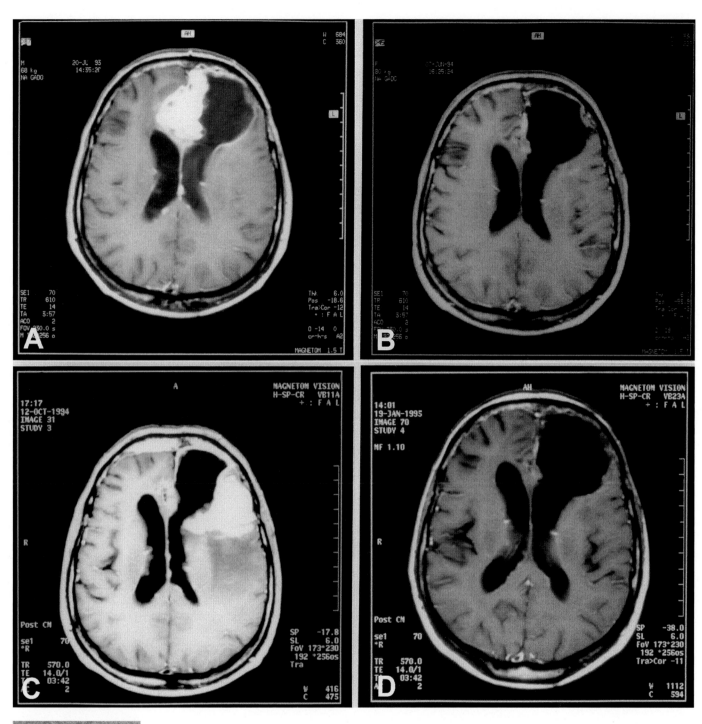

FIGURE 23-4 Contrast magnetic resonance imaging of recurrent oligodendroglioma. *A,* Intraventricular and subependymal recurrence of oligodendroglioma in a 45-year-old man. *B,* Partial tumor response with small residual tumor following six cycles of procarbazine CCNU vincristine (PCV) administration. *C,* Progressive disease after 15 months. *D,* Partial tumor response following two new cycles of PCV. The patient died 2 months later from progressive disease.

Temozolomide is a new orally administered alkylating agent that has been approved in the United States for the treatment of refractory anaplastic astrocytomas and in Europe for recurrent anaplastic astrocytomas and glioblastomas. In 54% of patients treated with temozolomide as first-line chemotherapy for recurrent oligodendrogliomas after RT, complete and partial responses were observed. At 12 months 40% of patients were still free from progression. Temozolomide was also effective and well tolerated as a second-line treatment following treatment with PCV. In this setting, objective responses were obtained in 26% to 40% of patients, with 32% to 51% of patients remaining free from progression at 6 months. Moreover, it was found that patients who did not respond to PCV may respond to temozolomide.

The loss of chromosome arm 1p seems to be indicative of the response to chemotherapy.[5] The combined loss of 1p and 19q was associated with both chemosensitivity and longer recurrence-free survival after treatment with chemotherapy. Tumors with TP53 mutations, generally lacking losses of 1p and 19q, usually do not respond to chemotherapy. Tumors with combined losses of 1p and 19q respond even better to chemotherapy than the tumors with losses on 1p alone. It is expected that refinements in molecular tumor diagnostics will provide tools to define oligodendroglial tumor subsets that will respond successfully to particular treatment modalities.

References

1. Bailey H, Bucy P: Oligodendrogliomas of the brain. J Pathol 32:735–750, 1929.
2. Berger MS, Deliganis AV, Dobbins J, et al: The effect of extent of resection on recurrence in patients with low grade cerebral hemisphere gliomas. Cancer 74:1784–1791, 1994.
3. Burger PC: What is an oligodendroglioma? Brain Pathol 12:257–259, 2002.
4. Cairncross G, Macdonald D, Ludwin S, et al: Chemotherapy for anaplastic oligodendroglioma. National Cancer Institute of Canada Clinical Trials Group. J Clin Oncol 12:2013–2021, 1994.
5. Cairncross JG, Ueki K, Zlatescu MC, et al: Specific genetic predictors of chemotherapeutic response and survival in patients with anaplastic oligodendrogliomas. J Natl Cancer Inst 90:1473–1479, 1998.
6. Daumas-Duport C, Varlet P, Tucker ML, et al: Oligodendrogliomas. Part I: Patterns of growth, histological diagnosis, clinical and imaging correlations: a study of 153 cases. J Neurooncol 34:37–59, 1997.
7. De la Monte SM: Uniform lineage of oligodendrogliomas. Am J Pathol 135:529–540, 1989.
8. Giannini C, Scheithauer BW, Weaver AL, et al: Oligodendrogliomas: reproducibility and prognostic value of histologic diagnosis and grading. J Neuropathol Exp Neurol 60:248–262, 2001.
9. Karim AB, Afra D, Cornu P, et al: Randomized trial on the efficacy of radiotherapy for cerebral low-grade glioma in the adult: European Organization for Research and Treatment of Cancer Study 22845 with the Medical Research Council study BRO4: an interim analysis. Int J Radiat Oncol Biol Phys 52:316–324, 2002.
10. Kros JM, Pieterman H, van Eden CG, et al: Oligodendroglioma: the Rotterdam-Dijkzigt experience. Neurosurgery 34:959–966; discussion 966, 1994.
11. Lacroix M, Abi-Said D, Fourney DR, et al: A multivariate analysis of 416 patients with glioblastoma multiforme: prognosis, extent of resection, and survival. J Neurosurg 95:190–198, 2001.
12. Lu QR, Park JK, Noll E, et al: Oligodendrocyte lineage genes (OLIG) as molecular markers for human glial brain tumors. PNAS 11:10851–10856, 1998.
13. Mason WP, Krol GS, DeAngelis LM: Low-grade oligodendroglioma responds to chemotherapy. Neurology 46:203–207, 1996.
14. Mueller W, Hartmann C, Hoffmann A, et al: Genetic signature of oligoastrocytomas correlates with tumor location and denotes distinct molecular subsets. Am J Pathol 161:313–319, 2002.
15. Olson JD, Riedel E, DeAngelis LM: Long-term outcome of low-grade oligodendroglioma and mixed glioma. Neurology 54:1442–1448, 2000.
16. Puduvalli VK, Hashmi M, McAllister LD, et al: Anaplastic oligodendrogliomas: prognostic factors for tumor recurrence and survival. Oncology 65:259–266, 2003.
17. Reifenberger J, Reifenberger G, Liu L, et al: Molecular genetic analysis of oligodendroglial tumors shows preferential allelic deletions on 19q and 1p. Am J Pathol 145:1175–1190, 1994.
18. Schiffer D, Dutto A, Cavalla P, et al: Role of apoptosis in the prognosis of oligodendrogliomas. Neurochem Int 31:245–250, 1997.
19. Smith MT, Ludwig CL, Godfrey AD, et al: Grading of oligodendrogliomas. Cancer 52:2107–2114, 1983.
20. Soffietti R, Ruda R, Bradac GB, et al: PCV chemotherapy for recurrent oligodendrogliomas and oligoastrocytomas. Neurosurgery 43:1066–1073, 1998.
21. van den Bent MJ, Kros JM, Heimans JJ, et al: Response rate and prognostic factors of recurrent oligodendroglioma treated with procarbazine, CCNU, and vincristine chemotherapy. Dutch Neuro-oncology Group. Neurology 51:1140–1145, 1998.
22. van den Bent MJ, Looijenga LH, Langenberg K, et al: Chromosomal anomalies in oligodendroglial tumors are correlated with clinical features. Cancer 97:1276–1284, 2003.
23. Yates AJ, Comas T, Scheithauer BW, et al: Glycolipid markers of astrocytomas and oligodendrogliomas. J Neuropathol Exp Neurol 58:1250–1262, 1999.

CHAPTER 24

MIXED GLIOMAS

W.K. Alfred Yung, Joann Aaron, and Kenneth D. Aldape

Malignant gliomas cause 2% of cancer deaths in Western countries, and as many as 25% are classified as mixed oligoastrocytoma (OA) or oligodendroglioma. OAs are also referred to as low-grade gliomas, a term that encompasses low-grade astrocytoma and neuroepithelial tumors such as oligodendroglioma and ependymoma. Of the various forms of mixed gliomas, OAs, which are classified as World Health Organization (WHO) grade II tumors, are the most prevalent and primarily affect young adults. Anaplastic OAs, classified as WHO grade III, or intermediate-grade gliomas, are less prevalent. Histologically, mixed gliomas are composed of more than a single type of neoplastic glial cell. Although the criteria for their diagnosis are not uniformly defined, it is generally accepted that phenotypic heterogeneity is their basic characteristic. Varying opinions exist for defining the minimum astroglial component for making the diagnosis of OA; they range from at least 1% and up to 25%, but some are as high as 50%. It has recently been suggested that the microscopic presence of even a single astrocytic cell in a single ×100 microscopic field of an oligodendroglial tumor is sufficient for assigning the diagnosis of OA rather than astrocytoma.[27] The existence of a meaningful classification scheme for mixed glioma is debatable and is likely to change as molecular criteria are added to the mix. Although patients with these tumors often have a reasonably long survival, most will ultimately die from their tumors. Slow-growing astrocytic neoplasms with a high degree of cellular differentiation that diffusely infiltrate nearby brain, they have a tendency to progress to higher grade astrocytomas, a process that occurs most rapidly in older patients[10] and dictates the ultimately poor survival[27] associated with mixed glioma.

Much debate surrounds the actual meaning and significance of a mixed glioma diagnosis. The optimal management of patients with OA remains to be precisely defined. The prognostic value of histologic factors and tumor grade is especially controversial. The same is true for how best to distinguish OA from pure oligodendroglioma, the benefit of the extent of surgical resection, the timing of surgical resection or debulking, the efficacy of postoperative radiation therapy, and the utility of standard chemotherapeutic regimens. This conundrum is partially due to studies that have examined the benefits of surgery and radiotherapy being retrospective, spanning many years, lacking uniformity of pathologic grades (often grouping both low- and high-grade tumors), and including differences in the extent of removal and radiation doses, ultimately making definitive comparisons challenging.[24]

EPIDEMIOLOGY, INCIDENCE, PREVALENCE

Determinations of the incidence of oligodendroglial tumors, including oligodendroglioma and OA, vary, ranging from 5% to 18% of all primary human brain tumors.[18] Other estimations for the occurrence of low-grade astrocytomas, including OAs, are approximately 15% of gliomas in adults and 25% of all gliomas of the cerebral hemispheres in children.[10] Interestingly, patients with OAs of the temporal lobe (mean age 36 years) were younger ($P < .05$, t test) than patients with nontemporal tumors (mean age 41 years). Within the temporal tumor group, patients with TP53 mutations (mean age 33 years) were younger than those without this alteration (mean age 38 years).[18]

LOCATION

OA and anaplastic OA can develop in any region of the central nervous system but usually develop supratentorially in the cerebrum of children and adults (Table 24-1). The brainstem is the next most common site, but these tumors do not typically occur in the cerebellum. Within the cerebrum they arise roughly in proportion to the relative mass of the different lobes; thus the frontal lobe is the most common location, followed by the temporal lobe. One group of investigators found that among the 203 gliomas they evaluated, 103 were located in the frontal, 53 in the temporal, 17 in the frontotemporal, 11 in the parietal, 6 in the parietotemporal, 7 in the ventricular, 3 in the occipitotemporal, and 1 in the occipital region; 2 were from the spinal cord.[18]

DIAGNOSIS

Initial Symptoms and Signs

Brain tumors produce clinical change either through regional parenchymal or diffuse intracranial effects. Regional parenchymal effects of brain tumors include compression, invasion, and destruction of surrounding brain. Hypoxia, arterial or venous competition for nutrients, altered transmitter metabolism and electrolyte concentration, and the spread of cytokines and free radicals alter the cellular environment, disrupting normal neural and glial cell function. Irritation (e.g., focal seizures) or depression (e.g., neurologic deficits) of neuronal function can be the

TABLE 24-1

Location of Oligoastrocytomas and Anaplastic Oligoastrocytomas in Brain

Tumor Type	WHO Grade	Location
Oligoastrocytoma	II	Frontal lobe (60%)
		Temporal lobe (33%)
Anaplastic oligoastrocytoma[20,21]	III	Frontal lobe (53%)
		Temporal lobe (38%)
Mixed glioma[22]		Frontal lobe alone (27%)
		Temporal lobe alone (27%)
		Parietal lobe (7%)
		Frontal lobe involvement (54%)
		Temporal lobe involvement (47%)

WHO, World Health Organization.

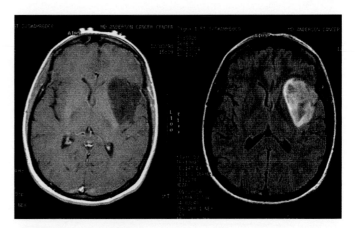

FIGURE 24-1 A magnetic resonance image showing typical presentation of low-grade glioma as a well-circumscribed, low-intensity area on a T1-weighted image in contrast to increased signal intensity corresponding with an increased relaxation time on a fluid attenuation inversion recovery (FLAIR) sequence.

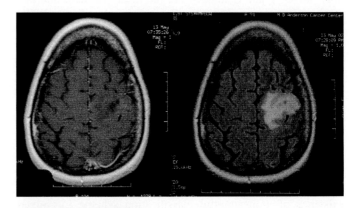

FIGURE 24-2 Magnetic resonance image shows an diffused area of increased fluid attenuation inversion recovery (FLAIR) signal and low intensity on a T1-weighted image with small speckles of contrast enhancement.

result. Elevated intracranial pressure mediates many clinical effects of brain tumors. A rapidly growing tumor is more likely to produce symptoms of elevated intracranial pressure than a slowly growing tumor of the same size.[25]

Common presenting symptoms of low-grade astrocytoma, including OA, are epilepsy, headache, mental changes, and focal neurologic deficits, which could include motor deficit, aphasia, or visual field deficits. Epilepsy is the presenting symptom in more than half of all cases. Oligodendrogliomas and mixed gliomas are vascular and have a greater tendency to hemorrhage than other tumors. Headache and focal neurologic deficits occur less frequently, and signs of raised intracranial pressure with papilledema are uncommon but are most likely to occur in children.[27] Other common presenting symptoms in glioma patients include anorexia, nausea, vomiting (particularly in children), lethargy, and drowsiness, most of which are likely related to increased intracranial pressure as well as alterations in the balance of cerebrospinal fluid (CSF) production and absorption caused by the gliomas themselves.[25] These symptoms also occur with tumor recurrence.[8] From a patient and family point of view, personality changes, mood disturbances, or decreased mental capacity and concentration may be as or more burdensome than some of the focal neurologic deficits.[8]

Imaging

In recent years the diagnostic procedures of choice have become computed tomography (CT) and magnetic resonance imaging (MRI). Pregadolinium and postgadolinium MRI, because of its ability to visualize brain anatomy and detect pathology in the brain, is the most sensitive test available to diagnose low- and intermediate-grade gliomas in most patients, although CT is more sensitive for identifying bone destruction, calcifications, and assessing acute changes such as subarachnoid hemorrhage and hydrocephalus. CT scanning typically reveals a nonenhanced lesion with a lower density than the sur-

rounding brain. A mass effect on surrounding ventricular structures is common. If enhancement occurs, it is generally faint and homogeneous and is likely to occur in higher grade oligodendroglioma or in oligodendroglioma mixed with astrocytic components. On MRI, the lesion typically presents as a low-intensity area on T1-weighted images, whereas there is almost always an increase in signal intensity corresponding with an increased relaxation time on T2-weighted images (Figure 24-1). The area of increased signal is usually homogeneous and well circumscribed with no evidence of hemorrhage or necrosis. Enhancement on MRI may also occur (Figure 24-2). Enhancement on CT or MRI occurs in 8% to 15% of cases. Unfortunately, CT and MRI are limited by the fact that the full extent of tumor extension into the surrounding brain cannot be accurately delineated with these techniques.[10,27] Even characteristic imaging appearances are misleading frequently enough to cause some to recommend an early tissue diagnosis for lesions that have the appearance of low-grade glioma.[25]

Recent years have brought advances to neuro-oncology imaging via dynamic imaging techniques used to assess perfusion, specifically dynamic susceptibility contrast mapping and arterial spin tagging. These techniques enhance the capability of MRI to map regional blood flow and regional cerebral blood flow in tumors. Different applications for these techniques are currently being evaluated. Other advances allow metabolites to be measured in brain tumors noninvasively through proton magnetic resonance spectroscopy.

The ability to functionally image eloquent areas of the central nervous system using functional MRI (fMRI) and positron-emission tomography (PET) enhances the safety of surgery and promises to become routinely employed in the resection of brain tumors, although MRI is not yet able to identify specific tumor types. fMRI records changes in the chemical makeup of areas of the brain or changes in fluid flow. Through detecting changes in blood flow to specific areas of the brain, an indirect measure of neuronal activity is revealed. Current techniques allow for the identification of speech and motor cortex and for the safe resection of some tumors near these cortical regions.[25]

There may also be a role for PET in diagnosis and treatment. A low-grade astrocytoma or OA will be hypometabolic and therefore "cold" on PET scanning.[10] PET is currently being used to determine the histologic grade of a lesion and to differentiate between tumor recurrence and radiation necrosis, as well as to monitor response to treatment.

PATHOLOGY

Because of the heterogeneity of low- and intermediate-grade OAs, grading is difficult to assess. Some investigators use the term *malignant* only for OAs with high cell density, pleomorphism, high nuclear or cytoplasmic ratio, necrosis, endothelial proliferation, and higher level of MIB-1 index.[2] There is general agreement that the term *oligoastrocytoma* is appropriate for tumors in which geographically distinct areas of oligodendroglioma and astrocytoma coexist. Although the percentages assigned to these areas vary widely, they are generally around 20%. It is, however, a matter of complexity to formulate an absolute diagnosis because of the considerable morphologic overlap of neoplastic cells and given the dearth of specific, routinely adopted markers that permit quantification of the proportion of oligodendroglial cells within OAs.[2]

The difficulty inherent in assigning a histologic diagnosis is highlighted in a study by Coons et al, who looked at interobserver concordance of the classification and grading of primary gliomas and noted difficulty in distinguishing diffuse astrocytoma from oligodendroglioma and OA.[7] The WHO recognizes two types of OA, the biphasic, in which discrete areas of oligodendroglial differentiation are seen adjacent to discrete astrocytic differentiation, and the intermixed, in which the two components are intimately related. The biphasic variant, shown in Figure 24-3, is perhaps less controversial in that areas of "classic" oligodendroglial histology and areas of "classic" astrocytic histology are seen in the same specimen. This variant, however, accounts for only a small proportion of all cases diagnosed as mixed glioma. Most cases encountered in daily practice that carry a diagnosis of OA are of the intermixed type. This is the more problematic and controversial and also more common of the two types. Cases in which the features are

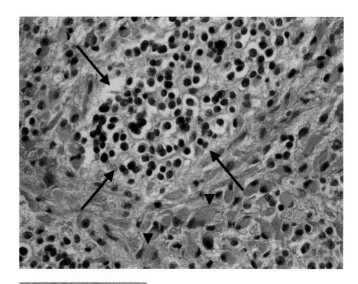

FIGURE 24-3 Biphasic oligoastrocytoma, showing areas of typical oligodendroglioma (arrows) surrounded by areas of typical gemistocytic astrocytoma.

intermediate between oligodendroglioma and astrocytoma can carry the diagnosis of mixed OA, which perhaps reflects the indeterminate nature of the histologic features, rather than a distinct clinicopathologic entity.

For the pathologist, the classic distinction between oligodendroglioma and OA is problematic because of the lack of clearly discriminating parameters. Furthermore, at the molecular level, the differences between morphologically defined oligodendroglioma and OA seem to disappear. Instead, a regional molecular heterogeneity emerges that can be used for molecular classification. A subclassification on molecular grounds provides a cogent approach to unifying previous findings about prognosis, behavior, and response to therapy in oligodendroglial and mixed gliomas. The emerging clinicogenetic associations suggest that oligodendroglial tumors will require molecular subdivision in the near future.[18] It remains to be seen whether molecular alterations will be identified that establish mixed glioma as an entity distinct from either pure astrocytomas or oligodendrogliomas, or, conversely, whether molecular genetic analysis will clarify and subdivide mixed gliomas into those with molecular signatures associated with either astrocytoma or oligodendroglioma.

Quantitative assessment of tumor proliferative activity by flow cytometry cell-cycle analysis or immunohistochemical methods that measure proliferation-associated nuclear proteins (Ki-67, proliferating cell nuclear antigen) or thymidine analog incorporation (bromodeoxyuridine [BrdU]) has been shown to have utility for the evaluation of gliomas. A clear role for flow cytometry cell-cycle analysis in assessing oligodendrogliomas and astrocytomas has been demonstrated. A strong relationship has been demonstrated between BrdU incorporation and histologic grade and survival of patients who have astrocytomas, with a similar association shown in a series of OAs. The applicability of BrdU labeling has, however, been limited by technical concerns related to the limited utility of the MIB-1 antibody for deletion of the Ki-67 antigen. Because the Ki-67 antigen is present in cells during proliferative phases of the cell cycle (G1, S, and G2-M phases) but not in the resting G0 phase,

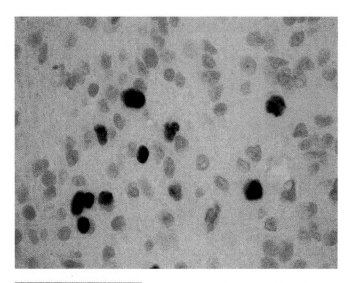

FIGURE 24-4 MIB-1 staining of oligoastrocytoma showing positive nuclei *(dark brown staining)*, indicative of proliferating cells.

it is a sensitive marker of the growth fraction and is an excellent alternative to BrdU labeling.[7] An example of MIB-1 staining in an anaplastic OA is shown in Figure 24-4.

When the correlation between the BrdU labeling index and MIB-1 and Ki-67 proliferating cell indices (PCIs) was evaluated in cerebral gliomas, including 15 mixed malignant gliomas, MIB-1 positive cells were detected easily in most cases. MIB-1 immunostaining was frequently superior to Ki-67 in individual tumors. The MIB-1 PCI was significantly higher than the Ki-67 PCI and the BrdU labeling index. Linear-regression analysis significantly correlated the three indices. The MIB-1 PCI was correlated with the BrdU labeling index in each group of the astrocytic tumors and mixed malignant gliomas; the MIB-1 PCI was approximately 2.4 to 2.8 times higher than the BrdU labeling index. The authors concluded that the close correlation between the MIB-1 PCI and in vivo BrdU labeling index suggests that MIB-1 immunostaining is a useful technique for analyzing the proliferative potential of individual gliomas.[19]

For tumors that are a lower grade than WHO grade IV tumors, particularly glioblastoma multiforme where labeling index has no particular usefulness, BrdU and MIB-1 labeling results are absolutely prognostic. Unsurprisingly, several studies proved that tumors with the greatest level of mitotic activity have the poorest prognosis. Low-grade astrocytomas, including OA, with a BrdU labeling index greater than 1% or a MIB-1 labeling index greater than 8% represent a subset with a poorer prognosis, although Ki-67 labeling was not found to correlate with prognosis.[10]

Another group of researchers evaluated 47 patients with gliomas to clarify the relationships between biologic and histologic classifications with the BrdU labeling index. The median age of the patients was 27.8 years at symptom onset and 31.8 years at labeling. Of the tumors, 45 were supratentorial, 30 were frontal, and 2 were cerebellar. Sixteen tumors were recurrent at the time of labeling. The median labeling index was 1% (range: 1:15; 1%). Forty-six tumors had oligodendroglial and astrocytic elements. The median labeling index was 4.4% in recurrent tumors and 1% in primary tumors. A higher BrdU labeling index correlated with an increased risk of and a shorter time to recurrence. These study findings corroborated the results of others that the BrdU labeling index and the grade of the oligodendroglial component of mixed gliomas have prognostic value.[26]

Ki-67 or MIB-1 immunochemistry was used to measure proliferative activity in 81 patients with oligodendrogliomas and OAs. The relationships between survival, proliferation, histologic features, and clinical variables were evaluated using a Cox proportional hazards regression analysis. After stratifying by histologic grade and adjusting for age at diagnosis, a significant association was found between the Ki-67 or MIB-1 labeling index (percentage of positive cells) and survival ($P = .04$). This association was illustrated further by the significantly different survivals of two groups based on labeling index ranges of less than or equal to 5 and greater than 5 ($P < .0001$).[7]

In summary, most research in this area confirms the prognostic usefulness of measuring cellular proliferation. Many investigators found MIB-1 to be the most promising approach. Currently available research data support the incorporation of such markers into the design of therapeutic protocols, which may produce a more accurate classification of tumors into treatment groups, as well as more accurate expectations regarding outcome. As their use is expanded, such markers may become an essential feature of histologic grading.[7]

Excellent technologies are available for assessing lesions and for obtaining tumor tissue for histologic assessment. Stereotactic biopsy is often used to make a histologic diagnosis in cases for which the benefits of surgical debulking are uncertain or are outweighed by the risks of the procedure. Frame-based biopsy allows a histologic diagnosis of most neoplastic intracranial lesions. Accuracy is usually limited by neuroimaging, because the mechanical accuracy of frame-based stereotaxy is often less than 1 mm. Except in rare cases in which stereotactic biopsy is precluded by tumor location or putative vascularity, diagnostic biopsy is accomplished most safely and effectively by a closed stereotactic procedure under local anesthesia. The choice of open operation versus biopsy depends on the location, size, gross characteristics (extent of demarcation, consistency, and vascularity), probable histology, and radiosensitivity of the tumor, as well as the neurologic and general medical condition of the patient.[25]

The difficulties inherent in making an absolute diagnosis of OA and anaplastic OA based on histologic characteristics presents practical problems, particularly because the traditional clinical practice and prognostications of neuro-oncology are based on an accurate and mutually accepted classification of tumors. The agreed-upon classification of tumors drives therapeutic decisions and positions given tumors for particular courses of clinical management. It is, however, becoming increasingly apparent that accepted histologic groupings, such as the WHO classification system, are best suited to the analysis of outcome in a series of cases but do not necessarily accurately predict response to therapy, tumor behavior, or survival for individual patients and their tumors. The advances in molecular biology and the increased understanding of the driving mechanisms behind gliomagenesis presage the development of an improved classification system for gliomas. Ultimately, tumors are likely to be classified according to their specific molecular makeup and inherent mutations so that individual therapies will be designed for individual patients and their individually characterized lesions. For example, chemotherapy may be an alternative to radiation therapy as the initial adjuvant treatment for a symptomatic progressing tumor with loss of heterozygosity of a gene, whereas if that loss is not present, radiotherapy might be preferable. Behind this promise is the fact that tumors, as classified today, are not homogeneous, but are as individual as the people who suffer from them. What is clearly needed for meaningfully classifying tumors is surrogate markers that will be able to predict the best kinds of therapies for individual tumors as well as being harbingers of a good or poor survival. Some theorize that the activation or silencing of particular protein pathways governs the phenotype of neoplastic subtypes that arise from specific precursor cells. The mechanisms behind the formation of the dual components of mixed astrocytomas have not yet been completely delineated nor have the genetic events leading to an undifferentiated state of neoplastic cells. The propensity of tumors to develop along given pathways will likely guide future treatments and tumor classifications.[16]

GENETIC PROFILING

Allelic losses in oligodendroglioma and OA occur preferentially on chromosomes 1p and 19q, affecting 40% to 80% of these tumor types,[16] although they occur significantly less frequently in temporal OAs, which have more TP53 mutations than OAs in other sites. This variance reflects the general problem of separating mixed OA from astrocytoma, and it could indicate that temporal OA not only differs with respect to the loss of heterozygosity of 1p and 19q but is possibly enriched by a fraction of tumors resembling astrocytoma. This argument is supported by the inverse association between the loss of heterozygosity of 1p and TP53 mutations found in OA. It is significant that the loss of heterozygosity of 1p and 19q is inversely associated with TP53 mutations. Because identical genetic alterations have been identified both in their astrocytic and oligodendroglial portions, it is likely that OAs have a clonal origin. Although it is generally assumed that the astrocytic component in OA implies a less favorable prognosis, this difference was not uniformly confirmed in all studies.[18]

The frequent loss of the 1p and 19q loci in low-grade, as well as anaplastic oligodendroglioma and OA, suggests that tumor suppressors are pivotal early in the history of oligodendroglial tumorigenesis. Although somatic deletions on the short arm of chromosome 1 (loss of heterozygosity of 1p) and the long arm of chromosome 19 (loss of heterozygosity of 19q) are typical of oligodendroglioma and OA, to date neither the 1p nor 19q gene has been identified. OAs may also display allelic losses of chromosome 17p; however, these losses are not often associated with TP53 mutations.[16]

Oligodendroglioma and OA can progress to either WHO grade III and anaplastic oligodendroglioma or anaplastic astrocytoma and sometimes to higher grade tumors with histologic features similar to glioblastoma multiforme. Anaplastic oligodendroglioma and OA can display allelic losses of chromosome 9p involving the CDKN2A gene and chromosome 10. It appears that allelic loss of chromosome 10 may be a common finding in high-grade malignant gliomas, whether their original lineage is astrocytic or oligodendroglial.[16]

In the quest for prognostic markers, one study sought to delineate the potential diagnostic and prognostic significance of 1p and 19q alterations in oligodendroglioma, astrocytoma,

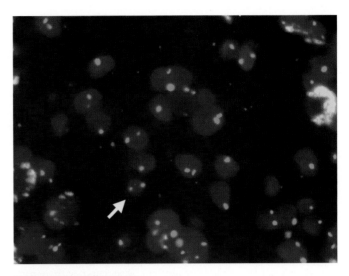

FIGURE 24-5 Fluorescent in situ hybridization (FISH) for chromosome 1p in an oligoastrocytoma. Dual-color FISH for a probe on chromosome 1q *(green)* and a probe at 1p36 *(red)*. Cell at arrow shows two green signals but only one red signal, indicative of loss at 1p.

and mixed OA. The results were that loss of the 1p or 19q loci combined with 1p and 19q common deletion regions were predominantly associated with the oligodendroglial rather than the OA phenotype. Although the frequencies of 1p and 19q alterations in mixed OA were intermediate between pure oligodendroglioma and pure astrocytoma, a combined loss of 1p and 19q was not found to be a statistically significant predictor of overall survival for grade IV astrocytoma or for patients with mixed OA. This category of tumors is, however, notoriously difficult to define, even among the most experienced neuropathologists.[23] An example of an OA with 1p loss by fluorescent in situ hybridization (FISH) is shown in Figure 24-5.

Taken together, existing data point to extensive genetic overlap between oligodendroglioma and OA in nontemporal sites. These tumors could represent variants of the same entity. One theory is that there are three molecular subsets of oligodendroglial tumors, which differ according to molecular rather than morphologic characteristics. A putative model of this phenotypic division would be composed of a set of predominately extratemporal oligodendroglial tumors with a loss of heterozygosity of 1p and 19q, and a set of predominately temporal lesions without these alterations. Each of these two sets would include morphologically defined oligodendroglioma and OA. A third potential set of OAs has TP53 mutations in the temporal lobe that are genetically similar to those found in astrocytoma. It is unknown, however, if OA and astrocytoma differ in other genetic alterations frequently described in astrocytomas such as CDKN2A deletions or a loss of heterozygosity of 22q.[23]

Although there are speculation and conflicting reports about the significance of 1p and 19q genetic alterations in relation to OAs, in vivo data will be required to draw firm conclusions regarding the effect of loss of heterozygosity of these elements. Further research will ultimately delineate exact molecular profiles for different tumor subtypes, and this clarification will likely lead to tailored genetic therapies for specific OAs and anaplastic OAs.

THERAPY

General Medical Therapy

Corticosteroids provide symptomatic improvement in most patients with increased intracranial pressure from edema. The effects of corticosteroids appear within 24 to 48 hours after the initial administration and usually peak at 1 week. Steroids produce a significant reduction in brain tumor volume and an even greater reduction in peritumoral edema, but they are not without pitfalls. The side effects of long-term glucocorticoids are well known and have the potential to cause disability greater than that produced by the tumor itself, particularly in the form of insomnia, steroid-induced (proximal) myopathy, facial adiposity, osteoporotic compression fractures, and non–dose-related risk of aseptic necrosis of the hip.[25]

Mannitol given as a bolus (0.25 to 1 g/kg every 4 to 6 hours) can acutely reduce symptoms associated with peritumoral edema. Unless followed by surgical debulking or successful cytotoxic therapy, its maximum length of benefit is usually measured in weeks. In general, the management of low-grade invasive gliomas is controversial, because the natural history of these lesions might include long periods of clinical quiescence.[25]

Seizures are prevalent in patients with glioma, particularly in slowly growing, low-grade gliomas, and require adequate management. Clinicians should recognize the possibility that seizures could be caused by hyponatremia, hypoglycemia, and hypocalcemia, as well as by mass effect. Seizures are generally managed with standard anticonvulsants, including phenytoin, phenobarbital, primidone, gabapentin, lamotrigine, carbamazepine, valproic acid, and clonazepam. Anticonvulsants, which are generally dose dependent, can interact with drugs that are commonly given to patients with brain tumors to produce adverse effects, some of which are drowsiness, dizziness, ataxia, nausea, vomiting, confusion, constipation, tremor, hypersalivation, and blurred vision.

Surgery

Currently, no short-term alternatives to open operation exist for alleviating the symptoms of brain tumors that have not responded to steroids and anticonvulsants. Surgery has several roles in the management of patients with anaplastic oligodendroglial and anaplastic OA, and current opinion favors early surgery for diagnosis and determination of appropriate adjuvant therapy for nearly all suspicious lesions.[25] Biopsy or resection provide tissue for classification, grading, and molecular characterization of the tumor. In symptomatic patients, surgical debulking can relieve symptoms of mass effect or neurologic deficits and can improve seizure control.[1] Additionally, many investigators found that total removal of tumor benefits patient survival or progression-free interval, whereas others do not agree with this approach.[5] Multivariate analyses in different retrospective series found that extent of resection is an independent prognostic factor for patients treated for oligodendroglioma or OA,[1] and maximal surgical resection has been associated with increased survival in essentially every large phase III study. In fact, survival data show that any degree of surgical resection larger than a biopsy improves patient survival.[5] Among infiltrative low-grade gliomas, optimal results are better achieved with complete rather than only partial tumor removal.

Similar considerations apply to recommendations for surgery for intermediate-grade gliomas (WHO grade III), with most but not all authors favoring maximal safe resection at initial diagnosis.[25] It appears that aggressive tumor resection improves the patient's neurologic function in addition to improving survival. Reported median survival times for anaplastic OA patients after surgery and high-dose radiation therapy are variable and range from 30 to 65 months.[2]

Surgery is also an option for people who have recurrent tumor. Recurrent growth after operative or adjuvant therapy occurs in most patients who have invasive glial tumors. Whether tumor growth is indicated by the patient's clinical deterioration or neuroradiographic studies, reoperation is often the cornerstone of therapy. The rationale for reoperation is the same as that for the original operation: confirmation of tumor histology and reduction of tumor mass without causing new neurologic deficits. In cases of infiltrative WHO grade II astrocytoma, oligodendroglioma, and mixed OA, it is also important to obtain confirmation or exclusion of malignant degeneration. If it occurs, additional therapy might be indicated.[25]

Radiation Therapy

Surgery followed by radiation therapy is the standard of care for most patients with malignant gliomas.[1] Some believe that postsurgical irradiation is the most effective treatment available for improving survival after surgery. Mounting evidence also suggests that additional radiation, given in the form of brachytherapy or radiosurgery, at initial diagnosis as a "boost" to standard radiation or at tumor recurrence, may improve patient outcome.[5]

Irradiation has been the cornerstone of therapy for malignant glioma patients since clinical trials published in the 1980s demonstrated improved survival outcome. Radiation is typically given following surgery, between 2 and 4 weeks after completion to allow for wound healing. Nevertheless, the role of radiation therapy in the treatment of OA and other low-grade astrocytomas remains controversial, ranging from finding a beneficial effect for patients with an otherwise poor prognosis, no beneficial effect for patients with low-grade astrocytoma, a slight survival advantage for those with incompletely resected tumors who received radiation therapy postoperatively, inconclusive findings, and the finding that the higher dose group has a lower quality of life.[10] However, few retrospective data exist regarding radiation dose or volume effects for anaplastic oligodendroglioma or mixed OA.

Some data suggest that there is an incremental benefit in survival when radiation is used to augment surgery and when chemotherapy is added to surgery plus radiation for patients who have anaplastic oligodendroglioma or mixed gliomas. The data also indicate that patients with pure anaplastic oligodendroglioma fare better than patients with anaplastic mixed gliomas when they are treated with the combination of surgery, radiation, and chemotherapy. Both groups do significantly better than patients who have pure anaplastic astrocytoma.[1]

The use of radiation therapy has to be carefully considered because of the risk of neurocognitive impairment in long-term survivors with WHO grade II tumors. It has been shown that radiation given in moderate doses (45 to 59 Gy) is unlikely to produce severe side effects in the short term, yet long-term results are unknown.[10]

Because of the high risk of cognitive impairment and other deleterious complications of radiation therapy, whole-brain irradiation, which has not been found to confer a survival advantage over focal radiation, is not used to treat OA or anaplastic astrocytoma.[5] Additionally, dose escalation combined with conventional radiation therapy techniques in high-grade or low-grade gliomas has produced increased toxicity with no improvement in survival.[1]

In an attempt to ameliorate the side effects of providing conventional doses of irradiation and to avoid unwanted sequelae, research strategies have been devised to modify the impact of the radiation dose used. These methods include radiation delivery either by dividing the daily dose (hyperfractionation) or by accelerated delivery. The goal of these approaches is to reduce toxic effects on normal tissue while delivering a higher total radiation dose.[5]

Brachytherapy and radiosurgery are radiation techniques that were developed in the hope of improving local disease control. Stereotactic radiosurgery is particularly suited to well-circumscribed lesions. Single-dose stereotactic radiosurgery can potentially produce high rates of local tumor control for such lesions. Low- and intermediate-grade gliomas are among the proposed targets of stereotactic radiosurgery, although improved outcomes have not been definitively shown for radiosurgery as a primary therapy or in the adjuvant setting. Surgery is likely to provide more rapid resolution of symptoms than radiosurgery.

Brachytherapy involves the placement of radioactive implants (i.e., interstitial brachytherapy) or the instillation of radioactive solutions or suspensions into preexisting cavities (i.e., intracavitary brachytherapy). Interstitial brachytherapy uses removable ^{125}I, ^{192}Ir, and ^{252}Cf sources placed directly into the tumor.[25] The interest in focal therapy has been driven by the knowledge that the principal pattern of treatment failure for malignant gliomas is tumor recurrence within 2 cm of the original tumor site, occurring in approximately 80% to 90% of patients. Brachytherapy and radiosurgery increase the focal doses of radiation to the tumor bed, whereas normal tissue tolerance limits the dose delivered by standard external-beam radiation therapy.[5]

Chemotherapy

Studies have shown that chemotherapy is useful for treating patients with primary oligodendroglioma or OA,[10] although more data support the use of adjuvant chemotherapy for patients with grade III tumors. The true effectiveness of chemotherapeutic treatment of anaplastic OA is, however, difficult to assess because of the small number of these tumors in the reported series. Almost all studies have evaluated mixed case groups composed of oligodendroglioma and OA.[2] Even though there is no standard of care for recurrent disease, chemotherapy is used to treat patients with tumor recurrence and, in the case of OA, after radiation therapy.[5]

A phase II study evaluated the benefits and toxicity of a combined regimen of procarbazine, lomustine, and vincristine (PCV) in 26 patients in the setting of low-grade oligodendroglioma and OA that were recurrent after being treated with surgery alone or with surgery and radiation therapy combined. Exclusion criteria were a histologic diagnosis of anaplastic oligodendroglioma or anaplastic OA (WHO grade III tumors). The study results suggested that PCV chemotherapy is effective in the treatment of recurrent low-grade oligodendroglioma and OA.[24]

For newly diagnosed low-grade oligodendroglioma and OA, the usefulness and timing of chemotherapy remain to be fully elucidated. Although responses to PCV have been reported, it is unknown if chemotherapy is superior to radiation therapy in symptomatic patients with measurable disease revealed by CT or MRI after surgery.[24]

Available data showing that anaplastic oligodendroglioma and anaplastic OA are chemosensitive with a favorable preirradiation response to chemotherapy are largely based on the fact that anaplastic oligodendroglioma and mixed OA are particularly sensitive to the combination of procarbazine, lomustine (CCNU), and vincristine, reported initially by Levin et al.[1,14] To date, adjuvant chemotherapy following irradiation with the three-drug regimen—PCV—has become a commonly accepted treatment for anaplastic astrocytoma, oligodendroglioma, and OA.[5]

Kirby et al[11] described the use of PCV neoadjuvant to radiation in a group of patients with malignant glioma. In a subset of patients with anaplastic astrocytoma or anaplastic OA, three out of seven patients responded to chemotherapy with a 58% 2-year survival. Jeremic et al[9] treated 23 patients with anaplastic mixed gliomas (WHO grade III) with PCV chemotherapy adjuvant to surgery and radiation. High response rates (83%) and a 5-year survival rate of 52% were seen in this group of patients also, as was a trend toward better survival among those with pure anaplastic oligodendrogliomas versus anaplastic mixed tumors.[1]

Other researchers found that at recurrence, a second course of PCV chemotherapy demonstrated a degree of efficacy, and reoperation was recommended as a favorable strategy to lengthen the survival time of anaplastic OA patients.[2]

Eventual relapse is almost an inevitability for patients with mixed glioma. For a total of 151 cycles in one study, the PCV regimen was administered every 8 weeks to patients with recurrent low-grade tumors as follows: lomustine, 110 mg/m^2 administered orally on day 1; procarbazine, 60 mg/m^2 administered orally on days 8 through 21; vincristine, 1.4 mg/m^2 administered intravenously (to a maximum of 2 mg) on days 8 and 29. PCV was discontinued after the sixth cycle, when the patient was responding, the disease was stable, or the tumor progressed. Most patients with either progressive disease while on PCV or recurrent tumor after discontinuation of PCV were treated with second-line chemotherapy or radiation therapy. Overall, the study results suggested that recurrent low-grade oligodendroglioma and OA, like anaplastic tumors, respond to PCV but eventually relapse.[24]

Levin et al recently analyzed findings from a phase III randomized study of post–radiation therapy chemotherapy that compared α-difluoromethyl ornithine; eflornithine (DFMO) plus PCV versus PCV for treating anaplastic gliomas, including patients with anaplastic OA. The addition of DFMO to the nitrosourea-based PCV regimen demonstrated a sustained benefit in survival for anaplastic glioma patients. Analyses after 10 years found that DFMO-PCV median survival of 6.3 years (49:114 events) was superior to the 5.1 years for PCV alone (55:114 events). The difference in survival over the first 2 years of study (hazard ratio 0.53, $P = .02$) supports the conclusion that DFMO adds to the survival advantage of PCV chemotherapy for anaplastic glioma and, in particular, anaplastic astrocytoma.[15]

Another study enrolled 32 patients with newly diagnosed anaplastic OA (median age 41 years; range 19 to 63; median Karnofsky score, 90; range 70 to 100). Patients were treated with cisplatin (109 mg/m^2) and BCNU (160 mg/m^2) on a regimen that began during the first week postsurgery. Treatment was administered every 6 weeks (5 scheduled cycles) for a total of 127 cycles. After the second cycle of chemotherapy, all patients received radiation therapy (56.5 Gy). The median time to tumor progression and the median survival time for the whole group of patients was 54.6 and 70.1 months, respectively, suggesting that the schedule of treatment provided a durable response in a selected group of anaplastic OA patients.[2] One concept driving the use of early postsurgical preirradiation cisplatin and BCNU chemotherapy is the opportunity to take advantage of alterations of the blood-brain barrier that occur immediately after tumor resection,[2] although it is possible that the presence of glioma per se disrupts the blood-brain barrier.

Boiardi et al[2] evaluated a group of 71 patients with anaplastic gliomas (WHO grade III) treated with neoadjuvant CCNU and cisplatin. The 30 patients with anaplastic OA or OA had a mean survival of 6 years, significantly better than patients with anaplastic astrocytoma (mean survival 3.2 years). No survival difference between patients with anaplastic OA or OA was noted.

Temozolomide is a relatively new alkylating agent that has demonstrated clinical antitumor activity and a relatively well-tolerated safety profile in phase I and II trials in patients with various advanced cancers, including malignant gliomas. Temozolomide is rapidly absorbed after oral administration and undergoes spontaneous hydrolysis and physiologic pH to its active metabolite 3-methyl-(triazen-1-yl)imidazole-4-carboxamide (MTIC).[29]

An open-label, multicenter phase II trial enrolled 162 patients (intent-to-treat [ITT] population). After central histologic review, 111 patients were confirmed to have had an anaplastic astrocytoma or anaplastic mixed OA. Chemotherapy-naive patients were treated with temozolomide, 200 mg/m^2/day. Patients previously treated with chemotherapy received temozolomide, 150 mg/m^2/day; the dose could be increased to 200 mg/m^2/day in the absence of grade 3 or 4 toxicity. Therapy was administered orally on the first 5 days of a 28-day cycle.[29]

Progression-free survival (PFS) at 6 months, the primary protocol endpoint, was 46% (95% confidence interval, 38% to 54%). The median PFS was 5.4 months, and PFS at 12 months was 24%. The median overall survival was 13.6 months, and the 6- and 12-month survival rates were 75% and 56%, respectively. The objective response rate determined by independent central review of gadolinium-enhanced MRI scans of the ITT population was 35% (8% complete response [CR], 27% partial response [PR]), with an additional 26% of patients with stable disease (SD). The median PFS for patients with stable disease was 4.4 months, with 33% progression free at 6 months. Maintenance of progression free status and objectively assessed response (CR/PR/SD) were both associated with health-related quality-of-life benefits. Adverse events were mild to moderate, with hematologic side effects occurring in less than 10% of patients. The investigators concluded that temozolomide demonstrated good single-agent activity and an acceptable safety profile, and they documented health-related quality of life benefits in patients with recurrent anaplastic astrocytoma.[29]

Additionally, there was no difference in efficacy in patients with anaplastic astrocytoma or anaplastic OA tumors. This is significant because the drug is effective in the more difficult-to-treat anaplastic astrocytoma histologic tumors, which have been less chemosensitive than anaplastic OA tumors.[29] Also, Chinot et al found an improved response to temozolomide in patients with anaplastic oligodendroglioma (AO) versus anaplastic OA. The authors found that temozolomide is safe and effective for treating recurrent AO and anaplastic OA.[6]

Temozolomide has a relatively nontoxic profile. Its most common adverse effects are nausea, vomiting, headache, fatigue, and constipation. The noncumulative toxicity and favorable adverse events profile of temozolomide make this agent a logical choice against recurrent malignant astrocytomas and suggest that, unlike nitrosoureas, it could be used effectively at relapse.[29]

Experimental cytotoxic and cytostatic agents are increasingly being developed and evaluated with the hopes of being able to abrogate the inevitable progression of gliomagenesis in patients with gliomas.

Table 24-2 illustrates the difficulties inherent in presenting a meaningful analysis of the available data in the literature and illustrates the fact that not much has changed since Shaw wrote about the "paucity of medical literature devoted to mixed gliomas of the central nervous system" nearly 10 years ago.[22] There are discrepancies in the literature regarding enrollment criteria, numbers of patients enrolled, histologic diagnoses, percentage of astrocytic or oligodendrogliomal cells in a specimen used to define a mixed glioma, treatments given, doses given, and all other parameters essential to ascertaining the statistical significance of study results.

PROGNOSIS

Despite uniform definitions of pure versus mixed oligodendroglioma, as well as the criteria for diagnosing high-grade (anaplastic) versus low-grade tumors remaining elusive from a prognostic standpoint the presence of an oligodendroglial component in a malignant glioma predicts longer survival times for patients treated with surgery and radiation therapy with or without chemotherapy.[1] In contrast, although it could be assumed that in OA the astrocytic component implies a less favorable prognosis, most studies could not confirm differences in outcome between oligodendroglioma and OA[18] (see Table 24-2).

Overall, the outlook for patients who have OA is likely somewhere between the outlook for those with low-grade astrocytoma and those who have pure oligodendrogliomal tumors. Although both pure oligodendroglioma and OA respond to chemotherapy, pure tumors are likely to be more chemosensitive. Thus the degree to which the tumor has oligodendroglioma cells probably dictates its chemosensitivity and prognosis.[27]

The median survival time of patients with OA after surgical intervention ranges from 6 to 8 years with marked variation. Shaw et al showed a median survival of 6.3 years and 5- and 10-year survival rates of 58% and 32%, respectively.[27] Harbingers of a longer survival include gross-total surgical removal of the tumor; lack of preoperative neurologic deficit; long duration of symptoms before surgery; seizures as a presenting symptom; and having had surgery in recent decades.[13] Almost all would agree, however, that young age at the time of

TABLE 24-2 Data from Various Studies

Authors	Study Type/Time	N	Age (yr)	Histologic Diagnosis	KPS	Previous RT	Previous Chemotherapy
Jeremic et al[9]	Phase II 1988–1993	23	≥18	AO = 18 AOA = 5	≥50	No	No
Shaw et al[22]	Retrospective 1960–1982	71	10–73	Mostly (>50%) astrocytoma 14:71 Mostly oligodendroglioma 28:71 (39%) Equal astrocytoma + oligodendroglioma 29:71 (41%)	—	—	—
Kyritsis et al[12]	Consecutive cases 1988–1992	544	—	AO = 22 AOA = 221 Mixed or low grade AOA = 31	—	Initial cases 2:12	—
Levin et al[15]	Phase II 1988–1992	90	18–67	AA = 69 AOA = 14 AO = 7	≥60	—	—
Buckner et al[4]	Phase II 1994–1998	31	23–62	Low-grade oligodendroglioma or mixed oligoastrocytoma	—	—	—
Winger et al[28]	Consecutive cases 1982–1987	285	≥18	GBM = 188 AA = 76 AG, mixed = 11 AO = 1—all newly diagnosed supratentorial tumors	—	Yes, 17 wk postsurgery	—
Bouffet et al[3]	Pilot study (chemotherapy) 1988	23	≥16	Oligodendroglioma Oligoastrocytoma	≥50	8:23	Acceptable for enrollment
Yung et al[29]	Phase II	162; 111 with acceptable histology	≥18	AA = 97 (60%) AOA = 14 (9%) Other histologies excluded from analysis	≥70	100% 162:162	Nitrosourea-based 97:162 (60%) Chemo-naïve 65:162 (40%)

Authors	Radiation Regimen	Chemotherapy Regimen	Surgery Performed	Overall Response	Complete Response
Jeremic et al[9]	60 Gy 30 daily fractions (30 days)	Given 2 wk after RT Procarbazine 60 mg/m² Days 1–14 CCNU 100 mg/m² Day 1 Vincristine 1.4 mg/m² Days 1 + 8 (max, 2 mg) 1 cycle = 6 wk (up to 6 cycles or progression; toxicity-limited)	100% (including biopsy)	83%	14 (61%)

TABLE 24-2	Data from Various Studies—cont'd				
Authors	Radiation Regimen	Chemotherapy Regimen	Surgery Performed	Overall Response	Complete Response
Shaw et al [22]	66:71 (93%)	—	100%	—	—
Kyritsis et al[12]	Initial AO 5:8 ACCF; 3:8 C Initial AOA 7:12 ACCF; 4:12 C 1:12 none Recurrent AO: 10:12 C; 2:12 ACCF Recurrent AOA: 5:6 C; 1:6 ACDCF	Initial AO = PCV 7:8 (3–6 cycles) 1:8 MTX and CTX Initial AOA = PCV 12:12 (2 to 7 cycles) Recurrent AO = PCV 9:12 1:12 PCV/DFMO 4:12 5-FU/CPL/PB Recurrent AOA; 10 different regimens	Initial AO 8:8 Initial AOA 12:12 Recurrent AO 12:12 Recurrent AOA 6:6	—	Initial AO 1:8 Initial AOA 2:12 Recurrent AO 1:12 Recurrent AOA 0:6
Levin et al[15]	60 Gy total dose (2-Gy fractions) Reduced after radiation effects to 57 Gy (1.9 fractions)	Given during RT Carboplatin 33 mg/m² IV 1.75 hr before RT; total dose = 990 mg/m² PCV 4 wk post-RT CCNU 110 mg/m² orally, day 1 Procarbazine 60 mg/m² orally, days 8–21 Vincristine 1.4 mg/m² IV, days 8 + 29 6 cycles every 6 wk	GTR 20:90 (22%) Subtotal resection 45:90 (50%) Biopsy 25:90 (28%)		
Buckner et al[4]	After chemotherapy (within 10 wk or disease progression) 50.4 Gy (1:8 Gy fractions/day) Then 9 Gy in 5 fractions 18 patients = 59 Gy 5 patients = 54 Gy 2 patients = 50.4 Gy 1 patient = 50.7 Gy	PCV CCNU 130 mg/m² orally, day 1 Procarbazine 75 mg/m² orally, days 8–21 Vincristine 1.4 mg/m² IV, days 8 + 29 6 cycles every 8 wk	Biopsy or subtotal resection	—	—
Winger et al[28]	Uniform for most patients 4400 cGy in 22 fractions to whole brain 1400 cGy in 8 fractions as focal boost over 6 wk Patients divided into those who received adequate (≥5000) cGy to tumor or those who did not	—	GTR Biopsy Subtotal resection Subtotal resection with lobectomy	—	—

TABLE 24-2 Data from Various Studies—cont'd

Authors	Radiation Regimen	Chemotherapy Regimen	Surgery Performed	Overall Response	Complete Response
Bouffet et al[3]	None	PCV CCNU 110 mg/m² orally, day 1 Vincristine 1.4 mg/m² days 8 and 29 Procarbazine 60 mg/m² orally, days 8–21 Ondansetron (8 mg), day 1 after CCNU and day 8 IV before procarbazine and vincristine Metroclopramide during procarbazine, but replaced by ondansetron if nausea/vomiting	—	16:23 (69%)	2:23 (9%)
Yung et al[29]	—	For chemo-naïve patients Temozolomide 200 mg/m² orally/day For patients with previous chemotherapy 150 mg/m² orally/day days 1–5 of 28-day cycle	110 patients at initial diagnosis; 30 patients at relapse	—	13:162 (8%) PFS range 11 mo to >2 yr 7 patients had CR >16 mo

Authors	Partial Response	Median Survival	1–15 Yr Overall Survival	1–15 Yr PFS Survival	Remarks
Jeremic et al[9]	5 (22%)	Not available	Yr 1 = 100% Yr 2 = 100% Yr 3 = 78% Yr 4 = 61% Yr 5 = 52%	Yr 1 = 100% Yr 2 = 100% Yr 3 = 70% Yr 4 = 52% Yr 5 = 52%	
Shaw et al[22]	—	5.8 yr	Yr 5 = 55% Yr 10 = 29% Yr 15 = 17%	—	
Kyritsis et al[12]	Initial AO 3:8 Initial AOA 3:12; SD 7:12 Recurrent AO 3:12; PD 5:12 Recurrent AOA 2:6	—	—	—	—
Levin et al[15]	—	All AG patients = 28.1 mo AA = 27.8 mo AO + AOA = 40 mo			
Buckner et al[4]	—	—	Yr 1 = 100% Yr 2 = 96% Yr 5 = 89%	Yr 1 = 91% Yr 2 = 62% Yr 5 = Unknown	
Winger et al[28]	—	Analysis by variable Age: 18–44 yr, 70:285, 107 wk Age 45–65 yr; 136:285, 42 wk Age ≥65 yr; 79:285, 23 wk Biopsy only, 19 wk Partial resection with or without lobectomy, 41 and 47 wk GTR, 76 wk Histology GBM = 32 wk AA = 63 wk AOA = 57 wk AO = 278 wk With RT = 48 wk Without RT = 17 wk	Yr 5 = 55% Yr 10 = 29%	—	

TABLE 24-2	Data from Various Studies—cont'd				
Authors	Partial Response	Median Survival	1–15 Yr Overall Survival	1–15 Yr PFS Survival	Remarks
Bouffet et al[3]	14:23 (61%)	17:23 patients survived with median follow-up of 17 mo 5:23 died of progressed disease 1 lost to follow-up	—	–	–

Yung et al[29]	44:162
	Median PFS = 11 mo
		ITT patients: 5.4 mo
		Eligible histology: 5.5 mo
			ITT patients
			  13.6 mo
			  6 mo = 75%
			  12 mo = 56%
			Eligible histology
			  14.5 mo
			  AA (78%); AOA
			  (79%)
				ITT patients
				  6 mo = 46%
				Eligible histology
				  6 mo = 48%
					Median PFS for pts with SD = 4.4 mo
					PFS at 6 mo for SD patients (33%)
					End point = PFS at 6 mo and safety profile
					≥20% oligodendroglial component defined mixed glioma (AOA)
					Only baseline KPS was significant prognostic factor

AACF, accelerated fractionated radiation therapy; AG, anaplastic glioma; AO, anaplastic oligodendroglioma; AOA, anaplastic oligoastrocytoma; C, conventional radiation therapy; CCNU, CTX, cytoxan; 5-FU, 5-fluorouracil; DFMO, α-difluoromethylornithine; GBM, glioblastoma multiforme; GTR, gross-total resection; IV, intravenously; KPS, Karnofsky performance scale score; MTX, methotrexate; PCV, procarbazine, lomustine, and vincristine; PD, progression; PFS, progression-free survival; pts, patients; RT, radiation therapy; SD, stable disease.

diagnosis is by far the most important factor that correlates with a long survival in OA, and seizures as a presenting symptom are correlated with a better prognosis. Focal deficits and changes in personality are indicative of a worse prognosis.[10]

QUALITY OF LIFE ASSESSMENTS

Long-term survival after diagnosis of anaplastic OA and OA is common, so the long-term impact of treatments on function and quality of life in these patients is of particular concern.[2] However, clinical trials of new anticancer agents do not adequately assess potential clinical benefits for patient function other than survival and time to tumor progression. The minimal survival benefit of existing treatments highlights the need for other measures of patient outcome, including ability to function and quality of life.[17] In the case of brain cancer, which is characterized by progressive impairments of mental function, a beneficial treatment may be one that stabilizes or slows the progression of worsening symptoms, whether or not overall survival is extended. A multifaceted assessment of the three components proposed by the WHO in 1980 to classify the effects of neurologic disease on the patient—impairment, disability, and handicap—can be used to document patient response to treatment, to distinguish the effects of tumor and treatment on brain function, and to provide a basis for implementing intervention strategies in patients with neurologic compromise.[17]

The major instrument used at The University of Texas MD Anderson Cancer Center for functional assessments of the status of patients with brain tumors is the Functional Assessment of Cancer Therapy Instrument (FACT-Br). This questionnaire is given to the patient to fill out and is based on a 5-level rating scale. The instrument assesses self-perceptions about the patient's physical well-being, social and family well-being, emotional well-being, and functional well-being and also includes a section dealing with additional concerns such as seizures; feelings of independence; changes in personality; and ability to read, write, and drive. Additional tests assess attention span (Digit Span; Wechsler, 1981); graphomotor speed (Digit Symbol; Wechsler, 1981); memory (Hopkins Verbal Learning Test); verbal fluency (Controlled Oral Word Association); visual-motor scanning speed (Trail Making Test Part A); executive function (Trail Making Test Part B); and Activities of Daily Living (ADL), Functional Independence Measure. These tests involve repeating numbers forward and backward, coding symbols for numbers, measuring immediate recall, recognition of actual words from distractors, connecting dots, placing pegs into holes as rapidly as possible, and other tasks.[17]

Instruments for measuring health-related quality of life also include the European Organization for Research and Treatment of Cancer Quality of Life Questionnaire (EORTC QLQ-C30) or the MOS Short-Form Health Survey (SF-36), a self-report questionnaire developed in the United States. This is made up of 36 items, organized into eight multi-item scales to assess physical functioning, limitations due to physical health problems, bodily pain, general health perception, vitality, social functioning, limitations due to emotional problems, and general mental health.[8]

References

1. Bauman GS, Cairncross JG: Multidisciplinary management of adult anaplastic oligodendrogliomas and anaplastic mixed oligo-astrocytomas. Semin Radiat Oncol 11:170–180, 2001.

2. Boiardi A, Eoli M, Salmaggi A, et al: Cisplatin and BCNU chemotherapy for anaplastic oligoastrocytomas. J Neurooncol 49:71–75, 2000.

3. Bouffet E, Jouvet A, Thiesse P, et al: Chemotherapy for aggressive or anaplastic high grade oligodendrogliomas and oligoastrocytomas: better than a salvage treatment. Br J Neurosurg 12:217–222, 1998.

4. Buckner JC, Gesme D Jr, O'Fallon JR, et al: Phase II trial of procarbazine, lomustine, and vincristine as initial therapy for patients with low-grade oligodendroglioma or oligoastrocytoma: efficacy and associations with chromosomal abnormalities. J Clin Oncol 21:251–255, 2003.

5. Burton EC, Prados MD: Malignant glioma. Curr Treat Options Oncol 1:459–468, 2000.

6. Chinot O-L, Honore S, Dufour H, et al: Safety and efficacy of temozolomide in patients with recurrent anaplastic oligodendrogliomas after standard radiotherapy and chemotherapy. J Clin Oncol 19:2449–2455, 2001.

7. Coons SW, Johnson PC, Pearl DK: The prognostic significance of Ki-67 labeling indices for oligodendrogliomas. Neurosurgery 41:878–885, 1997.

8. Heimans JJ, Taphoorn MJB: Impact of brain tumour treatment on quality of life. J Neurol 249:955–960, 2002.

9. Jeremic B, Shibamoto Y, Grujicic D, et al: Combined treatment modality for anaplastic oligodendroglioma: a phase II study. J Neurooncol 43:179–185, 1999.

10. Kaye AH, Walker DG: Low grade astrocytomas: controversies in management. J Clin Neurosci 7:475–483, 2000.

11. Kirby S, Macdonald D, Fisher B, et al: Pre-radiation chemotherapy for malignant gliomas in adults. Can J Neurol Sci 23:123–127, 1996.

12. Kyritsis AP, Yung WKA, Bruner J, et al: The treatment of anaplastic oligodendrogliomas and mixed gliomas. Neurosurgery 32:365–371, 1993.

13. Laws ER Jr: Neurosurgical management of low-grade astrocytoma of the cerebral hemispheres. J Neurosurg 61:665–673, 1984.

14. Levin VA, Edwards MS, Wright DC, et al: Modified procarbazine CCNU and vincristine (PCV-3) combination chemotherapy in the treatment of malignant brain tumors. Cancer Treat Rep 64:237–241, 1980.

15. Levin VA, Yung WKA, Bruner J, et al: Phase II study of accelerated fractionation radiation therapy with carboplatin followed by PCV chemotherapy for the treatment of anaplastic gliomas. Int J Radiat Oncol Biol Phys 53:58–66, 2002.

16. Louis DN, Holland EC, Cairncross JG: Glioma classification: a molecular reappraisal. Am J Pathol 159:779–786, 2001.

17. Meyers CA, Hess KR: Multifaceted end points in brain tumor clinical trials: cognitive deterioration precedes MRI progression. Neurooncol, 5:89, 2003.

18. Mueller W, Hartmann C, Hoffmann A, et al: Genetic signature of oligoastrocytomas correlates with tumor location and denotes distinct molecular subsets. Am J Pathol 161:313–319, 2002.

19. Onda K, Davis RL, Shibuya M, et al: Correlation between the bromodeoxyuridine labeling index and the MIB-1 and Ki-67 proliferating cell indices in cerebral gliomas. Cancer 74:1921–1926, 1994.

20. Reifenberger G, Kros JM, Burger PC, et al: Anaplastic oligoastrocytoma. In Kleihues P, Cavenee WK (eds): World Health Organization Classification of Tumours: Pathology & Genetics; Tumors of the Nervous System. Lyon, France, IARC Press, 2000.

21. Reifenberger G, Kros JM, Burger PC, et al: Oligoastrocytoma. In Kleihues P, Cavenee WK (eds): World Health Organization Classification of Tumors: Pathology & Genetics; Tumours of the Nervous System. Lyon, France, IARC Press, 2000.

22. Shaw EG, Scheithauer BW, O'Fallon JR, et al: Mixed oligoastrocytomas: a survival and prognostic factor analysis. Neurosurgery 34:577–582, 1994.

23. Smith JS, Perry A, Borell TJ, et al: Alterations of chromosome arms 1p and 19q as predictors of survival in oligodendrogliomas, astrocytomas, and mixed oligoastrocytomas. J Clin Oncol 18:636–645, 2000.

24. Soffietti R, Ruda R, Bradac GB, et al: PCV chemotherapy for recurrent oligodendrogliomas and oligoastrocytomas. Neurosurgery 43:1066–1073, 1998.

25. Tatter SB: Neurosurgical management of low- and intermediate-grade gliomas. Semin Radiat Oncol 11:113–123, 2001.

26. Wacker MRT, Hoshino DK: The prognostic implications of histologic classification and bromodeoxyuridine labeling index of mixed gliomas. J Neuro-Oncol 19:113–122, 1994.

27. Walker DG, Kaye A: Diagnosis and management of astrocytomas/oligodendrogliomas and mixed gliomas: a review. Australasian Radiol 45:472–482, 2001.

28. Winger MJ, MacDonald DR, Cairncross JG: Supratentorial anaplastic gliomas in adults: the prognostic importance of extent of resection and prior low-grade glioma. J Neurosurg 71:487–493, 1989.

29. Yung WKA, Prados MD, Yaya-Tur R, et al: Multicenter phase II trial of temozolomide in patients with anaplastic astrocytoma or anaplastic oligoastrocytoma at first relapse. J Clin Oncol 17:2762–2771, 1999.

CHAPTER 25

EPENDYMOMA

Allan H. Friedman, Roger E. McLendon, James N. Provenzale, and Henry S. Friedman

DEMOGRAPHICS

Ependymomas account for 2.5% of all intracranial gliomas. They are the most common brain tumor in children younger than age 5 and the third most common brain tumor in patients younger than age 20, accounting for 10% of all brain tumors in the pediatric population. Although usually occurring sporadically, they can be associated with neurofibromatosis type II.

Younger children have a worse prognosis. It is unclear whether this is because the tumors are intrinsically more malignant, because there is a delay of radiation therapy in the younger age group, or because of the greater numbers of lateral fourth ventricular tumors occurring in younger children.

Subependymomas demonstrate clumps of nuclei separated by abundant cell processes. Their cellular density is low with the histologic picture dominated by the sea of fibrillary processes. Microcysts are often present in lesions ringing the foramen of Monro. Dense calcifications are common; especially in lesions of the fourth ventricle, hyalinized blood vessels and Rosenthal fibers may be seen. Even in high-grade tumors, the predetermined pattern of recurrence is localized regrowth.

SIGNS AND SYMPTOMS

The symptoms produced by ependymomas most commonly arise from obstruction of cerebrospinal fluid (CSF) but may result from brainstem compression, focal cerebral infiltrations, or focal cerebral distortion.[18,30,34]

Headaches are the most common symptom reported. The headaches are usually episodic and may be worse in the morning, even waking the patient from a sound sleep. Although often nondescript, the classic headache occurs in the occipital area and may be associated with nuchal rigidity. Paroxysmal vomiting not associated with a particular time of day or posture is often present. Children younger than age 2 experience lethargy, whereas older children suffer a change in personality marked by withdrawal and indifference.

The most common signs are the result of CSF obstruction (e.g., papilledema or enlarging head circumference in younger children). Ataxia, nystagmus, and sixth nerve dysfunction are also common with posterior fossa tumors. Less common are lower cranial nerve palsies or torticollis, reflecting tonsillar herniation. Supratentorial tumor may manifest as focal neurologic deficits or seizures, reflecting the region of the brain infiltrated or compressed.

RADIOGRAPHIC IMAGING

Radiographic imaging of an ependymoma reflects the inhomogeneity of the tumor and the presence of necrosis, cysts, and calcifications. Calcification is seen in 60% of infratentorial tumors, and areas of necrosis or cysts are seen in 80% of tumors. These tumors are often surrounded by peritumoral edema. Tumors originating from the walls of the fourth ventricle are amorphous and poorly defined. The tumor may ooze through the foramen of Luschka and even surround the brainstem (Figure 25-1). Hydrocephalus may be apparent on imaging studies. Supratentorial tumors are usually extraventricular. They are commonly cystic and approximately half contain areas of calcification. Areas of hemorrhage are not common.

An uncontrasted computed tomography (CT) scan reflects the tumors' heterogeneity. Necrosis and cysts are hypointense, whereas calcifications and areas of hemorrhage are hyperintense. Tumors usually contrast in an inhomogeneous fashion, but if the center is necrotic, the tumor may appear as an enhanced ring.

The anatomy of a fourth ventricular ependymoma is best seen on a sagittal magnetic resonance imaging (MRI) scan. Unlike the more common medulloblastoma, a cleft of CSF is often visible sandwiched between the top of the tumor and the roof of the fourth ventricle (Figure 25-2). Tumors tend to be hypointense to isointense on T1 imaging, but areas of hemorrhage or cysts may be hyperintense. Areas of calcification of blood flow are hypointense. Contrast enhancement is moderate and usually is homogeneous. The tumors are usually mild to moderately hyperintense on T2-weighted images (Figure 25-3).

Subependymomas are seen as nodular masses protruding into the ventricle. They can arise from any ventricular surface but have a propensity to arise near the foramen of Monro and/or walls of the fourth ventricle. These tumors often contain calcifications and may be cystic. Generally, they manifest little contrast enhancement, but exceptions to this rule are seen with fourth ventricular tumors.

GROSS PATHOLOGY

Tumors usually occur in the posterior fossa in children younger than age 3. Supratentorial tumors become more common as children get older, accounting for 40% of ependymomas by the time patients reach their teenage years. In adults ependymomas

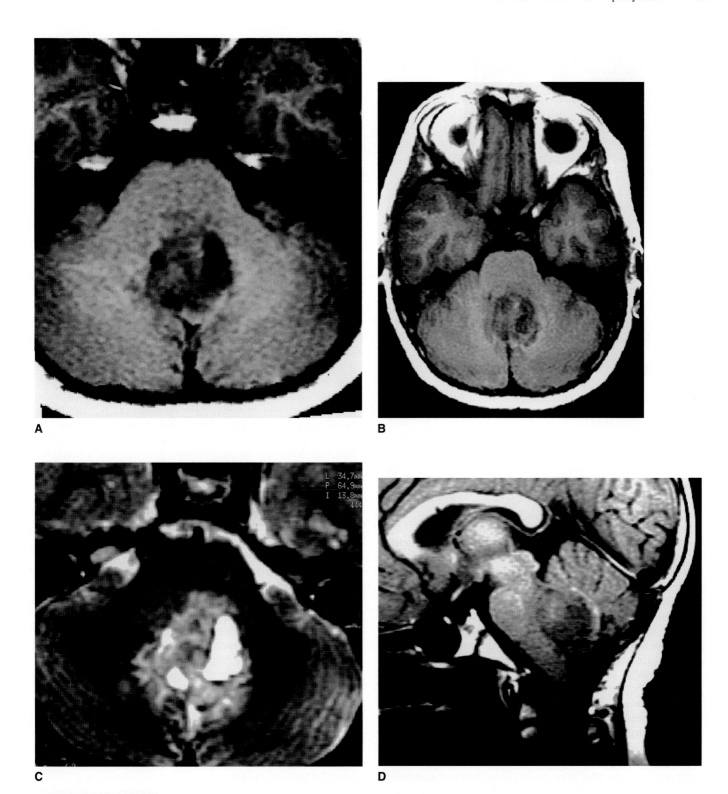

FIGURE 25-1 Fourth ventricle ependymoma in a 9-year-old girl with headache and vomiting. *A,* Axial unenhanced T1-weighted magnetic resonance (MR) image shows a mass filling the fourth ventricle. Note that the left half of the mass is hypointense, consistent with a cystic cavity. *B,* Axial contrast-enhanced T1-weighted MR image shows mild, inhomogeneous enhancement of the mass. *C,* Axial T2-weighted image of the mass shows that the mass is inhomogeneous and hyperintense to normal brain tissue. Note that the left half of the mass is markedly hyperintense, confirming that this portion of the mass is cystic. *D,* Sagittal contrast-enhanced T1-weighted MR image indicates that the mass fills the entire fourth ventricle and elevates the adjacent cerebellar vermis.

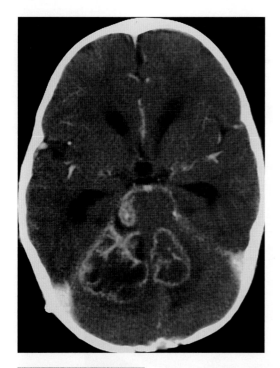

FIGURE 25-2 Extensive "anaplastic ependymoma" in a 2-year-old boy with intractable vomiting. Axial contrast-enhanced computed tomography image shows a rim-enhanced mass extending from the fourth ventricle through the foramen of Luschka and into the ambient cistern. Note the marked dilation of the temporal horns of the lateral ventricles.

are evenly split between those occurring along and those occurring below the tentorium.[1,9,10,13,17]

Fourth ventricular tumors most commonly originate from the caudal floor and project up into the ventricle. Rarely they originate from the lateral wall of that ventricle. These soft tumors mold themselves to the general shape of the fourth ventricle. They can originate from within the foramen of Luschka, spilling out into the cerebellopontine angle. Tumors can grow out from both foramen of Luschka and surround the brainstem. The tumors tend to be soft with a bosselated surface. Blood vessels and the lower cranial nerves may be trapped between lobules of tumor. Fortunately, these nerves and arteries are usually sandwiched between sheets of arachnoid.

Supratentorial tumors usually are in contact with a ventricular surface growing into the brain parenchyma but may arise from ependymal rests within the parenchyma. Supratentorial ependymomas tend to be relatively well demarcated from the surrounding brain. They often contain cysts, and approximately 50% contain calcium.

Subependymomas are usually incidentally discrete masses found protruding at the ventricular wall. Subependymomas can arise from any ventricular system but favor the lateral walls and roof of the fourth ventricle or the septum pellucidum close to the foramen magnum. These tumors tend to be more firm in consistency than ependymomas and have a lobulated surface that projects into the ventricle. Subependymomas often calcify.

Spinal seeding occurs in approximately 10% of patients. In less than 5% of patients the seeding is present at the time of the original diagnosis. A seeding is most likely to occur from tumors of the fourth ventricle or from anaplastic ependymomas. Disseminated disease is more common in pediatric patients. Horn[14] reported that 13% of 61 children had disseminated disease at diagnosis, and Pollock[27a] noted that 22% of patients had leptomeningeal disease at diagnosis.

HISTOLOGY

Light Microscopy

Ependymal cells are ciliated columnar epithelium of neuroectodermal origin that line the cerebral ventricles and the central canal of the spinal cord. These cells are embryologically related to astrocytes and oligodendroglia but at maturation demonstrate an epithelial appearance.

The World Health Organization (WHO) divides ependymomas into ependymomas (WHO grade II), anaplastic ependymomas (WHO grade III), subependymomas (WHO grade I), and myxopapillary ependymomas (WHO grade I). There are four histologic variants of WHO grade II ependymomas: cellular, papillary, clear cell, and tanycytic.

Ependymomas usually have uniform cells, infrequent mitosis, and little necrosis. The nuclei of ependymal cells are oval and contain dense clumps of chromatin as seen in other glial cells. Microscopic examination demonstrates a predominant glial pattern, studded with islands of cells demonstrating epithelial features, which make the diagnosis of ependymoma. Pseudorosettes are the most common epithelial feature seen. They appear as eosinophilic zones surrounding blood vessels. These eosinophilic zones are the result of cell processes containing cytoplasm lining up around blood vessels, with the cell nuclei ringing the cytoplasm peripherally. When sectioned along the axis of the blood vessel, these pseudorosettes appear as eosinophilic clefts. Rare true rosettes consist of cuboidal cells surrounding a clear lumen. On the luminal edge of the cells forming true rosettes, blepharoplasts, the phosphotungstic acid-hematoxylin (PTAH)-staining basal bodies of cilia may be seen under high-power microscopy. Although considered diagnostic of ependymomas, blepharoplasts usually only confirm a diagnosis that was already established from other features of the tumor.

A tanycyte is an immature, bipolar, glial fibrillary acidic protein (GFAP)-positive cell that may represent an intermediate phase in the development of an ependymomal cell. Tanycytic ependymomas comprise elongated bipolar cells. Microscopically, they appear as a sea of fibrillary processes separating isolated islands of nuclei.

Papillary ependymomas may be superficially difficult to distinguish from choroids plexus papilloma. Although the fronds of a choroids plexus papilloma consist of fingers of fibrosis tissue lined by a single layer of ependymal cells, the fronds of a papillary ependymoma contain ependymal cells sandwiched between the ependymal-coated surface.

Clear cell ependymomas have the same "fried egg" appearance as oligodendrogliomas. Light microscopy demonstrates small round nuclei surrounded by a clear halo of cytoplasm. Careful examination may reveal telltale surface-forming

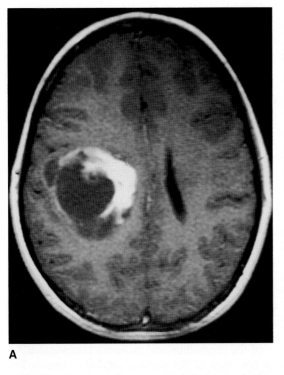

A

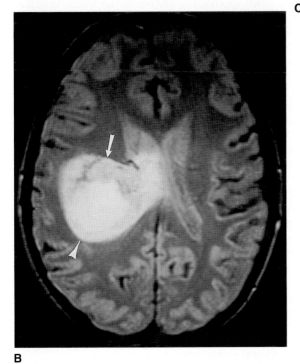

B

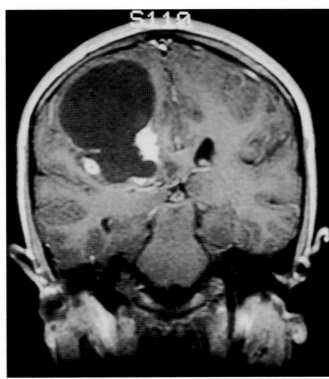

C

FIGURE 25-3 Supratentorial ependymoma in an 11-year-old girl with persistent headaches who was found to have papilledema on funduscopic examination. *A,* Axial contrast-enhanced T1-weighted magnetic resonance image shows a partially cystic, enhanced mass in the right frontal lobe. *B,* Axial fluid-attenuated inversion recovery (FLAIR) sequence of a cystic mass. *C,* Coronal contrast-enhanced T1-weighted magnetic resonance image shows a partially cystic, enhanced mass in the right frontal lobe.

epithelial structures. Electron microscopy demonstrates characteristic cilia, microvilli, and intracellular junctions.

As ependymal tumors become more aggressive, large areas of necrosis, nuclear pleomorphism, vascular proliferation, and frequent mitotic figures appear. These changes are more common in supratentorial tumors. In the WHO grading system, a grade III anaplastic astrocytoma is an ependymal tumor with evidence of anaplasia as defined by high cellularity, variable

nuclear atypia, marked mitotic activity, and prominent vascular proliferation. There are no quantitative criteria.

The lack of correlation between histologic grade and prognosis stems from a lack of a uniform grading system. Even using the 1993 WHO grading system, some authors have not found a difference in prognosis between grade II and grade III ependymomas. The literature does indicate that tumors with necrosis and an increased proliferative index associated with 10 mitoses in a high power field tend to have a worse prognosis.

Ho[13] used multivariate analysis of 13 histologic features and found that greater than 4 mitoses per high power field, necrosis, endothelial proliferation necrosis, and hypercellularity were significant in predicting an adverse outcome. The presence of two or more of these features predicted a worse patient survival. Others have noted that a higher level of GFAP staining and lower level of vimentin expression are associated with a better prognosis. It would appear that consistent correlation between histology and prognosis awaits a better definition of grade III ependymomas.

Electron Microscopy

Electron microscopy demonstrates cilia, basal bodies, tight intracellular junctions, and intracytoplasmic intermediate filaments. Intermediate filaments are present in small numbers in ependymal cells but become more abundant in ependymal tumor cells.

Immunohistochemistry

Positive staining for GFAP is usually, but not invariably, present in ependymomas. Staining for vimentin is usually positive, but staining for cytokeratin, Leu-7, and epithelial membrane antigen (EMA) is only occasionally positive.

MOLECULAR GENETICS

The most commonly reported genetic abnormalities in ependymomas are losses of chromosome 6q, 22q, and the X chromosome and gains of 1q or 9q. The fact that spinal ependymomas are more common in patients with neurofibromatosis type 2 (NF2) raises the possibility that ependymomas might harbor an abnormality in chromosome 22. The incidence of 22q abnormalities reported in the literature ranges from 16% to 60%, depending on tumor location and the age of the patient. The incidence of 22q abnormalities is much higher in spinal ependymomas. Of patients with allelic loss on 22q, those with mutations of the NF2 gene almost invariably harbor ependymomas of the spinal cord.[2,28]

Series looking at childhood tumors note that in 40% of cases no chromosomal imbalance is seen using comparative genomic hybridization. In cases with chromosomal imbalance, 6q is often lost. This abnormality has been noted in other cancers. The gain of 1q in childhood anaplastic ependymoma appears to be associated with posterior fossa tumors. Similarly, a loss of 17p was noted in 50% of tumors analyzed by microsatellite analysis.

DNA flow cytometry has not proven useful in predicting outcome in patients harboring an ependymoma, although Kotylo reported that the presence of a diploid DNA stemline predicted a worse outcome.

The intracerebral inoculation of newborn hamsters with simian virus 40 (SV-40) induces ependymomas and choroid plexus tumors. This simian virus was found to contaminate polio and adenovirus vaccines administered in 1955 to 1963. Large-scale epidemiologic studies have failed to show a correlation between polio virus vaccines and tumors. Using polymerase chain reaction (PCR), investigators have found evidence of the SV-40 genome in 0% to 90% of ependymomas sampled. The role of the virus in tumor induction is not known. The virus genome has been detected in various other tumors and in healthy individuals. Thus it is possible that the SV-40 virus can provide one step on the road to oncogenesis in ependymomas.

TREATMENT

Surgery

Although this chapter does not focus on the technical nuances of surgery, certain important points can be gleaned from the literature that will increase the success of a surgical resection. The goals of surgery are to make a histologic diagnosis, remove obstacles to CSF flow, and achieve a complete tumor resection. If the patient is lethargic from hydrocephalus, a ventriculostomy should be performed. A permanent shunt will not allow CSF drainage or pressure to be monitored. In almost half of patients with preoperative radiographic evidence for CSF obstruction, tumor resection will relieve the obstruction to CSF flow and obviate the need for placement of a permanent CSF shunt. Overdrainage of CSF through a ventriculostomy should be avoided because it can result in upward transtentorial herniation of the cerebellum and midbrain compression.*

Although resection of the inferior cerebellar vermis has been the standard approach to tumors of the fourth ventricle, this approach runs the risk of producing postoperation mutism. A better understanding of the anatomy of the inferior vermis and cerebellar tonsils has led surgeons to open the cerebellomedullary fissure bilaterally, freeing the tonsils from their attachment to the lower vermis and the medulla. This approach results in a large opening into the fourth ventricle and opens both foramen of Luschka. Surgery begins with a standard midline suboccipital craniotomy. Cervical laminectomy is done to expose tumor that extends through the foramen magnum into the cervical spine. The uvula, tonsillar, and medullotonsillar spaces are opened by lysing arachnoid adhesions. Supralateral retraction of the tonsils demonstrates attachment of the tela choroidea to the tenia along the foramen of Luschka. The posterior margin of the lateral recess is opened by cutting this membrane, freeing the tonsils from the medulla. Although the lower cranial nerves may appear hopelessly encased in tumor, it is not uncommon for these nerves to be preserved in a sandwich of arachnoid planes pushed ahead of the lobules of growing tumor. If these lobules are patiently decompressed respecting these arachnoid planes, the lower cranial nerves can be preserved by unfolding the arachnoid. More malignant tumors, which may invade the surface of the nerves, defy removal. Preoperative dexamethasone may reduce postoperative oropharyngeal motor apraxia.

The use of autologous material for watertight closure of the dura, as opposed to cadaveric material, reduces the incidence of postoperative aseptic meningitis and the need for a CSF shunt.

A review of the literature indicates that the perioperative mortality was approximately 8% by the late 1980s. Morbidity results from the technical problems inherent to surgery and damage to neurologic structures surrounding the tumor. Technical problems include infection, aseptic meningitis, CSF leak,

---

*References 3, 8, 10, 12, 15, 16, 20, 23, 29, 31, 33, and 34

pseudomeningocele, air embolism, stress gastric ulcers, and pressure injuries caused by patient position on the operating table. More specific to the surgery of fourth ventricular ependymoma are injuries to the floor of the fourth ventricle, brainstem arteries, and cranial nerves. Ependymomas are not encapsulated and often invade the obex of the fourth ventricle. Patients with injury to this area may manifest vocal cord paralysis, recurrent bouts of aspiration, pneumonia, difficulty swallowing, ataxia, or loss of respiratory drive in response to retained carbon dioxide. Injury to the floor of the fourth ventricle at the pontomedullary junction can produce a facial or abducent nerve palsy. A transient pseudobulbar palsy characterized by dysarthria, nystagmus, somnolence, emotional lability, mutism, and facial diplegia has been described. Injury of the midline structures of the cerebellum can result in a transient mutism with permanent scanning speech. Disruption of the spinal cerebellar tracts or cerebellar peduncles can produce ataxia and dysmetria. Although some surgeons have employed electrophysiologic monitoring of structures innervated by the cranial nerves to thwart dysfunctions, the efficacy of this strategy is unproven.

Although most reports in the literature are retrospective, in reviews of small series of patients the presence of residual disease seen on a postoperative imaging study has proven to be the most important negative prognostic factor (Table 25-1).

Tumor quantified on postoperative imaging is a better prediction of outcome than surgeon estimate of percentage of tumor removed. When a tumor recurs, it is most likely to recur locally, with fewer than 10% of cases manifesting a noncontiguous recurrence. Although complete resection is a laudable goal, it is accomplished in only 27% to 62% of patients. A complete resection is more commonly accomplished with supratentorial tumors than tumors of the fourth ventricle. Complete resection in young children of tumors spilling into the subarachnoid spaces around the brainstem may be particularly problematic. Secondary surgery can sometimes achieve a gross-total resection. Foreman accomplished a gross-total resection in four of five patients undergoing a second surgery.[8] Osterdoch attempted a second surgery in 12 of 16 patients with residual tumor.[21a] A gross-total resection was achieved in 10 patients at the cost of a single mortality and a second patient requiring a tracheostomy and gastrostomy. Some authors have commented that radiation therapy has made a second resection easier, although this observation has not been generally corroborated.

Radiation Therapy

It is often pointed out that a small number of tumors have been successfully treated without radiation therapy. The criteria for selecting patients who do not require postoperative radiation therapy have yet to be defined. Although no report of a randomized controlled study exists in the literature, a series of patients treated with radiation therapy demonstrates an improvement in survival when compared with historical controls. The literature indicates that more radiation is better in preventing tumor regrowth. However, higher doses of radiation are more likely to result in radiation necrosis of normal brain.

TABLE 25-1	Prognostic Factors and Degree of Surgical Resection			
Author (Year)	No. of Patients	Degree of Resection	Follow-up	Results
Sutton (1995)	45	>90%	5-yr PFS	60%
		<90%		21%
Rousseu (1993)	80	GTR	5-yr PFS	51%
		LGTR		26%
Perilongo (1997)	88	GTR	10-yr PFS	57%
		LGTR		11.8%
Healey (1991)	19	GTR	5-yr PFS	75%
		LGTR		0%
Pollack (1995)	37	GTR	5-yr PFS	68%
		LGTR		9%
Horn (1999)	83	GTR		60%
		LGTR		29%
Robertson (1998)	32	>1.5 cm	5-yr PFS	66%
		<1.5 cm		11%
Timmerman (2000)	55	GTR	3-yr PFS	83.3%
		LGTR		38.5%
Duffner (1998)	48	GTR	5-yr survival	61%
		LGTR		30%
Nazar (1990)	32	GTR	5-yr survival	86.7%
		LGTR		29.5%
Vanuytsel (1992)	93	GTR	5-yr PFS	58%
		LGTR		36%
Papadopoulus (1990)	26	GTR	5-yr survival	60%
		LGTR		30%

GTR, Gross-total resection; LGTR, less than gross-total resection; PFS, progression-free survival.

Studies reviewing dose-response data point to an optimal dose between 4500 and 5000 rads. This dose should be administered in 1.6- to 1.8-Gy fractions in fewer than 50 days. The issues being explored in radiation therapy are the size of the field to be treated and the consequences of delaying radiation therapy in young children.[4,5,18,19,22–26,30,32]

The volume of tissue to be treated has been debated in the literature. The need for whole neural axis radiation therapy has been challenged. Less than 15% of tumors disseminate, and most tumors recur locally. Merchant studied 104 patients who had no evidence of disseminated tumor before radiation therapy.[18] Of six failures seen at 17 months, five were within the radiated field. Paulino noted that of 17 patients with localized posterior fossa ependymomas that progressed following radiation therapy, 3 demonstrated distant metastases on recurrence that did not also manifest progression of the local tumor.[24] Robertson also found no cases with isolated distant relapses in patients who had no distal tumor seeding.[29] As a precautionary note, Rousseau[29a] did note that 4 of 43 patients receiving only local radiation failed with isolated spinal metastases, and Healey[12] found that disseminated disease was present at first relapse in 8 of 61 patients who initially had isolated tumors.

The risk of conformal field radiation is recurrence of tumor just beyond the radiation field. Merchant treated 36 patients with 56 to 60 Gy to 1.5 cm beyond the surgical resection site as residual tumor.[18] At mean follow-up of 14 months, there were two recurrences, both within the radiation field and with no margin of recurrence.

Nevertheless, the consensus from the literature appears to be that there is no advantage to treating more than the local tumor bed with radiation therapy in patients who do not have metastatic disease (Table 25-2).

The literature also states that patients treated with local radiation have better full-scale intelligence scores and verbal scores following therapy than patients treated with whole neural axis radiation and less musculoskeletal retardation and pituitary dysfunction. With three-dimensional planning and intensity-modulated and conformal radiation techniques, less radiation is administered to the normal brain, the hypothalamus–pituitary axis, and the cochlea. It is still the practice to treat patients harboring spinal metastases with craniospinal radiation, although the evidence that this is more effective than focal radiation to the radiographically defined disease is inconclusive.

Stereotactic radiosurgery is a promising adjuvant treatment for patients who have not had a complete surgical resection or who have recurrent disease. Aggrawal et al report progression-free survival at 14 to 40 months' follow-up in four of five patients with an incomplete tumor resection.[1a] Jawahar treated 22 patients harboring an anaplastic ependymoma with radiosurgery to a marginal dose of 32 Gy and found a reduction or stabilization of tumor in 68% and 5-year local control in 52%. Stafford treated 17 recurrent sites in 12 patients with a marginal dose of 12.24 Gy. Of three treatment failures, two were in field and one was marginal. Grabb et al noted fewer good results from stereotactic radiation.[10a] A few centers have advocated fractionated radiosurgery, but there are only very preliminary data available in the efficacy of this technique in the treatment of ependymomas. Similarly, low activity ^{125}I-seeds have been implanted at the time of surgery in a small number of patients.

The fractionated dose is most often given as 1.6 to 1.8 Gy per day. Based on the hypothesis that late adverse effects are based on fraction size, some institutions have initiated hyperfractionated therapy. Although this strategy has not proven efficacious in treating medulloblastomas or brainstem gliomas in children, encouraging results have been reported by Kovnar et al in children with ependymomas.

Chemotherapy

Ependymomas are more like glial tumors than medulloblastomas in that they tend to be chemoresistant. In younger children, response rates averaging 50% have been reported using vincristine and cyclophosphamide with or without etoposide.

TABLE 25-2	Focal versus Whole Neural Axis Radiation		
Author	**Type of Radiation**	**Follow-up**	**Result**
Salazar (1983)	Regional	5-yr survival	10%
	Craniospinal		50%
Goldwein (1991)	Regional	2-yr survival	40%
	Craniospinal		52%
Healey (1991)	Regional	10-yr PFS	31%
	Craniospinal		44%
Vanuytsel (1992)	Regional	10-yr PFS	31%
	Craniospinal		44%
Pollack (1995)	Regional	10-yr PFS	70%
	Craniospinal		39%
Perilongo (1997)	Regional	10-yr PFS	37%
	Craniospinal		32%
Schild (1998)	Regional	Spinal seeding	9%
	Craniospinal		24%
Huring (1999)	Regional	5-yr PFS	67%
	Craniospinal		40%

PFS, Progression-free survival.

Several researchers report having response rates of up to 65% using platinum agents. A lower response rate has been generally noted using nitrosourea-based chemotherapy. Controlled studies have failed to demonstrate a significant advantage to using radiation therapy plus lomustine, vincristine, and either prednisone or procarbazine to using radiation therapy alone. Chemotherapy with stem cell rescue has not proved to enhance survival. Newer studies suggest that agents such as temozolomide or etoposide administered in small daily doses are active in recurrent ependymomas. Nevertheless, the overall role of chemotherapy in the treatment of this tumor remains unidentified.[6,10,11,21,29]

PROGNOSIS

The overall prognosis of intracranial ependymomas is not good. Reported 5-year survival ranges from 40% to 80%, and only 25% to 50% of patients will enjoy a 5-year progression-free survival.[7,14,18,25,27,30,33,34]

Many series note that a young age is associated with a poorer survival, with the definition of *young* varying from age 2 to 5. Whether this worsening prognosis is due to a more aggressive histology, unfavorable tumor location, or the need to delay radiation therapy is debated. Based on the adverse effects seen after treating young children harboring a medulloblastoma with radiation therapy, radiation is not employed in treating ependymomas in children younger than age 3. Whether there is a deleterious effect of delaying radiation therapy while chemotherapy is given is not clear. Timmerman found no difference when treating 55 patients with either surgery or chemotherapy followed by radiation therapy or surgery and radiation therapy followed by chemotherapy. Robertson found no difference in administering craniospinal radiation before or after the induction of chemotherapy.[29] Duffner, Pollack, and Horn have noted a poor prognosis in patients diagnosed with an ependymoma before age 3.[3,14,27a] This poor survival has been attributed to withholding radiation therapy but could also be due to delay in diagnosis and more aggressive tumor biology.

Supratentorial ependymomas seem to have a better prognosis than the tentorial ependymomas. Infratentorial tumors centered in the foramen of Luschka have a worse prognosis than tumors centered in the central portion of the fourth ventricle.

Correlation between histology and prognosis remains unsettled. The literature is unclear whether a WHO grade III tumor has a worse prognosis than a WHO grade II tumor. The debate may arise from the pathologists' interpretation of WHO criteria, which is subjective and nonquantitative. Most series have reported that necrosis, more than 5 mitoses in a high power field, Ki-67 greater than 1%, and endothelial proliferation are associated with a poorer prognosis. Other histologic features indicating a worse prognosis include upgrade of erb-B2 or erb-B4 receptor, expression of GFAP at a lower level, expression of vimentin, and the presence of a diploid DNA stemline.

The most consistent factor found to correlate with prognosis is, again, the extent of tumor resection (see Table 25-1). A complete tumor resection as defined by a high-quality MRI scan appears to be the most relevant factor in predicting a good prognosis. It is unclear how much of the retained tumor is caused by the invasiveness of the tumor and how much is the result of the experience of the surgeon.

References

1a. Aggrawal R, Young D, Kumar P, et al: Efficacy and feasibility of stereotactic radiosurgery in the primary management of unfavorable pediatric ependymomas. Radiother Oncol 43:269–273, 1997.

1. Burger PC, Scheithauer BW, Vogel FS: Surgical Pathology of the Nervous System and its Coverings, 4th ed. New York, Churchill Livingstone, 2002.

2. Carter M, Nicholson J, Ross F, et al: Genetic abnormalities detected in ependymomas by comparative genomic hybridisation. Br J Cancer 86:929–939, 2002.

3. Duffner PK, Krischer JP, Sanford RA, et al: Prognostic factors in infants and very young children with intracranial ependymomas. Pediatr Neurosurg 28:215–222, 1998.

4. Duffner PK, Krischer JP, Horowitz ME, et al: Second malignancies in young children with primary brain tumors following treatment with prolonged postoperative chemotherapy and delayed irradiation: a Pediatric Oncology Group study. [Comment]. Ann Neurol 44:313–316, 1998.

5. Duffner PK, Horowitz ME, Krischer JP, et al: Postoperative chemotherapy and delayed radiation in children less than three years of age with malignant brain tumors. [Comment]. N Engl J Med 328:1725–1731, 1993.

6. Evans AE, Anderson JR, Lefkowitz-Boudreaux IB, Finlay JL: Adjuvant chemotherapy of childhood posterior fossa ependymoma: cranio-spinal irradiation with or without adjuvant CCNU, vincristine, and prednisone: A Childrens Cancer Group study. Med Pediatr Oncol 27:8–14, 1996.

7. Figarella-Branger D, Civatte M, Bouvier-Labit C, et al: Prognostic factors in intracranial ependymomas in children. [Comment]. J Neurosurg 93:605–613, 2000.

8. Foreman NK, Love S, Gill SS, Coakham HB: Second-look surgery for incompletely resected fourth ventricle ependymomas: technical case report. Neurosurgery 40:856–860; discussion 860, 1997.

9. Gerszten PC, Pollack IF, Martinez AJ, et al: Intracranial ependymomas of childhood. Lack of correlation of histopathology and clinical outcome. Pathol Res Pract 192:515–522, 1996.

10. Gornet MK, Buckner JC, Marks RS, et al: Chemotherapy for advanced CNS ependymoma. J Neurooncol 45:61–67, 1999.

10a. Grabb P, Lunsford L, Albright A, et al: Stereotactic radiosurgery for glial neoplasms of childhood. J Neurosurgery 38:696–701, 1996.

11. Grill J, Le Deley MC, Gambarelli D, et al: Postoperative chemotherapy without irradiation for ependymoma in children under 5 years of age: a multicenter trial of the French Society of Pediatric Oncology. J Clin Oncol 19:1288–1296, 2001.

12. Healey EA, Barnes PD, Kupsky WJ, et al: The prognostic significance of postoperative residual tumor in ependymoma. Neurosurgery 28:666–671; discussion 671–672, 1991.

13. Ho DM, Hsu CY, Wong TT, Chiang H: A clinicopathologic study of 81 patients with ependymomas and proposal of diagnostic criteria for anaplastic ependymoma. J Neurooncol 54:77–85, 2001.

14. Horn B, Heideman R, Geyer R, et al: A multi-institutional retrospective study of intracranial ependymoma in children: identification of risk factors. J Pediatr Hematol/Oncol 21:203–211, 1999.

15. Hukin J, Epstein F, Lefton D, Allen J: Treatment of intracranial ependymoma by surgery alone. Pediatr Neurosurg 29:40–45, 1998.

16. Matsushima T, Inoue T, Inamura T, et al: Transcerebellomedullary fissure approach with special reference to methods of dissecting the fissure. J Neurosurg 94:257–264, 2001.

17. McLendon RE, Enterline DS, Tien RD, et al: Tumors of central neuroepithelial origin. In Bigner DD, McLendon RE, Bruner JM, Russell DS (eds): Russell and Rubinstein's Pathology of Tumors of the Nervous System, 6th ed. New York, Oxford University Press, 1998.

18. Merchant TE: Current management of childhood ependymoma. Oncology (Huntingt) 16:629–642, 644; discussion 645–646, 648, 2002.

19. Merchant TE, Zhu Y, Thompson SJ, et al: Preliminary results from a Phase II trial of conformal radiation therapy for pediatric patients with localised low-grade astrocytoma and ependymoma. Int J Radiat Oncol Biol Phys 52:325–332, 2002.

20. Mussi AC, Rhoton AL, Jr: Telovelar approach to the fourth ventricle: microsurgical anatomy. J Neurosurg 92:812–823, 2000.

21. Needle MN, Goldwein JW, Grass J, et al: Adjuvant chemotherapy for the treatment of intracranial ependymoma of childhood. Cancer 80:341–347, 1997.

21a. Osterdoch RJ, Sanford RA, Merchant TE: Pediatric ependymomas presented at Pediatric Section Neurological Surgery (AANS/CNS) Dec. 5–9, 2000 Coronado, California.

22. Oya N, Shibamoto Y, Nagata Y, et al: Postoperative radiotherapy for intracranial ependymoma: analysis of prognostic factors and patterns of failure. J Neurooncol 56:87–94, 2002.

23. Palma L, Celli P, Mariottini A, et al: The importance of surgery in supratentorial ependymomas. Long-term survival in a series of 23 cases. Childs Nervous System 16:170–175, 2000.

24. Paulino AC: Radiotherapeutic management of intracranial ependymoma. Pediatr Hematol Oncol 19:295–308, 2002.

25. Paulino AC, Wen BC, Buatti JM, et al: Intracranial ependymomas: an analysis of prognostic factors and patterns of failure. Am J Clin Oncol 25:117–122, 2002.

26. Paulino AC, Wen BC: The significance of radiotherapy treatment duration in intracranial ependymoma. Int J Radiat Oncol Biol Phys 47:585–589, 2000.

27. Perilongo G, Massimino M, Sotti G, et al: Analyses of prognostic factors in a retrospective review of 92 children with ependymoma: Italian Pediatric Neuro-oncology Group. Med Pediatr Oncol 29:79–85, 1997.

27a. Pollack I, Gerszten P, Martinez A, et al: Intracranial ependymomas of childhood c long-term outcome and prognostic factors. Neurosurgery 37:655–667, 1995.

28. Reardon DA, Entrekin RE, Sublett J, et al: Chromosome arm 6q loss is the most common recurrent autosomal alteration detected in primary pediatric ependymoma. Genes Chromosomes Cancer 24:230–237, 1999.

29. Robertson PL, Zeltzer PM, Boyett JM, et al: Survival and prognostic factors following radiation therapy and chemotherapy for ependymomas in children: a report of the Children's Cancer Group. [Comment]. J Neurosurg 88:695–703, 1998.

29a. Rousseau P, Habrend JL, Sonafin D, et al: Treatment of intracranial ependymomas of children: review of 15-year experience. Int J Radiat Oncol Biol Physs 28:381–386, 1993.

30. Smyth MD, Horn BN, Russo C, Berger MS: Intracranial ependymomas of childhood: current management strategies. Pediatr Neurosurg 33:138–150, 2000.

31. Sutton LN, Goldwein J, Perilongo G, et al: Prognostic factors in childhood ependymomas. Pediatr Neurosurg 16:57–65, 1990.

32. Vanuytsel L, Brada M: The role of prophylactic spinal irradiation in localized intracranial ependymoma. Int J Radiat Oncol Biol Phys 21:825–830, 1991.

33. Verstegen MJ, Leenstra DT, Ijlst-Keizers H, Bosch DA: Proliferation- and apoptosis-related proteins in intracranial ependymomas: an immunohistochemical analysis. J Neurooncol 56:21–28, 2002.

34. Vinchon M, Soto-Ares G, Riffaud L, et al: Supratentorial ependymoma in children. Pediatr Neurosurg 34:77–87, 2001.

CHAPTER 26

CHOROID PLEXUS TUMORS

Alfredo Quinones-Hinojosa, Peter Jun, Jaque Jumper, Tarik Tihan, and Michael W. McDermott

Choroid plexus tumors (CPTs) are primary brain neoplasms originating from the epithelium of the choroid plexus, the fibrovascular tissue found within the ventricular system where the cerebrospinal fluid is formed. The first reported case of a CPT was of one found during autopsy in a 3-year-old female in 1832.[25] The first surgical attempt at resection in an adult was reported by Bielschowsky more than 70 years later.[7] Although this patient died, subsequent operations proved successful, and it was quickly realized that gross-total resection (GTR) of the tumor was necessary for a good long-term outcome. During the next century, our understanding, methods for diagnosis, and management of this rare tumor type have evolved. We now recognize two distinct tumor types: an indolent choroid plexus papilloma (CPP) and more aggressive choroid plexus carcinoma (CPC). The purpose of this review is to present an overview of the current understanding of diagnosis, management, and treatment of these tumors.

LOCATION

CPTs are most often located in the lateral ventricles; however, this varies with the patient's age at the time of diagnosis. Unlike most central nervous system (CNS) neoplasms, CPTs are found in progressively caudal locations with advancing age. A meta-analysis of 566 patients found that primary CPTs were often located supratentorially in infants and infratentorially in most other groups.[54] The median ages of patients harboring tumors in the lateral ventricles, third ventricle, fourth ventricle, and cerebellopontine angle are 1.5 years, 1.5 years, 22.5 years, and 35.5 years, respectively.[54] CPC is found more often in the lateral ventricles, whereas CPP is more common in the cerebellopontine angle.[54]

CPTs tend to metastasize along cerebrospinal fluid (CSF) pathways, but other rare sites include the abdomen, bone, and lung.[54] Thirty percent of patients are found to have metastases at the time of diagnosis or at autopsy, with tumors featuring a supratentorial location and a CPC histology being more likely to spread.[3,19,42,54] CPPs, which are considered benign tumors, are also capable of diffuse craniospinal seeding.[35]

EPIDEMIOLOGY

CPTs are considered pediatric malignancies because of their higher incidence in younger patients. Although the age at diagnosis can range from neonate to 72 years (mean age 3.5 years), 70% of patients are younger than 24 months.[8,19,54] Across all ages, CPTs constitute only 0.4% to 1.3% of intracranial tumors.[42,58] Within pediatric series, this rises to 2.9%, and in children younger than 1 year, CPTs account for 10% to 20% of CNS neoplasms.[19] There is a slight male gender preference with a male to female ratio of 1.2:1.[54]

DIAGNOSIS

Presentation

The clinical features depend on the age of the patient and location of the tumor. In infants, an enlarging head related to associated hydrocephalus may be the only sign. In children, symptoms of increased intracranial pressure, such as nausea, vomiting, irritability, and headache, secondary to hydrocephalus may be seen. Other findings include papilledema, hemiparesis, hyperreflexia, abducens nerve palsy, stupor, and coma.[6,19,45] Those with posterior fossa lesions are more likely to have brainstem and cerebellar findings, including cranial nerve abnormalities, pyramidal tract signs, and ataxia.[8] The duration of symptoms before diagnosis varies from 1 day to 4 years (median 4 weeks), with earlier symptom onset in younger patients and patients with CPC.[19,45]

Hydrocephalus is a near ubiquitous finding in those with CPTs, and several reasons for its development have been suggested, including obstruction of CSF pathways by the tumor, hypersecretion of CSF by the tumor, and blockage of CSF absorption from repeated tumor microhemorrhage or elevated CSF protein concentrations.[9,45] Of these, CSF overproduction is considered the principle mechanism with one series identifying a patient with CSF production almost doubling the norm.[45]

Diagnostic Studies

The diagnosis of CPTs relies on modern imaging modalities such as computed tomography (CT), magnetic resonance imaging (MRI), and magnetic resonance angiography (MRA). Laboratory studies have limited sensitivity and specificity in detecting or predicting this type of tumor. Studies examining CSF are of low diagnostic yield. Cytology from 24 patients was positive in only three cases.[6,8,42] Ten of 21 patients had xanthochromic fluid, whereas protein content ranged from 19 to

460 mg/100 mL (median 122 mg/100 mL).[19] The significance of these results is uncertain, but the risk of herniation from a lumbar puncture in patients with elevated intracranial pressure should direct physicians to initial CT and MRI studies.

Their unilaterality and peripheral lobulations can help distinguish CPTs from other tumors, including meningiomas, ependymomas, and metastasis.[32] CPP and CPC are generally isodense or hyperdense intraventricular masses on unenhanced CT scans. They show intense enhancement on contrast-enhanced CT images. CT is superior to MRI in detecting associated intratumoral calcifications (Figure 26-1). However, MRI is the imaging modality of choice because of its inherent superb anatomic detail, tissue contrast, ability to directly image in multiple planes, and increased sensitivity in determining tumor extent. The uncalcified portions of CPPs appear isointense or hypointense to normal brain parenchyma on T1-weighted images and hyperintense on T2-weighted images. If doubt remains about the imaging diagnosis with MRI, a simple non-contrast CT may improve diagnostic acumen because, in general, adult fourth ventricular CPPs will appear markedly calcified, whereas ependymomas will not. Contrast enhancement on MRI tends to be uniform and intense, and flow voids are common. MRA or conventional angiograph are not routinely necessary but may demonstrate enlarged choroidal arteries supplying the tumor (Figure 26-2).[45]

The distinction between CPP and CPC is not always possible on imaging studies.[36,51] Differentiation of the two is based on histology, not radiology. CPTs with a benign imaging appearance may be carcinomas histologically, and those with an aggressive imaging appearance may turn out to be papillomas. Nonetheless, proper imaging characterization of CPTs preoperatively may affect surgical approach to the tumor. CPCs tend to have more heterogeneous T1- and T2-weighted imaging and enhancement characteristics. This reflects the presence of more tumor necrosis due to the tumor's rapid growth rate. Extraventricular extension into brain parenchyma and presence of associated vasogenic edema favor CPC over CPP.[14] CSF dissemination can occur with CPP or CPC but is much more common with the latter.[1,20] The degree of hydrocephalus in CPC has been noted to be less than that seen with CPPs.[14] Functional imaging with positron-emission tomography (PET) may demonstrate increased metabolic activity in CPC.[28]

Seeding of the cerebrospinal fluid has been reported in both CPPs and CPCs. However, clinically significant seeding is much more common in patients with a CPC.[32] Therefore imaging of the spinal neural axis may be helpful in detecting CSF dissemination.

HISTOPATHOLOGY

In the current World Health Organization (WHO) classification, CPP is a WHO grade I neoplasm, whereas CPC corresponds to a WHO grade III neoplasm.

Macroscopic Features

CPTs are often soft to rubbery, having a cauliflower-like form, and may have a gritty texture due to calcifications. The tumors are often orange-brown, and an attachment to the normal choroid plexus or the ventricular wall may be present. Some CPCs, and rare CPPs, bleed profusely.

Microscopic Features

CPPs typically are uniform and lack significant architectural or cytologic atypia. The tumor faithfully recapitulates the choroid plexus with regular, cuboidal epithelial cells, well-developed underlying fibrovascular stroma, and lack of mitotic activity or aggressive features. The CPP has distinct epithelial features with cuboidal or "hobnail" cells in mostly single layers. The fibrovascular stroma is often well defined in larger papillae, but may not be obvious in smaller ones. Intraoperative smear preparations often contain papillary tissue fragments in CPPs and in some CPCs. Nuclear uniformity is typical of CPP with regular and distinct cytoplasmic borders. Similar to normal choroid plexus, CPPs often have regions with hyalinized vessels and "degenerative" changes (Figure 26-3A).

CPPs often display calcifications, clear cells, and xanthomatous cells.[30] There are reports of osseous, cartilaginous or chondroid metaplasia,[10,56] and acinar or tubular differentiation,[2] but these changes are less common. Melanin pigment with or without ultrastructural evidence of melanosomes is rare.[16,34,46,53] CPC, and less commonly CPP, can display ependymal differentiation and rosettes associated with long fibrillary, glial fibrillary acidic protein (GFAP)-positive processes. In some CPCs, hyaline droplets can be observed within the cells.

CPP and CPC differ in their degree of architectural complexity, solid nonpapillary growth, cytologic atypia, mitotic activity, atypical mitoses, and tumor necrosis. High cellularity, nuclear pleomorphism and hyperchromasia, mitoses, and necrosis are common features of CPCs. The distinction between CPP and CPC can be arbitrary, and some tumors may not be readily classified as one or the other. Some CPPs show varying degrees of cytologic atypia or architectural complexity. These tumors straddle the boundaries that separate CPP and CPC and have been termed "atypical" CPPs. Currently, there are no diagnostic criteria for this group of tumors.

Even though both CPP and CPC can invade surrounding neuropil, this feature appears more common in CPC and has a weak association with outcome.[44] Most CPCs display multilayer arrangement of papillae, and rare cases appear indistinguishable from metastatic papillary carcinoma (Figure 26-3B).

Immunohistochemical Features

Cytokeratins and vimentin are expressed by virtually all CPPs and most CPCs. GFAP can be found focally in approximately 25% to 55% of CPPs and 20% of CPCs.[31] Most of the GFAP-positive cells are simultaneously positive for cytokeratin.[33] S-100 protein is present in almost all cases of CPP and less commonly in CPCs. The staining for S-100 is often stronger and more diffuse compared with GFAP staining.[33] Synaptophysin has been used as a marker for choroid plexus epithelium, but staining of tumors with this marker is variable. Epithelial membrane antigen (EMA) is positive in tumor cells only focally, if at all. In addition, transthyretin is suggested as a reliable marker for choroid plexus and its tumors.[27]

A recent study suggested that immunohistochemical staining for prealbumin and carcinoma embryonic antigen (CEA) are of significant value for the differential diagnosis of CPPs and CPCs.[29] Staining for insulin-like growth factor II (IGF-II) is also suggested as a useful marker to distinguish normal choroid plexus and CPP from CPC.[5] Indirect indices of proliferation, such as the Ki-67 antibody, have been used to dis-

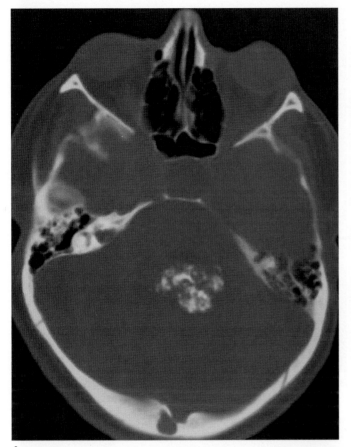

A

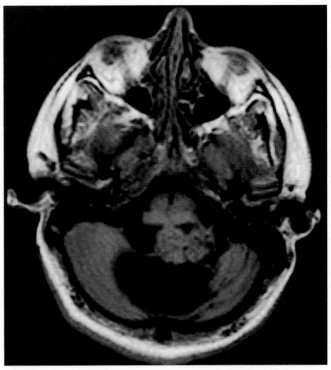

B

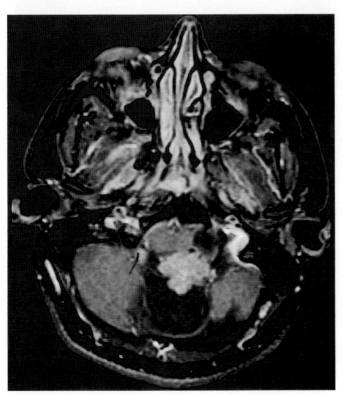

C

FIGURE 26-1 Noncontrast computed tomography (CT) (A) and precontrast and postcontrast T1-weighted axial magnetic resonance images (B and C) in a 21-year-old male with hydrocephalus and a choroid plexus papilloma in the fourth ventricle. CT shows the calcifications within the mass that are inconspicuous on magnetic resonance imaging. The papilloma demonstrates homogeneous enhancement after contrast administration.

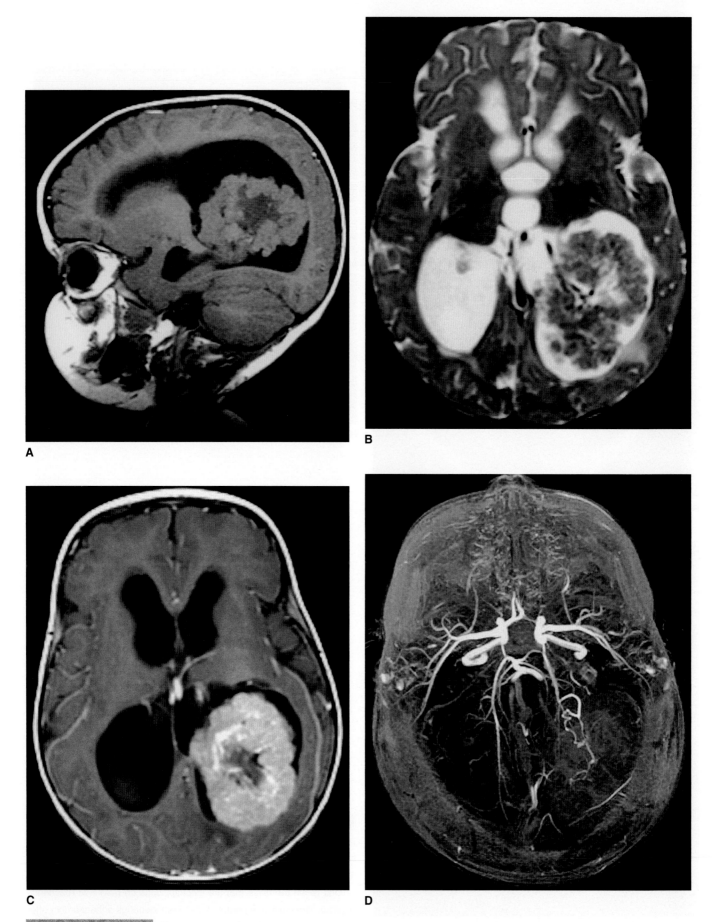

FIGURE 26-2 Eleven-year-old female with hydrocephalus and a choroid plexus papilloma in the atrium of the left lateral ventricle. T1-weighted sagittal *(A)* and T2-weighted axial magnetic resonance (MR) images *(B)* show a T1 isointense, T2 hyperintense mass with central flow voids and necrosis. There is intense enhancement on the postcontrast T1-weighted axial image *(C)*. Collapsed image from a three-dimensional time-of-flight MR angiogram *(D)* demonstrates an enlarged left posterior choroidal artery supplying the mass.

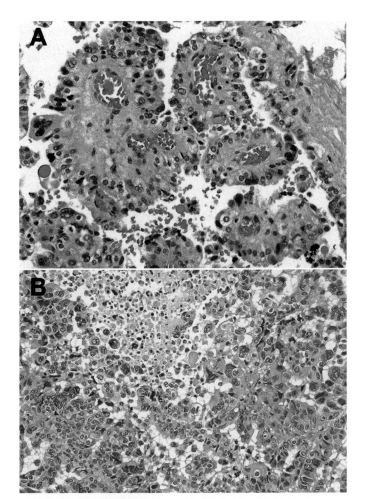

FIGURE 26-3 *A,* Microscopic appearance of choroid plexus papilloma. The tumor is characterized by well-formed papillae with centrally located fibrovascular cores, epithelioid cells with little or no pleomorphism. The tumors often lack significant mitoses or necrosis as in this case. (Original magnification ×200.) *B,* Microscopic appearance of choroid plexus carcinoma. The tumor exhibits marked anaplastic features, mitoses as well as necrosis. There is a vague papillary formation, but in some areas the tumor loses its papillary architecture and resembles an undifferentiated carcinoma. (Original magnification ×200.)

tinguish CPP from CPC.[11,15] The mean Ki-67/MIB-1 labeling index is often less than 2% for CPPs and 13.8% for CPCs. Immunohistochemical staining for p53 protein is found more often in carcinomas than papillomas.[23] Despite the elaborate studies mentioned previously, distinguishing some CPPs from CPCs is highly challenging.

Ultrastructural Features

Most CPPs exhibit apical microvilli and scattered cilia, apical junctional complexes, interdigitating lateral cell borders, presence of a basement membrane that separates the tumor cells from underlying stroma, and fenestrated capillaries. Cilia exhibit the 9 + 0 microtubule configuration characteristic of neuroepithelial cells. Some tumors also exhibit irregularly

shaped structures containing lipid droplets and filamentous material and microtubules, and they resemble the "silver bodies" of Biondi found in normal choroid plexus.[41] Even high-grade carcinomas often show epithelial features as well as cilia and microvilli. CPCs are often more varied in their ultrastructural appearance, and typical findings may be only focally present. They can show features of immature cellular characters such as polyribosomes, glycogen granules, and hypertrophied rough endoplasmic reticulum.[4]

MOLECULAR AND CYTOGENETIC FEATURES

In CPP recurrent abnormalities, including partial gains of chromosome 7, have been reported.[24] A recent comparative genomic hybridization study of a large number of choroid plexus tumors showed that +5q, +6q, +7q, +9q, +15q, +18q, and −21q were significantly more common in CPP, whereas CPCs were characterized by +1, +4q, +10, +14q, +20q, +21q, −5q, −9p, −11, −15q, and −18q.[47]

Choroid plexus neoplasms have been associated with the Li-Fraumeni and Aicardi syndromes.[49,52,57] Several reports have identified SV-40 virus genetic material within the tumor cells, yet the contribution of this virus to formation of choroid plexus tumors is unknown.[12,43,50]

SURGICAL TREATMENT

Surgery is the mainstay of treatment for CPPs and a necessary first step in diagnosis and treatment of CPCs. As noted previously, the younger the patient, the more likely it is that CPPs are found within the lateral or third ventricle, and as the patient approaches adulthood tumors in the fourth ventricle or cerebellopontine angle are more common. Also, the younger the patient, the more likely it is that the tumor will be associated with hydrocephalus.[26] Therefore the goals in the management of these patients are relieving hydrocephalus, establishing a tissue diagnosis, and complete tumor removal. Complete tumor removal is the goal with CPPs and can be achieved in most cases even if this requires more than one operation. However, with CPCs subtotal resection is more common.[39] The treatment of associated hydrocephalus and the surgical approaches to each of the ventricular sites are unique and beyond the scope of this text, but some general comments can be made.

Hydrocephalus associated with these tumors can usually be managed with an external ventricular drain as necessary before or at the time of definitive tumor removal. We avoid a permanent shunt system before tumor removal, because in many patients tumor removal can solve the problem, and intraventricular surgery is associated with postoperative blood products that need to be cleared from the ventricle over several days and may obstruct permanent systems. Ellenbogen et al found that after tumor removal in children, 63% did not require a permanent shunt.[19] In some patients, despite tumor removal, ventriculoperitoneal shunting may be necessary for communicating hydrocephalus, and some will require subdural to peritoneal shunting for subdural fluid collections that persist after transcortical approaches to tumors of the lateral ventricles.[8]

Surgery for these tumors is complicated by their extreme vascularity and an inability to preoperatively embolize the arteries supplying the tumor. The tumors are quite friable, and blood loss can be a limiting factor in achieving gross-total tumor removal in neonates and infants.[48] Staged surgery for CPPs is always an option. The blood supply to these tumors comes from the named choroidal arteries that normally supply the plexus, and these small vessels (anterior choroidal, posterior medial choroidal, posterior lateral choroidal, choroidal branch of the posterior inferior cerebellar artery) cannot be cannulated or embolized by interventional neuroradiologists for technical reasons (small caliber, distal arterial tree location) of risks of interference with blood supply to normal brain by the same artery (anterior choroidal, posterior inferior cerebellar). Ideally, once the tumor is exposed, interruption of the feeding artery before tumor resection is begun is recommended. Some authors have described en bloc removal of smaller tumors after doing just that.[26] In adults, fourth ventricular tumors may be heavily calcified at diagnosis and may be relatively avascular.

Tumors of the lateral ventricles (frontal horn, temporal horn, body) are approached either by an interhemispheric transcallosal approach (anterior to midbody of lateral ventricle; third ventricle) or a transcortical-transventricular route (temporal horn, posterior body to atrium). Transcortical incisions may be associated with ventriculo-subdural connections that account for the fluid collections requiring subdural to peritoneal shunting postoperatively. Most surgeons will attempt a sulcal splitting approach to limit the amount of subcortical white matter cut and to reduce the chance of fluid collections developing.[40]

For tumors of the fourth ventricle a midline suboccipital craniotomy is used, and planes of dissection between the cerebellum and brainstem can be developed that allow for adequate exposure without the need for splitting of cerebellar tissue.[37] Tumors of the cerebellopontine angle are approached by a retrosigmoid (more lateral) suboccipital craniotomy. In both cases, because of proximity to cranial nerves within the subarachnoid space, neurophysiologic monitoring of these nerves is routine to reduce the chance of nerve injury with exophytic or large tumors.

In general, complete removal of CPPs is possible in the majority of cases even if more than one operation is required. Complete removal holds the best chance for long-term tumor control or cure.[13,36,39] For CPCs, which are often disseminated at diagnosis and more often invading brain, subtotal removal is the norm.

ADJUVANT THERAPIES

Elucidating the exact role of radiation and chemotherapy has been hampered by our inability to conduct prospective, randomized clinical trials due to the rarity of this tumor type. Our current understanding is based on case reports and small series that vary in their radiation dosages and chemotherapy regimens. This has made it difficult to evaluate the effects of any one therapy on long-term patient survival. In general, adjuvant therapies are reserved for CPCs, which are difficult to resect completely and have a propensity to recur.[48]

Subtotally Resected Tumors

In subtotally resected CPCs, the use of adjuvant therapies has largely been ineffective. In 26 cases reviewed by Duffner, only 2 of 19 patients receiving either radiation, chemotherapy, or both survived.[17] One patient received a chemotherapy regimen consisting of 10 monthly cycles of "eight-drugs-in-1-day" without the need for radiation.[21] The other patient received an initial course of four cycles of cisplatin and etoposide daily for 5 days.[3] This was followed by the Pediatric Oncology Group (POG) regimen of 28-day cycles of vincristine plus cyclophosphamide and cisplatin plus etoposide.[17] Both patients were followed for more than 24 and 46 months, respectively.

Recent reports are consistent with these findings. Of Duffner's patients, four had partial resections and were placed on the POG regimen, of which two had long-term survival of more than 51 and 60 months.[17] One patient's disease progressed after 7 months of chemotherapy but was salvaged with radiation therapy. The other completed chemotherapy and received radiation therapy per protocol with no signs of progression. Berger et al reported 11 patients receiving adjuvant treatments after subtotal resection.[6] Of those, only one patient on the French Society of Pediatric Oncology (SFOP) regimen (consisting of carboplatin, procarbazine, etoposide, cisplatin, vincristine, and cyclophosphamide) had complete remission for more than 55 months without additional radiation. The rest had tumor recurrence between 2 and 23 months. Chow et al had three cases of subtotally resected CPCs, of which one patient had no evidence of disease for more than 23 months.[13] This patient received two cycles of cyclophosphamide, etoposide, and carboplatin, followed by another subtotal resection and radiation treatments. Greenberg was able to induce complete remission for longer than 15 months in a patient with ifosfamide, carboplatin, and etoposide (ICE regimen).[22] Pencalet et al had one case of incomplete resection in which the patient died 7 months later despite receiving an unknown chemotherapy and adjuvant radiation therapy.[45]

Chemotherapy may have a potential role in facilitating subsequent surgeries to achieve GTR in CPCs that are unresectable at time of diagnosis. Greenberg describes the use of the ICE regimen between surgeries to decrease tumor volume, vascularity, and friability.[22] Five patients underwent two to five cycles of chemotherapy following less than GTR. All had reoperation that was capable of achieving GTR. Of these five patients, two survived with no evidence of disease at more than 120 and 29 months. Histologically, tumor from the second surgery revealed marked fibrosis of the tumor and blood vessels compared with prechemotherapy sections.

Gross-Totally Resected Tumors

The necessity of adjuvant therapies in patients with GTR is less clear. Duffner's review found 13 of 18 cases where GTR of CPCs was accomplished with good outcome.[17] Of these surviving cases, nine (69%) received adjuvant treatment: five received radiation therapy, three received chemotherapy, and one received both. In the five cases with poor outcome, radiation treatment was attempted in one, chemotherapy in two, and no adjuvant treatment in the last two.

If adjuvant therapy is used, the current trend is to delay radiation therapy for as long as possible. Frequent dissemination of CPCs have required large doses of radiation directed on the neuraxis to achieve adequate coverage, often causing long-term neurologic and endocrinologic sequelae.[17] Initial treatment is usually with chemotherapy followed by radiation therapy as an option if the tumor progresses. The main variation in administration has been the timing: immediately following surgery or waiting until recurrence.

In the postoperative setting, Duffner et al had four patients on the POG regimen after GTR.[17] Of these patients, two progressed and were successfully salvaged with radiation therapy. Two patients without relapse declined radiation, which was part of the study protocol. Of these four patients, three had good outcomes for longer than 48, 48, and 69 months, respectively. One patient declining radiation died from a histologically distinct malignancy at the same location. In Packer's series, two patients with GTR received adjuvant therapy.[42] One died while receiving intrathecal methotrexate and systemic lomustine and vincristine. The sole survivor received radiation only. Pencalet et al report on eight patients with GTR, of which seven received chemotherapy (either nitrosourea or a multidrug regimen of carboplatin, etoposide, procarbazine, and cyclophosphamide) and one received radiation.[45] Two developed recurrence and died; each was on one of the two chemotherapy regimens. Of Berger's eight patients with GTR, one received radiation therapy and seven received chemotherapy (six receiving the SFOP regimen, one receiving lomustine monthly, and one receiving etoposide and carboplatin).[6] Of these patients, only one relapsed after 2 months while on SFOP. Chow's seven patients all received chemotherapy.[13] Six patients survived on various combinations of carboplatin, cyclophosphamide, etoposide, and vincristine. Two received radiation in addition to their chemotherapy. One died after progressing after 13 months of therapy failing salvage using radiation.

There are only a few cases in which adjuvant therapy was delayed until time of recurrence. Ellenbogen et al waited to treat three patients who relapsed after GTR with vincristine and cisplatin.[19] In addition to chemotherapy, two had good outcomes and were operated on achieving GTR of the recurring tumor. In one patient GTR was not achieved and he died 6 weeks later.

To summarize, when adjuvant therapy is administered after GTR, it usually follows the operation. From the series that we reviewed, out of 29 patients receiving an adjuvant, 23 (79%) survived. Of these, 21 received chemotherapy, 3 received radiation therapy, and 5 received both (radiation following progression while on chemotherapy).

The importance of complete tumor resection in CPC patients cannot be overemphasized. Even when GTR is achieved and adjuvant therapy employed, the tumor can recur, suggesting that radiation and chemotherapy are not enough to provide definite cure. In his literature review, Greenberg suggested that disease-free status at 2 years may be predictive of a good long-term outcome.[22] The latest recurrence in Greenberg's review occurred at 23 months after surgery. New technologies, such as radiosurgery, including the Gamma Knife® and modified or dedicated linear accelerator, are able to target small tumor volumes while limiting irradiation of surrounding normal tissues.[38] Because there are only a few cases reported in the literature, results of this treatment are difficult to summarize, although it can be said that radiosurgery is used widely for both benign and malignant recurrent tumors.[18] Radiosurgery may have future application in treatment of CPCs.

OUTCOME AND QUALITY OF LIFE ASSESSMENTS

In either CPP or CPC, the best long-term outcomes are realized when GTR is achieved. Wolff et al conducted a meta-analysis of 566 CPT patients, finding that CPP patients with GTR have a 10-year survival rate of 85% compared with 56% in those with subtotal resections.[54] Patients with CPCs fared worse, having a 2-year survival rate of 72% and 34% in GTR and subtotal resections, respectively. Wolff et al also studied survival using adjunctive therapies and were able to conclude only that the use of radiation therapy after surgery improved survival in patients with CPC regardless of whether it is completely resected.[54,55] Of course, they cautioned against this practice in younger patients.

Patient morbidity was documented in several studies. The major postoperative morbidity reported by Ellenbogen et al were seizures.[19] Ten children who did not have preoperative seizures experienced one or more seizures postoperatively. Other reported deficits include hemiparesis, hemianopsia, and strabismus.[13,19,45] Neurologic outcome was documented by Pencalet et al. They noted that 68% of CPP patients were fully independent; however, only 44% of CPC patients reached this level, with 56% requiring some form of daily assistance.[45]

CONCLUSION

CPTs are relatively rare tumors that primarily affect pediatric patients. They have been divided into two classifications by the WHO, including benign CPPs and malignant CPCs. Although CPPs are considered cured after complete removal, CPCs are known to recur despite GTR. This has encouraged physicians to use radiation therapy, chemotherapy, or both to impede tumor growth and limit recurrence. Neither adjuvant therapies can guarantee cure, but it appears that neoadjuvant chemotherapy may provide a chance for second surgery to achieve GTR in a previously unresectable tumor. Further studies are needed on the optimum adjuvant therapy regimen for the best long-term outcome in this tumor type.

References

1. Aguzzi A, Brandner S, Paulus W: Choroid plexus tumours. In Kleihues P, Cavanee W (eds): Pathology and Genetics of Tumours of the Nervous System. Lyon, France, IARC, 2000.
2. Ajir F, Chanbusarakum K, Bolles JC: Acinar choroid plexus adenoma of the fourth ventricle. Surg Neurol 17:290–292, 1982.
3. Allen J, Wisoff J, Helson L, et al: Choroid plexus carcinoma—responses to chemotherapy alone in newly diagnosed young children. J Neurooncol 12:69–74, 1992.
4. Anguilar D, Martin JM, Aneiros J, et al: The fine structure of choroid plexus carcinoma. Histopathology 7:939–946, 1983.

5. Asano K, Sekiya T, Hatayama T, et al: A case of endolymphatic sac tumor with long-term survival. Brain Tumor Pathol 16:69–76, 1999.

6. Berger C, Thiesse P, Lellouch-Tubiana A, et al: Choroid plexus carcinomas in childhood: clinical features and prognostic factors. Neurosurgery 42:470–475, 1998.

7. Bielschowsky M, Unger E: Kenntinis der primaren Epithelgeschwultse der Adergeflechte des Gehirns. Arch Klin Chir 81:61–82, 1906.

8. Boyd MC, Steinbok P: Choroid plexus tumors: problems in diagnosis and management. J Neurosurg 66:800–805, 1987.

9. Buxton N, Punt J: Choroid plexus papilloma producing symptoms by secretion of cerebrospinal fluid. Pediatr Neurosurg 27:108–111, 1997.

10. Cardozo J, Cepeda F, Quintero M, et al: Choroid plexus papilloma containing bone. Acta Neuropathol (Berl) 68:83–85, 1985.

11. Carlotti CG, Jr, Salhia B, Weitzman S, et al: Evaluation of proliferative index and cell cycle protein expression in choroid plexus tumors in children. Acta Neuropathol (Berl) 103:1–10, 2002.

12. Chen J, Tobin GJ, Pipas JM, Van Dyke T: T-antigen mutant activities in vivo: roles of p53 and pRB binding in tumorigenesis of the choroid plexus. Oncogene 7:1167–1175, 1992.

13. Chow E, Reardon DA, Shah AB, et al: Pediatric choroid plexus neoplasms. Int J Radiat Oncol Biol Phys 44:249–254, 1999.

14. Coates TL, Hinshaw DB, Jr., Peckman N, et al: Pediatric choroid plexus neoplasms: MR, CT, and pathologic correlation. Radiology 173:81–88, 1989.

15. Coons S, Johnson PC, Dickman CA, Rekate H: Choroid plexus carcinoma in siblings: a study by light and electron microscopy with Ki-67 immunocytochemistry. J Neuropathol Exp Neurol 48:483–493, 1989.

16. Dobin SM, Donner LR: Pigmented choroid plexus carcinoma: a cytogenetic and ultrastructural study. Cancer Genet Cytogenet 96:37–41, 1997.

17. Duffner PK, Kun LE, Burger PC, et al: Postoperative chemotherapy and delayed radiation in infants and very young children with choroid plexus carcinomas. The Pediatric Oncology Group. Pediatr Neurosurg 22:189–196, 1995.

18. Eder HG, Leber KA, Eustacchio S, Pendl G: The role of gamma knife radiosurgery in children. Childs Nerv Syst 17:341–346; discussion 347, 2001.

19. Ellenbogen RG, Winston KR, Kupsky WJ: Tumors of the choroid plexus in children. Neurosurgery 25:327–335, 1989.

20. Enomoto H, Mizuno M, Katsumata T, Doi T: Intracranial metastasis of a choroid plexus papilloma originating in the cerebellopontine angle region: a case report. Surg Neurol 36:54–58, 1991.

21. Gianella-Borradori A, Zeltzer PM, Bodey B, et al: Choroid plexus tumors in childhood. Response to chemotherapy, and immunophenotypic profile using a panel of monoclonal antibodies. Cancer 69:809–816, 1992.

22. Greenberg ML: Chemotherapy of choroid plexus carcinoma. Childs Nerv Syst 15:571–577, 1999.

23. Griffiths PD, Blaser S, Boodram MB, et al: Choroid plexus size in young children with Sturge-Weber syndrome. AJNR Am J Neuroradiol 17:175–180, 1996.

24. Grill J, Avet-Loiseau H, Lellouch-Tubiana A, et al: Comparative genomic hybridization detects specific cytogenetic abnormalities in pediatric ependymomas and choroid plexus papillomas. Cancer Genet Cytogenet 136:121–125, 2002.

25. Guerard M: Tumeur fongeuse dans le ventricle droit du cerveau chez une petite fille de trois ans. Bull Soc Anat Paris 8:211–214, 1832.

26. Gupta N, Jay V, Blaser S, et al: Choroid plexus papillomas and carcinomas., in Youmans JR (ed) Neurological Surgery. Philadelphia, WB Saunders, 1996.

27. Herbert J, Cavallaro T, Dwork AJ: A marker for primary choroid plexus neoplasms. Am J Pathol 136:1317–1325, 1990.

28. Itoh Y, Kowada M, Mineura K: Choroid plexus carcinoma. Report of a case with positron emission tomographic study. Neuroradiology 28:374, 1986.

29. Kato T, Fujita M, Sawamura Y, et al: Clinicopathological study of choroid plexus tumors: immunohistochemical features and evaluation of proliferative potential by PCNA and Ki-67 immunostaining. Noshuyo Byori 13:99–105, 1996.

30. Kepes JJ: "Xanthomatous" changes in a papilloma of the choroid plexus. Acta Neuropathol (Berl) 16:367–369, 1970.

31. Kimura T, Budka H, Soler-Federsppiel S: An immunocytochemical comparison of the glia-associated proteins glial fibrillary acidic protein (GFAP) and S-100 protein (S100P) in human brain tumors. Clin Neuropathol 5:21–27, 1986.

32. Koeller KK, Sandberg GD: From the archives of the AFIP. Cerebral intraventricular neoplasms: radiologic-pathologic correlation. Radiographics 22:1473–1505, 2002.

33. Kouno M, Kumanishi T, Washiyama K, et al: An immunohistochemical study of cytokeratin and glial fibrillary acidic protein in choroid plexus papilloma. Acta Neuropathol (Berl) 75:317–320, 1988.

34. Lana-Peixoto MA, Lagos J, Silbert SW: Primary pigmented carcinoma of the choroid plexus. A light and electron microscopic study. J Neurosurg 47:442–450, 1977.

35. Leblanc R, Bekhor S, Melanson D, Carpenter S: Diffuse craniospinal seeding from a benign fourth ventricle choroid plexus papilloma. Case report. J Neurosurg 88:757–760, 1998.

36. Levy ML, Goldfarb A, Hyder DJ, et al: Choroid plexus tumors in children: significance of stromal invasion. Neurosurgery 48:303–309, 2001.

37. Matsushima T, Inoue T, Inamura T, et al: Transcerebellomedullary fissure approach with special reference to methods of dissecting the fissure. J Neurosurg 94:257–264, 2001.

38. McDermott MW, Sneed SK, Chang SM, et al: Results of radiosurgery for recurrent gliomas. In Kondziolka D (ed): Radiosurgery 1995. Boston, Karger, 1996.

39. McEvoy AW, Harding BN, Phipps KP, et al: Management of choroid plexus tumours in children: 20 years experience at a single neurosurgical centre. Pediatr Neurosurg 32:192–199, 2000.

40. Nagib MG, O'Fallon MT: Lateral ventricle choroid plexus papilloma in childhood: management and complications. Surg Neurol 54:366–372, 2000.

41. Navas JJ, Battifora H: Choroid plexus papilloma: light and electron microscopic study of three cases. Acta Neuropathol (Berl) 44:235–239, 1978.

42. Packer RJ, Perilongo G, Johnson D, et al: Choroid plexus carcinoma of childhood. Cancer 69:580–585, 1992.

43. Palmiter RD, Chen HY, Messing A, Brinster RL: SV40 enhancer and large-T antigen are instrumental in development of choroid plexus tumours in transgenic mice. Nature 316:457–460, 1985.

44. Paulus W, Janisch W: Clinicopathologic correlations in epithelial choroid plexus neoplasms: a study of 52 cases. Acta Neuropathol (Berl) 80:635–641, 1990.

45. Pencalet P, Sainte-Rose C, Lellouch-Tubiana A, et al: Papillomas and carcinomas of the choroid plexus in children. J Neurosurg 88:521–528, 1998.

46. Reimund EL, Sitton JE, Harkin JC: Pigmented choroid plexus papilloma. Arch Pathol Lab Med 114:902–905, 1990.

47. Rickert CH, Wiestler OD, Paulus W: Chromosomal imbalances in choroid plexus tumors. Am J Pathol 160:1105–1113, 2002.

48. St Clair SK, Humphreys RP, Pillay PK, et al: Current management of choroid plexus carcinoma in children. Pediatr Neurosurg 17:225–233, 1991.

49. Uchiyama CM, Carey CM, Cherny WB, et al: Choroid plexus papilloma and cysts in the Aicardi syndrome: case reports. Pediatr Neurosurg 27:100–104, 1997.

50. Van Dyke TA, Finlay C, Miller D, et al: Relationship between simian virus 40 large tumor antigen expression and tumor formation in transgenic mice. J Virol 61:2029–2032, 1987.

51. Vazquez E, Ball WS, Jr, Prenger EC, et al: Magnetic resonance imaging of fourth ventricular choroid plexus neoplasms in childhood. A report of two cases. Pediatr Neurosurg 17:48–52, 1991.

52. Vital A, Bringuier PP, Huang H, et al: Astrocytomas and choroid plexus tumors in two families with identical p53 germline mutations. J Neuropathol Exp Neurol 57:1061–1069, 1998.

53. Watanabe K, Ando Y, Iwanaga H, et al: Choroid plexus papilloma containing melanin pigment. Clin Neuropathol 14:159–161, 1995.

54. Wolff JE, Sajedi M, Brant R, et al: Choroid plexus tumours. Br J Cancer 87:1086–1091, 2002.

55. Wolff JE, Sajedi M, Coppes MJ, et al: Radiation therapy and survival in choroid plexus carcinoma. Lancet 353:2126, 1999.

56. Yap WM, Chuah KL, Tan PH: Choroid plexus papilloma with chondroid metaplasia. Histopathology 31:386–387, 1997.

57. Yuasa H, Tokito S, Tokunaga M: Primary carcinoma of the choroid plexus in Li-Fraumeni syndrome: case report. Neurosurgery 32:131–133; discussion 133–134, 1993.

58. Zulch K: Biologie und pathologie der hirngeschwulste. In Olivercrona H, Tonnis W (eds): Handbuch der Neurochirurgie. Berlin, Springer-Verlag, 1956.

CHAPTER 27

ASTROBLASTOMA

Ivo W. Tremont-Lukats and Kenneth D. Aldape

The term *astroblastoma* has been in the literature since Percival Bailey and Harvey Cushing systematically classified 400 cases of gliomas seen at Johns Hopkins and the Peter Bent Brigham Hospital from 1903 through 1924.[1] Although 13 of these cases were called astroblastoma, inspection of a photomicrograph of an example of one of these cases reveals features more consistent with what most pathologists would consider a glioblastoma. Since then, there has been confusion as to the definition of this entity, even to the extent of skepticism of its existence. Adding to this problem is the fact that some of the histologic patterns of astroblastoma can be seen as elements within the more common infiltrating gliomas, such as astrocytoma and glioblastoma. However, following the introduction of definitive diagnostic criteria,[2] sufficient experience has been accumulated to warrant defining this tumor as a distinct clinicopathologic entity. As a reflection of this experience, the most recent World Health Organization (WHO) classification of central nervous system tumors includes astroblastoma as a defined entity.

LOCATION, CLINICAL PRESENTATION

Most astroblastomas are supratentorial, but exceptional cases have been reported in the cerebellum, optic nerve, brainstem, and cauda equina. Approximately 75% of supratentorial astroblastomas are in the frontal or parietal lobes. Any age group can be affected, but the highest frequency is in persons between 10 and 30 years old. Taking the contemporary series of astroblastomas together, there is a slight female predominance, and the most common symptom at presentation is headache, followed by seizures and focal neurologic deficits.[2,3,11]

IMAGING

Astroblastomas present usually as a large, single, and lobulated lesion located peripherally in a cerebral hemisphere. The mass has a mixed solid and cystic component with ring enhancement, soap-bubble appearance, and proportionately little edema in many, but not all cases.[3,10] On T1-weighted postcontrast magnetic resonance imaging (MRI), the solid component enhances heterogeneously, but the overall appearance may be nonspecific. Small astroblastomas can be confused with ependymoma and other tumors, but the lack of peritumoral edema and mass effect favors astroblastoma. On CT scan, the solid lesion is hyperdense and can include calcifications.

HISTOLOGIC AND ULTRASTRUCTURAL FEATURES

Astroblastoma is a tumor of uncertain histogenesis, although the evidence to date places its origin as glial. There are no gross pathologic features that definitely distinguish this lesion from other gliomas, although they may appear more discrete than the typical infiltrating glioma on gross examination. Microscopically, they show a tendency toward demarcation with respect to surrounding brain, similar to other noninfiltrating gliomas, such as pilocytic tumors and pleomorphic xanthoastrocytomas. A papillary appearance can be appreciated in some tumors. In addition, the typical cases are characterized by a specific perivascular arrangement of tumor cells, called a perivascular pseudorosette. Unlike the perivascular rosette of the more common ependymoma, which shows a tapering of glial processes toward the vascular lumen, the astroblastoma rosette shows no such tapering. The astroblastoma cellular processes are, in general, shorter and broader than the fibrillar processes of ependymoma. Cytologically, the tumor cells often have a polygonal shape, with an "epithelioid" appearance. Representative examples of astroblastoma histology are shown in Figure 27-1. An additional common feature is vascular hyalinization, which when extreme can be associated with dystrophic calcification. These changes are probably most pronounced in long-standing lesions and are histologic evidence of chronicity. It should be emphasized that the epithelioid morphology, distinctive pseudorosettes, and vascular hyalinization can be seen as focal patterns within more common tumors, such as astrocytoma or glioblastoma. Therefore the diagnosis of astroblastoma should be considered only in instances where these features represent the predominant histologic pattern, in conjunction with supporting imaging and clinical features. The immunohistochemical features are not exceedingly helpful in distinguishing astroblastoma from other tumors in the histologic differential diagnosis. The tumor cells are typically positive for GFAP and S-100. Although positivity for neuronal markers has been reported,[9] this has not been a universal finding.[6]

Electron microscopic examination of astroblastoma shows features most similar to those seen in ependymoma, including microvilli, cilia, and zipper-like junctions.[2] These findings have led to the hypothesis that astroblastoma arises from neoplastic

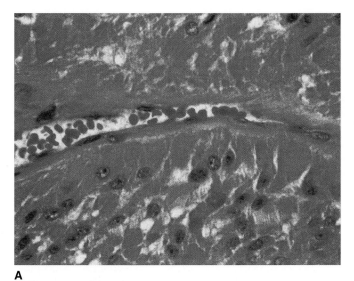 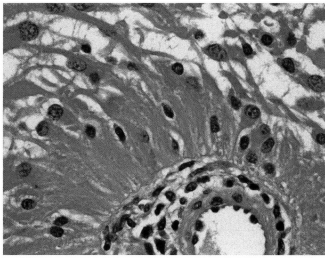

A   B

FIGURE 27-1 Astroblastoma histopathology. *A,* The broad-based processes typical of astroblastoma. *B,* A typical astroblastoma perivascular pseudorosette.

transformation of the tanycyte or subependymal glia. However, ependymoma-like features are not seen in all of the reported cases.[5,7] In general, although electron microscopy is not helpful to distinguish astroblastoma from ependymoma, it is of use in ruling out other entities with similar histology on light microscopy, such as a diffuse astrocytoma and papillary meningioma.

Although the WHO does not indicate criteria for the grading of astroblastoma, there is evidence that a relationship exists between histologic features and clinical behavior. Several studies indicate that anaplastic features are associated with poorer outcome.[2,11] Evidence of anaplasia in astroblastoma includes loss of papillary architecture, with a solid growth pattern, high cellularity, mitotic activity, and microvascular proliferation. In contrast to the diffuse gliomas, tumor necrosis does not appear to be of importance in grading. Given the suggested relationship between histologic features and outcome, it seems prudent to consider whether the tumor is of low or high histologic grade when deciding on the clinical management of patients with astroblastoma.

MOLECULAR GENETICS

Good evidence for the inclusion of astroblastoma as a distinct pathologic entity comes from cytogenetic studies. Conventional cytogenetic studies indicate that astroblastoma does not show the changes typical of either ependymoma or diffuse astrocytoma.[7,8] Comparative genomic hybridization, a technique that can detect gains and losses of genetic material at subchromosomal resolution, has been reported in seven cases. The most common changes were gains on chromosomes 19 and 20, which although seen in astrocytoma or glioblastoma, are not as common as other aberrations in these tumors.[3,4] These data, in addition to the distinctive histology and radiologic appearance, support the notion that astroblastoma arises by molecular alterations distinct from the more common gliomas.

CLINICAL MANAGEMENT

The rarity of astroblastomas has hindered the definition of the best treatment strategy. However, given the relative circumscription of these tumors, it makes sense to attempt a complete macroscopic resection whenever possible. If the resection is complete (on a gross level), and the tumor is well differentiated (low mitotic activity, lack of anaplastic features), external-beam radiation may be considered as adjuvant therapy, although all three patients with low-grade astroblastomas in the series from the Memorial Sloan-Kettering Cancer Center (MSKCC) had surgery alone and remained disease free for a mean of 29 months.[11]

If resection is subtotal, or the neurosurgeon achieves a gross total resection but the tumor is anaplastic, more intensive modalities may be prudent, even though the role of radiation and chemotherapy in the treatment of astroblastomas is unclear at present. Intensive chemotherapy regimens that included autologous bone marrow replacement have been tried, but the experience has not been promising, because three of the four patients with anaplastic astroblastoma in the MSKCC series treated with this intensive regimen died from toxicity or tumor progression. The only survivor in this group (median follow-up 76 months) received carboplatin and vincristine without further chemotherapy. An unreported case at the M. D. Anderson Cancer Center has been treated with procarbazine and CCNU for two courses before irradiation following a gross-total resection. After 2 years of follow-up, the patient is alive and recurrence free (Levin V., personal communication). The use of adjuvant chemotherapy against astroblastomas is fraught with anecdotal experience, and more experience is required to demonstrate that chemotherapy has benefit in the treatment of astroblastomas. Given the increasing recognition of this tumor as a distinct entity, it is likely that further study will help clarify the role, if any, of adjuvant therapy.

References

1. Bailey P, Cushing H: A classification of the tumors of the glioma group on a histogenetic basis with a correlated study of prognosis. New York, Sentry Press (Reprinted by Argosy-Antiquarian Ltd, 1971), 1926.
2. Bonnin JM, Rubinstein LJ: Astroblastomas: a pathological study of 23 tumors, with a postoperative follow-up in 13 patients. Neurosurgery 25:6–13, 1989.
3. Brat DJ, Hirose Y, Cohen KJ, et al: Astroblastoma: clinicopathologic features and chromosomal abnormalities defined by comparative genomic hybridization. Brain Pathol 10:342–352, 2000.
4. Burton EC, Lamborn KR, Feuerstein BG, et al: Genetic aberrations defined by comparative genomic hybridization distinguish long-term from typical survivors of glioblastoma. Cancer Res 62:6205–6210, 2002.
5. Cabello A, Madero S, Castresana A, et al: Astroblastoma: electron microscopy and immunohistochemical findings—case report. Surg Neurol 35:116–121, 1991.
6. Husain AN, Leestma JE: Cerebral astroblastoma: immunohistochemical and ultrastructural features. Case report. J Neurosurg 64:657–661, 1986.
7. Jay V, Edwards V, Squire J, et al: Astroblastoma: report of a case with ultrastructural, cell kinetic, and cytogenetic analysis. Pediatr Pathol 13:323–332, 1993.
8. Mierau GW, Tyson RW, McGavran L, et al: Astroblastoma: ultrastructural observations on a case of high-grade type. Ultrastruct Pathol 23:325–332, 1999.
9. Pizer BL, Moss T, Oakhill A, et al: Congenital astroblastoma: an immunohistochemical study. Case report. J Neurosurg 83:550–555, 1995.
10. Port JD, Brat DJ, Burger PC, et al: Astroblastoma: radiologic-pathologic correlation and distinction from ependymoma. AJNR Am J Neuroradiol 23:243–247, 2002.
11. Thiessen B, Finlay J, Kulkarni R, et al: Astroblastoma: does histology predict biologic behavior? J Neurooncol 40:59–65, 1998.

CHAPTER 28

GLIOMATOSIS CEREBRI

Justin S. Smith, Susan M. Chang, Kathleen R. Lamborn, Michael D. Prados,
Mitchel S. Berger, and G. Edward Vates

Gliomatosis cerebri (GC) is an uncommon and enigmatic diffuse glioma. Its most consistent characteristic is the diffuse infiltration of malignant cells throughout large regions of the central nervous system. The term *gliomatosis cerebri* was introduced by Nevin in 1938,[18] and since then, nearly 200 cases have been reported in the literature. The current World Health Organization (WHO) classification of brain tumors describes GC as a diffuse glial tumor infiltrating the brain extensively, involving two or more lobes, commonly bilaterally, and often extending to infratentorial structures.[15] Despite active investigation into the cytogenesis and classification of GC, it is unclear whether GC is a distinct pathologic entity or simply an extreme form of diffusely infiltrating glioma. Regardless of its classification, GC carries a grim prognosis, and details regarding its etiology, clinical behavior, and therapeutic options remain limited due to its rarity and the only recent ability to provide antemortem diagnosis.

LOCATION

GC has been reported in nearly every location within the central nervous system. In 1994 Jennings et al summarized the localization of disease in cases of GC from the world literature, with the primary source of data from postmortem examination, rather than by magnetic resonance imaging (MRI) and surgical biopsy.[13] The most commonly involved sites included the cerebral hemispheres (76%), midbrain (52%), pons (52%), thalamus (43%), basal ganglia (34%), cerebellum (29%), and corpus callosum (25%). Sites less commonly involved included medulla oblongata (13%), hypothalamus (9%), and optic nerve or chiasm (9%). Leptomeningeal and spinal cord involvement were identified in 17% and 9%, respectively.

Vates et al reported 22 cases of GC identified using MRI and biopsy.[20] The most common locations included the cerebral hemispheres (100%), thalamus and basal ganglia (95%), midbrain (36%), and pons (27%) (Table 28-1). Seventy-seven percent of patients had bilateral disease, and 23% had unilateral disease (80% right side and 20% left side). The reason for the asymmetry observed in unilateral disease is unclear.

DIAGNOSIS

Initial Symptoms

The symptoms and signs of patients with GC are nonspecific, reflecting the diffuse and infiltrative nature of this neoplasm. Interestingly, signs and symptoms are often minimal given the widespread areas of brain infiltrated with tumor. In the report by Jennings et al, the interval from onset of symptoms to diagnosis varied from days to 23 years, with 65% of the patients symptomatic for fewer than 24 months before diagnosis; the authors noted that the delay in diagnosis of the more protracted cases made it difficult to distinguish presenting symptoms and signs from those consistent with progressive disease.[13] The most common findings included corticospinal tract deficits (58%), dementia (44%), headache (39%), seizures (38%), cranial neuropathy (37%), papilledema or increased intracranial pressure (34%), spinocerebellar dysfunction (33%), mental status changes (20%), behavioral changes or psychosis (19%), sensory deficits or paresthesias (18%), and visual alterations (17%), including blindness, hemianopsia, or obscurations. Less commonly identified were back pain or radicular pain (3%) and myelopathy (1.4%).

In the more recent report by Vates et al, the most common presenting complaints included changes in mental status (77%), seizures (46%), headaches (41%), nausea (36%), gait changes (36%), weakness (36%), visual changes (23%), and decreased dexterity (23%) (Table 28-2).[20] Changes in mental status were often subtle and included decreased memory or personality changes. Six of the ten patients with seizures had initial grand mal seizures, with two of these patients in status epilepticus. The remaining four patients had partial complex seizures initially, with two of these patients having occasional generalized seizures. No specific pattern of headache was identified. Although some patients had sudden-onset headaches that precipitated work-up, most of the patients with headache had long-standing symptoms (>2 months).

Neurologic Examination

Vates et al reported that the most common deficit on formal neurologic testing was dementia (68%) (see Table 28-2).[20]

Other deficits included corticospinal deficits (36%), gait abnormalities (36%), papilledema (27%), dysphasia (23%), visual alterations (23%), cranial neuropathies (5%), and paresthesias (5%). Most of the patients with dementia had memory disturbances, but two were obtunded. Corticospinal tract abnormalities were varied and ranged from mild pronator drift or mild diffuse hyperreflexia to profound weakness. Speech findings were predominantly word-finding abnormalities, although two patients were obtunded with complete aphasia. The one patient with a cranial neuropathy (excluding cranial nerve I and II) had decreased oculocephalic activity and a right facial droop.

Kim et al reported the neurologic findings in 16 GC patients.[14] The most common disturbances were papilledema (63%), decreased visual acuity or visual field deficit (33%), facial palsy (25%), trigeminal nerve dysfunction (19%), extraocular movement disturbance (13%), lower cranial nerve dysfunction (6%), and hearing deficit (6%).

Laboratory Evaluations

Laboratory findings are mostly normal and primarily helpful in excluding infectious or inflammatory disease. Before the advent of noninvasive imaging, laboratory investigation of GC patients was limited primarily to electroencephalography (EEG), which typically demonstrated diffuse slowing, polyspike activity, and progression over time.

Cerebrospinal fluid (CSF) analyses are not useful for the diagnosis of GC, although are helpful in excluding infectious or inflammatory diseases. Artigas et al reviewed 10 cases of GC and reported that the CSF protein level was elevated to 50 to 95 mg/dL in a third of their cases.[1] In a review of 160 cases of GC from the world literature, Jennings et al identified only one case in which CSF cytology was diagnostic of a neoplasm.[13] Herrlinger et al performed CSF analyses on five GC patients; none of the samples demonstrated pathologic findings, including cytology.[11] Thus a consistent feature of GC is normal CSF cytology and serology.

EPIDEMIOLOGY

Although the number of diagnosed cases of GC has increased as noninvasive imaging modalities have become more sensitive, it remains an uncommon diagnosis, representing approximately 1% of the infiltrative glial neoplasms of the brain. The most comprehensive analysis of the epidemiology of GC remains the report by Jennings et al, reviewing 160 cases reported in the world literature.[13] The age at diagnosis was reported for 151 patients and ranged from infancy to 83 years, with a peak incidence between the ages of 40 and 50. The male-to-female ratio was 1.07 : 1 for 147 patients, and symptom onset for women was at a somewhat younger age. Of the 22 GC cases reported by Vates et al, 50% were male, and the median age at presentation was 49 years (range 7 to 79 years).[20]

Although no clear risk factors have been identified for GC, an association has been made with neurofibromatosis type 1

TABLE 28-1

Prevalence of MR Image Findings in the Study Population

MR Image Finding	N	%
No. of lobes:		
2	10	45
3	7	32
4	5	23
Location:		
Cerebral hemisphere	22	100
Dienc/BG	21	95
Midbrain	8	36
Pons	6	27
Cerebellum	0	0
Medulla	1	5
Spinal cord	1	5
Left	1	5
Right	4	18
Bilateral	17	77
Mass effect	12	55
Dominant mass	13	59
Enhancement	12	55
Cyst	2	9
Hydrocephalus	2	9
MRS	7	32

%, Percentage of total patients; Dienc/BG, diencephalon or basal ganglia; MR, magnetic resonance; MRS, magnetic resonance spectroscopy; N, number of patients.

TABLE 28-2   Prevalence of Patient Complaints and Deficits Found on Examination in the Study Population

Patient Complaint	N	%	Presenting Deficits	N	%
Mental status changes	17	77	Dementia	15	68
Seizures	11	50	Corticospinal deficits	8	36
Headache	9	41	Gait abnormalities	8	36
Nausea	8	36	Papilledema	6	27
Gait changes	8	36	Dysphasia	5	23
Weakness	8	36	Visual alterations	5	23
Visual changes	5	23	Cranial neuropathies	1	5
Decreased dexterity	5	23	Paresthesias	1	5

%, Percentage of total patients; N, number of patients.

(NF1). At least 9.4% of 139 GC patients retrospectively reviewed by Jennings et al were also diagnosed with NF1.[13]

NEUROIMAGING

Magnetic Resonance Imaging

MRI has enabled antemortem diagnosis of GC and, in combination with brain biopsy, has become the primary means of diagnosing GC in current clinical practice. On T1-weighted images, GC is typically isointense to hypointense compared with brain and poorly defined, whereas T2-weighted images usually show high-intensity signal abnormalities with diffuse mass effect. Hyperintensity on T2-weighted images observed in white matter tracts most likely reflects tumor spread but may also represent secondary destruction of myelin along axonal fibers. Because T2-weighted changes are often the most prominent feature of GC, imaging sequences that accentuate these changes are helpful in delineating the full extent of disease. Fluid-attenuated inversion recovery (FLAIR) produces heavily T2-weighted images but suppresses the distracting brightness of T2 signal arising from CSF in the ventricles and subarachnoid space (Figure 28-1). This approach reduces gray-to-white matter contrast and improves visualization of lesions adjacent to CSF, enabling better delineation of periventricular, subpial, and callosal infiltration.[7] FLAIR imaging has become a routine MRI sequence in the assessment of cerebral pathologies and is superior to conventional imaging for demonstrating the full extent of disease.

Although contrast enhancement on T1-weighted images is not a prominent finding in most reports, Vates et al found contrast enhancement in 55% of their patients (see Table 28-1).[13] When enhancement is present, it is generally nodular, associated with minor mass effect and perifocal edema, and without evidence of necrosis. Areas of focal enhancement likely represent anaplastic transformation and are typically disproportionately limited relative to the extensively infiltrative presence of the lesion.

Another MRI technique, dynamic contrast-enhanced T2-weighted perfusion MRI (perfusion MRI), enables a noninvasive assessment of tissue vascularity.[21] Conventional contrast-enhanced MRI cannot provide this information for GC, because it relies on breakdown of the blood-brain barrier, a feature not prominent in these tumors. The role of perfusion MRI in the clinical management of GC remains unproved; however, the finding of normal regional cerebral blood volume (rCBV) in a region with significant T2 abnormality may lend further support to a diagnosis of GC. Although not yet clearly demonstrated, another potential use may be in monitoring for malignant transformation during treatment, since secondary transformation to glioblastoma has been reported.

The MRI findings of GC are not unique; other diseases may produce similar findings and must be considered. The differential diagnosis includes ischemic or infectious diseases, demyelinating diseases such as leukoencephalopathy or multiple sclerosis, and other tumor processes, including diffusely infiltrating astrocytomas or multicentric glioblastoma multiforme. The acuity of onset of clinical symptoms generally enables differentiation of ischemic disease from GC, whereas it may be very difficult, if not impossible, to distinguish some infectious diseases, such as viral encephalitis. As a general rule, leukoencephalopathy is uncommon in the setting of deep or superficial gray matter involvement. Multiple sclerosis plaques are typically more circumscribed than the signal abnormalities of GC. It can be difficult to differentiate GC from a multicentric glioma, although the latter tends to demonstrate a different MRI pattern, including necrosis, heterogeneous contrast enhancement, vasogenic edema, and extension along white matter tracts. The distinction of other diffusely infiltrating gliomas from GC remains debatable. Astrocytomas and oligodendrogliomas tend to be more limited, to be associated with a

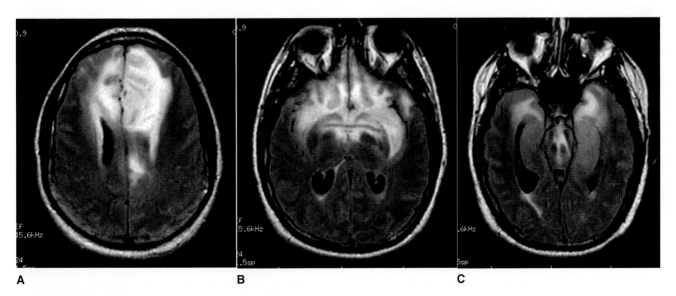

A   **B**   **C**

FIGURE 28-1 *A through C,* Axial fluid-attenuated inversion recovery magnetic resonance imaging sequences showing abnormal gray and white matter T2 prolongation in the frontal and temporal lobes and the deep gray matter and brainstem before biopsy in a representative patient with gliomatosis cerebri. (Reprinted from Vates GE, Chang S, Lamborn KR, et al: Gliomatosis cerebri: a review of 22 cases. Neurosurgery 53:261–271, 2003.)

dominant mass, exhibit a contiguous extension, and produce more symptoms. In addition, the brainstem, which is commonly involved in GC, is less commonly involved in other diffuse gliomas. Nonetheless, these associations remain relatively nonspecific, and clinical and pathologic correlations are necessary.

Computed Tomography

Multiple studies have demonstrated the superiority of MRI over computed tomography (CT) imaging for the characterization of GC.[8] CT imaging of GC generally shows an isodense to hypodense lesion with a diffuse mass effect and lack of contrast enhancement. The findings tend to be subtle and nonspecific and are commonly misinterpreted. Furthermore, CT imaging occasionally fails to detect lesions or to accurately show their extent. Therefore CT is useful only to demonstrate an abnormality in the brain and to rule out immediately life-threatening diseases but does not provide much more diagnostic information. In addition, a normal CT scan should not preclude an MRI scan for more sensitive and specific evaluation of a patient's symptoms.

Magnetic Resonance Spectroscopy

Magnetic resonance spectroscopy (MRS) is a noninvasive biochemical assay that helps to distinguish normal and pathologic brain tissue.[2,9] The relative amounts of several biomolecules are assessed with MRS, including choline (Cho), creatinine (Cr), N-acetyl aspartate (NAA), and lactate. Relative to normal tissue, tumor tissue exhibits increased Cho/Cr and Cho/NAA ratios. This is thought to be secondary to an increase in Cho, reflective of increased membrane turnover in tumors and to a decrease in NAA and Cr, reflecting replacement of neurons with tumor cells.

Several reports have suggested that grading of GC is of great importance for prognosis and possibly for therapy. Accurate grading of GC is complicated, however, because the lesion is typically quite diffuse, and conventional MRI has been shown to be unreliable for grading of gliomas. Thus biopsy planning based solely on MRI may be misleading and not yield representation of the highest-grade tumor tissue. Recently, attempts have been made to correlate specific MRS-derived brain chemical signatures with particular glioma tumor grades to guide brain biopsy. An association between the level of Cho/Cr and Cho/NAA elevation and tumor grade has been shown for gliomas, with high-grade gliomas exhibiting the highest ratios. Thus the area of maximum elevation may aid in the overall grading of the tumor and help determine the optimal site for representational biopsy.

It is important to note that a small percentage of nonneoplastic lesions may also exhibit elevated Cho and decreased NAA and Cr, including encephalitis, demyelination, and organizing hemorrhage. This underscores the need to obtain histologic diagnosis and not to rely solely on noninvasive imaging.

Positron-Emission Tomography

Positron-emission tomography (PET) remains primarily a research tool with regard to GC, although preliminary reports suggest that it may prove clinically useful. Both [^{18}F]-fluorodeoxyglucose (FDG) PET and [^{11}C]-methionine PET have been applied to GC. FDG PET is essentially a measure of metabolic activity, and low-grade lesions have demonstrated marked reduction in FDG uptake, whereas high-grade lesions have shown increased uptake. These findings are consistent with a higher level of metabolic activity in high-grade lesions and may provide a better means of estimating tumor grade with noninvasive imaging. Thus FDG PET may aid in biopsy targeting and in providing more meaningful patient prognosis, although further investigation is necessary before such gains may be realized.[6]

In contrast to FDG PET, [^{11}C]-methionine PET measures amino acid uptake, which is increased in both low- and high-grade lesions. Limited studies have suggested that C^{11} methionine PET of GC patients demonstrates a more extensive lesion than does MRI. This has been confirmed in a single case with autopsy correlation. Thus the sensitivity of [^{11}C]-methionine PET may be better than MRI in some cases.[17,19] It must be remembered, however, that neither PET nor MRI demonstrates the true extent of GC lesions, because tumor cells are inevitably seen beyond the boundaries of imaging abnormalities on pathologic specimen.

HISTOPATHOLOGY

Gross examination of the GC-afflicted brain demonstrates generalized enlargement of significant portions of the brain. The brain is typically heavy, and the disease may be evident on the surface through swollen and flattened gyri. The gray matter exhibits increased firmness and the white matter is conspicuously absent in the affected regions.

Microscopic examination reveals a more extensive process than is recognized by either gross inspection or noninvasive imaging. Both gray and white matter areas are extensively infiltrated by neoplastic cells, although the underlying neuronal architecture is generally preserved, except in areas with the densest cellular proliferation and infiltration. Demyelination is a prominent feature that correlates with the extent of neoplastic invasion, and tumor cells are often arranged in a perineuronal, perivascular, and subpial distribution. Although there may be areas of high mitotic activity and microvascular proliferation, these are usually limited to areas with a focal mass of tumor where the neoplasm has presumably progressed to a higher grade lesion.

The histopathology of reported GC cases is heterogeneous, and there are no specific histologic, immunologic, or genetic markers. Most cases demonstrate astrocytic tumor cells, but occasional reports describe tumors with oligodendroglial or ependymal components. Ultrastructural studies have suggested that GC is a neoplastic process of glial cells in all stages of development, from glioblasts to mature astrocytes and transitional forms of oligodendrocytes.[4] Varying grades of neoplastic elements have been described, ranging from WHO grade I to grade III or IV. In addition, in some cases there are slender, wavy cells with elongated nuclei that have been considered to represent diffuse infiltration by microglial elements. These latter cells have been reported to be glial fibrillary acidic protein (GFAP) negative, whereas a subset of the glial elements are GFAP positive.[10]

Cases of GC are classified as either primary or secondary. Primary GC is further subdivided into two groups: type I is the classic, diffusely infiltrative glioma without an apparent tumor mass, and type II exhibits a diffusely infiltrative component as well as a tumor mass. Secondary GC is a contiguous infiltration of tumor cells from a previously diagnosed glioma.

It is important to recognize that the diffuse nature of GC, coupled with the typically limited biopsy sampling, may complicate the histologic diagnosis, and it is imperative to be aware of other processes that may share GC's appearance. Histologically, the differential diagnosis includes astrocytic and oligodendroglial neoplasms, multicentric glioma, inflammatory and infectious conditions, and a rare form of neoplastic transformation of microglial cells, termed *microgliomatosis*. Astrocytic neoplasms are also highly infiltrative lesions that may exhibit elongated neoplastic cells. However, astrocytomas typically exhibit a significant focal mass, tend to be destructive processes, and may demonstrate necrosis, features not characteristically associated with GC. In addition, the extent of tumor cell dissemination is greater in GC than in infiltrating glioma.

Like GC, oligodendrogliomas may infiltrate both gray and white matter and form secondary structures. Oligodendroglioma cells typically exhibit a characteristic appearance, with round nuclei surrounded by a clear halo. Similar-appearing cells may also be found in GC. However, the degree of dissemination and the presence of elongated, undifferentiated cells help to distinguish GC.

Multicentric gliomas may be distinguished from GC based on GC's lack of contiguous dissemination, as well as specific microscopic features. Multicentric well-differentiated glioma may pose a particularly challenging differential diagnosis. Multicentricity, however, is almost always seen with high-grade lesions. In addition, the elongated, undifferentiated cells that are commonly observed in GC may also assist in distinguishing these two processes.

Inflammatory and infectious reactions may lead to proliferation of microglial cells and thus may be mistaken for GC. Certain features of inflammatory and infectious conditions may suggest the diagnosis, including perivascular lymphocytic infiltration, meningeal inflammation, and, in some cases, direct identification of the infectious agent.

Microgliomatosis presents a histologic appearance very similar to GC. Both are diffuse processes without predominant focal masses. In addition, both feature relative preservation of underlying structure and demonstrate cells of similar morphology. Immunohistochemistry can help distinguish these two conditions, because microgliomatosis has been reported to be immunoreactive for macrophage markers and not reactive to GFAP; the opposite is generally true of GC.

The extremely diffuse nature of GC has led to two main hypotheses regarding its formation: (1) GC forms in the simultaneous transformation of wide fields of cells, and (2) GC arises from a single clone of cells that subsequently proliferates and extensively migrates. The former is known as the oligoclonal origin hypothesis, and the latter is known as the monoclonal origin hypothesis. If GC represents a monoclonal lesion, it may provide a potentially powerful model to help elucidate the mechanisms by which the more common diffuse gliomas invade and migrate through surrounding structures and thus aid in designing novel therapies.

Two recent molecular genetic studies have provided insight into the origin of GC. Kros et al randomly selected tissue samples from 24 locations throughout the brain from a single autopsy of a GC patient.[16] These samples were subjected to comparative genomic hybridization, a genome-wide screening technique designed to identify gross chromosomal deletions, amplifications, and rearrangements. In addition, DNA sequencing of the TP53 tumor-suppressor gene was performed for each sample. A similar pattern of genetic alterations was identified in a widespread distribution of the biopsy samples, including the same base-pair mutation of TP53. These results provide a strong argument favoring the monoclonal origin hypothesis of GC development.

Herrlinger et al studied neoplastic tissue from 13 GC patients and evaluated several tumor-suppressor genes and oncogenes known to be altered in the more common diffuse gliomas.[11] These included TP53, PTEN, CDK4, MDM2, and CDKN2A. The pattern of alteration observed in GC patients resembled that of the diffuse gliomas, suggesting that GC is a subset of the more common diffuse gliomas.

THERAPY

Surgery

Surgical biopsy remains essential for the antemortem diagnosis of GC, because other processes may present with similar clinical and radiographic features. Stereotactic biopsy provides the least invasive means of diagnosis. However, in the early stages of GC, the limited density of neoplastic cells may prove difficult to distinguish from reactive gliosis. When stereotactic biopsy is employed, targeting is typically guided by MRI and MRS (see previous discussion). In cases that demonstrate contrast enhancement, the center of the enhancement and the immediate periphery are typically selected for biopsy. For cases without contrast enhancement, the center of the diffuse infiltrative lesion is typically selected.

The alternative to stereotactic biopsy is open biopsy. Although this approach is more invasive, it provides the opportunity to obtain multiple biopsy samples over a broader range of brain tissue. Open biopsy not only facilitates diagnosis but may also be used for decompression in patients with symptoms of increased intracranial pressure and either a focal tumor mass or a region of noneloquent brain that is heavily infiltrated by tumor.

Radiation Therapy and Radiosurgery

Surgical treatment is primarily restricted to diagnosis and decompression; it plays little role in decreasing tumor burden because of the diffuse and widespread infiltration of neoplastic cells, often into functional brain regions. Due to the limitations of the surgical treatment approach, radiation therapy may offer a beneficial treatment option.

Horst et al reviewed the literature on radiation therapy in GC from 1985 to 2000; they identified a total of 17 reported cases and presented data for three new cases.[12] Therapy ranged from local irradiation to whole-brain irradiation, and the total dose of radiation ranged from 22 to 64.8 Gy (mean 51.2 Gy). Three patients received combined radiation and chemotherapy; however, the limited number of cases available for analysis precluded any conclusions regarding the effectiveness of chemotherapy. For the 18 patients with available clinical follow-up, 13 (72%) had improvement of symptoms and 9

(50%) had stable improvement at 6 months after irradiation. Mean overall survival from onset of symptoms for the 17 patients with available data was 22.8 months (range 8 to 42 months).

Since the review of Horst et al, there have been several reports regarding the use of radiation therapy in GC. Kim et al performed a retrospective analysis of 15 GC patients treated with radiation therapy.[14] One patient died secondary to rapid disease progression after receiving 2700 cGy of radiation therapy. The remaining 14 patients completed the full course of radiation therapy, with doses ranging from 4680 cGy to 6300 cGy (mean 5700 cGy), with a daily radiation fraction of 180 cGy. Eight patients received whole-brain and seven patients received regional-brain radiation. For the latter cases, the field of radiation covered the area of high signal intensity on T2-weighted MRI. The median duration of follow-up was 17 months and the range of survival was 50 days to 46 months. At the time of analysis, 6 patients had died and 10 remained alive. Median survival time for all 16 patients was 38.4 months from the time of operation and 40.4 months from the onset of symptoms. Survival rates at 1 and 2 years were 77% and 58%, respectively, and the median Karnofsky Performance Scale (KPS) score for those patients still alive was 80 (range 40 to 100). Kim et al concluded that radiation therapy might be a good treatment modality. It is important to recognize, however, that the survival of GC patients receiving only palliative care varied from months to more than 10 years.[14] Thus radiation therapy may provide relief of neurologic symptoms, but studies with longer follow-up are necessary to confirm this. In addition, this study did not include patients who were not treated with radiation and thus had no comparison group.

Vates et al also reported a retrospective analysis of 22 GC patients.[20] Initial therapy consisted of radiation for 13 patients and radiation and chemotherapy for an additional 3 patients. For all but 2 patients, between 5400 cGy and 6100 cGy was delivered using routine fractionated plans over 4 to 6 weeks. One patient progressed despite radiation therapy and received only 1000 cGy, and a pediatric patient received 3000 cGy secondary to age. There was no significant difference in survival between treatment with radiation alone and radiation combined with chemotherapy, but because 60% of the 22 patients remain alive, and thus censored from survival analysis, no firm conclusions regarding the effectiveness of radiation therapy could be made. In addition, the patients who did not receive any kind of therapy were older and had lower initial KSs; therefore selection bias makes interpretation of this data limited.

It is difficult to predict the optimal radiation dose or configuration for GC patients at present. However, considering the possibility of high-grade elements and the possibility of sampling error, higher doses may be indicated and extensive involved-field therapy or whole-brain radiation therapy appear to be most appropriate.[5]

Thus based on the available literature, it appears that radiation may, in some GC patients, stabilize the clinical condition and reverse neurologic symptoms. Whether the prolonged survival observed with radiation therapy in some studies represents effective treatment is unclear because of the limited number of patients observed and the lack of studies with extended follow-up time. In addition, because technical advances in imaging have enabled earlier diagnosis of GC,

some proposed gains in survival attributed to radiation therapy in studies without internal negative control groups may be compromised by lead-time bias.

Chemotherapy

Reports describing the use of chemotherapy in GC are very limited and consist of case reports or small series of patients. Herrlinger et al reported 13 cases of GC. Six of these patients were treated with procarbazine, carmustine, and vincristine (PCV) chemotherapy; three received PCV treatment as initial therapy, and three received PCV treatment after either whole-brain radiation therapy or focal radiation.[11] One patient demonstrated partial remission, two patients demonstrated minor response, and one patient had stable disease. In addition, three patients received temozolomide chemotherapy; all three of these patients had progressive disease. The limited number of patients analyzed precluded meaningful survival analysis.

In the series of 22 patients reported by Vates et al, five patients were treated with chemotherapy, either PCV or temozolomide.[20] There was no significant difference from treatment with radiation alone.

Benjelloun et al reported a single case of GC that was responsive to temozolomide chemotherapy.[3] At the time of report, the patient had received 12 cycles of temozolomide and had experienced resolution of symptoms, including lethargy, memory disturbance, and seizures. In addition, MRI showed significant shrinkage of the lesion, and on spectroscopic profile, Cho had decreased, NAA had increased, and the lactate-lipid peak returned to normal.

Experimental Therapies

Because of the rarity of GC and the unproven benefit of traditional neuro-oncology therapies, these patients are not included in most trials of experimental therapies.

OUTCOME

Length of survival for GC patients is variable, with the reported range from days to decades. Stratification of these patients based on survival could help provide meaningful prognosis and assist with treatment planning. In the study by Vates et al, the following factors were correlated with increased length of survival on multivariate analysis: KPS score 70 or better, absence of enhancement on MRI, lower tumor grade, and treatment. Notably, age at symptom onset was not predictive of length of survival.[20]

In a univariate comparison of Kaplan-Meier survival curves, Kim et al suggested that a Ki-67 labeling index (a measure of cellular proliferation) of greater than 1.0 had a significantly unfavorable impact on survival.[14] In addition, a KPS score of less than score 70 was associated with poor survival, although statistical significance was not definite. Several other factors were evaluated but not found to be associated with survival, including TP53 labeling index, age at diagnosis, presenting symptoms, duration of symptoms, type of surgical procedure (decompression versus biopsy), cytologic categorization, and amount of radiation received.

References

1. Artigas J, Cervos-Navarro J, Iglesias JR, et al: Gliomatosis cerebri: clinical and histological findings. Clin Neuropathol 4:135–148, 1985.
2. Bendszus M, Warmuth-Metz M, Klein R, et al: MR spectroscopy in gliomatosis cerebri. Am J Neuroradiol 21:375–380, 2000.
3. Benjelloun A, Delavelle J, Lazeyras F, et al: Possible efficacy of temozolomide in a patient with gliomatosis cerebri. Neurology 57:1932–1933, 2001.
4. Cervos-Navarro J, Artigas J, Aruffo C, et al: The fine structure of gliomatosis cerebri. Virchows Arch A 411:93–98, 1987.
5. Cozad SC, Townsend P, Morantz RA, et al: Gliomatosis cerebri: results with radiation therapy. Cancer 78:1789–1793, 1996.
6. Dexter MA, Parker GD, Besser M, et al: MR and positron emission tomography with fluorodeoxyglucose in gliomatosis cerebri. AJNR 16:1507–1510, 1995.
7. Essig M, Schlemmer H-P, Tronnier V, et al: Fluid-attenuated inversion-recovery MR imaging of gliomatosis cerebri. Eur Radiol 11:303–308, 2001.
8. Freund M, Hähnel S, Sommer C, et al: CT and MRI findings in gliomatosis cerebri: a neuroradiologic and neuropathologic review of diffuse infiltrating brain neoplasms. Eur Radiol 11:309–316, 2001.
9. Galanaud D, Chinot O, Nicoli F, et al: Use of proton magnetic resonance spectroscopy of the brain to differentiate gliomatosis cerebri from low-grade glioma. J Neurosurg 98:269–273, 1003.
10. Galatioto S, Marafioti T, Cavallari, et al: Gliomatosis cerebri: clinical, neuropathological, immunohistochemical and morphometric studies. Zentralbl Pathol 139:261–267, 1993.
11. Herrlinger U, Felsberg J, Küker W, et al: Gliomatosis cerebri: molecular pathology and clinical course. Ann Neurol 52:390–399, 2002.
12. Horst E, Micke O, Romppainen ML, et al: Radiation therapy approach in gliomatosis cerebri. Acta Oncol 39(6):747–751, 2000.
13. Jennings MT, Frenchman M, Shehab T, et al: Gliomatosis cerebri presenting as intractable epilepsy during early childhood. J Child Neurol 10:37–45, 1995.
14. Kim DG, Yang HJ, Park IA, et al: Gliomatosis cerebri: clinical features, treatment, and prognosis. Acta Neurochir (Wien) 140:755–763, 1998.
15. Kleihues P, Cavenee WK (eds): Pathology and Genetics of Tumours of the Nervous System. Lyon, France, IARC Press, 2000.
16. Kros JM, Zheng P, Dinjens WNM, et al: Genetic alterations in gliomatosis cerebri support monoclonal tumorigenesis. J Neuropathol Exper Neurol 61:806–814, 2002.
17. Mineura K, Sasajima T, Kowada M, et al: Innovative approach in the diagnosis of gliomatosis cerebri using carbon-11-L-methionine positron emission tomography. J Nucl Med 32:726–728, 1991.
18. Nevin S: Gliomatosis cerebri. Brain 61:170–191, 1938.
19. Shintani S, Tsuruoka S, Shiigai T: Serial positron emission tomography (PET) in gliomatosis cerebri treated with radiotherapy: a case report. J Neurolog Sci 173:25–31, 2000.
20. Vates GE, Chang S, Lamborn KR, et al: Gliomatosis cerebri: a review of 22 cases. Neurosurgery 53:261–271, 2003
21. Yang S, Wetzel S, Cha S: Dynamic contrast-enhanced T2*-weighted MR imaging of gliomatosis cerebri. AJNR 23:350–355, 2002.

CHAPTER 29

CHORDOID GLIOMA OF THE THIRD VENTRICLE

Gary L. Gallia, Martin G. Pomper, and Alessandro Olivi

Chordoid glioma of the third ventricle, described by Brat et al[1] in 1998 as a distinct clinicopathologic entity, is a rare, slowly growing glial tumor, located in the third ventricle of adults. This tumor has been provisionally assigned a grade II in the latest World Health Organization classification of tumors of the nervous system.[8] Since the initial description, fewer than 35 cases have been detailed in the English language.[1-7,11-14,16-18] This chapter highlights the clinical, neuroradiologic, and pathologic features, as well as the treatment and prognosis, of these rare lesions.

CLINICAL FEATURES

Chordoid gliomas have been described almost exclusively in adult patients with a mean age at presentation of 46 years (range 31 to 70 years). One case has been reported in a 12-year-old child.[3] The initial report of eight cases by Brat et al[1] reported a 7:1 female-to-male ratio. As more cases have accumulated, chordoid gliomas appear to be only slightly more common in females with a female-to-male ratio of 1.4:1.

Chordoid gliomas arise in the region of the hypothalamus and the anterior third ventricle, and presenting signs and symptoms are related to their location in this region of the brain. The most common symptom is headache. Other clinical manifestations of these tumors are (1) obstructive hydrocephalus with signs of elevated intracranial pressure including nausea, vomiting, somnolence, memory deficits, and ataxia; (2) visual disturbances secondary to compression of the optic chiasm; and (3) endocrine abnormalities such as diabetes insipidus, hypothyroidism, and amenorrhea.

NEUROIMAGING

Neuroimaging features of chordoid gliomas are remarkably uniform.[2,12,17] These tumors are well circumscribed, ovoid, and located in the region of the hypothalamus and the anterior third ventricle. On computed tomography (CT) scans, chordoid gliomas are hyperdense to gray matter with homogeneous enhancement after contrast administration (Figure 29-1A and B). On magnetic resonance imaging (MRI), tumors are typically isointense on T1-weighted sequences, isointense to hyperintense on T2-weighted images, and enhance homogeneously following gadolinium administration (Figure 29-1C and D).

Obstructive hydrocephalus is a common finding. Vasogenic edema, when present, tends to be bilaterally symmetric and may involve the optic tracts, basal ganglia, posterior limb of internal capsule, and lateral geniculate ganglia of thalamus.[1,12,17] These lesions are typically solid, although cystic components (both central and peripheral) have been noted in approximately 15% to 20% of cases.[1,6,12,17]

PATHOLOGY

The histopathologic and immunohistochemical features of adult chordoid gliomas are also remarkably consistent. Histopathologic hallmarks of chordoid gliomas include (1) cords and clusters of oval-to-polygonal epithelioid cells with abundant eosinophilic cytoplasm, (2) basophilic mucinous stroma, and (3) lymphoplasmacytic infiltrate with plasma cells containing frequent Russell bodies (Figure 29-2A). There is no significant infiltration of the surrounding brain, and adjacent brain tissue often exhibits reactive changes with gliosis and Rosenthal fibers. Vascular proliferation and necrosis are absent. These lesions lack whorl formation, psammoma bodies, nuclear pseudoinclusions, and physaliphorous cells.

The proliferative potential of chordoid gliomas corresponds to a low-grade glioma. Mitoses are rare or absent. The proliferation index is low, with MIB-1 labeling values usually less than 1.5% and uniformly less than 5%.

Immunohistochemically, chordoid gliomas stain strongly for glial fibrillary acidic protein (GFAP) and vimentin (Figure 29-2B). These tumors may also demonstrate focal expression of CD34, S-100, epithelial membrane antigen (EMA), and cytokeratin. Estrogen and progesterone receptors have not been demonstrated in these lesions. Interestingly, Wanschitz et al[19] described a 24-year-old woman with a solid, third ventricular tumor with similar histologic and immunohistochemical features. The authors described nests and cords of cuboid cells, a myxoid vacuolated matrix, a prominent lymphoplasmacytic infiltrate, and immunoreactivity for GFAP. Although the authors concluded that the tumor represented a meningioma with a peculiar expression of GFAP, this case probably represents a chordoid glioma.

The only reported case of a chordoid glioma occurring in a child shared many histologic features with adult chordoid gliomas, including cords and clusters of epithelioid tumor cells embedded in a mucinous matrix, low-grade histology, relative

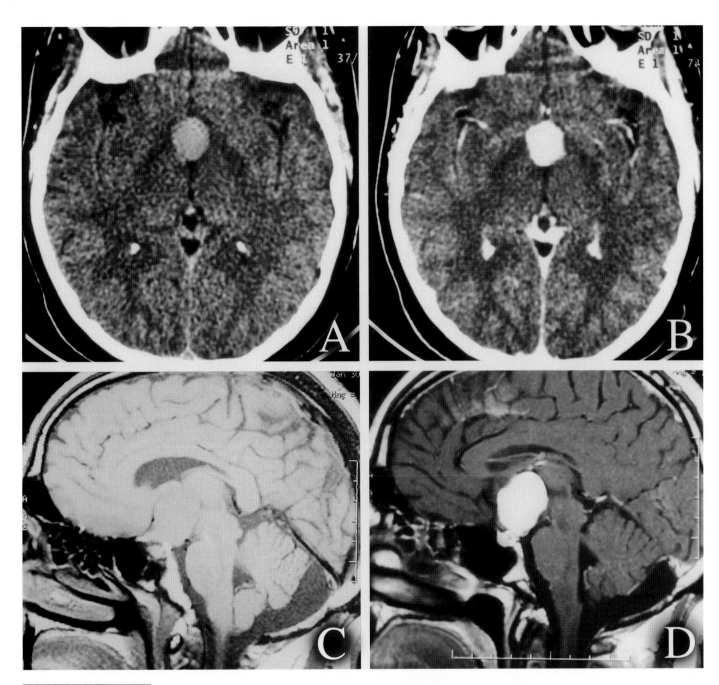

FIGURE 29-1   *A* and *B,* Computed tomography (CT) scans of a patient with a chordoid glioma. Unenhanced axial CT scan reveals a hyperdense mass in the suprasellar region *(A),* which enhances uniformly after contrast administration *(B). C* and *D,* Magnetic resonance images of a patient with a chordoid glioma. Unenhanced sagittal T1-weighted image demonstrating an isointense mass in the hypothalamus and third ventricular regions *(C),* which enhances homogeneously after gadolinium administration *(D).* (Used with permission from Pomper MG, Passe TJ, Burger PC, et al: Chordoid glioma: a neoplasm unique to the hypothalamus and anterior third ventricle. Am J Neuroradiol 22:464–469, 2001. © American Society of Neuroradiology.)

circumscription, and strong GFAP immunostaining.[3] In addition, this case has several distinct features. More specifically, this tumor contained islands and sheets of cells with cartilaginous differentiation intermixed with the glial component. A graded morphologic transition was noted between chordoid and chondroid regions, and cells in both regions were GFAP and S-100 positive. Also, in contrast to the prominent lym-

phoplasmacytic infiltrate and Russell bodies found in adult chordoid gliomas, this case demonstrated only scattered plasma cells without Russell bodies.[3]

Although the cell of origin of chordoid gliomas remains uncertain, several reports suggest an ependymal derivation. Ultrastructural examination of these tumors demonstrated that the majority of tumors contained abundant cytoplasmic

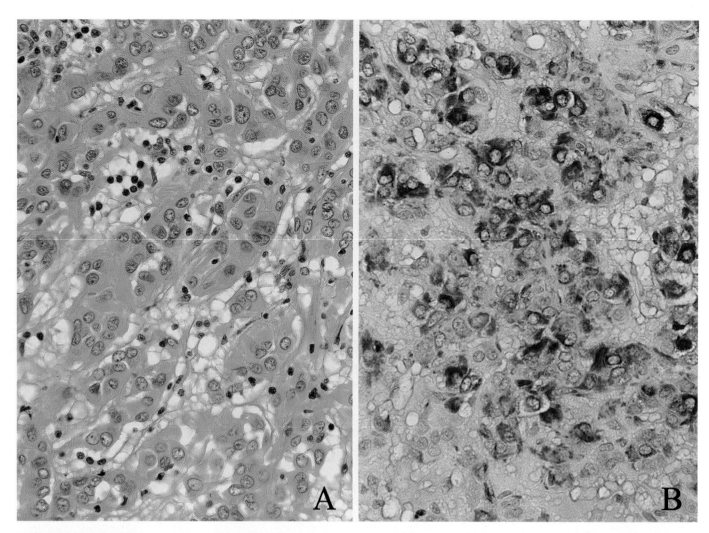

FIGURE 29-2 Histopathologic features of chordoid gliomas. *A,* Cords or clusters of large neoplastic epithelioid cells embedded in a vacuolated mucin-rich stroma with a lymphoplasmacytic infiltrate. *B,* Tumor cells are immunoreactive for glial fibrillary acidic protein.

intermediate filaments, intermediate junctions, focal basal lamina formation, and focal microvilli; sparse juxtanuclear abnormal cilia have also been reported.[1,4,11,14] Features suggestive of meningioma, such as complex cell membrane interdigitations, were absent. Two additional reports support an ependymal origin. In the case report of Ricoy et al,[14] part of the tumor surface was covered with ependyma, and the neoplasm was thought to have developed from the subependymal tissue. In addition, Cenacchi et al[4] observed ultrastructural similarities between chordoid glioma cells and ependymomas, such as an apical pole with microvilli and a basal pole with many hemidesmosome-like structures connecting the cell membranes to the underlying basal lamina. Moreover, they observed ultrastructural similarities between chordoid gliomas and specialized secretory ependymal cells of the subcommissural organ (SCO), a circumventricular organ located in the dorsocaudal region of the third ventricle. More specifically, Cenacchi et al[4] described a submicroscopic cell body zonation with perinuclear, intermediate, subapical, and apical regions and the presence of secretory granules. Similar ultrastructural findings have been described for the SCO,[15] suggesting that

chordoid gliomas may represent a subtype of ependymoma whose cells resemble the highly specialized ependyma of the subcommissural organ.[2]

DIFFERENTIAL DIAGNOSIS

The differential diagnosis includes other contrast-enhancing solid tumors arising within or preferentially involving the hypothalamic, suprasellar, or anterior third ventricular regions.[10] From a histopathologic viewpoint, chordoid glioma must be distinguished from two other chordoid lesions, chordoid meningiomas and chordomas. Chordoid gliomas can be distinguished from chordoid meningiomas by the lack of cellular whorls, psammoma bodies, and nuclear pseudoinclusions. In addition, in contrast to chordoid gliomas, chordoid meningiomas are immunophenotypically reactive for EMA and negative for GFAP. Chordoid gliomas can be distinguished from chordomas by the lack of physaliphorous cells in the former. Moreover, chordomas express EMA and cytokeratin and are only rarely positive for GFAP.

MOLECULAR GENETICS

Analysis of four chordoid gliomas by comparative genomic hybridization (CGH) did not reveal any chromosomal imbalances.[13] Additional genetic analysis revealed neither aberrations of the TP53 and CDKN2A tumor-suppressor genes nor amplification of the epidermal growth factor receptor (EGFR), CDK4, and MDM2 proto-oncogenes. The absence of detectable alterations of these genes, which are often aberrant in diffuse astrocytomas,[9] suggests that the molecular pathogenesis of chordoid gliomas differs from that of astrocytomas. In addition, the absence of deletions on chromosome 22q by CGH coupled with the strong expression of schwannomin or merlin suggests that inactivation of the neurofibromatosis 2 (NF2) gene, an alteration found in many meningiomas,[20] is not involved in the pathogenesis of chordoid gliomas.[13]

TREATMENT AND PROGNOSIS

The current treatment of choice for chordoid glioma is surgical resection with the goal of complete tumor removal. The location of these tumors within the third ventricle and their attachment to hypothalamic and suprasellar structures presents a formidable challenge to neurosurgeons and often precludes a total resection. Indeed, gross-total resections were achievable in less than 40% of reported cases.

Follow-up is available in only 20 of the reported cases to date. Of these patients, 11 were alive without evidence of recurrence with a mean of 22.5 months (range 6 to 68 months). Four patients, all of whom had a subtotal resection, had a recurrence at a mean of 24.8 months (range 5 to 48 months). Three of these patients with recurrent disease died, one from massive tumor regrowth and two from medical complications. In addition, five patients died in the postoperative period (four from pulmonary embolism and one from pneumonia).

The role of adjuvant radiation therapy or chemotherapy for chordoid gliomas following a subtotal surgical resection is unclear. Five of the reported patients underwent radiotherapy after a subtotal resection; three of these experienced tumor regrowth. No patient reported to date has been treated with adjuvant chemotherapy. With the limited number of cases, more experience will be necessary to help define the prognosis and optimal treatment strategy for patients with chordoid gliomas.

References

1. Brat DJ, Scheithauer BW, Staugaitis SM, et al: Third ventricular chordoid glioma: a distinct clinicopathologic entity. J Neuropathol Exp Neurol 57:283–290, 1998.
2. Castellano-Sanchez AA, Recine MA, Restrepo R, et al: Chordoid glioma: a novel tumor of the third ventricle. Ann Diagn Pathol 4:373–378, 2000.
3. Castellano-Sanchez AA, Schemankewitz E, Mazewski C, et al: Pediatric chordoid glioma with chondroid metaplasia. Pediatr Dev Pathol 4:564–567, 2001.
4. Cenacchi G, Roncaroli F, Cerasoli S, et al: Chordoid glioma of the third ventricle: an ultrastructural study of three cases with a histogenetic hypothesis. Am J Surg Pathol 25:401–405, 2001.
5. Galloway M, Afshar F, Geddes JF: Chordoid glioma: an uncommon tumour of the third ventricle. Br J Neurosurg 15:147–150, 2001.
6. Grand S, Pasquier B, Gay E, et al: Chordoid glioma of the third ventricle: CT and MRI, including perfusion data. Neuroradiology 44:842–846, 2002.
7. Hanbali F, Fuller GN, Leeds NE, et al: Choroid plexus cyst and chordoid glioma: report of two cases. Neurosurg Focus 10:1–6, 2001.
8. Kleihues P, Cavenee WK (eds): World Health Organization Classification of Tumors. Pathology and Genetics. Tumors of the Nervous System. Lyon, France, IARC Press, 2000.
9. Nagane M, Huang HJ, Cavenee WK: Advances in the molecular genetics of gliomas. Curr Opin Oncol 9:215–222, 1997.
10. Osborn AG, Maack J (eds): Diagnostic Neuroradiology. St Louis, Mosby, 1994.
11. Pasquier B, Péoc'h M, Morrison AL, et al: Chordoid glioma of the third ventricle: a report of two new cases, with further evidence supporting an ependymal differentiation, and review of the literature. Am J Surg Pathol 26:1330–1342, 2002.
12. Pomper MG, Passe TJ, Burger PC, et al: Chordoid glioma: a neoplasm unique to the hypothalamus and anterior third ventricle. Am J Neuroradiol 22:464–469, 2001.
13. Reifenberger G, Weber T, Weber RG, et al: Chordoid glioma of the third ventricle: immunohistochemical and molecular genetic characterization of a novel tumor entity. Brain Pathol 9:617–626, 1999.
14. Ricoy JR, Lobato RD, Báez B, et al: Suprasellar chordoid glioma. Acta Neuropathol 99:699–703, 2000.
15. Rodríguez EM, Rodríguez S, Hein S: The subcommissural organ. Microsc Res Techn 41:98–123, 1998.
16. Taraszewska A, Matyja E: Immunohistochemical studies in diagnosis of the uncommon cases of tumors of the central nervous system. Folia Histochem Cytobiol 40:207–208, 2002.
17. Tonami H, Kamehiro M, Oguchi M, et al: Chordoid glioma of the third ventricle: CT and MR findings. J Comput Assist Tomogr 24:336–338, 2000.
18. Vajtai I, Varga Z, Scheithauer BW, et al: Chordoid glioma of the third ventricle: confirmatory report of a new entity. Hum Pathol 30:723–726, 1999.
19. Wanschitz J, Schmidbauer M, Maier H, et al: Suprasellar meningioma with expression of glial fibrillary acidic protein: a peculiar variant. Acta Neuropathol (Berl) 90:539–544, 1995.
20. Zang KD: Cytological and cytogenetical studies on human meningiomas. Cancer Genet Cytogenet 6:249–274, 1982.

CHAPTER 30

MIXED NEURONAL AND GLIAL TUMORS

Richard A. Prayson, Lilyana Angelov, and Gene H. Barnett

Gangliogliomas are the most commonly encountered glial-neuronal neoplasm. These tumors are defined by two histologic components: atypical ganglion cells and neoplastic glial cells. Incidence rates for gangliogliomas have been variably reported to be 0.4% to 6.25% of all primary brain tumors in adults and up to 10% of primary brain tumors in children. The apparent wide variability in incidence is likely related to the histologic diversity of the tumors and individual pathologist bias in interpreting the histology.[7] The age of affected individuals is quite variable and ranges from infancy to 80 years of age. The majority of cases present during the first 2 or 3 decades of life, and there appears to be a slight male predominance in cases reported from several large series.[13,17,22]

LOCATION

Gangliogliomas may arise throughout the neuroaxis, with the majority of supratentorial tumors originating in the temporal lobe. One possible reason for this is that the granular neurons continue to be produced postnatally in the subgranular zone of the dentate gyrus. Hence this area may have a greater susceptibility to a mixed neuronal-glial neoplastic transformation resulting in a ganglioglioma. Less common locations for ganglioglioma include the cerebellum, basal ganglia, pineal gland, hypothalamus, spinal cord, brainstem, and pituitary gland. Optic nerve gangliogliomas arising in the setting of neurofibromatosis type I have been described in children.

CLINICAL PRESENTATION

Signs and symptoms at the time of presentation depend on the location of the neoplasm. Most supratentorial lesions present with seizures, with the semiology related to the tumor location. Specifically, temporal lobe–based tumors usually present with medically intractable partial complex seizures. The duration of seizures prior to diagnosis may be quite extensive, often on the order of years (mean of 14 years, range 1 to 38 years in one study).[17] Further, long-standing seizures in children, or the anticonvulsants used to treat them, may result in developmental delay, learning disabilities, and behavioral problems. Most gangliogliomas do not present with evidence of raised intracranial pressure, because their growth is typically indolent. Cerebellum-based tumors often present with ataxia and headaches caused by hydrocephalus from fourth ventricular compression. Spinal cord tumors may present with progressive weakness. Tumors arising in the spinal cord and brainstem generally have a shorter interval of symptoms before diagnosis (approximately 1 to 1.5 years) than do temporal lobe neoplasms.

IMAGING CHARACTERISTICS

Magnetic resonance imaging (MRI) provides the best diagnostic modality for tumor detection and is more sensitive than computed tomography (CT). It is unable, however, to reliably differentiate between different tumor types and, in particular, ganglioglioma. This is due, in part, to the fact that gangliogliomas do not have a single "diagnostic" radiographic appearance. MRI also has the added benefit of being a good screening tool for other pathologies often encountered in the chronic epilepsy setting such as cortical dysplasia and hippocampal sclerosis. Imaging studies of gangliogliomas usually show a relatively circumscribed mass (hypointense on T1-weighted images and hyperintense on T2-weighted images), which may be either solid or cystic (Figure 30-1).[3] Enhancement is variable and may range from none to marked. On CT scan, the most common appearance is that of a cystic isodense or hypodense tumor with a mural nodule that is calcified in approximately half of the tumors studied. Edema and mass effect are often not present. The lesions typically are avascular on angiography. Because gangliogliomas often involve the cortical surface, inner-table indentation can at times be seen on CT scan. Rarely, anaplastic gangliogliomas are infiltrative (i.e., less circumscribed in appearance). Increased enhancement and peritumoral edema have also been more commonly described in higher grade tumors.

Low-grade gangliogliomas, evaluated by positron-emission tomography with ^{18}F-fluorodeoxyglucose (FDG-PET) by Kincaid et al, showed tumor hypometabolism; high-grade tumors were marked by increased ^{201}T1-single-photon emission computed tomography (SPECT) activity in contrast to low-grade gangliogliomas.[10]

NEUROPHYSIOLOGY

In patients with chronic epilepsy, electroencephalography (EEG) is helpful in defining seizure type and site of origin. In

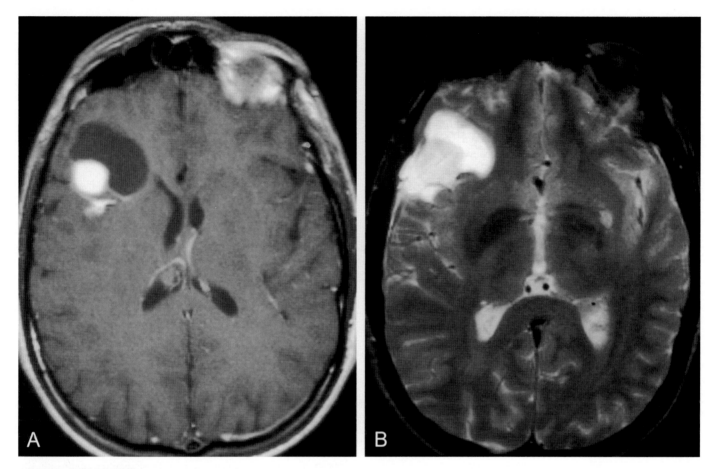

FIGURE 30-1 Axial contrast-enhanced T1-weighted *(A)* and nonenhanced T2-weighted *(B)* magnetic resonance images of a right supratentorial ganglioglioma with a prominent mural nodule and cystic component.

most cases, the interictal EEG focus corresponds to the true location of the tumor. A minority of patients may demonstrate a second interictal focus or widespread interictal activity. Seizures may arise at a site distant from the epileptogenic zone. In many instances the tumor itself is electrically silent, and the seizure activity appears to be generated from the surrounding parenchyma. This finding may be related to the high incidence of coexisting cortical dysplasia (malformations of cortical development), a well-recognized cause of chronic epilepsy.[17,22]

HISTOPATHOLOGY

Ganglioglioma

Histologically, the tumor is marked by an admixture of atypical-appearing neuronal or ganglion cells intermixed with a glioma-like component, most often resembling an astrocytoma (Figure 30-2). The neuronal cell component commonly is unevenly distributed throughout the neoplasm; therefore sampling of the tumor is important for arriving at an accurate diagnosis. Neurons are considered to be neoplastic if they occur in a heterotopic location or demonstrate cytologic atypia. Binucleate neurons are a common finding. The glial component of the tumor may demonstrate variable degrees of hypercellularity

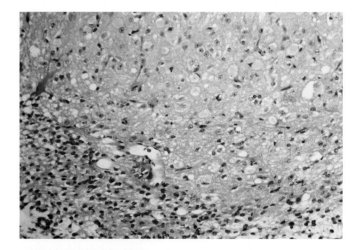

FIGURE 30-2 Ganglioglioma is histologically marked by an atypical ganglion cell component and a glioma component. (Hematoxylin and eosin, original magnification ×200.)

and nuclear pleomorphism. Mitotic activity is difficult to identify in the ordinary low-grade ganglioglioma, in contrast to anaplastic ganglioglioma where mitotic activity may be readily identifiable. Focal vascular proliferative changes and hypervascularity are also common findings in these tumors and may account for the enhancement seen radiographically. Microcystic degeneration may be focally identified in a subset of lesions. The cyst wall of those lesions associated with a large cystic component is often composed of non-neoplastic, compressed brain parenchyma. Calcification was observed in slightly less than half of tumors in one series.[17] Eosinophilic granular bodies can be observed in a majority of cases, as can vessels with perivascular lymphocytic infiltrates. Necrosis is a distinctly uncommon feature in ordinary gangliogliomas, but is more commonly observed in anaplastic tumors. Focal leptomeningeal extension of tumor may also be present but does not appear to adversely affect outcome.

The precise criteria for distinguishing anaplastic ganglioglioma from ordinary low-grade ganglioglioma are not well defined. Most of the literature on the subject consists of isolated case reports. In anaplastic ganglioglioma, the malignant features usually occur in the glioma component of the tumor and resemble a high-grade astrocytoma (glioblastoma multiforme). This tumor is marked by a variable constellation of findings, including prominent hypercellularity, readily identifiable mitotic activity, and necrosis. Ancillary testing with cell proliferation markers may be useful in identifying those tumors with a particularly high rate of cell proliferation.

Variants

A few histopathologic variants of ganglioglioma deserve mention. Occasional tumors contain islands or geographic areas marked by prominent numbers of small, round neuronal cells resembling neurocytoma. The tumors tend to be similarly well-circumscribed and are focally contrast enhanced. Histologically, these neurocytoma-like areas may be intermixed with areas that resemble a more conventional-appearing ganglioglioma. Occasionally, mitotic activity may be somewhat prominent in these regions. The terms *gangliocytoma* or *ganglioneurocytoma* have been historically applied to these neurocytoma-like lesions. The small cellular component of the tumor is marked with immunostains to synaptophysin and neurofilament, indicating neuronal differentiation. Distinction of this lesion from an oligodendroglioma or mixed glioma should be made because of the more aggressive behavior of the latter two tumors. There is no known behavioral difference, however, from ganglioglioma associated with this histologic variant.[5]

Another rare variant of ganglioglioma is the papillary glioneuronal tumor. The neoplasm is characterized by pseudopapillary architectural pattern in which the papillae are lined by cuboidal cells with intervening solid areas comprising cells with rounded nuclei and scant cytoplasm that demonstrate evidence of neural differentiation.[11] Mature gangliocytic cells are generally not present. Although the literature is limited on this tumor type, it appears to behave in a relatively benign fashion.

A small percentage of gangliogliomas have a particularly spindled-cell appearance and are associated with a collagenous stroma. This particular subset is generally referred to as the *desmoplastic infantile ganglioglioma*. These tumors are more superficially located, most commonly arising in the frontotemporal lobe region, and classically present as cystic, dural-based masses in the first 2 years of life.[21] Occasionally, aggregates of poorly differentiated cells may be observed in the tumor. These cells may demonstrate appreciable mitotic activity. Although the reported number of cases of this variant is relatively small, there is a suggestion that with gross-total resection, long-term survival is the usual outcome.

One other recently described variant deserves brief mention. In 1999 Teo et al described a morphologically distinct tumor arising in adults that was marked by the presence of neuropil-like "rosetted" islands.[20] The neuropil-like islands demonstrate evidence of neural differentiation in the background of what otherwise resembles a World Health Organization grade II or III astrocytoma. Experience with these tumors is limited but indicates a variable outcome, particularly when associated with worrisome histologic features, including necrosis and prominent mitotic activity.

Cortical Dysplasia

Recognition of an association of ganglioglioma with cortical dysplasia has also emerged in the past decade. In a series of intracranial gangliogliomas, evidence of adjacent cortical architectural abnormalities (cortical dysplasia) was identified in 50% of cases in which there was sufficient amount of adjacent tissue suitable for evaluation.[17] There have also been reports of an association of ganglioglioma with other low-grade glioneuronal tumors, some of which are, likewise, associated with cortical dysplasia; these include pleomorphic xanthoastrocytomas and dysembryoplastic neuroepithelial tumors.[15,16] These associations raise interesting questions regarding the relationship between cortical dysplasia and these other developmental neoplasms and ganglioglioma. Whether a subset of gangliogliomas represent a tumoral form of dysplasia, arise out of dysplasia, or are similarly derived from abnormalities of cortical development remains to be elucidated.

Immunohistochemistry, Proliferation Indices, and Molecular Diagnosis

Because of the variability of the ganglion cell component of these tumors, immunohistochemistry can be occasionally helpful in delineating the neuronal cells from their glial counterparts. Markers of neural differentiation such as synaptophysin can be helpful in highlighting the atypical ganglion cells.[18] One must be careful, however, not to overinterpret normal, resident neuronal cells as representing part of the neoplasm. Further, normal neurons in the spinal cord may stain positive with synaptophysin, making the pathologic diagnosis more challenging when gangliogliomas arise in the spinal cord. The astrocytic component of the tumor generally stains positively with antibody to glial fibrillary acidic protein (GFAP).

Not surprisingly, rates of cell proliferation, as determined by cell proliferation markers such as Ki-67 or MIB-1, are low, with labeling indices (percentage of positive staining tumor cells) often less than 1%.[17,22] In contrast, the anaplastic ganglioglioma often demonstrates higher cell proliferation labeling indices. Utilization of cell proliferation markers in the routine evaluation of these tumors is probably not warranted. In a case of suspected anaplastic ganglioglioma, use of a cell proliferation marker may corroborate the pathologist's impression that the lesion is higher grade, yielding a labeling index that is often in the range observed with anaplastic gliomas.

Currently, the role for genetic or molecular biologic evaluation of gangliogliomas remains undefined. Increased p53 immunoexpression has been described in association with recurrent and higher grade tumors. A variety of genetic abnormalities have been described in association with gangliogliomas, including abnormalities on the short arm of chromosome 9; trisomies of chromosomes 5, 6, and 7; deletions on chromosome 6; and ring chromosome 1.[14,23] Rare cases of ganglioglioma with malignant transformation that have been studied show a variety of karyotypic abnormalities involving multiple chromosomes. There has also been some suggestion in the literature that mutations associated with the tuberous sclerosis 2 (TSC2) gene on chromosome 16p13 may confer a predisposition to ganglioglioma.[2]

MANAGEMENT

Surgery

Surgery is the treatment of choice in these lesions. The tumors are often well circumscribed and therefore have the potential for complete resection, which results in greater than 90% 5-year survival.[6,13] The location of the lesion dictates the surgical approach. Because the majority of these tumors are located in the temporal lobe, a temporal or pterional craniotomy is used to approach the lesion. Whereas aggressive resection is the goal, the sylvian and perforating vessels, cerebral peduncle, and cranial nerves III and IV must be recognized and carefully preserved in this approach. Similarly for lesions in other locations, local and regional anatomy must be considered. If the lesion is on the cortical surface, the gyri typically appear pale, swollen, and discrete from the normal brain across a sulcus. These lesions are usually avascular and can at times be visibly calcified. Given the often long-standing seizure history associated with gangliogliomas, intraoperative electrocorticography (ECoG) is an important surgical adjunct and often guides the extent of resection beyond the radiographic or visuotactile boundaries of the tumor.

Because the epileptogenic focus is not always the tumor, the extent of resection may be variable and is an issue of some debate. In an analysis of tumors associated with chronic epilepsy, Awad et al noted that the seizure focus was within the structural lesion in 23% of patients, contiguous but extending to at least 2 cm beyond the lesion in 38% of patients, and remote or noncontiguous in the remainder.[1] The surgical decision is whether resection of the tumor alone is sufficient to treat the seizures or whether resection of the tumor with adjacent epileptogenic cortex is required. Although there are substantial data associating resection of the tumor alone with good seizure outcome, some have recommended that resection of the adjacent cortical cortex be performed to improve seizure outcome, using ECoG or subdural electrodes.[9] In cases where the tumor is relatively inaccessible and the epileptogenic zone is not localized with the tumor, a surgical approach limited to resection of the epileptogenic zone has been suggested by some. This approach often provides some improvement in seizure frequency and severity but does not usually provide seizure-free outcome.[4] With satisfactory pharmacologic management of patients, however, one could argue in favor of delaying surgical intervention, given the low-grade nature of most gangliogliomas. Others would counter that early surgery allows for an accurate histologic diagnosis and identification of those tumor types that might be more likely to undergo malignant transformation or degeneration over time, most notably diffuse or fibrillary astrocytomas, oligodendrogliomas, and mixed gliomas (oligoastrocytomas). Often, seizures are well controlled postoperatively, and consideration can be given to discontinuing anticonvulsants.

Adjuvant Therapy

There appears to be little support in the literature for routine use of adjuvant radiation therapy or chemotherapy in the management of these tumors. With a complete resection, patients do not receive follow-up radiation therapy. Even with incomplete resections, the role of radiation therapy in the treatment of benign gangliogliomas remains uncertain, with some reports suggesting that neither conventional radiation therapy nor radiosurgery provide significant tumor control.[6,8,13] Moreover, besides the adverse effects of radiation therapy on the developing central nervous system in a child, there is also the risk of inducing malignant transformation in an otherwise low-grade neoplasm.[19] Furthermore, even with subtotal resection, relapse is reported as being uncommon even in the absence of adjuvant therapy.[3,12] Radiation therapy is thus generally reserved for recurrent tumors not amenable to further resection or malignant tumors.

Similarly, chemotherapy, which is generally nitrosourea-based, appears to have a limited role, with some studies suggesting it be used after surgery and radiation therapy have failed or as a way to defer radiation therapy in a young child with an aggressive tumor.[3] Newer agents, such as the oral alkylating agent temozolomide, have been used with some success where complete resection is not possible and have resulted in radiologic stabilization of the lesion, although further studies are needed (Barnett, unpublished data).

ANAPLASTIC GANGLIOGLIOMAS

These malignant gangliogliomas are relatively uncommon and histologically present with grade III and IV features in the glial compartment, often with high MIB-1 and TP53 labeling indices. These tumors tend to arise in young patients and are inherently more aggressive behaving and have a significantly worse prognosis than their benign counterpart. Anaplastic gangliogliomas can arise because of malignant degeneration in a previously resected or irradiated ganglioglioma or can present as de novo lesions. Surgical resection continues to play a role in these cases. Adjuvant therapy, though less well defined in this subset of tumors, may play a role in their management. Specifically, radiation, conventional chemotherapy, intracavitary radioactive monoclonal antibodies, and autologous chemotherapy have all been used. Patients, however, ultimately succumb to their disease despite aggressive treatment.

Acknowledgments

The authors wish to thank Ms. Martha Tobin for her assistance with the preparation of this manuscript. This work was supported, in part, by the Rose Ella Burkhardt Endowment.

References

1. Awad IA, Rosenfeld J, Ahl J, et al: Intractable epilepsy and structural lesions of the brain: mapping, resection strategies and seizure outcome. Epilepsia 32:179–186, 1991.
2. Becker AJ, Löbach M, Klein H, et al: Mutational analysis of TSC1 and TSC2 genes in gangliogliomas. Neuropathol Appl Neurobiol 27:105–114, 2001.
3. Castillo M, Davis PC, Takei Y, Hoffman JC: Intracranial ganglioglioma: MR, CT and clinical findings in 18 patients. AJNR 11:109–114, 1990.
4. Fish D, Andermann F, Olivier A: Complex partial seizures and small posterior temporal or extratemporal structural lesions: surgical management. Neurology 41:1781–1784, 1991.
5. Giangaspero F, Cenacchi G, Losi L, et al: Extraventricular neoplasms with neurocytoma features: a clinicopathological study of 11 cases. Am J Surg Pathol 21:206–212, 1997.
6. Haddad SF, Moore SA, Menezes AH, VanGilder JC: Ganglioglioma: 13 years of experience. Neurosurgery 31:171–178, 1992.
7. Hamburger C, Büttner A, Weis S: Ganglioglioma of the spinal cord: report of two rare cases and review of the literature. Neurosurgery 41:1410–1416, 1997.
8. Im S-H, Chung CK, Cho B-K, et al: Intracranial ganglioglioma: preoperative characteristics and oncologic outcome after surgery. J Neurooncol 59:173–183, 2002.
9. Khajavi K, Comair YG, Prayson RA, et al: Childhood ganglioglioma and medically intractable epilepsy. Pediatr Neurosurg 22:181–188, 1995.
10. Kincaid PK, El-Saden SM, Park S-H, Goy BW: Cerebral gangliogliomas: preoperative grading using FDG-PET and ^{201}T1-SPECT. AJNR 19:801–806, 1998.
11. Komori T, Scheithauer BW, Anthony DC, et al: Papillary glioneuronal tumor. A new variant of mixed neuronal-glial neoplasm. Am J Surg Pathol 22:1171–1183, 1998.
12. Krouwer HGJ, Davis RL, McDermott MW, et al: Gangliogliomas: a clinicopathological study of 25 cases and review of the literature. J Neurooncol 17:139–154, 1993.
13. Lang FF, Epstein FJ, Ransohoff J, et al: Central nervous system gangliogliomas. Part 2: Clinical outcome. J Neurosurg 79:867–873, 1953.
14. Neumann E, Kalousek DK, Norman MG, et al: Cytogenetic analysis of 109 pediatric central nervous system tumors. Cancer Genet Cytogenet 71:40–49, 1993.
15. Perry A, Giannini C, Scheithauer BW, et al: Composite pleomorphic xanthoastrocytoma and ganglioglioma: report of four cases and review of the literature. Am J Surg Pathol 21:763–771, 1997.
16. Prayson RA: Composite ganglioglioma and dysembryoplastic neuroepithelial tumor. Arch Pathol Lab Med 123:247–250, 1999.
17. Prayson RA, Khajavi K, Comair YG: Cortical architectural abnormalities and MIB-1 immunoreactivity in gangliogliomas: a study of 60 patients with intracranial tumors. J Neuropathol Exp Neurol 54:513–520, 1995.
18. Quinn B: Synaptophysin staining in normal brain. Importance for the diagnosis of gangliogliomas. Am J Surg Pathol 22:550–556, 1998.
19. Rumana CS, Valadka AB: Radiation therapy and malignant degeneration of benign supratentorial gangliogliomas. Neurosurgery 42:1038–1043, 1998.
20. Teo JGC, Gultekin SH, Bilsky M, et al: A distinctive glioneuronal tumor of the adult cerebrum with neuropil-like (including "rosetted") islands. Am J Surg Pathol 23:502–510, 1999.
21. Vandenberg SR, May EE, Rubinstein LJ, et al: Desmoplastic supratentorial neuroepithelial tumors of infancy with divergent differentiation potential ("desmoplastic infantile gangliogliomas"). J Neurosurg 66:58–71, 1987.
22. Wolf HK, Müller MB, Spänle M, et al: Ganglioglioma: a detailed histopathological and immunohistochemical analysis of 61 cases. Acta Neuropathol 88:166–173, 1994.
23. Yin X-L, Hui AB-Y, Pang JC-S, et al: Genome-wide survey for chromosomal imbalances in ganglioglioma using comparative genomic hybridization. Cancer Genet Cytogenet 134:71–76, 2000.

CHAPTER 31

NEURONAL TUMORS

Scott R. VandenBerg

Tumors composed of neoplastic neuronal cells as either the sole or predominant population are heterogeneous with respect to both the spectrum of histopathologic features and the range of biologic behavior. Neoplasms constituted by well-differentiated or "mature" neuronal cells as the sole component include two types, both of which have hamartomatous and neoplastic features. The first, designated as *gangliocytoma*, are lesions predominantly composed of cells resembling pyramidal neurons or "ganglion" cells. The second, designated as *dysplastic gangliocytoma* of the cerebellum (Lhermitte-Duclos disease), contains a more heterogeneous population of well-differentiated neurons and is associated with the phakomatosis of Cowden's disease.

The second group of tumors has a predominantly neuronal phenotype but may exhibit some bipotential differentiation with highly variable astrocytic differentiation. These are relatively cellular neoplasms composed of smaller cells displaying a spectrum of neuronal phenotypes. The first type is the central neurocytoma, and the second type, a more recently described entity that was previously classified as a variant of medulloblastoma, is the cerebellar liponeurocytoma.

GANGLIOCYTOMAS

Incidence, Age, and Sites

The term *gangliocytoma* denotes a spectrum of rare tumors in which neuronal cell populations are the sole neoplastic constituents. As the designation implies, the neoplastic cells typically display ganglionic or a pyramidal neuronal cytoarchitecture. In addition to the conspicuous neuronal population, there is a highly variable, but usually negligible, presence of non-neoplastic glia (astrocytes) as the stroma of the lesion. The true incidence of gangliocytomas, in distinction from gangliogliomas that have a predominant neuronal component, is not well documented. Estimates range from 0.1% to 0.5% of all brain tumors.[21,120] The sites for these rare lesions include the cerebrum, hypothalamus adjacent to the floor of the third ventricle, pituitary, pineal region, brainstem, and cervicothoracic spinal cord.* Within the cerebral hemispheres, the temporal lobe, either alone or in combination with frontal or parietal regions, appears to be the slightly favored site.[3,20,25,44,49,50,102] Tumors confined to the cerebellum may also occur as dysplastic

gangliocytomas (Lhermitte-Duclos disease, see following discussion).

Most lesions within the cerebrum and the spinal cord become clinically symptomatic within the first 3 decades,[3,20,25,29,49,50,72,88,102] with a reported average of 25 years; however, clinical presentation may span into the sixth decade.[12,21,25,47,57] The duration of clinical symptoms preceding surgical intervention typically spans approximately 3 to 4 years,[3,20,21,25,29,44,49,50,102] with a range from 6 weeks to 18 years[25]; seizures and headache are the most common neurologic manifestations.[3,25] For tumors arising in the pineal and adjacent to the third ventricle, hydrocephalus may be present,[12,21,57] whereas spinal cord lesions usually produce slowly evolving long-tract signs. Gangliocytomas of the pituitary may develop in coincidence with adenomas (Figure 31-1).

Neuroimaging Studies and Macroscopic Appearance

Gangliocytomas tend to be macroscopically discrete lesions with calcification and variable cyst formation,[12,21,49,57,88] and a distinct dissection plane at the interface with adjacent tissue is variably noted.[29,50] Conspicuous mass effects are uncommon.[3,20,25,29,50] The inconsistent density of intervening neuropil that is dispersed between the cellular elements of these lesions markedly affects their discrimination by neuroimaging. Computed tomography (CT) typically shows variable focal calcification and cyst formation and regional heterogeneity within the lesion that varies from isodense to hyperdense compared with surrounding tissue.[3,20,21,25,29,44,49,88] T1-weighted magnetic resonance imaging (MRI) usually demonstrates a mixed, heterogeneous image with intermediate to decreased signal intensity, and gadolinium infusion typically demonstrates moderate heterogeneous enhancement. Punctate calcification may be visualized with T2-weighted images that usually have variable signal intensities, ranging from decreased to increased levels,[29,92] whereas the signal intensity on proton-weighted sequences tends to be increased.

Histopathology, Immunohistochemistry, and Ultrastructure

The hallmark histopathologic feature of gangliocytomas is a population of disordered neuronal cells with greater cellularity compared with the neuronal populations that normally constitute the region. The neoplastic neurons typically have large

---

*See references 3, 6, 12, 15, 20, 21, 25, 29, 44, 47, 49, 50, 57, 72, 88, 89, 102.

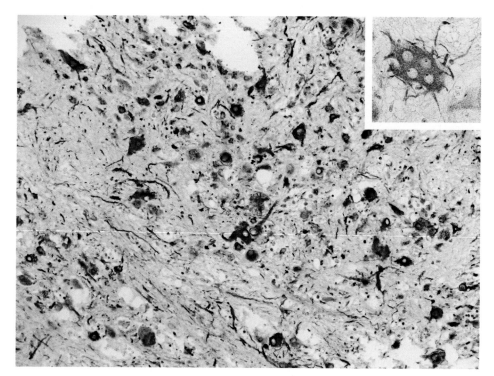

FIGURE 31-1 Gangliocy-
toma. This gangliocytoma of the pituitary
is composed of randomly oriented, dysmorphic neurons embedded in a fibrillary
matrix without an intervening astrocytic
proliferation. The majority of neoplastic
neurons are well-differentiated ganglionic
cells, many with an aberrant cytoarchitecture, including multiple nuclei *(inset)*. The
gangliocytoma in this case is intimately
adjacent to a growth-hormone-producing
pituitary adenoma. SMI-33 (phosphoryla-
tion-independent NF:H/M epitope)–avidin-
biotin complex linked immunoperoxidase
technique.

vesicular nuclei, conspicuous nucleoli, and a well-defined soma with abundant cytoplasm and a variety of aberrant cytoarchitectural features, including swollen, dysplastic multipolar processes and binucleated or multinucleated forms (see Figure 31-1). These anomalous neurons are nonrandomly grouped with anomalous orientations in a scarcely cellular "stroma" that is usually a variable combination of an ill-defined web of neuronal processes, sparse nonreactive glia, and a delicate reticulin network.[21,25,29,44,49,50,88] Within the pineal region, the stroma may notably contain melanotic cells. Whereas these neurons may share the features of cytomegaly and cytoskeletal pathology with certain types of cortical dysplasias,[69] the aberrant ganglion cells within gangliocytomas typically have a far greater degree and range of pleomorphism, including the presence of bizarre vacuolated and multinucleate forms. Silver impregnation techniques readily reveal abnormal neuritic morphology and numerous cytoplasmic granules.[12,25,57]

Immunohistochemical studies detect synaptophysin, neurofilament epitopes (M/H) and a variable array of neuropeptide and biogenic amines in the neuronal cell bodies, including immunoreactive somatostatin, met-enkephalin, leu-enkephalin, corticotrophin-releasing hormone, vasogenic intestinal peptide, β-endorphin, calcitonin, and serotonin.[25,29,102] In addition, there is a more variable distribution of chromogranin and synaptophysin that suggests neuritic terminal zone differentiation.[25,29]

An apparent variant of the gangliocytoma that contains a wider range of neuronal phenotypes with a conspicuous and more cellular admixture of both ganglionic and smaller, more neurocytic cells has occurred in two patients, aged 30 and 67 (unpublished data). The ganglionic cells display a typically large, vesicular nucleus with frequent binuclear forms, whereas the smaller neurons tend to comprise a more homogeneous cell population with round to slightly lobulated nuclei and less coarse chromatin. Both cell types are dispersed in a densely fibrillary matrix. The small cells are irregularly distributed throughout the neoplasm, including clusters of higher cellularity. No mitotic activity, nuclear pleomorphism, or endothelial proliferation is apparent.

Immunohistochemical studies of these variants demonstrate synaptophysin, microtubule-associated protein 2 (MAP2), and medium-high molecular weight neurofilament protein (NF-H/M) epitopes in both types of neuronal populations. Glial fibrillary acidic protein (GFAP) immunoreactivity is conspicuously confined to rare stromal astrocytes, consistent with the neuronal nature of gangliocytomas. The low level of MIB-1 (Ki-67) immunolabeling, which is confined to the small cell population, reflects the low growth potential of these variants.

Ultrastructural studies emphasize the dysmorphic and degenerative properties of the ganglion cells that constitute this lesion. There are a variety of abnormal cytoplasmic and neuritic inclusions, including curvilinear bodies, concentric laminated bodies, and branched tubular structures. Cytoarchitectural evidence of ganglionic maturation, including prominent nucleoli, a well-developed rough endoplasmic reticulum, abundant free ribosomes, neuritic microtubular arrays, and dense core and clear vesicles are common. Synaptic contacts, as suggested by membrane-associated punctate synaptophysin reactivity,[29] may be present but are not a conspicuous feature.[44,49,77]

Biologic Behavior and Therapy

These tumors are World Health Organization (WHO) grade I. Tumor recurrence after surgical resection, always at the original site, is extremely rare[25,50] and appears to be associated with an incomplete removal.[12,50] One notable exception is a series of nine cases in which two patients required second operations to remove additional tumor after a postoperative period of 7 to 8 years. The histologic composition of the recurrences, with respect to excluding gangliogliomas, however, was not specifically addressed.[25]

Histogenesis

There is considerable debate concerning the hamartomatous or neoplastic nature of gangliocytomas, because these lesions, by definition, contain well-differentiated but atypical neuronal cell lineages without a neoplastic glial component. The bizarre neuronal morphology, including binucleate and enlarged forms that may be present in large cortical lesions as hemimegalencephaly, which occur with aberrant neuronal migration,[19,73,106] challenges the notion that a simple set of neuronal cytoarchitectural criteria, devoid of a clinicopathologic context, can exclusively discriminate all gangliocytomas, as neoplastic lesions, from hamartomas. A partial explanation for this overlap is that, regardless of origin, both types of neuronal cell populations would be chronically subjected to common pathophysiologic influences, including abnormal extrinsic cues during neurocytogenesis, abnormal intercellular relationships including disconnection from normal afferent activity, seizure activity, and chronic reactive astrocytosis. The more common appearance of the bizarre neuronal morphology in larger hamartomas may simply reflect the greater disruption of normal cues that would be present in most neoplastic gangliocytic lesions.

The phenotypic similarities between the neuronal cell populations in some large hamartomas and gangliocytomas may also suggest that both types of abnormal neuronal lineages may arise from a similar mechanism of abnormal focal somatic mosaicism in the developing ventricular matrix[73] before neoplastic transformation in one or more of the lineages that ultimately give rise to gangliocytomas. Immunohistochemical characterization of the diverse spectrum of neuroendocrine markers that are expressed by the neoplastic neuronal cell lineages in gangliocytomas and gangliogliomas that may not be normally expressed by regional neurons may provide an additional mode by which to discriminate neoplastic from hamartomatous lineages. In contrast to the typically homogeneous and morphologically bland, often scarce astroglial component of gangliocytomas, the astrocytic population within the large hamartomatous lesions usually displays a greater range of pleomorphic and reactive changes. More definitive criteria to discriminate between dysplastic and neoplastic neuronal lineages awaits a greater understanding of the biologic mechanisms involved with origin, differentiation, and vulnerability to neoplastic transformation of the neuronal progenitors and neuronal lineages within the adult central nervous system (CNS).[40,104]

DYSPLASTIC GANGLIOCYTOMA OF THE CEREBELLUM (LHERMITTE-DUCLOS DISEASE)

Incidence, Age, and Associated Lesions

Dysplastic gangliocytoma of the cerebellum (Lhermitte-Duclos disease)[61] is a rare lesion that usually arises in a hemisphere but also may involve the vermis, usually by extension.* The lesions usually become clinically apparent between the third and fourth decades, with a reported mean age of 34 years,[111] but there is a wide age range without gender predilection, spanning the neonatal period to 74 years. The multitude of diverse designa-

tions previously applied to this lesion, including granular cell hypertrophy, granomolecular hypertrophy of the cerebellum, diffuse hypertrophy of the cerebellar cortex, and gangliomatosis of the cerebellum and ganglioneuroma, vividly signify the problem of whether the fundamental nature of this lesion is malformative or neoplastic. Regardless of histogenesis, the progressive cerebellar lesions ultimately require surgical resection, and postsurgical recurrence has been reported in at least seven cases.[11,37,64,83,96,117]

The progressive clinical manifestations of the cerebellar lesion have a mean chronicity of 46 months before diagnosis and are usually related to the effects of chronically elevated intracranial pressure from hydrocephalus or to a progressive cerebellar syndrome.[111] Less commonly, there may be cranial nerve deficits or long-tract signs caused by compressive rotation of the brainstem by the mass effect.[62] The duration in individual cases, however, may vary significantly, from less than 1 year in approximately 30% of cases with an occasionally acute onset of symptoms to more than 10 years in approximately 20% of cases. Although most neurologic symptoms result from the mass effect of the cerebellar lesion, there are a variable number of associated developmental lesions, including megalencephaly, neuronal heterotopias in the white matter, hypertrophy of the olivary nuclei, hydromyelia, a cervical syrinx, and vascular malformations, that may be accompanied by intellectual impairment or seizure disorders.[111]

More recent studies have linked the occurrence of dysplastic gangliocytomas of the cerebellum to an autosomal dominant syndrome, Cowden's disease, leading to the development of multiple hamartomas and the predisposition for carcinomas of the breast.[1,23,51,85,111,112,115] The autosomal-dominant Cowden's disease has been linked in some families to a germline mutation of PTEN[86,100] and has the hallmark mucocutaneous manifestations of trichilemmomas, related follicular malformations, and a distinctive type of hyalinizing, mucinous fibroma,[98] in addition to acral keratoses and oral papillomas.[97] A significant number of patients also have thyroid adenoma or multinodular goiter, fibrocystic disease of the breast, gastrointestinal polyps (colon, gastric, and esophageal), and ovarian cysts or polyps.[17,86,97] Approximately 40% of patients with Lhermitte-Duclos disease appear to have the clinical manifestations of Cowden's disease; however, the actual percentage of cases is most likely much higher. Carefully studied families have multiple members with both diseases.[23,80,86] This significant association of these two rare diseases has prompted the hypothesis that Lhermitte-Duclos and Cowden's diseases are a single phakomatosis.[80,86,100] There may be an additional association between dysplastic cerebellar gangliocytomas and the rare Bannayan-Zonana syndrome that also has a germline PTEN mutation. One family has been identified with individuals showing either Bannayan-Zonana syndrome or Cowden's disease.[105] The development of the cerebellar lesions in adolescents may herald the presence of these diseases with germline PTEN mutations that usually do not more fully develop until the second to third decades.[115]

Neuroimaging Studies and Macroscopic Appearance

Neuroimaging provides a relatively precise assessment of these sharply defined lesions.[8,35,41,68,92,93] The MRI scan of the dys-

---

*See references 1, 23, 60, 63, 74, 80, 85, 86, 100, 111, 112, 115.

plastic gangliocytoma is distinctive and highlights the abnormally laminated, folial, or striated pattern of the lesion. This pattern corresponds to the enlarged folia that preserve a macroscopic gyriform pattern. The T1-weighted images are typically more heterogeneous and either isointense or hypointense, whereas the proton and T2-weighted images are homogeneous with a high signal intensity. There is no vascular enhancement following administration of gadolinium contrast. CT imaging demonstrates an ill-defined, hypodense lesion without vascular enhancement or prominent calcification. The broadened posterior fossa, thinned occipital bone, and erosion of the dorsum sellae highlight the effects of chronic intracranial pressure. Although the neuroimaging features of the dysplastic cerebellar gangliocytomas are relatively specific, medulloblastomas rarely mimic these features, so pathologic diagnostic confirmation is imperative.[18] Metabolic imaging studies may provide more specific supplemental data reflecting both the hamartomatous and unique neoplastic nature of these dysplastic gangliocytomas. Positron-emission tomography (PET) alone or combined with fluorodeoxyglucose (FDG) demonstrates hyperperfusion and hypermetabolism in a corresponding pattern; however, ^{99m}Tc-L,L-ethyl cysteinate dimer (ECD) singlephoton emission computed tomography (SPECT) imaging indicates that this lesion has a normal blood-brain barrier function, in contrast to most tumors.[54,76]

The remarkably invariable histopathologic composition (see following discussion) of the dysplastic gangliocytoma confers a number of common features to its overall macroscopic appearance.[4,74] The lesions are firm, rubbery, poorly circumscribed masses that may be immediately beneath a relatively normal-appearing surface. The greatest expanse of the lesion is composed of significantly thickened, enlarged, pearlygray folia with multiple foci of myelination in the outer zones

in the site of the molecular layer with a thickening of the underlying gray matter. In contrast, the deep white matter adjacent to the lesion is comparatively attenuated. The abnormal regions gradually decrease in extent such that there is no discrete macroscopic border between normal cerebellum and the lesion, analogous to the ill-defined microscopic transitional zones.[84]

Histopathology and Immunohistochemistry

Two histopathologic features predominate in the enlarged and abnormal folia. The first is an inner layer of abnormal ganglion cells that occupies the deep portion of the folium and replaces the normal Purkinje cell layer or disrupts all but the deepest zone of the internal granular cells. In some cases these abnormal ganglion cells may focally replace the entire Purkinje cell and internal granular cell layers (Figure 31-2). In the adjacent deep white matter, edema and axonal swelling accompany variable demyelination. The second conspicuous feature is an upper layer of large, abnormally myelinated processes that distends and variably fills the molecular layer. Ultrastructural studies reveal that the myelin is incompletely developed and disproportionately thin for the size of the 3- to 7-μm-diameter axons.[82,84] Silver impregnation readily demonstrates that the axons, attributed to the subjacent population of abnormal ganglion cells, tend to travel in parallel arrays beneath the pial surface in zones where the numbers of abnormal fibers are highest and in a perpendicular orientation in the peripheral transition zones where there are less prominent myelinated processes and variable, smaller numbers of dysplastic neurons adjacent to normal cortex.[4] Abnormal subpial blood vessels may be also variably associated with the lesion.[96]

Despite the rarity of Lhermitte-Duclos disease, the morphologic and immunohistochemical features of the anomalous

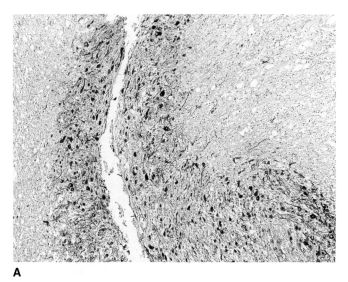

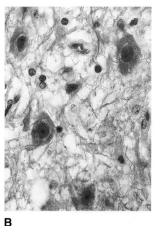

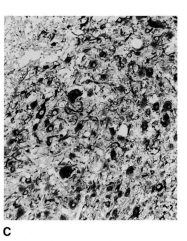

A   **B**   **C**

FIGURE 31-2   Gangliocytoma of the cerebellum (Lhermitte-Duclos disease). Populations of variably sized dysplastic ganglion cells with abnormal cytoarchitecture and neuritic processes replace both the molecular and granular layers in this dysplastic gangliocytoma of the cerebellum. The subjacent white matter was significantly diminished and demyelinated. This lesion comprised zones of macroscopically thickened folia (A). Higher magnification (B and C) reveals the heterogeneous cytoarchitecture of the neuronal cells, some of which are large pyramidal cells with markedly aberrant cell processes. Note the absence of a glial stroma. In this lesion, only a scant number of ganglionic cell processes near the deep white matter are abnormally myelinated with thin sheaths. A and C, SMI-33-avidin-biotin complex linked immunoperoxidase technique. B, Hematoxylin and eosin.

neuronal population has been carefully described.* The atypical but well-differentiated neurons comprise a heterogeneous morphologic population. Two principal morphologic types appear to be unequally admixed. The first is a large polygonal ganglion cell with a prominent macronucleolus, numerous mitochondria, and cell processes with densely packed coarse intermediate filaments and neurotubules. Golgi are present and moderately developed in contrast to an inconspicuous Nissl substance and small numbers of free ribosomes and polysomes. The second type, with smaller and more hyperchromatic nuclei, contain fewer mitochondria and increased numbers of free ribosomes and are often multipolar with tangled processes. Both types contain clear and dense-core vesicles and apparently form only modest numbers of synaptic contacts that are principally axodendritic. Other studies have also provided data that suggest axosomatic contacts.[27,37,91] Golgi silver impregnation[4,27] has highlighted a unique cytoarchitecture in some cells, compared with both cerebral and cerebellar gangliogliomas. These include long, distended neurites with multiple branches forming claw-shaped terminals.[27] Despite this aberrant neuritic geometry, immunohistochemical examination of phosphorylation-dependent and dephosphorylation-dependent neurofilament epitopes suggested that the majority of these neurons have a normal pattern of neurofilament (NF) expression and phosphorylation, comparable to cerebellar granule cells.

Immunohistochemical studies of Purkinje cell–associated epitopes, including the leu-4 epitope,[91] the calcium-binding protein PEP-19,[37,119] and Purkinje cell specific promotor gene (L7),[37,75] also support the concept that the aberrant ganglionic cell population is heterogeneous, containing neurons related to either granule cell or Purkinje cell lineages. The lineages related to granule cells appear to predominate in the cases where this question has been specifically addressed.[24,37,84,91,118] One apparently congenital case, diagnosed in a neonate, adds support to this hypothesis that the lesion is, in part, associated with aberrant granule cell development.[87] In the cerebellar regions containing dysplastic neurons, the external granular layer was depleted. A second case,[110] apparently present at birth, showed progressive development of the hallmark mass lesion over 10 years. This is consistent with FDG- and methionine-uptake studies also suggesting that Lhermitte-Duclos disease is an active and evolving disease[81]. Another case with a careful postmortem study of the cerebellum[13] suggests that the process of aberrant proliferative expansion and cellular hypertrophy of the granular cell progenitors can occur at their site of origin, along their migratory paths, or within zones of their ultimate destination within the granular layer. It is important to note that, in addition to the large macroscopic lesion, the whole cerebellum was affected with numerous smaller foci of cortical disorganization consistent with multiple stages in the development of this disease process.

PTEN Inactivation and Histogenesis

At present, the most reasonable conclusion about histogenesis is that the dysplastic gangliocytoma of the cerebellum is an indolent, hyperplastic cellular lesion that arises because of a loss of PTEN function and a corresponding increase in Akt activation because of a germline mutation in PTEN with Cowden's disease and to somatic PTEN mutations in the sporadic cases of Lhermitte-Duclos disease[9,10,42,59] in a postmitotic neuroblast, leading to an "expansion" of neuroblast population by reduction or loss of the normal levels of developmental apoptosis, migratory defects, and increases in soma size. In combination, these defects, affecting the entire cerebellum, could account for the apparent "progressive" nature of the lesions in the absence of active cell proliferation.

Biologic Behavior and Therapy

Dysplastic gangliocytomas show either very rare or no mitotic activity[4,13,37,70,74] and are designated as WHO grade I. Even the analysis of a "recurrent" case using both immunohistochemistry (proliferating cell nuclear antigen) and Feulgen staining with flow cytometry failed to detect a proliferative cell population.[37] Decompression of the posterior fossa with complete gross surgical resection of the lesion is the preferred treatment. Complications include necessity for permanent postsurgical shunt drainage.[74]

CENTRAL NEUROCYTOMA

Incidence, Age, and Sites

The rates of incidence for central neurocytoma are not known, because it occurs uncommonly, and it has been definitively recognized for only 2 decades. More than 200 cases have been described in the literature, and in three inclusive surgical series its incidence ranges from 0.1% to 0.5% of all CNS tumors. The majority of tumors develop, without gender predilection, between the third and fourth decades (mean 29 years), but ages range from 8 to 69 years.[38,66,67] Central neurocytomas are tumors that arise most commonly within the ventricular wall or septum pellucidum. More than half of cases develop in the lateral ventricles adjacent to the foramen of Monro, whereas approximately 15% involve both the lateral and third ventricles or are bilateral.[55] More uncommonly, these tumors may arise in the fourth ventricle, although one report of cases treated within a serial 6-year period describes the majority of tumors arising at this site.[7] Tumors that share some histologic similarity to central neurocytomas have been reported to develop at "atypical locations" beyond the "central" ventricular system, including the spinal cord[65,103] and parietal lobes[7]; however, these tumors should not be considered within the clinicopathologic entity of central neurocytomas.[109]

The initial clinical course is commonly short (mean 3 months).[55] Most patients seek medical attention because of symptoms of obstructive hydrocephalus or mass effect, including headache, visual disturbances, frontal lobe syndrome, and hormonal disturbances (from large lesions that may impinge on the hypothalamus). Intratumoral hemorrhage[46,79] or complete ventricular obstruction may precipitate severe clinical symptoms or death.

Neuroimaging Studies and Macroscopic Appearance

CT imaging of central neurocytomas typically gives a heterogeneous, multicystic hyperintense mass with clumped, amor-

---

*See references 4, 14, 24, 26, 27, 31, 37, 82, 84, 87, 91, 118.

phous foci of calcium in approximately 50% of cases. MRI of central neurocytomas reveals a well-circumscribed, intraventricular mass that is heterogeneous but overall isointense, commonly with a lobulated pattern on T1-weighted sequences with heterogeneously moderate to marked vascular enhancement by gadolinium. T2-weighted sequences have a variable signal intensity ranging from low to hyperintense, compared with cerebral cortex.[48,55,92] Neuroimaging of biologic parameters of these tumors is limited. Proton magnetic resonance spectroscopy (H-MRS) and thallium-201 SPECT (TI-SPECT) of several tumors demonstrated high choline peaks, compared with N-acetyl aspartate and creatine phosphate, and significant thallium uptake in all tumors irrespective of MIB-1 immunohistochemical proliferative indices.[48] The high choline in the tumors is confirmed by high-pressure liquid chromatography (HPLC) in frozen tissue.[99] FDG uptake with PET is typically low, but increased FDG uptake has been detected in an atypical central neurocytoma (see following discussion) with an elevated MIB-1 labeling index (7.0%).[78]

Histopathology, Immunohistochemistry, and Ultrastructure

The hallmark histologic features of central neurocytomas reflect a relatively homogeneous tumor cell population within an irregular microvascular stroma. These relatively small cells with round to slightly lobulated nuclei and finely speckled chromatin form a conspicuously fibrillated matrix with poorly defined cell borders (Figure 31-3). The delicate microvasculature forms an open branching network in a pattern slightly reminiscent of oligodendrogliomas. The uniform cells, finely fibrillated matrix, and typical microvessels are readily appreciated on smear preparations of fresh tissue and are distinct from oligodendrogliomas and pineal tumors. Variably sized anuclear islands composed of a dense fibrillary matrix that alternates with more cellular zones are a consistent and characteristic feature of these tumors. A small number of neurocytomas show

low levels of mitoses, nuclear atypia, and scant microfoci of necrosis; however, significant nuclear pleomorphism or endothelial proliferation are not typically present, compared with atypical central neurocytomas (see following discussion).

The predominant neuronal phenotype of the tumor is confirmed by immunohistochemistry for synaptophysin, MAP2, neuronal cytoskeletal proteins, neuron-defined epitopes, and neuron-associated adhesion molecules.[28,34,36,39,66,113] Retinal-S-antigen, leu-encephalin, calcineurin, and somatostatin have also been documented in a number of tumors.[34,66] High levels of the neurotransmitter γ-aminobutryric acid (GABA), also a neuronal marker, have been detected by analytical gas chromatography-mass spectroscopy (GC-MS) and HPLC in one tumor.[99] In addition, one study documented the production of neuromelanin in tumor cells that also contained dense-core vesicles,[71] suggesting biogenic amine production. The presence of epitopes that are found in both primitive (class III β-tubulin, embryonal immunoglobin superfamily neural cell adhesion molecule [NCAM]) (approximately 100% of cases), and differentiating neuronal lineages[107] (tau and high or medium molecular weight [NF-H/M] neurofilament proteins; 14% to 60% of cases) suggests that these tumors are composed of both immature and differentiating neuronal cell lineages. Despite neuron-specific enolase (NSE) immunoreactivity, chromogranin A is not detected, and these tumors do not appear to have a neurosecretory phenotype, such as in olfactory neuroblastomas or paragangliomas. GFAP immunoreactivity and astrocytic differentiation has been described in small fractions of tumor cells in approximately 10% to 12% of cases,[7,66,95,108,113] but care must be taken to distinguish tumor cells from reactive stromal astrocytes.[39]

Ultrastructural features, including clear and dense-core vesicles, cellular processes filled with parallel microtubular arrays, and synapses, definitively confirm the diagnosis of central neurocytomas.[38,39,113]

A variant of central neurocytomas, designated as *atypical central neurocytomas*, have histopathologic features suggestive of increased anaplasia, including increased occurrence of micro-

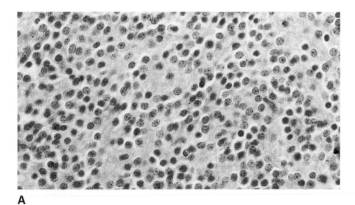

A

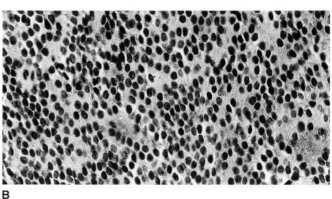

B

F IGURE 3 1 - 3   Central neurocytoma. Central neurocytomas typically consist of homogeneous cell populations with round nuclei and delicately dispersed chromatin. The cells have indistinct borders and produce a moderately delicate fibrillary matrix of densely packed neuritic processes. These make up the anuclear zones that often show the most prominent immunohistochemical reaction for synaptophysin *(B)* and neuronal cytoskeletal proteins. The microvascular stroma is variably prominent and commonly forms an open, delicately arborizing webwork. *A,* Hematoxylin and eosin. *B,* SY38 (synaptophysin)-avidin-biotin complex linked immunoperoxidase technique with hematoxylin counterstain.

vascular hyperplasia, necrosis, and increased mitoses.[7,56,95] A higher recurrence rate in these cases was associated with an overall higher proliferative activity (MIB-1 index of more than 2%). Elevation of MIB-1 indices also correlated with the histopathologic feature of microvascular hyperplasia ("vascular proliferation").[56,95]

Biologic Behavior and Therapy

Central neurocytomas are designated as WHO grade II, and overall these tumors are generally considered to have a favorable long-term prognosis after gross-total surgical resection. Surgical management is accepted as the primary therapeutic approach. Tumor-free survival as long as 17 years after total-gross resection alone has been reported.[66] The rates of recurrence are difficult to accurately access because of a combination of variables, including degree of resection and the highly variable proliferative rate of individual tumors. However, the overall recurrence rate appears to be as high as 22% in long-term follow-up (>12 years).[95] In one retrospective series, most regrowth occurs within 25 months, (9 to 25 months, 17.5 months mean)[5]; however, late regrowth may occur after 3 years.[67] Adjuvant treatment in uncomplicated cases with total macroscopic resection of tumors with an MIB labeling index less than 2 is probably not warranted on the basis of current data. However, in the cases of tumor recurrences with or without atypia, several reports have described the efficacy of radiation therapy,[7,58,90] including Gamma Knife® radiosurgery.[5,58] There appears to be an overall local control rate of 80% at 5 years, either by further surgery or radiation therapy.[67]

Histogenesis

The histogenesis of central neurocytomas is unclear. The predominant phenotype of most tumor cells is neuronal, with varying degrees of maturation. The existence of this spectrum of neuronal differentiation, the variable mitotic activity, the presence of GFAP in a low percentage of tumors,[114] and the rare bipotential phenotypic differentiation of tumor cells that express neuronal and glial epitopes in cell culture[43,116] suggest that these tumors may arise from neural progenitor lineages that retain a degree of bipotential phenotypic plasticity in the subventricular zone (SVZ).[104] The spectrum of neurotransmitters that have been detected in these tumors is consistent with an SVZ origin.[99] The clinical implications are that these tumors, although commonly exhibiting indolent growth and extremely low invasive potential, have a potential for local recurrence and rapid regrowth. A more precise means to prospectively fully identify what regulates this potential awaits further investigation.

CEREBELLAR LIPONEUROCYTOMA

Incidence, Age, and Sites

Cerebellar liponeurocytomas are very rare tumors arising in the cerebellum of adults.[45] The tumors may develop in a hemisphere or in the vermis and were initially designated as a variant of medulloblastoma (lipomatous medulloblastoma) with a good prognosis when arising in adults.[16,22,32,94] Tumors with an identical histopathologic, ultrastructural, and biologic behavior can

apparently arise within supratentorial sites typically associated with central neurocytomas.[30] The age at the first clinical manifestation of these tumors appears to be generally older than with central neurocytomas (mean 50 years); however, the range varies from 36 to 77 years.[2,45,101]

Neuroimaging Studies and Macroscopic Appearance

CT scanning of cerebellar liponeurocytoma demonstrates a well-demarcated tumor that is hypodense to isodense compared with brain parenchyma and has a moderate, heterogeneous contrast enhancement.[2] MRI with T1-weighted sequences shows areas of focal high signal intensity within an overall hypo-intense tumor, consistent with lipid within the tumor. Gadolinium enhancement of T1-weighted images is minimal, irregular, and heterogeneous, whereas T2-weighted and proton density–weighted images are heterogeneously, slightly hyperintense compared with cortex. Variable peritumoral edema is present.[2,92,101] The tumors tend to be demarcated from adjacent structures with a surgical cleavage plane. The macroscopic appearance of tumors is marked by patchy bright yellow areas admixed with the typically soft, gray-reddish tissue.[2,101]

Histopathology, Immunohistochemistry, and Ultrastructure

All liponeurocytomas have the hallmark biphasic feature of relatively uniform small cells with scant cytoplasm and round to oval hyperchromatic nuclei intermingled with varying amounts of lipidic cells. The former cells recalled the histologic features of primitive cell populations of medulloblastomas. Mitoses are low in number, and in initial tumors, necrosis and microvascular hyperplasia are inconspicuous or absent.

Immunoreactivity for synaptophysin, MAP2, and NSE can be readily detected in both the small cell and lipidic cell populations. Tumor cells that are immunoreactive for GFAP, S-100, and vimentin are always present but more variable in number and distribution.[53,94] Striated muscle differentiation has also been described.[33] No chromogranin immunoreactivity has been documented.[101]

Ultrastructural studies demonstrate mitochondria, scant rough endoplasmic reticulum, and moderate numbers of polyribosomes. Variable numbers of cells with a higher degree of cellular maturation show evidence of neuronal differentiation, including processes with bundles of microtubules, dense-core vesicles, and rare synaptic junctions. Astrocytic cell processes packed with intermediate filaments are present but not conspicuous. The tumor cells contain cytoplasmic lipid, which also appears to coalesce into large macrodroplets.[45,94]

Biologic Behavior and Therapy

The overall proliferative activity of these tumors appears to be comparatively low, ranging from 1% to 6%,[52] with a mean of approximately 3%. The number of cases is yet too low for the establishment of meaningful prognostic criteria and adjuvant therapy. However, a significant number of patients enjoy recurrence-free survivals of longer than 5 years, and the longest survival time is approximately 18 years with 2 recurrences.[2,45]

References

1. Albrecht S, Haber RM, Goodman JC, Duvic M: Cowden syndrome and Lhermitte-Duclos disease. Cancer 70:869–876, 1992.

2. Alkadhi H, Keller M, Brandner S, et al: Neuroimaging of cerebellar liponeurocytoma. J Neurosurg 95:324–331, 2001.

3. Altman NR: MR and CT characteristics of gangliocytoma: a rare cause of epilepsy in children. Am J Neuroradiol 9:917–921, 1988.

4. Ambler M, Pogacar S, Sidman R: Lhermitte-Duclos disease (granule cell hypertrophy of the cerebellum). Pathological analysis of the first familial cases. J Neuropathol Exp Neurol 28:622–647, 1969.

5. Anderson RC, Elder JB, Parsa AT, et al: Radiosurgery for the treatment of recurrent central neurocytomas. Neurosurgery 48:1231–1237; discussion 1237–1238, 2001.

6. Asa SL, Scheithauer BW, Bilbao JM, et al: A case for hypothalamic acromegaly: a clinicopathological study of six patients with hypothalamic gangliocytomas producing growth hormone-releasing factor. J Clin Endocrinol Metab 58:796–803, 1984.

7. Ashkan K, Casey ATH, D'Arrigo C, et al: Benign central neurocytoma: a double misnomer? Cancer 89:1111–1120, 2000.

8. Ashley DG, Zee C-S, Chandrasoma PT, Segall HD: Lhermitte-Duclos disease: CT and MR findings. J Comput Assist Tomogr 14:984–987, 1990.

9. Backman S, Stambolic V, Mak T: PTEN function in mammalian cell size regulation. Curr Opin Neurobiol 12:516–522, 2002.

10. Backman SA, Stambolic V, Suzuki A, et al: Deletion of PTEN in mouse brain causes seizures, ataxia and defects in soma size resembling Lhermitte-Duclos disease. Nature Genet 29:396–403, 2001.

11. Banerjee AK, Gleadhill CA: Lhermitte-Duclos disease (diffuse cerebellar hypertrophy): prolonged postoperative survival. Ir J Med Sci 148:97–99, 1979.

12. Beal MF, Kleinman GM, Pjemann RG, Hochberg FH: Gangliocytoma of third ventricle: hyperphagia, somnolence, and dementia. Neurology 31:1224–1228, 1981.

13. Beuche W, Wickboldt J, Friede RL: Lhermitte-Duclos disease: its minimal lesions in microscopic data and CT findings. Clin Neuropathol 2:163–170, 1983.

14. Beuche W, Wickboldt J, Friede RL: Lhermitte-Duclos disease (granule cell hypertrophy of the cerebellum). Pathologic analysis of the first familial cases. J Neuropathol Exp Neurol 28:622–647, 1983.

15. Bevan JS, Asa SL, Rossi ML, et al: Intrasellar gangliocytoma containing gastrin and growth hormone-releasing hormone associated with a growth hormone-secreting pituitary adenoma. Clin Endocrinol 30:213–214, 1989.

16. Budka H, Chimelli L: Lipomatous medulloblastoma in adults: a new tumour type with possible favorable prognosis. Hum Pathol 25:730–731, 1994 (Letter).

17. Carlson GJ, Nivatvong S, Snover DC: Colorectal polyps in Cowden's disease (multiple hamartoma syndrome). Am J Surg Pathol 8:763–770, 1984.

18. Chen KS, Hung PC, Wang HS, et al: Medulloblastoma or cerebellar dysplastic gangliocytoma (Lhermitte-Duclos disease)? Pediatr Neurol 27:404–406, 2002.

19. Dom R, Brucher JM: Unilateral cerebral cortex hamartoblastoma (diffuse gangliocytoma) associated with a sudanophilic degeneration of the white matter in the opposite side. Revue Neurologique 120:307–318, 1969.

20. Duchowny MS, Resnick TJ, Alvarez L: Dysplastic gangliocytoma and intractable partial seizures in childhood. Neurology 39:602–604, 1989.

21. Ebina K, Suzuki S, Takahashi T, et al: Gangliocytoma of the pineal body. A case report and review of the literature. Acta Neuropathol (Berl) 74:134–140, 1985.

22. Ellison DW, Zygmunt SC, Weller RO: Neurocytoma/Lipoma (neurolipocytoma) of the cerebellum. Neuropathol Appl Neurobiol 19:95–98, 1993.

23. Eng C, Murday V, Seal S, et al: Cowden syndrome and Lhermitte-Duclos disease in a family: a single genetic syndrome with pleitrophy. J Med Genet 131:458–461, 1994.

24. Faillot T, Sichez J-P, Brault J-L, et al: Lhermitte-Duclos disease (dysplastic gangliocytoma of the cerebellum). Report of a case and review of the literature. Acta Neurochir (Wien) 105:44–49, 1990.

25. Felix I, Bilbao JM, Asa SL, et al: Cerebral and cerebellar gangliocytomas: a morphological study of nine cases. Acta Neuropathol (Berl) 88:246–251, 1994.

26. Ferrer I, Isamat F, Acebes J: A Golgi and electron microscopic study of a dysplastic gangliocytoma of the cerebellum. Acta Neuropathol (Berl) 47:163–165, 1979.

27. Ferrer I, Marti E, Guionnet N, et al: Studies with the Golgi method in central gangliogliomas and dysplastic gangliocytoma of the cerebellum (Lhermitte-Duclos disease). Histol Histopathol 5:329–336, 1990.

28. Figarella Branger D, Pellisier JF, Daumas-Duport C, et al: Central neurocytomas. Critical evaluation of small-cell neuronal tumour. Am J Surg Pathol 16:97–109, 1992.

29. Furie DM, Felsberg GJ, Tein RD, et al: MRI of gangliocytoma of cerebellum and spinal cord. J Comput Assist Tomogr 17:488–491, 1993.

30. George DH, Scheithauer MD: Central liponeurocytoma. Am J Surg Pathol 25:1551–1555, 2001.

31. Gessaga EC: Lhermitte-Duclos disease (diffuse hypertrophy of the cerebellum). Report of two cases. Neurosurg Rev 3:151–158, 1980.

32. Giangaspero F, Cenacchi G, Roncaroli F, et al: Medullocytoma (lipidized medulloblastoma). A cerebellar neoplasm of adults with favorable prognosis. Am J Surg Pathol 20:656–664, 1996.

33. Gonzalez-Campora R, Weller RO: Lipidized mature neuroectodermal tumour of the cerebellum with myoid differentiation. Neuropathol Appl Neurobiol 24:397–402, 1998.

34. Goto S, Nagahiro S, Ushio Y, et al: Immunocytochemical detection of calcineurin and microtubule-associated protein 2 in central neurocytoma. J Neuro-Oncol 16:19–24, 1993.

35. Grand S, Pasquier B, le Bas JF, Chirossel JP: Case report: magnetic resonance imaging in Lhermitte-Duclos disease. Br J Radiol 67:902–905, 1994.

36. Gultekin SH, Dalmau J, Graus Y, et al: Anti-Hu immunolabeling as an index of neuronal differentiation in human brain tumors: a study of 112 central neuroepithelial neoplasms. Am J Surg Path 22:195–200, 1998.

37. Hair LS, Symmans F, Powers JM, Carmel P: Immunohistochemistry and proliferative activity in Lhermitte-Duclos disease. Acta Neuropathol (Berl) 84:570–573, 1992.

38. Hassoun J, Soylemezoglu F, Gambarelli D, et al: Central neurocytoma: a synopsis of clinical and histological features. Brain Pathol 3:297–306, 1993.

39. Hessler RB, Lopes MBS, Frankfurter A, et al: Cytoskeletal immunohistochemistry of central neurocytomas. Am J Surg Path 16:1031–1038, 1992.

40. Hitoshi S, Tropepe V, Ekker M, van der Kooy D: Neural stem cell lineages are regionally specified, but not committed, within distinct compartments of the developing brain. Development 129:233–244, 2002.

41. Hulcelle P, Dooms G, Vermonden J: Lhermitte-Duclos disease. A case report. J Neuroradiol 21:40–45, 1994.

42. Iida S, Tanaka Y, Fujii H, et al: A heterozygous frameshift mutation of the PTEN/MMAC1 gene in a patient with Lhermitte-

Duclos disease—only the mutated allele was expressed in the cerebellar tumor. Int J Mol Med 1:925–929, 1998.

43. Ishiuchi S, Nakazato Y, Lino M, et al: In vitro neuronal and glial production and differentiation of human central neurocytoma cells. J Neurosci Res 51:526–535, 1998.

44. Itoh Y, Yagishita S, Chiba Y: Cerebral gangliocytoma. An ultrastructural study. Acta Neuropathol (Berl) 74:169–178, 1987.

45. Jackson TR, Regine WF, Wilson D, Davis DG: Cerebellar liponeurocytoma. J Neurosurg 95:700–703, 2001.

46. Jamshidi J, Izumoto S, Yoshimine T, Maruno M: Central neurocytoma presenting with intratumoral hemorrhage. Neurosurg Rev 24:48–52, 2001.

47. Kalyanaraman UP, Henderson JP: Intramedullary ganglioneuroma of spinal cord. A clinicopathologic study. Hum Pathol 13:952–955, 1982.

48. Kanamori M, Kumabe T, Shimizu H, Yoshimoto T: (201)Tl-SPECT, (1)H-MRS, and MIB-1 labeling index of central neurocytomas: three case reports. Acta Neurochir (Wien) 144: 157–163; discussion 163, 2002.

49. Kawamoto K, Yamanouchi Y, Suwa J, et al: Ultrastructural study of a cerebral gangliocytoma. Surg Neurol 24:541–549, 1985.

50. Kernohan JW, Learmonth JR, Doyle JB: Neuroblastomas and gangliocytoma of the central nervous system. Brain 55:287–310, 1932.

51. King MA, Coyne TJ, Spearritt DJ, Boyle RS: Lhermitte-Duclos disease and Cowden disease: a third case. Ann Neurol 32:112–113, 1992.

52. Kleihues P, Cavenee WK: Tumours of the Nervous System: Pathology and Genetics. World Health Organization Classification of Tumours. Lyon, France, IARC Press, 2000.

53. Kleihues P, Louis DN, Scheithauer BW, et al: The WHO classification of tumors of the nervous system. J Neuropathol Exp Neurol 61:215–225, 2002.

54. Klisch J, Juengling F, Spreer J, et al: Lhermitte-Duclos disease: assessment with MR imaging, positron emission tomography, single-photon emission CT, and MR spectroscopy. Am J Neurorad 22:824–830, 2001.

55. Koeller KK, Sandberg GD: Cerebral intraventricular neoplasms: radiologic-pathologic correlation. Radiographics 22:1473–1505, 2002.

56. Kuchiki H, Kayama T, Sakurada K, et al: Two cases of atypical central neurocytomas. Brain Tumor Pathol 19:105–110, 2002.

57. Kudo M: Hypothalamic gangliocytoma. Selective appearance of neurofibrillary changes, granulovacuolar degeneration, and argentophilic bodies. Acta Pathologica Japonica 36:1225–1229, 1986.

58. Kulkarni V, Rajshekhar V, Haran RP, Chandi SM: Long-term outcome in patients with central neurocytoma following stereotactic biopsy and radiation therapy. Br J Neurosurg 16:126–132, 2002.

59. Kwon CH, Zhu X, Zhang J, et al: PTEN regulates neuronal soma size: a mouse model of Lhermitte-Duclos disease. Nature Genet 29:404–411, 2001.

60. Leech RW, Christopherson LA, Gilbertson RL: Dysplastic gangliocytoma (Lhermitte-Duclos disease) of the cerebellum. J Neurosurg 47:609–612, 1977.

61. Lhermitte J, Duclos P: Sur un ganglioneurome diffus du coertex du cervelet. Bull Assoc Fr Etud Cancer 9:99–107, 1920.

62. Lobo CJ, Mehan R, Murugasu E, Laitt RD: Tinnitus as the presenting symptom in a case of Lhermitte-Duclos disease. J Laryngol Otol 113:464–465, 1999.

63. Maccombe WBA: A case of Lhermitte-Duclos disease. Clin Exp Neurol 19:120–122, 1983.

64. Marano SR, Johnson PC, Spetzler RF: Recurrent Lhermitte-Duclos disease in a child. J Neurosurg 69:599–603, 1988.

65. Martin AJ, Sharr MM, Teddy PJ, et al: Neurocytoma of the thoracic spinal cord. Acta Neurochir (Wien) 144:823–828, 2002.

66. Mena H, Morrison AL, Jones RV, Gyure KA: Central neurocytomas express photoreceptor differentiation. Cancer 91:136–143, 2001.

67. Metellus P, Alliez JR, Dodero F, et al: Central neurocytoma: 2 case reports and review of the literature. Acta Neurochir (Wien) 142:1417–1422, 2000. (Erratum 143:320, 2001.)

68. Milbouw G, Born JD, Martin D, et al: Clinical and radiological aspects of dysplastic gangliocytoma (Lhermitte-Duclos disease): a report of two cases with review of the literature. Neurosurgery 22:124–128, 1988.

69. Mischel PS, Nguyen LP, Vinters HV: Cerebral cortical dysplasia associated with pediatric epilepsy. Review of neuropathologic features and proposal for a grading system. J Neuropathol Exp Neurol 54:137–153, 1995.

70. Nelson JS, Kjellstrom Ch, Dalianis T, Bogdanovic C: Examination of Lhermitte-Duclos disease (LDD) for PCNA, Ki67, and p53 expression and JC/BK papova virus DNA. Hum Pathol 25:136A, 1994.

71. Ng TH, Wong AY, Boadle R, Compton JS: Pigmented central neurocytoma: case report and literature review. Am J Surg Pathol 23:1136–1140, 1999.

72. Ng TH, Fung CF, Goh W, Wong VCN: Ganglioneuroma of the spinal cord. Surg Neurol 147–151, 1991.

73. Norman MG, McGillivray BC, Kalousek DK, et al: Congenital Malformations of the Brain. Pathologic, Embryonic, Clinical, Radiologic and Genetic Aspects. New York, Oxford University Press, 1995.

74. Nowak DA, Trost HA, Porr A, et al: Lhermitte-Duclos disease (dysplastic gangliocytoma of the cerebellum). Clin Neurol Neurosurg 103:105–110, 2001.

75. Oberdick J, Leventhal F, Levinthal C: A purkinje cell differentiation marker shows a partial DNA sequence homology to the cellular sis/PDGF2 gene. Neuron 1:367–376, 1988.

76. Ogasawara K, Yasuda S, Beppu T, et al: Brain PET and technetium-99m-ECD SPECT imaging in Lhermitte-Duclos disease. Neuroradiology 43(11):993–996, 2001.

77. Ohta M, Nishio S, Kosaka H, et al: The ultrastructure of a gangliocytoma. NoTo Shinkei 33:817–824, 1981.

78. Ohtani T, Takahashi A, Honda F, et al: Central neurocytoma with unusually intense FDG uptake: case report. Ann Nucl Med 15:161–165, 2001.

79. Okamura A, Goto S, Sato K, Ushio Y: Central neurocytoma with hemorrhagic onset. Surg Neurol 43:252–255, 1995.

80. Padberg GW, Schot JD, Vielvoye GJ, et al: Lhermitte-Duclos disease and Cowden disease: a single phakomatosis. Ann Neurol 29:517–523, 1991.

81. Pirotte B, Goldman S, Baleriaux D, Brotchi J: Fluorodeoxyglucose and methionine uptake in Lhermitte-Duclos disease: case report. Neurosurgery 50:404–407; discussion 407–408, 2002.

82. Pritchett PS, King TI: Dysplastic gangliocytoma of the cerebellum: an ultrastructural study. Acta Neuropathol (Berl) 42:1–5, 1978.

83. Reeder RF, Saunders RL, Fratkin JD, Cromwell LD: Magnetic resonance imaging in the diagnosis and treatment of Lhermitte-Duclos disease. Neurosurgery 23:240–245, 1988.

84. Reznik M, Schoenen J: Lhermitte-Duclos disease. Acta Neuropathol (Berl) 59:88–94, 1983.

85. Rimbau J, Isamat F: Dysplastic gangliocytoma of the cerebellum (Lhermitte-Duclos disease) and its relation to the multiple hamartoma syndrome (Cowden disease). J Neurooncol 18:191–197, 1994.

86. Robinson S, Cohen AR: Cowden disease and Lhermitte-Duclos disease: characterization of a new phakomatosis. J Neurosurg 46:371–383, 2000.

87. Roessmann U, Wongmongholrit T: Dysplastic gangliocytoma of the cerebellum in a newborn. J Neurosurg 60:845–847, 1984.

88. Russo CP, Katz DS, Corona RJ, Winfield JA: Gangliocytoma of the cervicothoracic spinal cord. Am J Neuroradiol 16:889–891, 1995.

89. Saeger W, Puchner MJ, Ludecke DK: Combined sellar ganglio-cytoma and pituitary adenoma in acromegaly or Cushing's disease. A report of 3 cases. Virchows Arch 425:93–99, 1994.

90. Schild SE: Benign central neurocytoma: a double misnomer? Cancer 94:284, 2002 (Letter).

91. Shiurba RA, Gessaga EC, Eng LF, et al: Lhermitte-Duclos disease. An immunohistochemical study of the cerebellar cortex. Review of Reported Cases. Acta Neuropathol (Berl) 75:474–80, 1988.

92. Shin JH, Lee HK, Khang SK, et al: Neuronal tumors of the central nervous system: radiologic findings and pathologic correlation. Radiographics 22:1177–1189, 2002.

93. Siddiqi SN, Fehlings MG: Lhermitte-Duclos disease mimicking adult-onset aqueductal stenosis. Case report. J Neurosurg 80:1095–1098, 1994.

94. Soylemezoglu F, Soffer D, Onol B, et al: Lipomatous medulloblastoma in adults: a distinct clinicopathologcal entity. Am J Surg Pathol 20:413–418, 1996.

95. Soylemezoglu F, Scheithauer BW, Esteve J, Kleihues P: Atypical central neurocytoma. J Neuropathol Exp Neurol 56:551–556, 1997.

96. Stapleton SR, Wilkins PR, Bell BA: Recurrent dysplastic cerebellar gangliocytoma (Lhermitte-Duclos disease) presenting with subarachnoid hemorrhage. Br J Neurosurg 6:153–156, 1992.

97. Starink TM: Cowden's disease: analysis of fourteen new cases. J Am Acad Dermatol 11:1127–1141, 1984.

98. Starink TM, Meijer CJLM, Brownstein MH: The cutaneous pathology of Cowden's disease: new findings. J Cutan Pathol 12:83–93, 1985.

99. Sugita Y, Yamada S, Sugita S, et al: The biochemical analysis of neurotransmitters in central neurocytomas. Int J Mol Med 7:521–525, 2001.

100. Sutphen R, Diamond TM, Minton SE, et al: Severe Lhermitte-Duclos disease with unique germline mutation of PTEN. Am J Med Genet 82:290–293, 1999.

101. Taddei GL, Buccoliero AM, Caldarella A, et al: Cerebellar liponeurocytoma: immunohistochemical and ultrastructural study of a case. Ultrastruct Pathol 25:59–63, 2001.

102. Takahashi H, Wakabayashi K, Kawai K, et al: Neuroendocrine markers in central nervous system neuronal tumors (gangliocytoma and ganglioglioma). Acta Neuropathol (Berl) 77:237–243, 1989.

103. Tatter SB, Borges LF, Louis DN: Central neurocytomas of the cervical spinal cord. Report of two cases. J Neurosurg 81:2882–2893, 1994. (Erratum 82:706, 1995.)

104. Temple S, Alvarez-Buylla A: Stem cells in the adult mammalian central nervous system. Curr Opin Neurobiol 9:135–141, 1999.

105. Tok Celebi J, Chen FF, Zhang H, et al: Identification of PTEN mutations in five families with Bannayan-Zonana syndrome. Exp Dermatol 8:134–139, 1999.

106. Townsend JJ, Neilson SL, Malamud N: Unilateral megalencephaly: hamartoma or neoplasm. Neurology 251:448–453, 1975.

107. Trojanowski JQ, Tohyama T, Lee V M-Y: Medulloblastoma and related primitive neuroectodermal brain tumors of childhood recapitulate molecular milestones in the maturation of neuroblasts. Mol Chem Neuropathol 17:121–135.

108. Tsuchida T, Matsumoto M, Shirayama Y, et al: Neuronal and glial characteristics of central neurocytoma: electron microscopical analysis of two cases. Acta Neuropathol (Berl) 91:573–577, 1996.

109. Vallat-Decouvelaere AV, Gauchez P, Varlet P, et al: So-called malignant and extra-ventricular neurocytomas: reality or wrong diagnosis? A critical review about two overdiagnosed cases. J Neurooncol 48:161–172, 2000.

110. Verdu A, Garde T, Madero S: [Lhermitte-Duclos disease in a ten-year-old child: clinical follow-up and neuroimaging data from birth]. Revista de Neurologia 27:597–600, 1998.

111. Vinchon M, Blond S, Lejeune JP, et al: Association of Lhermitte-Duclos and Cowden Disease: report of a new case and review of the literature. J Neurol Neurosurg Psychiatry 57:699–704, 1994.

112. Vital A, Vital C, Martin-Negrier ML, et al: Lhermitte-Duclos type cerebellum hamartoma and Cowden disease. Clin Neuropathol 229–231, 1994.

113. von Deimling A, Janzer R, Kleihues P, Wiestler OD: Patterns of differentiation in central neurocytoma. An immunohistochemical study of eleven biopsies. Acta Neuropathol (Berl) 79:473–479, 1990.

114. von Deimling A, Kleihues P, Saremaslani P, et al: Histogenesis and differentiation potential of central neurocytomas. Lab Invest 64:585–591, 1991.

115. Wells GB, Lasner TM, Yousem DM, Zager EL: Lhermitte-Duclos disease and Cowden's syndrome in an adolescent patient. J Neurosurg 81:133–136, 1994.

116. Westphal M, Stavrou D, Nausch H, et al: Human neurocytoma cells in culture show characteristics of astroglial differentiation. J Neurosci Res 38:698–704, 1994.

117. Williams DW, Elster AD, Ginsberg LE, Stanton C: Recurrent Lhermitte-Duclos disease: report of two cases and association with Cowden's disease. Am J Neuroradiol 13:287–290, 1992.

118. Yachnis AT, Trojanowski JQ, Memmo M, Schlaepfer WW: Expression of neurofilament proteins in the hypertrophic granule cells of Lhermitte-Duclos disease: an explanation for the mass effect and the myelination of parallel fibers in the disease state. J Neuropath Exp Neurol 47:206–216, 1988.

119. Ziai R, Pan Y-CE, Hulmes JD, et al: Isolation, sequence and developmental prolife of a brain-specific polypeptide, PEP 19. Proc Natl Acad Sci USA 83:8420–8423, 1986.

120. Zülch KJ: Brain Tumours: Their Biology and Pathology, 3rd ed. Berlin, Springer-Verlag, 1986.

CHAPTER 32

DYSEMBRYOPLASTIC NEUROEPITHELIAL TUMOR

Walter A. Hall and H. Brent Clark

The dysembryoplastic neuroepithelial tumor (DNT) is usually a supratentorial cortical tumor that is found in children and young adults. This tumor is called *dysembryoplastic* because several features indicate its origin is in dysembryogenesis, including the presence of foci of cortical dysplasia, the young age of most patients at the onset of symptoms, and the evidence of bony deformity adjacent to the tumor on imaging studies such as computed tomography (CT).[9] This tumor is relatively new to neuro-oncology, with the first description being published in 1988.[2] In young patients who were followed long term, recurrence-free survival was noted.[2]

TUMOR LOCATION

Even though the DNT is usually cortical in its site of origin, it can also arise in various locations that correspond to the secondary germinal layers. The presence of foci of cortical dysplasia in these tumors suggests that they develop during the formation of the cortex.[2] Based on their primarily cortical locations in the temporal and frontal lobes, the subpial granular layer is thought to be the most likely site of origin.[2] After the temporal lobe, the frontal lobe is the most commonly involved supratentorial region.[2] Most DNTs are identified when surgery is performed for epilepsy; therefore they are usually found in the temporal lobe in the mesial structures and often involve the amygdala and hippocampus.[5] Less than 50% of these tumors arise in the temporal lobe, and they have also been found in the caudate nucleus, cerebellum, pons, and near the third ventricle.[2,8] If these tumors indeed arise from secondary germinal layers, that would explain their occasional occurrence in the cerebellum.[2]

DIAGNOSIS

A DNT is usually diagnosed in patients with long-standing seizures (range 2 to 18 years; mean 9 years; median 7 years) or intractable epilepsy.[2,5,8] The seizures may be drug resistant and partial with secondary generalization. Up to 75% of patients with DNT will have one or more seizures per day.[2] The seizures usually develop before the age of 20 but late-onset seizures can develop. Neurologic examination results in patients with DNT are normal between seizures. Occasionally, patients with DNT can present with headache. Papilledema has been seen in patients with DNT.

The characteristic clinical features of DNT have been described as intractable partial complex seizures with onset before 20 years of age, lack of significant interictal neurologic deficit, and no stigmata of phakomatosis.[2]

EPIDEMIOLOGY

The incidence of this tumor varies depending on whether it is studied in the general population or in epilepsy patients. It is an uncommon tumor with fewer than 100 cases reported worldwide.[9] In general, the DNT represents less than 1.0% of all brain tumors in adults, with a slightly higher incidence in patients under the age of 20.

NEUROIMAGING

Magnetic resonance imaging (MRI) demonstrates the cortical origin of these tumors better than CT. They are hypointense on T1-weighted images and hyperintense on T2-weighted images (Figure 32-1). A heterogeneous appearance for DNTs has been reported on MRI.[7] On CT, they are either hypodense or isodense and can demonstrate calcifications. Contrast enhancement can be seen in up to one third of patients on CT or MRI. Poorly defined tumor borders can be seen on CT or MRI.[7] Hemorrhage has been identified in DNTs on CT and MRI.[7] These tumors can appear cystic or contain single or multiple cysts on CT and MRI.[7] Large cysts measuring 10 mm to 30 mm have been reported on MRI.[7] Generally, mass effect and peritumoral edema is not present. Bone deformity such as thinning of the inner table of the skull can be seen on CT adjacent to the DNT in up to one third of patients.[2] The size of these tumors has ranged from 10 mm to 70 mm, with a mean tumor size of 37 mm in one report.[5,7] In one third of DNTs followed with serial CT or MRI studies over a 13-year period, slow but definite growth was discernable.[4]

When DNTs have been examined with positron-emission tomography using ^{18}F-fluorodeoxyglucose, they have uniformly shown glucose hypometabolism.[6] ^{123}I-N-isopropyl-p-iodoamphetamine (IMP) and ^{99m}Tc-hexamethyl propylene amine oxime (HMPAO) single-photon emission computed

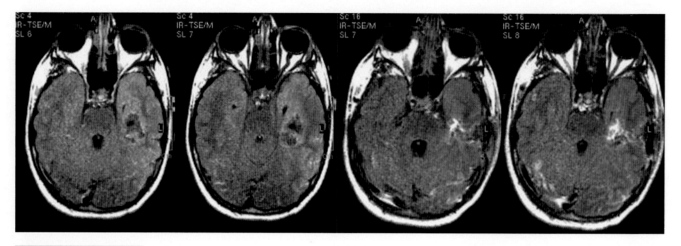

FIGURE 32-1 Axial contrast-enhanced, T1-weighted magnetic resonance imaging scan of the brain demonstrating a left temporal cystic tumor that was found to be a dysembryoplastic neuroepithelial tumor on pathologic examination.

tomography (SPECT) imaging demonstrated hypoperfusion of the DNT on cerebral blood flow images.[1] Thallium-201 SPECT showed no uptake by the DNT.[1] It is hoped that the use of these nuclear medicine imaging studies may help to distinguish low-grade gliomas from DNTs. The identification of a low-grade glioma on these nuclear medicine blood flow studies could indicate that additional postoperative adjuvant radiation therapy or chemotherapy is indicated in the presence of residual disease.

TUMOR GRADE

The DNT is considered a World Health Organization (WHO) grade I tumor with the international classification of diseases for oncology (ICD-O) code 9413/0. It has been seen in patients with neurofibromatosis type 1.

TUMOR HISTOLOGY

Although the term DNT was not introduced until the 1980s, it had long been recognized by neuropathologists who had experience with cortical resections for epilepsy that there was a distinctive tumor type seen in patients with intractable seizure disorders. These tumors had many features of oligodendroglioma but tended to be cortically based and often had a distinctive multinodular pattern. They often were diagnosed as oligodendrogliomas but with the understanding that they had a different, even more indolent, behavior than the typical oligodendroglioma and usually were cured by surgical resection.

The DNT is considered a benign neoplasm despite being characterized by excessive proliferation of cells, in most instances a sizable mass; patients have long-standing symptoms, epilepsy being their only clinical manifestation; and long-term follow-up discloses neither clinical nor radiologic signs of tumor recurrence.[2] The differential diagnosis includes low-grade gliomas and gangliogliomas.[9] The concept of DNT has been clouded in the past decade by attempts to include neoplasms with other histologic patterns under DNTs' terminology. These other tumors often have the appearance of more typical gliomas, gangliogliomas, or gangliocytomas but radiographically have cortically based appearances that are suggestive of DNT and occur in patients with childhood onset of seizures. They have a good prognosis after treatment by surgical resection alone.

DNTs typically arise in the cerebral hemispheres. There may be bosselation of the surface of the brain that sometimes is associated with thinning or remodeling of the overlying calvarium. The tumor usually involves the cerebral cortex, and on cut surface, a nodular pattern can sometimes be appreciated within the cortex. A gray mucinous consistency may be present, at least focally. At low magnification, the nodularity of the tumor within the cortex often is readily apparent in classical examples. These nests of tumor cells are composed primarily of monomorphic small cells, suggestive of the cells seen in oligodendrogliomas, often with perinuclear "clearing" and immunoreactive with antibodies against S-100 protein. A second element of the nodules are mature neurons that often appear to "float" in pools of an Alcian-blue-reactive mucopolysaccharide-containing matrix.

Intermixed with nodular areas are more diffusely cellular zones that are composed of cells similar to the oligodendrocyte-like component of the nodules. Within these more diffuse areas there typically are columnar aggregates of synaptophysin-immunoreactive neurites that are oriented perpendicular to the pial surface. These columnar aggregates (termed the *specific glioneuronal element*) are accompanied by the oligodendrocyte-like cells and may have a myxoid matrix surrounding them (Figure 32-2). In addition to the nodular areas and the specific glioneuronal element, there often are other patterns of growth, usually with an astrocytic component that may be composed of spindled, piloid cells. This pattern may mimic the histology of juvenile pilocytic astrocytoma. A feature sometimes associated with DNTs is the presence of areas of focal cortical dysplasia (i.e., maloriented cortical neurons, with or without glial proliferation, adjacent to the neoplastic foci).

Features that are correlated with anaplastic behavior in other glial neoplasms may be encountered in DNTs but do not have the same prognostic implications. Pleomorphism, glomeruloid vascular proliferation, and even necrosis have been described in these tumors with no obvious effect on prognosis. Mitotic activity usually is minimal, and in most instances

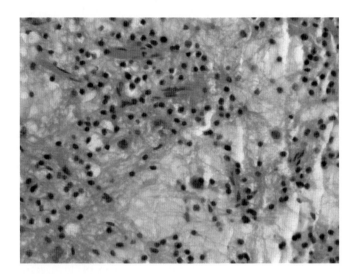

FIGURE 32-2 Dysembryoplastic neuroepithelial tumor containing areas of small dark oligodendrocyte-like cells and pale mucinous pools with several "floating" neurons.

proliferation indices using such markers as Ki-67 (MIB-1) are low, although cases with higher indices have been described, again without prognostic significance.[3]

THERAPY

Because DNTs are benign lesions, they can often be followed radiographically with sequential MRI if patients are asymptomatic or their epilepsy is well controlled with anticonvulsant therapy. Partially or completely surgically resected lesions that are followed for years have often demonstrated no progression or recurrence, respectively, on successive CT and MRI.

If the DNT is in a surgically accessible area of the brain, an attempt at complete surgical resection should be made. Recent advances in neurosurgery that now allow for more extensive tumor resections include neuronavigation using frameless stereotaxy and intraoperative MRI. Frameless stereotaxy does not allow the neurosurgeon to make adjustments for brain shift because the images are obtained preoperatively, before the craniotomy is performed. Intraoperative MRI-guided tumor resections are performed in near real time so that the neurosurgeon can react to dynamic changes in the operative site.[10] The advantages to intraoperative magnetic resonance–guidance for DNT are the ability to perform a radiographically complete surgical resection that should prove curative and to exclude the presence of intraoperative hemorrhage in the resection cavity before leaving the surgical suite.

Because many patients with DNT have seizures, they are often treated on an epilepsy surgery protocol. The majority of patients (30 : 39, or 77%, in one series) are seizure free after resection of their DNT.[2] Intraoperative electrocorticography has been performed during surgical resection of DNT to exclude the presence of any perilesional spike waves that would indicate residual epileptogenic foci.[8] A lesionectomy is usually curative of the epilepsy in patients with DNT, although some require a more extensive resection,[8] which provides the pathologist with a larger tumor sample to assure that an accurate diagnosis is made. If residual abnormal tissue is present on postoperative MRI, sequential MRI is all that is necessary to follow the DNT. Long-term follow-up in partially resected DNTs showed neither clinical nor radiologic evidence for progression in patients over a mean duration of 9 years (range 1 to 18 years).[2,8]

Postoperative adjuvant external-beam radiation therapy is not necessary for patients with residual tumor.[2] The deleterious effects of radiation therapy and chemotherapy can be avoided in patients with DNT after surgery. Patients have a normal life expectancy after removal of DNTs.[9] Only a single case of malignant transformation to a glioblastoma multiforme has ever been reported in a DNT of the complex form.[4] This patient was followed for 11 years after the initial resection and had received no postoperative adjuvant therapy. The authors reported the case as a warning to clinicians and stressed the importance of maximizing the surgical resection.

References

1. Abe M, Tabuchi K, Tsuji T, et al: Dysembryoplastic neuroepithelial tumor: report of three cases. Surg Neurol 43:240–245, 1995.
2. Daumas-Duport C, Scheithauer BW, Chodkiewicz JP, et al: Dysembryoplastic neuroepithelial tumour: a surgically curable tumour of young patients with intractable partial seizures. Neurosurgery 23:545–556, 1988.
3. Daumas-Duport C: Dysembryoplastic neuroepithelial tumors. Brain Pathology 3:283–295, 1993.
4. Hammond RR, Duggal N, Woulfe JM, Girvin JP: Malignant transformation of a dysembryoplastic neuroepithelial tumor. Case report. J Neurosurg 92:722–725, 2000.
5. Honavar M, Janota I, Polkey CE: Histological heterogeneity of dysembryoplastic neuroepithelial tumor: identification and differential diagnosis in a series of 74 cases. Histopathology 34:342–356, 1999.
6. Lee DY, Chung CK, Hwang YS, et al: Dysembryoplastic neuroepithelial tumor: radiological findings (including PET, SPECT, and MRS) and surgical strategy. J Neurooncol 47:167–174, 2000.
7. Ostertun B, Wolf HK, Campos MG, et al: Dysembryoplastic neuroepithelial tumors: MR and CT evaluation. AJNR Am J Neuroradiol 17:419–430, 1996.
8. Taratuto AL, Pomata H, Sevlever, et al: Dysembryoplastic neuroepithelial tumor: morphological, immunocytochemical, and deoxyribonucleic acid analyses in a pediatric series. Neurosurgery 36:474–481, 1995.
9. Tatke M, Sharma A, Malhotra V: Dysembryoplastic neuroepithelial tumour. Childs Nerv Syst 14:293–296, 1998.
10. Tummala RP, Chu RM, Liu H, et al: High-field functional capabilities for magnetic resonance imaging-guided brain tumor resection. Tech in Neurosurg 4:319–325, 2002.

CHAPTER 33

PINEOCYTOMA

Andrew T. Parsa and Jeffrey N. Bruce

CLINICAL FEATURES

The clinical syndromes associated with pineal region tumors relate directly to normal pineal anatomy as well as tumor histology. The pineal gland develops during the second month of gestation as a diverticulum in the diencephalic roof of the third ventricle. It is flanked by the posterior and habenular commisures in the rostral portion of the midbrain directly below the splenium of the corpus callosum. The velum interpositom is found rostral and dorsal to the pineal gland and contains the internal cerebral veins that join to form the vein of Galen.[31,55] The principal cell of the pineal gland is the pineal parenchymal cell or pineocyte. This cell is a specialized neuron related to retinal rods and cones. The pineocyte is surrounded by a stroma of fibrillary astrocytes that interact with adjoining blood vessels to form part of the blood-pial barrier.

The pineal gland is richly innervated with sympathetic noradrenergic input via a pathway originating in the retina and coursing through the suprachiasmatic nucleus of the hypothalamus and the superior cervical ganglion.[31] Upon stimulation, the pineal gland converts sympathetic input into hormonal output by producing melatonin, which in turn has regulatory effects on hormones such as luteinizing hormone and follicle-stimulating hormone.[16] The pineal gland can be considered a neuroendocrine transducer that synchronizes hormonal release with phases of the light-dark cycle by means of its sympathetic input. However, the exact relationship between the pineal gland and human circadian rhythm remains unclear and is an active area of investigation.

In their 1954 pineal tumor study, Ringertz and colleagues defined the pineal region as being bound by the splenium of the corpus callosum and telachoroidea dorsally, the quadrigeminal plate and midbrain tectum ventrally, the posterior aspect of the third ventricle rostrally, and the cerebellar vermis caudally.[58] Mass lesions that compress these adjacent structures will result in typical clinical syndromes. One of the most common presentations is headache, nausea, and vomiting caused by aqueductal compression and resultant obstructive hydrocephalus.[15] Untreated, hydrocephalus may progressively lead to lethargy, obtundation, and death. Compromise of the superior colliculus either through direct compression or tumor invasion will result in a syndrome of vertical gaze palsy that can be associated with pupillary or oculomotor nerve paresis. This eponymic syndrome was first described by the French ophthalmologist Henri Parinaud in the late 1800s and has become virtually pathognomonic for lesions involving the quadrigeminal plate. Further

compression of the periaqueductal gray region may cause mydriasis, convergence spasm, pupillary inequality, and convergence or refractory nystagmus. Impairment of down gaze becomes more pronounced in children with tumor involving the ventral midbrain.[54] Patients can also have motor impairment such as ataxia and dysmetria resulting from compromise of cerebellar efferent fibers in the superior cerebellar peduncle.[15]

Endocrine malfunction in children with pineal region tumors can present with diabetes insipidus secondary to hydrocephalus or concurrent suprasellar tumor.[15,33] More specific endocrine syndromes can arise from secretion of hormones by germ cell tumors. Pseudoprecocious puberty caused by beta human chorionic gonadotropin (BHCG) can be observed with germ cell tumors in either the pineal or suprasellar region.[44,81] In a large series of germ cell tumor patients with suprasellar involvement, 93% of girls older than 12 years had secondary amenorrhea, and 33% of patients younger than 15 years of age had growth arrest.[72]

Pineal apoplexy has been described as a rare presenting feature of pineal region tumors.[19,70] Hemorrhage into a vascular-rich pineal tumor can occur preoperatively and is a well described postoperative complication.[14]

DIAGNOSTIC CONSIDERATIONS

The symptoms of pineal region tumors can be as varied as their diverse histology with prodromal periods lasting from weeks to years. A rigorous and uniform preoperative work-up is therefore a requisite for all children suspected of harboring a pineal region tumor. Any endocrine abnormalities revealed during medical evaluation should be investigated before surgery. Patients with signs and symptoms of raised intracranial pressure must receive a head computed tomography (CT) scan or magnetic resonance imaging (MRI) scan to assess the need for emergent management. Subsequent nonemergent work-up of a child with a pineal region tumor can be divided into radiologic and laboratory studies.

Radiologic Diagnosis

High-resolution MRI with gadolinium is necessary in the evaluation of pineal region lesions. Tumor characteristics such as size, vascularity, and homogeneity can be assessed as well as the anatomic relationship with surrounding structures.[73] Irreg-

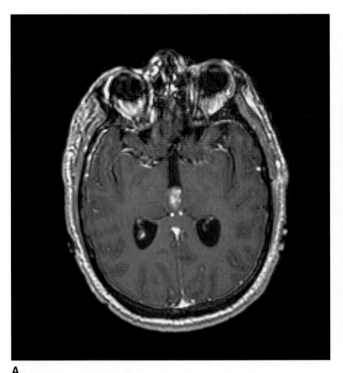
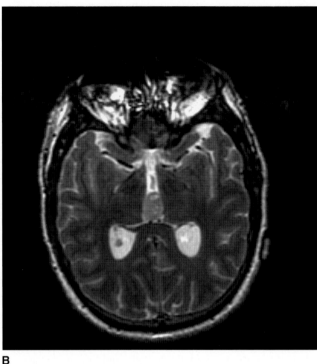

A

B

FIGURE 33-1   Pineocytomas and pineoblastomas are typically hypointense to isointense on T1-weighted images with increased signal on T2. They demonstrate homogeneous enhancement.

ular tumor borders can be suggestive of tumor invasiveness and associated histologic malignancy. Although the type of tumor cannot be reliably determined from the radiographic characteristics alone, there are some radiographic patterns associated with specific tumors.

Non–germ cell tumors consist of tumor derived from pineal parenchymal cells as well as surrounding tissue. Pineocytomas and pineoblastomas are typically hypointense to isointense on T1-weighted images with increased signal on T2 and demonstrate homogeneous enhancement (Figure 33-1). Pineoblastomas can be distinguished by their irregular shape and large size (i.e., some >4 cm).[65] Astrocytomas that arise from the glial stroma of the gland and surrounding tissue are also hypointense on T1 and hyperintense on T2. Astrocytomas have variable enhancement patterns. Calcium may be present in either pineal cell tumors or astrocytomas. Meningiomas typically enhance homogeneously with smooth borders. Tentorial meningiomas can have a dural tail of enhancement and are anatomically distinguished by their dorsal location relative to the deep venous system.

Germinomas are isointense on T1-weighted MRI studies and slightly hyperintense on T2 with strong homogeneous enhancement.[73,79] Calcification surrounds the pineal gland as the germinoma grows in contrast to the intratumoral calcium within a pineocytoma.[21] Intratumoral cysts can exist as well.[17] In contrast to germinomas, teratomas can contain tissue from all three germinal layers, resulting in a heterogeneous signal. They are well-circumscribed benign tumors characterized by their heterogeneity, multilocularity, and irregular enhancement. Contrast enhancement of teratomas can also be ring enhanced. In some cases a well-circumscribed teratoma can have areas of

low attenuation that correlate with adipose tissue, which serves to further distinguish it from other pineal region tumors.[50] Malignant nongerminomatous germ cell tumors can also have a heterogeneous appearance because of a mixture of benign and malignant germ cell components.[73,79] Areas of intratumoral hemorrhage may distinguish specific subtypes, such as choriocarcinoma.[80]

In addition to MRI, angiography is sometimes used in cases of suspected vascular anomalies. However, the anatomic and vascular information provided by MRI has largely circumvented the need for routine angiogram in the evaluation of pineal region neoplasms.

Laboratory Diagnosis

Measurements of serum and cerebrospinal fluid (CSF) tumor markers are a valuable component of the preoperative evaluation.[18] As with radiographic studies, they can be suggestive of tumor type but are only occasionally diagnostic.[62] Markers have been most helpful in the work-up of children with germ cell tumors. In addition to their histologic characteristics, germ cell tumors retain molecular characteristics of their primordial lineage. As a result, the expression of embryonic proteins such as alpha-fetoprotein (AFP) and BHCG are indicative of malignant germ cell elements.[2,42] Serum and CSF measurements can be used for diagnostic purposes or for monitoring a response to therapy.[3,78] In general, CSF measurements are more sensitive than serum measurements, and a CSF to serum gradient may be consistent with an intracranial lesion. However, there is still active debate in the literature regarding the diagnostic value of CSF and serum measurements.[1]

Pineal parenchymal cell tumor markers are less well characterized than their germ cell counterparts and include melatonin and the S-antigen.[31] Neither of these proteins has proved valuable in the diagnosis of pineal parenchymal cell tumors. However, some authors report the use of melatonin levels in the follow-up after surgical treatment of patients with pineocytoma.[51]

PATHOLOGIC FEATURES

Tumors of the pineal region have varied histology that can be generally divided into germ cell and non–germ cell derivatives. Most tumors are a result of displaced embryonic tissue, malignant transformation of pineal parenchymal cells, or transformation of surrounding astroglia. Pineal region tumors make up 0.4% to 1.0% of intracranial tumors in adults and 3% to 8% of brain tumors in children.[17] Symptom onset for most children occurs between 10 and 20 years of age, with the average age of presentation being 13 years.[29,38]

Non–germ cell tumors of the pineal region arise from the pineal gland or its surrounding tissue. The rarity of pineal cell lesions and the lack of an extracranial correlate have complicated the classification of these tumors. Currently, pineal parenchymal tumors are divided into high- and low-grade variants based on the extent of differentiation. The primitive pineoblastoma and the differentiated pineocytoma exist at opposite ends of the spectrum with intermediate-grade variants between. Russell and Rubinstein have described a more specific classification such that pineoblastomas include types without differentiation; types with pineocytic differentiation; and types with neuronal, glial, or retinoblastic differentiation.[60] Similarly, pineocytomas have been divided into types without further differentiation, types with only neuronal differentiation, types with only astrocytic differentiation, and types with divergent neuronal and astrocytic differentiation (i.e., the ganglioglioma).[60]

The pineocytoma is significantly less aggressive than the pineoblastoma. It usually presents during adolescence and rarely seeds the subarachnoid space. Pineocytomas consist of small cells similar to those of the pineoblastoma; however, they appear more spread out, more lobular, and are further distinguished by large hypocellular zones containing fibrillary stroma.[63,65] At the ultrastructural level these fibrils contain microtubules and dense-core granules.[49] The normal pineal gland tissue contains lobular cells of uniform size with an easily identified astroglial stroma, two features that can be used to distinguish normal gland from pineocytoma.[31]

TREATMENT CONSIDERATIONS

Management of patients with pineal region tumors should be directed at treating hydrocephalus and establishing a diagnosis. Preoperative evaluation should include (1) high-resolution MRI scan of the head with gadolinium, (2) measurement of serum and CSF markers, (3) cytologic examination of CSF, (4) evaluation of pituitary function if endocrine abnormalities are suspected, and (5) visual-field examination if suprasellar extension of tumor is noted on MRI. The ultimate management goal should be to refine adjuvant therapy based on tumor pathology.[13,18]

The treatment of hydrocephalus can be effectively accomplished temporarily with the placement of an external ventricular drain or permanently with ventriculoperitoneal (VP) shunt placement or third ventriculostomy. For symptomatic patients with hydrocephalus, preoperative third ventriculostomy is extremely effective and often eliminates the need for shunt placement. Successful resection of the lesion may remove the obstruction and allow free flow out of the third ventricle, obviating the need for any form of CSF diversion.[30,77]

Patients with hydrocephalus and radiographic evidence of a malignant pineal region tumor may have their hydrocephalus treated with third ventriculostomy or VP shunt before biopsy or resection. The staged procedure allows for definitive control of the hydrocephalus before surgical resection of lesions suspected of being malignant. A similar strategy may be employed for patients with marked, symptomatic hydrocephalus and benign-appearing lesions. The timing of the second procedure can vary according to the surgeon's preference. Peritoneal seeding with shunting is a rare but well-documented complication in these patients.[8,9,24,28,37,57] The use of a filter to decrease the incidence of seeding, however, has been associated with frequent shunt malfunctions and is generally not recommended, particularly because third ventriculostomy is a better option.[59]

Improved endoscopic techniques have made third ventriculostomy an easy and reliable method to divert CSF.[30,32,77] Third ventriculostomy is performed freehand or stereotactically with an endoscope passed via a burr hole into the right lateral ventricle and through the foramen of Monro. The floor of the third ventricle is then fenestrated to provide an alternate route for CSF flow and subsequent absorption. As with all CSF diversion procedures, CSF may be acquired and sent for cytologic and biochemical analysis during the case. Third ventriculostomy has the added advantage of potentially allowing for a biopsy by endoscopic guidance during the procedure. This provides the opportunity to make an intraoperative diagnosis with subsequent tailoring of further therapy.

The decision to perform biopsy versus an open procedure has been debated extensively in the pineal region tumor literature.[1a,11,13,18,27] Although the ultimate choice of procedure will be based to some extent on the surgeon's personal bias and experience, there are some distinct advantages and disadvantages to each of these procedures. Stereotactic biopsy has been described as the procedure of choice for obtaining a tissue diagnosis in certain situations such as widely disseminated disease, clearly invasive malignant tumor, or patients with multiple medical problems. Early experience with stereotactic biopsies encountered morbidity and mortality specifically related to targeting periventricular structures adjacent to the deep venous system. More recent studies, however, have shown stereotactic biopsy to be a safe and efficient means of obtaining a tissue diagnosis. In their 1996 series, Regis and colleagues revealed a mortality rate of 1.3% and a less than 1.0% morbidity rate in 370 stereotactic biopsies of pineal region tumor patients.[56] The study included data from 15 French neurosurgical centers and documented statistical homogeneity among the different centers. In a similar study Kreth and colleagues retrospectively evaluated the risk profile, diagnostic accuracy, and the therapeutic relevance of the stereotactic approach in 106 patients.[45] They showed a morbidity rate of 2:106, mortality rate of 9:106, and a definitive tissue diagnostic rate of 103:106 patients. Although stereotactic biopsy can clearly be performed safely and effectively at centers familiar with the technique, it falls short of one main operative goal that may be advantageous to some patients, namely, the complete or near-complete resection of tumor.

Open resection has been shown to benefit patients postoperatively by removal of most, if not all, of the tumor.[13,18] For patients with benign lesions, the surgical resection can prove to be curative. In patients with malignant-tumor components, evidence suggests that surgical debulking may improve the response to postoperative adjuvant therapy.[64] Gross-total tumor resection also provides ample tissue specimen to the neuropathologist for diagnosis. This circumvents the potential problems of sampling error and erroneous diagnosis associated with the small volume of tissue provided by stereotactic biopsy. The bulk of evidence provided by the current literature is derived from retrospective analyses, including cases performed a decade ago. Several advances have been made over the past decade that will likely lower the morbidity and mortality associated with open procedures as well as stereotactic biopsy.

Tissue diagnosis is a vital part of management in most patients with pineal region tumor. However, nonoperative management of patients with positive tumor markers is a reasonable option for some patients. A markedly elevated level of AFP and BHCG is pathognomonic for germ cell tumor with malignant components. New strategies currently under study have been aimed at minimizing surgical intervention before ascertaining whether a tumor is responsive to radiation or chemotherapy. In their 1998 retrospective study, Choi and colleagues described the treatment of 107 patients with primary intracranial germ cell tumor, including 60 patients with tumors in the pineal region.[22] Thirty of the patients with pineal tumors were managed without surgery on the basis of radiologic findings and tumor markers. Univariate analysis of a response to trial radiation and chemotherapy was shown to be correlative with outcome, justifying the administration of trial chemotherapy or radiation therapy without tissue biopsy in this subgroup of patients. These findings match well with a 1997 study by Sawamura and colleagues evaluating the necessity of radical

resection in patients with intracranial germinomas.[61] Twenty-nine patients treated with radiation or chemotherapy were studied retrospectively, including 10 with solitary pineal region masses. The results showed no significant difference in outcome related to extent of surgical resection, with an overall tumor-free survival rate of 100% at a follow-up of 42 months. This retrospective evidence is quite compelling in favor of withholding surgical treatment of children with marker-positive germ cell tumors.

SURGICAL MANAGEMENT

Improvements in surgical techniques and neuroanesthesia have significantly lowered the morbidity and mortality associated with pineal region surgery. For those patients for whom primary surgical resection is the best therapeutic and diagnostic option, there are several well-described approaches currently in use.[18] In general, surgical approaches to the pineal region can be divided into supratentorial, infratentorial, and most recently a combined supratentorial-infratentorial approach. Supratentorial approaches include the parietal-interhemispheric approach described by Dandy and the occipital-transtentorial approach originally described by Horrax and later modified by Poppen.[25,39,53]

POSTOPERATIVE STAGING

Gross-total resection of a well-differentiated pineocytoma has the potential of being curative (Figure 33-2). However, if malignant components are encountered, the physician is obligated to evaluate the patient for spinal metastasis.[12,68] Before widespread use of MRI, patients were staged postoperatively with CT-myelogram. Currently, the most sensitive radiographic modality for

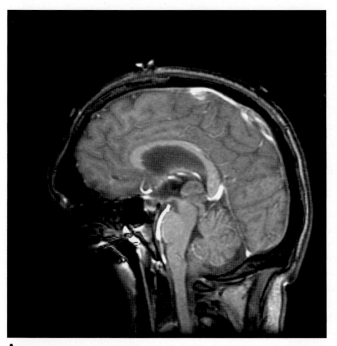

A

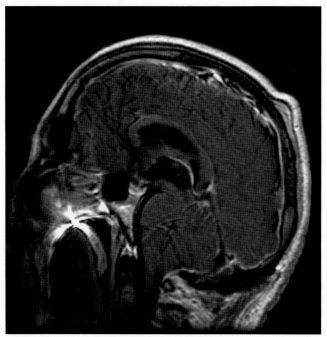

B

FIGURE 33-2   Gross-total resection of a well-differentiated pineocytoma has the potential of being curative.

screening is a complete spinal MRI scan with and without gadolinium.[13] The first MRI scan should be timed at least 2 weeks after surgery, because spinal canal enhancement can occur in the early postoperative period.[68] Equivocal findings on the initial postoperative scan warrant a repeat scan within 1 to 2 weeks. Radiographic artifacts secondary to surgery regress, whereas drop metastases remain stable or increase in size over time. The role for postoperative lumbar puncture and subsequent CSF analysis for cytology is questionable.[74,75] The presence of abnormal cells postoperatively does not correlate well with spinal metastasis caused by spillage during surgery.

The timing for follow-up cranial MRI varies depending on tumor histology and degree of resection. To estimate the amount of tumor removed it is advantageous to acquire a postoperative brain MRI within 48 hours of performing surgery. Postoperative enhancement unrelated to residual tumor may be seen on scans done later. The significance of residual tumor depends on tumor histology and the efficacy of available adjuvant therapy. The radioresponsive germinoma is a good example of this phenomenon. Series of patients treated with adjuvant radiation are reported to have a 100% tumor-free survival up to 4 years after diagnosis.[22] This survival rate has been shown to be unrelated to the extent of tumor resection. In contrast, much of the literature evaluating tumor resection and malignant pineal cell tumors and nongerminomatous germ cell tumors suggests that larger resections facilitate adjuvant therapy and long-term survival.[15,18] Regardless of tumor histology, long-term follow-up is required for all patients with pineal region tumors because recurrences several years after remission are possible. Accordingly, patients with pineocytomas should be followed on a regular basis.

ADJUVANT THERAPY

In general, patients with pineocytomas without malignant components and no evidence of dissemination do not require adjuvant therapy. However, aggressive therapy may be warranted in pineocytoma patients with highly mitotic tumors or cellular components that resemble pineoblastoma.

Radiation Therapy

Current treatment protocols for patients with malignant pineal region tumors include radiation therapy. Early clinical trials with series of patients treated with radiation therapy had significant mortality.[35,66] Even low doses of radiation can have significant long-term effects on a child's cognitive development.[5,7] Radiation-induced deficits are an important consideration because many children with pineal region tumors enjoy prolonged survival. Potential complications include hypothalamic and endocrine dysfunction, cerebral necrosis, new tumor formation, and progression of disease. There have been at least 35 cases of radiation-induced meningioma in children after radiation therapy for pineal region tumors reported in the literature since 1953.[67] Standard radiation therapy protocols for children with malignant pineal cell tumors use 4000 cGy of whole-brain radiation followed by 1500 cGy to the pineal region.[13,34,43] The dose is given in 180 cGy daily fractions. Whole-brain radiation can cause significant morbidity in prepubescent patients, limiting the recommended initial extended field to between 2500 cGy and 3000 cGy. An additional dose directed at the tumor

bed can subsequently be given. Several studies have shown that patients receiving less than 5000 cGy are at risk for recurrence, strongly suggesting that this is the optimal total dose of radiation. For children with malignant germ cell tumors, standard treatment is focal radiation therapy followed by radiation to the ventricular field.

The application of radiation therapy depends on the histology of the tumor being treated. Germinomas are among the most radiosensitive tumors, with patient response rates and long-term tumor-free survival greater than 90% in most published series. Nongerminomatous malignant germ cell tumors are significantly less responsive to radiation, with a 5-year survival rate of between 30% and 40% using this treatment alone.[34,41] Patients with low-grade pineocytomas can be cautiously followed after complete surgical resection without any adjuvant radiation. There is no clear evidence that radiation therapy benefits patients with low-grade lesions.[68] The morbid side effects of radiation can be avoided by carefully following these patients with serial MRI scans to assess tumor recurrence or progression.

The use of prophylactic spinal irradiation is controversial. Early recommendations for postoperative spinal irradiation have been preempted by reports showing the incidence of drop metastasis into the spine to be relatively low.[26,47] The propensity of a pineal region tumor to metastasize to the spine varies with tumor histology. Estimates of spinal seeding with pineal cell tumors are in the range of 10% to 20%, with significantly higher rates noted for pineoblastoma than for pineocytoma.[63] The incidence of spinal metastasis for germinomas has been reported to be as high as 11%; for endodermal sinus tumors, up to 23%.[46,52,71,76] Craniospinal radiation therapy for nongerminomatous germ cell tumors is controversial but routinely used in some countries.[20] As modern improvements in surgical and adjuvant therapy are reflected in present day long-term survival, the rates of spinal metastasis will likely drop significantly, making the need for spinal irradiation obsolete. Currently, a reasonable approach is to give spinal irradiation only for documented seeding. For patients with pineoblastomas, some authors suggest the use of preemptive spinal radiation therapy even if the postoperative surveillance MRI scan is negative.[43]

Chemotherapy

Chemotherapy has evolved as an attractive means to minimize the amount of radiation needed to effectively treat children with pineal region tumors. As with radiation therapy, the response to chemotherapy for patients with pineal region tumors varies according to tumor histology. Germ cell tumors have been historically more sensitive to chemotherapy than pineal cell tumors.

The reported effectiveness of chemotherapeutic regimens for children with pineal cell tumors is limited to anecdotal case reports and reported series involving small numbers of patients.[40] No dominant agent has evolved as the drug of choice, and treatment regimens have included various combinations of vincristine, lomustine, cisplatin, etoposide, cyclophosphamide, actinomycin D, and methotrexate. Recently high-dose cyclophosphamide has been advocated as a single agent protocol in the treatment of children with pineoblastomas.[4] In their 1996 study Ashley and colleagues demonstrated that children treated with high-dose cyclophosphamide had stable or diminishing disease while on protocol. Impaired pulmonary function and thrombocytopenia were notable side effects.[4]

Radiosurgery

Stereotactic radiation or radiosurgery is being increasingly applied to patients with central nervous system disease.[6,10,36] Currently, the experience with radiosurgery for pineal region tumor patients is limited. Manera and colleagues have described 11 patients with pineal region tumors treated with stereotactic radiosurgery, all of whom showed a response to treatment without preemptive whole-brain radiation.[48] In the pediatric population, radiosurgery is an attractive potential first-line treatment that merits further investigation. Radiosurgery is currently optimized for targets 3 cm or less, which would preclude treatment of some patients with larger pineal region tumors. As experience with radiosurgery grows, it might become a useful modality in treating tumor recurrence.

FOLLOW-UP, PROGNOSIS, AND MANAGEMENT OF RECURRENCES

Life-long follow-up of patients with pineal region tumors is required.[13,43] These tumors can recur locally or appear distally as late as 5 years after diagnosis. In addition, patients can present later in life with new tumor formation (e.g., meningioma).[67] MRI scans should be obtained on a periodic basis as determined by tumor histology of original diagnosis, extent of resection, and presence of metastasis at time of diagnosis. Tumor marker studies for patients with germ cell tumors should also be performed on a periodic basis even if markers were normal at diagnosis. The prognosis depends on tumor histology and is subject to change as more effective adjuvant therapy is developed. In general, patients with intracranial germinomas have an excellent prognosis because of the radiosensitivity of these tumors. Patients with nongerminomatous germ cell tumors have a significantly worse prognosis than patients with germinomas, as do children with pineal cell tumors. There is no conventional approach to managing recurrence. Chemotherapy, radiation therapy, or radiosurgery can be applied if maximal doses have not already been administered. A second surgical procedure is generally reserved for patients with benign lesions who demonstrate recurrence several years later.[13,69] Recurrent germ cell tumors have been shown to respond to chemotherapy as have some pineal cell tumors, although to a lesser degree.[22] Radiosurgery may be a consideration for all recurrences less than 3 cm in diameter.

CONCLUSION

Pineal region tumors represent a rare but challenging problem in neuro-oncology. Therapeutic and diagnostic advances in several disciplines have significantly improved the prognosis of patients with these lesions. Patients with low-grade pineocytomas can be effectively cured with gross-total resection. Regular long-term follow-up of these patients should be standard practice.

References

1. Allen JC: Controversies in the management of intracranial germ cell tumors. Neurol Clin 9:441–452, 1991.
1a. Allen JC, DaRosso RC, Donahue B, Nirenberg A: A phase II trial of preirradiation carboplatin in newly diagnosed germinoma of the central nervous system. Cancer 74:940–944, 1994.
2. Allen JC, Nisselbaum J, Epstein F, et al: Alphafetoprotein and human chorionic gonadotropin determination in cerebrospinal fluid. An aid to the diagnosis and management of intracranial germ-cell tumors. J Neurosurg 51:368–374, 1979.
3. Arita N, Ushio Y, Hayakawa T, et al: Serum levels of alpha-fetoprotein, human chorionic gonadotropin and carcinoembryonic antigen in patients with primary intracranial germ cell tumors. Oncodev Biol Med 1:235–240, 1980.
4. Ashley DM, Longee D, Tien R, et al: Treatment of patients with pineoblastoma with high dose cyclophosphamide. Med Pediatr Oncol 26:387–392, 1996.
5. Avizonis VN, Fuller DB, Thomson JW, et al: Late effects following central nervous system radiation in a pediatric population. Neuropediatrics 23:228–234, 1992.
6. Backlund EO: Radiosurgery in intracranial tumors and vascular malformations. J Neurosurg Sci 33:91–93, 1989.
7. Bendersky M, Lewis M, Mandelbaum DE, Stanger C: Serial neuropsychological follow-up of a child following craniospinal irradiation. Dev Med Child Neurol 30:816–820, 1988.
8. Berger M, Baumeister B, Geyer J, et al: The risks of metastases from shunting in children with primary central nervous system tumors. J Neurosurg 74:872, 1991.
9. Blasco A, Dominguez P, Ballestin C, et al: Peritoneal implantation of pineal germinoma via a ventriculoperitoneal shunt [letter]. Acta Cytol 37:637–638, 1993.
10. Brada M: Radiosurgery for brain tumours. Eur J Cancer 27:1545–1548, 1991.
11. Broggi G, Franzini A, Migliavacca F, Allegranza A: Stereotactic biopsy of deep brain tumors in infancy and childhood. Childs Brain 10:92–98, 1983.
12. Bruce DA, Allen JC: Tumor staging for pineal region tumors of childhood. Cancer 56:1792–1794, 1985.
13. Bruce J: Management of pineal region tumors. Neurosurgery Q 3:103–119, 1993.
14. Bruce J, Stein B: Supracerebellar approaches in the pineal region. In Apuzzo M (ed): Brain Surgery: Complication, Avoidance, and Management. New York, Churchill-Livingstone, 1993.
15. Bruce J, Stein B, Fetell M: Tumors of the pineal region. In Rowland L (ed): Merrit's Textbook of Neurology. Baltimore, Williams & Wilkins, 1995.
16. Bruce J, Tamarkin L, Riedel C, et al: Sequential cerebrospinal fluid and plasma sampling in humans: 24 hour melatonin measurements in normal subjects and after peripheral sympathectomy. J Clin Endocrinol Metab 72:819–823, 1991.
17. Bruce JN, Stein BM: Pineal tumors. Neurosurg Clin N Am 1:123–138, 1990.
18. Bruce JN, Stein BM: Surgical management of pineal region tumors. Acta Neurochir 134:130–135, 1995.
19. Burres K, Hamilton R: Pineal apoplexy. Neurosurgery 4:264–268, 1979.
20. Calaminus G, Andreussi L, Garre ML, et al: Secreting germ cell tumors of the central nervous system (CNS). First results of the cooperative German/Italian pilot study (CNS sGCT). Klin Padiatr 209:222–227, 1997.

21. Chang T, Teng MM, Guo WY, Sheng WC: CT of pineal tumors and intracranial germ-cell tumors. AJR Am J Roentgenol 153:1269–1274, 1989.

22. Choi JU, Kim DS, Chung SS, Kim TS: Treatment of germ cell tumors in the pineal region. Childs Nerv Syst 14:41–48, 1998.

23. Colombo F, Benedetti A, Alexandre A: Stereotactic exploration of deep-seated or surgically unamenable intracranial space-occupying lesions. J Neurosurg Sci 24:173–177, 1980.

24. Cranston PE, Hatten MT, Smith EE: Metastatic pineoblastoma via a ventriculoperitoneal shunt: CT demonstration. Comput Med Imaging Graph 16:349–351, 1992.

25. Dandy W: Operative experience in cases of pineal tumor. Arch Surg 33:19–46, 1936.

26. Dattoli MJ, Newall J: Radiation therapy for intracranial germinoma: the case for limited volume treatment. Int J Radiat Oncol Biol Phys 19:429–433, 1990.

27. Dempsey PK, Kondziolka D, Lunsford LD: Stereotactic diagnosis and treatment of pineal region tumours and vascular malformations [see comments]. Acta Neurochir 116:14–22, 1992.

28. Devkota J, Brooks BS, el Gammal T: Ventriculoperitoneal shunt metastasis of a pineal germinoma. Comput Radiol 8:141–145, 1984.

29. Edwards MS, Hudgins RJ, Wilson CB, et al: Pineal region tumors in children. J Neurosurg 68:689–697, 1988.

30. Ellenbogen RG, Moores LE: Endoscopic management of a pineal and suprasellar germinoma with associated hydrocephalus: technical case report. Minim Invasive Neurosurg 40:13–15, 1997; discussion 16.

31. Erlich SS, Apuzzo ML: The pineal gland: anatomy, physiology, and clinical significance. J Neurosurg 63:321–341, 1985.

32. Ferrer E, Santamarta D, Garcia-Fructuoso G, et al: Neuroendoscopic management of pineal region tumours. Acta Neurochir 139:12–20, 1997.

33. Fetell MR, Stein BM: Neuroendocrine aspects of pineal tumors. Neurol Clin 4:877–905, 1986.

34. Fuller BG, Kapp DS, Cox R: Radiation therapy of pineal region tumors: 25 new cases and a review of 208 previously reported cases. Int J Radiat Oncol Biol Phys 28:229–245, 1994.

35. Griffin BR, Griffin TW, Tong DY, et al: Pineal region tumors: results of radiation therapy and indications for elective spinal irradiation. Int J Radiat Oncol Biol Phys 7:605–608, 1981.

36. Goodman ML: Gamma knife radiosurgery: current status and review. South Med J 83:551–554, 1990.

37. Gururangan S, Heideman RL, Kovnar EH, et al: Peritoneal metastases in two patients with pineoblastoma and ventriculoperitoneal shunts. Med Pediatr Oncol 22:417–420, 1994.

38. Hoffman HJ, Yoshida M, Becker LE, et al: Experience with pineal region tumours in childhood. Neurol Res 6:107–112, 1984.

39. Horrax G: Treatment of tumors of the pineal body. Experience in a series of twenty-two cases. Arch Neurol Psychiatry 64:227–242, 1950.

40. Jakacki RI, Zeltzer PM, Boyett JM, et al: Survival and prognostic factors following radiation and/or chemotherapy for primitive neuroectodermal tumors of the pineal region in infants and children: a report of the Childrens Cancer Group. J Clin Oncol 13:1377–1383, 1995.

41. Jennings MT, Gelman R, Hochberg F: Intracranial germ-cell tumors: natural history and pathogenesis. J Neurosurg 63:155–167, 1985.

42. Jooma R, Kendall BE: Diagnosis and management of pineal tumors. J Neurosurg 58:654–665, 1983.

43. Kang JK, Jeun SS, Hong YK, et al: Experience with pineal region tumors. Childs Nerv Syst 14:63–68, 1998.

44. Krabbe K: The pineal gland, especially in relation to the problem on its supposed significance in sexual development. Endocrinology 7:379–414, 1923.

45. Kreth FW, Schatz CR, Pagenstecher A, et al: Stereotactic management of lesions of the pineal region. Neurosurgery 39:280–289, 1996; discussion 289–291.

46. Levin CV, Rutherfoord GS: Metastasizing pineal germinoma. A case report and review. S Afr Med J 68:36–39, 1985.

47. Linstadt D, Wara WM, Edwards MS, et al: Radiotherapy of primary intracranial germinomas: the case against routine craniospinal irradiation. Int J Radiat Oncol Biol Phys 15:291–297, 1988.

48. Manera L, Regis J, Chinot O, et al: Pineal region tumors: The role of stereotactic radiosurgery. Stereotact Funct Neurosurg 66:164–1673, 1996.

49. Min KW, Scheithauer BW, Bauserman SC: Pineal parenchymal tumors: an ultrastructural study with prognostic implications. Ultrastruct Pathol 18:69–85, 1994.

50. Muller-Forell W, Schroth G, Egan PJ: MR imaging in tumors of the pineal region. Neuroradiology 30:224–231, 1988.

51. Neuwelt EA, Mickey B, Lewy AJ: The importance of melatonin and tumor markers in pineal tumors. J Neural Transm Suppl 21:397–413, 1986.

52. Ono N, Isobe I, Uki J, et al: Recurrence of primary intracranial germinomas after complete response with radiotherapy: recurrence patterns and therapy. Neurosurgery 35:615–620, 1994; discussion 620–621.

53. Poppen J: The right occipital approach to a pinealoma. J Neurosurgery 3:1–8, 1966.

54. Posner M, Horrax G: Eye signs in pineal tumors. J Neurosurg 3:15–24, 1946.

55. Quest D, Kleriga E: Microsurgical anatomy of the pineal region. Neurosurgery 6:385–390, 1980.

56. Regis J, Bouillot P, Rouby-Volot F, et al: Pineal region tumors and the role of stereotactic biopsy: review of the mortality, morbidity, and diagnostic rates in 370 cases. Neurosurgery 39:907–912, 1996; discussion 912–914.

57. Rickert CH: Abdominal metastases of pediatric brain tumors via ventriculo-peritoneal shunts. Childs Nerv Syst 14:10–14, 1998.

58. Ringertz N, Nordenstam H, Flyger G: Tumors of the pineal region. J Neuropathol Exp Neurol 13:540–561, 1954.

59. Robinson S, Cohen AR: The role of neuroendoscopy in the treatment of pineal region tumors. Surg Neurol 48:360–365, 1997; discussion 365–367.

60. Russell DS, Rubinstein LJ: Tumours of specialized tissues of central neuroepithelial origin. In Russell DS, Rubinstein LJ (eds): Pathology of Tumours of the Nervous System. Baltimore, Williams & Wilkins, 1989.

61. Sawamura Y, de Tribolet N, Ishii N, Abe H: Management of primary intracranial germinomas: diagnostic surgery or radical resection? J Neurosurg 87:262–266, 1997.

62. Sawaya R, Hawley D, Tobler W, et al: Pineal and third ventricle tumors. In Youmans J (ed): Neurological Surgery. Philadelphia, WB Saunders, 1990.

63. Schild SE, Scheithauer BW, Schomberg PJ, et al: Pineal parenchymal tumors. Clinical, pathologic, and therapeutic aspects. Cancer 72:870–880, 1993.

64. Shokry A, Janzer RC, Von Hochstetter AR, et al: Primary intracranial germ-cell tumors. A clinicopathological study of 14 cases. J Neurosurg 62:826–830, 1985.

65. Smirniotopoulos JG, Rushing EJ, Mena H: Pineal region masses: differential diagnosis. Radiographics 12:577–596, 1992.

66. Smith NJ, El-Mahdi AM, Constable WC: Results of irradiation of tumors in the region of the pineal body. Acta Radiol Ther Phys Biol 15:17–22, 1976.

67. Starshak RJ: Radiation-induced meningioma in children: report of two cases and review of the literature. Pediatr Radiol 26:537–541, 1996.

68. Stein BM, Bruce JN: Surgical management of pineal region tumors (honored guest lecture). Clin Neurosurg 39:509–532, 1992.

69. Stein BM, Fetell MR: Therapeutic modalities for pineal region tumors. Clin Neurosurg 32:445–455, 1985.

70. Steinbok P, Dolmen C, Kaan K: Pineocytomas presenting as subarachnoid hemorrhage, report of two cases. J Neurosurg 47:776–780, 1977.

71. Takakura K: Intracranial germ cell tumors. Clin Neurosurg 32:429–444, 1985.

72. Takeuchi J, Handa H, Nagata I: Suprasellar germinoma. J Neurosurg 49:41–48, 1978.

73. Tien RD, Barkovich AJ, Edwards MS: MR imaging of pineal tumors. AJR Am J Roentgenol 155:143–151, 1990.

74. Ueki K, Tanaka R: Treatments and prognoses of pineal tumors: experience of 110 cases. Neurol Med Chir (Tokyo) 20:1–26, 1980.

75. Waga S, Handa H, Yamashita J: Intracranial germinomas: treatment and results. Surg Neurol 11:167–172, 1979.

76. Wolden SL, Wara WM, Larson DA, et al: Radiation therapy for primary intracranial germ-cell tumors. Int J Radiat Oncol Biol Phys 32:943–949, 1995.

77. Wong TT, Lee LS: A method of enlarging the opening of the third ventricular floor for flexible endoscopic third ventriculostomy. Childs Nerv Syst 12:396–398, 1996.

78. Yamashita J, Handa H: Diagnosis and treatment of pineal tumours. Kyoto University experience (1941–1984). Acta Neurochir Suppl 42:137–141, 1988.

79. Zee CS, Segall H, Apuzzo M, et al: MR imaging of pineal region neoplasms. J Comput Assist Tomogr 15:56–63, 1991.

80. Zimmerman R: Pineal region masses: radiology. In Wilkins R, Rengachary S (eds): Neurosurgery. Vol 1. New York, McGraw-Hill, 1985.

81. Zondek H, Kaatz A, Unger H: Precocious puberty and choriepithelioma of the pineal gland with report of a case. J Endocrinol 10:12–16, 1953.

CHAPTER 34

PINEOBLASTOMA

Susan M. Chang, Fred G. Barker II, and Tarik Tihan

LOCATION

The pineal region consists of a pineal body, posterior wall of the third ventricle, tela choroidea, and velum interpositum. Pineal parenchymal tumors (PPTs) arise from the body of the pineal gland and represent a spectrum of tumors from the well-differentiated pineocytes, or pineocytoma (45%), to the primitive parenchymal cells, or pineoblastoma (45%).[7] PPTs can also be composed of both well-differentiated pineocytes as well as primitive cells (mixed pineocytoma and pineoblastoma) or of cells of intermediate histologic features. These two types make up 10% of PPTs.

The pineoblastoma and tumors of intermediate histology have a propensity to spread along the cerebrospinal pathways and can disseminate along the leptomeninges. Very rarely, hematogenous dissemination with systemic metastases may also occur.

EPIDEMIOLOGY, INCIDENCE, AND PREVALENCE

Pineal region tumors, which account for 0.4% to 1% of intracranial tumors, are 10 times more common in children than in adults.[1] The PPTs represent 11% to 28% of these tumors. Of the types of primary parenchymal tumors, pineocytoma (45% of PPTs) tends to be widely distributed, from young patients in the 10- to 14-years age group to older patients in the 65- to 69-years age group. In contrast, pineoblastoma (45% of PPTs) shows the highest incidence in the 0- to 4-years age group and decreases in incidence with age. The largest series of adults with pineoblastoma was reported by Lutterbach et al, where the age range was 17 to 77 years.[13]

Familial pineoblastoma has been reported in the absence of signs of any other heritable tumor susceptibility syndrome. Because these families are so rare, it is difficult to determine whether the disease occurrence is caused by an unidentified germline mutation in a tumor-suppressor gene or a common environmental exposure. Children with bilateral retinoblastoma have germline mutations of the tumor-suppressor gene Rb at the chromosomal band 13q14 and are at an increased risk for the development of other forms of cancer, specifically pineoblastoma (trilateral retinoblastoma).[10]

DIAGNOSIS

Clinical Presentation

Because of the central location and its proximity to the central nervous system (CSF) pathways, patients with malignant PPTs most commonly have symptoms related to hydrocephalus. These include headache, blurred vision, nausea, and vomiting. If there has been dissemination throughout the CNS, symptoms may be present depending on the location of the disseminated disease. Symptoms suggesting metastatic spread in the spine (e.g., back pain, radiculopathy or sensory changes, and bowel and bladder dysfunction) may be present.

Neurologic examination often confirms the presence of raised intracranial pressure with signs of papilledema and visual disturbances. Parinaud's syndrome, characterized by loss of voluntary upward gaze, may also be found at the time of clinical evaluation.

Neuroimaging

Once a patient has signs and symptoms of raised intracranial pressure, neuroimaging studies are done for further evaluation.[14] In the emergency setting, a computed tomography (CT) scan may be done as the first study. In the case of a PPT, the mass located in the pineal region is seen usually with resulting obstruction to cerebrospinal fluid (CSF) flow and hydrocephalus. Calcification or hemorrhage may also be seen. Because of the multiplanar images acquired with magnetic resonance imaging (MRI), there has been marked improvement in the preoperative delineation of benign and malignant pineal masses and in distinguishing true pineal masses from parapineal masses impinging into the region of the gland.[3] Other tumor types that involve the pineal region include germ cell tumors (the most common histology in the pineal region), astrocytic tumors, metastatic disease, and meningioma.

The reports of imaging findings for PPTs vary greatly, and the specific histologic diagnosis is not possible on MRI. Pineal neoplasms are lobulated solid masses that enhance densely following gadolinium administration. There may be a cyst present in conjunction with the solid component. Generally, pineoblastomas are isointense to gray matter on T2-weighted images, reflecting their high cellularity. Brain invasion and surrounding cerebral edema may also be seen with pineoblastomas. It is important to assess the entire brain for any evidence of remote metastatic spread to other structures, especially leptomeningeal involvement.

Patients who have a diagnosis of retinoblastoma, symptoms of hydrocephalus, and a pineal mass need close evaluation of their orbits to determine the status of their disease. Rarely, the intracranial mass is diagnosed before the retinal tumor. Because of the increased incidence among patients with germline Rb, screening for intracranial disease in these patients is thought beneficial by some.

If the imaging characteristics are consistent with a PPT, further staging of the neuroaxis with a contrast MRI scan of the entire spine is important before any surgical intervention is performed. This is important not only for staging the disease and determining prognosis but also to guide treatment decisions (e.g., the aggressiveness of the extent of surgical intervention). Staging the neuroaxis following a craniotomy can be difficult because of postoperative changes that could confound the staging evaluation. If staging is not performed preoperatively, a period of at least 2 to 3 weeks should pass before evaluation with an MRI scan of the spine because of the blood products that can interfere with the imaging studies. This could delay the start of therapy and adversely affect the treatment planning.

Tumor Histology and Cytogenetics

Macroscopic Features

Pineoblastomas are soft, gelatinous, and often hemorrhagic and necrotic masses. They can be focally distinct from the surrounding normal parenchyma, but are often not amenable to gross-total resection.

Microscopic Features

Pineoblastomas are considered the most aggressive form of the PPT spectrum. Histologically, the pineoblastoma is a small-blue-round-cell tumor that shows little differentiation toward pineocytes and is mitotically active. The neoplasm often exhibits necrosis with apoptotic cells in addition to mitoses. In some tumors, vascular endothelial proliferation can be easily identified. The tumor cells have typically scant cytoplasm and hyperchromatic nuclei. Homer Wright or Flexner-Wintersteiner type rosettes (retinoblastoma) are often the hallmark of the microscopic pattern and are often present.[16] Even though the majority of the tumor is poorly differentiated, there is a variable amount of better-differentiated regions in each case with evidence of "retinal" differentiation. In rare instances, there can be focal glial as well as neuronal differentiation that produces a fibrillary background.

Histologic grade of PPTs is considered to be a significant independent prognostic factor.[5] The current World Health Organization (WHO) grading of PPTs includes three categories: pineocytoma, PPT of intermediate differentiation, and pineoblastoma. The grading of PPTs is done with respect to the area of highest grade. Mixed tumors with foci of both intermediate differentiation and pineoblastoma are considered to be pineoblastoma. There is little evidence that such grading underscores a progressive pathway, yet pineal tumors showing a mixed pattern of grades suggest that at least some tumors may progress to higher grade lesions. Another approach to grading uses two criteria, the mitotic count and the presence or absence of staining for neurofilament protein.[9]

Immunohistochemical Features

Pineoblastomas are only focally positive for synaptophysin and neurofilament protein, especially in the center of pineocytomatous or Homer Wright rosettes and in the fine neuropil-like areas.[9,16] Other proteins such as tau protein, glial fibrillary acidic protein (GFAP), and retinal S-antigen may also be focally positive in some cases. The MIB-1 labeling index is often high in pineoblastomas and can be greater than 50%.

Ultrastructural Features

Pineoblastoma cells can have microtubules and neurofilaments, but glial intermediate filaments and definite synapses are not usually identifiable. Some cells in tumors contain dense-core vesicles, "vesicle-crowned rods" ("synaptic ribbons"), microtubules, and the so-called fibrous filaments.

Molecular and Cytogenetic Features

There is a well-documented relationship between germline mutations of Rb and the occurrence of pineoblastoma, but the mutational status of Rb in sporadic pineoblastomas has not been well studied. There have been studies describing a very limited number of genetically evaluated pineoblastoma. There was one report of a mutation of the hSNF5 gene on chromosome 22q11, a gene that is also mutated in familial and sporadic rhabdoid tumors, a malignant tumor of infants. The hSNF5 protein is important for chromatin remodeling during cell division. Although histologically these tumors are similar to primitive neuroectodermal tumors, the isochromosome i17q, usually thought to be a cytogenetic characteristic of medulloblastoma, is not commonly seen in pineoblastoma, suggesting that these tumors are genetically distinct.

A recent study on cytogenetic alterations in pineoblastomas identified five high-level gains found on 1q12-qter, 5p13.2-14, 5q21-qter, 6p12-pter, and 14q21-qter. In this study, the genetic imbalances in higher grade tumors mainly included gains of 12q and losses of chromosome 22.[18]

Pathologic Differential Diagnosis

Distinguishing pineal parenchymal neoplasms from normal pineal parenchyma or parenchyma incorporated in the wall of a pineal cyst is the principal issue in the differential diagnosis. Other small-blue-round-cell tumors, especially medulloblastoma, is also a possibility, but the issue is easily resolved on clinical and radiological grounds. The histologic distinction, albeit more challenging, can also be made based on the presence of Flexner-Wintersteiner rosettes and absence of pale islands in a typical pineoblastoma. Differential diagnosis based on clinical features may be more challenging when confronted with a germ cell tumor, metastatic melanoma, pilocytic astrocytoma, or a rare meningioma in the pineal region, yet the pathologic evaluation can readily differentiate such lesions from a PPT.

THERAPY

Because of the rarity of the disease, much of the literature on the treatment of pineoblastoma is retrospective. The resulting heterogeneity of management makes it difficult to evaluate the efficacy of therapies.[7,13] There are no large prospective randomized studies evaluating the various treatment modalities in pineoblastoma. In general, therapy has been developed based on treatment for other supratentorial primitive neuroectodermal tumors (PNETs) and the age of the patient. The Childrens Cancer Group conducted a randomized study in children (18 months to 22 years) with PNETs in which 17 patients of the entire cohort of 304 patients had pineoblastoma.[4,8] In this study all patients received a combination of radiation therapy and chemotherapy following definitive surgery. With this multimodality therapy that involved surgery, radiation to the craniospinal axis, and systemic chemotherapy, the 3-year survival and progression-free survival rates of children with pineoblastoma was 73% ± 12% and 61% ± 13%, respectively. For infants, for whom radiation therapy is withheld, the prognosis is dismal, with a median time to progression of 4 months and death by 2 to 14 months. The majority of studies describe the experience in children given the higher incidence in this patient population, but a recent review of the management in adults was recently published. The accepted prognostic factors include age (worse outcome in infants), grade, and stage of disease. The current information on the disease's management in adults is reviewed.

Surgery

Although surgical resection alone cannot cure a pineoblastoma, surgery can potentially play several roles in pineoblastoma treatment. Many patients with pineoblastomas require CSF diversion for treatment of hydrocephalus. Either open or endoscopic surgery can provide evidence of tumor dissemination through CSF pathways. A biopsy or resection can provide a definitive diagnosis to guide further therapy. Finally, many surgeons believe that pineoblastomas should be completely resected, when possible, as the initial cytoreductive step in a multimodality treatment plan.

Biopsy

Biopsies of tumors in the pineal region and posterior third ventricle are usually performed in one of two ways: stereotactically or endoscopically. For stereotactic biopsy, a frame-based method is usually chosen, using local anesthesia.[17] Although frameless stereotactic biopsy techniques have been described, the accuracy demanded for biopsy of the centrally located pineal region is probably still best provided by a frame-based method.

The risks of stereotactic biopsy of a pineal region mass are higher than the low rate characteristic of most intracranial lesions.[6,17] Pineal region tumors are surrounded by the internal cerebral veins and the basal veins of Rosenthal, and injury to these veins must be scrupulously avoided. Added to the risk of potential injury to the deep veins, intratumoral hemorrhage is a potential cause of serious morbidity or death. Pineoblastomas seem to have a higher risk of this complication than other pineal region tumors. Finally, stereotactic biopsy provides a negative or inconclusive result in approximately 5% of cases, and additional inaccuracy resulting from sampling error (given the intrinsic heterogeneity of pineal tumors) is present as well.

Endoscopic biopsy is usually performed through a third ventricular route using a flexible endoscope.[15] Although some surgeons believe this procedure to be safer than stereotactic biopsy, intraventricular hemorrhage is still a significant risk.

The specimen is normally much smaller than one from a stereotactic biopsy, and both the difficulty of achieving a correct diagnosis and the chance of sampling error are correspondingly higher. The advantages of this technique are the ability to perform a third ventriculocisternostomy for CSF diversion (see following discussion) at the same procedure and the opportunity to inspect the third ventricle for disseminated tumor that may be below the detection threshold of imaging studies.

Cerebrospinal Fluid Access and Diversion Procedures

Many patients with pineoblastoma have symptomatic hydrocephalus because of obstruction of the sylvian aqueduct in the dorsal midbrain, and these patients usually require either temporary or permanent CSF diversion. A ventriculostomy tube can be used to drain the lateral ventricles for temporary relief of hydrocephalus. A unilateral procedure usually suffices, because blockage of the foramina of Monro is unusual. For patients who require permanent CSF diversion because of obstructive hydrocephalus, the preferred procedure is third ventriculocisternostomy, or the creation of an opening through the floor of the third ventricle into the basal cisterns.[15] Usually a biopsy of the tumor is performed at the same procedure, as described previously.

For patients who are not suitable for third ventriculocisternostomy, a ventriculoperitoneal shunt is placed. This has a small risk of seeding the peritoneum with tumor cells when the tumor has the potential to spread through CSF pathways.

CSF for cytology and tumor marker studies is always obtained during either CSF diversion procedure. However, ventricular CSF cytology is less sensitive than using a lumbar CSF specimen, and negative ventricular cytology should prompt a lumbar puncture for adequate staging. The relative sensitivity of ventricular and lumbar CSF for tumor markers (important in the diagnosis of germ cell tumors of the pineal region) is not known.

Chronic access to the intraventricular space is sometimes useful when patients require intrathecal chemotherapy to treat a tumor with CSF dissemination. This is achieved by placing a ventriculostomy into the frontal horn of the lateral ventricle and connecting it to a subcutaneous reservoir, which can be tapped percutaneously.

Resection

There are three main reasons to resect a pineoblastoma. The first is to provide adequate tissue for an accurate pathologic diagnosis to guide further therapy with radiation, chemotherapy, or both. Stereotactic and, particularly, endoscopic biopsy specimens of pineal region masses are very small and can be challenging to the pathologist. In addition, heterogeneity within pineal region tumors is well known, and entities such as the mixed pineoblastoma-pineocytoma tumor have been described that may be diagnosed inaccurately and treated inadequately if the entire mass is not available for study.

The second reason to resect a pineoblastoma is to relieve symptomatic mass effect. Symptoms of a pineal mass can include those of increased intracranial pressure, either from hydrocephalus or a large tumor, as well as Parinaud's syndrome or other disorders of gaze, ataxia, or tetraparesis. Although pineoblastomas are often sensitive to radiation therapy and chemotherapy, surgery provides the most rapid relief of symptoms from a local mass.

The third benefit of resecting a pineoblastoma is cytoreduction of a nondisseminated tumor in preparation for other therapies (radiation or chemotherapy). Before proposing a resection for cytoreduction, negative staging of the spinal axis and CSF should be demonstrated. The true benefit of surgical cytoreduction of pineoblastomas has not been rigorously demonstrated and remains somewhat controversial.[13]

Resection of pineal region masses is a complex topic, and a full treatment is beyond the scope of this chapter. The most common surgical approach is the supracerebellar-infratentorial route. An alternative approach, useful when the tumor extends into the supratentorial compartment, is the occipital transtentorial approach. For more details on these and other surgical approaches, the interested reader is referred to specialized treatises.[2,19]

Whenever possible, to reduce perioperative morbidity to a minimum, resection should be performed by a surgeon with extensive experience in pineal tumor surgery. In the modern neurosurgical era, the usual sequelae of a pineal resection mass are limited to a possible temporary deficiency of up gaze and, less commonly, temporary disturbances of cognition. More serious complications are usually the result of hemorrhage, either during the resection or from a postoperative tumor remnant, or to injury of the deep veins that surround the tumor.

Radiation Therapy

Pineoblastoma is radiosensitive, and objective responses are seen with radiation therapy. The propensity for cerebrospinal axis dissemination has led to the standard approach in older children of using craniospinal axis radiation at doses of 2400 to 3600 cGy to the axis and 5400 to 6000 cGy to the pineal region.[4] The side effects of this therapy include developmental delay, neurocognitive abnormalities, growth retardation, and neuroendocrine dysfunction. Attempts at various radiation therapy schedules to abrogate the effects on normal tissue (e.g., hyperfractionation) have been tested in small numbers of patients, making it difficult to assess efficacy. Radiation therapy is withheld in infants (<3 years) because of the risk to the developing brain. Current strategies of neoadjuvant high-dose chemotherapy followed by involved-field radiation therapy are being tested for this high-risk group. Management of patients with trilateral retinoblastoma presents an especially difficult challenge because of the risk of the development of secondary malignancy such as radiation-associated sarcoma.

Radiosurgical Treatment of Pineoblastomas

Like surgical resection, radiosurgical treatment of pineoblastomas has a purely local effect and is usually considered when a small primary or recurrent pineoblastoma, or postoperative residual disease, is present in the absence of distant tumor dissemination.[12] This should be confirmed with recent staging of the spine and CSF before treatment. There are several commonly used methods of delivering stereotactic radiation (linear accelerator, Gamma Knife®, or proton beam), and none has yet been demonstrated to be superior. The treatment dose is chosen based on tumor size and proximity to surrounding critical structures (thalamus, midbrain), with the dose to the tumor margin usually ranging from 12 to 20 Gy.

Many pineoblastomas are responsive to radiosurgery, although the reported number of cases is too small to estimate the response rate or the durability of responses reliably.[12,11] Whether the responses achieved extend survival is unclear, because many patients die of disseminated disease, but some patients may have palliation of symptomatic mass effect. Complications of treatment include radiation-related changes in the thalamus and dorsal midbrain; symptoms are often but not always relieved by corticosteroids and may resolve with time. The treatment can sometimes be repeated, but the risk of complications is higher for a second treatment to the same or closely adjacent targets.

Chemotherapy

Pineoblastomas, like the other PNETs, are potentially chemosensitive. This appears to be less likely in infants, where minimal responses are seen using a variety of agents. Even with more intensive chemotherapy, the 2-year progression-free survival rate for infants is only 9% ± 9%.[7] In older children the timing of chemotherapy has traditionally been given as an adjuvant to the craniospinal axis (CSA) radiation and consists of PNET regimens, most commonly CCNU, cisplatin, and vincristine in combination. Other active agents include cyclophosphamide, ifosfamide, and etoposide. The side effects of chemotherapy are drug specific but also a result of the effect on normally dividing cells. Delivery of full doses can be limited by increased toxicity because of prior exposure to CSA radiation. Attempts to intensify the dose of the chemotherapeutic regimen using high-dose regimens and stem cell or bone marrow support have been reported but remain to be fully evaluated. This strategy not only allows for dose intensification but may also allow for lower doses of radiation to be administered to the CSA.

Management at Recurrence

Unfortunately, the pattern of recurrence in this disease is not only local but also with dissemination throughout the craniospinal axis. Systemic spread has also been reported. There is therefore a limited role for further surgical intervention, and radiosurgery can be used only if the recurrence is small and localized. In general, chemotherapy is used as salvage therapy, but responses are low and transient at best. Multiple agents, mainly alkylating drugs, have been used, but time to death is short, regardless of the salvage therapy used.[7]

PROGNOSIS AND OUTCOME

Prognosis is determined by several factors, including histologic differentiation and stage of disease. Patients with tumors of intermediate histology or of mixed elements have a better prognosis than those with pineoblastoma. Patients with localized disease without evidence of CSF dissemination also have a better prognosis. Without treatment, the disease rapidly progresses, with a median survival of a few months. With current treatment modalities, the projected 1-year, 3-year, and 5-year survival rates are 88%, 73%, and 58%, respectively.[7] Infants have a worse prognosis mainly because of the limitation of the use of craniospinal axis radiation. For patients with trilateral retinoblastoma, prognosis is worse.

References

1. Ashwal S, Hinshaw DB, Jr, Bedros A: CNS primitive neuroectodermal tumors of childhood. Med Pediatr Oncol 12:180–188, 1984.
2. Bruce JN, Stein BM: Surgical management of pineal region tumors. Acta Neurochir (Wien) 134:130–135, 1995.
3. Chiechi MV, Smirniotopoulos JG, Mena H: Pineal parenchymal tumors: CT and MR features. J Comput Assist Tomogr 19:509–517, 1995.
4. Cohen BH, Zeltzer PM, Boyett JM, et al: Prognostic factors and treatment results for supratentorial primitive neuroectodermal tumors in children using radiation and chemotherapy: a Childrens Cancer Group randomized trial. J Clin Oncol 13:1687–1696, 1995.
5. Fauchon F, Jouvet A, Paquis P, et al: Parenchymal pineal tumors: a clinicopathological study of 76 cases. Int J Radiat Oncol Biol Phys 46:959–968, 2000.
6. Field M, Witham TF, Flickinger JC, et al: Comprehensive assessment of hemorrhage risks and outcomes after stereotactic brain biopsy. J Neurosurg 94:545–551, 2001.
7. Jakacki RI: Pineal and nonpineal supratentorial primitive neuroectodermal tumors. Childs Nerv Syst 15:586–591, 1999.
8. Jakacki RI, Zeltzer PM, Boyett JM, et al: Survival and prognostic factors following radiation and/or chemotherapy for primitive neuroectodermal tumors of the pineal region in infants and children: a report of the Childrens Cancer Group. J Clin Oncol 13:1377–1383, 1995.
9. Jouvet A, Saint-Pierre G, Fauchon F, et al: Pineal parenchymal tumors: a correlation of histological features with prognosis in 66 cases. Brain Pathol 10:49–60, 2000.
10. Kivela T: Trilateral retinoblastoma: a meta-analysis of hereditary retinoblastoma associated with primary ectopic intracranial retinoblastoma. J Clin Oncol 17:1829–1837, 1999.
11. Kobayashi T, Kida Y, Mori Y: Stereotactic gamma radiosurgery for pineal and related tumors. J Neurooncol 54:301–309, 2001.
12. Kondziolka D, Hadjipanayis CG, Flickinger JC, et al: The role of radiosurgery for the treatment of pineal parenchymal tumors. Neurosurgery 51:880–889, 2002.
13. Lutterbach J, Fauchon F, Schild SE, et al: Malignant pineal parenchymal tumors in adult patients: patterns of care and prognostic factors. Neurosurgery 51:44–55; discussion 55–46, 2002.
14. Nakamura M, Saeki N, Iwadate Y, et al: Neuroradiological characteristics of pineocytoma and pineoblastoma. Neuroradiology 42:509–514, 2000.
15. Pople IK, Athanasiou TC, Sandeman DR, et al: The role of endoscopic biopsy and third ventriculostomy in the management of pineal region tumours. Br J Neurosurg 15:305–311, 2001.
16. Raisanen J, Vogel H, Horoupian DS: Primitive pineal tumor with retinoblastomatous and retinal/ciliary epithelial differentiation: an immunohistochemical study. J Neurooncol 9:165–170, 1990.
17. Regis J, Bouillot P, Rouby-Volot F, et al: Pineal region tumors and the role of stereotactic biopsy: review of the mortality, morbidity, and diagnostic rates in 370 cases. Neurosurgery 39:907–912; discussion 912–904, 1996.
18. Rickert CH, Simon R, Bergmann M, et al: Comparative genomic hybridization in pineal parenchymal tumors. Genes Chromosomes Cancer 30:99–104, 2001.
19. Yamamoto I: Pineal region tumor: surgical anatomy and approach. J Neurooncol 54:263–275, 2001.

CHAPTER 35

MEDULLOBLASTOMA

Geoffrey R. Barger, James G. Douglas, William J. Kupsky, Andrew E. Sloan, and Imad T. Zak

DEFINITION AND EPIDEMIOLOGY

Medulloblastomas in adults are uncommon but not rare. Medulloblastoma is a malignant and invasive embryonal tumor of the cerebellum, corresponding histologically to World Health Organization (WHO) grade IV, that has sometimes been referred to as an infratentorial primitive neuroectodermal tumor, or PNET.[21] Although medulloblastoma is the most common histologic type of malignant central nervous system (CNS) tumor in childhood (0 to 19 years), accounting for 17.2% of these tumors, they account for only 0.7% of all malignant CNS tumors in adults (age ≥20).* The incidence of this tumor steadily decreases with increasing age after a peak occurrence at age 6 (Figure 35-1).* It is estimated that only 29% of medulloblastomas in the United States occur in patients age 20 or older.* This tumor rarely occurs after the age of 50. Sixty-two percent of patients are male (61% age <20 and 63% age ≥20).* The total number of medulloblastoma cases (ICD-O-2 histology codes 9470-9472) reported to the Central Brain Tumor Registry of the United States (CBTRUS) by 12 state cancer registries for 1995 to 1999 was 444: 315 in children ages 0 to 19 and 129 in adults 20 years and older. Of these, 398 were medulloblastoma (ICD-O-2 code 9470/3), while 44 were desmoplastic nodular medulloblastoma (9471/3).* An estimated 448 new cases of medulloblastoma (9470-9472) were expected to be diagnosed in the United States in 2003. Of these 448 cases, an estimated 318 cases were expected in children up to 19 years of age, and an estimated 130 cases were expected in adults 20 years or older. (Estimates were calculated using CBTRUS 1995 to 1999 data and 2003 U.S. census population estimates [www.census.gov] for 5-year age groups).*

THE PROBLEM

The low incidence of this tumor in adults makes it more difficult for the clinician to diagnosis it preoperatively. Because of the high proclivity for metastasis within the CNS, all patients require staging. Because posterior fossa (PF) surgery leads to postoperative changes in the spine that can be seen very early postoperatively and that can be misinterpreted as metastatic tumor deposits, the ideal time to perform staging magnetic res-

onance imaging (MRI) of the spine is before craniectomy and tumor resection. This is seldom done in adults with medulloblastoma, because the patient is usually seen by a nonpediatric neurosurgeon and because the index of suspicion is low. Contributing to the lowered index of suspicion is the fact that adult medulloblastomas are more often eccentric to the midline or laterally placed in the cerebellum than in children and that the MRI appearance of medulloblastomas in adults may differ from the typical homogeneously contrast-enhanced midline tumor seen in childhood.

HISTORY

Adults are usually excluded from medulloblastoma clinical trials. Whereas most children with newly diagnosed medulloblastoma are entered on prospective phase II or phase III clinical trials, the majority of reported cases of adult medulloblastoma are single-institution retrospective series that span decades. Patients have been imaged, operated upon, and treated with radiation and chemotherapy in a variety of ways without prospective data collection. It is therefore difficult to draw firm conclusions about the best treatment regimen. Nonetheless, certain principles of treatment are clear, as is the need for clinical trials in the adult population to address and clarify the two most pressing clinical treatment questions: (1) is craniospinal axis radiation therapy in good-prognosis (average risk) patients adequate initial treatment, and (2) does adding chemotherapy to craniospinal axis radiation therapy improve survival?

CLINICAL PRESENTATION

The clinical presentation of PF tumors is similar in adults and children, and many signs and symptoms are related to hydrocephalus caused by obstruction of cerebrospinal fluid (CSF) flow by the tumor. Early in the course of disease, complaints of nonspecific headache, fatigue, slight imbalance, and personality changes may occur. As the disease progresses, signs and symptoms of increased intracranial pressure predominate, especially headache. These headaches are usually present on awakening in the morning and improve or resolve after rising and as the day progresses. Headaches may become persistent if the tumor is not diagnosed and treated. Nausea and vomiting are also common. Sixth cranial nerve palsies and diplopia, caused by increased intracranial pressure, are not uncommon. Focal

---

*Personal communication with Bridget McCarthy, PhD, principal investigator, CBTRUS, Chicago, May 2003.

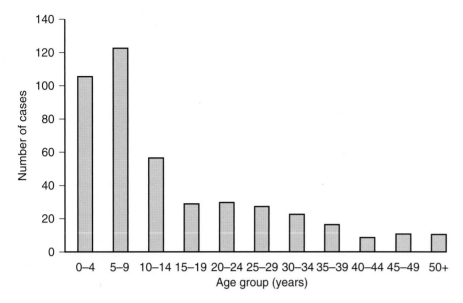

FIGURE 35-1 Total number of cases of medulloblastoma (ICD-O-2 codes 9470–9472) 1995–1999 reported to CBTRUS by age. (Personal communication with Bridget McCarthy, PhD, principal investigator. Courtesy of CBTRUS, Chicago, May 2003, www.cbtrus.org.)

neurologic deficits caused by pressure on or infiltration of the brainstem, cranial nerves, or cerebellar structures also occur. Dizziness or other cerebellar dysfunction occurs in most patients, and the pattern of deficits is related to the location of tumor in the PF. Lesions occurring in the midline are likely to cause truncal and gait ataxia, whereas limb ataxia is more common in lesions involving the lateral cerebellar hemispheres. Other focal neurologic deficits such as hemiparesis, hearing loss, and seventh cranial nerve palsies occur less often. Seizures are rarely seen in children or adults with PF tumors unless extension into the supratentorial cortex occurs. Alterations of consciousness may occur late in the course of the disease. Hemorrhage into the PF mass may cause acute loss of consciousness and coma.

NEUROIMAGING

Adult medulloblastoma is radiologically distinct from the childhood variety. Although central vermian location, homogeneity, and uniformly intense contrast enhancement is the rule in children, this appearance is much less common in adults.[2,28,38]

Because of its exquisite contrast resolution, MRI is the imaging modality of choice in the preoperative work-up for infratentorial tumors and for the evaluation of leptomeningeal metastasis. Once medulloblastoma is suspected on imaging or confirmed cytologically or pathologically, MRI of the brain and entire spine before and after administration of gadolinium contrast becomes necessary. The goal of this imaging is to determine whether there are demonstrable metastases in the craniospinal axis because of the significant impact these metastases have on management and prognosis.

It is estimated that approximately one half of adult patients with medulloblastoma have their tumors originate peripherally in the cerebellum (paramedian and lateral locations) (Table 35-1). On rare occasions, a medulloblastoma presents as an exclusively extra-axial mass in the cerebellopontine angle and may be mistaken for a meningioma or vestibular schwannoma on computed tomography (CT) and MRI scans.[2,38] Multifocal cerebellar adult medulloblastoma is extremely rare: only three cases

have been reported in the literature.[27] The classic childhood presentation in the midline of the vermis occurs in only one half of adult patients.

Adult medulloblastoma is typically heterogeneous on CT and can appear hypodense or hyperdense to gray matter and have variable patterns of enhancement.[2,6] The more common peripheral tumors are poorly enhanced with contrast (Figure 35-2), whereas the less common vermian central tumors tend to be intensely enhanced with contrast. On MRI, tumors show hypointense signal on T1- and hyperintense signal on T2-weighted images (Figure 35-3A and B). Contrast-enhanced T1 sequences best demonstrate the heterogeneity of these tumors (Figure 35-3C). Small cysts are commonly encountered in the peripheral tumors, whereas a predominantly cystic medulloblastoma is rare.[6,34,38] Melanotic medulloblastoma is a rare form of medulloblastoma that can potentially demonstrate high T1 signal on the unenhanced T1 sequences.[22,60] This high signal can suggest or be confused with hemorrhage. A rare entity in the adult literature, "lipidized" or "lipomatous" medulloblastoma has been provisionally reclassified by WHO as cerebellar liponeurocytoma (9506/1) and can also demonstrate high signal on unenhanced T1 sequences. MRI of the brain and spine is useful in assessing response to treatment, stability, tumor progression, and metastatic disease. MRI of the entire spine with and without gadolinium contrast enhancement has become the study of choice for evaluating drop metastases (Figure 35-4). Positron-emission tomography (PET) and magnetic resonance spectroscopy are sometimes useful in differentiating recurrent tumor from radiation necrosis (Figure 35-5).

PATHOLOGY

The gross appearance and histology of medulloblastoma occurring in adults overlap substantially with the features of pediatric medulloblastoma. The histology includes the five principal patterns: undifferentiated or classic medulloblastoma, desmoplastic nodular medulloblastoma, medulloblastoma with neuroblastic or neuronal differentiation, large cell or anaplastic medulloblastoma, and medulloblastoma with glial differentiation.[7,21] The

TABLE 35-1	Patient Characteristics in Ten Adult Contemporary Series						
Authors	No. of Patients	Disease Limited to PF	M Stage	Location within PF	Chemotherapy	Initial Site of Failure	Extent of Resection
Giordana[28]	44	NR	NR	17 midline 15 lateral or both	0/44	NR	13 GTR 19 STR
Frost[20]	48	25	21 M_0 2 M_1 1 M_2, M_3 1 M_4	16 midline 14 lateral 18 both	1/48	14 PF 3 ST 2 Spine 6 Other	22 GTR 26 STR
Carrie[8]	156	81	14 M+	75 central 71 lateral	75/156	22 PF 11 Spine 12 ST	101 GTR 50 STR
Prados[55a]	47	27	2 M_1 3 M_2 7 M_3 1 M_4	15 midline 31 lateral 1 CP angle	32/47	9 PF 7 PF + other 5 Spine 2 Bone 5 Other	36 GTR 11 STR
Kunscher[41]	28	25	2 M_1 1 M_2	33% central 50% lateral 17% diffuse/multifocal	6/28	6 PF 2 Bone 1 Spine	15 GTR 12 STR 1 Bx
Peterson[53]	45	31	3 M_1 7 M_3 4 M_3 (no PF mass)	17 midline 12 lateral 2 multifocal	18/45	2 PF 11 Spine/ST 2 Bone	30 GTR 10 STR 5 Bx
Abacioglu[1]	30	27	3 M_3	14 central 16 lateral	10/30	5 PF 1 PF + spine 1 ST + spine 2 Spine 1 Spine + bone 2 Bone	20 GTR 10 STR
Chan[9]	32	25	1 M_1 4 M_2 3 M_3	13 midline 14 lateral	24/32	12 PF 2 Spine 3 Bone	17 GTR 11 STR 4 Bx
Greenberg[30]	17	10	1 M_1 1 M_3 5 M_2, M_4	10 central 7 lateral	17/17	8 PF 5 Spine 1 ST 5 Bone	8 GTR 9 STR
Malheiros[45]	15	13	13 M_0	4 midline 5 lateral 6 both	11/13	2 PF	8 GTR 4 STR 3 Bx

Bx, Biopsy only; CP, cerebellopontine angle; GTR, gross-total resection; M+, metastatic disease; NR, not reported; PF, posterior fossa; Spine, CSF-positive or sub-arachnoid disease; ST, supratentorial; STR, subtotal resection.

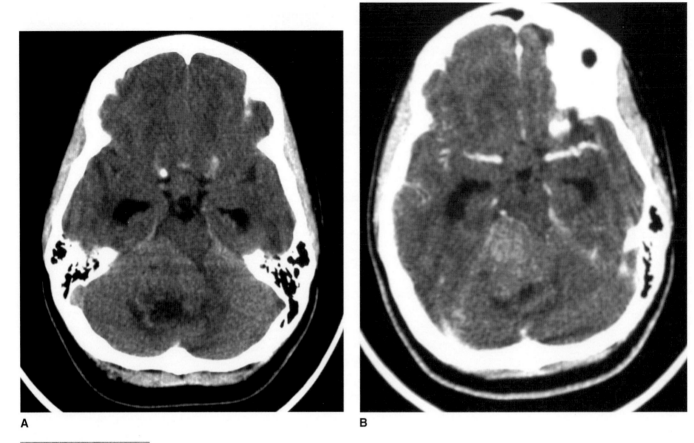

A　　　　　　　　　　　　　　　　　　　　　　**B**

FIGURE 35-2　Computed tomography scan in a 22-year-old woman shows a 4 cm heterogeneous paramedian right cerebellar tumor with mass effect on the fourth ventricle *(A)*. There is poor and incomplete enhancement following the administration of intravenous contrast material *(B)*.

other variant forms such as medullomyoblastoma and melanotic medulloblastoma are rare in the adult population,[44,57] as are the forms containing more heterogeneous differentiation.

Undifferentiated or "classic" medulloblastoma, consisting of patternless masses of monotonous small cells, comprises the majority of medulloblastomas in both adult and pediatric groups. Evidence of neuronal differentiation by hematoxylin and eosin (H&E) staining in some cases includes the formation of neuroblastic rosettes and, occasionally, the presence of ganglion cells. Despite the common lack of evidence of differentiation by routine H&E staining, evidence of neuronal differentiation may be demonstrable by immunohistochemical staining for synaptophysin or other neuronal markers or by the electron microscopic demonstration of neurites, synaptic structures, or neurosecretory granules. The findings of necrosis, apoptosis, calcification, infiltrative behavior, intratumoral hemorrhage, and tumor extension into the overlying leptomeninges occur in both pediatric and adult cases.

The nodular or desmoplastic variety, defined by the presence of prominent nodules or "pale islands" of tumor of lower cellularity in a background of collagen-rich, highly proliferative tumor, occurs more often in the older population.[1,23,33,45,56] Grossly, desmoplastic medulloblastoma is typically more discrete than classic medulloblastoma and is often located in the cerebellar hemispheres. Histologically, the nodules generally consist of larger cells with rounded, uniform nuclei in a vari-

ably abundant background of fine fibrillary processes (Figure 35-6). Collagen and reticulin fibers are sparse within the islands but abundant in the internodular tumor (Figure 35-7). The abundance of connective tissue fibers may be apparent on H&E-stained sections and is readily demonstrable with connective tissue stains, such as reticulin stains (Figure 35-8). The cell islands generally show strong immunoreactivity to synaptophysin (Figure 35-9), but synaptophysin immunostaining may be sparse in the internodular areas.[36] Electron microscopy shows that the "pale islands" often contain abundant neurite-like cytoplasmic processes containing parallel arrays of microtubules, synaptic formations, and dense-core vesicles. Cell proliferation markers generally demonstrate a higher labeling index within the collagen-rich internodular areas than in the islands. Diffuse desmoplasia, in the form of a diffuse increase in collagen or reticulin fibers between tumor cells, occurs in occasional classic medulloblastomas. Such tumors are not classified as "desmoplastic medulloblastoma" in the absence of the nodular growth pattern. Studies comparing the prognoses of classic and desmoplastic medulloblastomas have yielded contradictory results, possibly reflecting variation in application of criteria for the diagnosis of desmoplastic medulloblastoma. In recognition of these characteristics and issues, the third edition of the *International Classification of Diseases for Oncology* (ICD-O-3) now uses "desmoplastic nodular medulloblastoma" (code 9471/3) as the preferred term to describe this tumor. A

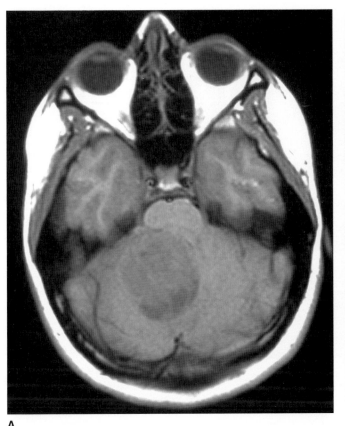

A

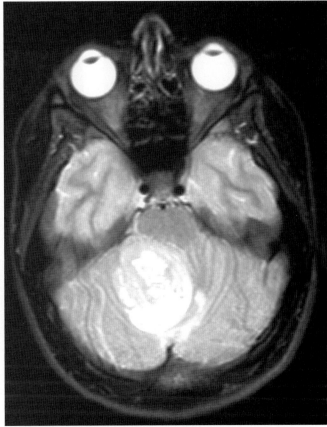

B

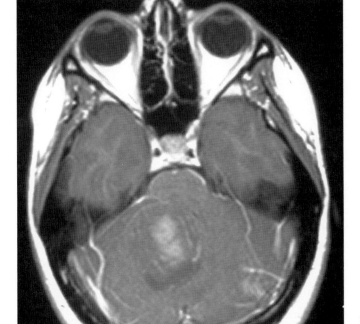

C

FIGURE 35-3   T1-weighted magnetic resonance imaging examination shows a 4 cm heterogeneous mass in the right cerebellar hemisphere *(A)*. Heterogeneous bright signal on T2-weighted image *(B)*. Gadolinium-enhanced T1-weighted sequence best demonstrates heterogeneity of the tumor with small cystic components *(C)*.

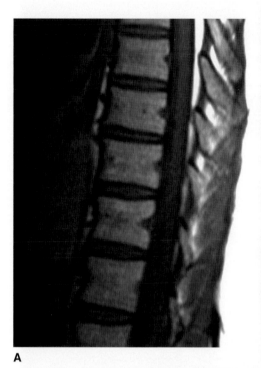

A

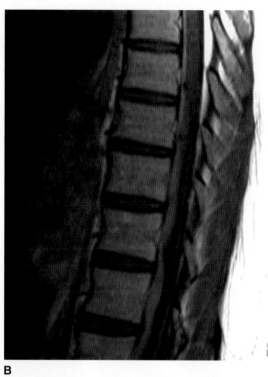

B

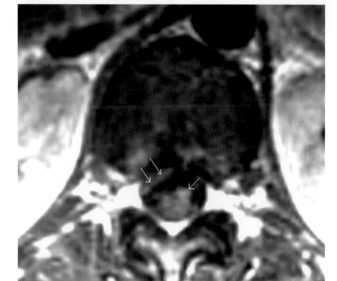

C

FIGURE 35-4   Magnetic resonance image of the spine of the patient in Figure 35-3 demonstrates subtle signal abnormality anterior to the lower thoracic spinal cord on the unenhanced T1 sagittal sequence *(A)*. Post-gadolinium contrast T1 sagittal *(B)* and axial *(C)* images demonstrate drop metastases on the surface of the cord and inner side of the dura *(arrows)*.

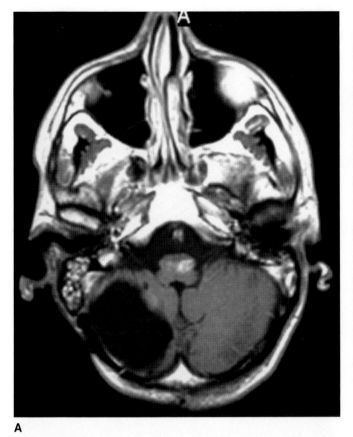

A

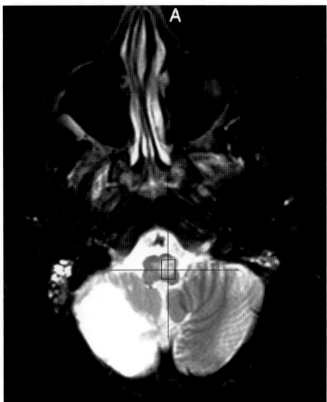

B

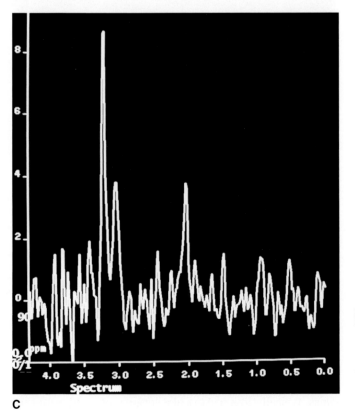

C

FIGURE 35-5 Magnetic resonance spectroscopy (MRS) in a 26-year-old man who had been treated for a peripheral right cerebellar medulloblastoma with tumor excision, radiation therapy, and chemotherapy. He subsequently developed a new enhancing mass in the medulla *(A and B)*. A single-voxel MRS shows a high choline peak consistent with tumor recurrence rather than radiation necrosis *(C)*.

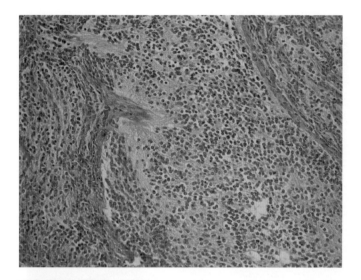

FIGURE 35-6 Characteristic large "pale islands" of uniform cells in desmoplastic nodular medulloblastoma from a 34-year-old man. (Hematoxylin and eosin, ×50 original magnification.)

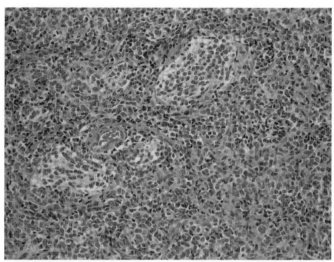

FIGURE 35-7 Area of intense desmoplasia with small cell islands and abundance of internodular primitive cells in a collagenous stroma from a 35-year-old man. (Hematoxylin and eosin, ×50 original magnification.)

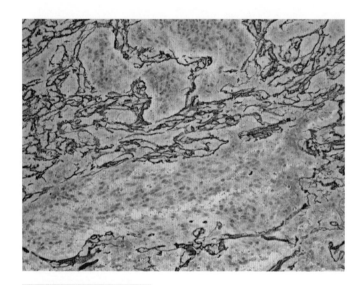

FIGURE 35-8 Reticulin stain demonstrates the abundant meshwork of reticulin fibers and outlines cell islands. (Reticulin, ×50 original magnification.)

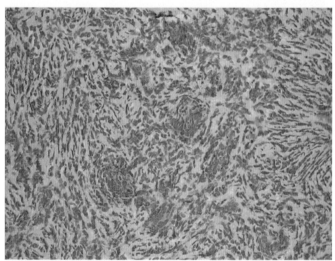

FIGURE 35-9 Synaptophysin immunoreactivity is most prominent in cell islands. (Synaptophysin, ×50 original magnification.)

rare variant medulloblastoma with extensive nodularity and neuronal differentiation associated with a more favorable prognosis is more common in the pediatric population.[17,24]

Medulloblastoma with neuroblastic or neuronal differentiation, characterized by extensive nodularity and differentiation toward neurocytes or ganglion cells and referred to by some authors as "cerebellar neuroblastoma," is an uncommon variant and occurs primarily in infants and very young children. Large cell or anaplastic medulloblastoma, characterized by populations of larger, more pleomorphic tumor cells than those in classic medulloblastoma, is also an uncommon variant occurring predominantly in the pediatric population and is often associated with an unfavorable outcome.[16,25]

Glial rather than neuronal differentiation in medulloblastoma has been reported in up to one third of cases of medulloblastoma occurring in older individuals. Mature glial cells, identified by the presence of eosinophilic cytoplasm and cell processes, may be difficult to identify in H&E-stained sections (Figure 35-10). By immunohistochemical staining for glial fibrillary acidic protein (GFAP), immunoreactive fibrillated cells can be identified in most pediatric[11] and adult medulloblastomas, typically in a perivascular location or at the periphery of the tumor. Although such cells have commonly been considered entrapped reactive astrocytes rather than tumor cells, similar cells have been observed in metastatic medulloblastoma in nonbrain sites, suggesting that they are actually tumor cells.

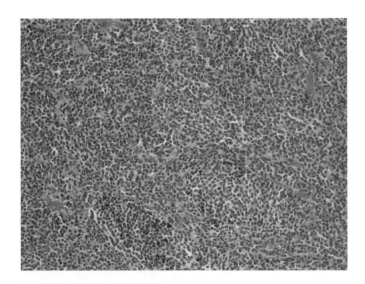

FIGURE 35-10 Glial differentiation is not readily apparent in hematoxylin and eosin (H&E)-stained sections of a "classic" medulloblastoma from a 46-year-old man. (H&E, ×50 original magnification.)

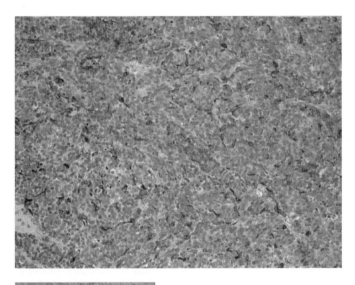

FIGURE 35-11 Immunostaining for glial fibrillary acidic protein (GFAP) demonstrates abundant population of GFAP-immunoreactive tumor cells and cell processes throughout the tumor. (GFAP, ×50 original magnification.)

Glial differentiation in tumor cells, usually defined by the finding of glial fibrillary acidic protein-immunoreactivity in the perikaryon or short cell processes of cells with distinctively neoplastic nuclear features (Figure 35-11), has been described in a small percentage of medulloblastomas, particularly in the adult population. GFAP-immunoreactive cells have also been noted within the nodules and in the internodular tumor cell population of desmoplastic nodular medulloblastomas. Studies investigating the prognostic significance of glial differentiation have yielded contradictory results.[11,29,35]

In addition to studies correlating tumor histology and tumor stage with clinical outcome, a number of investigators

TABLE 35-2

Chang Staging System for Metastasis

Stage	Definition
M_0	No evidence of gross subarachnoid or hematogenous metastasis
M_1	Microscopic tumor cells found in cerebrospinal fluid
M_2	Gross nodular seedings demonstrated in the cerebellar, cerebral subarachnoid space, or in the third or lateral ventricles
M_3	Gross nodular seeding in spinal subarachnoid space
M_4	Extraneuroaxial metastasis

have looked at other parameters such as tumor cell proliferation indices, apoptotic index, and various genetic and molecular markers. Studies of cell proliferation markers and apoptosis have shown variations between adult and pediatric tumors and among medulloblastoma variants but have not correlated well with outcome.[58] In the pediatric population, suggestions of correlations between genetic markers and prognosis such as cytogenetic studies of chromosome 17 and others, p53 overexpression, studies of ErbB2 receptors, high TRKC receptor expression, amplification of MYC, and abnormalities in the sonic hedgehog (SHH)–PTCH pathway have been noted, with the best correlations occurring in the large cell–anaplastic variant.[17,42,65] In adult medulloblastoma, a recent study correlated overexpression of MDM2 with shorter survival.[27a,28]

More recently, cDNA-based gene-expression profiling has demonstrated that medulloblastomas are distinct from primitive neuroectodermal tumors and that the "classic" and desmoplastic subtypes are distinct.[54] These studies confirmed earlier observations about high TRKC receptor expression and amplification of MYC. These studies have also strongly supported the hypothesis that medulloblastomas are derived from cerebellar granular cells through the activation of the SHH pathway and suggested various novel prognostic markers related to SHH pathway activation. However, more extensive investigation will need to be carried out to verify the utility of the various genetic and molecular markers in assessing prognosis, especially in the forms of medulloblastoma more commonly encountered in the adult population such as desmoplastic nodular medulloblastoma. Furthermore, a parallel between pediatric and adult tumors cannot be assumed.

STAGING

The Chang staging system (Table 35-2), which was published in 1969,[10] evaluates tumor size, local extension, and the presence or absence of metastases. The tumor (T) staging portion of the staging system may no longer have the same prognostic value that it once had. Several pediatric studies have shown that the amount of residual disease, age, and M stage are more predictive of outcome than T stage.[39,66] It was initially based on the surgeon's intraoperative observations; however, in the modern era of neuroimaging, preoperative and postoperative scans provide similar if not better information. The Chang metastasis (M) stage (M_0 denotes local disease only, M_1 denotes positive CSF cytology, M_2 denotes tumor present beyond the primary site but within the brain, M_3 denotes gross nodular seeding in the spinal subarachnoid space, and M_4 denotes extracranial spread) has consistently been related to outcome in pediatric studies, although this is less clear in adult series.

Evaluation for the purpose of staging includes preoperative MRI scans of the cranial vault and entire spine. CSF sampling should be performed before surgery or 10 to 14 days postoperatively to avoid a false positive related to surgery. Postoperative MRI scans of the brain should be obtained within 24 to 48 hours after resection to minimize postoperative imaging changes and accurately evaluate the extent of resection. If a preoperative MRI scan of the spine was not performed, it should be performed 2 weeks after surgical resection to allow for resolution of postoperative blood and protein artifacts that may be misinterpreted as metastatic tumor.

Over the past 10 to 15 years, sequential studies carried out by the Children's Cancer Group (CCG) and the Pediatric Oncology Group (POG)[18,19,49,51] have revealed two risk categories defined by age, extent of surgical resection, and M stage. Patients are considered to be average or standard risk if they are older than 3 years, have no more than 1.5 cm^2 of residual tumor after surgical resection, and have no CSF or spinal involvement (M_0).[66] All other pediatric medulloblastoma patients are considered to be poor or high risk. Although recent data suggest that a histologic variant showing moderate to severe anaplasia may have an adverse prognosis in pediatric tumors,[16] this and other possible genetic and histopathologic prognostic variables have not yet been used in prospective risk categorization, and need to be verified in other studies.[17,27a,28,42,65]

SURGERY

Surgery plays an integral and important role in the management of adults with medulloblastoma. The goals of surgical therapy are threefold: histologic diagnosis, maximal safe tumor resection, and restoration of patency of CSF pathways. Because medulloblastomas commonly present with some degree of hydrocephalus, the first surgical decision often pertains to management of this condition. Tumor resection alleviates hydrocephalus in up to 90% of patients in most modern series,[63] and avoids shunt-related complications such as upward herniation of the brainstem, intratumoral hemorrhage, and CSF dissemination. Thus prompt, definitive surgical resection with use of steroids to control edema is preferred to a staged approach of shunting followed by resection. If steroids fail or urgent ventricular drainage is required, a nondominant ventriculostomy is preferred over a shunt, because it allows more precise control of intracranial pressure and drainage. Care should be taken to measure opening pressure and drain slowly at 20 cm of CSF or higher, and resection should be accomplished promptly.

Numerous studies have demonstrated the relationship between extent of resection and prognosis[41]; thus optimization of the surgical procedure is critical. This is achieved in part by meticulous preoperative preparation and by using stereotactic computer-aided navigation (CAN) tools, intraoperative ultrasound, and in some cases, brainstem evoked-potential monitoring. Surgery is more often performed with patients prone to avoid the risk of air embolism and subdural hematoma associated with sitting. The patient is managed preoperatively with antibiotics, corticosteroids, mannitol, and moderate hyperventilation. A ventriculostomy is usually performed at the time of surgery if it has not already been performed and is managed as noted previously.

After a generous craniotomy or craniectomy centered over the tumor, the cisterna magna is opened to drain CSF. Although invasive, the tumor usually is surrounded by a pseudocapsule facilitating identification and removal from the surrounding brain. CAN and ultrasound are also helpful in this regard. Using microsurgical techniques, the tumor is internally debulked using an ultrasonic aspirator and a self-retaining retractor to minimize cerebellar retraction. The surgeon must anticipate the location of critical structures such as the posterior inferior cerebellar artery, inferior vermian veins, cranial nerves (in the case of laterally placed tumors), the dentate nuclei, the cerebellar peduncles, and the floor of the fourth ventricle. Often, the tumor can be gently peeled from these structures without damaging the pial membrane. The surgeon places cottonoids along the cisterna magna and along the roof and floor of the fourth ventricle to prevent iatrogenic dissemination of tumor along CSF pathways as these structures are exposed. Invasive tumor is aggressively resected from the cerebellum and, if required, a single cerebellar peduncle. However, aggressive resection of tumor invading the floor of the fourth ventricle or the second cerebellar peduncle is avoided to reduce unacceptable postoperative morbidity.

After as complete a gross resection consistent with good neurologic function has been achieved, the resection cavity is reinspected using microscopic magnification, CAN, and ultrasound to identify and then resect any residual tumor, cerebellar hematoma, or retraction injury. Meticulous hemostasis minimizes postoperative nausea, vomiting, and hydrocephalus. A watertight closure of the dura is performed using tisseal or fibrin glue to avoid CSF leak, pseudomeningocele, and chemical meningitis. Postoperatively, the ventriculostomy is drained until the blood clears, and then the patient weaned from ventricular drainage if possible. Postoperative MRI with and without contrast is done within 48 hours postoperatively, both as a baseline and to assess extent of resection. MRI of the spinal axis should be performed approximately 2 weeks after surgery if it has not been done preoperatively. If significant resectable residual neoplasm is seen or the patient requires a ventriculoperitoneal shunt, prompt reoperation is indicated to avoid delay of postoperative radiation therapy and chemotherapy. Operative mortality should be well under 1%; morbidity is 5% to 10% in most series.[41] Most common complications are transient, including ataxia, nystagmus, and dysmetria. Cranial nerve palsies are related to manipulation along the floor of the fourth ventricle. Cerebellar mutism may also be induced by damage to the dentate nuclei. It is advisable to wait 10 to 14 days after surgery before beginning radiation therapy to ensure adequate wound healing and minimize the possibility of wound dehiscence.

RADIATION THERAPY

The inadequacy of surgery alone or surgery plus local irradiation was first conclusively demonstrated in Harvey Cushing's seminal report from 1930 in which only 1 of 61 patients survived 3 years after surgery alone ($n = 30$) or surgery plus limited field irradiation ($n = 31$).[12] In 1936, Cutler reported on 20 children with medulloblastoma who were treated with surgical resection followed by radiation therapy to the brain and spine. Cutler concluded, "Roentgen therapy to the ventricular system and the entire spine, as well as to the cerebellum, is essential."[13] In 1969, Bloom[5] reported a 5- and 10-year survival rate of 40% and 30%, respectively, in 71 patients treated with craniospinal irradiation (CSI).[5] Since that time, numerous studies have reinforced the importance of neuraxis radiation therapy for the successful treatment of medulloblastoma in both adults and children.

When radiation therapy is used in newly diagnosed patients, the standard dose delivered to the craniospinal axis is 35 to 36 Gy if patients have no evidence of neuraxis dissemination (M_0). The PF is then boosted for an additional 18 to 20 Gy so that the total dose to the PF is approximately 54 to 56 Gy. If CSF cytology is positive (M_1), the recommended dose to the CSA according to the pediatric experience is still only 36 Gy. If nodular disease in the subarachnoid space (M_2 or M_3) is present, a boost is delivered immediately following CSI to the site of the original metastatic disease (M_2 to M_3) up to a total dose of 45 Gy. The fractionation scheme used most often in the United States is 1.8 Gy daily, 5 days per week.

Because of the endocrinologic and neurocognitive toxicity of CSI in children, a CCG and POG randomized trial compared treatment with a CSI dose of 23.4 Gy to the standard CSI dose of 36 Gy; both groups received a boost to the PF to 54 Gy. The study was closed prematurely because an early analysis showed an increased incidence of failures in the low-dose group.[14] Of the 126 patients enrolled, 81 were evaluable for the final analysis. This longer-term follow-up showed marginally significant differences at 5 years (5-year event-free survival [EFS] 52% [reduced dose] vs. 67% [standard dose], $P = .08$). However, with follow-up reported at 8 years, there is no statistically significant difference in EFS (8-year EFS 52% vs. 67%, $P = .141$).[62] It thus appears from this study that a lower CSI dose results in earlier failures, but with time there is no statistically significant difference between the two dose regimens. Comparable data are lacking for the adult population of medulloblastoma patients.

There are clear data regarding the dose necessary for control of the primary PF tumor, with a dose relationship clearly seen for doses greater than 50 Gy. The current standard therapy is to boost the entire PF to a total dose of 54 to 55.8 Gy at a fractionation of 1.8 Gy per day using high-energy photons (x-rays). There are no convincing data that administering higher doses to the PF by conventional fractionation or hyperfractionated treatment schedules improves outcomes,[55] although boosting residual disease with a stereotactic radiosurgical boost has shown promise in a limited number of patients.[52,64]

The duration of radiation therapy may also influence outcomes. Taylor et al[61] showed a statistically significant reduction in overall survival and EFS if the time from the first radiation treatment to the last radiation treatment was more than 50 days. In this study, there was no difference in the mean or median duration of radiation therapy between those patients treated with radiation therapy alone and those treated with chemotherapy followed by irradiation. It is advisable to complete radiation therapy without breaks.

Complications associated with radiation therapy can be divided into two time frames: acute effects occurring during or shortly after treatment, and late effects occurring months to years after completion of treatment. Acute side effects in adults are usually more pronounced than in children and consist of nausea, vomiting, fatigue, alopecia, skin erythema, significant bone marrow suppression, soreness in the back of the throat with resultant dysphagia, transient loss of taste, transient xerostomia, and occasionally wound dehiscence (usually when there is not an adequate 10- to 14-day interval between surgery and initiation of radiation therapy). Late effects are generally less prominent in adults than in children and include potential pituitary dysfunction, possible infertility, effects on cognition, and possible induction of second malignancies. Although the neurocognitive effects in treated adults have not been studied as extensively as in children, there are data to suggest that cranial doses of 30 to 36 Gy may have an impact on cognitive function in survivors, especially on memory, reasoning, visual-spatial ability, and arithmetic calculation skills.[40]

CHEMOTHERAPY

The usefulness of chemotherapy has been established in the pediatric medulloblastoma population. However, for adults with medulloblastoma, the role of chemotherapy is not yet established. The most commonly used regimen is the Packer regimen, which consists of weekly vincristine during CSI and eight cycles of CCNU, cisplatin, and vincristine (CCV) after CSI for children with medulloblastoma. This has become the standard against which all other chemotherapy regimens are measured in the United States.[49] There has not been a preradiation chemotherapy combination used in a randomized trial that has shown better efficacy as measured by overall survival or progression-free survival, although a recently reported study by Taylor et al describes EFS at 5 years that is comparable.[61] The most notable dose-limiting side effects of this CCV-chemotherapy combination are peripheral neuropathy, hearing loss, renal insufficiency, and myelosuppression. As with most chemotherapy regimens, occasional patients succumb to overwhelming infection. Less serious side effects include nausea, vomiting, constipation, obstipation, and elevated transaminases.

Hundreds of children have been treated with this combination, but there is little in the literature to describe the tolerance that adults have to the same combination. Whereas the thrust of recent pediatric trials has been to add chemotherapy to decrease the dose of craniospinal axis radiation and thereby decrease the harmful effects of radiation on neurocognitive and endocrine function such as low full-scale intelligence quotients (IQs) and short stature, there has not been a comparable effort in treating adults for several reasons. These reasons include the fact that there is an approximate 60% 5-year progression-free survival rate with surgery and CSI alone,[8] a belief that there is less harm to giving standard radiation doses to adults than children, and a less convincing case for a survival benefit to receiving chemotherapy as part of initial therapy. As a result, there is a perception among many clinicians that one can safely rely more on radiation and omit chemotherapy. However, there has been little formal investigation of neuropsychologic sequelae in adults who are long-term survivors of medulloblastoma. In one recent study of 10 such adults, the authors concluded that adults may also suffer significant cognitive deficits, including below-average IQs and specific deficits in memory, reasoning, visuospatial ability, and arithmetic skills.[40] The causes of these deficits include whole-brain radiation therapy, tumor location, perioperative complications, hydrocephalus, and possibly chemotherapy. In recent years, there has also been an increasing recognition of the CNS neurotoxicity caused by irradiation of adults in a variety of settings. The drug most notorious for causing CNS neurotoxicity is methotrexate, but it is seldom used in the treatment of medulloblastoma. The drugs most often used to treat patients with medulloblastoma have not been strongly implicated in causing CNS neurotoxicity. For these reasons, and a belief that medulloblastoma in children is more similar to than different from that in adults and that it should therefore be treated in the same way, many neuro-oncologists have concluded that adults are as likely to benefit from treatment with chemotherapy as children.

Because of these conflicting views, patients have been treated in a variety of ways, mainly involving maximal safe surgical resection followed by CSI with or without chemotherapy. In the largest series of adult patients reported to date, a retrospective analysis involving 156 patients treated at 13 institutions in France, Carrie et al concluded that 5- and 10-year EFS rates of 61% and 48%, respectively, were similar to those observed in children. Multivariate analysis identified a postoperative performance status score of less than 2, spinal axis radiation dose of more than 30 Gy, lack of involvement of the floor of the fourth ventricle, and desmoplastic histologic subtype as factors significantly correlated with EFS.[8] Among the patients, 79 were treated with radiation therapy without chemotherapy, 75 patients were treated with both radiation therapy and one of a variety of types of chemotherapy, and 2 patients had no postoperative treatment: 1 died after surgery and 1 refused treatment. Although there was better 5- and 10-year EFS in the group treated with chemotherapy (66% and 52% vs. 57% and 43%), this did not reach statistical significance. An interesting subgroup of the total was a group of nine patients treated with a combination of ifosfamide, cisplatin, and vincristine as well as CSI. This subgroup had a 5-year and 7-year EFS rate of 87% (10-year point not yet reached). Carrie et al also concluded that chemotherapy in general appeared to be more toxic in adults than in children; five patients in their series died of complications related to treatment and all had received chemotherapy. Their ultimate conclusion was that radiation therapy at the usual dose without chemotherapy should be considered the standard postoperative treatment in adults with medulloblastoma.

Greenberg et al[30] retrospectively analyzed a group of adults diagnosed between 1991 and 1997 who were treated at one of three institutions with chemotherapy consisting of the Packer regimen[51] or a POG protocol consisting of preradiation chemotherapy with cycles of cisplatin and etoposide alternating with cyclophosphamide and vincristine[15] followed by CSI. Ten patients were treated according to the Packer regimen and seven were treated according to the POG protocol. The original Chang T and M classification system was used to assign risk categories. Despite more patients being classified as poor risk on the POG protocol (6/7 vs. 6/10 on the Packer regimen), the estimated median survival of the patients treated on the POG protocol was 57 months, whereas the estimated median survival of the patients treated with the Packer regimen was 36 months, approaching but not reaching statistical significance ($P = .058$). In addition, most complications of the two chemotherapy regimens were more common in the Packer regimen and included nausea, vomiting, or abdominal pain; peripheral neuropathy; hearing loss or tinnitus; nephrotoxicity; and thrombocytopenia. Adults treated with the Packer regimen also required dose reduction of CCNU and cisplatin more often than children. Although this is a small, retrospective study and

these results may have more to do with risk factors that were not accounted for, it suggests that adults may be more susceptible to the toxicities of the Packer regimen and that preradiation chemotherapy in adults may be worthy of further consideration.

In the most recent adult series reported, Malheiros et al[45] reviewed treatment response and survival in 15 adult patients with medulloblastoma treated and followed at their university-based hospital between January 1991 and December 2000. Two patients refused postoperative adjuvant treatment and died 10 and 15 months later. The remaining 13 patients all received CSI. Of the 13, 11 received one to five cycles of ifosfamide, carboplatin, vincristine, and etoposide. Excluding the two patients who refused postoperative treatment, the estimated 5- and 10-year progression-free survival rates were 93% and 74%, respectively.

In the most recently reported randomized study of children with nonmetastatic medulloblastoma, Taylor et al[61] report significantly better EFS ($P = .0366$) with a vincristine, etoposide, carboplatin, and cyclophosphamide regimen preceding CSI than with CSI alone.

There is agreement among those who have written about the management and treatment of medulloblastoma in adults that patients should have maximal safe tumor resection followed by CSI. The role of and type of chemotherapy that should be employed and when it should be used remains less clear. Most neuro-oncologists would agree that patients with poor-risk medulloblastoma should also be treated with chemotherapy as part of initial therapy, but there is not agreement about its use in average-risk patients. There is a suggestion that combinations of cyclophosphamide or ifosfamide plus carboplatin or cisplatin plus vincristine with or without etoposide may be as effective and less toxic to adults than the Packer CCV regimen. Clinical trials in the adult population would help clarify the role of chemotherapy, especially in patients with average-risk disease.

PROGRESSION AND RECURRENCE

Recurrence in adult medulloblastoma patients occurs in 20% to 50% of patients by 5 years (see Table 35-1). The most common site of first failure is in the PF and accounts for approximately 50% of all recurrences (see Table 35-1). Only approximately 40% (see Table 35-1) of adults receive chemotherapy as first-line treatment in addition to radiation therapy. In contrast, the pattern of relapse reported in pediatric patients is primarily that of spinal dissemination, with or without simultaneous PF failure,[39,49,61] and almost all children now receive chemotherapy as part of their initial treatment regimen. These two major differences between adults and children suggest that different approaches might be considered for recurrent disease.

Patients who suffer a local, isolated PF failure, whether children or adults, might benefit from therapy directed locally, such as surgery or directed radiation therapy. Patrice et al[52] reported treating 11 patients with recurrent, isolated PF medulloblastoma with stereotactic radiosurgery (SRS). The median survival was 10 months (range 5 to >59 months), and no patients failed within the SRS-treated volume. The site of failure predominately was dissemination elsewhere in the CNS. Other approaches have included surgical resection with placement of ^{125}I radioactive seeds along the resection cavity. The long-term survival despite effective local-control strategies, however, remains dismal, with almost all patients experiencing eventual recurrence elsewhere in the CNS or at distant, non-CNS sites. The addition of systemic agents should be considered in these patients, although even with the addition of systemic therapy survival remains extremely poor.

Patients relapsing with disseminated disease, either confined to the CNS or other distant sites, require systemic therapy, and the role of local therapy is limited. Patients who have previously been treated with chemotherapy as part of their initial therapy are particularly challenging to manage. Generally, phase I or phase II studies are reasonable approaches because the patients may be less likely to respond to drugs with which they have been previously treated. High-dose chemotherapy with stem cell transplants have also shown limited success in this patient cohort.[46] For patients who have not been previously treated with chemotherapy (approximately 60% of adults), the use of one or more of the known active agents, including CCNU, vincristine, cisplatin, carboplatin, VP-16 (etoposide), cyclophosphamide, and ifosfamide, is the most rational approach and may prolong survival.

OUTCOME

The ability to categorize patients by risk factors has led to specific tailoring of treatment for the pediatric population,[66] and it is against these results that adult studies need to be compared. Since the initial encouraging reports describing the use of combination chemotherapy and reduced-dose radiation therapy by Packer et al[51] in the early 1990s, this approach has become the standard of care at most pediatric institutions. In 1999, Packer et al[49] reported the results of a CCG study using a reduced craniospinal dose (23.4 Gy) of irradiation given with weekly vincristine followed by chemotherapy consisting of CCNU, vincristine, and cisplatin for eight cycles following CSI for average-risk patients between the ages of 3 and 10 years. The total dose to the PF remained at 55.8 Gy. The progression-free survival rates were 86% at 3 years and 79% at 5 years, which were more favorable than historical comparisons from previous CCG or POG studies. In 2003, Taylor et al[61] reported the results of a European prospective randomized trial in which pediatric patients with M_0 and M_1 disease were randomized to radiation therapy alone versus preradiation therapy chemotherapy with vincristine, etoposide, carboplatin, and cyclophosphamide. The radiation therapy consisted of 35 Gy CSI in 1.67 Gy daily fractions followed by a PF boost of 20 Gy for a total PF dose of 55 Gy in both treatment arms. The EFS was superior in the patients who received preradiation chemotherapy, with EFS at 5 years of 74% versus 59.8% in the patients who received radiation therapy alone.

Improvements in imaging modalities, surgical techniques, and the precision of radiation therapy delivery, as well as the addition of systemic chemotherapy over the past 2 decades, have contributed to the increased overall survival in pediatric series. It is more difficult to assess improvement in the outcome of adults with medulloblastoma because of the paucity of patients and lack of prospective or randomized adult trials. However, as displayed in Figure 35-12, the Surveillance, Epidemiology, and End Results (SEER) data* suggest a significant

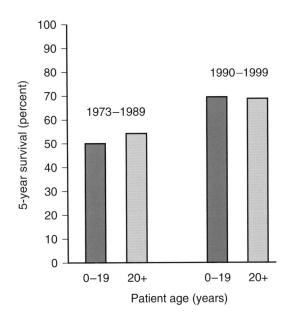

*Personal communication with Bridget McCarthy, PhD, principal investigator, CBTRUS, Chicago, May 2003.

FIGURE 35-12   Five-year survival by patient age and year of diagnosis. (Personal communication with Bridget McCarthy, PhD, principal investigator. Courtesy of CBTRUS, Chicago, May 2003, www.cbtrus.org.)

improvement in the survival of both children and adults when comparing patients diagnosed from 1973 through 1989 with those diagnosed from 1990 through 1999. It is most likely that the improvement in survival of these groups is related most to the improvements in surgical techniques, radiation therapy, and imaging and probably less to the improvements in the addition of chemotherapy, at least in the adult population.

Table 35-3 summarizes the results of 10 adult contemporary series.

Survival

Overall survival ranges from 25% to 84% at 5 years with 10-year survival rates ranging from 35.6% to 51%.

Progression-Free Survival

The 5-year progression-free survival in these studies ranges from 45% to 65% with a 10-year progression-free survival of 38% to 52%. The rather large variation in outcomes between the studies most certainly reflects the heterogeneity of both the patient cohorts and the treatment techniques. These results are inferior to those reported in the contemporary pediatric literature as mentioned previously.

Patterns of Failure

The most common initial site of relapse is the PF, which alone accounts for more than 50% of treatment failures. The primary tumor bed is most commonly involved in those series that report specific sites of relapse within the PF. Spinal dissemination, either in the subarachnoid space or involving CSF, is the second most common site of failure, followed by supratentorial sites and then bone sites.

TABLE 35-3   Result Summaries of Ten Adult Contemporary Series

Authors	No. of Patients	Years Diagnosed	Median Age (Range in years)	5-Year Overall Survival	5-Year Progression-Free Survival	10-Year Overall Survival	10-Year Progression-Free Survival
Giordana[28]	44	1952–1990	32.5 (18–62)	40%	NR	35.6%	NR
Frost[20]	48	1958–1988	25 (16–48)	62%	47%	41%	38%
Carrie[8]	156	1975–1991	28 (18–58)	70%	61%	51%	48%
Prados[55a]	47	1975–1991	28 (16–56)	60%	50%	NR	NR
				good risk = 81%	good risk = 58%		
				poor risk = 54%	poor risk = 32%		
Kunscher[41]	28	1978–1998	26 (18–57)	84%	62%	NR	NR
					(no difference high risk vs. low risk)		
Peterson[53]	45	1981–1995	24 (15–62)	NR	51% †	62% †	NR
Abacioglu[1]	30	1983–2000	27 (16–45)	65%	63%	51%*	50%*
Chan[9]	32	1986–1996	25.5 (16–47)	83%	57%	45%*	40%*
Greenberg[30]	17	1991–1997	23 (18–47)	25%	45%	NR	NR
Malheiros[45]	15	1991–2000	34 (23–48)	72.7%	80%	72.7%	68.6%

*8-year data.
†Crude rate.
NR, Not reported.

In contrast to these results, the most recently reported CCG study[49] showed that out of 14 recurrences only 2 were confined to the PF (14%), whereas 9 had simultaneous PF and disseminated CNS disease, and 3 had nonprimary site recurrences. In the previously mentioned European study,[61] a total of only 22 out of 90 patients relapsed in the chemotherapy arm: 5 in the PF alone (23%), 6 in the neuraxis alone, 10 in the PF and neuraxis, and 1 in a distant site. Kortmann et al[39] reported a 47% distant CNS progression rate in 52:184 patients. Only 17% of failures were confined to the PF, with the remaining patients failing simultaneously in the PF and distant CNS sites.

FUTURE DIRECTIONS

In Children

Children's Oncology Group (COG) study A9961 compares the standard Packer (vincristine, CCNU, cisplatin) regimen with a regimen containing vincristine, cyclophosphamide, and cisplatin in children with average-risk medulloblastoma. The study is designed to determine whether there is any benefit, either in improved outcome or reduced complications, from the substitution of cyclophosphamide for CCNU. Preliminary findings from this study show equal efficacy of these two regimens; at a median follow-up interval of 36 months, the EFS in both arms is almost identical, at 84% and 82% (personal communication, Packer R, Sposto R, COG, Arcadia, Calif, March 26, 2003). In an effort to further reduce the neurocognitive, endocrine, and oto-toxicities of radiation therapy for average-risk children, the next randomized COG study (ACNS0331), which opened for accrual in April 2004, compares a reduced CSI dose of 18 Gy with 23.4 Gy in children ages 3 to <8 years. Older children (ages 8 to 21 years) will receive 23.4 Gy CSI. All children (ages 3 to 21 years) will then be randomized to treatment with a whole PF boost versus a more limited volume

boost dose to the postoperative primary tumor site, which has been found to be as effective as a whole PF boost in recent studies.[13a,63a] All patients will receive weekly vincristine during radiation therapy, followed by three courses of a chemotherapy regimen consisting of two cycles of CCV, followed by one cycle of vincristine, cyclophosphamide, and mesna. It is hypothesized that by further reducing the CSI dose and the amount of normal CNS volume included in the high-dose boost field, the neurocognitive, endocrinologic, and otologic complications can be reduced while maintaining the excellent EFS and overall survival shown in previous studies. It is also hoped that by adding cyclophosphamide to the Packer CCV regimen in this fashion, chemotherapy will be more effective.

In Adults

The variability in patient ages, staging, preoperative imaging, immediate postoperative imaging to assess extent of resection, definition of risk categories, variability in radiation dosing to the craniospinal axis and PF boost, and the extreme variability in the types, duration, and indications for chemotherapy in reported series of adults with medulloblastoma makes it exceedingly difficult to make definitive recommendations regarding treatment in this patient population based on these results alone. However, based on the available pediatric and adult studies, we believe that some recommendations can be made. Patients should be staged completely with neuraxis imaging and CSF analysis and have as complete a resection of PF tumor as is consistent with good neurologic function, followed by CSI. For patients with no evidence of neuraxis dissemination (M_0) or only positive CSF cytology (M_1), CSI to a dose of 36 Gy plus a PF boost of 18 Gy to 19.8 Gy (for a total of 54 Gy to 55.8 Gy) seems prudent. In patients with nodular neuraxis dissemination (M_2 or M_3), pediatric studies suggest that a higher dose of 45 Gy is required to the nodular spinal disease and 36 Gy to the remainder of the spine, in addition to systemic chemotherapy. If there is nodular supratentorial disease, it should also receive a radiation boost.

The large U.S. pediatric trials have showed the efficacy of vincristine during and CCNU, cisplatin, and vincristine chemotherapy following CSI in improving overall and progression-free survival in children with average- and poor-risk medulloblastoma. Comparable trials in adults have yet to be done. However, there is suggestive evidence that chemotherapy with carboplatin, vincristine, and ifosfamide or cyclophosphamide with or without etoposide may be quite active in children and adults and less toxic than the Packer CCV regimen. One needs to keep abreast of pediatric studies as they are reported for any recommended changes in radiation doses and planning technique and to guide one in the use of chemotherapy, until results of prospective trials in adults are available. We should encourage patients to participate in clinical trials for this patient population as they become available. To our knowledge, the only cooperative group trial open at present for adults is the Eastern Cooperative Oncology Group (E4397) phase II trial for adults with poor-risk medulloblastoma, primitive neuroectodermal tumors, and disseminated ependymoma. The trial is investigating preradiation cisplatin, VP-16, vincristine, cyclophosphamide, and mesna, with scheduled filgrastim (G-CSF) to prevent prolonged neutropenia. Cycles of chemotherapy are repeated every 4 weeks for a total of three cycles followed by 36 to 42 Gy CSI (depending on M stage), plus a boost to any spinal or supratentorial deposits of tumor, plus a boost to 53.4 to 54 Gy to the PF in adults (age >18) with poor-risk medulloblastoma.[47a]

The protocol was activated based on very promising pilot data from Vanderbilt and Emory universities,[47] where eight adults, including five with poor-risk medulloblastoma and three with disseminated ependymoma, were treated. Four of these five poor-risk medulloblastoma patients achieved a complete response, and one had a partial response during induction chemotherapy. One patient with disseminated ependymoma had a complete response, and two had stable disease.

An exciting recent advance for both adults and children is the gene-expression characterization of medulloblastomas by Pomeroy et al. They have demonstrated distinct differences in gene expression in classic medulloblastomas, desmoplastic medulloblastomas, supratentorial PNETs, atypical teratoid and rhabdoid tumors, normal cerebella, and malignant gliomas. In addition, they reported that the clinical outcome of children with medulloblastoma was predictable based on gene-expression profiles from tumor tissue obtained at the time of diagnosis. If these results are substantiated, it will allow for gene-expression profiles to be incorporated into the current clinical staging system. This and other recent work characterizing molecules and pathways that are important to the malignant behavior of medulloblastoma should enable us to begin to use novel therapies that target specific genes, gene products, and pathways involved in this malignancy.*

References

1. Abacioglu U, Uzel O, Sengoz M, et al: Medulloblastoma in adults: treatment results and prognostic factors. Int J Radiat Oncol Biol 54:855–860, 2002.
2. Becker RL, Backer AD, Sobel DF: Adult medulloblastoma: review of 13 cases with emphasis on MRI. Neuroradiology 37:104–108, 1995.
3. Berman DM, Karhadkar SS, Hallahan AR, et al: Medulloblastoma growth inhibition by hedgehog pathway blockade. Science 297:1559–1561, 2002.
4. Reference deleted in proofs.
5. Bloom HJG, Wallace MB, Henk JM: The treatment and prognosis of medulloblastoma in children: a study of 82 verified cases. Am J Roentgenol Rad Ther Nucl Med 105:43–62, 1969.
6. Bourgouin PM, Tampieri D, Grahovac SZ, et al: CT and MR imaging findings in adults with cerebellar medulloblastoma: comparison with findings in children. Am J Radiol 159:609–612, 1992.
7. Burger PC, Scheithauer BW, Vogel FS: Surgical Pathology of the Nervous System and Its Coverings. New York, Churchill Livingstone, 2002.
8. Carrie C, Lasset C, Alapetite C, et al: Multivariate analysis of prognostic factors in adult patients with medulloblastoma. Cancer 74:2352–2360, 1994.
9. Chan AW, Tarbell NJ, Black PM, et al: Adult medulloblastoma: prognostic factors and patterns of relapse. Neurosurgery 47:623–632, 2000.
10. Chang CH, Housepain EM, Herbert CJ: An operative staging system and a megavoltage radiotherapeutic technic for cerebellar medulloblastomas. Radiology 93:1351–1359, 1969.
11. Coffin CM, Mukai K, Dehner LP: Glial differentiation in medulloblastomas. Am J Pathol 7:555–565, 1983.
12. Cushing H: Experience with the cerebellar medulloblastomas. ACTA Pathol Microbiol Scand 7:1–86, 1930.
13. Cutler EC, Sosman MC, Vaughan WW: The place of radiation in the treatment of cerebellar medulloblastomata. Am J Roentgenol Rad Ther Nucl Med 35:429–445, 1939.
13a. Douglas JG, Barker JL, Ellenbogen RG, Geyer JR: Concurrent chemotherapy and reduced-dose cranial spinal irradiation followed by conformal posterior fossa tumor bed boost for average-risk medulloblastoma: efficacy and patterns of failure. Int J Radiat Oncol Biol Phys 58:1161–1164, 2004.
14. Duetsch M, Thomas PRM, Krischer J: Results of a prospective randomized trial comparing standard dose neuraxis irradiation (3,600 cGy/20) with reduced neuraxis irradiation (2,340 cGy/13) in patients with low-stage medulloblastoma. Pediatr Neurosurg 24:167–177, 1996.
15. Duffner PK, Horowitz ME, Krischer JP, et al: Postoperative chemotherapy and delayed radiation in children less than three years of age with malignant brain tumors. N Engl J Med 328:1725–1731, 1993.
16. Eberhart CG, Kepner JL, Goldthwaite PT, et al: Histopathologic grading of medulloblastoma. Cancer 94:552–560, 2002.
17. Ellison D: Classifying the medulloblastoma: insights from morphology and molecular genetics. Neuropathol Appl Neurobiol 28:257–282, 2002.
18. Evans AE, Jenkin RDT, Sposto R, et al: The treatment of medulloblastoma. J Neurosurg 72:572–582, 1990.
19. Freeman CR, Taylor RE, Kortmann R, et al: Radiotherapy for medulloblastoma in children: a perspective on current international clinical research efforts. Med Pediatric Oncology 39:99–108, 2002.
20. Frost PJ, Laperriere NJ, Shun Wong C, et al: Medulloblastoma in adults. Int J Radiat Oncol Biol Phys 32:951–957, 1995.

*See references 3, 17, 26, 28, 32, 37, 43, 48, 54, 59.

21. Giangaspero F, Bigner SH, Kleihues P, et al: Medulloblastoma. In Kleihues P, Cavenee WK (eds): Pathology and Genetics of Tumors of the Nervous System. Lyon, France, IARC Press, 2000.

22. Giangaspero F, Cenacchi G, Roncaroli F, et al: Medullocytoma (lipidized medulloblastoma). Am J Surg Pathol 20:656–664, 1996.

23. Giangaspero F, Chieco P, Ceccarelli C, et al: "Desmoplastic" versus "classic" medulloblastoma: comparison of DNA content, histopathology and differentiation. Virchow Arch 418:207–214, 1991.

24. Giangaspero F, Perilongo G, Fondelli MP, et al: Medulloblastoma with extensive nodularity: a variant with favorable prognosis. J Neurosurg 91:971–977, 1999.

25. Giangaspero F, Rigobello L, Badiali M, et al: Large cell medulloblastoma: a distinct variant with highly aggressive behavior. Am J Pathol 16:687–693, 1992.

26. Gilbertson R, Wickramasinghe C, Herman R, et al: Clinical and molecular stratification of disease risk in medulloblastoma. Br J Cancer 85:705–712, 2001.

27. Giliemorth J, Kehler U, Knopp U, et al: A multifocal cerebellar and supratentorial medulloblastoma in an adult. Acta Neurochir (Wien) 140:723–724, 1998.

27a. Giordana MT, Duo D, Gasverde S, et al: MDM2 Overexpression is associated with short survival in adults with medulloblastoma. Neuro-oncology 4:115–122, 2002.

28. Giordana MT, Schiffer P, Lanotte M, et al: Epidemiology of adult medulloblastoma. Int J Cancer 80:689–692, 1999.

29. Goldberg-Stern H, Gadoth N, Stern S, et al: The prognostic significance of glial fibrillary acidic protein staining in medulloblastoma. Cancer 68:568–573, 1991.

30. Greenberg HS, Chamberlain MC, Glantz MJ, et al: Adult medulloblastoma: multiagent chemotherapy. Neuro-oncology 3:29–34, 2001.

31. Haie-Meder C, Song PY: Medulloblastoma: Differences in adults and children—regarding Frost et al: IJROBP 32: 951–957; 1995 and Prados et al: IJROBP 32:1145–1152; 1995. Int J Radiat Oncol Biol Phys 32:1255–1257, 1995.

32. Hernan R, Fasheh R, Calabrese C, et al: ERBB2 up-regulates S100A4 and several other prometastatic genes in medulloblastoma. Cancer Res 63:140–148, 2003.

33. Hubbard JL, Scheithauer BW, Kispert DB, et al: Adult cerebellar medulloblastomas: the pathological, radiographic, and clinical disease spectrum. J Neurosurg 70:536–544, 1989.

34. Hyman AD, Lanzieri CF, Solodnik P, et al: Cystic adult medulloblastoma. CT. J Compute Tomogr 10:139–143, 1988.

35. Janss AJ, Yachnis AT, Silber JH, et al: Glial differentiation predicts poor clinical outcome in primitive neuroectodermal brain tumors. Ann Neurol 39:481–489, 1996.

36. Katsetos CD, Herman MM, Frankfurter A, et al: Cerebellar desmoplastic medulloblastomas. A further immunohistochemical characterization of the reticulin-free pale islands. Arch Pathol Lab Med 113:1019–1029, 1989.

37. Kim JY, Sutton ME, Lu DJ, et al: Activation of neurotrophin-3 receptor TrkC induces apoptosis in medulloblastomas. Cancer Res 59:711–719, 1999.

38. Koci TM, Chiang F, Mehringer CM, et al: Adult cerebellar medulloblastoma: imaging features with emphasis on MR findings. AJNR: Am J Neuroradiol 14:929–939, 1993.

39. Kortmann RD, Kuhl J, Timmerman B, et al: Postoperative neoadjuvant chemotherapy before radiotherapy as compared to immediate radiotherapy followed by maintenance chemotherapy in the treatment of medulloblastoma in childhood: results of the German prospective randomized trial HIT 91. Int J Radiat Oncol Biol Phys 46:269–279, 2000.

40. Kramer JH, Crowe AB, Larson DA, et al: Neuropsychological sequelae of medulloblastoma in adults. Int J Radiat Oncol Biol Phys 38:21–26, 1997.

41. Kunschner LJ, Kuttesch J, Hess K, et al: Survival and recurrence factors in adult medulloblastomas: the MD Anderson Cancer Center Experience from 1978 to 1998. Neuro-oncology 3:167–173, 2001.

42. Leonard JR, Cai DX, Rivet DJ, et al: Large cell/anaplastic medulloblastomas and medullomyoblastomas: clinicopathological and genetic features. J Neurosurg 95:82–88, 2001.

43. MacDonald TJ, Brown KM, LaFleur B, et al: Expression profiling of medulloblastoma: PDGFRA and the RAS/MAPK pathway as therapeutic targets for metastatic disease. Nat Genet 29:143–152, 2001.

44. Mahapatra AK, Sinha AK, Sharma MC: Medullomyoblastoma: a rare cerebellar tumor in children. Childs Nerv Syst 14:312–316, 1998.

45. Malheiros SM, Franco CM, Stavale JN, et al: Medulloblastoma in adults: a series from Brazil. J Neurooncol 60:247–253, 2002.

46. Millot F, Delval O, Giraud C, et al: High-dose chemotherapy with hematopoietic stem cell transplantation in adults with bone marrow relapse of medulloblastoma: report of two cases. Bone Marrow Transplant 24:1347–1349, 1999.

47. Moots PL, Jennings MT, Bowen MG, et al: Multiagent chemotherapy followed by craniospinal radiation (CSRT) for adults with poor risk medulloblastoma (MBL) and ependymoma with subarachnoid dissemination (D.E.). Neurology 50:A380 Abstract, 1998.

47a. Moots PL, O'Neill A, Barger GR, et al: Toxicities associated with chemotherapy followed by craniospinal radiation for adults with poor-risk medulloblastoma/PNET and disseminated ependymoma: a preliminary report of ECOG 4397. Annual Meeting Proceedings of the American Society of Clinical Oncology, 23(Abst 1573):125, 2004.

48. Newton HB: Review of the molecular genetics and chemotherapeutic treatment of adult and pediatric medulloblastoma. Expert Opin Investig Drugs 10:2089–2104, 2001.

49. Packer RJ, Goldwein J, Nicholson HS, et al: Treatment of children with medulloblastomas with reduced-dose craniospinal radiation therapy and adjuvant chemotherapy: a Children's Cancer Group study. J Clin Oncol 17:2127–2136, 1999.

50. Packer RJ, Sutton LN, Elterman R, et al: Outcome for children with medulloblastoma treated with radiation and cisplatin, CCNU, and vincristine chemotherapy. J Neurosurg 81:690–698, 1994.

51. Packer RJ, Sutton LN, Goldwein JW, et al: Improved survival with the use of adjuvant chemotherapy in the treatment of medulloblastoma. J Neurosurg 74:433–440, 1991.

52. Patrice SJ, Tarbell NJ, Goumnerova LC, et al: Results of radiosurgery in the management of recurrent and residual medulloblastoma. Pediatr Neurosurg 22:197–203, 1995.

53. Peterson K, Walker RW: Medulloblastoma/primitive neuroectodermal tumor in 45 adults. Neurology 45:440–442, 1995.

54. Pomeroy SL, Tamayo P, Gassenbeek M, et al: Prediction of central nervous system embryonal tumor outcome based on gene expression. Nature 415:436–442, 2002.

55. Prados MD, Edwards MS, Chang SM, et al: Hyperfractionated craniospinal radiation therapy for primitive neuroectodermal tumors: results of a phase II study. Int J Radiat Oncol Biol Phys 43:279–285, 1999.

55a. Prados MD, Warnick RE, Wara WM, et al: Medulloblastoma in adults. Int J Radiat Oncol Biol Phys 32:1145–1152, 1995.

56. Ramsay DA, Bonnin J, MacDonald DR, et al: Medulloblastomas in late middle age and the elderly: report of 2 cases. Clin Neuropathol 14:337–342, 1995.

57. Rao C, Friedlander ME, Klein E, et al: Medullomyoblastoma: a population-based study of 532 cases. Cancer 65:157–163, 1990.

58. Sarkar C, Pramanik P, Karak AK, et al: Are childhood and adult medulloblastomas different? A comparative study of clinicopathological features, proliferation index, and apoptotic index. J Neurooncol 59:49–61, 2002.

59. Segal RA, Goumnerova LC, Kwon YK, et al: Expression of the neurotrophin receptor TrkC is linked to a favorable outcome in medulloblastoma. Proc Natl Acad Science USA 91:12867–12871, 1994.

60. Soylemezoglu F, Soffer D, Onol B, et al: Lipomatous medulloblastoma in adults. Am J Surg Pathol 20:413–418, 1996.

61. Taylor RE, Bailey CC, Robinson K, et al: Results of a randomized study of preradiation chemotherapy versus radiotherapy alone for nonmetastatic medulloblastoma: The International Society of Pediatric Oncology/United Kingdom Children's Cancer Study Group PNET-3 Study. J Clin Oncol 21:1581–1591, 2003.

62. Thomas PRM, Deutsch M, Kepner JL, et al: Low-stage medulloblastoma: final analysis of trial comparing standard-dose with reduced-dose neuraxis irradiation. J Clin Oncol 18:3004–3011, 2000.

63. Tomita T, Rosenblatt S: Management of hydrocephalus secondary to posterior fossa tumors. In Matsumoto S, Tamaki N (eds): Hydrocephalus: Pathogenesis and Treatment. Tokly, Springer-Verlag, 1991.

63a. Wolden SL, Dunkel IJ, Souweidane MM, et al: Patterns of failure using a conformal radiation therapy tumor bed boost for medulloblastoma. J Clin Oncol 21:3079–3083, 2003.

64. Woo C, Baldassarre S, Lulu B, et al: The use of stereotactic radiosurgical boost in the treatment of medulloblastoma. Int J Radiat Oncol Biol Phys 37:761–764, 1997.

65. Woodburn RT, Azzarelli B, Montebello JF, et al: Intense p53 staining is a valuable prognostic indicator for poor prognosis in medulloblastoma/central nervous system primitive neuroectodermal tumors. J Neurooncol 52:57–62, 2001.

66. Zeltzer PM, Boyett JM, Finlay JL, et al: Metastasis stage, adjuvant treatment, and residual tumor are prognostic factors for medulloblastoma in children: conclusions from the Children's Cancer Group 921 randomized phase III study. J Clin Oncol 17:832–845, 1999.

CHAPTER 36

ADULT SUPRATENTORIAL PRIMITIVE NEUROECTODERMAL TUMORS

Marc C. Chamberlain, Thomas Chen, Sara H. Kim, and Deborah L. Cummins

Primitive neuroectodermal tumor (PNET) is an undifferentiated neoplasm arising from the germinal matrix of the primitive neural tube.[3] In 1973 Hart and Earle[4] introduced the term *primitive neuroectodermal tumor* describing embryonal neoplasms outside the cerebellum and morphologically similar to medulloblastoma.[4] In 1993 the World Health Organization (WHO) classification of brain tumors defined all primitive neuroectodermal tumors of the central nervous system (CNS) as PNETs, regardless of location, and when supratentorial, divided them into several types including retinoblastoma, esthesioneuroblastoma (or olfactory neuroblastoma), pineoblastoma, neuroblastoma, and supratentorial PNET not otherwise specified.[6] This review concerns only neuroblastoma and supratentorial PNET not otherwise specified and only in adults. The majority of the literature regarding PNET, however, has dealt with children (discussed in other chapters), in whom this tumor is quite common. In adults less than 0.5% of all primary brain tumors are supratentorial PNETs (S-PNETs), and consequently the literature is dominated by case reports and one small series.[1,5,7–9]

PRESENTATION

Clinical

The majority of patients are young adults (20 to 30 years old) who have symptoms of raised intracranial pressure manifested as an altered level of consciousness, new-onset and evolving headache, nausea, vomiting, diplopia, visual obscuration, or gait instability. In addition, patients may present with new-onset and often evolving focal neurologic symptoms such as hemiparesis, visual field defects, and partial seizures. This symptom complex is not dissimilar from nor does it differentiate S-PNET from other supratentorial primary brain neoplasms. Occasionally, patients may demonstrate evidence of cerebrospinal fluid (CSF) dissemination and neoplastic meningitis resulting in cranial neuropathy, encephalopathy, or spinal cord symptoms. This presentation of CSF-disseminated disease is characteristic of only a few primary brain tumors (primary CNS lymphoma, primary CNS germ cell tumor, PNETs of other types and locations, and ependymoma) and if found, is highly suggestive of a PNET. Neurologic examination usually reveals papilledema, homonymous hemianopsia,

abductor paresis, hemiparesis, hemisensory loss, or gait ataxia reflective of a supratentorial mass lesion with associated vasogenic edema.

Neuroradiography

Adult S-PNETs more often are found in the parietal-occipital region (nearly 50%) or temporal lobes (approximately 30%) and less often in the frontal lobes (10%). Rarely, tumors are in the thalamus, are multicentric at presentation, or present with spinal cord drop metastasis. By precontrast computed tomography (CT), these tumors are isodense or hyperdense, the latter suggesting tumor hypercellularity. Intratumoral calcification (either globular or multiple and small) is seen in nearly half of all S-PNETs. On postcontrast CT, the tumors measure 3 to 8 cm in their longest dimension (mean 5 cm), demonstrate peritumoral edema, and homogeneously enhance. Intratumoral cysts, necrosis, or hemorrhage are not uncommon (30%, 25%, 15%, respectively).[10] On precontrast magnetic resonance imaging (MRI), the solid tumor component has heterogeneous signal on T1- and T2-weighted images. Postcontrast MRI demonstrates homogeneous enhancement of the solid portion of the tumor with good demarcation between tumor and normal brain.[2] Magnetic resonance spectroscopy (MRS) shows the nonspecific primary brain tumor spectra of elevated choline, decreased *N*-acetyl aspartate, and elevated lactate peaks. Because of the proclivity of these tumors to spread by way of CSF, whole-spine contrast-enhanced MRI is indicated as is CSF cytology. Ideally, spine imaging is performed before surgery; however, it is most often performed following surgery because of preoperative diagnostic uncertainty. MRI identifies spinal or intracranial metastases of S-PNETs by demonstrating either leptomeningeal enhancement or contrast-enhancing subarachnoid nodules, so-called M+ disease. Because of blood artifacts found in the spine following surgery, a 2- to 3-week delay is often recommended before performing spine MRI and CSF cytology.

PATHOLOGY

PNETs are WHO grade IV embryonal neoplasms that are composed of undifferentiated or poorly differentiated neuroepithelial cells, which show evidence of divergent differentiation along neuronal or glial lines. Evidence for photoreceptor and muscular differentiation have also been described.[3,8]

The terminology used to classify these tumors has not been completely standardized. The WHO[6] suggests *supratentorial PNET* and uses the names *cerebral neuroblastoma* and *cerebral ganglioneuroblastoma* for a subset of these tumors with demonstrable neuroblastic and neuronal differentiation, respectively. The semantic problem of how much evidence of neuroblastic differentiation is needed to change the diagnosis from simply supratentorial PNET to cerebral neuroblastoma is somewhat arbitrary, because evidence of neuronal differentiation in the form of synaptophysin positivity is often found in very undifferentiated-appearing tumors. A reasonable approach is that taken by the WHO. Clear-cut evidence of neuronal differentiation by light or electron microscopy (described later) is required to make the diagnosis of neuroblastoma or ganglioneuroblastoma. Tumors that show only immunohistochemical evidence of neuronal differentiation would be considered PNETs, not otherwise specified (NOS).

Gross Appearance

The gross appearance of adult PNETs is nonspecific. They are generally tan-pink, soft, and may or may not have cysts and areas of hemorrhage. The degree of demarcation from the surrounding brain and the size of the mass is also variable.

Microscopic Appearance

The most undifferentiated of PNETs are small-blue-cell tumors and thus on routine, light microscopic examination are similar or identical to other primitive tumors, including medulloblastoma, small cell carcinoma of the lung, and small cell glioblastoma multiforme (GBM). Undifferentiated PNETs are highly cellular tumors (Figure 36-1). The cells are typically small with a very high nuclear to cytoplasmic ratio; generally, little cytoplasm can be appreciated. The nuclei are round to somewhat

angulated. The nuclear chromatin is dense and evenly dispersed, and nucleoli are usually absent. Mitotic figures are numerous, as are apoptotic cells. The cellularity is so high that there is only scant stroma. There may or may not be areas of confluent necrosis. The only evidence for differentiation in these tumors may be found with electron microscopy or, more typically, with immunohistochemistry. Electron microscopy generally reveals a poorly differentiated tumor, but evidence for neuronal differentiation may be indicated by the presence of microtubules or dense-core granules. The latter feature is considered by the WHO to be diagnostic of neuroblastoma. Glial filaments, indicative of astrocytic differentiation, may also be found. Immunohistochemically, tumors are often positive for synaptophysin, even those that appear very undifferentiated (Figure 36-2). Glial fibrillary acidic protein (GFAP) positivity, indicative of glial differentiation, may be present. When found in a tumor containing cells with more abundant cytoplasm and increased nuclear pleomorphism, differentiating the tumor from a GBM can be difficult. Some tumors may show desmin positivity, indicative of muscular differentiation.

Routine histologic evidence of more advanced neuronal differentiation, justifying the diagnosis of cerebral neuroblastoma, can be found in the presence of Homer-Wright rosettes. In these structures tumor cell nuclei form a circle or wreath surrounding a core filled with fibrillary processes. Other evidence supporting the diagnosis of neuroblastoma includes a fibrillar stroma resembling neuropil (typically synaptophysin positive) and the streaming or palisading of tumor cells. As the tumor becomes more differentiated, ganglion cells are found (ganglioneuroblastoma). Ganglion cells often stain positively for neurofilament protein. Ultrastructural features found in these more differentiated tumors include microtubules, intermediate filaments, dense-core granules and synaptic vesicles. True synapses are rarely seen.

Occasional PNETs will show evidence of photoreceptor differentiation in the form of Flexner-Wintersteiner rosettes,

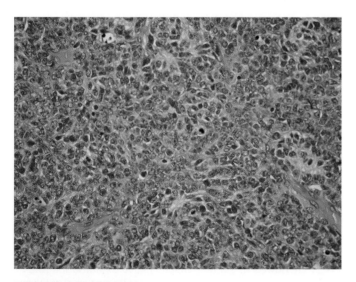

FIGURE 36-1   A typical undifferentiated adult S-PNET showing dense cellularity, a high nuclear-to-cytoplasmic ratio, frequent mitoses, and apoptotic cells. Hematoxylin and eosin, ×250.

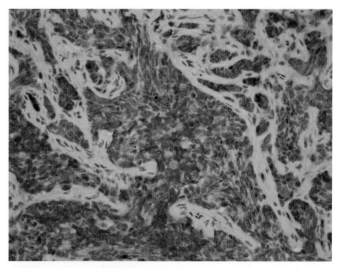

FIGURE 36-2   The brown staining indicates diffuse positivity of this adult S-PNET for synaptophysin, a neuronal marker. Blood vessels are negative for this marker. Immunohistochemical stain for synaptophysin, ×250.

such as are found in retinoblastomas. Flexner-Wintersteiner rosettes are round, well formed and have small, circular, empty lumens lined by terminal bars and apical protuberances.

Few studies have examined proliferation markers such as the Ki-67 labeling index in adult S-PNETs. However, there is limited evidence to suggest that very high labeling indices (e.g., >30%) portend a worse prognosis.

TREATMENT

Surgery

Preoperative Considerations

The decision to perform an open craniotomy for resection versus stereotactic biopsy for adults with S-PNET should be predicated on the degree of certainty of the preoperative diagnosis, the amount of mass effect at the time of presentation, and the location of the tumor. If the diagnosis of a tumor is uncertain or a chemosensitive tumor (i.e., lymphoma) is a possibility, a stereotactic biopsy should first be employed. If the patient does not have increased intracranial pressure, a stereotactic biopsy may also be performed to obtain a diagnosis. Finally, if the location is surgically inaccessible for an open craniotomy (i.e., thalamus), a biopsy should also be performed. In most circumstances an open craniotomy is the surgery of choice, in which case preoperative functional MRI may be beneficial in determining the site of initial corticectomy. Because S-PNETs are often cortically located tumors, it is important preoperatively to determine whether any important functional areas of the brain are involved to aid preoperative surgical planning. If preoperative functional MRI demonstrates speech function close to the tumor, then an awake craniotomy should be considered for mapping speech or motor function.

Operative Procedure

There have been no large series published on the surgical management of S-PNET, and as a consequence the prognostic importance of complete tumor resection is unknown. Regardless, attempted image-verified complete resection is desirable based on extrapolation of the literature regarding medulloblastoma. Many institutions perform tumor resection using a neuronavigational system to help tailor the craniotomy flap and to localize the tumor intraoperatively. The surgery is performed using an operating microscope, and a microscopic excision of the tumor is performed. S-PNETs tend to be soft and vascular. They are often lobulated and purplish-gray or pinkish. They are usually easily distinguished from normal brain, unlike other intrinsic tumors such as gliomas. Once the lesion is localized, bipolar cautery is used to establish a pseudocapsule and develop it between the brain and the tumor, with resection of the tumor itself. The chance of a postoperative neurologic deficit can be minimized even in functionally important regions of the brain if care is taken to make the initial corticectomy and incision in a functionally noneloquent region, with careful dissection toward the tumor.

If there is sufficient concern from preoperative assessment (MRI scan, functional MRI scan) that the tumor is in a functionally important region of the brain, an awake craniotomy with speech or motor intraoperative testing should be considered.

Postoperative Care

Postoperative care usually consists of an overnight stay in the intensive care unit and a day in the ward the following day. Patients are discharged on postoperative day 2 or 3 barring unforeseen complications. All patients receive a postoperative MRI scan the day after surgery to determine the extent of resection. If an incomplete resection is performed and the lesion is surgically accessible, the patient is offered another surgery to remove the tumor before radiation therapy.

Radiation Therapy

PNETs show a high propensity for CSF dissemination, at both diagnosis and time of recurrence. As a consequence, treatment to the entire neuraxis is required. Additional radiation is given as a boost to the primary tumor. Opposed lateral fields are used to treat the whole brain and upper cervical spinal canal. A posterior field encompassing the entire spinal subarachnoid space is matched to the lateral brain fields. The inferior border of the spinal field is at either S2 or the inferior aspect of the lumbar thecal sac as defined by MRI, whichever is lower. The superior border is placed between C5 and C7. The lateral field borders are 1 cm lateral to the pedicles. To counteract daily set-up inaccuracies and provide a homogeneous dose, it is important to feather the gap by shifting the anatomic junction site by at least 5 mm every 7 fractions. Lateral opposed beams encompassing both the intracranial contents and the upper cervical spinal canal are used to treat the craniocervical field. After a dose of 36 Gy in 20 fractions to the neuraxis, the primary tumor receives a boost of 19.8 cGy in 11 fractions for a total tumor dose of 55.8 Gy in 31 fractions. The volume radiated should be the primary tumor plus a minimum of 1-cm margin.

In patients with no evidence of metastasis (M_0) and tumor confined to the site of surgery, craniospinal irradiation (CSI) is administered (36 Gy to the neuraxis and 55.8 Gy to the tumor) in conventionally fractionated daily doses (200 cGy). In patients with M+ disease, again CSI is administered (36 Gy to the neuraxis); however, all sites of metastasis and tumor receive 55.8 Gy. The role for conformal radiation therapy directed at visible tumor is under investigation as is the role for stereotactic radiation therapy boosts following conventional CSI.

Chemotherapy

Because of the rarity of adult S-PNET, there are no randomized clinical trials or for that matter any series that address the issue of adjuvant chemotherapy. As a consequence, the approach in adults has been similar to that developed for pediatric S-PNET using chemotherapeutic agents found effective primarily against medulloblastoma. The most often used regimens are PCV (CCNU, procarbazine, vincristine) or the so-called Packer protocol (CCNU, cisplatin, vincristine). Data regarding outcome (response rate, duration of response) following adjuvant chemotherapy is anecdotal at best. Pilot studies for pediatric S-PNET (reviewed in another chapter) have explored the role of adjuvant dose-intensive chemotherapy followed by autologous peripheral stem cell transplant. The results are encouraging; however, confirmation and larger studies are required.

In patients with metastatic disease, so called M+ disease, the role of intra-CSF chemotherapy has not been determined, because all patients are treated with CSI (see previous discussion), a therapy with proven efficacy against CSF disseminated disease. However, in patients with M+ disease, confirmation of response (CSF cytology and neuraxis neuroimaging) is necessary, because patients failing CSI would be candidates for intra-CSF chemotherapy.

Lastly, chemotherapy has a salvage role for recurrent disease. Regimens based on the treatment of medulloblastoma have, again, been used, most often a platinum-based or an oxazaphosphorine-based therapy (cyclophosphamide or ifosfamide). Response rates are not generally known, however, and therefore these patients would seem to be excellent candidates for experimental therapeutics.

OUTCOME

Adult S-PNETs appear to have a similar or slightly better survival than pediatric S-PNETs excluding pineoblastoma. In the only large series of adult S-PNETs ($n = 12$), Kim reported a mean survival of 86 months and a 3-year survival of 75%. A report of pediatric S-PNETs from the same institution ($n = 28$), reported a 68-month mean survival and a 73% 3-year survival.[5] A larger study of pediatric S-PNETs from the Children's Cancer Group study ($n = 52$) reported a 3-year survival of 57%. Because adult S-PNETs are rare, the prognostic significance of neuronal or glial differentiation, proliferation indices such as Ki-67 labeling index, and extent of surgical resection are unclear.

References

1. Bellis EH, Salcman M, Bastian FO: Primitive neuroectodermal tumor in a 57-year-old man. Surg Neurol 20:30–35, 1983.
2. Figeroa RE, el Gammal T, Brooks BS, et al: MR findings on primitive neuroectodermal tumors. J Comput Assist Tomogr 13:773–778, 1989.
3. Gould VE, Rorke LB, Jansson DS, et al: Primitive neuroectodermal tumors of the central nervous system express neuroendocrine markers and may express all classes of intermediate filaments. Hum Pathol 21:245–252, 1990.
4. Hart MN, Earle KM: Primitive neuroectodermal tumors of the brain in children. Cancer 32:890–897, 1973.
5. Kim DG, Lee DY, Paek SH, et al: Supratentorial primitive neuroectodermal tumors in adults. J Neuro Oncol 60:43–52, 2002.
6. Kleihues P, Burger PC, Scheithauer BW: The new WHO classification of brain tumors. Brain Pathol 3:255–268, 1993.
7. Kuratsu J, Matsukado Y, Seto H, et al: Primitive neuroectodermal tumor arising from the thalamus of an adult-case report. Neurol Med Chir (Tokyo) 26:30–34, 1986.
8. Louis DN, Hochberg FH: Cerebral primitive neuroectodermal tumor in an adult, with spinal cord metastasis after 18-year dormancy. J Neurooncol 9:77–80, 1990.
9. Miyazawa T, Ueno H, Hatashita S: "Undifferentiated" cerebral primitive neuroectodermal tumor in a young adult-case report. Neurol Med Chir (Tokyo) 34:759–762, 1994.
10. Pickuth D, Leutloff U: Computed tomography and magnetic resonance imaging findings in primitive neuroectodermal tumors in adults. Br J Radiol 69:1–5, 1996.

CHAPTER 37

LIPOMATOUS TUMORS

Jason S. Weinstein, Bette K. Kleinschmidt-DeMasters, and Kevin O. Lillehei

The lipomatous tumors are an uncommon group of tumors within the central nervous system (CNS). Although they are classically separated into four relatively distinctive subtypes—lipoma, angiolipoma, hibernoma, and intracranial liposarcoma—lipomas are by far the most commonly encountered member of the group and as such will be the main focus of this chapter. Lipomas may be found intracranially as well as intra- and extra-axially along the spinal cord. In this discussion the intra-axial variants will be emphasized. Small incidental intracranial lipomas, typically near the falx or brainstem, are regularly identified by neuroradiologists during the course of neuroimaging studies in patients who have unrelated problems. As such, small lipomas usually do not prompt neurosurgical intervention. On the other hand, large intracranial and intraspinal lipomas are removed with some regularity by neurosurgeons who treat pediatric patients.

Lipoma, angiolipoma, and the exceedingly rare hibernoma are all benign entities, whereas the equally rare intracranial liposarcoma is malignant like its extracranial counterpart. Some authors argue that the lipomas and angiolipomas should not be considered as separate tumor types, but rather represent either a spectrum within lipomas of variable degrees of vascularity or are capillary hemangiomas with large amounts of accompanying fat. Whereas the semantic debate is not important, lipomas with a conspicuous vascular component should be recognized for their potential to hemorrhage. Hence in this chapter angiolipomas will be discussed as a separate entity to underscore their potentially differing clinical and neuroimaging presentations.

Most lipomatous tumors share overlapping clinical presentations and appearances on neuroimaging studies because of the distinctive signal of fat on both computed tomography (CT) and magnetic resonance imaging (MRI). Neuroimaging studies further distinguish between different types of intracranial lipomas, based on whether the lipoma is or is not associated with other brain findings. Intracranial lipomas can be separated into three general groups: isolated lipomas not associated with significant developmental anomalies of the surrounding brain and soft tissues; lipomas associated with developmental anomalies (Table 37-1); and lipomas that occur as part of a genetic syndrome (Table 37-2). Understanding these very different co-associated conditions is particularly important when called upon to make management decisions regarding neurosurgical intervention. The source of the patient's symptoms may often be attributable to the co-associated malformations and not to the lipoma at all.

Even in cases where lipomas are the source of symptomatology, resection may not be indicated. In cases where spinal nerves are enveloped within the lipoma, judicious use of surgery is necessary to avoid postoperative morbidity. Likewise, resection of a lipoma that invests a cranial nerve may alleviate symptoms attributable to that cranial nerve, but the surgical morbidity associated with this procedure may be unacceptably high. Resection of an intracranial lipoma associated with severe developmental anomalies is also not likely to benefit patients except in select cases involving lower cranial nerves. Resection is also not generally indicated for patients with genetic syndromes. Management decisions regarding spinal cord lipomas and lipomyelomeningoceles will be discussed in their respective sections.

This chapter will attempt to provide answers to the following basic questions:

- Is there an embryologic explanation for where and why lipomatous tumors occur in the CNS axis?
- Are there genetic syndromes or specific anomalies associated with intra-axial lipomatous tumors that the clinician should be aware of, particularly in pediatric patients?
- Are the neuroimaging characteristics of lipomatous tumors sufficiently distinctive to provide a definite preoperative diagnosis?
- Are there unifying treatment principles that may be applied to benign intracranial lipomatous tumors?

INTRACRANIAL LIPOMA

Embryologic Origin

Theories regarding the pathogenesis of intracranial lipomas have evolved since the first report of a chiasmatic lipoma by Meckel in 1818.[23] A contemporary consensus holds that intracranial lipomas result from the "abnormal persistence and maldifferentiation of the *meninx primitiva* during the development of the subarachnoid space."[20] This theory, first proposed by Verga in 1929 and well summarized and further supported by Truwit and Barkovich in 1990,[20] accounts for several of the distinctive features of intracranial lipomas: the subarachnoid, cisternal locations of intracranial lipomas; the commonly associated parenchymal malformations (see Table 37-1); and the incorporation of, and respect for, intracranial vessels and nerves.

TABLE 37-1

Anomalies Associated with Intracranial Lipomas

Agenesis or hypogenesis of surrounding neural tissue (e.g., corpus callosum)
Frontal bone defects; facial dysplasia or hypoplasia
Absent, tortuous, or dilated blood vessels; aneurysms
Cranial nerve absence or duplication; unusual branching patterns of nerves

(Modified from Wilkins RH, Rengachary SS: Neurosurgery, ed 2. New York, McGraw-Hill, 1996.)

TABLE 37-2

Genetic Syndromes that Manifest Intracranial Lipomas

Genetic Syndrome	Associated Features
Bannayan	Macrocephaly, hemangiomas (intracerebral and bony)
Gorlin-Goldenhar	Mandibular hypoplasia, macrostomia, upper vertebral anomalies, and epibulbar dermoids
Encephalocutaneous lipomatosis	Soft scalp masses with overlying alopecia, papular skin lesions over face and eyes, and progressive intracranial calcifications
Frontonasal dysplasia	Midline craniofacial anomalies, hypertelorism, cranium bifidum, cleft lip or nose, and mental retardation
Neurofibromatosis variants	Café-au-lait lesions, neurofibromas, Lisch nodules, plexiform neuromas

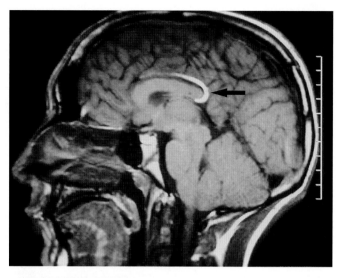

FIGURE 37-1 Sagittal, T1-weighted magnetic resonance image demonstrates the characteristic bright signal image of a curvilinear, pericallosal lipoma *(arrow)* associated with partial agenesis of the posterior corpus callosum. (Image courtesy of the Neuroradiology Division, Department of Radiology, University of Colorado Health Sciences Center.)

The *meninx primitiva*, first described by Salvi, is a mesenchymal derivative of the neural crest. Between days 32 and 44 of embryogenesis, the *meninx* dissolves, giving rise to the subarachnoid spaces.[20] The dissolution of *meninx primitiva* occurs in a stepwise fashion, regressing first in the region of the ventral brainstem (eventually to form the prepontomedullary cisterns), then dorsally (sites of the future perimesencephalic and dorsomesencephalic cisterns), and finally cephalad (to form the supratentorial cisterns).[20,23] This genetic patterning, in conjunction with the predilection for lipoma formation at areas of flexion or at sites of redundant *meninx*, accounts for the observed distribution of intracranial lipomas.

The vast majority (80% to 95%) of intracranial lipomas are found along or near the midline.[6] Approximately 50% of all intracranial lipomas are found within the pericallosal cistern; 20% in the ambient, quadrigeminal plate and chiasmatic cisterns combined; 12% in the cerebellopontine angle (CPA) or internal auditory canal (IAC); and 7% along the convexities of the brain. Other types and locations include rare intradural cervical lipomas, which can spread into the posterior fossa,

and multiple intracranial lipomas. Lipomas have also been described in the choroid plexus, interpeduncular cistern, septum pellucidum, and pineal region.[6,15,19,23] Lipomas of the choroid plexus are usually extensions of callosal lipomas, and lipomas of the interpeduncular cistern often contain bone within their matrix. Lipomas containing bone are referred to as osteolipomas.

Pericallosal lipomas account for approximately half of all intracranial lipomas, with two distinct subtypes of pericallosal lipomas recognized based on their configuration: the tubulonodular and curvilinear. The pathogenesis outlined by Truwit and Barkovich[20] helps account for the features of these two subtypes. Tubulonodular lipomas are generally found anteriorly within the pericallosal cistern. Because they form early in embryogenesis, they are usually large, round, or cylindrical and associated with more severe anomalies of the corpus callosum, frontal lobes, and surrounding soft tissue and bone.[6,23] In contrast, curvilinear lipomas occur more posteriorly, are usually smaller than tubulonodular lipomas, and form thin, ribbon-like structures (Figure 37-1). These lipomas are more often asymptomatic and are unassociated with severe anomalies. Curvilinear lipomas are thought to form later in embryogenesis, and therefore they do not grow as large and are less likely to disturb callosal or frontal lobe formation. Other anomalies of the neighboring parenchyma, soft tissue and bone, blood vessels, cranial nerves, and various body parts may be associated with intracranial lipomas, depending on their location or as a part of a genetic syndrome.

Clinical Presentation

More than 30% of patients with intracranial lipomas are asymptomatic.[23] The vast majority of the remaining patients have signs and symptoms not attributable to the lipoma but secondary to the associated developmental anomalies. Approximately 30% of patients with supratentorial lipomas have a seizure disorder. The seizure disorder is reportedly "often severe, is focal or generalized, and has an average onset age of 15 years. Recurrent headaches are a presenting symptom in 25 percent, and . . . 10 to 15 percent have behavioral problems and/or mental retardation."[23] Other reported signs and symptoms include "fainting spells, vomiting, episodic leg weakness, blurred vision, sleepwalking, diencephalic disturbances such as adiposogenital dystrophy and hypothermia, and even transient ischemic attacks."[6] Presenting signs and symptoms of patients with infratentorial lipomas may include hydrocephalus, cerebellar ataxia, motor weakness, sleep apnea, and cochleovestibular symptoms such as hearing loss, vertigo, otalgia, trigeminal neuralgia, hemifacial spasm, and tinnitus.[6,19,23]

The cited incidence of intracranial lipomas ranges from 0.08% to 0.21% of all patients who come to autopsy and 0.06% to 0.30% of all patients studied by CT scans.[6,23] However, there are a few autopsy reports that suggest the incidence may be as high as 2.6%.[22] Although large MRI series have not been reported, MRI scans might be predicted to yield an even higher overall incidence of lipomas when very small asymptomatic lesions are included. Intracranial lipomas represent 0.1% to 1.3% of all recognized intracranial tumors.[6] There have been hundreds of reports of pericallosal lipomas in the world literature since 1818, whereas lipomas of the cerebellopontine angle represent only 0.14% of all tumors seen in this region. A recent report and review of the literature revealed 98 reported cases of lipomas of the CPA or IAC.[19]

The epidemiology of intracranial lipomas is significant in that there appears to be no age or sex-specific differences with the following exceptions: CPA lipomas are twice as common in males than females, and lipomas in the pediatric population are more commonly localized to the pericallosal cistern.[6,19,23] As previously mentioned, several syndromes may also manifest intracranial lipomas, including Bannayan syndrome, an autosomal dominant disorder amenable to genetic counseling; Gorlin-Goldenhar syndrome, encephalocraniocutaneous lipomatosis, neurofibromatosis variants, and frontonasal dysplasia[23] (see Table 37-2).

Neuroimaging

Neurological examination may occasionally be helpful for gross localization of intracranial lipomas, but the diagnosis is generally made with neuroimaging studies. In the past, pneumoencephalography, carotid angiography, and plain radiographs were useful adjuncts to the physical examination of a patient with an intracranial lipoma. In the current age of CT, MRI, and advanced nuclear imaging techniques, the previously used tools find limited utility.

CT is a fast and accurate means to diagnose most intracranial lipomas because of the low attenuation value of fat (−40 to −100 Hounsfield units); however, MRI is the study of choice.[23] Lipomas, in general, do not enhance with contrast and do not cause perilesional edema.[23] On T1-weighted, nonenhanced MRI scans, lipomas appear homogeneous and hyperintense to brain. On T2-weighted, nonenhanced MRI scans, they are isointense to hypointense to brain. With fat suppression techniques, their signal is absent. MRI is also superior to CT for the characterization of associated brain anomalies and

intralesional vessels and nerves. The presence of a chemical shift artifact on MRI is pathognomonic for lipoma.[23]

Gross and Microscopic Appearance

Intracranial lipomas appear as dark-yellow lesions on gross inspection. The *meninx primitiva* contains within it "primitive perivascular reticuloendothelium,"[6] which may become specialized in the storage of fat, and this may account for the histology of intracranial lipomas. Early precapillary parenchyma may also differentiate into fat cells. Microscopic examination reveals that these lesions are composed of mature adipose cells with peripheral, sometimes indented, small bland nuclei. A collagenous capsule that is intimately associated with adjacent brain often surrounds the lipoma. In general, no cleavage plane exists between the tumor and surrounding brain tissue. Histologically, although mature fat is the predominant element, variable amounts of fibrovascular tissue, bone, and calcification can also be present. Adjacent parenchymal calcifications and bone formation may occur, although the exact percentage of lipomas showing these changes is not well documented. Bone formation within lipomas appears to be unique to lipomas of the central nervous system[6,19,23] and is particularly characteristic in the suprasellar variants (as seen in the previously discussed osteolipomas).

Therapeutic Options

Therapeutic considerations for patients with intracranial lipomas must be made within a risk-benefit analysis. Although there are limited data on the treatment of intracranial lipomas, surgical resection versus observation alone has been the standard of care. There are no reports of attempts to treat intracranial lipomas with radiation or chemotherapy. Because intracranial lipomas are benign entities whose contribution to the patient's underlying symptomatology is often unclear, the indications for surgical removal must be strong. Although there are case reports of intracranial lipomas increasing in size and causing symptom progression,[19,23] this appears to be the exception rather than the rule.

Intracranial lipomas are congenital lesions and hence the associated malformations, often the source of the actual symptoms, occur early in development and are not amenable to treatment. In general, surgical resection of intracranial lipomas should be the last resort. Hydrocephalus, if present, should be treated appropriately by shunting. Attempts to manage seizure disorders with medications should be made, because there is no strong evidence that surgical resection of pericallosal or sylvian fissure lipomas leads to seizure reduction. Lipomas of the CPA or IAC, likewise, should not be operated on except in cases of medical treatment failure or rehabilitation failure. A review by Tankere et al[19] highlights the danger of surgical resection of these lesions.

Tankere et al studied 54 patients with CPA or IAC lipomas who underwent surgical resection. Approximately 50% had improvement of their initial complaint; however, more than half those patients complained of multiple new deficits after surgery, and 65% suffered postoperative hearing loss.[19] With regard to surgical technique, the translabyrinthine approach appears to provide the best chance for total resection, but hearing loss is virtually assured. Use of the middle and posterior fossa approaches provides more hearing preservation (26%) but less chance for total resection.[19] As stated previously, Tankere et al concluded that surgical resection of CPA or IAC lipomas should be restricted to patients who have failed all medical and rehabilitative options or those with severe trigeminal neuralgia or hemifacial spasm.[19]

Little recurrence or outcome data exist regarding intracranial lipomas. The available reports suggest that these lesions remain stable over time and do not recur following surgical resection. Standard vestibular rehabilitation may be useful for some patients, and many authors recommend periodic surveillance of these lesions with MRI or magnetic resonance angiography.

In summary, intracranial lipomas range from relatively common "incidentalomas" on neuroimaging studies, to rare isolated lesions unassociated with other brain abnormalities, to even rarer lesions associated with congenital anomalies. Regardless of the co-associated conditions, most are found in the midline. They may be diagnosed with MRI because of their characteristic hyperintense signal on T1-weighted images and null signal with fat-suppression techniques. Management strategies for these lesions should be conservative, including medical therapy for seizure and cochleovestibular symptom control; vestibular rehabilitation; ventricular shunting for hydrocephalus; and cosmetic surgery for associated frontal bone anomalies. Surgical resection of intracranial lipomas or cranial nerve decompression or vestibular nerve transection should be done only in selected cases where other management strategies have failed.

INTRASPINAL LIPOMA

It is imperative to clarify the nomenclature regarding lipomatous tumors of the spinal cord. This becomes of utmost importance when discussing treatment options and outcomes data. The lipomatous tumors of the spinal cord may be subdivided into three types: intradural or intramedullary spinal cord lipomas not associated with spinal dysraphism; lipomyelomeningoceles (often termed lumbosacral lipomas) associated with spinal dysraphism; and filum terminale lipomas. Similar to their intracranial counterparts, intraspinal lipomas may be isolated lesions or associated with significant developmental abnormalities.

Intradural Intramedullary and Intradural Extramedullary Lipomas Unassociated with Spinal Dysraphism

Spinal cord intradural, intramedullary lipomas are rare entities, usually found along the dorsal aspect of the thoracic spine and in the midline.[12,23] In one early report, they were found in decreasing frequency over the cervical-thoracic spine and over the cervical spine. In addition, there are eight reports of intramedullary spinal cord lipomas affecting nearly all levels of the spinal cord, known as holocord lipomas.[12]

Patients with spinal cord lipomas most often have slowly progressive signs of spinal cord compression. The most commonly reported presenting symptoms are those of an ascending spastic motor weakness in one or both legs.[10,12,23] The clinical presentation and examination findings reflect the location and size of the spinal cord lipoma.

Spinal cord lipomas are uncommon, with approximately 200 reported cases, predominantly of the intradural or extramedullary type, having been identified in the cervical and upper thoracic spine since the first report by Gowers in 1876.[12] Spinal cord lipomas account for 0.6% to 1% of all intraspinal tumors.[10,12] They are found with equal frequency in males and females and are presumed to be present from birth. However, because of their benign, slow-growing nature, these lesions often do not present until the second or third decades of life.[12,23] As with other lipomatous tumors, the diagnosis may be suggested with the use of plain radiographs, but CT or MRI is the study of choice.

The pathogenesis of spinal cord lipomas may be related to the incorporation of multipotential mesodermal cells present between days 18 and 27 of embryogenesis.[23] Like intracranial lipomas, spinal cord lipomas are composed of mature adipocytes with a collagenous matrix and capsule, which is reflected in their appearance on CT and MRI. Spinal cord lipomas have also been noted to enlarge and regress with changes in total body fat.[23] Dietary modification has been proposed as a treatment modality for spinal cord lipomas, but surgical debulking remains the mainstay of therapy, if needed.

Given their characteristic location, spinal cord lipomas are commonly accessible by way of a posterior approach. The goal of surgery is not total resection, because multiple authors have noted the lack of identifiable planes between the lipoma and the spinal cord tissue. Instead, the goal should be decompression and subtotal resection, with careful attention to the spinal cord elements. Multilevel laminectomies, covering the area of involvement, are performed. There are no reports of radiation therapy or chemotherapy used as adjuncts in the treatment of spinal cord lipomas. Recurrence is rare, because these tumors do not contain neoplastic elements, and there are no reports of malignant transformation.

Outcome data are limited, but in a report on eight patients with spinal cord lipomas who underwent surgical decompression, all patients demonstrated improved muscle strength, one third had improved sensation, one fourth had improved pain, and one fourth had improved bladder function.[3] These improvements stand in sharp contrast to the postoperative outcomes seen in patients with lipomyelomeningoceles, discussed later.

Lipomas of the Spinal Cord Associated with Spinal Dysraphism

The term *lipomyelomeningocele* refers to a congenital lesion of the meninges or spinal cord plus meninges and the presence of benign fat, both of which exist with a dysraphic spinal column. Depending on the classification system used, these lesions may be divided into as many as five subtypes as they appear on neuroimaging.[2] In general, a lipomyelomeningocele is recognized on MRI as a caudally descended conus medullaris invested in fat. Arai et al, using conventional myelogram and MRI, define lipomyelomeningocele as a "low lying tethered spinal cord [that] enters a subcutaneous cystic meningeal sac and terminates in the lipomatous mass on the wall of the meningeal sac."[2] The lipoma and meningocele may appear together or on opposite sides of the spinal canal. The asymmetric variety is less common and is generally associated with more severe deformities of the sacrum and lower extremities.[23] Lipomyelomeningoceles may also be associated with a "syringomyelia, tethered spinal cord, dermal sinus tract, dermoid tumor, menigocele manqué, diastematomyelia, and neurenteric cyst."[23] Greater than 90% of these lesions will present with lumbosacral cutaneous anomalies such as "dermal sinus tracts, atretic meningocele, hemangioma, and focal hirsutism."[23] As such, there is generally little difficulty in making the diagnosis.

Lipomyelomeningoceles are not uncommon, and there is a female-to-male predominance of approximately 1.5:1.[23] They are thought to result from mistakes in posterior canalization between days 28 and 48 of embryogenesis.[23] Their histology is similar to other types of lipomatous tumors, with the lipomatous portion made up of mature adipocytes.

Most patients experience symptom onset early in life and many are diagnosed in utero using ultrasound. Of those not recognized or treated at birth, clinical manifestations generally progress slowly over months to years and may include motor weakness and sensory changes in the lower extremities, bladder incontinence, and pain.[2,3,23] Lipomyelomeningoceles may present with both upper and lower motor neuron signs, and "asymmetrical weakness of the feet and legs is a hallmark of this condition."[23] The acuity and degree of impairment depends on the nature of the lesion, but most authors agree that neurologic deterioration, over time, is assured in these patients.

Controversy exists regarding the timing of surgical repair in asymptomatic patients. The likelihood that patients will develop neurologic problems is high (88%), given a long enough period of follow-up, whereas the risk of complications during operative procedures is less than 10%.[2,3,23] It is important in surgical planning to know whether the tethered cord lies within the spinal canal. The goals of surgery are to remove as much of the lipoma as possible while preserving nervous tissues, release the tethered cord, and attempt to prevent retethering.[2,23] Refer to Management of Spinal Cord Lipomas and Lipomyelomeningoceles[23] for further details on operative approaches.

Compared with intradural or intramedullary lipomas and lipomas of the filum terminale (discussed later), the prognosis for patients with lipomyelomeningoceles is not as favorable. In the report by Bulsara et al,[3] only 29% of patients with lipomyelomeningocele had improved motor function postoperatively, and there was very little improvement (7%) in bladder function or sensation. There was also little reported significant improvement in bowel function, pain, or scoliosis. They did note, however, that "younger patients tended to have better motor outcomes."[3] It has been stated that "the longer and more complete the deficit [in motor, sensory, or bowel or bladder function], the less likely it is to resolve following surgical intervention."[23] This would suggest that patients with lipomyelomeningoceles should be operated on early in the hopes of avoiding neurologic deterioration. It may also be concluded that early detection of these cases, by way of recognition of cutaneous stigmata, is critical to good clinical outcomes in this patient population.[3]

Lipomas of the Filum Terminale without Spinal Dysraphism

Lipomas of the filum terminale occur at the caudal tip of the spinal canal. These malformations are more common than lipomyelomeningoceles and greater than 90% are recognizable on CT or MRI.[23] The finding of a thickened filum terminale and a caudally descended conus medullaris are sufficient for the diagnosis.[23]

Patients with lipomas of the filum terminale may have similar symptoms to patients with lipomyelomeningocele and other tethered cord syndromes, including motor weakness, sensory disturbances, bladder and bowel malfunction, and pain. Their imaging and histologic characteristics are as described for other lipomatous tumors.

Surgical resection and untethering of the spinal cord are the mainstays of treatment for symptomatic lipomas of the filum terminale. Outcome data for these patients are similar to patients with spinal cord lipomas, with the majority showing improved motor, bowel, and bladder function and decreased pain.[3] Recurrence of these lipomas has not been reported. However, recurrent tethering of the spinal cord may occur and should be suspected when recurrent or progressive symptoms are noted.

ANGIOLIPOMA

The first spinal angiolipoma was described by Berenbruch in 1890.[1,13] Andaluz et al have recently reviewed the subject of angiolipomas within the CNS.[1] They reported 94 documented cases: 86 within the spinal canal (predominantly extradural) and 8 found intracranially.[1] Table 37-3 outlines the 8 reported intracranial angiolipomas.

The majority of cases of spinal angiolipomas are found in the posterior epidural compartment. This is in contrast to the infiltrating angiolipomas that occur more commonly in the anterior epidural space. More than 75% of the reported spinal canal cases occurred along the thoracic spine, the majority involving three or more spinal segments.[1,13] The intracranial angiolipomas appear too infrequently to make any generalizations regarding their most common locations (see Table 37-3).

The presentation of angiolipomas both intracranially and within the spinal canal may be more acute than that of the spinal cord lipomas and intracranial lipomas. Most patients seek treatment less than 1 year after the onset of symptoms. Long and fluctuating courses, however, are not unheard of, making the diagnosis more difficult. The acute precipitation of symptoms, in the case of angiolipomas, is likely related to complications within their vascular component, such as hemorrhage, thrombosis, vascular engorgement, and vascular steal.[1,13] Pregnancy has also been noted to precipitate symptoms from spinal and intracranial angiolipomas.[1] Like other mass lesions of the CNS, the size and location of the angiolipoma will dictate neurologic signs and symptoms.

The epidemiology of angiolipomas is difficult to trace because there are no clear-cut diagnostic criteria to define them. Some authors have suggested that if "lipomas and hemangiomas truly represent the limits of the same pathologic spectrum, angiolipoma, angiolipoma with erosion, and infiltrating angiolipoma may represent intermediate steps."[13] In addition, it would appear that some pathologists may use the term *angiolipoma* for capillary hemangiomas with a lipomatous component, whereas others diagnose highly vascularized lipomas as angiolipomas. According to the available published data, angiolipomas, as a group, account for 0.14% to 1.2% of all spinal tumors.[1,13] Based on the list accumulated by Andaluz et al,[1] it appears that angiolipomas are found more commonly in women

TABLE 37-3	Intracranial Angiolipomas Reported to Date		
Study	**Patient Age and Sex**	**Location**	**Presenting Symptoms**
Takeuchi, 1980	72-yr-old female	Suprasellar or parasellar	Acute subarachnoid hemorrhage and associated aneurysms
Wilkins, 1987	60-yr-old female	Parasellar	Seizures
Lach, 1994	65-yr-old female	Suprasellar	Hypopituitarism, cranial nerve deficit
Shuangshoti, 1995	25-yr-old male	Thalamic	Acute hemorrhage
Prabu, 1995	26-yr-old female	Frontoparietal	Seizures
Prabu, 1995	28-yr-old male	CPA	Deafness, ataxia, lower cranial nerve deficits
Murakami, 1997	31-yr-old male	Internal auditory canal	Recurrent acute hearing loss
Andaluz, 2000	29-yr-old female	Frontal	Seizures

CPA, Cerebellopontine angle.
(Modified from Andaluz N, Balko G, Bui H, Zuccarello M: Angiolipomas of the central nervous system. J Neurooncol 49:219–230, 2000.)

than men (1.65:1), presenting most commonly in the fourth or fifth decades of life. The mean age of presentation was 43 years in both the infiltrating and noninfiltrating spinal angiolipoma groups. No statistical analysis was performed on the intracranial angiolipoma group given the small sample size.

As mentioned previously, lipomatous tumors have a characteristic appearance on CT and MRI and angiolipomas are no exception. However, variations in the appearance of these tumors may be related to their intense vascularity, with their individual appearance on MRI dependent on the relative contributions of adipose tissue and vasculature within the tumor. Interestingly, angiolipomas tend not to show flow voids on MRI. This may be related to the relatively high density of slow-flow capillary and venous channels within them. Infiltrating angiolipomas may produce trabeculated patterns within vertebral bodies, in some cases resembling hemangiomas; however, angiolipomas do not show late enhancement with contrast.[1]

Therapy has generally consisted of surgery, by way of a posterior approach, as in the case of intraspinal lipomas. There are no documented cases of radiation therapy or chemotherapy used for treatment of these benign lesions. Recurrence has not been documented to occur. Once the tumor is removed, the prognosis is generally good, with most patients achieving near-complete or complete recovery.[1,13]

HIBERNOMA

Hibernomas are rare tumors composed of brown adipose tissue that recapitulates the microvesicular storage seen within special fat deposits in hibernating animal species. Hibernomas were first described by Merkel in 1906 and named by Gery in 1914.[4] There are occasional reports in the literature of "pure" hibernomas within the CNS. Shuangshoti and Menakanit[17] reported a 14-year-old boy with an intradural, extramedullary hibernoma extending from L3 to L5. Chitoku et al[4] reported the case of a 35-year-old woman who had an intradural, extramedullary hibernoma at the level of C7. In 1972 Vagn-Hansen and Osgard reported the case of a 33-year-old woman with a parasagittal hibernoma; to our knowledge this is the only reported case of an intracranial hibernoma.[21]

Clinical presentations were as expected for mass lesions at the lumbosacral and cervical cord levels. The 14-year-old boy had lower back pain extending into the calves, whereas the 35-year-old woman had motor weakness and numbness of the left upper extremity.[4,17] The 33-year-old woman with the parasagittal hibernoma had partial motor seizures.[21]

Radiographic imaging of hibernomas is similar to other lipomatous tumors. The L3 to L5 lesion was discovered on myelogram in the pre-CT era, and the cervical lesion was noted to be highly vascular, appearing more like an angiolipoma. This latter lesion was noted to be hyperintense on both T1- and T2-weighted MRI scans and markedly contrast enhanced. The intracranial hibernoma was suspected on carotid angiography.

Grossly, hibernomas are well encapsulated and slightly dark-yellow to red-brown. Surgical specimens are required to make the correct final diagnosis.[4,21] Histologically, hibernomas are composed of brown adipose tissue, considered to be an immature form of white adipose tissue. These tumors are generally positive for S-100 protein as are normal fat cells. Combined hibernoma and lipomas are probably more common than pure hibernomas.[4]

Therapy for hibernomas consists of surgical resection. In contrast to intracranial and intraspinal lipomas, these tumors are easily separable from the surrounding tissue. Recurrence is rare, given their benign nature. However, there is one questionable report of a malignant hibernoma.[21] Standard postoperative follow-up is likely adequate.

INTRACRANIAL LIPOSARCOMA

Primary intracranial liposarcomas, like hibernomas, are a very rare tumor type within the lipomatous tumor group. There is a paucity of case reports in the literature. Kothandaram[11] reported a case in a 4-month-old girl, Sima at al[18] reported a case in a 70-year-old woman, and Cinalli et al[5] identified a case of a liposarcoma related to a subdural hematoma in a 6-month-old girl. There is also a letter to the editor from Shuangshoti in which he mentions two additional cases. One of these cases was described as occurring in the CPA and extending through the ipsilateral jugular foramen to an extracranial location.[16]

Initial signs and symptoms were consistent with mass lesions within the skull. The 4-month-old girl had macrocranium and was vomiting,[11] and the 70-year-old woman had dizziness and ataxia.[18] Both of these cases were reported in the pre-CT era and were correctly diagnosed only after surgical resection. The 6-month-old girl had partial seizures following trauma to the head, and a CT revealed subdural bleeding. This same patient was readmitted 2 years later for vomiting and decreased consciousness. MRI scans at that time revealed a subdural fluid collection plus contrast-enhanced nodules.[5] These nodules subsequently proved to be liposarcomas in the subdural space. These few reported cases involve tumors that are predominantly dural-based. MRI is the study of choice for these lesions.

Liposarcomas, in general, may be classified into five histologic subtypes. These include well-differentiated, myxoid, round-cell, pleomorphic, and mixed type, which may be further subdivided into predominantly well-differentiated and myxoid types with round-cell or pleomorphic areas. These subtypes have a definite prognostic significance for systemic liposarcomas, with the best prognosis associated with the well-differentiated liposarcomas and the worst prognosis associated with the pleomorphic liposarcomas.[18,24] In contrast to the benign lipomatous tumor types discussed previously, the liposarcomas are malignant and, depending upon their subtype, show the variable presence of mitotic figures, hemorrhage, and necrosis.

Therapeutic considerations for primary intracranial liposarcomas are different than for other lipomatous tumors of the CNS because of their malignant behavior. More aggressive surgical resection plus radiation therapy and chemotherapy should be employed to manage these tumors. However, given their rarity, no clinical protocols have been established for their treatment. Ifosfamide, carboplatin, and etoposide were used with some efficacy in the pediatric patient who initially experienced a subdural hematoma and was later diagnosed with dural-based intracranial liposarcomas.[5] In a large study of systemic liposarcomas not primary within the CNS, it was concluded that surgery plus radiation therapy is more effective for liposarcomas than surgery alone.[24] The efficacy of radiation therapy in the CNS, however, must be weighed against its potential morbidity, especially in the pediatric population.

In general, the prognosis for patients with intracranial liposarcomas, like patients with liposarcomas at other sites,

may be related to patient age, tumor size, and tumor subtype.[24] Two of the three reported cases of primary intracranial liposarcoma illustrate this. Of the two patients with high-grade variants of liposarcomas, the 4-month-old girl who had macrocranium and was vomiting survived for only 28 months after diagnosis. The second pediatric patient, who had a subdural fluid collection, lived for only 14 months after diagnosis.

Like other primary malignant tumors of the CNS, recurrence of intracranial liposarcomas is to be expected. These patients, therefore, need close follow-up and repeated imaging studies to watch for signs of recurrence. In addition, the consideration must always be given that the lesion may be metastatic rather than primary, although this is rare. In a recent study from Memorial Sloan Kettering Cancer Center, less than 1% of all soft tissue sarcomas metastasized to brain, with 21 brain metastases occurring in 3829 patients. However, of these few metastatic soft tissue sarcomas to the brain, liposarcomas were the second most common type, accounting for 5 of the 21 cases.[7]

LIPOMATOUS CHANGE IN NEUROCYTOMAS, EPENDYMOMAS, ASTROCYTOMAS, AND MENINGIOMAS

Finally, lipomatous change can be found either focally or as a widespread feature within more common types of brain and dural neoplasms. It is useful to be aware of these admittedly rare entities, because the neuroimaging signal characteristics, intraoperative impression, and histopathologic features will be that of a lipid-containing tumor. Lipomatous differentiation has been reported in ependymomas, neurocytomas, medulloblastomas (although many of these tumors have been reclassified as less aggressive cerebellar liponeurocytomas), cerebellar and spinal cord astrocytomas, and primitive neuroectodermal tumors.[14] Central liponeurocytomas[8] and lipomatous change in meningiomas[9] have also been described.

References

1. Andaluz N, Balko G, Bui H, Zuccarello M: Angiolipomas of the central nervous system. J Neurooncol 49:219–230, 2000.
2. Arai H, Sato K, Okuda O, et al: Surgical experience of 120 patients with lumbosacral lipomas. Acta Neurochir 143:857–864, 2001.
3. Bulsara KR, Zomorodi AR, Villavicencio AT, et al: Clinical outcome differences for lipomyelomeningoceles, intraspinal lipomas, and lipomas of the filum terminale. Neurosurg Rev 24:192–194, 2001.
4. Chitoku S, Kawai S, Watabe Y, et al: Intradural spinal hibernoma: case report. Surg Neurol 49:509–513, 1998.
5. Cinalli G, Zerah M, Carteret M, et al: Subdural sarcoma associated with chronic subdural hematoma. J Neurosurg 86:553–557, 1997.
6. Donati F, Vassella F, Kaiser G, Blumberg A: Intracranial lipomas. Neuropediatrics 23:32–38, 1992.
7. Espat NJ, Bilsky M, Lewis JJ, et al: Soft tissue sarcoma brain metastases. Prevalence in a cohort of 3829 patients. Cancer 94:2706–2711, 2002.
8. George DH, Scheithauer BW: Central liponeurocytoma. AJSP 25:1551–1555, 2001.
9. Jesionek-Kupnicka D, Liberski PP, Kordek R, et al: Metaplastic meningioma with lipomatous change. Folia Neuropathol 35:187–190, 1997.
10. Klekamp J, Fusco M, Samii M: Thoracic intradural extramedullary lipomas: report of three cases and review of the literature. Acta Neurochir 143:767–774, 2001.
11. Kothandaram P: Dural liposarcoma associated with subdural hematoma. J Neurosurg 33:85–87, 1970.
12. McGillicuddy GT, Shucart W, Kwan ESK: Intradural spinal lipomas. Neurosurgery 21:343–346, 1987.
13. Pagni CA, Canavero S: Spinal epidural angiolipoma: rare or unreported? Neurosurgery 31:758–764, 1992.
14. Ruchoux MM, Kepes JJ, Dhellemmes P, et al: Lipomatous differentiation in ependymomas. AJSP 22:338–346, 1998.
15. Saatci I, Aslan C, Renda Y, Besim A: Parietal lipoma associated with cortical dysplasia and abnormal vasculature: case report and review of the literature. AJNR 21:1718–1721, 2000.

16. Shuangshoti S: Primary intracranial liposarcomas. J Neurosurg 55:1011, 1981.

17. Shuangshoti S, Menakanit W: Intraspinal hibernoma. Br J Surg 61:580–582, 1974.

18. Sima A, Kindblom LG, Pellettieri L: Liposarcoma of the meninges. Acta Pathol Microbiol Scand A 84:306–310, 1976.

19. Tankere F, Vitte E, Martin-Duvemeuil N, et al: Cerebellopontine Angle lipomas: Report of four cases and review of the literature. Neurosurgery 50:626–632, 2002.

20. Truwit CL, Barkovich AJ: Pathogenesis of intracranial lipoma: an MR study in 42 patients. Am J Roentgenol 155:855–864, 1990.

21. Vagn-Hansen PL, Osgard O: Intracranial hibernoma. Acta Pathol Microbiol Scand A 80:145–149, 1972.

22. Valenca MM, Valenca LP, Menezes TL: Computed tomography scan of the head in patients with migraine or tension-type headache. Arquivos de Neuro-Psiquiatria 60:542–547, 2002.

23. Wilkins RH, Rengachary SS: Neurosurgery, ed 2. New York, McGraw-Hill, 1996.

24. Zagars GK, Goswitz MS, Pollack A: Liposarcoma: outcome and prognostic factors following conservation surgery and radiation therapy. Int J Radiat Oncol Biol Phys 36:311–319, 1996.

CHAPTER 38

FIBROUS TUMORS

Egon M.R. Doppenberg, J. Chris Zacko, Michael Y. Chen,
and William C. Broaddus

Fibrous tumors are neoplasms arising from mesenchymal parenchyma and composed predominantly of fibroblasts. Fibroblasts are one of the principal cells derived from mesenchyme. They are responsible for synthesis and maintenance of the extracellular material (ground substance, fibers including collagen, and structural glycoproteins). This subset of neoplasms is rare in the central nervous system (CNS). Fibrous tumors can form in bones or soft tissues because both are mesenchymal-derived tissue. In the World Health Organization (WHO) classification of brain tumors they are classified among mesenchymal, nonmeningothelial tumors of the meninges.

Mesenchyme is embryonic tissue originating from mesoderm, which is one of the three germ cell layers resulting from gastrulation. After formation, mesenchyme migrates from the original mesodermal germ layer to various regions of the body to form specialized tissues. Mesenchyme can be thought of as a primordial loose embryonic connective tissue consisting of mesenchymal cells, usually in stellate form, supported in interlaminar jelly—the gelatinous material between ectoderm and endoderm that serves as the substrate on which mesenchymal cells migrate.

Sources of mesenchymal cells within the cranial cavity are dura, pial, or adventitial fibroblasts covering perforating blood vessels deep in the cerebral white matter, tela choroidea, and the stroma of the choroids plexus.

This chapter reviews the following subtypes of fibrous tumors:

- Solitary fibrous tumor
- Fibrosarcoma
- Benign and malignant fibrous histiocytoma

SOLITARY FIBROUS TUMOR OF THE MENINGES

Solitary fibrous tumors (SFTs) have only recently been described as a separate entity of tumor involving the CNS, with only 35 cases being reported to date.[6] They are a relatively rare and discrete, collagen-rich, spindle-cell neoplasm, now known to be of mesenchymal origin, which have been benign in all but one case.[6]

Location

These types of tumors are most commonly found outside the CNS. Historically, they are most commonly associated with the pleura. However, they may also occur paracranially (orbit, nose, paranasal sinuses), attached to the peritoneum, or in the kidney, liver, lung, and bone. When related to the neuraxis, they occur more commonly in the cranium than in the spine. Of note is that paracranial SFTs may extend into the intracranial compartment from an origin in the infratemporal fossa or nasal cavity.

Generally, SFTs of the CNS have sites of predilection quite similar to those of meningiomas. However, SFTs are more commonly located in the posterior fossa and in the spinal compartment when compared with meningiomas. Intracranial SFTs almost exclusively originate from dura, whereas 8 of the 12 described spinal SFTs were not related to dura. Furthermore, one of these spinal SFTs was strictly intramedullary.[6]

Diagnosis

The signs and symptoms resulting from these lesions are those of a slowly evolving mass.

Typically, these tumors have an indolent course, usually manifested by a slowly progressive neurologic deficit. Whereas general symptoms may include headaches and seizures, focal deficits may occur, and these depend on the location of the tumor. They include cranial nerve dysfunction, hemiparesis, unsteadiness, and cognitive dysfunction.

Epidemiology

Thirty-five cases of SFT of the meninges have been reported to date. The age range thus far has been from 11 to 73 years old (mean 48.6), but only three have occurred in patients under age 20. There is a slight male preponderance. The male-to-female ratio is 3:2. There have been no cases with a traceable family history and only one case showing prior history of radiation therapy for another neoplasm.[6]

Neuroimaging

In general, the imaging characteristics of SFTs are similar to those of meningiomas.

On computed tomography (CT), these lesions appear isodense to normal brain tissue and are usually brightly enhancing with contrast administration. On magnetic resonance imaging (MRI), these lesions are typically well defined. They are isointense on the T1 sequence and hypointense on T2. They are brightly enhanced and rather homogeneous to moderately heterogeneous with administration of gadolinium. Those regions within the mass that display both hypointensity and hyperintensity are thought to correspond to those areas within the tumor that demarcate boundaries between the collagenous and hypercellular areas of the tumor. Calcifications are uncommon. Other features include thickened dural tails, focal reactive hyperostosis or erosion of the inner table of the skull, mass effect on surrounding tissue, moderate peritumoral edema, capping cysts, and rarely, invasive behavior.[6]

Histology

Gross, microscopic, immunohistochemical, and ultrastructural characteristics of solitary fibrous tumor within the CNS are, not surprisingly, similar to those of solitary fibrous tumors of other tissues. There is no single diagnostic feature, and pattern variation is the rule; however, the typical appearance is an unencapsulated but well-circumscribed spindle-cell neoplasm composed of moderately cellular areas with relatively uniform cell morphology interlaced with densely collagenous bands. The collagen bands are similar to fibrous meningioma but less uniformly distributed. There is usually no necrosis or hemorrhage, and tumoral cyst formation has been described in only one case.

Macroscopically, the neoplasm is white to tan, firm but slightly rubbery, and has a smooth, unencapsulated surface. It has only recently been recognized as a dural-based neoplasm distinct from fibrous meningioma, because gross appearance is very similar. In all reported cases, the tumor has been found to compress surrounding CNS parenchyma, but only four cases demonstrate parenchymal invasion. Invasion of dural venous sinuses by intracranial SFTs is relatively common. Focal infiltration of overlying bone has been noted.[3] Overall, they are moderately vascular, but an array has been reported, from virtually avascular to quite vascular on inspection.[6] Blood vessels are classically thin walled and ectatic with variable concentration of distribution. These blood vessels lack hyalinization (as seen in meningioma and schwannoma), and only one case has shown the classic "staghorn" pattern seen with hemangiopericytoma.

Some cases depart from the typical pattern and contain tumor cells in alternative arrangements—such as storiform (a pattern of cellular arrangement seen in certain fibrous tumors when the elongated cells intersect or intertwine at various angles so as to resemble the weaving of a doormat), herringbone, or patternless. Giant cells, although seen in one case, are not typical, and probably represent a degenerative process without malignant potential. As with many tumors, immunohistochemical staining is critical in making the final diagnosis of SFTs. They have strong and diffuse cytoplasmic immunopositivity for CD34, vimentin, bcl-2, reticulin, factor XIIIa, and scattered immunoreactivity to Leu-7. They are variably immunopositive for progesterone and estrogen receptors. There is no strong nuclear staining, but weak staining for p53 is seen. The MIB-1 index ranges from 1% to 18%, with an average of 1.1%.[6] Electron microscopy demonstrates neoplastic cells with ultrastructural characteristics of fibroblasts. Ultrastructural features associated with smooth muscle or meningothelial differentiation have not been identified. It was these light and electron microscopic characteristics, as well as their distinct immunohistochemical profile, that led to the conclusion that SFTs originate from fibroblasts or primitive mesenchymal cells. These primitive cells are thought to have features of multidirectional differentiation, which explains the rare cases with positive staining for markers of neural and muscle differentiation. The cells were primarily elongate or angular with evenly distributed chromatin.[3] Nucleoli varied, from ovoid to irregularly indented with small chromocenters, and sometimes were not prominently observed at all. Cytoplasm was moderate and contained abundant dilated rough endoplasmic reticulum (RER), occasional mitochondria, lipid droplets, scattered lamellar mitosis, intermittent microfilaments, and a small number of intermediate filaments.[3] The occasional psammoma bodies seen in spinal SFTs are unusual and may represent incorporation of arachnoid membrane.

Until recently, all cases of SFTs of the meninges were benign. However, one case of malignant primary meningeal SFT and one case of metastatic meningeal SFT have been reported. The malignant case was locally aggressive with many atypical features, having invaded the falx cerebri, superior sagittal sinus, and brain. Mitotic index in this case was 6 phf. Immunochemistry was the same as in benign cases, with the addition of weak membranous positivity for anti-Ewing's sarcoma MIC-2.[6]

The histopathologic differential diagnosis of SFT of the meninges centers on other spindle cell tumors that arise in the meninges. This neoplasm should be considered for any meningeal mass with a fibrous component. The differential diagnosis includes fibrous meningioma, schwannoma, hemangiopericytoma, leiomyoma, various meningeal sarcomas, meningeal myofibroblastoma, anaplastic meningioma, malignant fibrous histiocytoma, and other benign fibrous and fibrohistiocytic lesions of the meninges. As with any poorly differentiated tumor, cell lineage must be extensively investigated using immunohistochemistry and electron microscopy. CD34 immunostaining is helpful in distinguishing SFTs from other neoplasms. SFTs display diffuse, strong CD34 expression, in contrast to other entities in the differential diagnosis, where CD34 staining is mostly limited to the vascular bed.[7]

Therapy

Surgical resection is the mainstay of treatment of these lesions, with the intention of gross-total resection. Radiation therapy has been reported as successful in selected cases outside the CNS; however, the role of radiation therapy in the treatment of these tumors arising from the meninges is not well established and may potentially be considered in tumors that are not amenable to surgical resection or in patients who are poor surgical candidates. Overall, the rare incidence of these tumors has prevented thorough evaluation of adjuvant therapy.[6]

Recurrence and Outcome

Again, generalizations regarding recurrence and outcome are made with reservation, considering the paucity of reported cases, and we base our recommendations mostly on the behavior of pleural SFTs. It can be said that SFTs in the pleura behave benignly. Of pleural SFTs, 30% have some atypical features, and 15% to 20% show local invasion, intrathoracic spread, or distant metastasis. Reviewing CNS cases, invasion occurred in only four cases and complete resection has been possible in most.

Recurrence has been reported in only 4 of the 35 known cases; 2 of the 23 reported intracranial cases and 2 of the 12 spinal cases.[6]

Although an understanding of the behavior of SFT of the meninges is limited by the small number of reported cases, the evidence gathered thus far indicates that its behavior is much like that of SFT of other tissues, with a largely benign course. The extent of resection and level of invasion or metastasis are the most prognostic measures, with the most important being resectability and tumor size. No single histologic feature has been associated with malignant tendencies or poor prognosis. Anaplastic features such as high cellularity, mitotic figures, and pleomorphism are poor prognostic indicators unless the lesion is completely resectable.[6]

FIBROSARCOMA

Fibrosarcomas are discrete spindle cell neoplasms of mesenchymal origin comprising malignant fibroblasts in a background of collagen. These tumors are a subset of the larger category of neoplasms, meningeal sarcomas, the distinction being that fibrosarcomas are sarcomas (neoplasm of mesenchymal origin) that have differentiated along the fibroblastic cell line.

Location

Fibrosarcomas can appear in three situations in the CNS: as part of a gliosarcoma, following irradiation of tumors like pituitary adenomas, or rarely, as a primary tumor.

A primary fibrosarcoma in the CNS is either dural based or arises within the brain, possibly from leptomeningeal infoldings. The fibrosarcomas that arise de novo are associated with varying patient demographics in regard to age, localization, and microscopic features. Some are discrete dural masses with a tendency to infiltrate adjacent bone, whereas others are diffuse leptomeningeal lesions.

Although primary fibrosarcomas arise de novo, a minority of cases are secondary and develop from preexisting lesions, such as fibrous dysplasia, benign tumors, bone infarcts, pagetic bone, and chronic osteomyelitis, and previous fields of radiation. Those that are attributed to irradiation most often arise in the sellar region after treatment of a pituitary adenoma. Extensive involvement of the bone, dura, leptomeninges, and brain generally obscures a precise origin. The latency period between onset of radiation treatment and the discovery of sarcomas ranges from 5 to 12 years. Histologically, these tumors resemble a fibrosarcoma at any other body site. The origin of the tumor still raises some controversy; although most authors have proposed a meningeal origin, others have suggested that the vascular endothelium is the site of origin for these tumors.

Diagnosis

Symptoms vary with size, location, and extent of spread of the tumor. They include headaches, signs of increased intracranial pressure, seizures, or hemiparesis. Those located at the base of the skull might cause cranial nerve deficits.

Epidemiology

Primary fibrosarcomas of the dura mater are very rare and make up less than 0.5% to 2.7% of all intracranial neoplasms.

Although primary fibrosarcomas of the dura occur at any age, most often patients are between 30 and 50. The more poorly differentiated fibrosarcomas tend to occur in the older patients. There is an equal sex distribution, and no racial predilection seems to exist.

Infantile fibrosarcoma is the most common soft tissue sarcoma found in children younger than 1 year of age, but location within the CNS is still an uncommon site. They carry a better overall prognosis than adult cases, even with metastasis present, and can be treated successfully with surgery and chemotherapy.[2,4,10]

Neuroimaging

MRI will generally show an intensely enhanced lesion after administration of contrast. These lesions may also contain foci of hemorrhage. CT scans are useful to delineate bony involvement or destruction.

Histology

Gross specimens reveal large, hemorrhagic, tan-white masses that destroy bone and invade soft tissue. The cells segregate into a firm, discrete mass. They are typically soft, unencapsulated (as opposed to fibromas), infiltrative, "fish-flesh" masses. Note that they may appear encapsulated if well differentiated. They routinely have areas of hemorrhage and necrosis. These tumors vary in aggressiveness, but at diagnosis generally carry a low to intermediate grade. The degree of cellular differentiation between tumors varies widely, with virtually the entire range of possibilities existing. It is the cellular differentiation that determines the amount of collagen and cytologic atypia. Immunocytochemistry is positive for vimentin, but not for glial fibrillary acidic protein (GFAP), S-100 protein, or epithelial membrane antigen (EMA).

The configuration of malignant fibroblasts is described as a herringbone pattern demonstrating an entwining pattern of sheets of spindle-shape fibroblasts in a collagen background. High-grade lesions are very cellular with marked anaplasia, pleomorphism, cellular atypia, mitotic activity, and necrosis that may bring to mind the histologic features of malignant fibrous histiocytoma.

Ultrastructural features include prominent bipolar cells, nuclei with coarse chromatin, and rough endoplasmic reticulum with dilated cristae. There is no basement membrane, and rarely are there cytoplasmic intermediate filaments and dense bodies.

Differential diagnosis includes fibrous dysplasia, benign and malignant fibrous histiocytoma, desmoid tumors, malignant schwannoma, osteosarcoma, Paget's sarcoma, and high-grade osteosarcoma. The distinction between fibroblastic collagen-producing sarcomas of bone, fibrosarcoma, and malignant fibrous histiocytoma is based on somewhat arbitrary morphologic criteria. If a tumor is dura based, it may be difficult to say whether the sarcoma has arisen de novo or it represents a sarcomatous change in a meningioma. The herringbone arrangement of fibroblasts will suggest fibrosarcoma rather than meningioma.

Therapy

Information regarding optimum treatment of primary fibrosarcomas arising intracranially is limited because of their rarity, and the best form of therapy is not yet known. Furthermore, no recommendation can be made regarding differences in therapy between primary and secondary intracranial fibrosarcomas. Treatment is based on the patient's age, overall health, the extent of the disease upon diagnosis, and the estimation of disease progression. Currently, the primary treatment consists of a combination of surgical resection, chemotherapy, and radiation therapy.

Recurrence and Outcome

Gaspar et al described nine patients with primary intracranial fibrosarcomas, 78% of which were high grade. The median survival time was 7.5 months. Local recurrence developed in eight patients and distant recurrence in six. Systemic metastases developed in four patients (50%) and meningeal seeding in four patients (50%). Longer survival was observed in superficially located tumors compared with intracerebral tumors. This clearly indicates that this type of tumor has a very poor prognosis despite multimodality therapy.[4]

BENIGN FIBROUS HISTIOCYTOMA AND MALIGNANT FIBROUS HISTIOCYTOMA

Fibrous histiocytomas are a rare and diverse group of pleomorphic lesions composed predominantly of two cell types of variable proportion: atypical fibroblasts and histiocytes. They are fibroblastic, hence mesenchymal, collagen-producing sarcomas of bone and soft tissues. There is a benign fibrous histiocytoma (BFH) and a malignant fibrous histiocytoma (MFH). Because of the dual cell composition and varied microscopic appearance, these tumors have been historically difficult to classify. As a result, they have either been incompletely identified or prematurely designated as a different entity such as dermatofibroma, sclerosing hemangioma, xanthogranuloma, fibroxanthoma, or nodular subepidermal fibrosis.

Location

These tumors can be attached to the dura or seated in the parenchyma. The benign variant is more often dural based, although MFH occurs equally in the parenchyma as well as attached to the dura. The malignant occurrences can arise as a primary or metastatic lesion of the skull. Outside the CNS, MFH occurs most commonly in the soft tissues of extremities, followed by the retroperitoneum. Like fibrosarcoma, it has been reported to arise from preexisting lesions such as areas of irradiation, bone infarction, trauma, Paget's disease, and fibrous dysplasia.

Diagnosis

Symptoms caused by these lesions vary with size, location, and extent of spread of the tumor. They include headaches, signs of increased intracranial pressure, seizures, or hemiparesis. Those located at the base of the skull might cause cranial nerve deficits.

Epidemiology

Primary BFH of the CNS is an extremely rare entity with fewer than 10 case reports described in the literature. They have been described in men and women as well as children.

After review of the literature, Akimoto presented a total of 22 documented cases of primary MFHs. Seventeen of these cases were described, and 14 of these patients were male.[1] To date, fewer than 30 primary MFHs of the brain have been reported. As far as secondary or radiation-induced MFH is concerned, their exact incidence and prevalence is unknown.

Neuroimaging

The MRI findings are nonspecific and include a well-delineated oval mass with low signal intensity on T1-weighted images and high signal intensity on T2-weighted images and marked heterogeneous contrast enhancement, with possibly dural tail signs mimicking meningioma. CT can further delineate bony involvement. No specific findings are present to predict this diagnosis with high likelihood.

Histology

Both the benign and malignant variant of fibrous histiocytoma have been described as firm, circumscribed, and sometimes invading the surrounding tissue with various degrees of peritumoral edema. As previously stated, these tumors can be either dural based or arising in the parenchyma. Microscopically, they show spindle-shaped fibroblast-like cells and more rounded cells with clear, oval nuclei, consistent with histiocytes, possessing abundant vacuolated cytoplasm. The malignant variant shows a high number of mitoses, necrotic foci, and at times infiltration by inflammatory cells, such as neutrophils, into the surrounding brain. Immunohistochemically, these tumors are positive for histiocytic markers such as alpha-1-antitrypsin, alpha-1-antichymotrypsin, muramidase, and vimentin. They are negative for GFAP. Electron microscopic findings of an admixture of pleomorphic fibroblast-like and histiocyte-like cells is the most reliable finding.[8,9]

Therapy

For BFH, surgical resection alone is the therapy of choice. In reviewing the literature Akito found that surgical excision was performed in 16 of 17 cases of MFH. Radiation therapy was performed postoperatively in 9 of 13 cases; however, different doses and methods were used in this small patient group, and therefore no conclusions can be made as far as the optimal radiation therapy strategy. No studies have been done to clarify the efficacy of chemotherapy in treatment of MFH. A variety of regimens have been tried and reported anecdotally; however, their effectiveness remains unclear.[5]

Recurrence

Local recurrence is approximately 30% in some reports, with distant metastases in up to 18%. The tumor-free interval has been reported as approximately 7 months in these cases. The distant metastases were found in the lung and the axillary and inguinal lymph nodes. One-year survival of 46% has been reported in the literature, with only 23% survival at 2 years, despite currently available therapy.[1]

References

1. Akimoto J, Takeda Y, Hasue M, et al: Primary meningeal malignant fibrous histiocytoma with cerebrospinal dissemination and pulmonary metastasis. Acta Neurochir 140:1191–1196, 1998.

2. Bisogno G, Roganovic J, Carli M, et al: Primary intracranial fibrosarcoma. Childs Nerv Syst 18:648–651, 2002.

3. Castilla EA, Prayson RA, Stevens GH, et al: Brain-invasive solitary fibrous tumor of the meninges: report of a case. Int J Surg Pathol 10:217–221, 2002.

4. Gaspar LE, Mackenzie IR, Gilbert JJ, et al: Primary cerebral fibrosarcomas. Clinicopathologic study and review of the literature. Cancer 72:3277–3281, 1993.

5. Ham SJ, Hoekstra HJ, van der Graaf WT, et al: The value of high-dose methotrexate-based neoadjuvant chemotherapy in malignant fibrous histiocytoma of bone. J Clin Oncol 14:490–496, 1996.

6. Martin AJ, Fisher C, Igbaseimokumo U, et al: Solitary fibrous tumours of the meninges: case series and literature review. J Neurooncol 54:57–69, 2001.

7. Obara Y, Matsumoto M, Chiba K, et al: Solitary cervical fibrous tumor. Case illustration. J Neurosurg 98:111, 2003.

8. Paulus W, Slowik F, Jellinger K: Primary intracranial sarcomas: histopathological features of 19 cases. Histopathology 18:395–402, 1991.

9. Simpson RH, Phillips JI, Miller P, et al: Intracerebral malignant fibrous histiocytoma: a light and electron microscopic study with immunohistochemistry. Clin Neuropathol 5:185–189, 1986.

10. Tomita T, Gonzalez-Crussi F. Intracranial primary nonlymphomatous sarcomas in children: experience with eight cases and review of the literature. Neurosurgery 14:529–540, 1984.

CHAPTER 39

MELANOCYTIC TUMORS

Nezih Oktar, Tarik Tihan, and G. Evren Keles

Melanocytic lesions in the central nervous system (CNS) can be considered in two broad categories: lesions that are non-neoplastic or "hamartomatous," and those that are considered clearly neoplastic. The hamartomatous lesions include neurocutaneous melanosis or diffuse melanocytosis, which refer to the presence of melanin pigment in the cells of the CNS that normally produce little or no pigment. The coexistence of skin and leptomeningeal lesions define the term neurocutaneous melanosis. Leptomeningeal melanocytosis can also be associated with melanocytic neoplasms, suggesting that the two categories of lesions are closely related.[36,43,44] Despite its non-neoplastic nature, leptomeningeal melanomatosis or neurocutaneous melanocytosis is an often fatal condition associated with giant congenital pigmented nevi.[59]

The melanocytic lesions that will be covered in this chapter include neurocutaneous melanosis and diffuse melanocytosis, melanocytoma, and primary malignant melanomas.

NEUROCUTANEOUS MELANOSIS AND DIFFUSE MELANOCYTOSIS

Neurocutaneous melanosis was recognized in the latter half of the nineteenth century, and since its description, more than 100 cases have been reported.[36] Peak incidence was reported to be in the fourth decade, affecting both sexes equally.[26] Diffuse melanocytosis usually manifests in children and involves supratentorial and infratentorial leptomeninges. Symptomatic leptomeningeal melanosis with giant congenital nevi is more prevalent in the young.[26,28,59] Thirty percent of patients with giant pigmented nevi were reported to eventually develop leptomeningeal melanoma. Because intracranial melanocytic lesions were diagnosed using various criteria, objective assessment of their incidence and epidemiologic characteristics has not been possible. This lesion is most commonly recorded as sporadic and was considered as an example of a genetic disorder's autosomal lethal genes surviving in a mosaic state.[26,28,33]

Pathologic Features

On gross examination, the meninges of diffuse melanocytic lesions appear densely black and can involve the basal cisterns. The meningeal layer becomes diffusely thickened and pigmented, most noticeably in the brainstem and base of the brain. Neurocutaneous melanosis has been observed in cerebral and cerebellar convexities, the cerebellopontine angle, the quadrigeminal plate, Meckel's cave, or the pineal gland. Gross identification depends on the recognition of color change. These lesions typically are not mass lesions.

Histologically, neurocutaneous melanosis consists of an increased number of spindle to ovoid cells with granular, brown pigment distributed throughout the leptomeningeal layers. These cells sometimes resemble meningothelial cells and contain eosinophilic cytoplasm, large nucleoli, and oval nuclei.[43] Mitosis is typically absent, and the lesion does not form large cellular clusters. The lesions may contain areas of recent and old hemorrhage or reactive changes; however, by definition, no mass is recognized. Immunohistochemically, the pigmented cells are positive for antibodies against S-100 protein, melan-A, and HMB-45 antigens.[43,46] Staining for vimentin is often strongly positive. Staining for epithelial markers, cytokeratin, or glial fibrillary acidic protein (GFAP) are typically negative. On ultrastructural studies, the cells exhibit abundant cytoplasm with many dendrites, organelles, and melanosomes in different stages of melanogenesis.[46] Unlike meningiomas, intercellular junctions and basement membrane formation are not observed.

Neurocutaneous melanosis characteristically involves a combination of multiple focally or diffuse pigmented congenital cutaneous nevi in addition to accumulation of melanotic cells in the meninges. These nevi usually exhibit histologic features of typical congenital nevi. In cases where neurocutaneous melanosis is associated with a melanocytic neoplasm, the lesion is typically a malignant melanoma but also can be a melanocytoma.[17,27,36,37,52]

Clinical Features

Neurocutaneous melanosis is often associated with giant congenital pigmented nevi.[26,28] These nevi preferentially involve the midline in the head and neck region, as well as the scalp. Often, the distribution of melanosis is quite variable. They become most noticeable in the basal leptomeninges, cerebral and cerebellar convexities, and the cerebellopontine angle.

In the adult, neurocutaneous melanosis can be asymptomatic, and often, the pigmented leptomeningeal lesions are incidental findings on autopsy.[7] In children, however, they are associated with congenital cutaneous lesions that occur as multiple or giant hairy, pigmented nevi found in the head, neck, trunk, lower abdomen, pelvis, buttocks, or upper thighs.[14,60] These patients are considered to have neurocutaneous melanosis, a disorder that, when symptomatic, carries a poor prognosis even in the absence of malignancy. The children become neurologically symptomatic within the first decade of life and may have seizures, meningitis, cranial nerve palsies, and signs of hydrocephalus.[26,28,36,69] Children with neurocutaneous melanosis may have more than 15 congenital cutaneous pigmented lesions measuring up to 15 cm.[14,15,43,44,69] In some cases, diagnosis can be suggested by the presence of pigment in CSF or neuroimaging,[15] yet the definitive diagnosis requires histopathologic evaluation of leptomeningeal tissue.

Children with large congenital melanocytic nevi may have associated leptomeningeal melanocytosis with or without CNS melanomas.[29,62,72] The disease was also reported in association with von Recklinghausen's disease, Sturge-Weber syndrome, Dandy-Walker syndrome, and hydrocephalus with arachnoid cysts.[4,23,26,44,53,69]

For all histologic entities covered in this chapter, magnetic resonance imaging (MRI) is the standard and most helpful neuroradiologic method because lesions containing melanin have unusual paramagnetic properties on both T1- and T2-weighted scans. On T1-weighted MRI scans, the melanin pigment within the melanocytes appears hyperintense to white matter and appears isodense to gray matter. On T2-weighted scans, the melanin-containing lesions appear hypointense compared with both white and gray matter. After infusion of intravenous contrast agents, melanocytic lesions diffusely enhance with intensity corresponding to the level of melanin pigment contained within the lesion. Paramagnetic free radicals associated with melanin are thought to be responsible for its unique MR properties.[24] Although methemoglobin and fat have similar MR signal properties as melanin, enhancement on postcontrast MR images can help distinguish melanocytic lesions from other lesions.[24] On computed tomography (CT) images, melanocytic lesions are usually isodense to hyperdense and enhance after contrast infusion.

Diffuse melanocytosis appears as thickened enhancing leptomeninges on both CT and MR scans, best depicted on coronal MR images. Neoplastic cells often spread into Virchow-Robin spaces, and these can be visualized on transverse images without involvement of brain parenchyma. Neurocutaneous melanosis on MR shows homogeneous enhancement of the leptomeninges with greatest signal in the cerebral convexities and at the base of the brain. However, absence of meningeal enhancement in neurocutaneous melanosis has been reported.[75] Imaging alone cannot distinguish benign from malignant forms of neurocutaneous melanosis, and the appearance of these lesions on MR is not pathognomonic.[75] Marked enhancement of the leptomeninges can also be seen in a variety of conditions, including meningitis; fungal infections; metastatic lesions from breast, renal, and lung tumors; and primary tumors of the brain that can spread to the leptomeninges.

Treatment and Outcome

Patients with diffuse melanocytosis have a poor outcome regardless of histologic malignancy.[59] The prognosis for most patients is poor despite various treatment modalities including chemotherapy and surgery, and often these lesions are fatal within a few years.[7,14,59] Patients with large congenital melanocytic nevi are at increased risk for developing melanoma.[2]

There is also a significant increased risk for developing neurocutaneous melanosis.[12]

For patients with neurocutaneous melanosis, prognosis is poor once neurologic symptoms occur.[5,75] In a study describing five children with neurocutaneous melanosis who had either seizures or signs of raised intracranial pressure within the first decade of life, all children died within 2 years despite chemotherapy.[14] From 1961 to 1991, eight patients with neurocutaneous melanosis were reported from the Hospital for Sick Children.[3] Survival of these eight patients ranged from 1 month to 54 months after diagnosis.[3]

MELANOCYTOMA

Fewer than 50 cases of melanocytomas have been reported in the literature, with only a few cases diagnosed in patients younger than age 30.[13,21,61] The lesion commonly occurs during the fourth or fifth decade as a solitary mass and affects both sexes equally. An accurate assessment of the incidence and epidemiologic characteristics of this extremely rare neoplasm is lacking.

Pathologic Features

Melanocytomas exist as discrete, encapsulated lesions whose color ranges from jet black to reddish brown.[13,55] Melanocytomas are soft to rubbery masses adherent to the leptomeninges and do not involve the underlying cortex.[13,30,55]

Melanocytomas contain variably pigmented melanocytic cells often arranged in tight nests, sheets, or fascicles. The tumors are often composed of spindled to oval cells remotely resembling well-differentiated melanocytes containing varying levels of melanin pigment. Although most melanocytomas are composed entirely of either spindled or ovoid cells, some tumors can exhibit a mixture of both cell types (Figure 39-1). Brain parenchymal invasion, vascular abnormalities, and coagulative necrosis are usually absent, and their presence raises the possibility of a malignant melanocytic neoplasm. Mitosis is extremely rare. In general, melanocytomas are well-differentiated tumors that are less cellular, have a lower nuclear-to-cytoplasmic ratio when compared with primary malignant melanoma, and lack nuclear hyperchromasia.[52] At the ultrastructural level, melanocytoma has distinctive cellular features such as poorly formed pericellular basal lamina, lack of cell junctions, and abundant melanosomes showing different stages of melanogenesis.[13,46,55] Absence of desmosomes and interdigitating cytoplasmic processes can help to distinguish melanocytic tumors from pigmented meningioma.[47] Intermediate junctions (zonula adherens) are rarely seen in melanocytomas.

Immunohistochemical detection of antigens such as melan-A, HMB-45, and S-100 and absence of staining with epithelial membrane antigen (EMA) are helpful in identifying the lesion as a melanocytic neoplasm and excluding meningioma; however, a word of caution is in order, because staining with these markers can be focal and variable in intensity. Absence of staining with cytokeratins, lymphoid, and histiocytic markers is useful to exclude carcinomas, T-cell, and histiocytic lymphomas. Schwannomas can often be ruled out based on the immunohistochemical pattern, but electron microscopy may be needed to exclude a schwannoma.

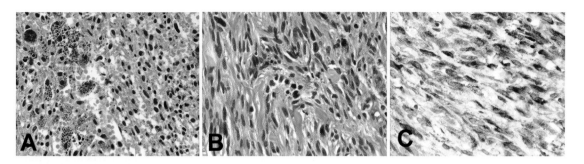

FIGURE 39-1   *A,* Microscopic image of a melanocytoma primarily composed of cells with round, oval, and occasionally spindle nuclei and abundant fine pigment deposition, typical of melanocytoma. (Original magnification ×400.) *B,* Microscopic appearance of a melanocytoma with predominantly spindled cells, collagenous background, and scattered pigment. These neoplasms can easily be confused with meningiomas or other stromal neoplasms. (Original magnification ×400.) *C,* Immunohistochemical staining for HMB-45, a melanocytic marker, is diffusely positive in this melanocytoma. The tumor is composed of primarily spindle cells as in *B.* (Original magnification ×400.)

Clinical Features

In contrast to diffuse melanocytosis and neurocutaneous melanosis, melanocytomas occur as solid masses, usually encapsulated, black or dark brown, and attached to the dura.[13,21,46,55,57] They often compress adjacent neural structures rather than infiltrate brain tissue.[13] They can occur throughout the CNS but have a predilection for the spinal canal and posterior fossa.[13,30,35,54,55,58] Occasional cases have been reported in Meckel's cave, the foramen magnum, and the pineal and suprasellar regions.[25,34] In almost all cases, the neoplasm appears extra-axial.[54]

Melanocytomas predominantly cause compression, either in the spinal cord or intracranially.[13] The duration of symptoms in patients with melanocytoma range from a few months to 10 years.[11,13,30,47,58,74] This range may be due in part to the slow rate of growth of the lesion as it eventually produces a mass effect; symptoms will depend on the site of the lesion.

On neuroradiologic studies, melanocytoma appears isodense with gray matter on CT scans, hyperintense on T1-weighted MR images, and hypointense on T2-weighted MR images.[24] The differential diagnosis for melanocytoma includes more common extra-axial tumors such as meningioma or schwannoma, partly because of the long duration of symptoms and their appearance on CT and MRI scans.[24,74]

Treatment and Outcome

In contrast to diffuse melanocytosis and neurocutaneous melanosis, melanocytomas occur as solid masses. The primary therapeutic modality is surgery. In surgery, melanocytoma usually appears as an encapsulated, black or dark brown mass attached to the dura.[13,47,49] They often compress adjacent neural structures rather than infiltrate brain tissue.[47,49]

The prognostic significance of various therapeutic modalities is not known. Although surgery is usually the initial approach in the management of most of these lesions, the effect of extent of resection and its ideal timing are not well defined. In the literature, the decision for adjuvant radiation treatment is primarily based on the extent of tumor resection. Most patients treated with radiation had lesions that were partially resected.[22] There is no convincing evidence regarding the effect of radiation therapy, and our knowledge is based on case reports.[42] Radiosurgery is a valuable mode of therapy when lesions are not amenable to surgical resection.[22] Melanocytomas are usually good candidates for radiosurgery, because they are discrete, and their slow proliferative rate allows prolonged relapse-free survival.[42]

Melanocytomas are usually low-grade melanocytic lesions that are often benign and are cured by total resection[13]; however, local recurrences have been reported, and therefore follow-up imaging studies are warranted even after total resection of lesions.[22] In various series, postoperative recurrence rate was calculated to range from 15% to 50.9%.[22,42,49,56] Although melanocytomas are usually diploid, cases with a significant population of aneuploid cells are more likely to exhibit an aggressive natural history.[31] The reported postoperative survival time ranges from 1 year to 28 years.[20,22] In a recent study, 11 of 17 melanocytoma lesions were surgically resected, and the remaining 6 lesions were partially resected.[13] Three of the six patients with subtotal resections also received radiation therapy (4500 to 5000 cGy). After a median follow-up of 36 months, none of the patients showed evidence of clinical or radiographic recurrence.[13] In a retrospective review, Rades et al concluded that complete resection was superior to partial resection alone or in combination with radiation. For patients with incompletely resected tumors, addition of radiation treatment showed a trend toward better survival.[56a]

MALIGNANT MELANOMA

Primary malignant melanoma of the CNS is not well characterized, and reports suggest an incidence of 1% or less compared with all melanomas.[32] There are fewer than 250 primary melanomas reported in the literature.[32,64,76] Peak incidence is in the fourth decade of life with a secondary peak in the first decade affecting both sexes equally. There is a strong association between primary melanoma and neurocutaneous melanosis, and such cases account for almost all melanomas in the pediatric population.[1-3,17,27,32,37,48,52,63,70,72] These rare tumors are extremely aggressive lesions.[3]

The prominent distinction between a primary and a metastatic melanoma is location. Even though it may not always be possible to distinguish all melanomas as primary or metastatic, a typical metastatic melanoma is a parenchymal lesion, whereas primary melanoma is associated with the meninges. Primary malignant melanoma can occur anywhere in the CNS, including the pineal, posterior fossa and cerebellopontine angle, and spinal cord.[3,6,61,76,77]

Pathologic Features

Malignant melanomas present a significant challenge to the surgical neuropathologist because they can show extreme variation in both morphologic and immunohistochemical features. Some tumors can easily be mistaken for glioblastoma, metastatic carcinoma, or even malignant peripheral nerve sheath tumor.[40] Histopathologic features other than location and multifocality cannot distinguish primary from metastatic melanomas. The only reliable method for the diagnosis of a primary melanoma is to exclude conclusively a primary site elsewhere in the body. In large series of melanomas, 60% to 80% of tumors occur as solitary lesions, whereas the remainder occur as multiple lesions at diagnosis.[9]

Macroscopically, both primary and metastatic melanomas are well-defined, dark lesions that are often friable, soft, and hemorrhagic. Typically, neurosurgeons find them easy to remove, because they can find a clear plane between the tumor and the parenchyma.

Malignant melanomas are poorly differentiated neoplasms with significant pleomorphism, large irregular nuclei with strikingly prominent nucleoli, numerous mitotic figures, and necrosis. The anaplasia encountered in most cases leaves no doubt as to the malignancy of the lesion. The histologic features of melanomas vary substantially and can include many subtypes such as pleomorphic, epithelioid, and spindle- and mixed-cell varieties. Rare examples also include the balloon-cell subtype, spindle cell subtype with microvilli, papillary, and a rhabdoid phenotype.[1,8,16,18] Approximately one third of melanomas do not contain detectable amounts of melanin on routine and special histochemical stains; however, most of these tumors display melanosomes in different stages of differentiation, making electron microscopy a very useful tool in identifying amelanotic melanomas. Typically, melanoma cells contain mature melanosomes and exhibit intracytoplasmic fine fibrils, whereas other tumor cells contain a small rim of ribosomal-rich cytoplasm, occasional premelanosomes, and no intracytoplasmic fibrils.[67] All tumors contain melanosomes, although the classic forms are more difficult to identify than the abnormal variant forms.[51]

Immunohistochemically, melanomas are often positive for one or more melanocytic markers, as well as S-100 protein and vimentin. Although not specific, HMB-45 immunoreactivity is often diagnostic of a malignant melanoma.[65] The combined panel of S-100 protein, HMB-45, and melan-A antibodies stains most melanomas. Interestingly, some primary and metastatic melanomas can stain for EMA or cytokeratins, further confounding the differential diagnosis.[10,66] Metastatic melanomas are found to stain with epithelial markers to a higher extent than primary lesions. Nevertheless, such examples constitute a minority of tumors, and exhibit strong positive staining with melanoma markers (HMB-45, melan-A).

Clinical Features

Primary melanoma of the CNS may occur either with localized intra-axial or extra-axial mass lesions or with meningeal spread, which carries a worse prognosis.[32] Primary leptomeningeal melanoma typically occurs in the young and in the setting of leptomeningeal melanosis. Patients with large congenital melanocytic nevi are at increased risk for developing melanomas.[12] The clinical presentation of primary malignant melanoma is variable and nonspecific and may include seizures, weakness, focal motor and sensory deficits, hydrocephalus, psychiatric changes, and cranial nerve palsies depending on the tumor location. A rare melanoma in the cerebellopontine angle can cause audiovestibular symptoms and facial nerve palsy.[45] The primary melanomas are usually solitary masses in contrast to multiple, small masses typical of metastatic melanoma. The diagnosis is often challenging, and primary melanomas can be confused with many non-neoplastic and neoplastic lesions. The neoplasms in the differential diagnosis include metastatic carcinoma, lymphoma, and primitive neuroectodermal tumor (PNET), as well as extra-axial tumors such as meningioma or schwannoma. CSF cytology may show melanin containing malignant or atypical cells, which suggest the diagnosis.[68] However, CSF cytology can be noninformative, even in cases with leptomeningeal dissemination.[50]

Malignant melanoma may vary in its imaging properties, because these lesions often have hemorrhagic, necrotic cores (Figure 39-2). They are typically hyperintense on T1-weighted images without contrast and uniformly hypointense on T-2 weighted images. Macroscopic and radiologic distinction between a melanocytoma and melanoma is extremely difficult, if not impossible.[13] Intraoperative impression is often that of a dural lesion, reminiscent of a meningioma, except for dark pigmented appearance.

Treatment and Outcome

The literature mostly consists of case reports with no high-quality evidence regarding the prognostic implications of various treatment options (i.e., surgery, radiation therapy, and chemotherapy).

The distinction between metastatic melanoma and primary melanoma of the CNS is important; total surgical resection of primary lesions has a relatively better prognosis than metastatic melanoma. Primary malignant melanomas have a higher level of local recurrence and a higher mortality rate, and their prognosis is more influenced by the extent of surgical resection of the lesion compared with the other melanocytic lesions.[13] Although malignant melanoma is considered to be resistant to radiation therapy, some disease control was achieved with the use of high-dose fractionated radiation.[38,41] Other treatment modalities for malignant melanoma, including chemotherapy, have also been tried with minimal success. DTIC [1-(4-amino-2-methyl-5-pyrimidinyl)-methyl-3-(2-chlororthyl)-3-nitrosourea], which is a common melanoma chemotherapy agent, as well as vincristine, cisplatin, and intrathecal methotrexate were not effective in halting disease progression.[3,73]

Although aggressive treatment with various modalities, including chemotherapy, radiation therapy, and surgery may help prolong survival, most patients die within a year.[13,39,71] The average survival rate for primary malignant melanomas is 5 to 10 months[3,39]; however, survival rates of up to 3 years have

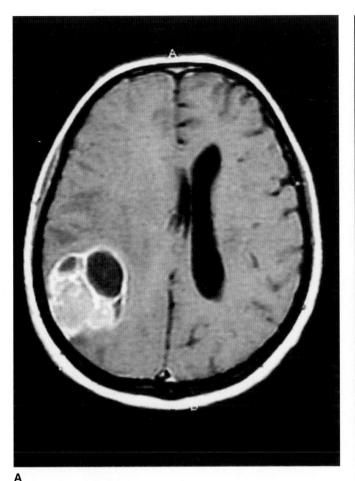

A

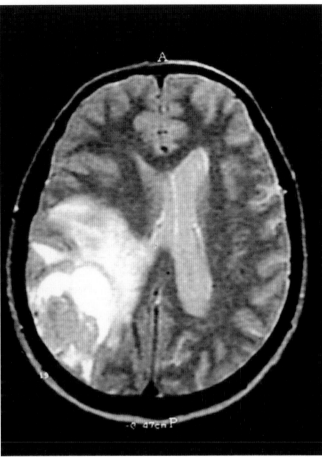

B

FIGURE 39-2 T1- *(A)* and T2- *(B)* weighted axial magnetic resonance images of a 54-year-old female patient with a right parietal primary malignant melanoma. The solid component of the tumor appears hyperintense on T1-weighted and hypointense on T2-weighted images. Progression-free survival was 8 weeks, and overall survival was 42 weeks with multiple resections, radiation therapy, and chemotherapy.

been reported after surgical resection.[76] In a recent study of 13 primary CNS melanomas, Brat et al reported a "cure" in 4 cases following complete resection, and 4 additional surviving cases following recurrences.[13] Their findings supported the suggestion that primary CNS melanomas have a better survival rate, and even "cure" may be achieved, in contrast with the dismal

outcomes of patients with melanomas metastatic to the CNS. The authors suggested complete surgical removal as the main goal of treatment in primary melanomas as well as melanocytomas.[13] Other case reports also support the suggestion of a better outcome in primary melanomas of the CNS in comparison with melanoma metastases.[64,71,76,77]

References

1. Adamek D, Kaluza J, and Stachura K: Primary balloon cell malignant melanoma of the right temporo-parietal region arising from meningeal naevus. Clin Neuropathol 14:29–32, 1995.
2. Akinwunmi J, Sgouros S, Moss C, et al: Neurocutaneous melanosis with leptomeningeal melanoma. Pediatr Neurosurg 35:277–279, 2001.
3. Allcutt D, Michowiz S, Weitzman S, et al: Primary leptomeningeal melanoma: an unusually aggressive tumor in childhood. Neurosurgery 32:721–729; discussion 729, 1993.
4. Alwatban J, Tampieri D, Salazar A, et al: MRI of leptomeningeal melanocytosis in a patient with neurofibromatosis. J Comput Assist Tomogr 21:38–40, 1997.
5. Arunkumar MJ, Ranjan A, Jacob M, Rajshekhar V: Neurocutaneous melanosis: a case of primary intracranial melanoma with metastasis. Clin Oncol (R Coll Radiol) 13:52–54, 2001.
6. Atkinson L: Melanoma of the central nervous system. Aust N Z J Surg 48:14–16, 1978.
7. Balmaceda CM, Fetell MR, O'Brien JL, Housepian EH: Nevus of Ota and leptomeningeal melanocytic lesions. Neurology 43:381–386, 1993.
8. Baloch ZW, Sack MJ, Yu GH, Gupta PK: Papillary formations in metastatic melanoma. Diagn Cytopathol 20:148–151, 1999.
9. Bar H, Schlote W: Malignant melanoma in the CNS, subtyping and immunocytochemistry. Clin Neuropathol 16:337–345, 1997.

10. Ben-Izhak O, Stark P, Levy R, et al: Epithelial markers in malignant melanoma. A study of primary lesions and their metastases. Am J Dermatopathol 16:241–246, 1994.

11. Biernat W: [Melanocytic tumors of the central nervous system (melanocytoma, melanoma malignum)]. Pol J Pathol 52(4 Suppl):173–175, 2001.

12. Bittencourt FV, Marghoob AA, Kopf AW, et al: Large congenital melanocytic nevi and the risk for development of malignant melanoma and neurocutaneous melanocytosis. Pediatrics 106:736–741, 2000.

13. Brat DJ, Giannini C, Scheithauer BW, Burger PC: Primary melanocytic neoplasms of the central nervous systems. Am J Surg Pathol 23:745–754, 1999.

14. Byrd SE, Darling CF, Tomita T, et al: MR imaging of symptomatic neurocutaneous melanosis in children. Pediatr Radiol 27:39–44, 1997.

15. Byrd SE, Reyes-Mugica M, Darling CF, et al: MR of leptomeningeal melanosis in children. Eur J Radiol 20:93–99, 1995.

16. Carstens PH, Hollander JL: Metastatic spindle cell malignant melanoma with prominent microvilli. Ultrastruct Pathol 16:587–591, 1992.

17. Chang CS, Hsieh PF, Chia LG, et al: Leptomeningeal malignant melanoma arising in neurocutaneous melanocytosis: a case report. Zhonghua Yi Xue Za Zhi (Taipei) 60:316–320, 1997.

18. Chang ES, Wick MR, Swanson PE, Dehner LP: Metastatic malignant melanoma with "rhabdoid" features. Am J Clin Pathol 102:426–431, 1994.

19. Chen CJ, Hsu YI, Ho YS, et al: Intracranial meningeal melanocytoma: CT and MRI. Neuroradiology 39:811–814, 1997.

20. Chow M, Clarke DB, Maloney WJ, Sangalang V: Meningeal melanocytoma of the planum sphenoidale. Case report and review of the literature. J Neurosurg 94:841–845, 2001.

21. Clarke DB, Leblanc R, Bertrand G, et al: Meningeal melanocytoma. Report of a case and a historical comparison [see comments]. J Neurosurg 88:116–121, 1998.

22. Classen J, Hehr T, Paulus W, et al: Suprasellar melanocytoma: a case of primary radiotherapy and review of the literature. J Neurooncol 58:39–46, 2002.

23. Craver RD, Golladay SE, Warrier RP, et al: Neurocutaneous melanosis with Dandy-Walker malformation complicated by primary spinal leptomeningeal melanoma. J Child Neurol 11:410–414, 1996.

24. Czarnecki EJ, Silbergleit R, Gutierrez JA: MR of spinal meningeal melanocytoma. AJNR Am J Neuroradiol 18:180–182, 1997.

25. Czirjak S, Vitanovic D, Slowik F, Magyar A: Primary meningeal melanocytoma of the pineal region. Case report. J Neurosurg 92:461–465, 2000.

26. DeDavid M, Orlow SJ, Provost N, et al: Neurocutaneous melanosis: clinical features of large congenital melanocytic nevi in patients with manifest central nervous system melanosis. J Am Acad Dermatol 35:529–538, 1996.

27. Ellis DS, Spencer WH, Stephenson CM: Congenital neurocutaneous melanosis with metastatic orbital malignant melanoma. Ophthalmology 93:1639–1642, 1986.

28. Foster RD, Williams ML, Barkovich AJ, et al: Giant congenital melanocytic nevi: the significance of neurocutaneous melanosis in neurologically asymptomatic children. Plast Reconstr Surg 107:933–941, 2001.

29. Frieden IJ, Williams ML, Barkovich AJ: Giant congenital melanocytic nevi: brain magnetic resonance findings in neurologically asymptomatic children. J Am Acad Dermatol 31(3 Pt 1):423–429, 1994.

30. Gardiman M, Altavilla G, Marchioro L, et al: Meningeal melanocytoma: a rare lesion of the central nervous system. Tumori 82:494–496, 1996.

31. Glick R, Baker C, Husain S, et al: Primary melanocytomas of the spinal cord: a report of seven cases. Clin Neuropathol 16:127–132, 1997.

32. Greco Crasto S, Soffietti R, Bradac GB, Boldorini R: Primitive cerebral melanoma: case report and review of the literature. Surg Neurol 55:163–168; discussion 168, 2001.

33. Hamm H: Cutaneous mosaicism of lethal mutations. Am J Med Genet 85:342–345, 1999.

34. Hirose T, Horiguchi H, Kaneko F, et al: Melanocytoma of the foramen magnum. Pathol Int 47:155–160, 1997.

35. Ibanez J, Weil B, Ayala A, et al: Meningeal melanocytoma: case report and review of the literature. Histopathology 30:576–581, 1997.

36. Kadonaga JN, Frieden IJ: Neurocutaneous melanosis: definition and review of the literature. J Am Acad Dermatol 24(5 Pt 1):747–755, 1991.

37. Kaplan AM, Itabashi HH, Hanelin LG, Lu AT: Neurocutaneous melanosis with malignant leptomeningeal melanoma. A case with metastases outside the nervous system. Arch Neurol 32:669–671, 1975.

38. Katz HR: The results of different fractionation schemes in the palliative irradiation of metastatic melanoma. Int J Radiat Oncol Biol Phys 7:907–911, 1981.

39. Keil FW, Starr LB, Hanson JL: Primary melanoma of two spinal cord. J Neurosurg. 18:616–629, 1961.

40. King R, Busam K, Rosai J: Metastatic malignant melanoma resembling malignant peripheral nerve sheath tumor: Report of 16 cases. Am J Surg Pathol 23:1499–1505, 1999.

41. Konefal JB, Emami B, Pilepich MV: Malignant melanoma: analysis of dose fractionation and radiation therapy. Radiology 164:607–610, 1987.

42. Kurita H, Segawa H, Shin M, et al: Radiosurgery of meningeal melanocytoma. J Neurooncol 46:57–61, 2000.

43. Lamas E, Diez Lobato R, Sotelo T, et al: Neurocutaneous melanosis. Report of a case and review of the literature. Acta Neurochir (Wien) 36:93–105, 1977.

44. Leaney BJ, Rowe PW, Klug GL: Neurocutaneous melanosis with hydrocephalus and syringomyelia. Case report. J Neurosurg 62:148–152, 1985.

45. Lesoin F, Leys D, Verier A, et al: [Primary melanomas of the central nervous system. Report of a melanocytic meningioma of the ponto-cerebellar angle]. Rev Otoneuroophtalmol 55:443–448, 1983.

46. Limas C, Tio FO: Meningeal melanocytoma ("melanotic meningioma"). Its melanocytic origin as revealed by electron microscopy. Cancer 30:1286–1294, 1972.

47. Litofsky NS, Zee CS, Breeze RE, Chandrasoma PT: Meningeal melanocytoma: diagnostic criteria for a rare lesion. Neurosurgery 31:945–948, 1992.

48. Makin GW, Eden OB, Lashford LS, et al: Leptomeningeal melanoma in childhood. Cancer 86:878–886, 1999.

49. Matsumoto S, Kang Y, Sato S, et al: Spinal meningeal melanocytoma presenting with superficial siderosis of the central nervous system. Case report and review of the literature. J Neurosurg 88:890–894, 1998.

50. Matsuno A, Hashizume K, Suzuki K, et al: [A case of primary intracranial malignant melanoma showing leptomeningeal dissemination]. No To Shinkei 44:935–939, 1992.

51. Mazur MT, Katzenstein AL: Metastatic melanoma: the spectrum of ultrastructural morphology. Ultrastruct Pathol 1:337–356, 1980.

52. Morris LL, Danta G: Malignant cerebral melanoma complicating giant pigmented naevus: a case report. J Neurol Neurosurg Psychiatry 31:628–632, 1968.

53. Narayanan HS, Gandhi DH, Girimaji SR: Neurocutaneous melanosis associated with Dandy-Walker syndrome. Clin Neurol Neurosurg 89:197–200, 1987.

54. Naul LG, Hise JH, Bauserman SC, Todd FD: CT and MR of meningeal melanocytoma. AJNR Am J Neuroradiol 12:315–316, 1991.

55. O'Brien TF, Moran M, Miller JH, Hensley SD: Meningeal melanocytoma. An uncommon diagnostic pitfall in surgical neuropathology. Arch Pathol Lab Med 119:542–526, 1995.

56. Oruckaptan HH, Soylemezoglu F, Kutluk T, Akalan N: Benign melanocytic tumor in infancy: discussion on a rare case and review of the literature. Pediatr Neurosurg 32:240–247, 2000.

56a. Rades D, Heidendreich F, Tatagiba M, et al: Therapeutic options for meningeal melanocytoma. Case report. J Neurosurg 95:225–231, 2001.

57. Reed WB, Becker SW Sr, Becker SW Jr, Nickel WR: Giant pigmented nevi, melanoma, and leptomeningeal melanocytosis: a clinical and histopathological study. Arch Dermatol 91:100–119, 1965.

58. Reidy JJ, Apple DJ, Steinmetz RL, et al: Melanocytoma: nomenclature, pathogenesis, natural history and treatment. Surv Ophthalmol 29:319–327, 1985.

59. Reyes-Mugica M, Chou P, Byrd S, et al: Nevomelanocytic proliferations in the central nervous system of children. Cancer 72:2277–2285, 1993.

60. Reyes-Mugica M, Alvarez-Franco M, Bauer BS, Vicari FA: Nevus cells and special nevomelanocytic lesions in children. Pediatr Pathol 14:1029–1041, 1994.

61. Rubino GJ, King WA, Quinn B, et al: Primary pineal melanoma: case report. Neurosurgery 33:511–515; discussion 515, 1993.

62. Sandsmark M, Eskeland G, Skullerud K, Abyholm F: Neurocutaneous melanosis. Case report and a brief review. Scand J Plast Reconstr Surg Hand Surg 28:151–154, 1994.

63. Sang DN, Albert DM, Sober AJ, McMeekin TO: Nevus of Ota with contralateral cerebral melanoma. Arch Ophthalmol 95:1820–1824, 1977.

64. Schneider F, Putzier M: Primary leptomeningeal melanoma. Spine 27:E545–E547, 2002.

65. Schwechheimer K, Zhou L: HMB45: a specific marker for melanoma metastases in the central nervous system? Virchows Arch 426:351–353, 1995.

66. Selby WL, Nance KV, Park HK: CEA immunoreactivity in metastatic malignant melanoma. Mod Pathol 5:415–419, 1992.

67. Silbert SW, Smith KR, Jr, Horenstein S: Primary leptomeningeal melanoma: an ultrastructural study. Cancer 41:519–527, 1978.

68. Singhal S, Singh K, Fernandes P, et al: Primary melanoma of the central nervous system: report of a case and review of the literature. Indian J Cancer 28:92–98, 1991.

69. Slaughter JC, Hardman JM, Kempe LG, Earle KM: Neurocutaneous melanosis and leptomeningeal melanomatosis in children. Arch Pathol 88:298–304, 1969.

70. Son YJ, Wang KC, Kim SK, et al: Primary intracranial malignant melanoma evolving from leptomeningeal melanosis. Med Pediatr Oncol 40:201–204, 2003.

71. Suzuki T, Yasumoto Y, Kumami K, et al: Primary pineal melanocytic tumor. Case report. J Neurosurg 94:523–527, 2001.

72. Theunissen P, Spincemaille G, Pannebakker M, Lambers J: Meningeal melanoma associated with nevus of Ota: case report and review. Clin Neuropathol 12:125–129, 1993.

73. Tosaka M, Tamura M, Oriuchi N, et al: Cerebrospinal fluid immunocytochemical analysis and neuroimaging in the diagnosis of primary leptomeningeal melanoma. Case report. J Neurosurg 94:528–532, 2001.

74. Uematsu Y, Yukawa S, Yokote H, et al: Meningeal melanocytoma: magnetic resonance imaging characteristics and pathological features. Case report. J Neurosurg 76:705–709, 1992.

75. Vanzieleghem BD, Lemmerling MM, Van Coster RN: Neurocutaneous melanosis presenting with intracranial amelanotic melanoma. AJNR Am J Neuroradiol 20:457–460, 1999.

76. Whinney D, Kitchen N, Revesz T, Brookes G: Primary malignant melanoma of the cerebellopontine angle. Otol Neurotol 22:218–222, 2001.

77. Yamane K, Shima T, Okada Y, et al: Primary pineal melanoma with long-term survival: case report. Surg Neurol 42:433–437, 1994.

CHAPTER 40

HEMANGIOBLASTOMAS

G. Edward Vates, Kurtis Ian Auguste, and Mitchel S. Berger

Hemangioblastomas are World Health Organization (WHO) grade I tumors of uncertain histologic origin that occur exclusively in the nervous system, most commonly in the posterior fossa.[4] Hemangioblastomas can occur sporadically or in association with other visceral tumors and cysts that have been grouped under the familial tumor syndrome von Hippel-Lindau (VHL) disease. The historical recognition of VHL disease has been described at length elsewhere and will not be reviewed here. Instead, this chapter reviews the epidemiology, presentation, treatment, and pathology of both the sporadic and inherited forms of this tumor and presents some of the new developments in our understanding of the gene responsible for von Hippel-Lindau disease.

LOCATION

Hemangioblastomas account for 2% of all intracranial tumors and approximately 10% of posterior fossa tumors.[2,4,6,19] They also constitute 2% to 3% of all intramedullary spinal cord tumors.[1,6] Rarely, hemangioblastomas occur in the conus medullaris, filum terminale, nerve roots, and peripheral nerves.[2,4,19] Approximately 25% of hemangioblastomas are associated with VHL disease, but this may be an artificially low estimate because some patients with hemangioblastomas do not undergo appropriate screening for VHL disease.[2,4,6,16]

DIAGNOSIS

Patients with sporadic hemangioblastomas seek treatment later than patients with VHL disease; most patients with sporadic tumors are diagnosed in their forties to fifties, whereas VHL-disease patients are diagnosed in their late twenties or early thirties. Sporadic hemangioblastomas predominantly occur in the cerebellum, but VHL-associated hemangioblastomas occur in the cerebellum, brainstem, or spinal cord, and VHL patients often have multiple hemangioblastomas at various sites. In fact, multiple tumors are nearly diagnostic of VHL disease. Typically, hemangioblastomas are slowly growing masses associated with cysts in the cerebellum or a syrinx in the brainstem or spinal cord.[2,6,16,19] In the posterior fossa, hemangioblastomas cause impaired cerebrospinal fluid (CSF) flow because of compression of the fourth ventricle, leading to increased intracranial pressure. Headache is the most common symptom, usually in the suboccipital region and worse in the mornings. Patients

with tumor located caudally in the posterior fossa can have compression of the brainstem as it passes through the foramen magnum; these patients may have neck stiffness or Lhermitte's sign. Vomiting is common and probably related to obstructive hydrocephalus, although a tumor originating in or compressing the floor of the fourth ventricle may irritate the vagal nucleus. If the tumor is located in the brainstem or middle cerebellar peduncle, adjacent to the vestibular nuclei, it can cause vertigo. Tumors in the cerebellum or pons can cause unstable gait and imbalance. Cerebellar hemispheric lesions cause limb ataxia, dysmetria, and intention tremor, whereas vermian lesions cause broad-based gait and truncal ataxia.

Patients with spinal cord hemangioblastomas typically have spinal pain, spasticity, weakness, sensory changes, hyperactive reflexes, and impaired urination consistent with an intramedullary tumor or syrinx.[1,6,16] Spinal cord lesions usually protrude through the pia mater at the dorsal root entry zone, which explains why patients with tumor in this location often have sensory symptoms, especially pain.[2] Some spinal hemangioblastomas are extramedullary and are attached to the posterior nerve roots, usually in the thoracic cord. Rarely, intracranial or spinal hemangioblastomas can cause intratumoral hemorrhage or even subarachnoid hemorrhage.[2,5,19] Supratentorial hemangioblastomas are rare, but they have been reported in the brain parenchyma of all cerebral lobes, in the corpus callosum or deep gray nuclei, within the ventricles, in the choroid plexus, and in the meninges.[4] Clinical presentation depends on the location of the tumor and whether the hemangioblastoma causes mass effect or hemorrhage. Hemangioblastomas can also occur in the prechiasmatic optic nerve, typically with visual deficits and with or without headache. Because patients with VHL disease can also have visual loss caused by retinal angiomas, visual loss must be correlated to the extent of retinal disease so that an optic nerve tumor is not missed.

Because improved neurosurgical technique has reduced the morbidity and mortality associated with cerebellar hemangioblastomas, extracranial manifestations of VHL disease have become a more important part of patient management. (This is reviewed in the discussion on related conditions.) Of note, however, polycythemia is a commonly discussed initial finding in patients with central nervous system (CNS) hemangioblastomas,[6,16] even though it is documented in less than 25% of cases and almost never in patients with exclusively spinal lesions. Erythrocytosis is caused by unregulated secretion of erythropoietin or an erythropoietin mimic by tumor cells[4,5,16]; this causes increased red cell synthesis and red cell iron turnover without splenomegaly, increased red cell turnover, or expansion of other cell types from the bone marrow.[19] Erythropoietin has been isolated from cyst fluid in some hemangioblastomas, and its secretion may be driven by the deregulated function of hypoxia-inducible factor 1 (HIF-1)-α (described in the discussion on Epidemiology). However, erythropoietin can also be secreted by renal tumors found in patients with VHL disease, so polycythemia in a patient with a CNS hemangioblastoma should trigger a rigorous work-up to rule out VHL disease (see later discussion on related conditions).

EPIDEMIOLOGY

Patients with sporadic hemangioblastomas typically seek treatment at age 40 to 50, whereas patients with VHL-disease-related hemangioblastomas seek treatment in their twenties or thirties.[4,16] Men are more commonly afflicted than women, although the absolute male-to-female ratio varies from 1.3:1 to 2:1.[1,2,4,6,16,19]

VHL disease is an autosomal dominant disorder that occurs at rates of 1:36,000 to 1:45,000.[4] Patients with VHL disease develop retinal angiomas, hemangioblastomas of the brain and spinal cord, clear cell renal cell carcinoma, pheochromocytomas, and visceral cysts.[14,16] The diagnostic criteria for VHL disease are (1) one or more hemangioblastomas within the CNS, (2) a CNS hemangioblastoma paired with one of the typical VHL-disease-associated tumors, or (3) a family history of VHL disease.[4] Table 40-1 lists many of the lesions associated with VHL disease. *Lindau's tumor* specifically refers to hemangioblastoma of the cerebellum, and *von Hippel's tumor* to angioma of the retina; histologically, these tumors are identical. Of the visceral tumors, clear cell renal carcinomas and pheochromocytomas are the most common.[5,19]

VHL disease is inherited as an autosomal dominant trait caused by mutations in the VHL gene.[5,8] The gene is located at chromosome 3p25-26, has three exons, and has a coding sequence of 639 nucleotides.[14] In the brain, VHL mRNA and protein expression is highest in Purkinje cells, Golgi type II cells, and dentate nucleus of the cerebellum; pontine nuclei; the inferior olivary nucleus of the medulla oblongata; and sympathetic ganglia, myenteric, and submucous plexus of the colon.[8] In the other target organs of VHL disease, the gene is highly expressed in the renal tubule system, the exocrine pancreas, the adrenal cortex, and liver parenchyma. The VHL protein is also expressed in organs not at risk for the disease, such as the eosinophilic cells of the pituitary gland, epithelial cells of the follicles of the thyroid, epithelial cells of the intestines, bile ducts, and bronchial epithelia. Immunohistochemistry does not reveal any differences in VHL protein levels in tumors obtained from VHL patients or tumors unrelated to VHL disease. Renal cell carcinomas, hemangioblastomas, and pheochromocytomas, either VHL-related or sporadic, demonstrate positive staining for the VHL protein, which suggests that the current antibodies recognize both normal and mutated VHL protein.

The mechanism by which inactivation of the VHL protein (pVHL) causes susceptibility to the disease and neoplastic transformation is unknown, although several lines of evidence indicate pVHL regulates angiogenesis, extracellular matrix formation, and the cell cycle, and that several signaling pathways may be involved.[22] The most important role of pVHL appears to be its interaction with HIF-1.[8,13,22] HIF-1 consists of two subunits (α and β); both are constitutively expressed in all cells, but in normoxic cells the HIF-1α subunit is rapidly degraded by ubiquitin-dependent pathways. In hypoxic cells, however, ubiquitin-dependent degradation of HIF-1α ceases, HIF-1α and β unite, and hypoxia-related gene expression increases. pVHL has two domains (also designated α and β). The α domain forms a complex with elongin B, elongin C, cullin-2, and Rbx1; these factors coordinate ubiquitin ligase activity, and the pVHLα domain regulates their targeting of cellular proteins for ubiquitination and proteasome-mediated degradation.[4,5,9] The second pVHL domain, the β domain, binds to HIF-1α; this binding occurs only when a specific proline residue on HIF-1α is hydroxylated, a modification that can only occur in normoxic cells.[11] Therefore, in normoxic cells, pVHL keeps levels of HIF-1α low by binding to it and bringing HIF-1α in proximity to ubiquitin-ligase components.[9,11,15] In hypoxic cells, or in pVHL-deficient cells, HIF-1α escapes the grasp of pVHL, binds with HIF-1β, and together the HIF-1α–β complex acts as a transcriptional activator of genes such as vascular endothelial growth factor (VEGF), the glucose transporter (GLUT-1), and carbonic anhydrase.[7] The constitutive overexpression of VEGF through this signaling pathway explains the intense vascularity of hemangioblastomas and other VHL-associated neoplasms.[8,9,15]

Additional functions of pVHL may contribute to the malignant evolution and phenotype of VHL-associated lesions. pVHL expression and subcellular localization is coordinated with stages of the cell cycle, and evidence suggests that pVHL is involved in the transition from G2 into quiescent G0 phase, possibly by preventing accumulation of the cyclin-dependent kinase inhibitor p27 and other cell-cycle regulators through ubiquitin-dependent degradation of these proteins.[22] pVHL may also directly regulate the intracellular signaling induced by activation of multiple growth factor pathways, including epidermal

---

TABLE 40-1

Lesions Associated with von Hippel-Lindau Disease

Central nervous system hemangioblastoma: cerebellar,* medullary,* spinal,* supratentorial

Retinal angiomatosis*

Pancreatic tumors: cysts,* adenoma, islet cell carcinoma, adenocarcinoma

Liver lesions: cyst, angioma, adenoma

Renal lesions: cyst,* angioma, adenoma, renal cell carcinoma* (unilateral or bilateral)

Spleen lesions: cyst, angioma

Lung lesions: cyst, angioma

Omental cyst

Adrenal lesions: cortical angioma, cortical adenoma, pheochromocytoma* (tends to be bilateral)

Epididymal lesions: cyst, adenoma

Ovarian lesions: cyst, carcinoma

Polycythemia*

---

*Common findings.

growth factor (EGF), hepatocyte growth factor, platelet-derived growth factor, transforming growth factor-α, and insulin-like growth factor-I.[4,5,8,11] pVHL may also modulate the ability of cells to produce extracellular matrix. Cells with defective pVHL show defective assembly of extracellular fibronectin and abnormal interactions with other extracellular matrix proteins.[22] pVHL may also down-regulate the activity of enzymes that degrade the extracellular matrix, through its effects on tissue inhibitor of metalloproteinase 2 (TIIMP-2) and urokinase-type plasminogen activator (uPA).

NEUROIMAGING

Magnetic Resonance Imaging

Magnetic resonance imaging (MRI) with administration of gadolinium-based contrast is the diagnostic method of choice.[5,6] MRI is more sensitive than computed tomography (CT), provides better imaging of posterior fossa and spinal cord lesions, and provides multiplanar anatomic definition. Cerebellar and supratentorial hemangioblastomas appear as a brilliantly contrast-enhanced nodule with an associated, sharply demarcated, nonenhanced smooth cyst in T1-weighted images (Figure 40-1). Hemangioblastomas in the fourth ventricle or based at the cervicomedullary junction are almost always solid and are enhanced brightly with contrast; spinal cord hemangioblastomas are also enhanced brightly with contrast and are associated with a cyst or syrinx in 50% of cases. Without contrast, the nodule is hypointense to isointense in T1-weighted images.

On T2-weighted images, the nodule is typically hyperintense, but this sequence is best used to differentiate edema from an adjacent cyst or, in the spinal cord, from an adjacent syrinx. Both T1- and T2-weighted images will often reveal serpiginous flow voids that correspond to large feeding arteries and draining veins. MRI is not only useful to evaluate a symptomatic lesion but is also best at detecting multicentric disease that is asymptomatic and is the best modality to detect CNS evidence of VHL disease.[6,22] Most surgeons advocate early screening for CNS manifestations of VHL disease for patients with a known VHL pedigree starting as early as 10 years of age or certainly by 20; in addition, any patient 50 years old or younger with a CNS hemangioblastoma should undergo a complete CNS survey with MRI to detect multicentric disease consistent with VHL (see later discussion on screening for VHL disease).

Conventional Angiography

Vertebral and spinal angiography can provide useful information for management of nervous system hemangioblastomas.[1] Although not useful as a screening tool, angiography can demonstrate the location of dominant feeding arteries and is particularly important for identifying feeding arteries that are deep to the lesion if surgical resection is considered. Typically, angiography shows the highly vascular tumor nodule with an avascular cyst, when a cyst is present. Superselective angiography with embolization of feeding arteries can be useful in select cases of hemangioblastomas as an adjunct to microsurgical or radiosurgical treatment, similar to the use of endovascular embolization for treating arteriovenous malformations.[1,6]

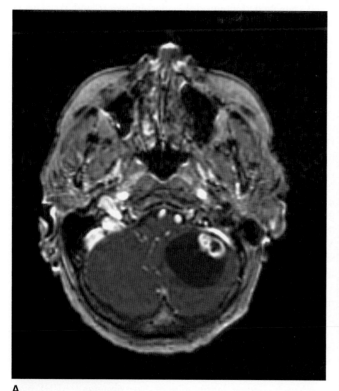

A

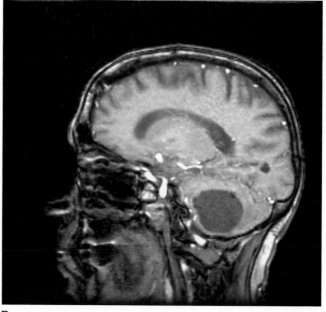

B

FIGURE 40-1 *A,* Axial T1-weighted magnetic resonance (MR) image with contrast showing a cystic cerebellar hemangioblastoma. The mural nodule and not the cyst wall is enhanced with contrast administration. *B,* Sagittal T1-weighted MR image with contrast of the same lesion.

TUMOR HISTOLOGY

Grossly, hemangioblastomas in all locations are the same and appear as cherry-red, well-circumscribed tumors.[1,2,4,6,19,22] Brainstem and spinal cord tumors are usually solid, but the majority of cerebellar tumors and a large portion of spinal cord tumors are associated with a cyst or syrinx, respectively; when a cyst is present, the neoplastic component is easily identified as a mural nodule generally close to the pial surface. The cyst wall is smooth and made up of glial cells and compressed neural tissue, without any tumor cells. The cyst contains clear, golden-yellow, and highly proteinaceous fluid that clots readily after removal. Hemangioblastomas may infiltrate the leptomeninges or the dura, but remain histologically benign.

Microscopically, hemangioblastomas consist of three cell types: endothelial cells lining capillary spaces, pericytes adjacent to the endothelial cells, and large round or polygonal stromal cells or "clear cells" (Figure 40-2).[1,2,4,19] The stromal cells are the neoplastic component of the tumor, and their nuclei may vary in size with occasional atypical and hyperchromatic nuclei. The stromal cells appear clear because the cytoplasm is filled with lipid-laden vacuoles. The tumor is filled with numerous capillary channels that form an anastomosing plexiform pattern lined by a single layer of endothelium. These channels are surrounded by reticulin fibers that are best demonstrated with reticulin stains. The pericytes are best identified on electron microscopy, where they appear adjacent to the endothelia, separated only by the periendothelial basement membrane. Cystic changes are common, but necrosis is unusual. The tumor edge is generally well demarcated, although small infiltrative nests of tumor tissue may be present. Mitotic figures are scarce, and the Ki-67 labeling index is usually less than 1%.

Because the stromal cells are typically "clear cells," they can be confused with metastatic clear-cell renal cancer; this confusion is easily settled by immunohistochemical survey for epithelial membrane antigen, which is expressed by clear cell renal cell carcinoma but not by stromal cells of hemangioblastoma.[2,4,19] Other immunohistochemical surveys of the stromal cells have not helped to narrow down the origin of these cells. Stromal cells lack endothelial-specific markers (von Willebrand factor and CD 34) and do not express endothelium-associated cell adhesion molecules (CD 31/platelet-endothelial cell adhesion molecule [PECAM]).[2,5,19] In addition, stromal cells express certain antigens that are absent from endothelial cells (neuron-specific enolase, neural cell adhesion molecule, and ezrin). Glial fibrillary acidic protein (GFAP) is not expressed in stromal cells, but can be found in reactive astrocytes within the nodule, and especially in the cyst wall. As mentioned previously, stromal cells in hemangioblastoma stain vibrantly for VEGF, and this undoubtedly explains the intense vascularity of these tumors; it is paired with high levels of VEGF receptor expression on the endothelial cells.[3] Erythropoietin is highly expressed in stromal cells, and lastly, pVHL (either wild type or mutant) and HIF are highly expressed as well.[4,5,19]

THERAPY

Surgery

Surgery with complete excision is the best avenue for obliteration of hemangioblastomas, and this is easily achieved in most patients with posterior fossa tumors. Tumors in the cerebellum are best approached through a suboccipital craniotomy or craniectomy, with the patient in a prone position, and with removal of the posterior elements of C1 and C2 as needed for exposure. We use intraoperative frameless stereotaxic navigation to find the shortest route to the tumor and, if present, the associated cyst. Once the tumor location is defined, the tumor nodule should be removed en bloc by dissecting along the gliotic margin. Piecemeal removal of the tumor is a tragic mistake that can quickly result in uncontrollable hemorrhage. If the tumor is associated with a cyst, the cyst wall should be left undisturbed, because it is not composed of tumor. Once the tumor nodule is removed, the dura should be closed water-tight using dural grafts if needed. Careful closure is critical, because in some patients with sporadic hemangioblastomas, and more often in patients with VHL disease, recurrence can occur. If further surgery in the posterior fossa is then required, careless closure the first time can make re-exploration treacherous for the surgeon and a significant risk for the patient.

Brainstem hemangioblastomas are different from their cerebellar counterparts and, depending on their location, can present surgical risks that make resection difficult.[1,2,6,19] Hemangioblastomas that occupy the fourth ventricle with minimal brainstem invasion most likely arise from the choroid plexus; they do not involve brainstem nuclei and can be resected with acceptable risk. Tumors that originate from the floor of the fourth ventricle at the cervicomedullary junction have a subpial attachment that makes finding a distinct, circumferential gliotic margin difficult. Resection of these tumors is associated with a high degree of neurologic morbidity and mortality, and in our experience attempts at resection of tumors with deep midline attachment to the medulla are invariably lethal. Therefore we do not recommended resection in these cases.

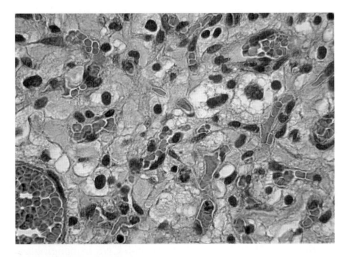

FIGURE 40-2 Hemangioblastomas consist of three cell types: endothelial cells lining capillary spaces; pericytes adjacent to the endothelial cells; and large, vacuolated stromal cells or "clear cells." (Hematoxylin and eosin stain, ×500). (Courtesy of Dr. Johan Kros, Erasmus University Medical Center, Rotterdam, Netherlands.)

Most spinal cord hemangioblastomas are located in the dorsal part of the spinal cord, near the dorsal root entry zone; they most often involve the thoracic spinal cord, followed next most commonly by the cervical cord.[1,6] Extramedullary intradural hemangioblastomas are usually attached to the posterior nerve roots and can be found in the filum terminale.[6] Fifty percent of intramedullary spinal cord hemangioblastomas are associated with a syrinx, analogous to the development of a cyst in cerebellar hemangioblastoma; T2-weighted MRI is best suited to differentiating between a syrinx and spinal cord edema. Because most spinal cord hemangioblastomas are situated dorsally, a wide laminectomy with resection of the medial portion of the facets provides adequate exposure for resection. More ventrally located tumors are best approached using a posterolateral trajectory, with laminectomy, facetectomy, resection of the pedicle, and gentle rolling of the spinal cord to reveal the lesion.[6] Anterior approaches to ventrally situated spinal cord hemangioblastomas have been described.[10] Ultrasound can be especially useful for locating the tumor if enlarged pial vessels do not provide a ready roadmap.[2,19] Like cerebellar hemangioblastomas, spinal cord tumors are embedded in a subpial plane with a clear gliotic margin that can be easily dissected from the adjacent spinal cord; once the mural nodule is freed by completely dividing the feeding vessels, it can be removed. As with cerebellar lesions, spinal cord hemangioblastomas should not undergo biopsies or be removed piecemeal, and the wall of the syrinx should be left undisturbed.

Radiation Therapy

There is growing evidence that radiation therapy, either conventional conformal external-beam or stereotactic radiosurgery, may have a role in the treatment of hemangioblastoma, either as an adjunct to surgical resection or as an alternative for treating lesions in sensitive brain structures.[6,12,18] External-beam radiation can be used to control incompletely resected solid lesions or multiple lesions in patients with VHL disease; it appears to either significantly reduce or retard the growth rate of lesions and improve the 5- and 10-year survival rates. Stereotactic radiosurgery may provide an even greater benefit, although even multicenter trials have reported on only a relatively small number of patients, and the benefit is probably greatest for VHL disease patients with recurrent disease or multiple tumors in the brainstem and spinal cord. As in other kinds of tumors treated with stereotactic radiosurgery, the risks of postirradiation edema and necrosis are highest when treating large lesions in the brainstem. Size is of particular concern in hemangioblastomas, where much of the tumor volume is a cyst that is probably not neoplastic.[18] The cyst can also be problematic, because, in many cases, it does not shrink after treatment and may even increase in size during the latency period after stereotactic radiosurgery. In cases where the cyst causes symptoms or becomes symptomatic after radiation treatment, an Ommaya reservoir may be implanted to allow cyst aspiration as needed.

Chemotherapy, Experimental Therapies, and Epilepsy Treatment

Because surgery is successful in treating most hemangioblastomas, there are few reports on the utility of chemotherapy or other experimental therapies in the treatment of these tumors. Also, the most common locations for these tumors are in brain regions where the tumor does not elicit cortical irritation that could cause seizures, so epilepsy is not a common problem; in those cases where seizures are a symptom, their treatment follows standard therapy.

OUTCOME AND QUALITY OF LIFE ASSESSMENTS

Patients not treated surgically for hemangioblastoma do poorly. In most series, outcomes after surgery are good; 50% to 80% of patients experience resolution of symptoms and are able to return to their premorbid lifestyle. Outcomes are less favorable in patients with medullary tumors or ventrally located spinal tumors, patients with multiple tumors, and in patients with VHL disease, although in these patients some morbidity is caused by non-CNS manifestations of VHL disease (see discussion on related conditions). For the purpose of predicting outcome, multifocal disease is likely equivalent to VHL disease. In one series, average lifespan in patients with non-VHL related hemangioblastomas was 63 years, whereas in patients with VHL disease, average lifespan was 46 years, and deaths were attributed equally to effects of CNS hemangioblastomas and renal tumors.[17]

RECURRENCE

Although hemangioblastomas are regarded as benign neoplasms, they may recur in up to 25% of cases. Recurrence has been correlated with younger age (i.e., younger than 30 years old at the time of diagnosis), VHL disease, and the presence of multicentric tumors of the CNS at initial diagnosis, whether or not VHL mutations were identified. Histopathologically, recurring hemangioblastomas were less likely to have associated cysts or lipid-laden stromal cells. The findings suggest that a particular constellation of clinical and pathologic features can be used to predict the likelihood of recurrence of a hemangioblastoma and therefore to identify patients in need of long-term follow-up or adjunctive therapy, although the specific predictive features have yet to be rigorously defined.[6]

RELATED CONDITIONS

Improved surgical techniques have made sporadic CNS hemangioblastoma a treatable disease with low neurologic morbidity and mortality. In VHL disease, CNS hemangioblastoma remains the most common cause of death because of higher incidence of recurrence and multicentric disease, although the survival rates have improved dramatically. As a consequence, detection of VHL disease in patients with CNS hemangioblastoma and the management of extracranial manifestations of VHL disease has assumed more importance. Most associated lesions in VHL disease are tumors or cysts in the viscera (see Table 40-1). Of the visceral tumors, clear cell renal cell cancer and pheochromocytomas are the most common and have the greatest importance to the neurosurgeon.

Renal Cell Carcinoma

Kidney lesions in patients with VHL disease are either benign cysts or clear-cell renal cell carcinoma (CCRCC). It is possible that these two entities are ends of a spectrum of disease, because the walls of cysts in patients with VHL disease often have foci of occult CCRCC, which is uncommon in patients in the general population with sporadic renal cysts. CCRCC is found in 25% of patients with VHL disease, although this may be an underestimation, because renal neoplasms remain occult in many patients; the percentage of patients with symptomatic CCRCC has increased as the treatment of CNS hemangioblastoma has improved.

CCRCC in patients with VHL disease differs from sporadic cases of CCRCC in a number of aspects: CCRCC in patients with VHL disease has earlier onset, occurs more often in men, and is more commonly multicentric and bilateral. The management of CCRCC in patients with VHL disease is still a matter of controversy and beyond the scope of this chapter. What is important to recognize, however, is that these lesions are best dealt with when discovered early. Therefore screening is essential, and most surgeons advocate abdominal CT scan or MRI with contrast to detect kidney lesions in patients 50 years old or younger with CNS hemangioblastoma (solitary or multicentric). In addition, patients in a known cohort of VHL disease should begin routine radiologic surveys for abdominal disease, and the care of teenagers should be coordinated by a multispecialist team that can address all the manifestations of VHL disease. Although flank pain, hematuria, and a palpable abdominal mass are a classic triad for kidney tumors, they are present in only approximately 10% of cases.

Pheochromocytoma

Approximately 10% of patients with VHL disease also have pheochromocytoma; conversely, almost a quarter of patients with pheochromocytoma will have either VHL disease or a multiple endocrine neoplasia syndrome (MEN). Unlike sporadic pheochromocytoma, patients with VHL disease tend to be younger and have bilateral tumors, so a VHL disease patient with unilateral pheochromocytoma is likely to develop another tumor in the contralateral adrenal gland. This also suggests that any patient with bilateral pheochromocytoma is very likely to have VHL disease, or one of the other heritable syndromes associated with pheochromocytoma (e.g., NF1, multiple endocrine neoplasia [MEN] syndromes). Ten percent of patients with pheochromocytoma have a malignant variant that cannot be distinguished histologically and can only be diagnosed by the appearance of metastatic disease.

The most common presenting symptoms of pheochromocytoma are episodic pounding headaches, diaphoresis, palpitations or tachycardia, nervousness, and tremor; these are all related to the excess catecholamine secretion from the tumor. Catecholamine excess can also cause impaired glucose tolerance and hypermetabolism. The best screening test for pheochromocytoma is a urinary metanephrine assay. If metanephrine values are elevated, a 24-hour urine specimen should be collected to detect metanephrine, vanillylmandelic acid, and catecholamines. Plasma catecholamine levels are unreliable, because excess catecholamine release can be paroxysmal. If a pheochromocytoma is suspected, then abdominal MRI is the most sensitive radiologic test. Surgical resection is generally curative, and because paroxysmal catecholamine excess can have dire consequences during any surgery, it is recommended that VHL-disease patients with both CNS lesions and pheochromocytoma undergo resection of the pheochromocytoma first.

SCREENING FOR VHL DISEASE

Based on many of the factors previously described, there are a number of reasons to screen for VHL disease.[6,20–22] We suggest the following screening guidelines:

1. Any patients younger than 50 years old with a CNS hemangioblastoma or any patient at any age with multicentric CNS hemangioblastoma should have full CNS MRI with contrast, ophthalmologic examination, abdominal CT scan with contrast, and single voided urine metanephrine assay.
2. Any patient with a VHL-disease pedigree should undergo routine CNS MRI (starting as early as age 10, no later than age 20) and ophthalmologic examination and should have routine abdominal CT scans with contrast (starting at 20 years of age).
3. Any patient suspected of VHL disease should have genetic analysis for germline mutations of the VHL gene.

References

1. Baumgartner BJ, Wilson C: Removal of posterior fossa and spinal hemangioblastomas. In Wilson C (ed): Neurosurgical Procedures: Personal Approaches to Classic Operations. Baltimore, Williams & Wilkins, 1992.
2. Berger MS, Kros JM: Sarcomas and neoplasms of blood vessels. In Youmans JR (ed): Neurological Surgery. Vol 4. Philadelphia, WB Saunders, 1996.
3. Bohling T, Hatva E, Kujala M, et al: Expression of growth factors and growth factor receptors in capillary hemangioblastoma. J Neuropathol Exp Neurol 55:522–527, 1996.
4. Bohling T, Plate KH, Haltia M, et al: von Hippel-Lindau disease and capillary haemangioblastoma. In Cavanee WK (ed): World Health Organization Classification of Tumours: Pathology and Genetics of Tumors of the Nervous System. Lyon, France, IARC Press, 2000.
5. Choyke PL, Glenn GM, Walther MM, et al: von Hippel-Lindau disease: genetic, clinical, and imaging features. Radiology 194:629–642, 1995.
6. Conway JE, Chou D, Clatterbuck RE, et al: Hemangioblastomas of the central nervous system in von Hippel-Lindau syndrome and sporadic disease. Neurosurgery 48:55–62; discussion 62–53, 2001.
7. Iliopoulos O, Levy AP, Jiang C, et al: Negative regulation of hypoxia-inducible genes by the von Hippel-Lindau protein. Proc Natl Acad Sci U S A 93:10595–10599, 1996.
8. Ivan M, Kaelin WG, Jr: The von Hippel-Lindau tumor suppressor protein. Curr Opin Genet Dev 11:27–34, 2001.

9. Ivan M, Kondo K, Yang H, et al: HIFalpha targeted for VHL-mediated destruction by proline hydroxylation: implications for O2 sensing. Science 292:464–468, 2001.

10. Iwasaki Y, Koyanagi I, Hida K, et al: Anterior approach to intramedullary hemangioblastoma: case report. Neurosurgery 44:655–657, 1999.

11. Jaakkola P, Mole DR, Tian YM, et al: Targeting of HIF-alpha to the von Hippel-Lindau ubiquitylation complex by O2-regulated prolyl hydroxylation. Science 292:468–472, 2001.

12. Jawahar A, Kondziolka D, Garces YI, et al: Stereotactic radiosurgery for hemangioblastomas of the brain. Acta Neurochir (Wien) 142:641–644; discussion 644–645, 2000.

13. Krek W: VHL takes HIF's breath away. Nat Cell Biol 2:E121–E123, 2000.

14. Latif F, Tory K, Gnarra J, et al: Identification of the von Hippel-Lindau disease tumor suppressor gene. Science 260:1317–1320, 1993.

15. Maxwell PH, Wiesener MS, Chang GW, et al: The tumour suppressor protein VHL targets hypoxia-inducible factors for oxygen-dependent proteolysis. Nature 399:271–275, 1999.

16. Neumann HP, Eggert HR, Weigel K, et al: Hemangioblastomas of the central nervous system. A 10-year study with special reference to von Hippel-Lindau syndrome. J Neurosurg 70:24–30, 1989.

17. Niemela M, Lemeta S, Summanen P, et al: Long-term prognosis of haemangioblastoma of the CNS: impact of von Hippel-Lindau disease. Acta Neurochir (Wien) 141:1147–1156, 1999.

18. Patrice SJ, Sneed PK, Flickinger JC, et al: Radiosurgery for hemangioblastoma: results of a multiinstitutional experience. Int J Radiat Oncol Biol Phys 35:493–499, 1996.

19. Rengachary SS, Blount JP: Hemangioblastomas. In Rengachary SS (ed): Neurosurgery. Vol I. New York, McGraw-Hill, 1996.

20. Wittebol-Post D, Hes FJ, Lips CJ: The eye in von Hippel-Lindau disease. Long-term follow-up of screening and treatment: recommendations. J Intern Med 243:555–561, 1998.

21. Zbar B: Von Hippel-Lindau disease and sporadic renal cell carcinoma. Cancer Surv 25:219–232, 1995.

22. Zbar B, Kaelin W, Maher E, et al: Third International Meeting on von Hippel-Lindau disease. Cancer Res 59:2251–2253, 1999.

CHAPTER 41

LYMPHOMAS AND HEMOPOIETIC NEOPLASMS

Enrico C. Lallana and Lisa M. DeAngelis

Primary central nervous system lymphoma (PCNSL) is defined as an extranodal lymphoma limited to the craniospinal axis without evidence of systemic involvement. It is found in the brain parenchyma in most cases but may present in the eyes, the leptomeninges, or rarely in the spinal cord. It accounts for approximately 3%[14] of all brain neoplasms and less than 1% to 4%[12,35] of all non-Hodgkin's lymphomas (NHLs).

Historically, the disease has been classified under a variety of synonyms, the first of which was *perithelial sarcoma*. Percival Bailey used the term in 1929 when he described two patients with brain tumors that appeared to be reticuloendothelial in origin and perivascular in location.[5] Succeeding authors classified the disease as a reticulum cell sarcoma, microglioma, and perivascular sarcoma in an effort to describe the histology or cell of origin. It was not until the 1970s that these tumors were recognized as histologically identical to systemic lymphomas. Almost a decade later, with the analysis of tumor cell surface immunoglobulins, PCNSL was established as an NHL of B-cell lineage with approximately 1% to 3% having a T-cell phenotype (Table 41-1).[12,26]

Metastatic systemic lymphoma is the most common cause of central nervous system (CNS) involvement by NHL and is easily distinguished from PCNSL. Metastatic lymphoma hematogenously spreads to the CNS late in the course of the disease and preferentially affects the leptomeninges. The syndrome is marked by diffuse involvement along the whole neuraxis and presents with symptoms of increased intracranial pressure, polyradiculopathy, or multiple cranial neuropathies. Brain parenchyma involvement is rare, occurring in less than 1% of all systemic lymphomas.

The origin of the malignant lymphocytes in PCNSL is unknown, because the CNS does not have lymph nodes or lymphatics. T cells normally traffic through the CNS, but B cells are not usually found there, and yet most PCNSLs are B-cell tumors. One hypothesis proposes that the lymphoma cells arise elsewhere in the body, then migrate into and preferentially reside in the CNS because of its immunologically privileged milieu; the systemic tumor cells are otherwise destroyed by the normal immune system. The absence of tumor in other immune-privileged sites, such as the testis, argues against this possibility. A corollary is that the transformed cells have homing receptors for cerebral endothelia, suggesting the presence of a unique cell surface marker that would induce migration into the CNS. No specific adhesion molecule has been identified so far that would support this explanation.[50] Another possibility is that a B cell attracted to a CNS inflammatory lesion becomes transformed within the CNS and proliferates there, giving rise to a neoplasm. This is similar to the development of mucosa-associated lymphoid tissue (MALT) lymphoma in the context of *Helicobacter pylori* gastritis.[49] In this situation, chronic antigenic stimulation leads to malignant transformation of B cells targeting the organism. However, the incidence of PCNSL is not increased in inflammatory disease states of the CNS such as multiple sclerosis, encephalitis, or bacterial infections, and no source of chronic antigenic stimulation has been identified in the CNS of PCNSL patients.

Like most diseases of the brain, the symptoms are dictated by the location of the lesion and the amount of local mass effect on surrounding areas. PCNSL usually presents as a brain tumor, with the most common complaints being headache and personality changes. Deficits in higher cortical functioning are common, and signs of increased intracranial pressure may appear. Focal neurologic deficits and epileptic phenomenon are seen as well. The average time to diagnosis from onset of symptoms is approximately 2 to 3 months.

The most common location of the tumor is in the cerebral hemispheres, usually in the frontal lobes, with a predilection for the periventricular white matter, basal ganglia, and corpus callosum (Table 41-2). PCNSL can be seen in the cerebellum, brainstem, and rarely in the spinal cord. The lesions are solitary in 60% to 70% of cases. Systemic dissemination is seen in approximately 7% to 8% of cases and occurs late in the course of the disease.[28] The usual sites of involvement are the lymph nodes of the abdomen and retroperitoneum. These metastatic sites are inconsequential in the course of the disease, and many are found only at autopsy, posing no additional morbidity to the patient.

Embryologically, the eyes are an extension of the nervous system and can be involved by PCNSL without being considered "systemic" disease. Ocular involvement is seen in 20% to 25% of PCNSL patients at diagnosis.[32,52] Occasional patients will have primary ocular lymphoma, the majority having binocular disease. Patients with pure ocular involvement will develop cerebral involvement in 60% to 80% of cases.[52]

EPIDEMIOLOGY

In immunocompetent individuals the incidence of PCNSL is approximately 0.28:100,000 person years, but the incidence

TABLE 41-1

Intracranial Hematopoietic Malignancies

Primary central nervous system lymphoma
Non-Hodgkin's lymphoma
  B cell
  T cell
Granulocytic sarcoma
Plasmacytoma

TABLE 41-2

Location of Primary Central Nervous System Lymphoma

Cerebral hemispheres	52.1%
Cerebellum	11.5%
Brainstem	2.3%
Spinal cord	0.6%
Multiple sites	33.5%

Source: Adapted from Murray K, Kun L, Cox J: Primary malignant lymphoma of the central nervous system. Results of treatment of 11 cases and review of the literature. J Neurosurg 65:600–607, 1986.

TABLE 41-3

Risk Factors for Primary Central Nervous System Lymphoma

Acquired immune deficiency syndrome
Chronic pharmacologic immune suppression
Postorgan transplantation
Myasthenia gravis
Vasculitis
Autoimmune disease
Rheumatoid arthritis
Systemic lupus erythematosus
Sarcoidosis
Sjögren's syndrome
Hereditary immune deficiency
Combined variable immunodeficiency
Immunoglobulin A deficiency
Hyperimmunoglobulin M syndrome
Severe combined immune deficiency
Wiskott-Aldrich syndrome

markedly increases among acquired immunodeficiency syndrome (AIDS) patients to 4.7:100,000 person years.[17] The average age of onset is 58 years for immunocompetent patients, and 43 years in patients with AIDS. The disease is rare in children and is usually associated with inherited immune deficiencies such as common variable immunodeficiency,[54] immunoglobulin A (IgA) deficiency, hyperimmunoglobulin M syndrome, severe combined immune deficiency, or Wiskott-Aldrich syndrome.[23]

The most obvious risk factor for PCNSL is alteration in a patient's immune system (Table 41-3). The disease has been reported to have increased incidence in patients with autoimmune diseases such as rheumatoid arthritis, systemic lupus erythematosus, sarcoidosis, and Sjögren's syndrome. Patients who have had renal and cardiac transplants are also at increased risk. AIDS is the most common immunodeficiency that predisposes patients to PCNSL. PCNSL occurs in approximately 5% of AIDS patients, although this incidence has markedly decreased with the introduction of highly active antiretroviral therapy (HAART).[25] PCNSL is an AIDS-defining illness. In all immunodeficient patients, PCNSL is an Epstein-Barr virus (EBV)-driven lymphoma. EBV is detected by polymerase chain reaction (PCR) in more than 85% of AIDS-related PCNSL compared with 11% to 54% in immunocompetent patients.[6,8,20] Latent EBV infection of B cells persists after all primary infections and immortalizes a subset of cells whose growth is controlled by T cells. When the T-cell control is lost because of compromise of the immune system, the EBV-infected B cells grow, leading to eventual monoclonal expansion and subsequent tumor formation.

Earlier reports found that PCNSL accounted for 0.85% to 3.3% of all intracranial tumors, but recent series have shown an increase in the incidence over the past 20 years, to as much as 4.1% between 1990 and 1994 according to the Central Brain Tumor Registry of the United States (CBTRUS) data.[13] Reasons for the increase are partly attributed to the increased incidence of AIDS, better imaging techniques, vastly improved histologic diagnosis of the disease, and increased survival of organ transplant recipients on immunosuppressive therapy. However, the initial increase was noted before the widespread use of computed tomography (CT) scanning and the AIDS epidemic. Furthermore, most cases occur in patients without any risk factors, and investigators have yet to fully account for the observed dramatic increase in incidence.

There is a slight male preponderance in immunocompetent patients in most large series, which mirrors the gender ratio in systemic lymphoma. In AIDS patients, the ratio is heavily skewed toward males because human immunodeficiency virus (HIV) infection in the United States affects mostly men. There are no known geographic or ethnic variations of PCNSL.

NEUROIMAGING

Magnetic resonance imaging (MRI) is invaluable in the initial evaluation of all brain tumors and should be the only modality used unless the patient cannot have an MRI scan. PCNSL in immunocompetent patients is characterized on both CT and MRI as a mass lesion with prominent homogeneous enhancement (Figure 41-1). Noncontrast CT scans show a hyperdense lesion with mass effect and surrounding vasogenic edema. The tumors are typically hypointense on T1-weighted magnetic resonance (MR) images and isointense to hyperintense on T2 sequences. The tumor is usually periventricular and may cross the midline. Necrosis, hemorrhage, or calcification is rare. Some patients will have a nonenhanced lesion on MRI,

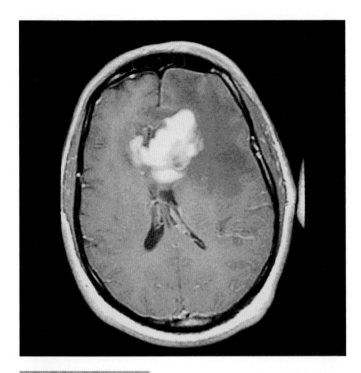

FIGURE 41-1 Primary central nervous system lymphoma. T1 postcontrast magnetic resonance imaging sequence showing the characteristic homogeneous enhancement of the lesions.

which may be confusing diagnostically, but nonenhanced disease is more characteristic of PCNSL in immunodeficient patients.

In AIDS patients, the typical lesion is multifocal with ring-like enhancement. There may be associated central necrosis or hemorrhage, and the lesions are commonly located more peripherally.

Positron-emission tomography (PET) and single-photon emission spectroscopy (SPECT) are ancillary imaging modalities that can help diagnostically in AIDS-related PCNSL. The imaging characteristics of toxoplasmosis and PCNSL are indistinguishable by MRI or CT; however, toxoplasmosis will have decreased metabolism on fluorodeoxyglucose (FDG)-PET scan, but hypermetabolism is seen in PCNSL.[57] Thallium-201 SPECT shows a similar increase in tracer uptake in PCNSL compared with decreased uptake in toxoplasmosis. Although these two modalities are quite sensitive and specific, false positives and false negatives may occur.

DIAGNOSIS

The diagnosis of a brain tumor is established by imaging, and the diagnosis of PCNSL by tissue histology. Stereotactic biopsy is the preferred approach in most patients and is safe and effective even for deep-seated lesions. Cerebrospinal fluid (CSF) cytology reveals tumor cells in approximately 15% of cases where a lumbar puncture is done.[42] A greater number of patients will have nonspecific abnormalities, such as an increased CSF protein concentration in approximately 75%.[28] In the occasional patient who refuses biopsy, CSF may establish the diagnosis. In addition to standard cytologic examination, CSF tumor

TABLE 41-4

Staging for Patients with Primary Central Nervous System Lymphoma

Cerebrospinal fluid cytology
Ophthalmologic (slit-lamp) examination
Computed tomography scan of chest, abdomen, and pelvis
Bone marrow biopsy
HIV test

markers, specifically beta-2 microglobulin, and immunophenotyping the CSF cells or demonstration of a clonal immunoglobulin gene arrangement can all increase the yield of CSF analysis. Vitrectomy can also establish the diagnosis and is necessary in patients with isolated ocular lymphoma. Identification of interleukin 10 levels in the vitreous fluid as well as immunophenotyping vitreous cells may establish the diagnosis.[66]

In the immunodeficient patient, detection of EBV DNA by PCR of the CSF is a reliable and specific diagnostic indicator of PCNSL. When EBV is identified in the CSF and the patient has a hypermetabolic lesion on PET or increased uptake on thallium-SPECT, there is 100% certainty that the lesion is PCNSL, and biopsy can be avoided.[4] This is important because biopsy of intracranial lesions, including PCNSL, is associated with an increased risk of significant CNS hemorrhage compared with brain biopsy in the immunocompetent host.[61] Therefore in AIDS and other immunosuppressed patients, the diagnosis can be established indirectly with certainty. These tests should replace empirical treatment for CNS toxoplasmosis as the first approach to an intracranial lesion in AIDS patients.

At diagnosis, staging with body CT scan, lumbar puncture, slit-lamp ophthalmologic examination, and bone marrow aspiration is performed to determine the extent of disease and to exclude systemic lymphoma (Table 41-4). Systemic staging identifies an extra-CNS site of lymphoma in less than 4%[47] of patients, so a comprehensive systemic evaluation may be eliminated[29] in some patients not enrolled in a clinical trial. Serology for HIV is imperative to rule out AIDS.

Corticosteroids may interfere with accurate diagnosis if given before biopsy of the lesion because of their potential for a direct cytotoxic effect on lymphoma cells.[18] There can be a manifest reduction in size or even disappearance of tumor after administration of corticosteroids.[60] A subsequent pathologic specimen may reveal normal or necrotic cells, and no lymphoma may be found. Some authors argue that a disappearing tumor in the wake of corticosteroid administration is pathognomonic of PCNSL, but diseases such as multiple sclerosis and neurosarcoidosis respond to steroids and can imitate the imaging and clinical characteristics of PCNSL. Prebiopsy administration of steroids should be avoided unless the patient is in imminent danger of cerebral herniation. Although the initial MRI scan of these patients can be quite dramatic, the majority are clinically stable and do well without corticosteroids while awaiting their biopsy. If corticosteroid administration is unavoidable and an inconclusive biopsy is obtained, the drug should be withdrawn promptly and timely rebiopsy of the lesion attempted. Close observation is warranted, because explosive tumor growth has been observed after discontinuation of corticosteroids.

TUMOR HISTOLOGY

Microscopic examination of PCNSL reveals perivascular lesions infiltrating small arteries, arterioles, and venules.[42] There is diffuse centrifugal invasion of the surrounding parenchyma with layering of neoplastic cells around the blood vessels. This angiocentric growth is characteristic, and follicular growth patterns are rarely encountered. The periphery of the tumor shows variable reactive gliosis and infiltration by reactive T lymphocytes. Leptomeningeal involvement is often evident in advanced disease,[28] even if CSF cytologic examination is negative for tumor.

Histologically, the majority of PCNSL tumors are typical B-cell NHLs. The cells consistently express monotypic immunoglobulin, commonly IgM kappa, and the B-cell restricted antigen CD20. Classified according to the International Working Formulation, roughly half would be diffuse large cell type, followed in decreasing frequency by diffuse large cell immunoblastic, diffuse small cleaved cell, unclassifiable, and diffuse small and large cell types.[49] Adoption of the Revised European-American Lymphoma (REAL) Classification in 1994 simplifies it further (Table 41-5), and approximately 90% of all PCNSLs are classified as diffuse large B-cell lymphoma (large cell variant).[12]

Primary T-cell lymphoma occurs in approximately 1% to 3% of all PCNSLs and is seen in both immunocompetent and immunocompromised patients.[12,26] A younger age at diagnosis has been observed and an infratentorial location more often reported. It is unclear if the biologic behavior and response to treatment is different from the usual B-cell PCNSL because of its rarity.

Ordinarily, morphology is adequate to establish the diagnosis, but occasionally immunophenotyping can improve diagnostic precision. Using morphology, immunophenotyping, and clinical features, agreement on classification by a panel of recognized experts is made 85% of the time in systemic NHL.[63]

TABLE 41-5

Histologic Classification of Primary Central Nervous System Lymphoma (REAL Classification)

Diffuse large cell	86%
Peripheral T cell	3%
Lymphocytic	2%
Lymphoplasmacytoid	1%
Burkitt lymphoma	1%
Hodgkin's disease	1%
Unclassified	2%

REAL, Revised European-American Lymphoma (REAL).
Source: Adapted from Camilleri-Broët S, Martin A, Moreau A, et al: Primary central nervous system lymphomas in 72 immunocompetent patients: pathologic findings and clinical correlations. Groupe Ouest Est d'étude des Leucénies et Autres Maladies du Sang (GOELAMS). Am J Clin Pathol 110:607–612, 1998.

Recent advances in molecular biology are being applied to classify systemic NHL based on genotype. Specialized DNA microarray technology was used to analyze the gene expression variations in diffuse large B-cell lymphoma (DLBCL).[3] Two different subtypes were identified among histologically identical tumors when gene expression during a specific stage in the differentiation of the B cell was investigated (the germinal center B-cell signature). The first subgroup, germinal center B-like DLBCL, showed close similarities with the gene expression of normal B cells. The other type, activated B-like DLBCL, lacked this expression and was found to have similarities with artificially activated peripheral blood B cells. Furthermore, germinal center B-like DLBCL was associated with a better clinical prognosis because of its response to chemotherapy. These findings indicate that within an apparently homogeneous phenotypic group, lymphomas will vary significantly in their genotypic make-up and biologic behavior. These techniques have not yet been applied to PCNSL, but we may anticipate similar findings.

THERAPY

Corticosteroids

As mentioned previously, some lymphomas are exquisitely sensitive to corticosteroids.[60] The lymphoma cells contain a glucocorticoid receptor that can trigger apoptosis, causing cell lysis and tumor reduction within hours to days of administration.[43] This is independent of the effect that dexamethasone may also have in reducing tumor-associated vasogenic edema. Tumor shrinkage is usually temporary; the tumor recurs several months later or soon after withdrawal of the drug. We have observed that at least 60% of PCNSL patients have a partial or complete response to dexamethasone. If corticosteroids have been withheld before biopsy, they may be initiated immediately after tissue has been obtained, to reduce neurologic symptoms.

Surgery

Henry et al reported a median survival of only 4.6 months in PCNSL patients treated with surgical excision alone.[28] Murray et al reviewed the literature in 1986 and found a median survival of 1 month for patients who had only resection.[44] Unlike most primary brain tumors, surgery is not helpful therapeutically, because most tumors are deeply situated and often widespread microscopically. Furthermore, attempted resection may lead to increased neurologic morbidity (Table 41-6).

The role of surgery in PCNSL is limited to diagnosis by stereotactic biopsy and emergency decompressive surgery in a patient with symptoms of acute herniation from mass effect. In cases where PCNSL was not suspected preoperatively, frozen section can indicate the correct diagnosis, and once sufficient tissue has been obtained for a final diagnosis, the planned resection can be aborted.

Radiation Therapy

Cranial irradiation achieves complete remission in most patients but recurrence develops approximately 1 year after therapy. Henry et al reported a median survival of 15.2 months for patients receiving cranial radiation in their published review

TABLE 41-6

Median Survival of Primary Central Nervous System Lymphoma

Supportive care	1–3 months
Surgery	1–4 months
WBRT	12–18 months
CHOP or CHOD + WBRT	8–16 months
IA MTX	40 months
IV MTX alone	33 months
IV MTX + WBRT	33–60 months

CHOD, Cyclophosphamide, doxorubicin, vincristine, and dexamethasone; CHOP, cyclophosphamide, doxorubicin, vincristine, and prednisone; IA, intra-arterial; IV, intravenous; MTX, methotrexate; WBRT, whole-brain radiation therapy.

of cases.[28] Murray et al observed a median survival of 17 months,[44] and in 1992 the Radiation Therapy Oncology Group (RTOG) conducted a prospective trial of whole-brain irradiation for PCNSL, finding a median survival of 12.2 months.[46] Cranial irradiation alone gives an overall survival of 12 to 18 months in almost all series, with less than 5% surviving after 5 years.

For PCNSL, radiation therapy must be delivered to the whole brain, because widespread infiltration of disease is present in all patients, even if only a single lesion is seen on neuroimaging. A recent study has evaluated the role of focal radiation therapy (RT) and found that patients who received a wide margin (4 cm) had better disease control than those treated with a standard focal RT port.[59] Current autopsy data identified microscopic tumor in multiple regions of the brain that are radiographically normal, including fluid-attenuated inversion recovery (FLAIR) sequences on MRI. Whole-brain doses of 30 to 50 Gy are effective, but there is no clear dose-response relationship for more than 30 Gy. In addition, there are no data to support using a tumor boost; it does not enhance local control. Some authors advocated craniospinal irradiation for disseminated disease, but this did not enhance outcome.[9]

Karnofsky Performance Scale score and age were identified as prognostic factors in the RTOG trial and other studies. In the RTOG study, a Karnofsky Performance Scale score of 70 or greater was associated with an improved survival to 21.1 months compared with 5.6 months in patients with a score of 60 or less.[46] Age younger than 60 was also associated with a significantly better prognosis for survival (median 23.1 months) compared with patients older than 60 years (median 7.6 months).

Present recommendations include whole-brain irradiation of 45 Gy without a boost. The eyes are not included in the port unless ocular involvement is present. The eyes receive approximately 36 to 40 Gy of radiation in the event of ocular lymphoma. Like brain lymphoma, recurrence is expected if only radiation therapy is used to treat the eyes; however, these patients may develop ocular or cerebral relapse.

Chemotherapy

PCNSL has attracted the interest of many investigators because of its rising incidence and relative chemosensitivity. Chemo-

therapy is efficacious in the treatment of systemic NHL, and standard systemic regimens have been tried in the treatment of PCNSL. Lachance et al were the first to report on cyclophosphamide, doxorubicin, vincristine, and prednisone (CHOP) combined with radiation therapy, but median survival was only 8.5 months.[36] Although CHOP induced a remission, rapid regrowth was often observed at sites in the CNS distant from the initial disease. The RTOG conducted a multicenter phase II trial of a similar regimen—CHOD (dexamethasone instead of prednisone)—before irradiation.[58] Their study had an overall survival of 16.1 months, and a significant number of patients experienced severe toxicity from the chemotherapy. O'Neill et al initiated a phase II trial of preirradiation CHOP with postirradiation high-dose cytosine arabinoside that can penetrate the blood-brain barrier and achieve therapeutic levels in the CNS; however, their study did not show a survival advantage over radiation therapy alone.[48] Most recently, Mead et al reported a randomized trial of whole-brain RT alone versus CHOP and whole-brain RT.[41] There was no difference in the outcome between the groups, and accrual had to be stopped, because they had difficulty enrolling patients in the study. The failure of CHOP or CHOD to improve outcome was partially due to the inability of the drugs to reach occult disease behind an intact blood-brain barrier. Initial responses are achieved because the observed bulky tumor has a defective blood-brain barrier, manifest by its generous uptake of imaging-contrast media. However, the microscopic disease that was protected by the blood-brain barrier continues to grow and is responsible for tumor progression.

Methotrexate is now recognized as the drug of choice for the initial treatment of PCNSL. It inhibits dihydrofolate reductase, an essential enzyme for folate reduction; reduced folate is a necessary coenzyme in the synthesis of purine and thymidine. The use of methotrexate in PCNSL is a consequence of the observation that NHL patients who received high doses of the drug had a lower incidence of CNS relapse. Early reports of successful treatment of recurrent PCNSL were first noted in the late 1970s. Loeffler et al observed a median survival of 44 months in 5 patients they treated with either intravenous or intrathecal methotrexate in addition to radiation therapy.[38] Gabbai et al used a dose of 3 g/m^2 and showed that complete and partial responses were achieved with the drug before irradiation, and that toxicities were minimal.[24] Glass et al used 3 to 5 g/m^2 of methotrexate followed by whole-brain irradiation and showed a median survival of 33 months in their 25 patients.[27] DeAngelis et al used 1 g/m^2 followed by whole-brain irradiation and high-dose cytarabine.[21] They treated 31 patients and observed a median survival of 41 months. A follow-up study by Abrey et al reported a median survival of 60 months in 52 patients using 3.5 g/m^2 of methotrexate with the addition of procarbazine and vincristine.[2]

Methotrexate is able to penetrate the intact blood-brain barrier when given in high doses (>1 g/m^2) and is thus able to treat microscopic disease that was previously inaccessible. It also achieves therapeutic levels in CSF at this dose. Rapid infusion over 2 to 3 hours achieves a significantly higher CSF level than an infusion over 24 hours,[31] obviating the need for intrathecal administration. Hence bulky, microinvasive, and leptomeningeal disease are all addressed with high-dose methotrexate. There are preliminary data to suggest that high-dose methotrexate may eliminate the need for supplemental intrathecal drugs in the treatment of PCNSL.[34]

Combined modality therapy has been shown to be the most effective way of controlling this disease. Chemotherapy is delivered before irradiation, so that initial response to the therapy can be observed and not masked by the effects of irradiation. With this scheme, nonresponders to chemotherapy can be identified early and an appropriate shift in management instituted before any significant toxicity from the drug is seen. In addition, administration of methotrexate before irradiation reduces the risk of neurotoxicity; however, despite sequencing the therapies in this fashion, significant neurotoxicity is still observed. Cranial irradiation and methotrexate are independently known to be neurotoxic and cause delayed leukoencephalopathy. Patients who receive brain irradiation for gliomas or metastases develop white matter changes related to demyelination and may develop clinical neurotoxicity.[19,53] However, whereas the radiographic changes are often seen, few have clinically significant effects, because radiation toxicity may be delayed and not evident unless the patient has long survival, a luxury not enjoyed by most patients with these diseases. Methotrexate by itself is neurotoxic and can cause transient neurologic symptoms such as seizures, cognitive deficits, and even motor dysfunction.[65] When given intrathecally, a chemical arachnoiditis may ensue and present as acute meningitis. The toxic results of combined therapy are synergistic, and patients older than 60 years are most vulnerable. Affected patients have progressive dementia, ataxia, urinary incontinence, and altered consciousness. Abrey et al observed that 25% of all patients and 83% of those older than 60 developed delayed toxicity.[2] In an effort to reduce neurotoxicity, patients were treated with chemotherapy alone and had radiation therapy deferred until relapse. They found a median survival of 33 months for the patients age 60 and older who deferred irradiation, identical to the median survival of 34 months in the same age group who received identical chemotherapy combined with whole-brain RT. Patients who deferred irradiation died mostly of progressive disease, whereas patients who underwent radiation therapy died from neurotoxicity, suggesting that irradiation helps with disease control but at an unacceptably high cost. Several other investigators have shown that delaying radiation therapy in older patients can be done without adversely affecting survival. Younger patients are more resilient but not immune from the sequelae of treatment. Initial reports showed preservation of quality of life in most patients, but other studies suggest that some degree of cognitive decline or physical deterioration is observed in all long-term survivors treated with combined therapy.

The increasing move to use chemotherapy alone to treat PCNSL in an effort to prevent or limit neurotoxicity has led to a single trial of high-dose chemotherapy with autologous stem cell rescue (ASCR) for newly diagnosed PCNSL patients.[1] Patients underwent induction therapy with high-dose methotrexate and only those with a partial response or better proceeded to high-dose therapy followed by stem cell rescue. Out of 28 enrolled patients, 14 (50%) proceeded to high-dose chemotherapy with ASCR; the other 14 patients had insufficient response to high-dose methotrexate to continue on the protocol. There was no transplant-related mortality, and only one patient had grade III or IV morbidity. Of the patients who had transplant, the median overall survival has not been reached after a median follow-up of 28 months, suggesting that this is a feasible approach that deserves further study.

Some authors advocate chemotherapy alone using blood-brain barrier disruption with a hyperosmolar agent followed by intra-arterial methotrexate. McAllister et al treated 111 patients with methotrexate-based therapy after blood-brain barrier disruption. They had a median survival of 40 months without significant late neurotoxicity.[39] Intra-arterial methotrexate does carry significant vascular and neurologic risks such as arterial dissection, seizures, and stroke. Using this form of drug delivery also requires a specialized center and unique competency that is of very limited availability.

Immunocompromised Patients

Effective therapy in immunocompromised patients, particularly in AIDS patients, is often limited by the patient's underlying systemic condition. Some patients are candidates only for palliative whole-brain RT, which can lead to increased survival, but the duration of response is usually 5 months or less; however, many of these patients die of a systemic process such as an opportunistic infection and not from progressive PCNSL. Chemotherapy is often not a viable option because of the immunocompromised status of the patient, but high-dose methotrexate has been used with good results in the minority of patients able to tolerate it.[15] Patients with a low viral load, a CD4 T-cell count greater than or equal to 200/mm^3, and no opportunistic infections are more likely to tolerate high-dose methotrexate-based therapy. Recent reports suggest that reconstitution of the immune system, primarily in AIDS patients, can also lead to PCNSL regression.[33] There are now several reports of AIDS patients with biopsy-proved PCNSL who had a complete tumor response when HAART was instituted in patients not previously taking antiretroviral therapy.[16,33,40] Many of these patients also received agents such as ganciclovir, directed against the EBV-stimulated growth.[55] Therefore this strategy should be incorporated into any treatment of PCNSL in AIDS patients, whether it is used as the sole therapeutic approach or in combination with more conventional treatments. In other immunocompromised patients, continuation of the immunosuppressives is required to maintain an organ transplant, and thus reversal of the immunocompromised state is not feasible.

Recurrent PCNSL

Despite the addition of methotrexate-based therapy, 40% to 60% of patients eventually relapse. For most patients, salvage therapy improves survival. Whole-brain RT may be used in patients who have not received cranial radiation as part of initial therapy. Several systemic and intrathecal drugs can be used at relapse: the procarbazine, lomustine, and vincristine (PCV) combination[2,56]; thiotepa[22]; high-dose cytarabine[56]; and ifosfamide, carboplatin, and etoposide.[2] Intrathecal therapy via an Ommaya reservoir is helpful in patients with leptomeningeal disease; this allows better distribution of drug compared with intrathecal administration via lumbar puncture. Patients with bulky leptomeningeal disease should have a radioisotope CSF flow study before drug is administered into the subarachnoid space. Abnormal studies signify obstruction leading to inhomogeneous distribution of drug, and if the drug is retained in the ventricle, leakage may occur around the catheter, resulting in localized necrotizing leukoencephalopathy.

The search for better therapies, whether to decrease the risk of neurotoxicity or to increase overall survival, continues. Rituximab is an anti-CD20 antibody that has excellent activity against systemic follicular and diffuse large cell lymphoma.[7] Approximately 90% of all PCNSLs express the CD20 antigen, and rituximab is being studied as an adjunct to existing methotrexate-based protocols. Initial case reports of intravenous and intrathecal administration show promising results,[51,56] and prospective trials in combination with methotrexate are under way.

Temozolomide is a cytotoxic alkylating agent that has activity against malignant glioma and is able to penetrate the intact blood-brain barrier readily. Some authors have reported good results when temozolomide is used in patients unable to receive high-dose methotrexate because of poor performance status or renal insufficiency.[30] Because of its relative tolerability and minimal potential for nephrotoxicity, temozolomide may emerge as a good alternative to methotrexate-based therapy in select patients[37] or prove to be a good salvage regimen at relapse.[56] Further studies are needed to elucidate the true efficacy of this drug.

There has been one study of high-dose chemotherapy and autologous stem cell transplantation in recurrent PCNSL. Soussain et al achieved a median survival of almost 3 years in relapsed PCNSL patients treated with high-dose busulfan and thiotepa and ASCR.[62] This is a good option in patients with a good performance status.

GRANULOCYTIC SARCOMA

Intracranial granulocytic sarcomas or chloromas are solid extramedullary manifestations of acute myelogenous leukemia (AML), and they occur in less than 1% of AML patients.[11] They can develop anywhere in the body, including the CNS and occasionally in the brain parenchyma but more commonly in the meninges (Figure 41-2). The clinical presentation depends on the location and amount of mass effect exerted by the tumor.

Most chloromas develop in patients with known AML, and they often have active disease. However, granulocytic sarcoma can be an isolated tumor without evidence of medullary leukemia. The definitive diagnosis of such tumors can be difficult because of the relative immaturity of the neoplastic cells.[45] Immunohistochemical staining and electron microscopy can be helpful to differentiate granulocytic sarcomas from malignant lymphomas in difficult cases; however, when a typical dural-based lesion develops in a patient with known AML, biopsy is rarely necessary for diagnosis, and appropriate treatment can be based on the radiographic findings alone. The tumors are managed with surgical excision if they are compressing a critical structure, followed by cranial irradiation. Initiation of systemic chemotherapy in patients with isolated chloroma is recommended by most authors because of the high incidence of developing systemic leukemia after local therapy alone, and initiation of chemotherapy reduces subsequent systemic disease.[11]

PLASMACYTOMA

Intracranial plasmacytoma is a solitary plasma cell tumor of the CNS that may affect the skull, meninges, or parenchyma (Figure 41-3). The majority are dural-based and often mimic meningiomas. Plasmacytomas are composed of monoclonal

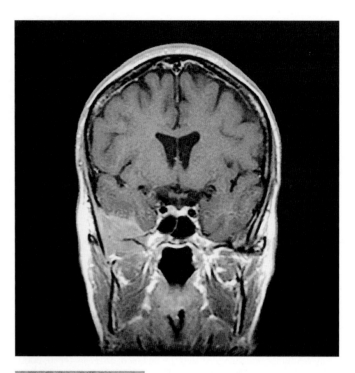

FIGURE 41-2 Granulocytic sarcoma or chloroma. A right temporal dural-based enhancing mass on magnetic resonance T1-weighted postcontrast imaging.

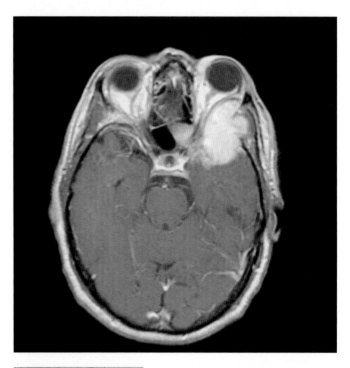

FIGURE 41-3 Plasmacytoma. T1-weighted postcontrast magnetic resonance image showing skull and dural invasion. (Courtesy of Sasan Karimi, MD, of Memorial Sloan-Kettering Cancer Center.)

plasma cells, which distinguish them from plasma cell granulomas and meningiomas. Transformation to multiple myeloma is common, especially in patients with calvarial lesions. Plasmacytomas that progress to multiple myeloma carry a worse prognosis than plasmacytomas that occur in isolation. A thorough systemic evaluation with bone marrow biopsy, serum and urine protein electrophoresis, quantitative immunoglobulin analysis, and skeletal survey is necessary for all patients with extramedullary intracranial plasmacytoma.[64] Treatment is surgical excision followed by cranial irradiation.[10] The tumors are radiosensitive, and local control is achieved in most cases.

Immunoglobulin measurements in the serum and CSF are useful in the follow-up of plasmacytoma, because decreasing levels often correlate with successful treatment. Calvarial and sinus-based lesions are approached with more caution because of their high incidence of progression to multiple myeloma. There are some data to suggest that adjuvant chemotherapy can delay progression to multiple myeloma, but there is no conclusive evidence that the incidence is decreased. At present, recommendations for the treatment of intramedullary plasmacytomas is complete surgical excision whenever possible followed by cranial irradiation.

References

1. Abrey LE, Moskowitz CH, Mason WP, et al: Intensive methotrexate and cytarabine followed by high-dose chemotherapy with autologous stem cell rescue in patients with newly diagnosed primary CNS lymphoma: an intent to treat analysis. J Clin Oncol 21:4151–4156, 2003.
2. Abrey LE, Yahalom J, DeAngelis LM: Treatment for primary CNS lymphoma: the next step. J Clin Oncol 18:3144–3150, 2000.
3. Alizadeh AA, Eisen MB, Davis RE, et al: Distinct types of diffuse large B-cell lymphoma identified by gene expression profiling. Nature 403:503–511, 2000.
4. Antinori A, De Rossi G, Ammassari A, et al: Value of combined approach with thallium-201 single-photon emission computed tomography and Epstein-Barr virus DNA polymerase chain reaction in CSF for the diagnosis of AIDS-related primary CNS lymphoma. J Clin Oncol 17:554–560, 1999.
5. Bailey P: Intracranial sarcomatous tumors of leptomeningeal origin. Arch Surg 18:1359–1402, 1929.
6. Bashir RM, Hochberg FH, Wei MX: Epstein-Barr virus and brain lymphomas. J Neurooncol 24:195–206, 1995.
7. Bendandi M, Longo DL: Biologic therapy for lymphoma. Curr Opin Oncol 11:343–350, 1999.
8. Bignon YJ, Clavelou P, Ramos F, et al: Detection of Epstein-Barr virus sequences in primary brain lymphoma without immunodeficiency. Neurology 41:1152–1153, 1991.
9. Brada M, Dearnaley D, Horwich A, Bloom HJ: Management of primary cerebral lymphoma with initial chemotherapy: preliminary results and comparison with patients treated with radiotherapy alone. Int J Radiat Oncol Biol Phys 18:787–792, 1990.
10. Bindal AK, Bindal RK, van Loveren H, Sawaya R: Management of intracranial plasmacytoma. J Neurosurg 83:218–221, 1995.
11. Byrd JC, Edenfield WJ, Shields DJ, Dawson NA: Extramedullary myeloid cell tumors in acute nonlymphocytic leukemia: a clinical review. J Clin Oncol 13:1800–1816, 1995.
12. Camilleri-Broët S, Martin A, Moreau A, et al: Primary central nervous system lymphomas in 72 immunocompetent patients: pathologic findings and clinical correlations. Groupe Ouest Est d'étude des Leucénies et Autres Maladies du Sang (GOELAMS). Am J Clin Pathol 110:607–612, 1998.
13. CBTRUS (1998). 1997 Annual Report. Published by the Central Brain Tumor Registry of the United States.
14. CBTRUS (2002). 2002 Statistical Report: Primary Brain Tumors in the United States, 1995–1999. Published by the Central Brain Tumor Registry of the United States.
15. Chamberlain MC: Long survival in patients with acquired immune deficiency syndrome-related primary central nervous system lymphoma. Cancer 73:1728–1730, 1994.
16. Corales R, Taege A, Rehm S, Schmitt S: Regression of AIDS-related CNS Lymphoma with HAART. XIII International AIDS Conference, 2000 (Abstract).
17. Coté TR, Manns A, Hardy CR, et al: Epidemiology of brain lymphoma among people with or without acquired immune deficiency syndrome. J Natl Cancer Inst 88:675–679, 1996.
18. DeAngelis LM: Primary CNS lymphoma: treatment with combined chemotherapy and radiotherapy. J Neurooncol 43:249–257, 1999.
19. DeAngelis LM, Delattre JY, Posner JB: Radiation-induced dementia in patients cured of brain metastasis. Neurology 39:789–796, 1989.
20. DeAngelis LM, Wong E, Rosenblum M, Furneaux H: Epstein-Barr virus in acquired immune deficiency syndrome and non-AIDS primary central nervous system lymphoma. Cancer 70:1607–1611, 2001.
21. DeAngelis LM, Yahalom J, Thaler HT, Kher U: Combined modality therapy for primary CNS lymphoma. J Clin Oncol 10:635–643, 1992.
22. De Smet MD, Vancs VS, Kohler D, et al: Intravitreal chemotherapy for the treatment of recurrent intraocular lymphoma. Br J Ophthalmol 83:448–451, 1999.
23. Filipovich AH, Grimley MS: Immunodeficiency and cancer. In Abeloff, MD, Armitage JO, Lichter AS (eds): Clinical Oncology, ed 2. Philadelphia, Churchill Livingstone, 2000.
24. Gabbai AA, Hochberg FH, Linggood RM, et al: High-dose methotrexate for non-AIDS primary central nervous system lymphoma. Report of 13 cases. J Neurosurg 70:190–194, 1989.
25. Gates AE, Kaplan LD: AIDS malignancies in the era of highly active antiretroviral therapy. Oncology (Huntingt) 16:657–665; discussion 665, 668–670, 2002.
26. Gijtenbeek JM, Rosenblum MK, DeAngelis LM: Primary central nervous system T-cell lymphoma. Neurology 57:716–718, 2001.
27. Glass J, Gruber ML, Cher L, Hochberg FH: Preirradiation methotrexate chemotherapy of primary central nervous system lymphoma: long-term outcome. J Neurosurg 81:188–195, 1994.
28. Henry JM, Heffner RR Jr, Dillard SH, et al: Primary malignant lymphomas of the central nervous system. Cancer 34:1293–1302, 1974.
29. Herrlinger U: Primary CNS lymphoma: findings outside the brain. J Neurooncol 43:227–230, 1999.
30. Herrlinger U, Küker W, Platten M, et al: First-line therapy with temozolomide induces regression of primary CNS lymphoma. Neurology 58:1573–1574, 2002.
31. Hiraga S, Arita N, Ohnishi T, et al: Rapid infusion of high-dose methotrexate resulting in enhanced penetration into cerebrospinal fluid and intensified tumor response in primary central nervous system lymphomas. J Neurosurg 91:221–230, 1999.
32. Hochberg FH, Miller DC: Primary central nervous system lymphoma. J Neurosurg 68:835–853, 1988.
33. Hoffmann C, Tabrizian S, Wolf E, et al: Survival of AIDS patients with primary central nervous system lymphoma is dramatically

improved by HAART-induced immune recovery. AIDS 15: 2119–2127, 2001.

34. Khan RB, Shi W, Thaler HT, et al: Is intrathecal methotrexate necessary in the treatment of primary CNS lymphoma? J Neurooncol 58:175–178, 2002.

35. Krol AD, Le Cessie S, Snijder S, et al: Primary extranodal non-Hodgkin's lymphoma (NHL): the impact of alternative definitions tested in the comprehensive cancer centre west population-based NHL registry. Ann Oncol 14:131–139, 2003.

36. Lachance DH, Brizel DM, Gockerman JP, et al: Cyclophosphamide, doxorubicin, vincristine, and prednisone for primary central nervous system lymphoma: short-duration response and multifocal intracerebral recurrence preceding radiotherapy. Neurology 44:1721–1727, 1994.

37. Lerro KA, Lacy J: Case report: a patient with primary CNS lymphoma treated with temozolomide to complete response. J Neurooncol 59:165–168, 2002.

38. Loeffler JS, Ervin TJ, Mauch P, et al: Primary lymphomas of the central nervous system: patterns of failure and factors that influence survival. J Clin Oncol 3:490–494, 1985.

39. McAllister LD, Doolittle ND, Guastadisegni PE, et al: Cognitive outcomes and long-term follow-up results after enhanced chemotherapy delivery for primary central nervous system lymphoma. Neurosurgery 46:51–60, 2000.

40. McGowan JP, Shah S: Long-term remission of AIDS-related primary central nervous system lymphoma associated with highly active antiretroviral therapy. AIDS 12:952–954, 1998 (Letter).

41. Mead GM, Bleehen NM, Gregor A, et al: A medical research council randomized trial in patients with primary cerebral non-Hodgkin's lymphoma. Cancer 89:1359–1370, 2000.

42. Miller DC, Hochberg FH, Harris NL, et al: Pathology with clinical correlations of primary central nervous system non-Hodgkin's lymphoma. The Massachusetts General Hospital experience 1958–1989. Cancer 74:1383–1397, 1994.

43. Molnar PP, O'Neill BP, Scheithauer BW, Groothuis DR: The blood-brain barrier in primary CNS lymphomas: ultrastructural evidence of endothelial cell death. Neuro-oncol 1:89–100, 1999.

44. Murray K, Kun L, Cox J: Primary malignant lymphoma of the central nervous system. Results of treatment of 11 cases and review of the literature. J Neurosurg 65:600–607, 1986.

45. Neiman RS, Barcos M, Berard C, et al: Granulocytic sarcoma: a clinicopathologic study of 61 biopsied cases. Cancer 48:1426–1437, 1981.

46. Nelson DF, Martz KL, Bonner H, et al: Non-Hodgkin's lymphoma of the brain: can high dose, large volume radiation therapy improve survival? Report on a prospective trial by the Radiation Therapy Oncology Group (RTOG): RTOG 8315. Int J Radiat Oncol Biol Phys 23:9–17, 1992.

47. O'Neill BP, Dinapoli RP, Kurtin PJ, Habermann TM: Occult systemic non-Hodgkin's lymphoma (NHL) in patients initially diagnosed as primary central nervous system lymphoma (PCNSL): how much staging is enough? J Neurooncol 25:67–71, 1995.

48. O'Neill BP, O'Fallon JR, Earle JD, et al: Primary central nervous system non-Hodgkin's lymphoma: survival advantages with combined initial therapy? Int J Radiat Oncol Biol Phys 33:663–673, 1995.

49. Paulus W: Classification, pathogenesis and molecular pathology of primary CNS lymphomas. J Neurooncol 43:203–208, 1999.

50. Paulus W, Jellinger K: Comparison of integrin adhesion molecules, expressed by primary brain lymphomas and nodal lymphomas. Acta Neuropathol 86: 360–364, 1993.

51. Pels H, Schultz H, Manzke O, et al: Intraventricular and intravenous treatment of a patient with refractory primary CNS lymphoma using rituximab. J Neurooncol 59:213–216, 2002.

52. Peterson K, Gordon KB, Heinemann MH, et al: The clinical spectrum of ocular lymphoma. Cancer 72:843–849, 1993.

53. Posner JB: Neurologic Complications of Cancer. Philadelphia, FA Davis Company, 1995.

54. Purtilo DT, Sakamoto K, Barnabei V, et al: Epstein-Barr virus-induced disease in boys with the X-linked lymphoproliferative syndrome (XLP). Am J Med 73:49–56, 1982.

55. Raez L, Cabral L, Cai JP, et al: Treatment of AIDS-related primary central nervous system lymphoma with zidovudine, gancyclovir, and interleukin 2. AIDS Res Hum Retroviruses 15:713–719, 1999.

56. Reni M, Ferreri AJ: Therapeutic management of refractory or relapsed primary central nervous system lymphomas. Ann Hematol 80(Suppl 3):B113–B117, 2001.

57. Roelcke U, Leenders KL: Positron emission tomography in patients with primary CNS lymphoma. J Neurooncol 43:231–236, 1999.

58. Schultz C, Scott C, Sherman W, et al: Preirradiation chemotherapy with cyclophosphamide, doxorubicin, vincristine, and dexamethasone for primary CNS lymphomas: initial report of radiation therapy oncology group protocol 88–06. J Clin Oncol 14:556–564, 1996.

59. Shibamoto Y, Hayabuchi N, Hiratsuka J, et al: Is whole-brain irradiation necessary for primary central nervous system lymphoma? Patterns of recurrence after partial-brain irradiation. Cancer 97:128–133, 2003.

60. Singh A, Strobos RJ, Rothballer AB, et al: Steroid-induced remission in CNS lymphoma. Neurology 32:1267–1271, 1982.

61. Skolasky RL, Dal Pan GL, Olivi A, et al: HIV-associated primary CNS morbidity and utility of brain biopsy. J Neurol Sci 163:32–38, 1999.

62. Soussain C, Suzan F, Hoang-Xuan K, et al: Results of intensive chemotherapy followed by hematopoietic stem-cell rescue in 22 patients with refractory or recurrent primary CNS lymphoma or intraocular lymphoma. J Clin Oncol 19:742–749, 2001.

63. The Non-Hodgkin's Lymphoma Classification Project: A clinical evaluation of the international lymphoma study group classification of non-Hodgkin's lymphoma. Blood 89:3909–3918, 1997.

64. Vujovic O, Fisher BJ, Munoz DG: Solitary intracranial plasmacytoma: case report and review of management. J Neurooncol 39:47–50, 1998.

65. Walker RW, Allen JC, Rosen G, Caparros B: Transient cerebral dysfunction secondary to high-dose methotrexate. J Clin Oncol 4:1845–1850, 1986.

66. Whitcup SM, Stark-Vancs V, Wittes RE, et al: Association of interleukin 10 in the vitreous and cerebrospinal fluid and primary central nervous system lymphoma. Arch Ophthalmol 115:1157–1160, 1997.

GERM CELL TUMORS

Masao Matsutani

Intracranial germ cell tumors characteristically include tumor subtypes with different histology. They are composed of cells resembling cells in embryonic stages of development: trophoblasts that appear as early as the stage involving blastocyte formation (choriocarcinoma), yolk sac endoderms (yolk sac tumor or endodermal sinus tumor), pluripotent stem cells of the embryo proper (embryonal carcinoma), embryonic differentiated cells (teratoma), and primordial germ cells (germinoma). Interestingly, choriocarcinoma, a cancer found primarily in females, can grow in the brains of males.

Germ cell tumors occur at various brain sites as a solitary mass or as multiple foci. Epidemiologically, the incidence of these tumors differs: Japan has the highest incidence. Germ cell tumors account for 3.0% of all primary brain tumors in Japan.[5] In the United States and Europe, in contrast, they account for less than 1.0%. Because of their differences from other neuroectodermal or embryonal tumors of the brain, germ cell tumors have attracted the special attention of neuropathologists and neurosurgeons.

HISTOLOGIC CLASSIFICATION

In the World Health Organization (WHO)[13] classification of tumors of the nervous system, germ cell tumors are categorized into five basic types (germinomas, teratomas, choriocarcinomas, yolk sac or endodermal sinus tumors, and embryonal carcinomas). Those that contain two or more components are designated mixed germ cell tumors.

Germinomas are composed of large polygonal cells with a pale eosinophilic or clear cytoplasm and small lymphocytes. Their cytoplasm stains positive for placental alkaline phosphatase (PLAP), and there is infiltration by small lymphocytes along the stroma of vascular connective tissue (Figure 42-1). Germinomas containing syncytiotrophoblastic giant cells (STGC) stain positive for human chorionic gonadotropin (HCG) (Figure 42-2).

Teratomas are divided into three subtypes according to the degree of tumor cell differentiation: mature teratomas, immature teratomas, and teratomas with malignant transformation. Mature teratomas contain three well-differentiated germ cell layers: ectoderm, endoderm, and mesoderm. Immature teratomas are composed of incompletely differentiated tissues resembling fetal tissue. Teratomas that, like carcinomas and sarcomas, contain elements exhibiting unequivocal malignant transformation are referred to as teratomas with malignant transformation.

Yolk sac or endodermal sinus tumors are composed of primitive epithelial cells that proliferate in a loose-knit reticular network or compact sheets. Diagnostic features are Schiller-Duval bodies and periodic acid-Schiff stain (PAS)-positive, cytoplasmic, and extracellular eosinophilic droplets immunopositive for α-fetoprotein (AFP) (Figure 42-3). Choriocarcinoma consists of two characteristic cell types, syncytiotrophoblasts and cytotrophoblasts, arranged in a two-layer pattern. These cells are strongly immunopositive for HCG (Figure 42-4). Embryonal carcinomas contain primitive epithelial cells growing in solid sheets or poorly formed glands (Figure 42-5). In mixed germ cell tumors, the component most often present is germinoma, followed by mature or immature teratomatous components.

The reported incidence of these pathologic subtypes differs. In a Tokyo University series[16] that examined 153 consecutive, histologically confirmed cases with primary intracranial germ cell tumors, 55 were germinomas (35.9%), 49 were mixed tumors (32.0%), 30 were teratomas (19.6%), 8 were STGC-germinomas (5.2%), 5 were embryonal carcinomas (3.3%), and 3 each (2.0%) were choriocarcinomas and yolk sac tumors. Of the 30 teratomas, 4 (13.3%) exhibited malignant transformation; in 3 of these the malignant element was epidermal carcinoma, in the other it was sarcoma. In the 49 mixed tumors, the component most often present was germinoma ($n = 37$, 75.5%); 36 of the tumors (73.5%) manifested teratomatous components and of these 36, 27 (75%) contained immature teratomatous elements. None of the mixed tumors exhibited a combination of germinoma and choriocarcinoma. The Tokyo series included 13 patients (8.5%) with multiple tumors; 8 were histologically diagnosed as germinomas, 2 as germinomas with STGC, and 3 as mixed tumors.

SEX AND AGE DISTRIBUTION

Of the 1127 patients with intracranial germ cell tumors registered in the Brain Tumor Registry in Japan between 1984 and 1993,[5] 865 (76.8%) were males and 262 (23.2%) were females. Only 34 patients (3.0%) were younger than age 5; 67 (5.9%) were older than age 35; 793 (70.4%) of the patients were between 10 and 24 years of age.

Jennings et al,[12] who analyzed 398 reported cases of germ cell tumor, found that the incidence of pineal tumors was low (6%) in females. Also, there appeared to be a male predominance with respect to tumors in the basal ganglia. This was not the case for tumors in the neurohypophyseal region; the

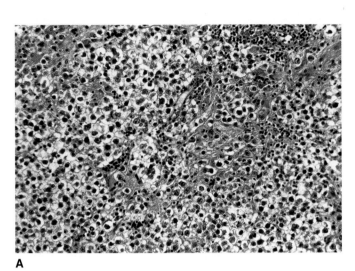

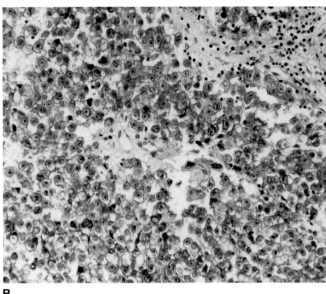

A

B

FIGURE 42-1 Germinoma. *A,* The tumor is composed of large polygonal cells with a pale eosinophilic or clear cytoplasm, and small lymphocytes. The lymphocytes infiltrate along the vascular connective tissue stroma (hematoxylin and eosin [H&E] stain). *B,* Large polygonal or spheroid cells show positive staining for placental alkaline phosphatase (PLAP stain).

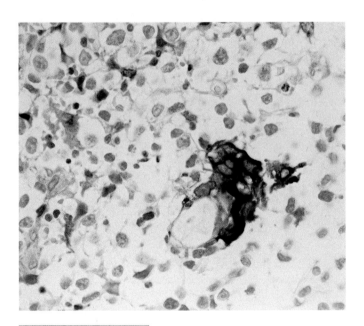

FIGURE 42-2 Germinoma with syncytiotrophoblastic giant cells. Large human chorionic gonadotropin–immunopositive cells are observed in the tumor.

male-to-female ratio was 43:57 in the series of Jennings et al,[12] 28:72 in that of Ho and Liu,[8] 25:75 in the pediatric patients reported by Hoffman et al,[9] and 46:54 in the Tokyo University series.[16] Although there was a male predominance among patients with choriocarcinoma and mature teratoma, it was not strong among cases with yolk sac tumors. Itoyama et al[10] reported that 4 of 6 patients with AFP-producing pineal tumors were females.

TUMOR LOCATION

The most common site of germ cell tumors is the pineal followed by the suprasellar region (Figures 42-6 and 42-7). Occasionally they are found in the basal ganglia and thalamus (Figure 42-8). There is magnetic resonance imaging (MRI) and autopsy evidence that suprasellar region tumors originate from the neurohypophysis; they grow intramedullarly along a line from the hypothalamus, pituitary stalk, and posterior pituitary lobe (neurohypophysis).[7] Pituitary function studies revealed decreased levels of anterior pituitary hormones (especially growth hormone [GH], follicle-stimulating hormone [FSH], and luteinizing hormone [LH]) and vasopressin and elevated prolactin titers, anomalies that manifest as panhypopituitarism because of neurohypophyseal dysfunction.[21] These anatomic and functional features of suprasellar germ cell tumors have led to the adoption of the term *neurohypophyseal tumor.*

In the Tokyo University series,[16] 78 of the 153 germ cell tumors (51.0%) were located in the pineal region, 46 (30.1%) in the neurohypophysis, 5 (3.3%) in the basal ganglia, 4 (2.6%) in the cerebellopontine angle, 3 each (2.0%) in the lateral ventricle and cerebellum (2.0%), and 1 (0.7%) in the corpus callosum. The other 13 patients (8.5%) manifested tumors at multiple sites.

Of the 153 patients, 87 (56.9%) were seen after the introduction of computed tomography (CT). Of these, 13 (14.9%) had multiple tumors that were primarily located in the pineal region (*n* = 5), the neurohypophysis (*n* = 7), or diffusely along the ventricular wall (*n* = 1).

Only 2 of 78 pineal tumors (2.6%) were found in females. None of the female patients had tumors in the basal ganglia; however, slightly more females than males (25 females versus 21 males) had tumors in the neurohypophysis. All but 1 of the 19 mature teratomas in the Tokyo University series of 153 germ cell tumors were found in males, and the preponderant site

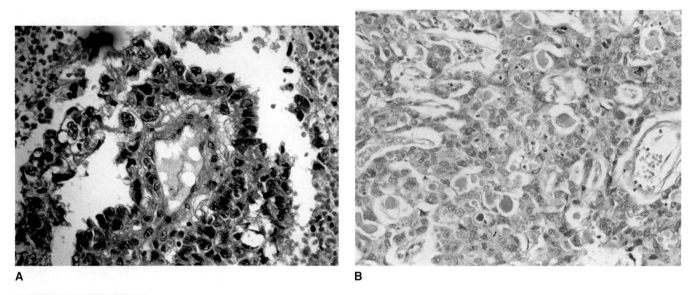

A

B

FIGURE 42-3 Yolk sac tumor. *A,* Schiller-Duval bodies in yolk sac tumor (hematoxylin and eosin stain). *B,* The tumor cells and globules show positive staining for α-fetoprotein (AFP stain).

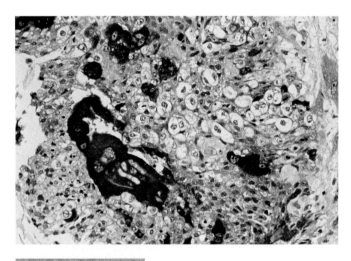

FIGURE 42-4 Choriocarcinoma. The giant syncytiotrophoblastic cells are positive for human chorionic gonadotropin (HCG) (HCG stain).

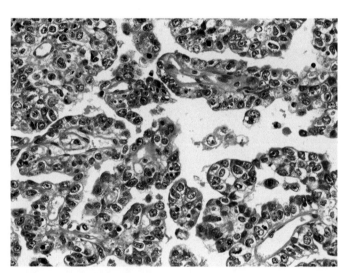

FIGURE 42-5 Embryonal carcinoma. The tumor forms clefts and spaces. (Hematoxylin and eosin stain.)

(17:19) was the pineal region. None of the female patients had histologically identified choriocarcinoma or yolk sac tumor. There were no statistical differences among the different histologic subtypes with regard to patient age, sex (males, 16.6 ± 8.5; females, 14 ± 6.4), or tumor location (pineal region, 14.6 ± 7, mean ± standard deviation (SD); neurohypophyseal region, 14.5 ± 5.4) .

Jennings et al[12] and Bjornsson et al[3] reported a higher incidence of suprasellar (neurohypophyseal) than pineal germinomas (58% vs. 37% and 49% vs. 38%, respectively). In contrast, Hoffman et al[9] and Ho and Liu[8] made the opposite observation; in their series more germinomas were located in the pineal than the neurohypophyseal area (62% vs. 32% and 47% vs. 30%, respectively). Overall, it appears that the incidence of germi-

nomas in the neurohypophyseal region tends to be similar to, or slightly higher than, their incidence in the pineal region.

Our search of the literature detected only two cases of pure mature teratoma in the parasellar region.

CLINICAL SYMPTOMS AND SIGNS

Patients with germ cell tumors manifest symptoms and signs attributable to the affected site. In general, tumors in the pineal region compress and obstruct the cerebral aqueduct, resulting in progressive hydrocephalus with intracranial hypertension. They also compress the tectal plate, producing the characteristic upward- and downward-gaze palsy (Parinaud's syndrome)

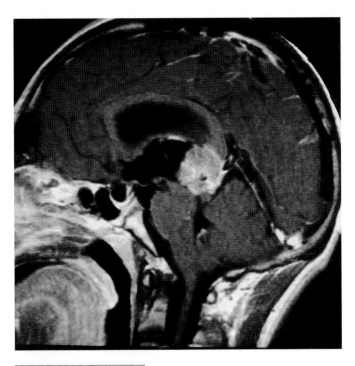

FIGURE 42-6 Pineal germinoma. The tumor is well enhanced by gadolinium.

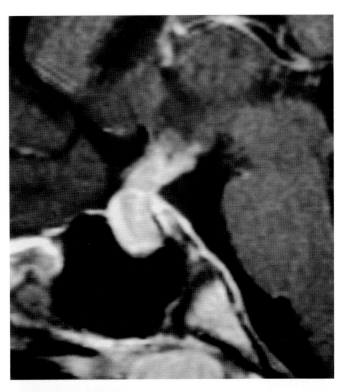

FIGURE 42-7 Neurohypophyseal germinoma. A less enhanced tumor grows in and infiltrates along the neurohypophysis; a well-enhanced pituitary anterior lobe is compressed by the tumor.

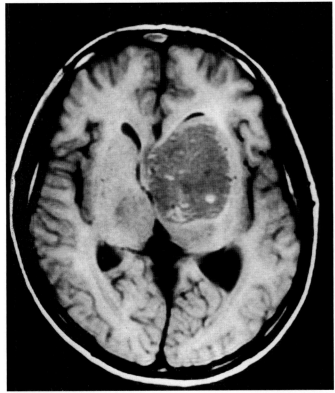

A

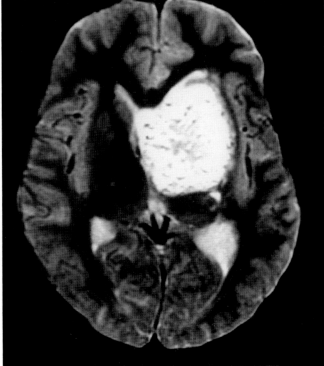

B

FIGURE 42-8 Embryonal carcinoma in the basal ganglia. The tumor is hypointense on T1-weighted image (A) and hyperintense on the T2-weighted image (B).

and Argyll-Robertson pupils. Suprasellar, or neurohypophyseal, tumors compress the optic chiasm, resulting in bitemporal hemianopsia and decreased visual acuity. Tumor invasion into the neurohypophysis produces panhypopituitarism and diabetes insipidus. The survey of pituitary function reveals lowered anterior pituitary hormones (especially GH, FSH, and LH) and vasopressin and elevated prolactin titer.[21] Tumors in the basal ganglia or thalamus invade the pyramidal tract and result in contralateral hemiparesis. However, with the exception of HCG-secreting tumors, the clinical signs and symptoms of the different histologic subtypes are not tumor specific. Some tumors secreting HCG manifest intratumoral hemorrhage that results in acute intracranial hypertension. In sexually immature males, they induce precocious puberty.

Of 79 patients with tumors in the pineal region in the Tokyo University series,[16] 75 (94.9%) manifested symptoms and signs of intracranial hypertension. Parinaud's syndrome and Argyll-Robertson pupil were observed in 57 patients (72.4%) and 33 (42.1%) of these patients, respectively; 19 (24.1%) complained of diplopia. The rare symptom of auditory impairment was noted in 3 patients (3.8%).

Of 50 patients with neurohypophyseal tumors, 43 (86.0%) presented with diabetes insipidus. Visual disturbance, including narrowing of visual field and decreased visual acuity, was observed in 43 (86.0%) of the patients. Of 14 females older than 12 years, 13 (92.9%) manifested primary or secondary amenorrhea. Growth retardation was noted in 10 of 33 patients (30.3%) younger than 15 years.

Increased intracranial hypertension was present in three of five patients with tumors in the basal ganglia; two suffered hemiparesis, and one had epilepsy. All four patients with tumors in the cerebellopontine angle had symptoms attributable to tumors in this region. In all patients with cerebellar tumors (n = 3) or tumors in the lateral ventricle (n = 3) there was evidence of marked intracranial hypertension; one patient suffered epilepsy, another hemiparesis. The patient with a corpus callosum tumor manifested diplopia, and seven patients with tumors in both the pineal and neurohypophyseal regions exhibited signs characteristic of tumors at these sites.

In general, the clinical signs and symptoms of the different histologic subtypes were not tumor specific. However, intratumoral hemorrhage was noted in all three patients with choriocarcinoma, in one with a germinoma with STGC, and in another patient who had a mixed tumor composed primarily of embryonal carcinoma.

Six patients under the age of 10 (five boys, one girl) exhibited precocious puberty. Their tumors were located in the pineal region (n = 4), the neurohypophysis (n = 1), and in both regions (n = 1). The histologic diagnosis in these six patients was choriocarcinoma (n = 1), immature teratoma (n = 2), mature teratoma (n = 2), and mixed tumor (n = 1). The serum HCG titer was assayed in four patients; it was elevated in two (one choriocarcinoma and one immature teratoma).

RADIOLOGIC FINDINGS

Because the histologic type determines treatment in patients with germ cell tumors, a differential diagnosis is important. MRI is useful not only for detecting tissue components of the tumor but also for revealing its anatomic relationships with neighboring critical structures, and they provide helpful infor-

mation for selecting surgical strategies. However, some tumor types have few characteristic features, making it impossible to establish a histologic diagnosis based on neuroradiologic findings alone.

Germinoma

On T1-weighted MRI, germinomas (Figure 42-9) are visualized as isointense or hypointense; on T2-weighted images they appear as isointense or hyperintense. They are mostly homogeneously and partly heterogeneously enhanced by gadolinium. They are round, square-round, or oval and usually regularly shaped. In some instances focal edema is seen. On CT scan, small-to-medium, sometimes multiple calcifications are noted in many pineal region tumors; they are rare in neurohypophyseal tumors. Small cysts may be seen.

The MRI pattern of germinomas with STGC is almost identical to that of pure germinomas except for the occasional presence of intratumoral hemorrhage. With current imaging technologies it is not possible to distinguish between pure germinomas and germinomas with STGC by CT and MRI studies alone.

Teratoma

Mature teratoma (Figure 42-10) is characterized by irregular shape, clear margins, mixed signals, and the common presence of large cysts and areas of calcification. MRI studies are useful for detecting fatty components.

The basic images of immature and malignant teratomas are identical to those of mature teratomas. However, their cystic components tend to be smaller, and areas of calcification are more rare. The demonstration of perifocal edema, a feature not observed in mature teratomas, is suggestive of immature or malignant components.

Choriocarcinoma

On T1-weighted MRI, choriocarcinomas appear isointense; on T2-weighted images they are isointense to hyperintense; this makes their appearance slightly different from germinomas. Most choriocarcinomas are intensely gadolinium enhanced. Only pineal region tumors appear with areas of calcification. CT scans are useful for detecting intratumoral hemorrhage.

Yolk Sac Tumor

On MRI, yolk sac tumors manifest as an irregularly shaped, isointense, hypointense, or hyperintense, homogeneously enhanced mass. Cystic component and perifocal edema are also observed.

Embryonal Carcinoma

On T1-weighted MRI, embryonal carcinoma tumors are visualized as hyperintense; they are well enhanced both homogeneously and heterogeneously. In some tumors cystic components can be seen.

Mixed Germ Cell Tumor

In mixed germ cell tumors the presence of a homogeneous, slightly hyperintense to hyperintense mass on MRI suggests a

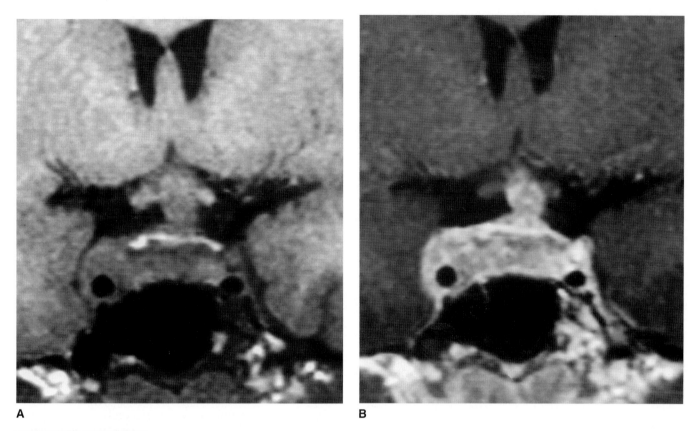

A   **B**

FIGURE 42-9   Germinoma in neurohypophysis (coronal view) The tumor with isointensity on T1-weighted image *(A)* infiltrates from hypothalamus to cavernous sinus via pituitary stalk. The tumor is slightly enhanced by gadolinium *(B)*.

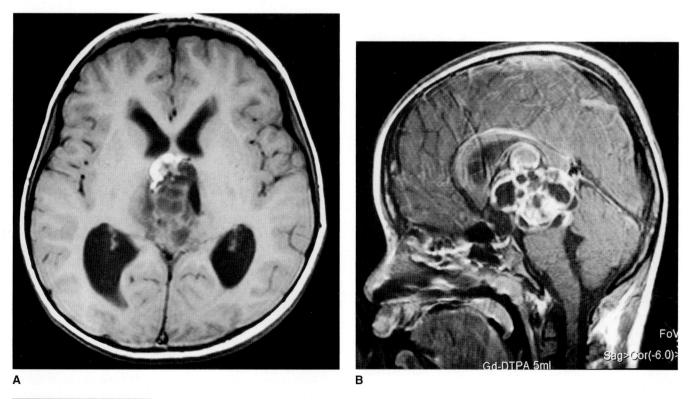

A   **B**

FIGURE 42-10   Immature teratoma. Heterogeneous tumor with hyperintensity, hypointensity, and isointensity on T1-weighted image occupies the third ventricle *(A)*. On gadolinium-enhanced images, the tumor contains multiple cysts *(B)*.

germinomatous component. In contrast, visualization of multiple calcified areas is strongly suggestive of teratomatous components. The existence of multiple medium- to large-size cysts is compatible with the identification of teratomatous components.

SERUM TITER OF AFP, HCG (HCG-β), AND PLAP

The serum and cerebrospinal fluid (CSF) titer of AFP, HCG, HCG-β, and PLAP is of clinical importance in diagnosing intracranial germ cell tumors. HCG (or HCG-β) is usually secreted by choriocarcinoma cells, STGC, and immature tumor cells; AFP, by yolk sac and immature tumor cells; and PLAP, by germinoma cells.

In the Tokyo University series,[16] the serum titer of AFP or HCG was elevated in 36 of 92 patients examined. None of the 29 patients with germinomas and 7 patients with mature teratomas had elevated titers; in 56 patients with tumors other than germinomas or mature teratomas, 27 (48%) did not have elevated titers. All three choriocarcinomas and one mixed tumor mainly consisting of choriocarcinoma had highly elevated serum HCG (2120 to 32,000 milli-international units per mL and 6000 milli-international units per mL, respectively). Tumors other than choriocarcinomas presented serum HCG titer less than 770 milli-international units per mL: 40 to 690 milli-international units per mL in all seven germinomas with STGC, 30 to 590 milli-international units per mL in four immature teratomas, and 61 to 770 milli-international units per mL in three mixed tumors. Highly elevated AFP titers were recorded in all 3 yolk sac tumors (2700 to 9500 ng/mL) and 3 mixed tumors mainly consisting of yolk sac tumors (3380-6700 ng/mL); lower elevated titers were observed in 3 immature teratomas (7.5 to 500 ng/mL), 2 embryonal carcinomas (183 to 700 ng/mL), and 11 mixed tumors containing a small part of immature teratoma, embryonal carcinoma, or yolk sac tumor (7.3 to 1810 ng/mL).

Surveys of tumor markers (AFP, HCG, HCG-ß, PLAP) have become an essential preoperative evaluation of patients with germ cell tumors but cannot determine precise histologic subtypes in most patients. HCG (or HCG-ß) and AFP proteins are sometimes secreted by immature teratomas or embryonal carcinomas. In some cases these markers reflect the number of cells secreting these proteins and are useful for differentiating tumors with predominant choriocarcinoma or yolk sac tumor from other kinds of marker-secreting tumors. Elevation of serum and CSF PLAP is characteristic of tumors composed wholly or in part of germinoma; the elevated PLAP can only suggest that the tumor contains germinoma.

SUMMARY OF BASIC CLINICAL DATA IN PATIENTS WITH INTRACRANIAL GERM CELL TUMORS

Analysis of clinical data disclosed characteristic features exhibited by these tumors.

1. Germ cell tumors in the brain are more prevalent in Asia than in Western countries.

2. They occur primarily in the young; 70% of tumors were found in patients between 10 and 24 years old.
3. Whereas pineal germ cell tumors are rare in females, there is a slight female predominance in neurohypophyseal tumors.
4. Tumors in the basal ganglia are observed mostly in males.
5. Germinomas occur as often in the neurohypophysis as in the pineal region.
6. Mature teratomas are rarely located in the neurohypophysis.
7. Fewer than 5% of the tumors arise in the posterior fossa.
8. There is a male predominance in choriocarcinomas and mature teratomas and a less strong male predominance in yolk sac tumors.
9. CT or MRI and tumor-marker (AFP and HCG or HCG-β) studies are not particularly helpful for differentiating between histologic subtypes.

SUMMARY OF PAST TREATMENT AND ANALYSIS OF CLINICAL BEHAVIOR OF DIFFERENT HISTOLOGIC SUBTYPES

Before 1981 radiation therapy to the whole brain (median tumor dose 50 Gy) was used in all patients except those with totally removed mature teratomas. Although effective radiation therapy produced excellent 10-year survival rates (>80%) in patients with pure germinomas, approximately 10% of patients experienced tumor recurrence or dissemination. Furthermore, in children, whole-brain irradiation with 50 Gy resulted in mental retardation and pituitary gland dysfunction in later life.

Nongerminomatous tumors proved refractory to conventional treatments with surgery and radiation. Jennings et al[12] analyzed the survival of 216 patients with intracranial germ cell tumors who had received conventional treatment and noted that most patients with nongerminomatous tumors did not survive beyond 3 years. Matsukado,[14] who presented the results of the Japanese Intracranial Germ Cell Tumor Study Group, reported a median survival of 18 months and a 45% rate of CSF dissemination or hematogenous metastasis in 33 patients with nongerminomatous tumors treated with postoperative irradiation.

After combination chemotherapy with cisplatin was confirmed to be effective in gonadal germ cell tumors, nongerminomatous germ cell tumors of the brain became candidates for chemotherapy. The first Japanese trial that delivered combination chemotherapy of cisplatin, vinblastine, and bleomycin (PVB) reported a 2-year survival rate of 67.7% for 30 patients with intracranial nongerminomatous tumors. This rate was an improvement over the 46.5% achieved in patients who received radiation therapy alone.[14] The second Japanese trial, using cisplatin and etoposide (PE) and carboplatin-etoposide (CE) combination therapy, had a 2-year survival rate for patients with nongerminomatous tumors of 48%.[24] These trials showed the comparable effectiveness of PVB and PE combination therapy in patients with intracranial germ cell tumors in the absence of serious complications and revealed that germinomas responded to combination chemotherapy.

Follow-up studies on 134 of the 153 patients included in the Tokyo University Study Group[16] showed that all patients were subjected to a consistent treatment policy consisting of surgical tumor removal followed by radiation therapy with or without chemotherapy. The study disclosed that treatment results differed among histologic subtypes, especially among mixed tumors. Chemotherapy consisting of cisplatin or carboplatin combinations was effective against moderately, but not highly, malignant tumors.[17] The high incidence of local failure (73.5%) in highly malignant tumors resulted in treatment failure, stressing the need for more aggressive, intensive therapy with radiation and chemotherapy with agents other than carboplatin or etoposide combinations directed at the primary tumor site.

Germinoma

Among germinoma patients ($n = 50$), the 5-, 10-, and 15-year survival rates were 95.4%, 92.7%, and 87.9%, respectively (Table 42-1). Of the 50 patients, 43 (86%) received postoperative radiation therapy ranging from 40 to 62 Gy (median 50 Gy) to (1) a generous local field encompassing the tumor site, the third and lateral ventricles, and the sellar and pineal regions ($n = 37$); (2) the tumor area (limited local field) alone ($n = 2$); or (3) the whole brain followed by boost irradiation to the tumor area ($n = 7$). In seven patients with neurohypophyseal tumors, combined chemotherapy (PE or CE) and local irradiation with a reduced dose of 30 Gy were used. In 19 of 23 (82.6%) patients who survived for more than 10 years, generous local irradiation resulted in their ability to pursue a good quality of life that included school attendance and work. Tumor recurrence or dissemination occurred in 3 of the 50 patients (6%) and was suspected in 3 others who died of unknown causes.

According to the literature, approximately 10% of germinoma patients suffer recurrence or dissemination. Some of the recurrent tumors developed within, others outside, the field of irradiation. These results suggest that pure germinomas seldom disseminate or metastasize and that irradiation of a generous local field encompassing the tumor site, the third and lateral ventricles, and the sellar and pineal regions is adequate. Jenkin et al[11] reported that children whose germinomas were treated by whole-brain irradiation experienced difficulties in school,

and others[6,22] also recommended local irradiation for germinomas. We previously reported long-standing anterior pituitary dysfunction in patients with neurohypophyseal germinomas.[15]

Germinoma with STGC

The clinical behavior of the special type of germinoma with STGC remains unclear. In the Tokyo University series,[16] 3 of 7 patients suffered recurrence within 4 years posttreatment; similarly, Utsuki et al[23] also reported 3 recurrences in 11 patients. Unlike pure germinomas, these tumors are not easily controlled by radiation therapy and require aggressive chemotherapy with radiation therapy.

Teratoma

Successful total removal of mature teratomas yields an excellent 10-year survival rate. In the Tokyo University series,[16] the 10-year survival rate for 11 patients with malignant teratoma including immature teratoma and teratoma with malignant transformation was 70.7%, which was better than predicted. Extensive surgery combined with radiation and chemotherapy succeeded in local control (4:5, 80%), whereas total removal alone or partial removal combined with radiation therapy resulted in a high rate of recurrence (5:6, 83%).

Nongerminomatous Tumors

Pure malignant germ cell tumors (choriocarcinoma, yolk sac tumor, and embryonal carcinoma) are refractory to radiation therapy; the median survival of 73 previously reported patients was 1.1 years (my calculation). In the Tokyo University series,[16] the 3-year survival rate of 11 patients with pure malignant germ cell tumors was poor (27.3%). None of the choriocarcinoma patients survived past 1 year, and the 1-year survival rate for patients with yolk sac tumors and embryonal carcinomas was 33.3% and 80.0%, respectively.

TABLE 42-1	Treatment Results of Tokyo University Series				
	Survival Rate (%)				
Histology* (Treated Cases)	1 yr	3 yr	5 yr	10 yr	15 yr
Germinoma[50]	100	95.4	95.4	92.7	87.9
Germinoma with STGC[7]	100	100	83.3	83.3	NC
Mature teratoma[16]	100	92.9	92.9	92.9	NC
Malignant teratoma[11]	100	70.7	70.7	70.7	NC
Pure malignant GCT[11]	45.5	27.3	27.3	NC	NC
Mixed tumors[39]	87.2	61	57.1	40.1	NC
Subtype of Mixed Tumors					
Germinoma and teratoma[17]	94.1	94.1	84.7	70.6	NC
Germinoma or teratoma[10]	80	70	52.5	35	NC
Mainly pure malignant elements[12]	83.3	9.3	9.3	NC	NC

*Histologic abbreviations are explained in the text.
GCT, Germ-cell tumor; NC, not calculable because of short period of follow-up or a small number of survivors; STGC, syncytiotrophoblastic giant cells.
Source: Matsutani M, Sano K, Takakura K, et al: Primary intracranial germ cell tumors: a clinical analysis of 153 histologically verified cases. J Neurosurg 86:446–455, 1997.

Although mixed tumors with more than two histologic elements represent 30% to 40% of intracranial gem cell tumors, treatment results for the different subgroups have not been analyzed individually. In the Tokyo University series,[16] the 5- and 10-year survival rates in 39 patients with mixed tumors were 57.1% and 40%, respectively. When these mixed tumors were divided into three subgroups according to their constituent tumor components (mixed germinoma and teratoma [MGT], mixed tumors primarily composed of germinoma or teratoma combined with a small portion of pure malignant tumors [MXB], and mixed tumors mainly consisting of pure malignant elements [MXM]), the 3- and 5-year survival rates were 94.1% and 84.7%, respectively, for MGT; 70.0% and 52.5%, respectively, for MXB; and 9.3% for both for MXM. The difference was statistically significant ($P = .0098$) (see Table 42-1), suggesting that histologic confirmation of the elements composing the mixed tumors is important for determining the most effective treatment. The median survival for 26 previously reported patients with malignant teratomas, MGT, and MXB was 2.6 years, according to my calculation.

The most recent 26 consecutive patients with nongerminomatous tumors in our series[17] (7 pure malignant tumors, 13 mixed tumors, and 6 malignant teratomas) received combination chemotherapy with cisplatin or carboplatin before or after radiation therapy. The 31 previous patients had received conventional radiation therapy alone (median tumor dose 50 Gy). Among patients with these moderately malignant tumors, the chemotherapy group showed a significantly better 5-year survival rate (92.9%) than the radiation group (62%). However, among patients with highly malignant tumors, the 3-year survival rate was 27.3% for the chemotherapy group and 10.2% for the radiation group; the difference was not statistically significant.

In the Tokyo University series,[16] 34 (55.7%) of 61 nongerminomatous germ cell tumors recurred or metastasized. The rate of recurrence increased with the degree of histologic malignancy. The sites of recurrence were the primary site alone ($n = 20$), the primary and a remote site ($n = 5$), the brain outside the primary site ($n = 3$), and the spinal cord alone ($n = 4$). Systemic metastasis alone was noted in two patients. Overall, 25 of the 34 patients (73.5%) suffered tumor recurrence at the primary site with or without recurrence at a remote site.

RECENT PROGRESS IN TREATING INTRACRANIAL GERM CELL TUMORS

Phase II Study of the Japanese Pediatric Brain Study Group

In 1995 a multi-institutional phase II study was started under the auspices of the Japanese Pediatric Brain Study Group.[18,19] Its aim was to establish a postoperative treatment regimen that included combination therapy comprising chemotherapy and radiation therapy to obtain a better quality of life for patients with germinomas and to prolong the survival of patients with nongerminomatous tumors.

Study Design

The study was organized by 14 neurosurgical clinics in Japan and consisted of 199 patients. The agreed treatment strategy

was to surgically debulk the tumor and to verify its histologic composition. Surgery in all cases in this phase II study was followed by preirradiation chemotherapy and subsequent radiation therapy. Treatment goals for patients in each group were set before the inception of the study, and prior informed consent was obtained from all participants.

In patients with germinomas, treatment was directed at reducing the radiation dose and target volume by combining chemotherapy. Efforts were focused on improving survival rate, quality of life, and pituitary function.

In patients with moderately malignant nongerminomatous tumors (intermediate prognosis group), combination chemotherapy with carboplatin-etoposide was followed by local radiation therapy to prolong survival time and to improve quality of life.

Patients with highly malignant tumors (poor prognosis group), received ifosfamide combination chemotherapy, because CE combinations or PVB combinations had failed to prolong survival time.

Two chemotherapy regimens were applied. In one, a CE combination (carboplatin-etopside [CARB-VP]) was used. This regimen consisted of carboplatin (450 mg/m^2) on day 1 and etoposide (150 mg/m^2) for 3 consecutive days (days 1 to 3). The other regimen consisted of an ifosfamide-carboplatin-etoposide combination (ICE). These patients received ifosfamide (900 mg/m^2), cisplatin (20 mg/m^2), and etoposide (60 mg/m^2) for 5 consecutive days (days 1 to 5). Each regimen was repeated every 4 weeks for three total courses as an induction therapy.

Radiation therapy consisted of a 4 MV linear accelerator x-ray delivered to the tumor area, the generous local area, or the whole brain and the whole spine. Radiation doses delivered to a generous local field encompassed the tumor site, the third and lateral ventricles, and the sellar and pineal regions.

Treatment Protocols

Patients with germinoma received three courses of CARB-VP chemotherapy followed by local radiation dose (24 Gy) delivered to the general local field. Our choice of the 24-Gy dose was based on data regarding the maximum dose protecting from radiation damage of the anterior pituitary gland in children.[20]

Patients in the intermediate prognosis group received three courses of CARB-VP chemotherapy followed by 30 Gy of radiation to a generous local field and 20 Gy to the tumor site. They then received additional CARB-VP chemotherapy every 3 to 4 months for a total of five cycles.

Patients in the poor-prognosis group received three courses of ICE chemotherapy followed by whole-brain and spinal irradiation of 30 Gy with a 30-Gy boost delivered to a generous local field. They received additional ICE chemotherapy every 3 to 4 months for a total of five cycles.

Results

The initial treatment, consisting of surgery, chemotherapy, and radiation therapy, was completed in 199 patients. These patients were subsequently evaluated for their initial response.

There were 118 patients with germinoma; in 14 (11.9%) the tumor recurred during a median follow-up of 5.1 years. None of the 26 patients with HCG-producing germinomas suffered recurrence. In 4 of 9 patients who refused subsequent radiation therapy and were, therefore, excluded from the study, the tumor recurred within 14 months, indicating that chemotherapy alone was not effective.

The 5-year survival rate of 35 patients in the intermediate-prognosis group was 94%; the 3-year survival rate of 20 patients in the poor-prognosis group was 69%. Their results were better than those obtained by conventional radiation therapy alone.

Of 84 patients in the germinoma group and the intermediate-prognosis group who were followed for more than 2 years, 65 (77.4%) had a Karnofsky Performance Scale score of not less than 90, indicating that their post-treatment quality of life was satisfactory.

International Central Nervous System Germ Cell Tumor Study Group

The International CNS Germ Cell Tumor Study Group[1] conducted a first trial to determine whether irradiation could be avoided by the delivery of four cycles of carboplatin, etoposide, and bleomycin. Following chemotherapy alone, 38 of 45 germinoma patients (84.4%) and 20 of 26 (76.9%) patients with nongerminomatous tumors experienced complete remission. During a median follow-up term of 31 months, 49% of the germinomas recurred. The 2-year survival rate was 84% for germinoma patients and 62% for patients with nongerminomatous tumors. This study clearly showed that in the absence of radiation treatment, chemotherapy was unable to control germinomas.

In their subsequent trial, this group tested the effectiveness and safety of two chemotherapy regimens that consisted of the administration of cisplatin, etoposide, cyclophosphamide, and bleomycin (regimen A) and of carboplatin, etoposide, and bleomycin (regimen B). Patients who did not manifest complete remission underwent salvage surgery with or without radiation therapy. The median follow-up was 6.3 years. Of 20 germinoma patients, 13 remained in complete remission; of these, 10 did not receive radiation. Of 19 patients with nongerminomatous tumors, 14 remained in complete remission; however, 4 died from treatment-related causes. The study concluded that although the results obtained in patients with nongerminomatous tumors were encouraging, the treatment protocol was associated with unacceptably high treatment-related morbidity and mortality rates. The results of this study are published in the abstracts from the 10th International Symposium on Pediatric Neuro-Oncology (2002).[12a]

French Society for Pediatric Oncology Study

The French Society for Pediatric Oncology (SFOP) conducted a study that combined chemotherapy (alternating courses of etoposide-carboplatin and etoposide-ifosfamide for a recommended total of four courses) with 40 Gy of local radiation to treat 57 patients with localized germinomas ($n = 57$).[4] The median follow-up was 42 months. In four patients (7%) there was recurrence within 9, 10, 38, and 57 months post-treatment; the estimated 3-year event-free survival was 96.4%.

In their earlier study,[2] this group had attempted to treat AFP and HCG-β secreting germ cell tumors with chemotherapy alone.[2] Patients ($n = 15$) received six cycles of chemotherapy (vinblastine, bleomycin, and carboplatin or etoposide-carboplatin or ifosfamide-etoposide) followed by salvage surgery. Focal radiation was to be delivered only in cases with viable residual tumor. However, because 12 of 13 patients with nonirradiated tumors relapsed, the authors concluded that these tumors were not curable with chemotherapy alone.

International Society of Pediatric Hematology and Oncology

The SIOP CNS GCT 96 trial by the International Society of Pediatric Hematology and Oncology (see abstracts of the 10th International Symposium on Pediatric Neuro-Oncology, 2002)[4a] and the Fifth Congress of the European Association for Neuro-Oncology (2002) used SFOP protocol to study treatment outcomes in 37 patients with germinomas. Their 5-year event-free survival rate was 85%. Patients with secreting germ cell tumors (AFP >25 ng/mL or HCG-β >50 international units per L) received four cycles of cisplatin, etoposide, and ifosfamide combination and radiation, delivered to the whole ventricle (54 Gy) or the whole neuraxis (30 Gy). The 5-year event-free survival rate in this group was 64%.

CONCLUSION

Based on our analysis of treatment outcomes obtained in the Tokyo University series,[16,17] we divided patients with intracranial germ cell tumors into three therapeutic groups: good, intermediate, or poor prognosis (Table 42-2). Our next step will be histologic verification of surgical specimens and, where possible, extensive mass reduction. In Japan, because of advances in microsurgical and radioimaging techniques, surgery for pineal tumors is now much safer, and the mortality rate is less than 1%. Patients with germinoma will receive combination

---

TABLE 42-2

Therapeutic Classification

Good-Prognosis Group
Germinoma, pure
Mature teratoma

Intermediate-Prognosis Group
Germinoma with STGC
Immature teratoma
Teratoma with malignant transformation
Mixed tumors mainly composed of germinoma or teratoma

Poor-Prognosis Group
Choriocarcinoma
Yolk sac tumor
Embryonal carcinoma
Mixed tumors mainly composed of choriocarcinoma, yolk sac tumor, or embryonal carcinoma

STGC, Syncytiotrophoblastic giant cells.

treatment with chemotherapy and a reduced dose of radiation to increase the cure rate while decreasing radiation-induced side effects, including anterior pituitary dysfunction. In patients with nongerminomatous malignant tumors, locally administered radiation therapy alone cannot control tumor progression.

In the intermediate-prognosis group, chemotherapy with a cisplatin or carboplatin combination followed by radiation therapy can be expected to control tumor growth. However, patients with the most highly malignant tumors (poor-prognosis group) will receive more aggressive chemotherapy.

References

1. Balmaceda C, Heller G, Rosenblum M, et al: Chemotherapy without irradiation—a novel approach for newly diagnosed CNS germ cell tumors: results of an international cooperative trial. J Clin Oncol 14:2908–2915, 1996.
2. Baranzelli MC, Patte C, Bouffet E, et al: An attempt to treat pediatric intracranial alphaFP and betaHCG secreting germ cell tumors with chemotherapy alone. SFOP experience with 18 cases. Societe Francaise d'Oncologie Pediatrique. J Neurooncol 37:229–239, 1998.
3. Bjornsson J, Scheithauer BW, Okazaki H, Leech RW: Intracranial germ cell tumors: pathological and immunohistochemical aspects of 70 cases. J Neuropath Exp Neurol 44:32–46, 1985.
4. Bouffet E, Baranzelli MC, Patte C, et al: Combined treatment modality for intracranial germinomas: results of multicentre SFOP experience. Societe Francaise d'Oncologie Pediatrique. Br J Cancer 79:1199–1204, 1999.
4a. Calaminus G: Germ cell tumours of the central nervous system. A multidisciplinary team approach. Educational Book of Postgraduate course, Fifth Congress of the European Association of Neuro-Oncology, Florence, Sept. 7, 2002.
5. The Committee of Brain Tumor Registry of Japan: Report of brain tumor registry of Japan (1969–1993). Neurol Med Chir (Tokyo) vol 40, Suppl, January, 2000.
6. Dattoli MF, Newall J: Radiation therapy for intracranial germinoma: The case for limited volume treatment. Int J Radiat Oncol Biol Phys 19:429–433, 1990.
7. Fujisawa I, Asato R, Okumura R, et al: Magnetic resonance imaging of neurohypophyseal germinomas. Cancer 68:1009–1014, 1991.
8. Ho DM, Liu H-C: Primary intracranial germ cell tumor. Pathologic study of 51 patients. Cancer 70:1577–1584, 1992.
9. Hoffman HJ, Otsubo H, Hendrick B, et al: Intracranial germ cell tumors in children. J Neurosurg 74:545–551, 1991.
10. Itoyama Y, Kochi M, Yamamoto H, et al: Clinical study of intracranial nongerminomatous germ cell tumors producing α-fetoprotein. Neurosurgery 27:454–460, 1990.
11. Jenkin D, Berry M, Chan H, et al: Pineal region germinomas in childhood. Treatment considerations. Int J Radiat Oncol Biol Phys 18:541–545, 1990.
12. Jennings MT, Gelman R, Hochberg F: Intracranial germ-cell tumors: natural history and pathogenesis. J Neurosurg 63:155–167, 1985.
12a. Kellie S, Boyce H, Lichtenbaum R, et al: Results of the second international CNS germ cell tumor (GCT) study group protocol. Neuro-Oncology 5:47, 2003 (abstract).
13. Kleihues P, Cavenee WK (eds): WHO classification of tumours. Pathology and Genetics of Tumours of the Nervous System. Lyon, France, IARC Press, 2000.
14. Matsukado Y: The Japanese Intracranial Germ Cell Tumor Study Group: cisplatin, vinblastine, bleomycin (PVB) combination chemotherapy in the treatment of intracranial malignant germ cell tumors—A preliminary report of phase II study. Jpn J Cancer Clin 32:1387–1393, 1986 (in Japanese).
15. Matsutani M, Sano K, Takakura K: Long-term follow-up of patients with primary intracranial germinomas. In Packer R, Bleyer WL, Pochedly C (eds): Pediatric Neuro-Oncology. London, Martin Dunitz, 1992.
16. Matsutani M, Sano K, Takakura K, et al: Primary intracranial germ cell tumors: a clinical analysis of 153 histologically verified cases. J Neurosurg 86:446–455, 1997.
17. Matsutani M, Sano K, Takakura K, et al: Combined treatment with chemotherapy and radiation therapy for intracranial germ cell tumors. Childs Nerv Syst 14:59–62, 1998.
18. Matsutani M, Ushio Y, Abe H, et al: Combined chemotherapy and radiation therapy for central nervous system germ cell tumors: preliminary results of a Phase II study of the Japanese Pediatric Brain Tumor Study Group. Neurosurg Focus 5: Article 7, 1998.
19. Matsutani M, The Japanese Pediatric Brain Tumor Study Group: Combined chemotherapy and radiation therapy for CNS germ cell tumors—The Japanese experience. J Neurooncol 54:311–316, 2001.
20. Rappaport R, Brauner R: Growth and endocrine disorders secondary to cranial irradiation. Pediatr Res 25:561–567, 1989.
21. Saeki N, Takami K, Murai H, et al: Long-term outcome of endocrine function in patients with neurohypophyseal germinomas. Endocr J 47:83–89, 2000.
23. Shibamoto Y, Abe Y, Yamashita J, et al: Treatment result of intracranial germinoma as a function of the irradiated volume. Int J Radiat Oncol Biol Phys 15:285–290, 1988.
23. Utsuki S, Kawano N, Oka H, et al: Cerebral germinoma with syncytiotrophoblastic giant cells: feasibility of predicting prognosis using serum HCG level. Acta Neurochir (Wien) 141:975–978, 1999.
24. Yoshida J, Sugita K, Kobayashi K, et al: Prognosis of intracranial germ cell tumours: effectiveness of chemotherapy with cisplatin and etoposide (CDDP and VP-16). Acta Neurochir (Wien) 120:111–117, 1993.

EXTRA-AXIAL AND
CRANIAL BASE TUMORS:
TUMORS OF THE CRANIAL
BASE WITH SPECIAL
CONSIDERATION OF
SKULL BASE TUMORS

Section Editor

Ossama Al-Mefty

CHAPTER 43

ACOUSTIC NEUROMAS (VESTIBULAR SCHWANNOMAS)

Cordula Matthies and Madjid Samii

The terminology for acoustic neuroma tumors has undergone several changes along with discoveries through pathology, specifically electron microscopy. The term *neuroma* refers to hyperplastic proliferation of nerve fibers and nerve sheaths induced by trauma and therefore is not adequate for these neoplasms. The term *neurilemoma* has been left, because the neurilemma is the Schwann cell *plasma membrane, its lamina, and connective tissue ground substance.*

Acoustic neuromas are correctly termed *vestibular schwannomas*. The Schwann cells of peripheral nerve segments give rise to *schwannoma* formation.

There are three cell types to be addressed that ensheathe neurites in the peripheral nervous system: the Schwann cell, the perineurial cell, and the fibroblast. The Schwann cell sheath starts at the point of pial penetration of the axons, whereas the proximal sheath close to the neuraxis is formed by neuroglia. The Schwann cell is supposed to be of neuroectodermal origin and is responsible for the myelin sheath formation in the peripheral nervous system.

INCIDENCE AND OCCURRENCE

Approximately 8% of all primary intracranial tumors are schwannomas. Their most common location is the cerebello-pontine angle, where 90% are vestibular schwannomas and only 10% are tumors of other histologic types. The sensory nerves are more often affected than the motor nerves, namely, the eighth and fifth nerves more often than the facial nerve.

There are further intraspinal schwannoma tumors of the nerve roots and peripheral nerve schwannomas.

ORIGIN

The origin of the vestibular schwannomas is the vestibular nerve; the superior part is presumed to be more often involved than the inferior part. The tumor is encapsulated, of firm consistency, and yellowish or sometimes white or slightly translucent. It may be cystic and may contain old hemorrhages.

On microscopic histologic investigation, long bipolar spindle cells are found that are arranged in bundles (Antoni A); in type B tissue the texture is more loose, and the tumor cells are separated by a special matrix filled with reticulin fibers.

Neurites are absent from the schwannomas with rare exceptions; in very rare cases nerve fibers have been identified by electron microscopy. Schwannomas also have angiogenic properties and thereby may induce enhanced vascularization and abnormalities such as telangiectatic formations, intratumoral thrombosis, or hemorrhage.

NEUROFIBROMATOSIS 2

Neurofibromatosis 2 (NF2) is characterized by bilateral acoustic neuromas, first detected and described by Wishart in 1822. It belongs to the group of phakomatoses comprising

321

tuberous sclerosis, morbus Bourneville-Pringle disease, Sturge-Weber-Krabbe syndrome, and Louis-Bar syndrome. Genetic disturbances in the differentiation of the ectoderm lead to "neurocutaneous syndromes." Increased rates of metaplasia and neoplasia are correlated with development of benign or malignant tumors in skin and nervous system.

NF2 is based on a genetic disorder with a mutation on chromosome 22, and the genetic transfer is mainly autosomal dominant or there is a new mutation; the disease penetration is very variable, with mild, very serious, or life-threatening manifestations. It is defined clinically by National Institutes of Health (NIH) criteria by occurrence of bilateral acoustic neuroma or by co-occurrence of unilateral acoustic neuroma and further by the presence of meningioma, glioma, and by affected first-line relatives.

Typically, NF2-afflicted patients have the following characteristics:

- Retinal disease with Lisch nodules
- Disturbed skin pigmentation with so-called café-au-lait spots
- Some subcutaneous schwannomas or neurofibromas
- Bilateral vestibular schwannomas
- Possibly further intracranial and intraspinal tumors, schwannomas, meningiomas, or gliomas

NF2 is to be differentiated from neurofibromatosis 1 (NF1). NF1 shows a mutation on chromosome 17 and presents with a more peripherally dominated tumor manifestation. There are very obvious subcutaneous tumors sometimes covering the whole body, optic gliomas, and spinal tumors.

TUMOR-SPECIFIC PRINCIPLES

Definition

Acoustic neuromas, or vestibular schwannomas, are benign neoplasms originating from the eighth cranial nerve and can be cured completely by microsurgical tumor resection with low morbidity and very low mortality rates.

Incidence

The incidence of acoustic neuroma is reported at 3% to 8%, and the main occurrence is in the fifth decade of life, with a slight preponderance in males. Ten percent of patients have bilateral acoustic neuroma exhibiting a rare genetic disorder, NF2, and showing a significantly earlier disease manifestation.

Tumor Development and Behavior

Acoustic neuromas originate from the eighth cranial nerve, the vestibulo-cochlear nerve, and specifically its vestibular part. The Schwann cells of the vestibular nerve form the initial tumor, either at the superior or the inferior nerve or both nerves, within the internal auditory canal (IAC), and gradually the whole nerve undergoes a tumorous change. The tumor enlarges within the IAC, causing widening of the meatus diameter and destruction of the posterior lip of the porus, and then grows into the cerebellopontine angle and toward the brainstem and the cerebellum. Once the cerebellopontine angle cistern is filled by tumor, it starts to expand toward the brainstem, compressing the cochlear nuclei, the facial nerve and nuclei toward the trigeminal nerve, the cerebellum, and also the caudal cranial nerves.

With further tumor growth, the brainstem compression becomes more and more serious because of the direct effect and because of the obstruction of the fourth ventricle. Obstructive hydrocephalus may develop at an advanced stage; that or the increasing cerebellum compression may be responsible for the cerebellar ataxia that develops.

Diagnosis

Clinical Presentation

Observations by the Patient. Initial symptoms, such as vertigo, dizziness, and tinnitus, result from irritation of the vestibular or the cochlear part of the eighth nerve. At the beginning these symptoms may be slight and temporary with several relapses occurring over weeks or months, or they may develop so slowly that they are neglected for a long time. Vestibular symptoms may be noticed by patients as a short intermittent feeling of being drawn to one side and almost losing their balance; mostly these symptoms are attributed to blood pressure disturbances. Acoustic symptoms include high-pitched (rarely low-pitched) tinnitus and decreasing hearing. Hearing loss may present as an acute attack with or without recovery or as a progression over a couple of years. Some patients become aware of their hearing problem only when using the phone on that ear. Then an otorhinolaryngologist is contacted.

Because of adaptation and often intermittent observations of eighth nerve symptoms, it is common for symptoms such as trigeminal hypesthesia, facial twitching or facial paresis, or swallowing difficulties—indicating irritation of neighboring cranial nerves—to be a cause for consultation of a neurologist. Severe unsteadiness of gait from compression of the cerebellum or headaches and vomiting resulting from increased cranial pressure from obstructive hydrocephalus occur in later stages.

Primary Diagnostic Measures

Primary diagnostic measures for this disease include the following:

- Clinical evaluation
- Tone audiometry
- Speech discrimination score
- Vestibular tests
- Neurologic examination
- Magnetic resonance imaging (MRI) with gadolinium contrast agent

The medical practitioner or family physician makes the diagnosis by evaluation of the hypacusis or deafness and the unsteadiness of gait; the medical consultant may also detect neurologic disturbances or symptoms of increased intracranial pressure such as headaches, nausea, vomiting, or visual disturbances. The medical consultant then transfers the patient to an otorhinolaryngologist and to a neurologist.

The otorhinolaryngologist is most often among the first to be contacted by patients for hearing disturbances. Typically, audiometry demonstrates hypacusis of high frequencies (above 1 kHz). Speech discrimination is found more affected than pure tone hearing. These two findings raise suspicion of a retrocochlear lesion and indicate the need for testing brainstem auditory evoked responses. These will demonstrate pathologic latency increases, specifically of waves III and in later stages of waves IV and V. Vestibular tests show decreased or lost caloric responses caused by impaired labyrinth excitability. The combination of these findings must prompt a radiologic investigation.

The neurologist investigates the cranial nerves, vestibular and cerebellar functions, and possible signs of increased cranial pressure such as papillary edema and characteristic headaches. Among the cranial nerves, the trigeminal-facial and the caudal cranial nerves are of special importance.

The neuroradiologist performs MRI of the skull base with infusion of contrast agent. In rare instances of incompatibility of the patient with a magnetic field, as with patients wearing pace makers or magnetizing osteosynthetic material, a contrast-enhanced cranial computed tomography (CT) scan is performed to demonstrate the tumor.

In acoustic neuroma in NF2, the symptom onset is much earlier in life, with more than 50% of patients seeking treatment between the ages of 15 and 25. Still, *unilateral acoustic neuroma* presentation at younger than 35 years of age raises suspicion of underlying NF2 and of the possibility of development of contralateral acoustic neuroma. The majority of NF2 patients, however, do exhibit bilateral tumors when first seen. The tumor development may be quite different on both sides, with such extremes as large tumor and good hearing on one side and small tumor and bad hearing on the other.

Treatment Options

Observation

Some suggest observing acoustic neuromas with clinical and MRI controls at 6- to 12-month intervals. They are slowly growing tumors that may sometimes stop growing for a year or longer. Observation is therefore a basic principle in managing small tumors presenting in patients 65 years or older and especially if serious medical illness such as cardiovascular or pulmonary disease or further oncologic illness limits the patient's general health.

However, some very small tumors that can be treated successfully with surgery may cause predominant vestibular disturbances and inability to walk.

There are also some ongoing studies of "spontaneous" tumor progression where all patients with small and medium tumors (i.e., those without life-threatening brainstem compression) are observed over months or even years. Tumor growth may vary from 0 to 4 mm per year and may be very variable.

However, the duration of acoustic nerve symptoms (i.e., of relevant nerve exposure to the tumor) is of importance regarding acoustic nerve function; slow or sudden hearing loss is

possible without documented tumor growth, and chances of hearing-conserving surgery decrease with the increasing duration of symptoms.

Stereotactic Radiosurgery

Two types of stereotactic radiosurgery are available, performed with the Gamma Knife® and the linear accelerator. Both therapies use gamma radiation and are based on a three-dimensional analysis of the tumor volume and a volume-based calculation of central and peripheral radiation doses that include the dose decrease at the isodose margins. The goal is delivery of a high dose to the tumor and a minimal dose to neighboring structures (i.e., cranial nerves, brainstem, and brainstem vessels).

Because schwannomas are benign tumors, radiation stops growth in most cases or at least provides some tumor reduction. Abolition of the tumor is an absolute exception.

Radiosurgery is possible in small tumors (up to 2 to 3 cm in diameter) equivalent to T_1 and T_2, sometimes T_{3A} extensions, in part because of the initial volume increase of the tumor after radiation therapy.

At the most experienced centers, tumor reduction is achieved in 65% to 81% of cases, with a temporary volume increase in approximately 25%; most such centers attain a 70% to 90% success rate in stopping growth. Rates of facial nerve lesions vary from 2.2% to up to 18%. Functional hearing preservation rates (in small tumors) are 50% or better, but hearing slowly deteriorates after 1 to 3 years.

In summary, the advantage for the patient is that stereotactic radiosurgery is done on an outpatient basis and that often a return to work is possible within days to weeks. The disadvantages include the following:

1. Persistent tumor
2. Persistent danger of deteriorating cranial nerve function remaining *after treatment*
3. Treatment options are limited to small tumors
4. Virtually nonexistent treatment options for radiation-induced nerve lesions, especially the trigeminal and facial neuropathies
5. Deteriorated conditions if surgical intervention becomes necessary

Therefore, radiosurgery may be an option for stopping tumor growth for selected patients, but it is not a definite cure.

Microsurgery

Acoustic neuroma can be cured by complete microsurgical tumor resection. Tumor resection is the only option for medium and large acoustic neuroma. The rate of mortality is less than 1%, and morbidity rates are decreasing with the refinement of techniques; these rates are better the earlier surgery is performed. The majority of patients will be able to return to work within weeks to months. The rate of recurrence is at 0.8% in non-NF2 patients.

When there is a genetic disposition from NF2, surgery is indicated in all cases of tumor progression and of tumor compression of the brainstem, and in conditions with a chance of hearing preservation. The rate of tumor recurrence is higher than in non-NF2 patients.

Preparation for Surgery

The general clinical status must be checked for operative contraindications or indications for preoperative special therapy. Specifically, serious noncompensated cardiovascular or pulmonary disease are contraindications. Previous cranial or cardiac infarction and previous thrombosis with or without emboli need presurgical consideration and treatment.

Chest x-ray and electrocardiogram (ECG) studies belong to the routine program in seemingly healthy patients. No thrombocyte aggregation inhibitors should be taken for 10 days before admission.

Neurologic examination is performed to control all cranial nerve functions, sensory and motor functions of long tracts, and vestibular and cerebellar functions, and to identify specific deficits that suggest increased risks, including the following:

■ *Papillary edema* may indicate increased pressure caused by obstructive hydrocephalus that can necessitate ventricular drainage or a shunt.
■ *Caudal cranial nerve palsies* are signs of large tumors or tumor of the jugular foramen and put the patients at risk for aspiration pneumonia.
■ *Trigeminal hypesthesia or trigeminal neuralgia* may hint of a large tumor and sometimes additional vascular nerve compression.
■ *Facial paresis* is rarely observed before surgery, whether in very large tumors, in cystic tumors, or after previous surgery or radiosurgery.

Otorhinolaryngologic preparation includes audiometric and vestibular testing, as mentioned previously. Vestibular function is very rarely normal, mostly decreased or lost on the tumor side. Audiometric function is determined based on pure tone audiometric loss and on speech discrimination scores; both parameters are considered for classification by standardized classification systems such as the Gardner-Robertson, Shelton-House, or Hannover grading systems.

Radiologic Preparation

X-ray examination of the cervical spine in anteflexion and retroflexion detects functional instabilities and may lead to further diagnostics to identify degenerative cervical disease or cervical disk protrusions.

Contrast-enhanced MRI or CT is performed with axial slices parallel to the skull base. The tumor location, extension, and effects on related structures are visible. By these means, the different tumor stages and possible implications are identified, and the surgical approach and technique can be planned (Figure 43-1). Four major stages of tumor development can be differentiated; T_1 is purely intrameatal; T_2 is partially extrameatal tumor; T_3 is intrameatal-extrameatal tumor with major parts filling the cerebellopontine angle cisterns; and T_4 is tumors with brainstem compression.

Bone window CT of the skull base is performed to demonstrate the details of the petrous pyramid, especially the positions of the semicircular canals and the auditory meatus and its widening on the tumor side.

Anesthesia

General anesthesia is induced by totally intravenous anesthesia (TIVA) with no or minimal muscle relaxation because control

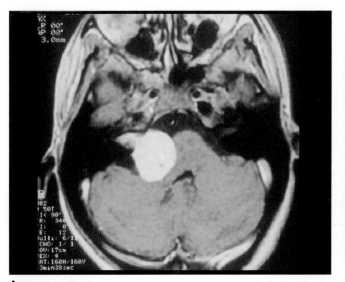

A

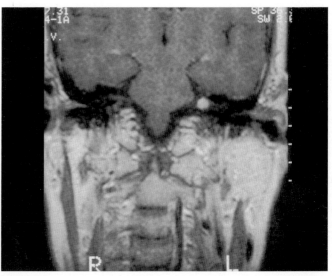

B

FIGURE 43-1   *A,* Large intrameatal-extrameatal acoustic neuroma with brainstem compression grade T_4. *B,* Intrameatal acoustic neuroma T_1.

of muscle function will be necessary during tumor resection. With large brainstem compressive tumors, the intubation is performed by fiberoptic endoscopy. Anesthesiologic monitoring includes, besides ECG, an arterial line for blood pressure control, oxy-shuttle, electroencephalography (EEG), and a precordial ultrasonography.

Surgery

Three different approaches have been standardized for surgical removal of acoustic neuroma: the translabyrinthine, the middle fossa, and the retrosigmoid suboccipital approaches.

The *translabyrinthine approach* traverses the mastoid and is favored by many otorhinolaryngologic surgeons because it is a transosseous approach (see Figure 43-1*A*). Small and large tumors thus can be resected. The disadvantages of this approach are the destruction of the labyrinth with resulting deafness, and furthermore control of the brainstem and its vascular supply is limited.

The *middle fossa approach* enters the IAC and cerebellopontine angle cistern from above (see Figure 43-1*B*). It gives a good overview of the nerves of the IAC but only limited access to the cerebellopontine angle; only small tumors up to 15 or 20 mm can be removed. The disadvantages are the limitation to small tumors, the retraction of the temporal lobe with a risk of epileptic fits, and the consideration that patients are prohibited from driving for 6 months.

The *retrosigmoid suboccipital approach* (see Figure 43-1*A*) is the only approach that simultaneously allows *radical resection of all tumor sizes* and of *functional nerve preservation* of all cranial nerves of the cerebellopontine angle.

Surgery of Acoustic Neuroma by the Suboccipital Approach

A craniotomy is performed in the angle between the transverse and the sigmoid sinuses. After the dura is opened, the cerebellum is lifted and the cisterna magna is opened to release the cerebrospinal fluid (CSF). Along the posterior aspect of the petrous pyramid, the view is opened to the cerebellopontine angle, porus (i.e., the entrance to the IAC), and tumor covering the (partially visible) cranial nerves (Figure 43-2*A*).

Tumor resection is performed in three steps:

- Tumor reduction by enucleation
- Tumor exposure in the IAC by removal of the posterior wall of the canal
- Complete tumor resection by removing the tumor capsule (Figure 43-2*B*) and the tumor origin (the tumorous vestibular nerve) and preservation of cranial nerves (Figure 43-2*C*)

Closure involves the following steps:

- Internal closure of the mastoid cells of the pyramid with fascia and muscle
- Watertight dura suture
- External closure by sealing the dura with fibrin glue and bone closure with a bone flap or plastic material (methylmethacrylate)

Monitoring

Intraoperative neurophysiologic monitoring provides a certain control of essential neurologic functions by recording far-field potentials from the scalp elicited by defined external stimuli.

Median or tibial nerve somatosensory evoked potentials are measured to control the long spinal tracts. This is important during positioning of the patient while the head is rotated and the neck is extended or flexed. Furthermore, it may be useful during dissection of an adherent tumor capsule at the brainstem.

Facial nerve electromyography of the orbicularis oculi and oris muscles is recorded continuously during tumor dissection. Various kinds of manipulations of the nerve during tumor dissection (such as stretching, touching, saline irrigation) cause nerve activation with resulting muscle activity. This is recorded and transferred by loudspeakers. The reactivity of the nerve during surgery gives feedback where the nerve is hidden behind the tumor and when the nerve is tolerating the manipulations or needs softer handling.

Auditory brainstem responses are registered at ear stimulation with click stimuli. The baseline recordings at the start of surgery give some insight into the functional changes that the auditory pathway has already undergone because of tumor compression. Further changes of waveforms during tumor dissection give information on the integrity of the pathway or endangered auditory function. Very fast reaction to certain critical changes is necessary to prevent nerve blockage, degeneration, and deafness. Along with fast reliable auditory brainstem response (ABR) monitoring, the rate and quality of hearing preservation can be improved considerably.

Special circumstances may speak in favor of subtotal tumor resection as the most sensible solution. This may be applicable for patients of advanced age or in NF2-afflicted patients for whom radical surgery is not practicable.

Postsurgical Treatment

Early Postoperative Therapy

The endotracheal tube is removed as early as possible in posterior fossa surgery, because awake patients are easier to monitor, and serious complications are easier to detect. The tube is removed while the patient is in the operating room or in the intensive care unit, not later than 2 hours after surgery.

Controls of the patient are monitored for 1 night in the intensive care unit. Wakefulness, pupillary reactions, and vegetative parameters are examined at 15-minute intervals for the first 2 hours and then at increasing intervals up to the next morning.

Medication includes 8 mg of dexamethasone administered four times in 24 hours and gastric protection by omeprazole or ranitidine.

Mobilization of the patient is undertaken on day 1 after surgery with the physiotherapist. Physiotherapy aims at training the patient's balance and reducing muscular tension. When the patient exhibits facial paresis, he or she learns and performs specific facial exercises.

Wound control is addressed every 1 to 2 days, and stitches are removed after 1 week.

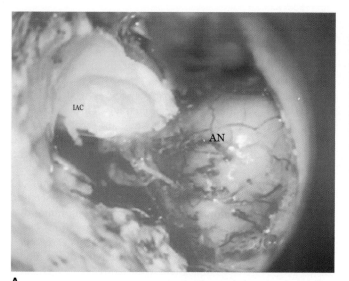

A

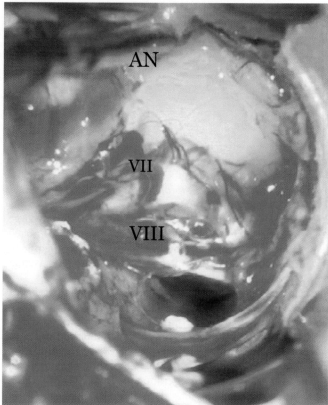

B

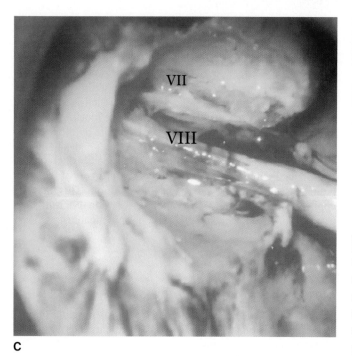

C

FIGURE 43-2 *A,* Suboccipital approach. Acoustic neuroma is exposed in the cerebellopontine angle and in the internal auditory canal (posterior wall is removed). *B,* After enucleation of the acoustic neuroma, the tumor capsule is pulled up, and cranial nerves VII and VIII are visible. *C,* After complete resection of the acoustic neuroma, the nerve bundle of VII and VIII is visible in the internal auditory canal (IAC).

Postoperative control evaluations include clinical neurologic examination with facial nerve grading, CT, and audiometry.

Complications

In general, the earlier a problem occurs after surgery, the more serious it is and the faster a remedy is needed. The clinical picture of an early postoperative complication is disturbed consciousness, either delayed awakening or decreasing alertness in the first hours. Various causes need to be differentiated.

Pneumoencephalos results from excessive loss of CSF and develops as air collection within the ventricular system or bifrontally at the skull base and over the hemispheres. It occurs somewhat more often after surgery when the patient is in a semi-sitting position rather than supine. It may cause apathy, drowsiness, or even unconsciousness and respiratory depression. Depending on the clinical status, surgical release of the air by drainage via a burrhole and replacement of CSF with saline may be necessary, but usually resorption occurs spontaneously.

Hemorrhage in the operative field may develop in 1% to 2% of cases. Especially in tumors with brainstem compression, bleeding in the cerebellopontine angle is a risk. A large hemorrhage with decreasing consciousness requires urgent surgical revision. In some patients, hemorrhage may develop so slowly and insidiously that the initial symptoms, such as irritability, are overlooked.

CSF fistulae occur in up to 9% of cases and present as rhinoliquorrhoea. The surgically opened mastoid cells from the site of craniotomy or at the IAC are sealed with a muscle and fascia layer at the end of surgery. However, CSF leaking into the mastoid and running through the eustachian tube will result in rhinoliquorrhoea. The internal fistula needs operative revision with sealing of the internal mastoid cells at the porus (2% to 3%). The external fistula rarely needs revision. CSF leakage is most often stopped by compressive external dressing and lumbar CSF drainage for 5 to 8 days.

Hydrocephalus may be present before or after surgery. In clinically symptomatic hydrocephalus (1% of cases), preoperative external drainage or ventriculo-peritoneal shunt implantation may be indicated and will improve the patient's condition for tumor surgery. Patients may also be asymptomatic regarding CSF circulation before surgery but develop postsurgical edema and an obstructed fourth ventricle. Temporary external drainage can overcome this critical period, but sometimes a permanent shunt becomes necessary after 1 to 2 weeks (in 1% to 2% of cases).

Death is a very rare complication, occurring in less than 1% of patients after tumor resection. The tumor-specific causes can be hemorrhage or aspiration pneumonia. Hemorrhage may be discovered late, if it develops very slowly, causing unconsciousness, and treatment options may be limited for hemorrhage into the brainstem. Aspiration pneumonia can develop because of caudal cranial nerve palsies, requiring temporary tracheostomy and specific antibiosis; nonetheless, it is life threatening. Furthermore, the general constitution of the individual patient, thrombosis, and embolism are relevant factors.

Functional Results and Rehabilitation

Postsurgical rehabilitation aims for functional recovery from neurologic deficits.

Vestibular function on the side operated on is completely lost in at least 90% of cases, although up to 10% of patients have some vestibular function preserved from a partially preserved superior or inferior vestibular nerve. Balance training is essential during the first days and, in many patients, the first weeks after surgery. Usually, within the first 3 days, dramatic improvement is seen, and eventually only slight unsteadiness in the dark or with eyes closed remains.

Auditory function on the side operated on may be preserved in up to 47% of cases, depending on the individual patient's preoperative function and tumor extension. With small tumors, some auditory function may be preserved in up to 74%, with 23% to 30% retaining a normal level. With very large tumors, 20% of patients may retain some function, with only 10% to 14% retaining good or normal function. Chances for auditory preservation are best for male patients and in cases that involve a short duration of symptomatology, tumor size no more than 25 mm in diameter, and preoperative hearing function no worse than a 40-dB loss. In recent years the refinement of functional neurosurgery has enabled increasing rates of hearing preservation, especially of good auditory quality (Tables 43-1 and 43-2). Hearing aids will help only if the interear functional difference is not too large.

TABLE 43-1

Hannover Audiological Classification

Class	Hearing Quality	Audiometry*	SDS Speech Discrimination
H1	Normal	0–20 dB	100–95%
H2	Useful	21–40 dB	90–70%
H3	Moderate	41–60 dB	65–40%
H4	Bad	61–80 dB	35–10%
H5	Nonfunctional	>80 dB	5–0%

*Average hearing loss at 1 to 3 kHz.

Cross rehabilitation equipment can be mounted to spectacles in case of unilateral deafness and allows the patient, via a receiver on the deaf side and a loudspeaker on the hearing side, to perceive noises and voices on the deaf side.

NF2's hallmark is the bilateral presence of acoustic neuroma. Compared with non-NF2, there are substantial differences to be considered.

Surgical Aspects. At surgery, the auditory nerve may be found to have undergone tumorous change. Furthermore, there may be multiple nerve origins of the tumor consisting of confluent grapelike tumors composed of several schwannomas of cranial nerves.

Under these conditions, complete tumor removal along with nerve preservation is impossible. Because a cure cannot be achieved in patients with NF2, not even by radical surgery, preservation of nerve function is regarded as more important than radical surgery. If a nerve with tumorous change still has useful clinical function, nerve preservation with subtotal tumor resection is a sensible compromise. Neurophysiologic monitoring is of great importance for intraoperative evaluation of nerve function. Subtotal tumor resection has enabled preservation of useful hearing in the remaining functioning ear in series of patients. Interestingly, despite some regrowth of tumor, auditory function was maintained at a useful level for periods as long as 12 years. This preserved function must be ascribed to the decompression that was obtained by bony opening of the IAC at surgery.

The general rule for NF2 patients is to operate as rarely as possible but as often as necessary to afford the patient a rather long-lasting good quality of life.

Auditory brainstem implants are designed for patients with NF2 who have bilateral hearing loss caused by bilateral destruction of the cochlear nerves from schwannomas. Implants initially give patients some perception of environmental sounds; patients then relearn to understand syllables, whole words, and finally sentences. With implants and lipreading, they achieve an understanding of 40% to 100% of conversation of an unknown context.

Facial nerve function is good in the majority of patients: 55% have completely normal function immediately after surgery, but impairment of various degrees occurs in up to 45% of patients in the early postoperative phase. Approximately 25%

TABLE 43-2	Hearing Preservation Rates in a Series of 1800 Tumors Depending on Preoperative Auditory Function and Tumor Extension		
Tumor Extension Incidences			
131 (7%)	266 (15%)	749 (42%)	654 (36%)
Preoperative Function	T1	T2	T3	T4
H1	74%	63%	65%	35%
H2	67%	77%	51%	25%
H3	41%	48%	36%	14%
H4	—	30%	18%	8%
H5*	6%	4%	3%	1%
Average	56% (65/115)	57% (123/216)	44% (262/592)	20% (79/392)

*Preservation in H5 signifies recovery from functional deafness to auditory function.

recover quickly and completely (House-Brackmann grades 1 and 2) within the first weeks and usually not later than the first 3 months. Some incomplete recovery is demonstrated in 20% who have a longer postsurgical rehabilitation. Recovery with continuous physiotherapy may take more than 1 to 2 years.

Facial nerve reconstruction is indicated in approximately 6% of cases for two different conditions:

- Whenever there is discontinuity of the facial nerve at surgery, the facial nerve may be reconstructed with a graft, usually from the sural nerve, which is interposed between the nerve stumps. Recovery will start approximately half a year afterward.
- When an anatomically preserved facial nerve does not show any reinnervation within 12 months, a reanimation procedure for the facial nerve is indicated. By hypoglossal-facial combination, reinnervation is enabled starting 6 to 9 months after reconstruction. At the beginning, the hypoglossal activity will animate the face; later, by cortical plasticity, facial movements become possible independent of the voluntary hypoglossal activity.

Up to 78% of reconstructed facial nerves will achieve a House-Brackmann grade 3 with good symmetry on rest, complete eye closure, and good control of the mouth.

These nerve reconstructive procedures provide results superior to any plastic techniques, because nerve reconstruction brings about functional and cosmetic recovery and emotional expressivity.

Facial Nerve in NF2. Compared with the non-NF2 facial nerve preservation rate of 94% to 95%, patients with NF2 have only 85% preservation. This is in part due to the higher rate of tumorous nerve changes with loss of nerve continuity at surgery, and furthermore there is a higher proportion of large tumors more than 30 mm in diameter (68%) as compared with tumors in non-NF2 patients (51%).

Recurrence

Recurrence rates in cases of complete tumor resection in non-NF2 patients are less than 1% during follow-up periods of 8 years.

In the case of subtotal tumor removal, for example with a tumor remnant left on the facial nerve, regrowth is likely; this concept of subtotal preservation is generally accepted only in elderly high-risk patients or in patients with NF2.

In NF2, even radical treatment will not bring about cure of the patient, because recurrence is possible from any cranial nerve in the cerebellopontine angle.

Outcome and Quality of Life

Acoustic neuroma can be cured by complete tumor resection via the suboccipital approach, and the patients will be able to return to their previous quality of life in most cases.

Facial nerve function is regarded as the most important outcome criterion by all patients. Some patients who show good recovery will nonetheless suffer from side effects such as synkinesia and aberrant innervation of tear secretion. Synkinesia can be treated successfully with specialized physiotherapy or with muscular injection of botulinum toxin at 4-month intervals.

The postoperative recovery period is highly variable. Based on a recovery recommended for 2 to 3 months, some patients feel eager and fit to take up their profession after as little as 4 to 6 weeks, whereas others continue to suffer from certain sequels, such as head and neck pains, tinnitus induced or worsened by noises and voices, dizziness, and general fatigue, for 6 months or even longer.

On close examination, head and neck pain are found to originate from occipital nerve irritation (rare) or preexisting cervical osteochondrosis. Tinnitus is less common in patients with some preserved hearing, whereas it is increased or more irritating to patients with postsurgical deafness. Balance disturbances resulting from the unilateral loss of vestibular nerve function (because of resection of its tumorous part) may persist in many patients when they are in the dark or have their eyes closed. The 10% of patients with partial preservation of vestibular function show a prolonged recovery course of their balance, possibly resulting from the increasing recuperating nerve function. Although this can be demonstrated clinically (by caloric, nystagmus, and Unterberger tests), this development may take 1 to 2 years with a very good final result.

Within a rather short period of medical history, the fate of patients with acoustic neuroma has changed dramatically, from suffering a life-threatening disease to a situation where cure and good quality of life are realistic goals.

CHAPTER 44

NONACOUSTIC SCHWANNOMAS OF THE CRANIAL NERVES

Samer Ayoubi and Ossama Al-Mefty

Schwannomas are tumors of Schwann cells. They may arise anywhere that a nerve has a Schwann cell sheath. With the exception of the optic nerves, which in fact are not nerves, the cranial nerves are myelinated by Schwann cells and are therefore potential sites for schwannomas.[4] Schwannomas of the cranial nerves are not common tumors (except for acoustic schwannomas). The most commonly affected nerve (a distant second to acoustic schwannomas) is the trigeminal nerve, followed by the glossopharyngeal nerve.[14] Involvement of the other cranial nerves is rare.

LOCATION

Nonacoustic schwannomas of the cranial nerves usually arise from the *intracranial* parts of the nerves, giving rise to intracranial tumors. These tumors follow the courses of the intracranial portions of the nerves. Rarely, schwannomas arise from the *extracranial* parts of the cranial nerves. These have been reported in the nasal cavity,[15] the orbit,[2,14] the infratemporal fossa, and other sites.

In the *nasal cavity*, it is often difficult to identify the origin of the tumor. The tumor in these cases can rise from the sensory branches of the ophthalmic and maxillary divisions of the trigeminal nerve, parasympathetic fibers from the sphenopalatine ganglion, and sympathetic fibers from the carotid plexus. It is also difficult to identify the origin of *intraorbital schwannomas*. They can arise from the ciliary, oculomotor, supraorbital, suborbital, or lacrimal nerves inside the orbit.

DIAGNOSIS

Symptoms and signs of nonacoustic intracranial schwannomas depend on the cranial nerve involved.

Schwannomas of the Oculomotor Nerves

Extraocular muscles are driven by cranial nerves III (oculomotor), IV (trochlear), and VI (abducens) and the autonomic efferent nerves. The major symptom of malfunction of any of these nerves is diplopia.

Because schwannomas have a particular proclivity for sensory nerves versus motor nerves, schwannomas of these nerves are rare.[9] For example, only 17 cases of trochlear nerve

neuromas are reported in the English medical literature.[12] The third cranial nerve is affected more often than the fourth, which is affected more often than the sixth.[9] Most oculomotor nerve schwannomas occur after the fourth decade of life.

The most common symptom is headache.[9] Diplopia, which draws attention to the oculomotor nerves, occurs in most but not all cases.[9,12] The nerves, particularly the fourth, can give rise to a tumor without demonstrated palsy of the nerve.[12] With enlargement of the tumor, other neighboring cranial nerves can be affected, particularly the fifth cranial nerve, with facial tingling, numbness, or pain. With even larger tumors, hemiparesis or symptoms of raised intracranial pressure can occur. Tung divided sixth nerve schwannomas into two types: Type I arises from the cavernous sinus portion of the sixth nerve. Patients predominantly have diplopia. Type II arises from the precavernous part of the sixth nerve. As well as diplopia, patients have symptoms and signs of posterior fossa tumor.[11]

On examination, if there is left abducens paresis, the left lateral rectus muscle cannot pull the left eye outward, and the patient will have double vision in left gaze.

The *fourth cranial nerve* innervates only the superior oblique muscle. Patients complain that objects seem tilted when they view them with an affected eye. If there is left trochlear paresis, greatest deviation is noted when the patient looks downward and to the right.

The *third cranial nerve* innervates all other ocular muscles. It also carries parasympathetic efferent fibers to the pupillary sphincter. Left oculomotor nerve lesions can cause a fixed dilated left pupil, ptosis, and an inability to adduct, elevate, or depress the left eye.

Trigeminal Schwannomas

Schwannomas that arise from the intracranial portion of the trigeminal nerve are rare, accounting for 0.8% to 8% of intracranial schwannomas.[1] Jefferson[6] classified these tumors into three types: (1) type A tumors are located mainly in the middle fossa that arise from the gasserian ganglion; (2) type B tumors are located predominately in the posterior fossa and arise from the root of the trigeminal nerve; and (3) type C tumors are dumbbell-shaped, or hourglass-shaped, tumors with significant components in both the middle and posterior fossae (Figure 44-1).

All patients will manifest trigeminal nerve dysfunction (sensory or motor deficit, or pain). The typical tic douloureux is manifested in only approximately 15% of patients.[1] Patients

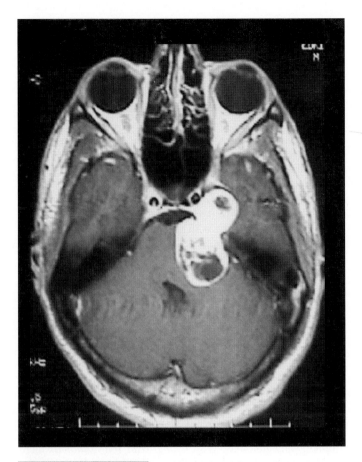

FIGURE 44-1   Dumbbell-shape trigeminal schwannoma involving both the middle and posterior fossa.

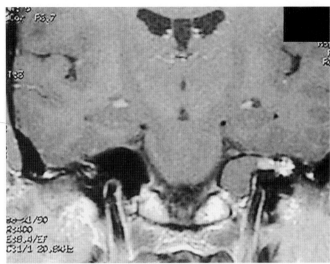

FIGURE 44-2   Facial nerve schwannoma.

may complain of retro-orbital or periorbital pain. Diplopia occurs as the tumor enlarges and involves the oculomotor nerves. With large tumors, half the patients will complain of diplopia. Headache, blurred vision, dizziness, imbalance, and hemiparesis are much less common symptoms.

The trigeminal nerve provides sensory innervation to the face and head and motor innervation to the muscles of mastication. When the nerve is affected, there may be reduced sensation—for touch, temperature, or pain—in one of the three somatotopic divisions of the nerve (ophthalmic, maxillary, or mandibular). The corneal reflex may be reduced. Motor weakness of the muscles of mastication—the temporalis, masseter, and medial and lateral pterygoid—is less commonly found than sensory signs on examination in patients with trigeminal schwannomas.

Facial Nerve Schwannomas

Schwannomas of the facial nerve can arise in the temporal bone proximal to the stylomastoid foramen or from the descending or tympanic segment of the nerve, occurring with facial palsy or oral polyp.[8] Because the Schwann cell sheath extends to within 1 mm of the brainstem, schwannomas can occur on the intracranial part of the nerve.

Facial nerve schwannomas are rare (Figure 44-2), accounting for approximately 2.5% of the cerebellopontine angle tumors,[8] and only 467 cases have been reported.[10] Tumors at

the geniculate ganglion level grow into the middle fossa, and those with proximal origin extend into the internal auditory meatus and cerebellopontine angle. Mean age of patients is approximately 40 years.[8,10] Facial palsy occurs in most, but not all, cases; it can be absent in up to one quarter. Severity of facial weakness ranges from mild paresis to total palsy. It is usually progressive, often proceeded by periods of facial twitching. Sensorineural deafness is usually present. It can be severe or total. However, it is conductive in some cases and rarely the patient can have intact hearing.[8] Other symptoms may include vertigo, tinnitus, or ear pain.[10] There is a long interval between onset of symptoms and diagnosis.

Facial nerve innervates the muscles of facial expression. It also innervates the stapedius muscle, salivary and lacrimal glands, and mucus glands of the nose, nasopharynx, and pharynx. It conveys taste sensation from the anterior two thirds of the tongue and carries somatic sensory fibers from the external ear. Signs of facial weakness depend on tumor location on the nerve. The tumor may be visible in the middle ear when the tympanic segment is involved. Signs of sensorineural deafness are usually present, with the tumor damaging the internal ear or compressing the cochlear nerve in the meatus. Signs of conductive hearing loss are less common, indicating involvement of the middle ear. Signs of raised intracranial pressure or signs of cerebellopontine angle syndrome may be present, with larger tumors causing mass effect.

Schwannomas of the Jugular Foramen Nerves

The jugular foramen forms an acute-angle triangle in the skull base. An anterior fibrous or bony band separates the jugular foramen into an anteromedial pars nervosa, which contains the glossopharyngeal nerve, and a posterolateral pars venosa, which contains the vagus and accessory nerves, as well as the jugular bulb.

Schwannomas of these nerves are very rare. They usually affect the glossopharyngeal nerve. The nerve of origin in the jugular foramen cannot always be identified (Figure 44-3).

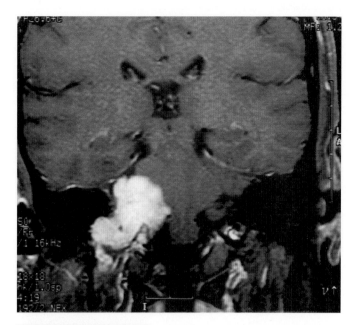

FIGURE 44-3   Lower cranial nerve schwannoma.

The most common symptom reported was hearing loss. Besides paresis of the nerves, patients can have vagoglossopharyngeal pain. Dysphagia, dysphonia, and persistent toothache have been reported. Schwannomas of the jugular foramen may mimic the clinical signs of glomus jugulare tumors in every aspect. Keye classified these tumors into three groups: (1) type A is confined to the intracranial compartment; (2) type B invades mainly the bone; and (3) type C is primarily extracranial.[7]

The glossopharyngeal nerve supplies motor innervation to the stylopharyngeus muscle and conducts sensory information from the pharynx, palate, eustachian tube, tympanic cavity, and posterior third of the tongue. It conveys taste sensation from the posterior third of the tongue. The motor innervation of the vagus includes most muscles of the palate and pharynx and the muscles of the larynx. The accessory muscle innervates both the trapezius and sternomastoid muscles.

On examination, patients with schwannomas of the jugular foramen nerves can show a reduced gag reflex, deviation of the uvula toward the intact side, a hoarse voice, or stridor. Signs of accessory nerve paresis include weakness in shrugging the shoulder or weakness in turning the head away from the muscle tested against resistance. With larger tumors, other cranial nerves can be involved and signs of raised intracranial pressure can be seen.

Intracranial Hypoglossal Schwannomas

Extracranial and intracranial schwannomas of the hypoglossal nerve are unusual.[3] These tumors usually cause unilateral lingual atrophy. Because of the minimal disability produced by the deficit, patients generally do not seek treatment until quite late, sometimes as late as 10 years after the nerve involvement had been noted.[13] With larger tumors, the other three lower cranial nerves (IX, X, XI) are often involved. Other cranial nerves (VII, VIII, V) are less often involved.

The hypoglossal nerve innervates the muscles of the tongue. With involvement of the hypoglossal nerve, there is deviation of the tongue toward the paretic side. With larger tumors there are signs of involvement of other cranial nerves, and there may be signs of cerebellar or brainstem compression or raised intracranial pressure.

RADIOLOGIC EXAMINATION

Schwannomas are slowly growing tumors that characteristically expand the thin bony confines of the cavities and foramina in which they arise. Although these radiologic signs can sometimes be seen on skull x-ray studies, they are much better seen on thin-slice bone-window computed tomography (CT) scans. With *nasal schwannomas*, there may be erosion of the floor of the frontal fossa with the tumor growing to reach the intracranial compartment.[15] With *orbital schwannomas*, there may be erosion of the bone of the orbital walls at the site of tumor development or erosion of the sphenoidal fissure as the tumor reaches the skull.[2] With *oculomotor schwannomas* bone erosion can be seen in the medial sphenoid wall, the posterior clinoid process, or the apex and anterior aspect of the petrous pyramid. There may be enlargement of the superior orbital fissure. Bone erosion is seen around the petrous apex and Meckel's cave in approximately 33% of cases of *trigeminal schwannomas*.[1] With *facial nerve schwannomas*, there may be enlargement of facial nerve canal, erosion into the middle fossa at the site of geniculate ganglion, or enlargement or erosion of the internal auditory meatus. Likewise, there may be enlargement or erosion of the *jugular foramen* with the jugular foramen schwannomas. With *hypoglossal schwannomas* there may be extensive erosion of the occipital bone lateral to the foramen magnum.[3]

Noncontrast CT scans usually show an isodense (sometimes hypodense) extra-axial mass that is homogeneously enhanced after intravenous administration of contrast agent.

Magnetic resonance imaging (MRI) is the method of choice in diagnosing nonacoustic schwannomas in all locations. The lesion is isointense or slightly hypointense on T1-weighted images, hyperintense on T2-weighted images, and homogeneously enhanced after administration of contrast agent. Magnetic resonance (MR) arteriography reveals the vascular anatomy of the area concerned, any narrowing or displacement of adjacent vessels, and any associated vascular lesions. MR venography visualizes the venous anatomy. This is important with schwannomas of the oculomotor nerves to see the cavernous sinus, with trigeminal schwannomas to see the vein of Labbé and the cavernous sinus, and with schwannomas of the jugular foramen to see the sigmoid sinus and jugular bulb.

HISTOLOGY

Nonacoustic schwannomas of the cranial nerves have the same histologic pattern as acoustic schwannomas. Macroscopically, the lesion is a discrete mass, which occasionally can be cystic. Microscopically, the lesion is composed of bundles of spindle cells, referred to as Antoni A tissue, and looser elements that produce sponginess, referred to as Antoni B. The distinctive palisading of nuclei may also be seen (Figure 44-4). S-100 staining is markedly positive in schwannomas, which helps distinguish them from meningiomas.

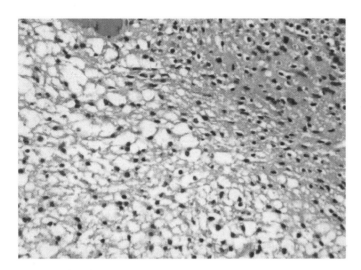

FIGURE 44-4 Antoni A tissue *(lower left)* and Antoni B tissue *(upper right).*

Cranial nerve schwannomas are overwhelmingly benign lesions with a biologic behavior of slow growth; only a few malignant cases have been reported.

TREATMENT

Surgery

Schwannomas are among the few tumors for which surgery can be curative while preserving function, even when large schwannomas displace surrounding neurovascular structures rather than engulfing them. Therefore total removal is believed to offer the best chance of cure. Subtotal removal is associated with a higher rate of recurrence and can be a source of postoperative bleeding from the tumor bed.

The surgical approach should be selected after a thorough study of each patient's preoperative radiologic findings and should be tailored to each case. Skull-base approaches have proved advantageous for large tumors, where more bone is removed to get a wider and shorter access to the tumor.

Surgery has been the mainstream of treatment for *oculomotor schwannomas*. Depending on the site and extension of the tumor, pterional, subtemporal, and suboccipital approaches have been used.[9,12,14] When the fourth nerve is resected, it may be possible to reanastomose the nerve and achieve good long-term nerve function recovery.[14] The sixth nerve is also a pure motor nerve and has a good chance of functional recovery after reconstruction. When the tumor involves the cavernous sinus, skull-base approaches are advantageous in removing these tumors.

The aim of treatment with *trigeminal schwannomas* should be total removal, even if the tumor is large and involves the cerebellopontine angle, petrous apex, or cavernous sinus.[1] With the introduction of microsurgical procedures, there has been a remarkable improvement in the ability to remove trigeminal schwannomas totally, with low risk of morbidity and mortality. The emphasis of treatment has shifted to the patient's quality of life through the preservation or improvement of cranial nerve

function, including that of the trigeminal nerve. Nontraumatic dissection of the trigeminal roots, ganglion, and divisions effectively preserves or even improves trigeminal nerve function. Compared with conventional approaches, skull-base approaches have been advantageous in reducing the percentage of residual or recurrent trigeminal schwannomas, reducing postoperative cranial nerve dysfunction, and improving clinical outcome.

Facial nerve schwannomas arising from the cerebellopontine angle are difficult to separate from schwannomas of the eighth nerve preoperatively. The nerve of origin is often established during surgery. Surgical approaches are similar to approaches for eighth nerve schwannomas.

Surgery is an effective strategy in most symptomatic cases, although sacrifice of a segment of the facial nerve is usually necessary and should be combined with interposition cable nerve graft, which should restore partial nerve function.[10]

Jugular foramen schwannomas are also removed surgically. These tumors are removed through the lateral suboccipital retrosigmoid route or the infratemporal posterior fossa approach. Special attention should be given to postoperative care, because temporary deficit of the lower cranial nerves is expected and can be associated with high morbidity, especially when there are pulmonary complications.

Hypoglossal schwannomas have been removed through suboccipital approaches, sometimes accompanied with a mastoid approach. A transcondylar skull-base approach is appropriate for large tumors.

Radiosurgery

The number of patients with nonacoustic schwannomas treated with radiosurgery remains relatively small because these lesions are rare. For *trigeminal schwannomas*, tumor shrinkage was achieved in 56% of treated patients and tumor growth in 44%.[5] Some authors recommend that radiosurgery be used as the primary treatment in patients with small and moderate-size trigeminal schwannomas. However, most authors believe that the best treatment is complete microsurgical removal of the lesion, reserving the use of radiosurgery as adjuvant therapy for residual or recurrent tumors that cannot be removed surgically, for patients unable to undergo surgery, and for patients who opt not to have surgery.[1]

Only very few patients with *facial nerve schwannomas* have been treated with radiosurgery. When patients had facial palsy, it was arrested or improved. Hearing was preserved. Radiosurgery should be considered as a treatment option in facial nerve schwannomas, but more experience is required to determine the control rates.[10]

OUTCOME

Because these lesions are benign, the recurrence rate depends on the extent of removal. Outcome of surgery is more favorable with small tumors that can be removed without damaging neighboring structures.

For *oculomotor schwannomas*, anastomosis of the fourth or sixth nerve, when possible, will yield better function. When reconstruction is not possible, strabismus surgery can help to correct diplopia.

With *trigeminal schwannomas*, preoperative levels of facial numbness improves in approximately 44% of patients, facial pain is alleviated in 73%, and trigeminal motor deficit improves in 80% of patients.[1] All other involved cranial nerve deficits improve within 4 to 6 months. Most surgically induced trigeminal nerve dysfunction and oculomotor nerve dysfunction will improve with time.

With *facial nerve schwannomas*, early diagnosis aids in the preservation of hearing, and it may benefit the outcome of facial nerve function, because the efficacy of grafting depends partially on the duration of paralysis.[10]

With *jugular foramen schwannomas*, the recurrence is also slow, coming 3 to 5 years after surgery in approximately 15% of cases.[14] The outcome of surgery is usually good.

References

1. Al-Mefty O, Ayoubi S, Gaber E: Trigeminal schwannomas: removal of dumbbell-shaped tumors through the expanded meckel cave and outcomes of cranial nerve function. J Neurosurg 96:453–463, 2002.
2. Cantore G, Ciappetta P, Raco A, et al: Orbital schwannomas: report of nine cases and review of the literature. Neurosurgery 19:583–588.
3. Dolan E, Tucker WS, Rotenberg D, et al: Intracranial hypoglossal schwannoma as an unusual cause of facial nerve palsy. J Neurosurg 56:420–423, 1982.
4. Fuller GN, Burger PC: Classification and biology of brain tumors. In Youmans JR (ed): Neurological Surgery, ed 4. Vol 4. Philadelphia, WB Saunders, 1996.
5. Huang CF, Kondziolka D, Flickinger JC, et al: Stereotactic radiosurgery for trigeminal schwannomas. Neurosurgery 45:11–16, 1999.
6. Jefferson G: The trigeminal neurinomas with some remarks on malignant invasion of the gasserian ganglion. Clin Neurosurg 1:11–54, 1955.
7. Kaye AH, Hahn JF, Kinney SE, et al: Jugular foramen schwannomas. J Neurosurg 60:1045–1053, 1984.
8. King TT, Morrison AW: Primary facial nerve tumors within the skull. J Neurosurg 72:1–8, 1990.
9. Leunda G, Vaquero J, Cabezudo J, et al: Schwannomas of the oculomotor nerves, report of four cases. J Neurosurg 57:563–565, 1982.
10. Sherman JD, Dagnew E, Pensak ML, et al: Facial nerve neuromas: report of 10 cases and review of the literature. Neurosurgery 50:450–456, 2002.
11. Tung H, Chen T, Weiss MH: Sixth nerve schwannomas: report of two cases. J Neurosurg 75:638–664, 1991.
12. Veshcehev I, Spektor S: Trochleare nerve neuroma manifested with intractable atypical pain: case report. Neurosurgery 50:889–892, 2002.
13. William JM, Fox JL: Neurinoma of the intracranial portion of the hypoglossal nerve. Review and case report. J Neurosurg 19:248–250, 1962.
14. Yasargil MG: Less common neurinomas: orbital, oculomotor, trigeminal, facial, glossopharyngeal, accessory, and hypoglossal. In Yassargil MG (ed): Microneurosurgery. Vol 4 B. New York, Thieme Verlag, 1996.
15. Zovickian, J, Barba D, Alksne JF: Intranasal schwannoma with extension into the intracranial compartment: case report. Neurosurgery 19:813–815, 1986.

CHAPTER 45

MENINGIOMAS

Ketan R. Bulsara, Ossama Al-Mefty, Dennis C. Shrieve, and Edgardo J. Angtuaco

In the words of Harvey Cushing, "Few procedures in surgery may be more immediately formidable than an attack upon a large tumor [meningioma] and that the ultimate prognosis hinges more on the surgeon's wide experience with the problem in all its many aspects than is true of almost any other operation that can be named."[11] "There is to-day nothing in the realm of surgery more gratifying than the successful removal of a meningioma with subsequent perfect functional recovery."[10] More than 80 years later, these words still stand true.

In 1922 the term *meningioma* was coined to describe a tumor proximal to the meninges.[10] These lesions were subsequently categorized by their site of origin by Cushing and Eisenhardt.[11] It is now known that meningiomas arise from arachnoidal cap cells. These are commonly associated with the arachnoid villi at the dural sinuses and their tributaries, cranial nerve foramina, cribriform plate, and medial middle fossa. Meningothelial cells in the choroid plexus and tela choroidea also give rise to meningiomas.

Meningiomas are more common in women; the male-to-female incidence ratio is approximately 1:1.4.[13] African Americans tend to have a higher predisposition than others for developing these tumors. The mean incidence of intracranial meningiomas is 20%, with the peak in the seventh decade of life. Overall, between 13% and 26% of primary intracranial tumors are meningiomas.[26] Of these, 85% to 90% are supratentorial. Approximately half of these are located along the base of the anterior and middle fossae.[13] Meningiomas in the pediatric population account for less than 2% of brain tumors and, interestingly, most occur in males.

ETIOLOGY

Meningiomas have been associated with radiation therapy and sex hormones. Radiation therapy, at a high or low dosage, can cause meningiomas several years after treatment.[27] These tumors are commonly atypical and multifocal with a propensity for higher proliferation indices and the tendency for recurrence and aggressive behavior. The role of sex hormones in the genesis of meningiomas is unclear. What is known is that, even though estrogen receptors are rarely detected, approximately two thirds of meningiomas express progesterone receptors.

Genetic susceptibility is a major etiologic risk factor. Meningiomas occur with neurofibromatosis type 2 (NF2) and are associated with an NF2 gene mutation or chromosome 22q loss.[27] There are some families without NF2 who have an increased susceptibility for developing meningiomas. This suggests that another gene locus may be involved. The most common cytogenetic finding in meningiomas is the monosomy of chromosome 22 (Figure 45-1). The progression of meningiomas to World Health Organization (WHO) grade II is associated with losses of chromosome 1p, 6q, 10q, 14q, and 18q. It is also associated with gains of 1q, 9q, 12q, 15q, 17q, and 20q.[27] Further progression to WHO grade III is seen with losses of chromosome 6q, 9p, 10, and 14q. This progression can also occur with the amplification of chromosome 17q, mutations of TP53 and PTEN, or deletions of CDKN2A.[27] The progression of chromosome aberrations may be mediated by both telomeric and centromeric instability.[30] Recurrent reciprocal translocations of 1;19 and q21;q13.3 are also seen.[31]

PRESENTING FEATURES: SYMPTOMS AND SIGNS

No single symptom or sign is specific for patients with intracranial meningiomas. Some patients are asymptomatic, and their tumors are detected incidentally. Other patients have symptoms such as headache, paresis, seizures, personality change or confusion, and visual impairment. Headache and paresis occur in 36% and 30% of patients, respectively.[13]

Meningiomas in some locations have a typical clinical presentation. Patients with olfactory groove meningiomas have anosmia and the Foster Kennedy syndrome (optic atrophy and scotoma in the ipsilateral eye with papilledema in the other eye). Tuberculum sellae meningiomas are usually associated with a chiasmal syndrome with ipsilateral optic atrophy and an incongruous bitemporal hemianopsia.[4] Cavernous sinus meningiomas may cause proptosis, diplopia, or primary aberrant oculomotor regeneration. Foramen magnum lesions may cause nuchal and suboccipital pain with stepwise appendicular sensory and motor deficits. In general, children show signs of increased intracranial pressure without further localizing features.

PATHOLOGY

Classification

In 1999 the working group that convened in Lyon, France, instituted the new WHO classification of central nervous system

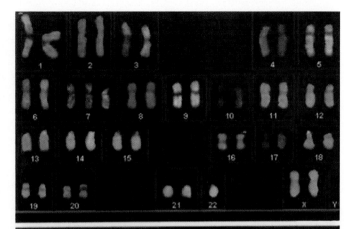

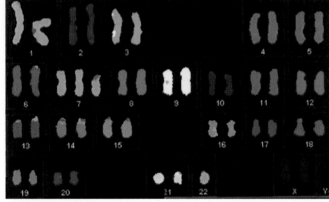

FIGURE 45-1   Spectral karyotyping demonstrating monosomy of chromosome 22.

TABLE 45-1

World Health Organization Classification of Meningiomas

Low Risk of Recurrence and Aggressive Growth
Grade I
Meningothelial meningioma
Fibrous (fibroblastic) meningioma
Transitional (mixed) meningioma
Psammomatous meningioma
Angiomatous meningioma
Microcystic meningioma
Lymphoplasmacyte-rich meningioma
Metaplastic meningioma
Secretory meningioma

Greater Likelihood of Recurrence, Aggressive Behavior, or Any Type with a High Proliferative Index
Grade II
Atypical meningioma
Clear cell meningioma (intracranial)
Chordoid meningioma

Grade III
Rhabdoid meningioma
Papillary meningioma
Anaplastic (malignant) meningioma

Adapted from Louis DN, Schiethauer BW, Budka H, et al: Meningiomas. In Kleihues P, Cavenee WK (eds): World Health Organization Classification of Tumours. Pathology and Genetics of Tumours of the Nervous System. Lyon, France, International Agency for Research on Cancer (IARC), 2000.

tumors.[27] Meningiomas with a greater likelihood of recurrence or aggressive behavior and a high proliferation index or tendency for brain invasion are assigned higher grades (Table 45-1). WHO grade I meningiomas are meningothelial meningiomas, fibrous meningiomas, transitional meningiomas, psammomatous meningiomas, angiomatous meningiomas, microcystic meningiomas, secretory meningiomas, lymphoplasmacyte-rich meningiomas, and metaplastic meningiomas. WHO grade II meningiomas are atypical meningiomas, clear cell meningiomas, and chordoid meningiomas. WHO grade III meningiomas are rhabdoid meningiomas, papillary meningiomas, and anaplastic meningiomas.

At the macroscopic level, most meningiomas have a firm consistency. They are usually well demarcated with broad dural attachments. Meningiomas usually compress adjacent brain, although invasion of brain parenchyma can occur. In some locations such as the sphenoid wing, meningiomas may grow as a flat mass, termed *en-plaque* meningiomas.

At the microscopic level, a wide range of histopathologies are present. The most common are meningothelial, fibrous, and transitional meningiomas (Figure 45-2). Meningothelial meningiomas have largely uniform oval nuclei that on occasion show central clearing. They form lobules surrounded by thin collagenous septae; whorls and psammoma bodies are not common.

Fibrous meningiomas have spindle-shaped cells in a parallel alignment that form interlacing bundles on a matrix of collagen and reticulin; whorl formation and psammoma bodies are not

common. Transitional meningiomas have features between those of meningothelial and fibrous meningiomas. Whorls and psammoma bodies are present. Psammomatous meningiomas have an abundance of psammoma bodies that may become confluent, forming irregular calcified and occasionally ossified masses.

Angiomatous meningiomas have numerous blood vessels in the background of a typical meningioma. Microcystic meningiomas are characterized by cells with elongated processes and by a loose mucinous background, giving the appearance of many small cysts. Secretory meningiomas have focal epithelial differentiation in the form of intracellular lumina containing PAS-positive eosinophilic material. Lymphoplasmacyte-rich meningiomas have extensive inflammatory infiltrates, often relegating the meningothelial component to the background. Metaplastic meningiomas have focal mesenchymal differentiation.

WHO grade II meningiomas include chordoid meningiomas. These contain regions that are histologically similar to chordoma with trabeculae of eosinophilic, vacuolated cells in a myxoid background. Clear cell meningiomas are often patternless meningiomas composed of polygonal cells with a clear, glycogen-rich cytoplasm. Atypical meningiomas have increased mitotic activity and can have increased cellularity, small cells with a high nucleus-to-cytoplasm ratio, prominent nucleoli, uninterrupted patternless or sheet-like growth, and foci of spontaneous or geographic necrosis (Figure 45-3).

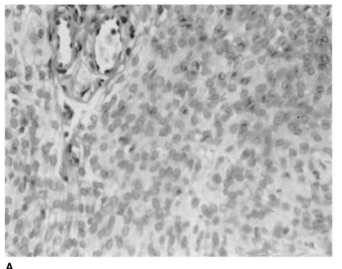

A

B

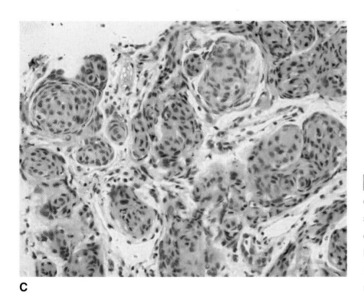

C

FIGURE 45-2 Example of histology of the three most common meningiomas. *A,* Hematoxylin and eosin (H&E) staining showing the histologic pattern of meningothelial meningiomas. Polygonal cells with ill-defined cytoplasm are noted. *B,* H&E stain showing fibroblastic meningioma formed of sheets of elongated meningothelial cells. *C,* H&E stain of transitional meningioma in which whorls as well as psammoma bodies are demonstrated.

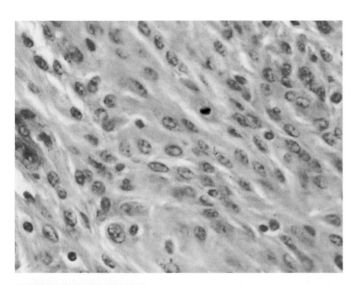

FIGURE 45-3 Hematoxylin and eosin stain of atypical meningioma. Mitotic figure is seen in the middle of the figure.

WHO grade III meningiomas include papillary meningiomas characterized by a perivascular pseudopapillary pattern in at least part of the tumor. Rhabdoid meningiomas contain patches with sheets of rhabdoid cells. These cells have eccentric nuclei often with a prominent nucleolus and prominent inclusion like eosinophilic cytoplasm composed of whorled intermediate filaments. Anaplastic (malignant) meningiomas exhibit histologic features of frank malignancies (Figure 45-4).

Brain invasion by meningiomas is characterized by irregular groups of tumor cells infiltrating the adjacent cerebral parenchyma without an intervening layer of leptomeninges. This often causes reactive astrocytosis. Brain invasion may occur with any meningioma. Its presence connotes a greater likelihood of recurrence. Higher grade meningiomas may metastasize. This typically occurs after surgery.

Vimentin positivity is found in all meningiomas. The majority of these lesions also stain for epithelial membrane antigen (EMA), although this staining is less consistent in atypical and malignant tumors. Immunohistochemical studies of S-100 protein have found varying positivity in meningiomas.[14]

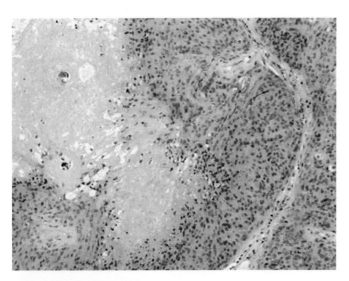

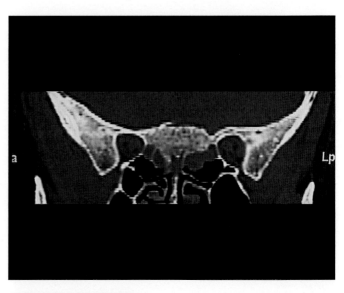

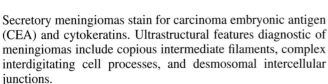

FIGURE 45-4   Hematoxylin and eosin stain of malignant meningioma with obvious malignant cytology and necrosis and a very high mitotic index.

FIGURE 45-5   Bone window computed tomography scan demonstrating hyperostotic bone invasion at the origin of the planum sphenoidale meningioma.

Secretory meningiomas stain for carcinoma embryonic antigen (CEA) and cytokeratins. Ultrastructural features diagnostic of meningiomas include copious intermediate filaments, complex interdigitating cell processes, and desmosomal intercellular junctions.

In general, tumor cell proliferation is related to meningioma histology, with anaplastic meningiomas having the fastest rate. The bromodeoxyuridine (BUdR) labeling index is inversely correlated with tumor doubling times. MIB-1 and Ki-67 indices may vary considerably among anaplastic meningiomas. The Ki-67 proliferation index may be the most important criterion for distinguishing the grade of the meningioma.[13] Flow cytometric studies have demonstrated significant correlations between aneuploid tumors and recurrence, pleomorphism, high cellular density, mitotic activity, and infiltration of brain and soft tissue.

RADIOLOGY

Modern imaging modalities of computed tomography (CT) and magnetic resonance imaging (MRI) readily diagnose and localize most meningiomas. Localization of an intracranial mass to an extra-axial intradural site points to this diagnosis. The excellent diagnostic map afforded by these imaging modalities gives the operating neurosurgeon the appropriate surgical approach to this usually readily treatable lesion. The deeper tumors involving the skull base offer a significant challenge to the operating neurosurgeon. Modern-day skull-base approaches in line with the excellent diagnostic localization afforded by current-day MRI and CT allow a safe removal of these tumors.

Computed Tomography

Nonenhanced CT of meningiomas usually shows a hyperdense mass relative to adjacent normal brain. In 25% of cases, intratumoral calcification is seen. Occasionally, cystic, fatty, or car-

tilaginous changes are seen. Close observation of the adjacent skull usually shows changes in the bone. In particular with tumors of the skull base, bone sclerosis of the primary site of origin of meningiomas may be shown. This finding is best observed with thin-section high-resolution studies afforded by helical CT scanners (Figure 45-5). Enhanced studies demonstrate marked contrast uptake by the tumors. Most meningiomas enhance homogeneously (like a light bulb), but occasionally, hypodensity can be seen within the tumor. Associated brain parenchymal reactive changes of surrounding vasogenic edema are quite variable. Larger tumors tend to incite this response, which may be due to the compressive effect, parasitization of pial arteries in the supply to the meningioma, or stasis of the compressed pial veins. In some cases, direct invasion by the tumor of the adjacent venous sinuses or venous thrombosis is seen.

Magnetic Resonance Imaging

On standard MRI sequences of T1- and T2-weighted images, most meningiomas exhibit a signal intensity similar to that of the adjacent gray matter. Contrast studies, however, demonstrate marked enhancement of the tumor, which makes it readily separable from the adjacent brain. In addition, a dural tail sign (dural enhancement crescent trail from the lesion) is often seen. This sign is often used to distinguish this mass from schwannomas, another common extra-axial tumor of the brain.

MRI is excellent in the diagnosis and localization of meningiomas. The precise localization of the tumor is easily demonstrated. In addition, the intense vascularity of meningiomas may be suggested by finding multiple flow voids within the lesion, intense enhancement of the lesion, or enlarged meningeal vessels that supply the tumor (Figure 45-6). In general, findings of enlarged branches of the middle meningeal artery may be shown on regular MRI sequences or on magnetic resonance (MR) angiography. In addition, encasement of adjacent vessels may be shown, as in meningiomas that involve the cavernous sinus and show a propensity for narrowing the cav-

MANAGEMENT

General Principles

The mainstay of treatment for meningiomas is surgical resection. The extent of surgical resection is affected by tumor location, size, consistency, vascular and neural involvement, and, in cases of recurrence, prior surgery or radiation therapy.

Anticonvulsant therapy is instituted for patients with supratentorial meningiomas. Decadron is administered before the operation. Pneumatic compression devices are placed on the legs when the patient is admitted to the hospital and they remain in use for the entire period of hospitalization. Perioperative antibiotics are used prophylactically for staphylococcal organisms in all patients, and a third-generation cephalosporin with activity against pseudomonal organisms and, at times, metronidazole are also used when surgery in the mouth, paranasal sinuses, ear, or mastoid is planned.

Using basal approaches wherever possible to resect meningiomas maximizes the general neurosurgical principle of removing bone to alleviate brain retraction.[3,4] At the time of primary meningioma surgery, in the vast majority of first operations for meningiomas, a layer of arachnoid separating the tumor from the brain parenchyma, cranial nerves, and blood vessels is usually found. Once the mass of the meningioma is removed, attention is focused on removing the dural tail and involved bone. Meningiomas with the greatest potential for total removal are those that overlie the cerebral convexities, because they can be excised with a wide dural margin.

Parasagittal and Falcine Meningiomas

Commonly, patients with parasagittal and falcine meningiomas in the anterior third of the falx experience headaches. Gradual progressive mental-status changes, seizures, or increased intracranial pressure can also occur. Focal seizures are often seen in patients with meningiomas of the middle third of the falx. They are initially evident in the contralateral foot and leg. Progressive mental decline, visual deterioration secondary to increased intracranial pressure, or generalized seizures can also occur. Meningiomas in the posterior third of the falx can have insidious symptoms. These include headaches, mental-status changes, and intracranial hypertension. A distinguishing feature is visual-field loss.

The primary consideration for the removal of these tumors is the extent of sagittal sinus involvement (Figure 45-7). Choosing the appropriate method of handling the involved sinus constitutes the most important decision in the treatment of falcine and parasagittal meningiomas. One or two walls of the sinus can be excised, and reconstruction still provides a good percentage of patency. Technically, total sinus replacement with a venous graft can be successful; however, the long-term results of this maneuver show patency of only 50%. The potential for delayed occlusion of a totally replaced sinus graft makes us hesitant to excise and replace a patent sinus in the posterior third or the posterior part of the middle third. Decisions regarding the sinus, however, should be individualized for each case according to several factors: the age and symptoms of the patient, the patency of the sinus, the location of the tumor, and the cortical venous collateral. A truly occluded sinus can be totally excised at any point. Preservation of collateral venous channels cannot be overemphasized, and this preservation

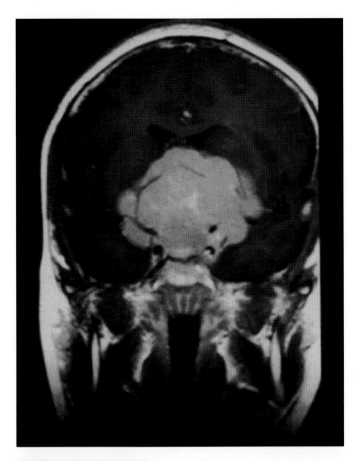

FIGURE 45-6 Coronal-cut magnetic resonance image of giant tuberculum sella meningioma showing homogeneous enhancement and flow void appearance of encased cerebral arteries.

ernous internal carotid artery. In cases where the tumor arises from the falx, MRI readily assesses the localization of the tumor and assesses the degree of sagittal sinus invasion. Additional MR sequences, such as MR venography, can detect the location and patency of the sagittal sinus. Primary intraosseous meningiomas have been reported and are seen as primary expansions of the inner and outer tables of the skull. Bone involvement is commonly associated with a large extra-axial mass that expands through the adjacent skull and involves the underlying soft tissues of the scalp. In tumors involving the skull base, an adjacent hyperostotic response is often seen and is primarily used to locate their site of origin.

Cerebral angiography is occasionally used in the diagnosis of meningiomas. In most cases, MRI studies provide a precise and incontrovertible diagnosis of meningiomas. Before MRI, cerebral angiography provided the most precise method of diagnosing meningiomas. The intense vascular blush, which appears early and leaves late, shown on these studies provided an important sign as to its presence. In addition, the findings of enlarged meningeal arteries, commonly the middle meningeal artery, showed the extra-axial location of these lesions. In tumors of the skull base, the enlarged meningeal feeders were the ophthalmic artery, meningohypophyseal branches of the cavernous internal carotid artery, or the posterior falx artery from the distal vertebral arteries. Preoperative embolization for decreasing intraoperative blood loss is sometimes performed.

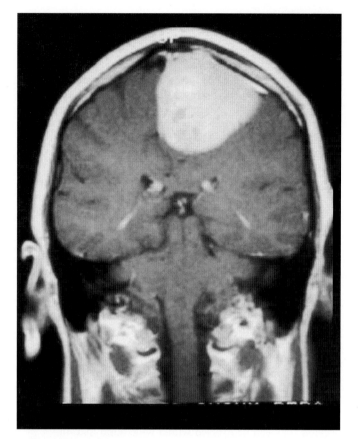

FIGURE 45-7 Magnetic resonance image of parasagittal meningioma involving one wall of a patent sagittal sinus.

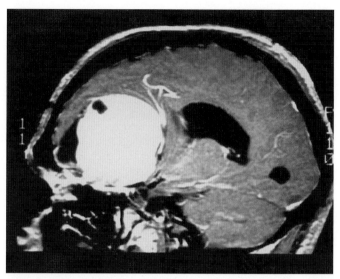

FIGURE 45-8 Sagittal magnetic resonance image of olfactory groove meningioma with displacement of anterior cerebral artery upward and posteriorly.

becomes a vital part of the operation. The anterior third of the sinus can be excised with or without a graft or replacement. Tumor infiltration of one wall can be repaired primarily after the tumor is removed from the sinus.

Olfactory Groove and Tuberculum Sellae Meningiomas

Olfactory groove and tuberculum sellae meningiomas are midline lesions (Figure 45-8). Their clinical presentation has been discussed previously. These lesions usually derive their blood supply from the ethmoidal branches of the ophthalmic artery, the anterior branch of the middle meningeal artery, and the meningeal branches of the internal carotid artery (ICA).[4] In the case of smaller tumors, the olfactory nerves can be preserved.

Sphenoid Ridge Meningiomas

The most common of the basal meningiomas occur along the sphenoid wing and are classified according to their origin along the sphenoid ridge.[2] Within this group is the meningioma *en plaque*. These meningiomas are characterized by marked hyperostosis of the sphenoid bone caused by diffuse tumor invasion (Figure 45-9). Progressive painless proptosis and occasionally diverse cranial neuropathies can occur. *En masse* lesions of the pterional third of the sphenoid ridge can be asso-

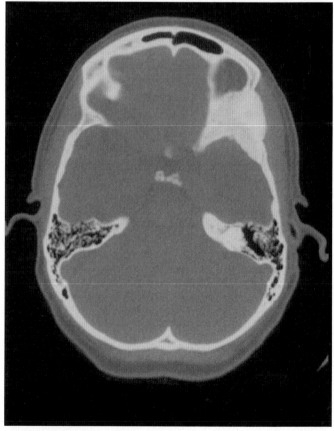

FIGURE 45-9 Computed tomography scan of hyperostosing meningioma of the sphenoid ridge.

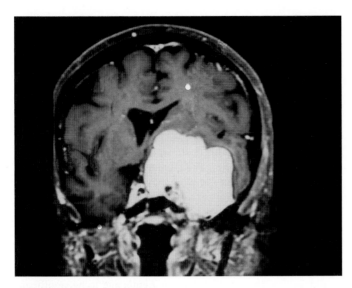

FIGURE 45-10 Coronal image of a clinoid meningioma with invasion of the cavernous sinus.

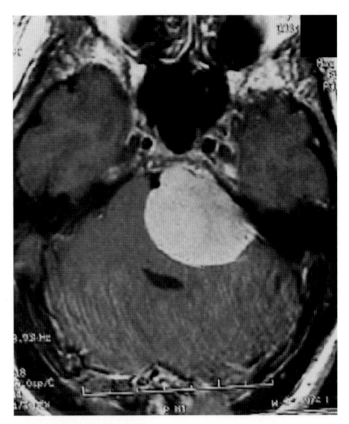

FIGURE 45-11 Axial cut of a petroclival meningioma that constitutes the greatest management challenge.

ciated with localized skull pain and frontal and temporal bone bulging. Seizures and contralateral hemiparesis can also occur. Complete removal of the involved greater and lesser sphenoid wings is the treatment of choice.

Clinoidal meningiomas can invade the cavernous sinus (Figure 45-10).[2] Involvement of the cavernous sinus does not preclude aggressive tumor removal. Progressive neurologic deficits or progressive enlargement of the tumor are indicators for resection.[13] In the senior author's experience, total removal of cavernous sinus meningiomas has been possible in 76% of patients. Major morbidity and mortality rates were 4.8% and 2.4%, respectively. Preoperative cranial nerve deficits improved in 14%, remained unchanged in 80%, and permanently worsened in 6%.[14]

Posterior Fossa Meningiomas

Posterior fossa meningiomas account for less than 10% of total intracranial meningiomas. Half of these are in the cerebellopontine angle; 40% occur at the tentorium or cerebellar convexity. Approximately 9% are clival and 6% occur at the foramen magnum. Petroclival meningiomas arising medial to the trigeminal nerve have a higher rate of surgical morbidity (Figure 45-11).[12] Meningiomas of the petrous pyramid can cause hearing loss, facial pain, and facial weakness. Headaches and ataxia are common with larger lesions.

Cerebellar convexity, or tentorial, meningiomas usually present with intracranial hypertension, headache, and progressive cerebellar signs. Large tentorial meningiomas may produce visual field deficits. The transverse sinus is the major venous consideration in the resection of these tumors. A totally occluded sinus can be excised with the rest of the meningioma. A transverse sinus can be sacrificed if temporary occlusion results in no swelling, venous engorgement, or rise in filling pressures.

Foramen magnum meningiomas are anterior or anterolateral to the cervicomedullary junction and are usually intimately involved with the lower cranial nerves (IX to XII), the cervi-

comedullary junction, and the vertebral artery and its branches, such as the posterior inferior cerebellar artery (PICA) (Figure 45-12). The typical clinical symptoms are suboccipital and neck pain, ipsilateral upper extremity dysesthesias, contralateral dissociated sensory loss, progressive limb weakness beginning in the ipsilateral upper extremity and progressing counterclockwise, and wasting of the intrinsic muscles of the hand.[12] The far lateral approach is usually used for tumor resection.

Primary jugular foramen tumors are probably one of the rarest subgroups of meningiomas. The most common presenting symptoms are hearing loss, swallowing difficulties, and weakness in the trapezius or sternocleidomastoid muscles. The senior author has successfully resected these tumors through either a suprajugular, transjugular, or retrojugular approach.[5] The most common dysfunction following surgery was transient deficit in ninth and tenth cranial nerve functions. Transient twelfth nerve deficits that resolved within a month were also noted.

Intraventricular Meningiomas

Intraventricular meningiomas account for fewer than 1% of all intracranial meningiomas. They arise from arachnoid cells contained in the choroid plexus and tela choroidea. They are almost always located in the trigone of the lateral ventricle. The vascular supply is usually from the anterior choroidal artery, although the posterior choroidal artery also contributes. Because all approaches to these lesions traverse the cerebral

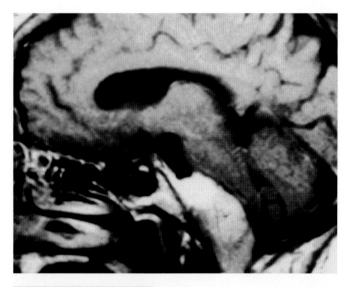

FIGURE 45-12 Sagittal magnetic resonance image of giant foramen magnum meningioma with expansion into the spinal canal and compression of the medulla.

cortex, the possibility of postoperative epilepsy is increased. Cortical dysfunction resulting from cerebral retraction may also occur. A midline section through the corpus callosum requires little retraction; however, it is contraindicated for patients with a right homonymous hemianopsia, because complete splenial section in this circumstance results in alexia without agraphia.

Pineal Meningiomas

Meningiomas of the pineal area arise from either the posterior velum interpositum or more commonly from the dura at the falcotentorial junction. Impaired upgaze and diminished pupillary reflexes are less common than with other pathologies. Signs of increased intracranial pressure and hydrocephalus bring the patient to medical attention. These lesions can be removed using the supracerebellar-infratentorial route and the supratentorial approach.

RADIATION THERAPY

Meningiomas have long been reputed to be "radioresistant," with early series reporting little clinical effect of radiation therapy.[22,33] However, over the past 25 years clear evidence to the contrary has emerged, and radiation therapy should be considered alongside surgery as appropriate and proven treatment for many clinical situations involving intracranial meningiomas.

The group at the University of California, San Francisco (UCSF) made a strong argument for the use of radiation therapy following incomplete resection of meningioma. Their initial study (1975) analyzed the outcome in 92 patients followed for 5 to more than 20 years following initial subtotal resection for benign meningioma.[36] Seventy-four percent of patients followed without postoperative radiation therapy had recurrence in the operative site, whereas 29% who had received postoper-

ative radiation therapy eventually had recurrence. A longer disease-free interval for the group of irradiated patients who had recurrence was reported as compared with those who had recurrence postoperatively without radiation therapy. As compared with 62% in the nonirradiated group, 47% of recurrences occurred within 5 years in the irradiated group.

Barbaro et al reported a series of patients treated more recently (1987) at UCSF.[6] Out of 30 patients, 18 (60%) had recurrence following subtotal resection alone compared with 17 of 54 (32%) treated with postoperative radiation therapy following subtotal resection. The median disease-free interval was nearly twice as long in the patients with recurrence following radiation therapy as compared with surgery alone: 125 months versus 66 months, respectively ($P < .05$).

Goldsmith et al reported on 117 patients who received postoperative radiation therapy for subtotally resected benign meningioma between 1967 and 1990.[19] The 10-year progression-free survival was 77%. Multivariate analysis revealed treatment date (before 1980) and patient's age to be significant prognostic factors. Seventy-seven patients treated after 1980 had a disease-free survival rate of 98%, as compared with 77% in 40 patients treated before 1980. The relative risk of progression was 0.09 for patients treated in the more recent era as compared with those treated earlier, presumably because of benefits of CT- and MRI-assisted treatment planning.

Single-institution reports support the finding that postoperative radiation therapy improves progression-free survival and lowers overall recurrence rates in patients undergoing subtotal resection of benign meningioma.[6,18,19,35,36] Recurrence rates at 5 years are 72% to 89% following radiation therapy and 43% to 59% following subtotal resection alone.

The use of radiation therapy following surgical recurrence of meningioma generally results in superior local control compared with re-excision alone. Wara et al reported on 43 patients with recurrent meningioma following initial resection.[36] Sixteen received radiation therapy alone or following surgery for recurrence. Eight patients (50%) were alive 1 to 9 years following treatment. Twenty-seven patients underwent reoperation without radiation therapy. Ten patients (37%) were living 1 to 23 years following surgery. Taylor et al reported results for 25 patients treated for recurrent benign meningioma.[34] All patients underwent resection of the recurrent tumor. Ten received postoperative radiation therapy, attaining 89% local control at 10 years as compared with 30% for 27 patients undergoing reresection without radiation therapy. A significant survival benefit was found for the group salvaged with surgery and radiation therapy: 90% at 10 years as compared with 45% for those patients salvaged with surgery alone. Sixteen patients treated with radiation therapy for recurrent meningioma at Massachusetts General Hospital (MGH) had a progression-free survival of 78% compared with 11% for patients treated with surgery alone.[29]

In cases where surgery is medically contraindicated, technically difficult, or high risk, primary radiation therapy may be considered as a definitive treatment option. Early studies from the Royal Marsden Hospital using doses of 50 to 55 Gy and wide fields demonstrated control rates of 53%, 47%, and 47% at 5, 10, and 15 years, respectively.[18] The Joint Center for Radiation Therapy series of 19 patients treated after simple biopsy or no surgery achieved a 4-year disease-free survival of 64%.[16] Carella et al reported 100% control at 3 to 6 years in 11 patients treated with doses of 55 to 60 Gy without histologic diagnosis.[7]

More recent series demonstrate control rates for primary radiation therapy similar to those found for irradiation of residual disease following biopsy or partial resection.[26] Refinements in imaging, precision of delivery of radiation therapy, and the use of radiation doses greater than 53 Gy are all associated with improved outcome.[19] Rates of local control of gross disease with fractionated radiation therapy in the modern era are similar to those reported for stereotactic radiosurgery.[17,23]

Although more than 90% of meningiomas are of benign histology, the WHO classification system also recognizes atypical and anaplastic or malignant meningioma.[37] These more aggressive histologies have a propensity for recurrence and infiltration of surrounding brain parenchyma, even following "gross-total resection." Jaaskelainen et al reported a recurrence rate at 5 years following surgical excision alone of just 3% for benign histology (21% at 25 years), but a recurrence rate of 38% for atypical and 78% for malignant meningiomas.[20] Given these high rates of recurrence following surgery, many centers offer postoperative radiation therapy for atypical meningiomas, and postoperative radiation therapy is considered the standard of care for malignant histologies. Goldsmith et al reported a 58% 5-year overall survival for 23 patients with malignant meningioma treated with postoperative radiation therapy.[19] Patients treated with doses greater than 53 Gy had a 5-year progression-free survival of 63% as compared with 17% for those receiving lower doses. Coke et al reported a 5-year survival of 60% for malignant histologies and 87% for atypical tumors.[9] Overall survival at 10 years was 60% for either histologic subtype.

It is reasonable to offer postoperative radiation therapy to patients with atypical histology and residual tumor. It is highly recommended to deliver postoperative radiation therapy to patients with malignant histology regardless of the extent of resection. Patients with complete resection and atypical histology have a high rate of recurrence and should be followed closely.

Conventional fractionation in radiation therapy refers to the delivery of a series of daily treatments of approximately 1.8 to 2.0 Gy. Goldsmith et al reported a 65% control rate for meningiomas treated with conventional fractionation to doses less than 53 Gy as compared with 93% for those treated with total doses of more than 53 Gy.[19] Stereotactic radiosurgery refers to the delivery of a large single dose of radiation to a well-defined small volume. According to findings available to date, radiosurgery appears to be safe and effective in producing a durable arrest of growth of small inoperable, recurrent or residual meningiomas. In a series of 97 patients with meningiomas reviewed by Loeffler et al, 67% of patients were treated for recurrence after their first operation.[25] Although the 2-year actuarial freedom from progression rate was 96%, 14 patients had complications, including cranial neuropathies in 5 patients and malignant edema in 5; 2 of those patients required reoperation. The complication rates were significantly higher for the larger or deep-seated lesions. The investigators concluded that fractionated radiation therapy might be preferable for this subset of lesions. Engenhart et al similarly showed excellent control rates (82%) but a high complication rate (42%) among patients who were treated radiosurgically for large meningiomas.[15] Kondziolka et al showed excellent 2-year control

rates (96%) and a low complication rate (6%) among patients treated with radiosurgery for small meningiomas.[23] Although these studies indicate that radiosurgery holds promise for the treatment of small meningiomas, patients must accrue in trials and be followed for several more years before its efficacy in comparison with surgery and radiation therapy can be judged definitively. Larger meningiomas (>3 cm) may be more safely treated with fractionated conformal radiation therapy.[17,26] The stereotactic and direct microsurgical implantation of radioactive seeds into meningiomas may be beneficial but has been tested in only a few patients.[34]

Summary—Radiation Therapy

Radiation therapy has become a valuable tool in the treatment of benign brain tumors.[35] For meningiomas, which may recur following surgery or may be unresectable, fractionated radiation therapy offers a safe and efficacious treatment. Local control rates of 80% to 95% have been reported in modern series with doses of fractionated radiation therapy of approximately 54 Gy. Radiosurgery with doses of approximately 15 Gy is an equally efficacious alternative to conventionally fractionated treatment, but should be reserved for lesions larger than 3 cm in diameter. The management of malignant meningioma remains difficult, but radiation therapy should be considered in all cases.

CHEMOTHERAPY

Chemotherapeutic agents have generally been ineffective against meningiomas. Adjuvant combined modality therapy in the treatment of malignant meningiomas using a combination of cyclophosphamide, adriamycin, and vincristine may improve survival, with a median of 5.3 years.[8] Although there was initially some interest in the use of tamoxifen and mifepristone, these agents are still under investigation. Recombinant interferon-α 2b has been shown to have some effect in preventing the growth of meningiomas.[21]

Hydroxyurea treatment has been reported for meningiomas. It is a chemotherapeutic agent with reversible and acceptable toxicity that can be administered chronically. It arrests meningioma cell growth in the S phase of the cell cycle and is also believed to induce apoptosis. Although tumor regression appears to occur seldom, hydroxyurea is being investigated for preventing progression of unresectable or recurrent benign meningiomas.[28] However, predicting which patients may benefit reliably from this treatment has not been accomplished.[32]

RECURRENCE

The only definitive cure for meningiomas is complete surgical resection. The more complete the resection, the less chance of recurrence. This principle was expressed in a landmark paper by Simpson in 1957[33] (Table 45-2). The lower the Simpson grade, the less the chance of recurrence. The anatomic location of the meningioma influences its rate of recurrence, because it determines the extent of tumor resection. The highest recurrence rates occur with sphenoid wing meningiomas,

TABLE 45-2	

Simpson Grade

Grade I	Macroscopically complete tumor removal with excision of the tumor's dural attachment and any abnormal bone
Grade II	Macroscopically complete tumor removal with coagulation of its dural attachment
Grade III	Macroscopically complete removal of the intradural tumor without resection or coagulation of its dural attachment or extradural extension
Grade IV	Subtotal removal of the tumor
Grade V	Simple decompression of the tumor

Source: Based on the principles of Simpson D: The recurrence of intracranial meningiomas after surgical treatment. J Neurochem 20:22–39, 1957.

followed by parasagittal meningiomas. Meningioma histology, as discussed previously, also influences the likelihood of recurrence.

CONCLUSION

Patients who have complete resection of their meningioma are cured of the tumor. The accomplishment and risks of resection depend on the tumor's location. Radiation therapy as fractionated or conventional irradiation or radiosurgery is used for growth control for aggressive, recurrent, residual, or unresected meningiomas. Even with complex meningiomas, patient satisfaction rates of up to 97% have been reported.[1] Ninety percent of the patients reported that their expectations had been met.

References

1. Akagami RNM, Sekhar LN: Patient-evaluated outcome after surgery for basal meningiomas. Neurosurgery 50:941–948, 2002.
2. Al-Mefty O: Clinoidal meningiomas. J Neurosurg 73:502–512, 1990.
3. Al-Mefty O, Fox JL, Smith RR: Petrosal approach for petroclival meningiomas. Neurosurgery 22:510–517, 1988.
4. Al-Mefty O, Smith RR: Tuberculum sellae meningiomas, In Al-Mefty O (ed): Meningiomas. New York, Raven Press, 1991.
5. Arnautovic KI, Al-Mefty O: Primary meningiomas of the jugular fossa. J Neurosurg 97:12–20, 2002.
6. Barbaro NM, Gutin PH, Wilson CB, et al: Radiation therapy in the treatment of partially resected meningiomas. Neurosurgery 20:525–528, 1987.
7. Carella RJ, Ransahoff J, Newall J: Role of radiation therapy in the management of meningioma. J Neurosurg 10:332–339, 1982.
8. Chamberlin MC: Adjuvant combined modality therapy for malignant meningiomas. J Neurosurg 84:733–736, 1996.
9. Coke CC, Corn BW, Werner-Wasik M, et al: Atypical and malignant meningiomas: an outcome report of seventeen cases. J Neurooncol 39:65–70, 1998.
10. Cushing H: The meningiomas (dural endotheliomas): their source and favoured seats of origin. Brain 45:282–316, 1922.
11. Cushing H, Eisenhardt L: Meningiomas: Their Classification, Regional Behaviour, Life History, and Surgical End Results. Springfield, Ill, Charles C Thomas, 1938.
12. DeMonte F, Al-Mefty O: Neoplasms and the cranial nerves of the posterior fossa. In Barrow DL (ed): Surgery of the Cranial Nerves of the Posterior Fossa. Park Ridge, Ill, American Association of Neurological Surgeons, 1993.
13. DeMonte F, Marmor E, Al-Mefty O: Meningiomas. In Kaye AH, Laws ER, Jr (eds): Brain Tumors: An Encyclopedic Approach. New York, Churchill Livingstone, 2000.
14. DeMonte F, Smith HK, Al-Mefty O: Outcome of aggressive removal of cavernous sinus meningiomas. J Neurosurg 81:245–251, 1994.
15. Engenhart R, Kimmig BN, Hover K, et al: Stereotactic single high dose radiation therapy of benign intracranial meningiomas. Int J Radiat Oncol Biol Phys 19:1021–1026, 1990.
16. Forbes AR, Goldberg ID: Radiation therapy in the treatment of meningioma: the Joint Center for Radiation Therapy Experience 1970 to 1982. J Clin Oncol 2:1139–1143, 1984.
17. Gademann G, Engenhart R, Schlegel W, et al: Results and comparison of single dose and fractionated stereotactic radiotherapy in 87 low grade meningiomas. Int J Radiat Oncol Biol Phys 27:153–154, 1993.
18. Glaholm J, Bloom HJG, Crow JH: The role of radiotherapy in the management of intracranial meningiomas: the Royal Marsden Hospital experience with 186 patients. Int J Radiat Oncol Biol Phys 18:755–761, 1990.
19. Goldsmith BJ, Wara WM, Wilson CB, et al: Postoperative irradiation of subtotally resected meningiomas. J Neurosurg 80:195, 1994.
20. Jaaskelainen J, Haltia M, Servo A: Atypical and anaplastic meningiomas: radiology, surgery, radiotherapy, and outcome. Surg Neurol 25:233–242, 1986.
21. Kaba SE, Demonte F, Bruner JM, et al: The treatment of recurrent unresectable and malignant meningiomas with interferon alpha-2B. Neurosurgery 40:271–275, 1997.
22. King DL, Chang CH, Pool JL: Radiotherapy in the management of meningiomas. Acta Radiol Ther Phys Biol 5:26–33, 1966.
23. Kondziolka D, Lunsford LD, Coffey RJ, et al: Stereotactic radiosurgery of meningiomas. J Neurosurg 74:552–559, 1991.
24. Kumar PP, Good RR, Patil AA, Leibrock LG: Permanent high-activity Iodine-125 in the management of petroclival meningiomas: case reports. Neurosurg 25:436–442, 1989.
25. Loeffler JS, Flickinger JC, Shrieve DC, et al: Radiosurgery for the treatment of intracranial lesions. In DeVita VT, Hellman S, Rosenberg SA (eds): Important Advances in Oncology. Philadelphia, JB Lippincott, 1995.
26. Loeffler JS, Shrieve DC, Alexander E, III, et al: Stereotactic radiotherapy for meningiomas. In Kondziolka D (ed): Radiosurgery 1995. Basel, Switzerland, Karger, 1996.
27. Louis DN, Schiethauer BW, Budka H, et al: Meningiomas. In K KPCW (ed): World Health Organization Classification of Tumours: Pathology and Genetics. Tumours of the Nervous System. Lyon, France, Internation Agency for Research on Cancer, 2000.
28. Mason WP, Gentili F, MacDonald DR, et al: Stabilization of disease progression by hydroxyurea in patients with recurrent or unresectable meningioma. J Neurosurg 97:341–346, 2002.
29. Miralbell R, Linggood RM, De la Monte S, et al: The role of radiotherapy in the treatment of subtotally resected meningiomas. J Neurooncol 13:157–164, 1992.

30. Sawyer JR, Husain M, Pravdenkova S, et al: A role for telomeric and centromeric instability in the progression of chromosome aberrations in meningioma patients. Cancer 88:440–453, 2000.

31. Sawyer JR, Thomas EL, Al-Mefty O: Translocation (1;19) (q21;q13.3) is a recurrent reciprocal translocation in meningioma. Cancer Genetics and Cytogenetics 134:88–90, 2002.

32. Schrell UMH, Rittig MG, Anders M, et al: Hydroxyurea for treatment of unresectable and recurrent meningiomas. II. Decrease in the size of meningiomas in patients treated with hydroxyurea. J Neurosurg 86:840–844, 1997.

33. Simpson D: The recurrence of intracranial meningiomas after surgical treatment. J Neurochem 20:22–39, 1957.

34. Taylor BW, Marcus RB, Friedman WA, et al: The meningioma controversy: postoperative radiation therapy. Int J Radiat Oncol Biol Phys 15:299–304, 1988.

35. Tsao MN, Wara WM, Larson DA: Radiation therapy for benign central nervous system disease. Semin Radiol Oncol 9:120–133, 1999.

36. Wara WM, Sheline GE, Newman H, et al.: Radiation therapy of meningiomas. Am J Roentgenol Radium Ther Nucl Med 123: 453–458, 1975.

37. Zulch KJ: Brain Tumors: The Biology and Pathology. New York, Springer-Verlag, 1986.

CHAPTER 46

MENINGEAL HEMANGIOPERICYTOMAS AND SARCOMAS

Samer Ayoubi and Ossama Al-Mefty

MENINGEAL HEMANGIOPERICYTOMAS

Hemangiopericytomas are located in the musculoskeletal system and the skin, rarely in intracranial locations. They represent 2% to 4% of meningeal tumors, thus accounting for less than 1% of all intracranial tumors.[1] Hemangiopericytomas are highly aggressive meningeal tumors with tendencies for recurrence and metastasis. In the current World Health Organization classification of central nervous system tumors, hemangiopericytoma is distinguished as an entity of its own, and classified with mesenchymal, nonmeningothelial tumors. These tumors arise from meningeal capillary pericyte or precursor cells with angioplastic tendencies.[5]

Location

Hemangiopericytomas are located in locations similar to those of meningiomas. Seventy percent are located supratentorially, 15% in the posterior fossa, and 15% in the spine.[3,12] Approximately half the spinal tumors are located in the cervical region. Very rarely the tumor is located in the pineal region.

Diagnosis

Symptoms and signs depend on the location of the tumor. The duration of symptoms is usually less than a year.[12] This can be explained by the tumor's rapid growth. The tumor usually presents with headache or focal deficit.[1,5] Sixteen percent of patients with supratentorial meningeal hemangiopericytomas have seizures.[12]

Unlike meningiomas, which are more common in females, meningeal hemangiopericytomas are more common in males. The average age at diagnosis is approximately 40 years.[4,12] Hemangiopericytomas are extremely rare in childhood.[23]

Radiology

Radiologically, hemangiopericytomas resemble meningiomas. On unenhanced computed tomography (CT) scans the lesion is more often hyperdense with focal areas of hypodensity.[4] With intravenous administration of contrast agent, there is heterogeneous enhancement. Mushrooming contrast enhancement or irregular border are signs of brain invasion and malignancy.[20]

Bone window CT scan shows bone erosion. The hyperostosis seen in meningiomas is not usually seen in hemangiopericytoma.[4]

Magnetic resonance imaging (MRI) usually shows an isointense lesion with prominent vascular flow voids on T1- and T2-weighted images.[1,4] There is heterogeneous enhancement on gadolinium-enhanced images (Figure 46-1). Dural tail sign, where there is extension of the tumor on the dura, is seen in nearly half the cases. Narrow-based dural attachment favors the diagnosis of hemangiopericytoma over meningioma, whereas hyperostosis favors the diagnosis of meningioma.

It is difficult to differentiate with certainty hemangiopericytomas from meningiomas even with gadolinium-enhanced MRI.[12] Positron-emission tomography (PET) may be useful in this differentiation, showing hot spots in hemangiopericytomas.

Characteristic arteriographic features include early filling vessels in a corkscrew vascular configuration, a significant internal carotid blood supply in half the patients, and early venous drainage in a few patients.[12,13,17] However, most cases are diagnosed preoperatively as meningiomas.

Histopathology

Macroscopically, hemangiopericytomas are lobulated, pink-gray to red, and usually firm.[5] These tumors adhere to the dura but do not usually invade the brain. They are extremely vascular and can bleed heavily during resection.[12,13] Unlike meningiomas, they do not spread *en plaque* and do not usually contain calcification.[4]

Microscopically, the tumor is very cellular with round to oval cells.[5] Tumor cells appear as sheets of cells with numerous vascular spaces that can assume a staghorn configuration, which is a distinguishing feature of hemangiopericytoma.[5] Mitosis, microcytes, necrosis, and papillary architecture may be seen.[12] Unlike meningiomas, in which reticulin envelops cell groups, giving the typical lobulated appearance, reticulin in hemangiopericytomas is abundant and envelops individual cells[5] (Figure 46-2).

Tumor markers (factor XIIIa, vimentin, HLD-DR, CD34, leu 7, S-100 protein) may be expressed in hemangiopericytomas. Expression of factor XIIIa helps in distinguishing hemangiopericytomas from meningiomas.[5]

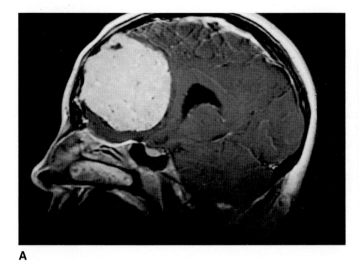

A

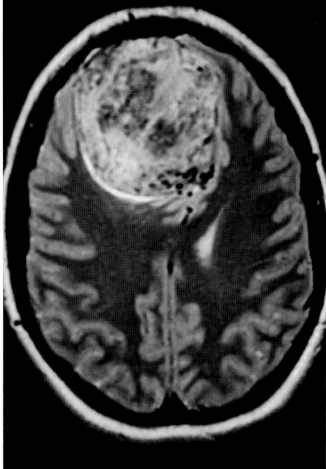

B

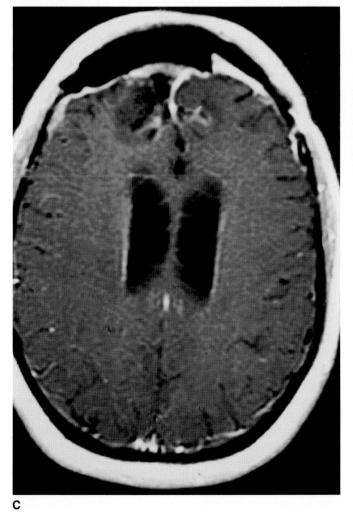

C

FIGURE 46-1   *A,* Sagittal contrast magnetic resonance image of a hemangiopericytoma demonstrating heterogeneous enhancement and skull erosion. *B,* Axial cut of T2-weighted image showing multiple areas of flow void hypointense vascular structures. *C,* Postoperative image total resection.

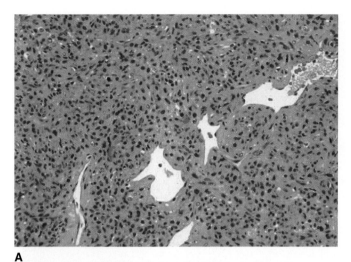

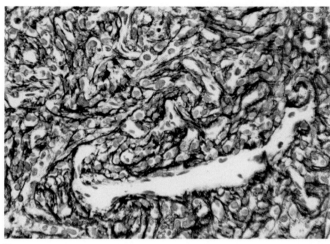

A   **B**

FIGURE 46-2   *A,* Hematoxylin and eosin staining of hemangiopericytoma composed of very cellular, round to oval cells with numerous vascular spaces with staghorn configuration. A distinguishing feature of hemangiopericytoma. *B,* Hemangiopericytoma with extensive reticulin stain enveloping individual cells.

Hemangiopericytomas are genetically distinct from meningiomas. Rearrangements of chromosome 12q13 are common in hemangiopericytomas but are not common in meningiomas. Conversely, mutations of neurofibromatosis 2 (NF2) tumor-suppressor gene, which is common in meningiomas, is not found in hemangiopericytomas.[14]

Treatment

Surgery

Surgery followed by radiation therapy of at least 5000 to 5500 cGy or radiosurgery is the treatment of choice.[5,6,15] Preoperative embolization can markedly reduce intraoperative bleeding. Removal of the tumor at initial surgery has the best chance of achieving total removal. Removal of recurrent tumor is more difficult. The aim of surgery should be total removal of the tumor and its basal attachment. This, however, may not always be possible.[12,13] Operative mortality has been relatively high, the main cause being heavy bleeding during surgery.[12,13] Improvement in surgical techniques and the use of preoperative embolization has made it possible to remove these tumors with low morbidity and mortality.[1,6]

Radiosurgery

Efficacy of radiosurgery for hemangiopericytomas has not been formally delineated.[5] Some authors recommend radiosurgery for small recurrent meningeal hemangiopericytoma.[6,9] Others recommend that when a residual tumor is identified after resection or radiation therapy, early radiosurgery should be considered.[21]

Outcome

Meningeal hemangiopericytomas have a tremendous tendency to recur, much more so than meningiomas.[1,5,12,15,21] The incidence of local recurrence varied from 26% to 80%, depending on the quality of resection, the length of follow-up, and particularly whether postoperative radiation therapy was administered.[6] Five-, ten-, and fifteen-year recurrence rates are approximately 65%, 76%, and 87%, respectively.[6] Recurrence can occur at the primary site or can occur as a diffuse leptomeningeal seeding.[15] Subsequent recurrences occur at shorter intervals.

Unlike other primary intracranial tumors, hemangiopericytomas often metastasize outside the central nervous system.[5] Bone, lung, and liver are the most common sites. Metastasis can appear years after patients apparently have had a tumor-free life.[15,23]

Five-, ten-, and fifteen-year survival is 67%, 40%, and 23%, respectively.[12] Survival is adversely affected by extracranial metastasis.

Postoperative radiation therapy improves survival time and reduces the risk of local recurrence, but it does not protect against neuraxis metastasis of hemangiopericytomas.[6]

MENINGEAL SARCOMAS

Sarcomas are defined as malignant tumors arising from mesenchymal tissue. The term sarcoma comes from the Greek terms *sarx,* meaning flesh, and *oma,* meaning tumor. Primary *de novo* meningeal sarcomas arise from intracranial mesenchymal cells. Secondary meningeal sarcomas arise in a preexisting meningioma. Sarcomas can also involve the meninges via direct extension from the skull base, the cranial vault, the sinuses, intracerebral sarcomas, or by distant metastasis. Meningeal sarcomas are rare, representing less than 3% of all brain tumors.[11] Like hemangiopericytomas, meningeal sarcomas are classified as mesenchymal, nonmeningothelial tumors. Related by their cellular differentiation, fibrosarcomas, leiomyosarcomas, rhabdomyosarcomas, chondrosarcomas, and malignant fibrous histiocytomas are included under meningeal sarcomas.

Diagnosis

Symptoms and signs depend on the location and size of the tumor. Meningeal sarcomas can present as space-occupying lesions with headache, vomiting,[2,24] somnolence, or papilledema[16,19] or with new-onset seizures, hydrocephalus, or symptoms of spinal cord compression.

Meningeal sarcomas usually present as a massive growth. The less differentiated group may seed in the subarachnoid space, giving rise to multiple tumors.

Differential diagnosis of primary meningeal sarcomas includes[22] meningeal metastasis from extracranial sarcomas, intracranial extension from extrameningeal sites, other malignant mesenchymal tumors such as hemangiopericytomas, malignant neuroectodermal tumors such as gliosarcomas, and malignant and nonmalignant meningeal tumors such as pleomorphic xanthoastrocytoma.

Cases of meningeal sarcomas have been associated with a medical history of trauma, previous surgery, previous subdural collection, previous irradiation,[26] neurofibromatosis, or AIDS. An etiologic cause-effect relationship is not clear in any of these cases.

Location

These tumors are rare. They occur in cranial and spinal locations. The cranial location is more common than the spinal,[8] with no preferential site of involvement.[28] Some locations and types, like the primary spinal intradural extramedullary gliosarcoma, are exceedingly rare.[28]

Incidence

Frequency of intracranial sarcomas in adults has been reported to range from 0.1% to 3%[18,22,28] and approximately 2% in children.[27]

Meningeal sarcomas can occur in patients of any age but are more common in the first decade of life, with the exception of malignant fibrous histiocytoma and fibrosarcomas, which occur preferentially in adults, and sarcomas with muscle differentiation, which occur preferentially in children.[2,22] No gender difference in incidence has been reported.[28]

Radiology

There is no specific radiologic profile of meningeal sarcomas. On CT scans sarcomas present as solitary or multiple lesions that are enhanced after administration of contrast material. Enhancement may be heterogeneous, and a cystic component may be seen. Bone erosion may be seen on bone-window CT scan, but hyperostosis is not usually present (Figure 46-3).

On MRI the mass is usually hypointense on T1-weighted images and hyperintense on T2-weighted images.[19] Liposarcomas may appear hyperintense on T1-weighted images because of tumor fat content. Severe edema may be seen with meningeal sarcomas.[19]

Histopathology

Macroscopically, meningeal sarcomas are demarcated from the adjacent brain in some places, whereas they lack a capsule and often infiltrate the brain in others.

Microscopically, meningeal sarcomas can be differentiated along several lines.[11,24,25] They can produce fibrous tissue (fibrosarcoma), cartilage (chondromas, chondrosarcomas),

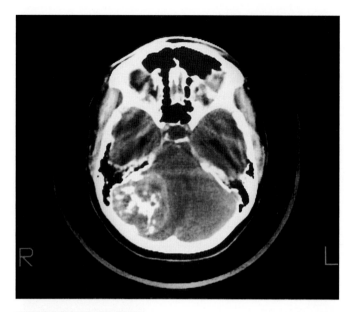

FIGURE 46-3 Computed tomography scan of chondrosarcoma with calcification.

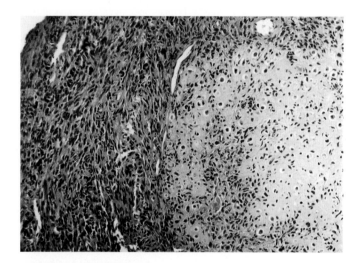

FIGURE 46-4 Hematoxylin and eosin staining of a mesenchymal chondrosarcoma showing a biphasic pattern. Part of the tumor is composed of undifferentiated spindle-shaped cells, whereas the other part reveals moderately well-differentiated cartilage.

smooth muscle (leiomyosarcomas), striated muscle (rhabdomyosarcomas), bone (osteosarcomas), adipose tissue (liposarcoma), or blood vessels (angiosarcomas).

Fibrosarcomas are characterized by bundles of spindle cells, giving a herringbone appearance with frequent mitosis and necrosis.[22] Meningeal seeding and metastasis occur in approximately 40% of fibrosarcomas.[10]

In *chondrosarcomas*, only cartilaginous elements are neoplastic. The tumor cells are stellate shaped and surrounded by abundant mucoid intercellular material.[11] In mesenchymal chondrosarcomas both cartilaginous and mesenchymal elements are neoplastic (Figure 46-4). What has been known as chondroid chordomas are thought to represent low-grade chondrosarcomas. The falx cerebri is the most common intracranial site.[8]

Leiomyosarcomas and *rhabdomyosarcomas* are more rare than other meningeal sarcomas. Immunohistologic techniques and electron microscopy are helpful in making the diagnosis.[22] Cases of diffuse meningeal rhabdomyosarcoma have been reported.[24] Other meningeal sarcomas, like liposarcomas, are even more rare.

Primary meningeal sarcomatosis refers to involvement of leptomeninges by sarcomatous spread in the absence of a localized tumor. This may totally encase the spinal cord. It must be differentiated from seeding or metastasis of other malignant tumors.

Some differentiation between the types of meningeal sarcomas may be apparent on light microscopic examination. However, periodic acid Schiff (PAS) stain, immunohistochem-istry, or electron microscope imaging is often needed to definitively differentiate them.

Treatment

Radical resection offers the best chance for long-term survival.[27] Most authors agree on the benefit of radiation therapy and chemotherapy. A multidisciplinary team approach is in the best interest of patients with meningeal sarcomas.

Outcome

Although the 5-year survival rate for patients with meningeal sarcomas is relatively low, some cases of long-term survival have been reported.[7] A favorable outcome is more likely after radical resection of a better differentiated, well-circumscribed tumor.

References

1. Alen JF, Lobato RD, Gomez PA, et al: Intracranial hemangiopericytoma: study of 12 cases. Acta Neurochirurgica 143:575–86, 2001.
2. Buttner A, Pfluger T, Weis S: Primary meningeal sarcomas in two children. J Neurooncology 52:181–188, 2001.
3. Cappabianca P, Mauri F, Pettinato G, et al: Hemangiopericytomas of the spinal canal. Surg Neurol 15:298–302, 1981.
4. Chiechi M, Smirniotopoulos J, Mena H: Intracranial hemangio-pericytomas: MRI and CT features. AJNR 17:1365–1371, 1996.
5. Cobbs CS, Guthrie BL: Meningeal hemangiopericytomas. In Kaye AH, Laws ER Jr (eds): Brain Tumors, 2nd ed. London, Churchill Livingstone, 2001.
6. Dufour H, Metellus P, Fuentes S, et al: Meningeal hemangiopericytoma: a retrospective study of 21 patients with special review of postoperative external radiotherapy. Neurosurg 48:756–762, 2001.
7. Ferracini R, Poggi S, Frank G, et al: Meningeal sarcomas with rhabdomyoplastic differentiation. Neurosurg 30:782–785, 1992.
8. Forbes R, Eljamel M: Meningeal chondrosarcomas: a review of 31 patients. Br J Neurosurg 12:461–464, 1998.
9. Galanis E, Buckner JC, Scheithauer BW, et al: Management of recurrent meningeal hemangiopericytoma. Cancer 82:1915–1920, 1998.
10. Gaspar L, Mackenzie I, Gilbert J, et al: primary cerebral fibrosarcomas: clinicopathologic study and review of the literature. Cancer 72:3277–3281, 1993.
11. Haddad GF, Al-Mefty O: Meningeal sarcomas. In Kaye AH, Laws ER, Jr (eds): Brain Tumors, 2nd ed. London, Churchill Livingstone, 2001.
12. Guthrie BL, Ebersold MJ, Scheithauer BW, et al: Meningeal hemangiopericytomas: histopathological features, treatment, and long-term follow-up of 44 cases. Neurosurgery 25:514–522, 1989.
13. Huisman TA, Bradner S, Niggli F, et al: Meningeal hemangiopericytoma in childhood. Eur Radiol 10:103–1075, 2000.
14. Jääskeläinen J, Servo A, Haltia M, et al: Intracranial hemangiopericytoma: radiology, surgery, radiotherapy and outcome in 21 patients. Surg Neurol 23:227–236, 1985.
15. Joseph J, Lisle D, Jacoby L, et al: NF 2 gene analysis distinguishes hemangiopericytoma from meningioma. Am J Pathol 147:1450–1455, 1995.
16. Katayama Y, Tsubokawa T, Meajima S, et al: Meningeal chondrosarcomatous tumor associated with meningocytic differentiation. Surg Neurol 28:385–380, 1987.
17. Kim JH, Jung HW, Kim YS, et al: Meningeal hemangiopericytomas: long-term outcome and biological behavior. Surg Neurol 59:47–53, 2003.
18. Lamszus K, Kluwe L, Matschke J, et al: Allelic losses at 1p, 9q, 10q, 14q, and 22q in the progression of aggressive meningiomas and undifferentiated meningeal sarcomas. Cancer Genet Cytogenet 110(2):103–110, 1999.
19. Lee Y, Van Tassel P, Raymond A: Intracranial dural chondrosarcoma. AJNR 9:1189–1193, 1988.
20. Marc J, Takei Y, Schecter MM, et al: Intracranial hemangiopericytomas: angiography, pathology, and differential diagnosis. Am J Roentgenol 125:823–832, 1975.
21. New PF, Hesselink JR, O'Carroll CP, et al: Malignant meningiomas: CT and histologic criteria, including a new CT sign. AJNR. 3:267–76, 1982.
22. Paulus W, Slowik F, Jellinger K: Primary intracranial sarcomas: histopathological features of 19 cases. Histopathology 18:395–402, 1991.
23. Reusche E, Rickels E, Reale E, et al: Primary intracerebral sarcoma in childhood: case report with electron microscope study. Neurology 237:382–384, 1990.
24. Smith MT, Armbrustmacher VW, Violett TW: Diffuse meningeal rhabdomyosarcoma. Cancer 47:2081–2086, 1981.
25. Surgita Y, Shigemori M, Harada H, et al: Primary meningeal sarcomas with leiomyoblastic differentiation: a proposal for a new subtype of primary meningeal sarcomas. Am J Surg Pathol 24:1273–1278, 2000.
26. Tiberin P, Maor E, Zaizov R, et al: Brain sarcoma of meningeal origin after cranial irradiation in childhood acute lymphocytic leukemia: case report. J Neurosurg 61:772–776, 1984.
27. Tomita T, Gonzalez-Crussi F: Intracranial primary nonlymphomatous sarcomas in children: experience with eight cases and review of the literature. Neurosurgery 14:529–540, 1984.
28. Zulch K: Brain Tumors: Their Biology and Pathology, 3rd ed. Berlin, Springer, 1986.

CHAPTER 47

PITUITARY ADENOMAS

Jeffrey J. Laurent, K. Michael Webb, John A. Jane, Jr.,
and Edward R. Laws, Jr.

More than any other neoplasm of the central nervous system (CNS), pituitary adenomas require a skilled team of caregivers across medical and surgical disciplines. The unique nature of these tumors stems from both their anatomic location and the role of the pituitary gland in maintaining hormonal homeostasis. The initial symptoms of a pituitary adenoma can vary greatly, depending on the cell population involved and the location and size of the tumor. Most patients with pituitary adenomas will first seek treatment from their primary care physician, and initial symptoms may be nonspecific or mimic other conditions. Delays in diagnosis can have disastrous consequences for the patient. These delays are all the more tragic because of the treatable nature of most pituitary lesions. In an era when health care resources and access to specialists are limited, it is important for all physicians to recognize the characteristics of these lesions and ensure prompt treatment.

Pituitary tumors account for 10% to 15% of intracranial neoplasms, placing them third in order of frequency after gliomas and meningiomas.[12] Epidemiologic studies indicate that the annual incidence of pituitary adenomas ranges between 0.4 and 18.7 cases per 100,000. The prevalence of pituitary tumors has been estimated to be around 20 cases per 100,000.[12] However, estimates of incidence and prevalence most likely underestimate the true frequency of pituitary tumors, because many asymptomatic tumors remain undetected. Toward this point, pituitary tumors have been discovered in up to 27% of autopsies.[13]

Overall, men and women are equally affected by pituitary tumors, although some tumor subtypes do show gender preference. Incidence increases with age, and pituitary tumors in children are relatively rare, representing only 2% to 5% of all pituitary tumors.[10]

Other patients at high risk are those known to have multiple endocrine neoplasia type 1 (MEN-1) syndrome, which is characterized by tumors of the pituitary, parathyroid, and pancreas. Approximately 25% of patients with MEN-1 will develop pituitary lesions.[13]

CLASSIFICATION AND CLINICAL PRESENTATION

Many classification schemes have been used to stratify pituitary tumors. These have included clinical, pathologic, and imaging-based classifications, many of which are still in use informally.

In an attempt to standardize reporting, the World Health Organization approved a five-tier classification based on (1) clinical presentation and secretory activity, (2) size and invasiveness (i.e., microadenoma versus macroadenoma), (3) histologic features, (4) immunohistochemical profile, and (5) ultrastructural features on electron microscopy.[7] This integrates many of the prior schemes and provides a practical, comprehensive method for describing pituitary tumors (Table 47-1).

Nonfunctioning adenomas account for 25% to 30% of pituitary adenomas seen in clinical practice. These tumors have also been referred to in the past as chromophobe adenomas, because they do not stain with hematoxylin and eosin (H&E).

Nonfunctioning pituitary tumors typically cause signs and symptoms of mass effect on surrounding structures. Bitemporal hemianopsia, loss of visual acuity, and chronic headache are all commonly described. A thorough visual-field examination is essential. Signs of cavernous sinus compression with facial pain, diplopia, and anisocoria may also occur.

These tumors do not secrete active hormones, and therefore signs of hormone excess are absent. Prolactin levels may be mildly elevated because of the "stalk effect," resulting from loss of tonic inhibition from the hypothalamus caused by compression or distortion of the pituitary stalk. Varying degrees of hypopituitarism may also be seen, and a full panel of hormone levels should be drawn. Signs of hormone insufficiency include decreased libido, fatigue, weakness, and hypothyroidism. It is essential to draw thyroid hormone levels in addition to thyroid-stimulating hormone (TSH) levels, because the patient with hypothyroidism of pituitary etiology will likely have a low TSH.

Prolactin-secreting tumors are the most common pituitary adenoma, responsible for approximately 27% of pituitary tumors.[5] They occur more often in women by nearly 2:1, but autopsy studies reveal an almost equal prevalence of prolactinomas in both sexes. Prolactinomas often cause amenorrhea or galactorrhea and infertility in women of childbearing age. In men, infertility, decreased libido, and impotence are seen. In both men and women, secondary endocrine dysfunction can occur (Table 47-2).

Serum prolactin levels at diagnosis are usually markedly elevated and correlate with tumor size. As mentioned previously, prolactin elevation from pituitary stalk compression alone is rarely greater than 150 ng/mL. In addition, most patients show evidence of secondary hypogonadism in addition to elevated prolactin values.

TABLE 47-1   World Health Organization Classification of Pituitary Tumors

I. Clinical Presentation and Secretory Activity

A. Endocrine Hyperfunction
1. Acromegaly/gigantism, elevated growth hormone levels
2. Hyperprolactinemia and sequelae
3. Cushing's disease, elevated serum ACTH and cortisol levels
4. Hyperthyroidism with inappropriate secretion of thyrotropin
5. Significantly elevated follicle-stimulating hormone and luteinizing hormone
6. Multiple hormonal overproduction

B. Clinically Nonfunctioning
C. Functional Status Undetermined
D. Endocrine Hyperfunction Due to Ectopic Sources
1. Clinical acromegaly secondary to ectopic GHRH overproduction
2. Cushing's disease secondary to ectopic CRH overproduction

II. Size and Invasiveness (e.g., Microadenoma)

A. Location
1. Intrasellar
2. Extrasellar extension
3. Ectopic

B. Size
1. Microadenoma (≤10 mm)
2. Macroadenoma (>10 mm)

C. Growth Pattern
1. Expansive
2. Grossly invasive of dura, bones, nerves, and brain
3. Metastasizing

III. Histologic Features
A. Adenoma
1. Typical
2. Atypical (pleomorphism, enhanced mitotic activity, high MIB-1 labeling index)
If growth pattern can be evaluated:
1. Expansive
2. Histologically invasive

B. Carcinoma
C. Nonadenoma
1. Primary or secondary nonadenohypophyseal tumors
2. Pituitary hyperplasia

IV. Immunohistochemical Profile

Principal Immunoreactivity	Secondary Immunoreactivity
1. GH	PRL, α-subunit, TSH, FSH, LH
2. PRL	α-Subunit
3. GH and PRL	α-Subunit, TSH
4. ACTH	LH, α-subunit
5. FSH/LH/alpha subunit	PRL, GH, ACTH
6. TSH	α-Subunit, GH, PRL
7. Rare hormone combinations	
8. Immunonegative	

V. Ultrastructural Features on Electron Microscopy

A. Growth Hormone
1. Densely granulated
2. Sparsely granulated

B. Prolactin
1. Sparsely granulated
2. Densely granulated

C. Growth Hormone–Prolactin
1. Mixed GH and PRL cell
2. Mammosomatotroph cell
3. Acidophil stem cell

D. ACTH
1. Densely granulated
2. Sparsely granulated
3. Crooke's cell variant

E. FSH/LH
1. Male type
2. Female type

F. Clinically Nonfunctioning
1. Nononcocytic
2. Oncocytic

G. Adenomas of Unknown Cell Derivation
1. Silent corticotroph adenoma subtype 1
2. Silent corticotroph adenoma subtype 2
3. Silent corticotroph adenoma subtype 3
4. Others (unclassified plurihormonal)

ACTH, Adrenocorticotropic hormone; CRH, corticotropin-releasing hormone; FSH, follicle-stimulating hormone; GH, growth hormone; GHRH, growth hormone–releasing hormone; LH, luteinizing hormone; PRL, prolactin; TSH, thyroid-stimulating hormone.
Source: Based on Kleihues P, Cavenee WK (eds): World Health Organization Classification of Tumours. Pathology and Genetics of Tumours of the Nervous System. Lyon, France: International Agency for Research on Cancer (IARC), 2000.

Somatotrophic adenomas are responsible for the manifestations of gigantism in children and adolescents and acromegaly in adults. The clinical characteristics of these conditions are due to an excess of growth hormone. Acromegaly is characterized by extensive soft-tissue swelling, particularly in the hands, feet, and tongue. This pathophysiology is responsible for the typical body habitus as well as complaints of excessive snoring, sleep apnea, and carpal tunnel syndrome.

In addition, acromegaly is associated with cardiomyopathies, hyperlipidemia, and abnormal serum glucose regulation, which pose significant health risks and morbidity if growth hormone hypersecretion is not corrected.

Corticotrophic adenomas constitute approximately 10% of pituitary adenomas in surgical series, and occur nearly five times more often in women than men.[5] Clinically, corticotrophic adenomas are responsible for Cushing's disease, characterized by pituitary-dependent hypercortisolism and a typical body habitus of moon facies, prominent supraclavicular fat pads, abdominal striae, centripetal obesity, acne, easy bruising, hirsutism, hypertension, glucose intolerance, and emotional lability (see Table 47-2).

Corticotrophic adenomas often present a diagnostic dilemma for clinicians, because their imaging characteristics and laboratory abnormalities are variable. Tumor size appears to have no correlation with severity of hypercortisolism, and the tumor is often not seen on imaging studies before surgery. Thus in all patients a thorough laboratory investigation must be performed to confirm the diagnosis preoperatively, especially where tumor is not obvious on imaging studies. Determinations of serum cortisol, adrenocorticotropic hormone (ACTH), 24-hour urine free-cortisol, high- and low-dose dexamethasone

suppression tests, and corticotropin-releasing hormone stimulation tests are most commonly used to make the diagnosis of Cushing's disease. These tests are used to differentiate Cushing's syndrome of pituitary origin from adrenal tumors and ectopic ACTH secretion, which appear similar (Table 47-3). If these tests are inconclusive or tumor is not seen on magnetic resonance imaging (MRI), inferior petrosal sinus sampling is used to confirm the diagnosis and provide a rough estimate of lateralization to guide surgical dissection.

Thyrotrophic adenomas are rare and account for only 1% of pituitary adenomas. They occur with equal frequency in all age groups, without male or female predominance. Two types of these tumors are commonly noted: those producing excessive TSH, causing clinical hyperthyroidism, and those occurring in the setting of thyrotroph hyperplasia caused by chronic hypothyroidism.[5]

IMAGING ANALYSIS

MRI is the imaging modality of choice for pituitary masses. MRI can give the physician information about the gland or mass as well as detail about surrounding structures such as the cavernous sinus and parasellar carotid arteries. Pituitary adenomas are usually hypointense on T1-weighted scans and hyperintense on T2-weighted scans. They usually are not enhanced with contrast administration, whereas the normal pituitary is enhanced brightly (Figure 47-1).

In patients unable to undergo MRI (e.g., a patient with a pacemaker), computed tomography (CT) is an alternative. Pituitary CT scans should include coronal reconstructions.

TREATMENT

Both medical and surgical therapies are available for the treatment of pituitary adenomas. Optimal treatment must take into account tumor type, clinical signs and symptoms, and general medical condition.

Medical Therapy

Great strides have been made in the medical treatment of hormonally active pituitary adenomas. The initial treatment for prolactinomas of any size is dopamine agonist therapy. The most commonly used dopamine agonists are bromocriptine and cabergoline, although pergolide is also used. These agents are effective at reducing prolactin levels and reducing the size of

---

TABLE 47-2

Common Clinical Presentations of Pituitary Adenomas

Hypersecretion
GH-secreting adenoma: acromegaly
ACTH-secreting adenoma: Cushing's disease; Nelson's syndrome
Prolactin-secreting adenoma: amenorrhea-galactorrhea
TSH secreting adenoma: secondary hyperthyroidism

Pituitary insufficiency
Symptoms: diminished libido, fatigue, weakness, hypothyroidism

Mass Effect
Optic chiasm: bitemporal visual-field deficit and possibly diminished acuity
Cavernous sinus: trigeminal nerve → facial pain; cranial nerves III, IV, VI → diplopia, ptosis, anisocoria
Dura or diaphragma sellae: headache
Hypothalamus: behavior, eating, and vigilance disturbances
Temporal lobe: complex partial seizures

Incidental
Evaluation for headaches, trauma, nasal sinus disorders

ACTH, Adrenocorticotropic hormone; GH, growth hormone; TSH, thyroid stimulating hormone.

TABLE 47-3 Cushing's Disease versus Ectopic ACTH

Source of Increased Cortisol	ACTH Level	Low-Dose Dex Supp	High-Dose Dex Supp
Increased pituitary secretion of ACTH (Cushing's disease)	Mild elevation	No suppression	Suppression
Ectopic ACTH production (usually paraneoplastic origin)	High elevation	No suppression	No suppression
Adrenal tumor	Low	No suppression	No suppression

ACTH, Adrenocorticotropic hormone; Dex Supp, dexamethasone suppression.

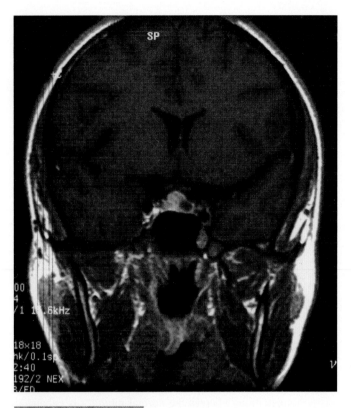

FIGURE 47-1 T1-weighted magnetic resonance image with coronal enhanced image of a hypointense pituitary macroadenoma. Note impingement on the optic nerves by tumor.

prolactinomas. In women, fertility can usually be restored with dopamine agonist therapy with no increased incidence of birth defects or miscarriage.[1] Visual deficits can be reversed as well, and surgical decompression for visual symptoms is rarely necessary.[11]

Recent advances in somatostatin analogues and growth hormone receptor antagonists have made medical treatment of acromegaly a viable option for patients with persistent disease postoperatively. Long-acting somatostatin analogues such as octreotide are used to reduce elevated growth hormone levels in acromegaly. Octreotide has been shown to reduce insulin-like growth factor 1 (IGF-1) to normal levels in approximately 60% of patients with persistent acromegaly following surgery as well as in *de novo* patients.[4] Pegvisomant, a growth hormone receptor antagonist, has shown promising initial results in normalization of IGF-1 levels.[15] There are relatively few clinical studies regarding the use of somatostatin analogues as primary therapy, and surgery remains the initial procedure of choice for most patients with acromegaly.

Although surgery is the mainstay of treatment for Cushing's disease, for patients in whom surgery has been unsuccessful or those unable to tolerate the procedure, some agents have been effective in controlling the manifestations of hypercortisolism. The most effective of these drugs is keto-conazole, which blocks adrenal steroid synthesis. Its utility is limited by occasional hepatotoxicity or transaminase elevation. Other agents that are used include metyrapone, mitotane, cyproheptadine, and aminoglutethimide. It is important to note that although these drugs may decrease cortisol levels, none of them acts to decrease ACTH production by the pituitary, and ACTH levels remain elevated.

Surgical Treatment

Despite these advances in medical therapy, surgical resection remains the first-line treatment for most pituitary adenomas. Prolactinomas are the exception. Treatment of nonfunctioning adenomas is largely based on the effects of the mass on surrounding structures. The most worrisome sign is visual loss, which is a common indication for surgical decompression of nonfunctioning adenomas. In addition, patients may also experience diplopia or facial numbness caused by compression of the third, fourth, and fifth cranial nerves in the cavernous sinus. In some cases, surgical decompression of nonfunctioning tumors may be performed for debilitating headache, although a thorough discussion with the patient regarding the reasonable expected outcomes should be undertaken before surgery.

Pituitary apoplexy, caused by hemorrhage into a preexisting tumor or acute necrosis of a pituitary tumor with edema, is characterized by sudden, severe headache associated with rapid loss of vision, ophthalmoplegia, and endocrine insufficiency. Its treatment remains immediate steroid replacement and surgical decompression.

Surgical resection of pituitary tumors is most often performed via the transsphenoidal route. In the past, a sublabial incision was commonly used to develop the corridor of approach, but the sublabial incision has largely been supplanted by less traumatic and less invasive endonasal approaches. In addition, the development of neuroendoscopic techniques has allowed surgeons to further reduce nasal trauma from the transsphenoidal approach and has improved visualization of the sella and surrounding structures during resection. This enhanced visualization may improve the extent of resection and reduce associated risks such as inadvertent vascular injury.

In the past, the preferred approach to pituitary lesions was through a subfrontal or pterional craniotomy. Although this approach may still be used when the circumstances warrant it, it has largely been supplanted by transsphenoidal techniques.

Results of surgical treatment vary by tumor type. For nonfunctioning adenomas, tumor recurrence depends on the size and invasiveness of the tumor as well as the extent of resection. Representative rates of recurrence for nonfunctioning adenomas are 2% to 18% with postoperative radiation therapy and 12% to 32% without postoperative radiation therapy.[16]

Patients with prolactinomas refractory to medical therapy are also surgical candidates. Prolactin levels were normalized in 70% to 87% of prolactin-secreting microadenomas treated surgically. As might be expected, surgery for prolactin macro-adenomas is somewhat less successful in normalization of serum prolactin, with 30% to 50% of patients developing remission. For all tumor sizes, nearly 18% of patients ultimately develop recurrent hyperprolactinemia.[14]

Studies have reported between 60% and 70% rates of early remission following surgery for patients with growth hormone–secreting adenomas.[8] A long-term follow-up study in the Netherlands showed 40% of patients still in remission without adjuvant medical therapy 16 years after surgery.[2] Recurrence seems to increase with time, as evidenced by two large clinical studies showing recurrence rates of 1.1% and 19% at mean follow-up periods of 33 months and 16 years, respectively.[2,8]

Important factors affecting recurrence in patients with Cushing's disease are the presence of tumor on MRI and tumor size. Transsphenoidal surgery for Cushing's disease results in a 70% to 90% rate of remission of hypercortisolism.[3] Recurrence rates following surgery are generally between 5% and 10%, and are directly proportional to tumor size, with 36% of patients with macroadenomas developing recurrence in one series.[3] Patients in whom refractory hypercortisolism occurs after surgery may be offered total hypophysectomy. These patients must be aware that they will require lifelong hormone replacement therapy. Occasionally, bilateral adrenalectomy may be performed, which sometimes results in Nelson's syndrome, caused by excessive circulating ACTH from the pituitary adenoma.

Although transsphenoidal surgery is very well tolerated, it is not without complications. Surgical morbidity and mortality rates are 2.2% and 0.5%, respectively. Repeat surgery is associated with greater risks. Complications include new hypopituitarism and diabetes insipidus, both of which may be transient or permanent. In patients with normal hormone levels preoperatively, the risk of new anterior hypopituitarism is 3% for microadenomas and 5% for macroadenomas.[9]

Anatomic complications that can occur include damage to the optic chiasm, carotid artery perforation, and cerebrospinal fluid (CSF) leak, which may result in meningitis. Nasal septal perforations and persistent sinus problems also can occur.

PATHOLOGY AND HISTOLOGY

Grossly, pituitary tumors are distinguished by a soft, creamy texture that contrasts with the firmness of the normal gland. Color ranges from white to purple. At the cellular level, normal pituitary architecture shows different cell types arranged in an acinar pattern. Adenomas will display a loss of the acinar architecture and cellular monomorphism (Figure 47-2).

Tissue should be stained with H&E and the standard immunohistochemical battery, which can help classify the

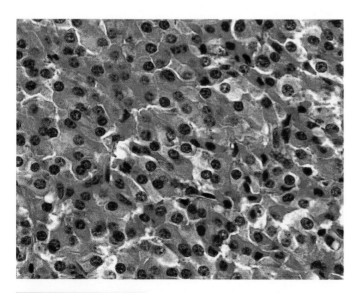

FIGURE 47-2   Hematoxylin and eosin stain of somatotroph adenoma. Notice the cellular monomorphism and loss of acinar structures.

secretory nature of the tumor. The immunohistochemical panel should include reactions for prolactin, ACTH, growth hormone, luteinizing hormone (LH), follicle-stimulating hormone (FSH), TSH, and α-subunit.

The combination of light microscopy and hormone immunohistochemistry is usually sufficient for diagnosis. However, sometimes further classification is aided by ultrastructural features seen on electron microscopy. Cell size and shape and the distribution and morphology of secretory granules are some of the features used to further classify these tumors.

ADJUVANT THERAPIES

Because recurrence rates for pituitary tumors are in general not insignificant, it is important for physicians to have a strategy for dealing with recurrences. As mentioned, the extent of resection is an important factor affecting recurrence. However, the surgeon cannot always safely achieve a total resection, and in these cases both radiation therapy and medical treatments may be warranted.

Both conventional irradiation and Gamma Knife® radiosurgery have been shown to be effective adjuvant treatments for secretory pituitary tumors. Radiosurgery has the advantage of being a single-dose modality and is thus much more convenient for the patient. In addition, some studies suggest a more rapid response to radiosurgery than to conventional techniques.[6] Both modalities are associated with development of hypopituitarism as well. A recent study showed new endocrine deficits in 21% to 36% of patients who underwent radiosurgery with at least 12 months of follow-up review. Conventional irradiation is associated with new endocrinopathies in 50% of patients at 10-year follow-up review. Longer follow-up studies of patients receiving radiosurgery are needed because the number of new endocrinopathies are likely to increase with time.

Patients with acromegaly who do not respond to initial surgical therapy will achieve remission with repeat surgery 48% of the time.[6] Somatostatin analogues and newer growth hormone receptor antagonists can, when combined with surgery, normalize IGF levels and halt tumor growth in 50% to 100% of patients. Radiation therapy has been associated with IGF normalization and remission in up to 70% of patients at 10 years. Remission increases over time but seems to occur sooner with radiosurgery, with a mean of 1.4 years as compared with 7.1 for conventional techniques.[6]

Radiation therapy has also proved to be an effective adjuvant therapy for patients with Cushing's disease. Radiosurgery and conventional techniques can provide remission in more than 70% of patients. The time until remission is less than with acromegaly. In patients who continue to experience hypercortisolism, medical treatment with ketoconazole may be an option. It is important to monitor liver enzymes when using this drug. One should also realize that ACTH levels will remain high, because there is no medical treatment that addresses the increased ACTH levels. Bilateral adrenalectomy can also be considered.

Patients with prolactinomas who have not responded to either medical or surgical treatment also benefit from radiation therapy, albeit less than those with Cushing's disease or acromegaly. Up to 50% of patients with prolactinomas have normalization of prolactin levels following radiation therapy at a mean of 8.5 years of follow-up review.

As mentioned, patients with incompletely resected non-functioning adenomas have lower recurrence rates with post-operative radiation treatment.

CONCLUSION

Because of the wide array of symptoms and the many medical problems associated with pituitary neoplasms, it is important to have a multidisciplinary team to take care of these patients. To provide the very best treatment, a center should have neuro-surgeons, endocrinologists, and radiation oncologists with experience in dealing with pituitary tumors. Patients with pituitary tumors must learn that although they suffer from a benign condition, they are likely to require close observation and follow-up for years to come. Hormone abnormalities may persist and new deficits that require treatment may occur. Tumor recurrence is not rare but if caught early is also treatable. It is also important that this team of specialists keep the patient's primary care physician well informed about the patient's condition and treatment. Good communication by all members of the health care team will allow problems to be recognized sooner and dealt with appropriately.

References

1. Aron DC, Howlett TA: Pituitary incidentalomas. Endocrinol Metab Clin North Am 29:205–221, 2000.
2. Biermasz NR, van Dulken H, Roelfsema F: Long-term follow-up results of postoperative radiotherapy in 36 patients with acromegaly. J Clin Endocrinol Metab 85:2476–2482, 2000.
3. Blevins LS, Jr, Christy JH, Khajavi M, Tindall GT: Outcomes of therapy for Cushing's disease due to adrenocorticotropin-secreting pituitary macroadenomas. J Clin Endocrinol Metab 83:63–67, 1998.
4. Colao A, Ferone D, Marzullo P, et al: Long-term effects of depot long-acting somatostatin analog octreotide on hormone levels and tumor mass in acromegaly. J Clin Endocrinol Metab 86:2779–2786, 2001.
5. Horvath E, Scheitauer BW, Kovacs K, Lloyd R: Regional neuropathology: hypothalamus and pituitary. In Graham DI, Lantos PL (eds): Greenfield's Neuropathology. New York, Oxford University Press, 1997.
6. Jane JA Jr., Woodburn CJ, Laws ER, Jr: Stereotactic radiosurgery for hypersecreting pituitary tumors: part of a multimodality approach. Neurosurg Focus 14:5, 2003.
7. Kovacs K, Stefaneanu L, Ezzat S, Smyth HS: Prolactin-producing pituitary adenoma in a male-to-female transsexual patient with protracted estrogen administration. A morphologic study. Arch Pathol Lab Med 118:562–565, 1994.
8. Kreutzer J, Vance ML, Lopes MB, Laws ER, Jr: Surgical management of GH-secreting pituitary adenomas: an outcome study using modern remission criteria. J Clin Endocrinol Metab 86:4072–4077, 2001.
9. Laws ER, Jr, Thapar K: Pituitary surgery. Endocrinol Metab Clin North Am 28:119–131, 1999.
10. Mindermann T, Wilson CB: Pituitary adenomas in childhood and adolescence. J Pediatr Endocrinol Metab 8:79–83, 1995.
11. Molitch ME: Medical treatment of prolactinomas. Endocrinol Metab Clin North Am 28:143–169, vii, 1999.
12. Monson JP: The epidemiology of endocrine tumours. Endocr Relat Cancer 7:29–36, 2000.
13. Thapar K, Laws ER: Pituitary tumors. In Kaye AH, Laws ER (eds): Brain Tumors. New York, Churchill Livingstone, 2001.
14. Thomson JA, Gray CE, Teasdale GM: Relapse of hyperprolactinemia after transsphenoidal surgery for microprolactinoma: lessons from long-term follow-up. Neurosurgery 50:36–39, 2002.
15. Trainer PJ, Drake WM, Katznelson L, et al: Treatment of acromegaly with the growth hormone-receptor antagonist pegvisomant. N Engl J Med 342:1171–1177, 2000.
16. Turner HE, Stratton IM, Byrne JV, et al: Audit of selected patients with nonfunctioning pituitary adenomas treated without irradiation: a follow-up study. Clin Endocrinol (Oxf) 51:281–284, 1999.

CHAPTER 48

CHORDOMAS AND CHONDROSARCOMAS OF THE CRANIAL BASE

Ossama Al-Mefty, Benedicto O. Colli, Edgardo J. Angtuaco, and Eugen B. Hug

Chordomas and chondrosarcomas are unusual slow-growing neoplasms; they are pathologically distinct but are similar in their biologic behavior, radiologic features, location, and surgical treatment. The sacrum and the clivus are their preferential sites. Chordomas presumably originate from remnants of the primitive notochord, and chondrosarcomas possibly have their origin from mesenchymal cells or from embryonic rests of the cartilaginous matrix of the cranium.[15,16] Virchow in 1846 described small soft, jelly-like tissues arising from the synchondrosis spheno-occipitalis that he supposed to be a lesion belonging to the group of the cartilaginous tumors. This lesion was constituted by characteristic large, vesicular, plant-like cells, which he called *physaliferous cells*. He denominated this lesion as *ecchondrosis physaliphora*. Muller in 1858 ascribed the origin of these tumors to the remnants of the notochord and called them *chordomas* or *ecchordosis*. Coenen in 1925 distinguished the incidental "benign" form, or ecchordosis (nonaggressive, possibly even heterogeneic rests of the notochord without intrinsic growth potential), from the clinically important "malignant" form, or chordoma (tumor).

Despite the improvement in diagnostic and surgical techniques, treatment of patients with chordomas and chondrosarcomas of the skull base is still a challenge for neurosurgeons. Because the tumor originates from the bone at the base of the skull, the recurrence rate of these lesions, even after exceptionally complete resection, remains high.[20]

INCIDENCE, ORIGIN, AND PATTERNS OF EXTENSION

Chordomas and chondrosarcomas occur in 0.1 to 0.5 per 100,000 persons per year, are found in approximately 0.5% of patients with intracranial tumors, and become symptomatic in the third to fifth decade.* They are slow-growing tumors, and the mean duration from first symptom to diagnosis generally lasts more than 12 months.[21] Computed tomography (CT) and magnetic resonance imaging (MRI) has allowed more precocious diagnosis of these tumors. Some series presented a male predominance,[16,28,35] and others showed female predominance

---

*See references 1, 2, 12, 14, 16, 20, 21, 28, 34, 35.

or no sex differences.[1,8,12,14,26] Chondrosarcomas predominate in men and occur more commonly during the second and third decades of life.[8,14] Although remnants of the notochord may persist anywhere along the axial skeleton, the sacrococcygeal (approximately 50% of cases) and clivus regions (in 25% to 36% of cases) are the preferential sites for chordomas. Another 15% of cases are distributed in the rest of spine.[16,21]

Typically, chordomas of the skull base are tumors of the midline, and the synchondrosis spheno-occipital is claimed to be the place of origin of the tumor. Chordomas can extend from the clivus to the parasellar region (23% to 60%), prepontine (36% to 48%), middle fossa (32.1%), nasopharynx (10% to 25%), and into the posterior fossa (78.5%).[1,23] Chondrosarcomas are most likely to locate off-midline.[23] Chordomas limited to the petrous apex region or to the nasopharynx have been reported in the literature. These atypical locations possibly occur because, during the developing period, several branches originated from the notochordal cells and penetrated the base of the skull in different directions. Pure intradural tumors have been reported, but no plausible explanation was given as to their intradural origin.

PATHOLOGY

The chordomas usually are tumors varying from one to several centimeters in diameter. When in soft tissues, they appear pseudocapsulated by fibrous strands, which can create lobulations, but demarcation from normal tissue is not present in the bone. The lobules have two appearance characteristics[16]: a sheet of cells and a pool of mucin. The sheet of vacuolated physaliferous cells contains cytoplasmic mucin, varying from a small amount to a quantity that ruptures the cells. Pools of mucin-containing cords of eosinophilic syncytial cells can be found. These cords often attach peripherally to the septa and project toward the center, giving an impression of a continuum from polyhedral cells containing little mucin (Figure 48-1). A chondroid subtype in which the stroma resembles hyaline cartilage with neoplastic cells in lacunae has been described.[16] The patterns range from small scattered foci with cartilaginous differentiation in a chordoma background to the reverse, in which a chondroid component dominates. A better survival rate is ascribed to this subtype,[14,16] but this statement has been questioned.[8,24]

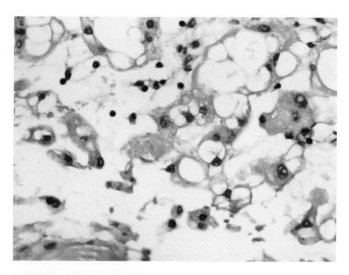

FIGURE 48-1 A high-power view showing a chordoma's typical vacuolated (physaliferous) cells.

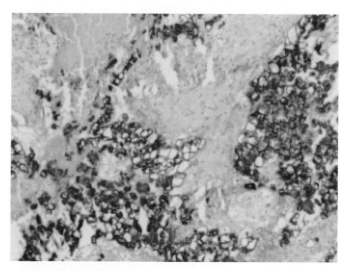

FIGURE 48-3 A positive cytokeratin stain confirming the diagnosis of chordoma.

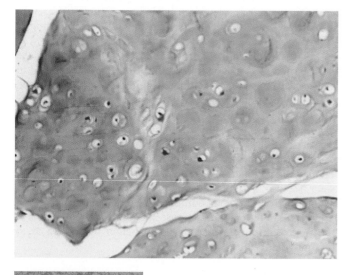

FIGURE 48-2 A high-power view demonstrating a chondrosarcoma's atypical chondrocytes arranged in a background hyaline cartilage matrix.

Chondrosarcomas are classified as classic, mesenchymal, and dedifferentiated.[23] Classic chondrosarcoma, the most common type, is constituted of large cells with single or multiple nuclei within a variable abundance of chondroid matrix. According to their mitotic rates, cellularity, the nuclear size of cells, and the amount of chondroid matrix, the classic chondrosarcomas are divided into grades I, II, or III.[11] Grade I resembles benign cartilaginous tumors (Figure 48-2), and grades II and III have more mitoses and less chondroid matrix. Low-grade chondrosarcomas are less aggressive and have minimal potential to metastasize.[15] Mesenchymal chondrosarcomas are composed of areas of undifferentiated mesenchymal cells and areas of cartilage. Dedifferentiated chondrosarcomas have the characteristics of anaplastic sarcoma. The low-grade type of chondrosarcomas probably are more common than other types.[15]

Immunohistochemistry

The advent of immunohistochemical techniques improved the differentiation of chordomas, mainly the chondroid variant and the myxoid variant of chondrosarcomas. Chordomas originate from the remnants of the notochord, and its epithelial phenotype is manifested through expression of positive markers for cytokeratin (CK) and epithelial membrane antigen (EMA) (Figure 48-3). Chondroid and classic chordomas are positive for CK, and many are also positive for EMA and carcinoembryonic antigen (CEA); chondrosarcomas do not stain for CK, EMA, or CEA, and vimentin (VIM) and S-100 protein are positive for most classic and chondroid chordomas and chondrosarcomas.[24] Nevertheless, the presence of a strong background to chordomas with areas of chondroid patterns and immunonegative CK staining is more consistent for chondroid chordoma than chondrosarcoma. Tumors with a predominantly chordoid pattern or with equal volumes of the chondroid and chordoid components and tumors that are CK- and EMA-positive or positive in the chordoid areas should be classified as chondroid chordomas. Otherwise, predominately cartilaginous tumors with small chordoid elements and negative stain in both areas are classified as chondrosarcomas.

CLINICAL MANIFESTATIONS

Symptoms of chordomas and chondrosarcomas of the skull base, like other intracranial tumors, depend on the specific sites of their extension (i.e., sellar, parasellar, clival, foramen magnum, C1 and eventually retronasopharyngeal, or sphenoid sinus). The most common initial signs are visual disturbances and headaches, followed by lower cranial nerve palsies.[1,8,15–17,20–24,26,28,29] The headaches are usually located in the occipital and occipitocervical areas and may be aggravated by changes in neck position. Tumors located in the basisphenoid most likely cause dysfunction of the upper cranial nerves and of the endocrine system. Lesions arising from the basiocciput more commonly compromise the lower cranial nerves, long tracts, and the cerebellum. Large tumors can give signs of upper and lower cranial nerve palsies. Permanent or intermittent diplopia is the first symptom in most patients, generally the result of compromising of the sixth cranial nerve.[1,8,16] Other symptoms include those related to other cranial nerve palsies, such as decreased visual acuity, facial numbness, facial weakness, hearing loss, dysphasia, dysarthria, hoarseness, and difficulty with speech and swallowing, as well as symptoms of brainstem or cerebellar compression such as dysmetria, gait ataxia, motor weakness, and memory disturbances. Local tumor extension into the retropharyngeal space or into the nasal cavity may occur, and nasopharyngeal symptoms, such as nasal obstruction or discharge, eustachian tube obstruction, throat fullness, dysphasia, or epistaxis, may occur, occasionally being the only symptoms.[1,16,20,21] Physical examination often discloses optic nerve dysfunction or extraocular palsies, particularly when the tumor involves the upper clivus.[8,20,21] Cranial nerve palsies, mainly of the sixth cranial nerve, are found in 40% to 90% of cases of chordomas, and more than half these patients have a retropharyngeal mass.[8,20,21]

DIAGNOSIS

A combination of clinical history, examination findings, and radiologic features raises suspicion of chordomas and chondrosarcomas of the skull base. These tumors should be suspected in patients with skull-base neoplasms, especially with nasopharyngeal extension and destruction of the basal cranium, mainly the clivus. Physical examination and biopsy of the nasopharynx can anticipate the diagnosis, because extension of chordomas to this cavity can occur in 10% to 25% of cases.[1,23]

In the past the radiographic assessment of intracranial chordomas consisted of skull radiographs and cerebral angiography. These studies provided an indirect assessment of the presence and extent of lesion. The advent of modern-day imaging studies of CT and MRI has improved the diagnostic assessment of this rare and hard to manage tumor of the skull base. The complementary role of these diagnostic procedures provides crucial information for the operating surgeon and radiation oncologist to plan for control of this difficult disease.

High-Resolution Computed Tomography

High-resolution CT (HRCT) imaging provides a sensitive method for detecting the destructive effects of intracranial chordomas. High-resolution thin-section CT slices (1-mm contiguous sections) allow exact delineation of the extent of clival involvement. Reformatted images and three-dimensional-volume–rendered studies of this volumetrically acquired data allow a clear assessment of extent of the effects of this tumor on the bone. In addition, the acquired data can be studied both with soft tissue and bone algorithms, which further delineate the associated soft-tissue extension of this skull-base tumor. CT characteristics of chordomas demonstrate a centrally located, well-defined, expansile, soft-tissue mass within the clivus, with extensive lytic bone destruction. The associated soft-tissue mass is usually slightly hyperdense in relation to adjacent brain structures and is enhanced following intravenous administration of iodine-based contrast agents. Calcifications within the soft-tissue mass may be seen and are thought to represent the sequestra from destroyed bone rather than dystrophic calcification within the tumor (Figure 48-4). In addition, sclerotic

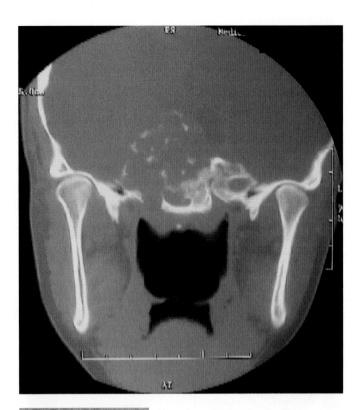

FIGURE 48-4 Coronal computed tomography scan of chordoma demonstrating bone destruction of the clivus and calcification within the tumor believed to represent the bony sequestra from destroyed bone.

regions around the lytic destructive areas are also seen on these high-resolution studies, which represent the permeative nature of tumor involvement.

Magnetic Resonance Imaging

MRI is the best diagnostic modality for studying intracranial chordomas. The major advantage of MRI is its unique ability to demonstrate the tumor's soft tissue component, which is a problem on CT scans because of associated bone artifacts in posterior fossa CT studies. The multiplanar capability of MRI with direct sagittal and coronal studies allows exact delineation of extent and associated involvement of adjacent tissues. The multitude of MRI sequences demonstrate the various characteristics of this tumor together with its effects on adjacent vital neural and vascular structures. On T1-weighted images, intracranial chordomas show intermediate to low signal and can be recognized within the background of the normal high-intensity signal of the fatty clivus. On T2-weighted images, most chordomas are hyperintense, which reflects the high fluid content of the vacuolated cellular components. Associated calcification, hemorrhage, and highly proteinaceous mucous pool within the tumor appear hypointense and heterogeneous on T2-weighted images. The multilobulated appearance of the tumor's gross morphology is shown on T2-weighted images as regions of septations of low signal intensity separating high-signal lobules. Following intravenous administration of gadolinium-based compounds, most chordomas show moderate to marked heterogeneous enhancement. Occasionally, the enhancement is absent. On postcontrast studies, fat-suppressed studies are performed to accentuate the enhancing mass within the normally fatty clivus (Figure 48-5).

An additional advantage of MRI is its ability to demonstrate the large vascular structures located within or around the skull base. The location of the petrous internal carotid and vertebrobasilar arteries either within or adjacent to the skull base make these vessels susceptible to displacement, encasement, or occlusion. One study shows that these vessels are involved in 79% of cases.[23] These intracranial arteries are visualized as flow voids on T1- or T2-weighted spin echo images. Additional sequences such as magnetic resonance angiography (MRA) provide a more exact demonstration of the abnormalities surrounding these vessels and have obviated in most instances the need for performing cerebral angiography. Magnetic resonance venography (MRV) shows the major venous sinuses within the skull base, a factor necessary for safe skull-base surgery.

Cerebral Angiography

Angiographic evaluation of intracranial chordomas is nonspecific. Abnormal tumor vascularity or staining is rare. Angiographic evaluation is reserved for cases where there is demonstrable involvement of the internal carotid or vertebral arteries on MRA. Balloon occlusion during angiography to evaluate collateral circulation and cerebral reserve may be performed if presurgical evaluation shows a need for possible sacrifice of the internal carotid artery.

Most chondrosarcomas have off-midline center points.[23] Differentiation between chordomas and chondrosarcoma based on the radiologic findings is not easy, and histologic analysis

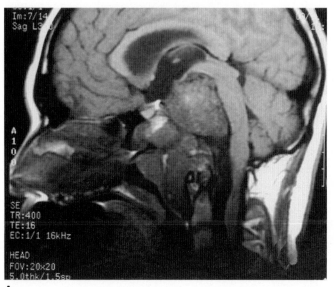

A

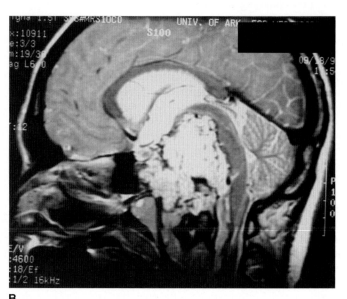

B

C

FIGURE 48-5 Magnetic resonance image of chordoma. A, T1-weighted image. B, T2-weighted image depicting hyperintensity of the tumor. C, Gadolinium enhancement demonstrating the enhancement of chordoma.

and immunohistochemical staining are the only ways to perform an effective diagnostic evaluation.

TREATMENT

Treatment of patients with chordomas or chondrosarcomas of the skull base is a challenge for neurosurgeons. Because of the origin of the tumor from the bone at the base of the skull, only exceptionally complete surgical removal of these tumors can be achieved. Microscopic "total removal" of chordomas often is followed by the finding of residual tumor in the postoperative CT or MRI scans (see Figures 48-2 and 48-3).

Surgical Treatment

The deep localization of chordomas at the middle of the skull base makes them difficult to access surgically. The patterns of spread of skull base chordomas preclude the use of only one surgical approach. Approaches to chordomas of the skull base should be based on the characteristics of growing in each case, and sometimes two or more skull-base procedures may be necessary to achieve a radical removal. Radical surgical removal has a well-known place in the treatment of skull-base chordomas, many authors considering that most cases of chordoma can be suspected based on clinical history, examination findings, and radiologic features, and that they are best approached with intent to resect rather than just to perform a biopsy.[1,6,12,20,21,33,34,35]

Survival

Survival rates for total or near-total tumor resection of craniocervical chordomas and chondrosarcomas range from 62% to 78%.[8,12,14,20,33,34,35] The estimated overall 5- and 10-year survival rates for patients with chordomas surgically treated are 13% to 51% and 18% to 35%, respectively.[12,35] Frequencies of recurrence for patients with chordomas and chondrosarcomas range from 12% to 60% with median follow-up from 1.9 to 30 years.[12,35] Overall recurrence-free survival rates at 5 years for patients with chordomas and chondrosarcomas submitted to total or near-total resection and to subtotal or partial resection range respectively from 55% to 84% and from 15% to 100%.[8,12,16,35] The estimated disease-free survival rates at 5 years range from 33% to 76%, and at 10 years the rate is 24%.[12,14] Patients previously operated on have a worse survival rate than patients not previously operated on (respectively, 64% and 93% recurrence-free survival rates at 5 years).[14,33] Patients with chordomas not previously operated on have better chances for radical resection and better recurrence-free estimates than patients previously operated on (Figure 48-6).[8,14]

Complications

Transient or permanent postoperative cranial nerve deficits occur in 0% to 80% of the patients, but cerebrospinal fluid (CSF) leak is reported as the main complication of surgical treatment of patients with chordomas and chondrosarcomas (7.9% to 30%), and some of these patients develop meningitis (0% to 10%).[8,14,20,33–35] Colli and Al-Mefty[8] reported postoper-

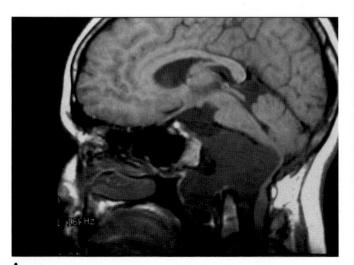

A

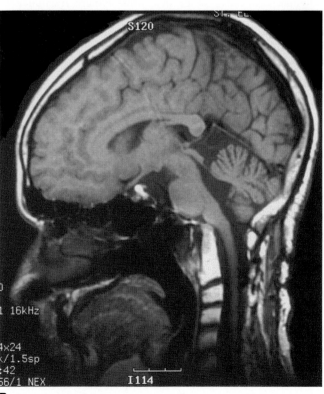

B

FIGURE 48-6   Magnetic resonance (MR) image of a patient who underwent radical surgical removal with long-term control. *A,* Preoperative sagittal MR image. *B,* No evidence of recurrence at 4.5-year follow-up review.

ative cranial nerve palsies in 58.7% of cases. They also observed that 30% of the preoperative cranial nerve palsies improved after surgery.

Mortality

The mortality rate for patients with chordomas varies according to duration of the follow-up (14% to 67% in 1.9- to 5-year median follow-up),[8,14] and operative mortality ranges from 0% to 7.8%.[12,33–35] Mortality among patients with chondrosarcomas is less than mortality among patients with chordomas, and patients who had previous surgery have higher mortality rate and increased risk of recurrence than patients not previously surgically treated.[8,14,33] In our study, previous surgery or previous radiation therapy increases the risk of death in both postoperative and follow-up periods.

Radiation Therapy

Chordomas and chondrosarcomas are historically considered "radioresistant" tumors, because the radiation doses required to successfully treat them are higher than tolerance doses of critical normal tissues close to the skull base. Conventional photon radiation therapy (RT) (i.e., radiation treatment preceding the era of three-dimensional radiation treatment planning and delivery) was unable to separate radiation delivered to the tumor from the dose given to brain, brainstem, upper cervical spine, optic nerves, and chiasm. Tolerance doses of these critical organs, defined as the radiation dose resulting in a likelihood of less than 5% risk of serious complications, is by and large less than 60 Gy. Considering that the majority of mesenchymal, connective tissue neoplasms require fractionated doses in excess of 60 Gy for control of microscopic disease and between 70 and 80 Gy for reasonable chance of gross disease control, it was not surprising that long-term outcome data following conventional radiation treatment have been disappointing.[5,13]

RT has undergone a silent revolution over the past decade. The advent of three-dimensional treatment planning systems as well as computerized beam-delivery systems has permitted target definition and radiation delivery accuracy previously available only in specialized treatment centers. The following is a review of state-of-the-art radiation treatment modalities for low-grade chondrosarcomas and chordomas. Only in selected centers were data prospectively collected. At present, no randomized trial has been performed to compare the different radiation modalities or radiation treatments with surgery or observation only. Comparison of data is even more difficult, because studies with few patients often report jointly on chordomas and chondrosarcomas. However, several authors have convincingly established that chordomas and chondrosarcomas are indeed two pathologically separate disease entities.[30]

Radiation Treatment Modalities

Three-dimensional treatment planning and conformal beam delivery for fractionated photon RT have reached a degree of sophistication that in many instances parallels the degree of high-dose conformity of radiosurgery or particle therapy. The exception remains highly irregular lesions, for which particle therapy continues to offer the tightest dose distribution.[36]

Advantages of three-dimensional conformal photon RT and intensity modulated RT are widespread availability (i.e., a technology that is no longer restricted to major academic centers only). This technology is not limited by tumor size, and treatment volumes are not restricted to only the gross tumor volume (GTV). A larger area of potential microscopic disease can be included as a separate clinical target volume (operative bed, operative excess route, and anatomic compartment). A wide range of fractionation schemes are used, ranging from only a few fractions (hypofractionated stereotactic RT, or SRT) to a protracted course of conventional doses of 1.8 to 2 Gy per fraction per day. At present, daily reproducibility for the majority of noninvasive immobilization systems is quoted as approximately 2 mm, slightly less than the invasive radiosurgery device.

At present, few data have been published. However, considering the widespread use of these new technologies, additional data are expected soon. Debus et al[10] from University of Heidelberg, Germany, reported on 37 patients with chordomas and 8 patients with chondrosarcomas of the skull base who underwent fractionated SRT. With mean doses of 64.9 Gy for chondrosarcomas and 66.6 Gy for chordomas and a mean follow-up of 27 months, actuarial 5-year local control rates were 100% for chondrosarcomas and 50% for chordomas. This translated into 5-year survival rates of 100% for chondrosarcomas and 82% for chordomas.

Proton Radiation Therapy or Particle Therapy

Protons are highly adaptable to the irregular tumors of the skull base. Because protons deposit the dose within the tumor by use of a spread-out Bragg peak and do not have an exit dose, dose distributions are highly conformal in all three dimensions. All reported proton data are based on a course of fractionated RT, either using protons exclusively or as combination of proton and photon RT.

Outcome data on more than 800 patients have been reported from groups at Massachusetts General Hospital (MGH),[19,25] Loma Linda University Medical Center (LLUMC),[18] Lawrence Berkeley Laboratory,[3] and more recently, Centre de Protontherapie d'Orsay, France.[27] Patients treated with particle therapy constitute the largest series worldwide. Local recurrence-free survival rates at 3 and 5 years following radiation doses between 65 and 79 cobalt gray equivalent (CGE) (mean 70.7 CGE) used at LLUMC[18] and 66 to 83 CGE at MGH[19,25] ranged from 94% to 98% for chondrosarcomas and 67% to 73% for chordomas. This translated into overall survival rates at 5 years of 91% to 100% for chondrosarcomas and 79% to 80% for chordomas. At 10 years, the long-term outcome data from MGH demonstrated an even greater difference between chondrosarcomas and chordomas: 94% local control and 88% survival for patients with chondrosarcomas as compared with 54% and 54%, respectively, for patients with chordomas.[19] Symptomatic, severe toxicities were observed in 5% to 13% of patients.

Carbon ion therapy combines the physical properties of protons with an increased radiobiologic effectiveness of carbon ions in tumor tissue. An early report of the Heavy Ion Research Facility in Heidelberg, Germany, on carbon ions in 13 patients with chondrosarcomas and 24 with chordomas revealed progression-free survival at 2 years of 100% for chondrosarcomas and 83% for chordomas. No major toxicity was reported.[32]

Radiosurgery

Most neuro-oncology centers have Gamma Knife® or linear accelerator (LINAC)-based radiosurgery systems available. Despite its widespread use for intra-axial tumors and selected skull base neoplasms, few published reports are available on radiosurgery for chordomas and chondrosarcomas. Muthukumar et al[26] reported on cobalt-60 Gamma Knife therapy for 15 patients with chordomas or chondrosarcomas of the base of the skull. With tumor volumes ranging between 0.98 mL and 10.3 mL (mean 4.6 mL), doses to the tumor margin of 12 to 20 Gy (median 18 Gy) were delivered. Two patients were treated without histologic tumor confirmation. At the median follow-up point of 40 months, two patients had died of disease, two patients had succumbed to intercurrent disease, and one other patient had developed tumor progression. Neither actuarial local control nor actuarial survival data were presented. Crockard et al[9] used a combined regimen of fractionated RT to 50 Gy followed by a radiosurgical boost to 10 to 15 Gy for histopathologically aggressive, subtotally resected skull base chordomas. Five-year actuarial survival rates of 65% were reported in this series of 36 patients.

Patients with skull-base neoplasms are increasingly considered for stereotactic radiosurgery. At present, too few reports on radiosurgery contain sufficient numbers of patients and statistical analysis of patterns of failure to permit drawing definitive conclusions about effectiveness and feasibility of radiosurgery as compared with other advanced technology alternatives.

Summary—Radiation Therapy and Radiosurgery

Chondrosarcomas of the skull base have a significantly better response to high-dose RT than chordomas. Long-term data suggest that radiation doses of approximately 70 Gy can achieve lasting tumor control and thus possibly cure in the majority of patients. If these doses can be delivered, there appears to be no difference between patients with prior gross-total tumor resection as compared with patients with subtotal resection only.

Patients with skull-base chordomas can be divided into good-prognosis and poor-prognosis groups depending on several factors. Outcome depends on tumor volume. The good-prognosis group includes patients in whom maximum surgery achieved either gross-total resection or only reduced tumor size. Other positive prognostic factors include being male and the absence of tumor compression of critical dose-limiting structures (i.e., brainstem, optic nerve, and chiasm). In these patients radiation doses of approximately 75 Gy offer a chance of durable tumor control. For patients in the high-risk group (i.e., patients with a large residual disease, compression of brainstem, optic nerve, optic chiasm [resulting in regional tumor dose deficit], and those who are female), even high doses of radiation appear to only temporarily halt tumor growth. Although 5-year local control and survival data after high doses of 75 to 80 Gy are better than with conventional radiation doses, survival curves continue to decline at 10 and 15 years.[19,25] These patients should be considered for aggressive surgical resection first to accomplish maximum tumor reduction and decompression of critical structures. It remains to be seen if further dose escalation will improve the outcome for these patients or if other, systemic adjuvant modalities are needed.

The excellent survival rates with low-grade chondrosarcomas and good-prognosis chordomas of the skull base have been achieved by targeting not only gross residual disease but also an anatomic volume harboring potential microscopic disease. We therefore recommend including not only gross tumor in the target volume but also the preoperative volume (i.e., operative bed and the entire anatomic compartment). Because of the low incidence rate of lymph-node involvement and an approximate 5% risk of seeding within the surgical access route for chordomas, we currently do not routinely include draining lymphatics or the surgical access route. Severe complications following high-dose conformal RT appear to be within acceptable range considering the high doses delivered and given the major morbidity associated with uncontrollable tumor growth in such patients.

In summary, high-dose RT such as can be delivered by modern radiation technologies following maximum skull-base surgery appears to be the best management policy currently available for patients with subtotally resected skull-base chordomas and chondrosarcomas.

PROGNOSTIC FACTORS

The average survival of patients with untreated chordomas is estimated as being 28 months after the onset of symptoms.[21] Surgery or radiation therapy, or both, increase by two to three times the survival rate compared with untreated chordomas, but all tumors are seen to recur with time.[28,29] In a few patients, cure can be achieved.[21] On average, recurrence occurs from 2 to 3 years after primary treatment, but sometimes tumor recurs more than 10 years after initial treatment.

Patients with chondrosarcomas have much better prognosis than those with chordomas when treated with surgery or adjuvant proton beam therapy.[6,14,17] Aside from pathologic patterns, patient's age, certain clinical manifestations, the extent of tumor removal, and the use of adjuvant postoperative irradiation has been suggested to be related to prognosis of these tumors.

Age of Patient

There is controversy regarding age of patients as a prognostic factor for adult patients with chordomas. Some authors suggest that the prognosis for patients younger than 40 years is significantly better than that for older patients,[12] but this was not confirmed by recent data.[8] A significantly worse prognosis was demonstrated for patients younger than 5 years because of the extreme diversity and malignant pathologic appearance of the tumors in this group.[4,7]

Diplopia

Diplopia has been suggested to have significance in the prognosis of chordomas, being that the tumor size is important.[12] Diplopia is the most common symptom of skull-base chordoma, and small and localized tumors can precociously present it. Probably the better prognosis for patients with diplopia could not be attributed to this symptom, because many tumors could be small, and certainly they are more feasible for surgical resection and growth control by radiation therapy.

Extension of Resection

Despite its association with a considerable complication rate, radical surgical removal has a well-known place in the treatment of skull base chordomas. Forsyth et al[12] observed that survival rates at 5 and 10 years were better for patients who underwent subtotal resection than for patients who underwent biopsy. More recently, some authors found that patients with total or subtotal removal had a better 5-year recurrence-free survival rate than did patients with partial resection.[8,14] It was also demonstrated that more extensive removal was correlated with a lower risk of recurrence.[14]

Adjuvant Radiation Therapy

Adjuvant radiation therapy, especially charged-particle irradiation, has been found to prolong survival or local control of the disease in patients with skull base chordomas.[1,2,8,12,17] This favorable outcome was more evident in patients younger than 40 years.[14]

Cytogenetic Analysis

Cytogenetic abnormalities have been described in patients with chordomas and chondrosarcomas, and they may be of prognostic value.[8,24,31] Similar proportions of diploid and tetraploid populations of cells were found in patients with typical and chondroid chordomas, and although aneuploidy was occasionally found in chondroid chordomas but not in typical chordomas, both types of tumor demonstrate similar clinical behavior.[24] Abnormal karyotype was found to be more common among patients with chordomas than with chondrosarcomas.[8]

No difference was found between karyotypes of patients with typical chordomas and chondroid chordomas, but patients with abnormal karyotypes had significantly higher probability of tumor recurrence.[8] In addition, chordomas with loss of tumor suppressor loci on 1q and 13q seem to be related to aggressive tumor behavior.[31]

CONCLUSION

Histopathologic findings of chordomas of the skull base often are not directly related to patient outcome. Benign tumors might have a fulminating evolution with precocious recurrence, but histologic findings of malignancy invariably have a fulminating evolution. Because of their rarity, few neurosurgeons become familiar with the surgical treatment of chordomas of the skull base and, alternatively, other therapeutic modalities have been used for them, with variable results. The development of skull-base surgery made possible the radical removal of chordomas.

There is still controversy about the treatment of chordomas of the skull base. The reviewed data suggest that prognostic factors that influence the recurrence-free survival for patients with chordomas and chondrosarcomas of the craniocervical junction are histologic features (chordoma or chondrosarcoma), previous treatment (surgery and possibly conventional radiation therapy), extension of resection, adjuvant radiation therapy with heavy particles, and normal karyotype. The current management for patients with chordomas of the craniocervical junction is the most extensive resection possible and adjuvant proton-beam therapy for residual tumor or recurrence.

References

1. Al-Mefty O, Borba LA: Skull base chordomas: a management challenge. J Neurosurg 86:182–189, 1997.
2. Austin-Seymour M, Munzenrider J, Goitein M, et al: Fractionated proton radiation therapy of chordoma and low-grade chondrosarcoma of the base of the skull. J Neurosurg 70:13–17, 1989.
3. Berson AM, Castro JR, Petti P, et al: Charged particle irradiation of chordoma and chondrosarcoma of the base of skull and cervical spine: the Lawrence Berkeley Laboratory experience. Int J Radiat Oncol Biol Phys 15:559–565, 1988.
4. Borba LAB, Al-Mefty O, Mrak RE, et al: Cranial chordomas in children and adolescents. J Neurosurg 84:584–591, 1996.
5. Catton C, O'Sullivan B, Bell R, et al: Long-term follow-up after radical photo irradiation. Radiother Oncol 41:67–72, 1996.
6. Chang SD, Martin DP, Lee E, et al: Stereotactic radiosurgery and hypofractioned stereotactic radiotherapy for residual or recurrent cranial base and cervical chordomas. Neurosurg Focus 10: Article 5, 1–7, 2001.
7. Coffin CM, Swanson PE, Wick MR, et al: Chordoma in childhood and adolescence. A clinicopathologic analysis of 12 cases. Arch Pathol Lab Med 117:927–933, 1993.
8. Colli B, Al-Mefty O: Chordomas of the craniocervical junction: long-term follow-up review and prognostic factors. J Neurosurg 95:933–943, 2001.
9. Crockard HA, Steel T, Plowman N, et al: A multidisciplinary team approach to skull base chordomas. J Neurosurg 95:175–183, 2001.
10. Debus J, Schulz-Ertner D, Schad L, et al: Stereotactic fractionated radiotherapy for chordomas and chondrosarcomas of the skull base. Int J Radiat Oncol Biol Phys 47:591–595, 2000.
11. Finn DG, Goeffert HG, Batsakis JG: Chondrosarcoma of the head and neck. Laryngoscope 94:1539–1543, 1985.
12. Forsyth PA, Cascino TL, Shaw EG, et al: Intracranial chordomas: a clinicopathological and prognostic study of 51 cases. J Neurosurg 78:741–747, 1993.
13. Fuller DB, Bloom JG: Radiotherapy for chordoma. Int J Radiat Oncol Biol Phys 15:331–339, 1988.
14. Gay E, Sekhar LN, Rubinstein E, et al: Chordomas and chondrosarcomas of the cranial base: results and follow-up of 60 patients. Neurosurgery 36:887–896, 1995.
15. Hassounah M, Al-Mefty O, Akhtar M, et al: Primary cranial and intracranial chondrosarcoma a survey. Acta Neurochir (Wien) 78:123–132, 1985.
16. Heffelfinger MJ, Dahlin DC, MacCarty CS, et al: Chordomas and cartilaginous tumors at the skull base. Cancer 32:410–420, 1973.
17. Hug EB: Review of skull base chordomas: prognostic factors and long-term results of proton-beam radiotherapy. Neurosurg Focus 10:Article 11, 1–5, 2001.
18. Hug EB, Loredo LN, Slater JD, et al: Proton radiation therapy for chordomas and chondrosarcomas of the skull base. J Neurosurg 91:432–439, 1999.
19. Liebsch NJ, Munzenrider JR: High-precision, combined proton and photon radiation therapy for skull base chordomas and chondrosarcomas. In Harsh G, Janecka I, Mankin HJ, et al (eds): Chordomas and Chondrosarcoma of the Skull Base and Spine. New York, Thieme Publishers, 2003.
20. Menezes AH, Gantz BJ, Traynelis VC, et al: Cranial base chordomas. Clin Neurosurg 44:491–509, 1997.

21. Menezes AH, Traynelis VC: Tumors of the craniocervical junction. In Youmans JR (ed): Neurological Surgery, Vol 4, 4th ed. Philadelphia, WB Saunders, 1996.

22. Meyer JE, Oot RF, Lindfors KK: CT appearance of clival chordomas. J Comput Assist Tomogr 10:34–38, 1986.

23. Meyers SP, Hirsch WL, Jr, Curtin HD, et al: Chordomas of the skull base: MR features. AJNR 13:1627–1636, 1992.

24. Mitchell A, Scheithauer BW, Unni KK, et al: Chordoma and chondroid neoplasms of the spheno-occiput. An immunohistochemical study of 41 cases with prognostic and nosologic implications. Cancer 72:2943–2949, 1993.

25. Munzenrider JE, Liebsch NJ: Proton therapy for tumors of the skull base. Strahlenther Onkol 175(Suppl II):57–63, 1999.

26. Muthukumar N, Kondziolka D, Lunsford LD, et al: Stereotactic radiosurgery for chordoma and chondrosarcoma: further experiences. Int J Radiat Oncol Biol Phys 41:387–392, 1998.

27. Noel G, Jauffret E, Crevoisier RD, et al: Radiation therapy for chordomas and chondrosarcomas of the base of the skull and cervical spine. Bull Cancer 89:713–723, 2002.

28. Raffel C, Wright DC, Gutin PH, et al: Cranial chordomas: clinical presentation and results of operative and radiation therapy in twenty-six patients. Neurosurgery 17:703–710, 1985.

29. Rich TA, Schiller A, Suit HD, et al: Clinical and pathologic review of 48 cases of chordoma. Cancer 56:182–187, 1985.

30. Rosenberg AE, Nielsen GP, Keel SB, et al: Chondrosarcoma of the base of skull: a clinicopathologic study of 200 cases with emphasis on its distinction from chordoma. Am J Surg Path 23:1370–1378, 1999.

31. Sawyer JR, Husain M, Al-Mefty O: Identification of isochromosome 1q as a recurring chromosome aberration in skull base chordomas: a new marker for aggressive tumors? Neurosurg Focus 10:Article 6, 1–6, 2001.

32. Schultz-Ertner D, Haberer T, Jaekel O, et al: Radiotherapy for chordomas and low-grade chondrosarcomas of the skull base with carbon ions. Int J Radiat Oncol Biol Phys 53:36–42, 2002.

33. Sekhar LN, Pranatartiharan R, Chanda A, et al: Chordomas and chondrosarcomas of the skull base: Results and complications of surgical management. Neurosurg Focus 10:Article 2, 1–4, 2001.

34. Sen C, Triana A: Cranial chordomas: results of radical excision. Neurosurg Focus 10:Article 3, 1–7, 2001.

35. Tamaki N, Nagashima T, Ehara K, et al: Surgical approaches and strategies for skull base chordomas. Neurosurg Focus 10:Article 9, 1–7, 2001.

36. Verhey LJ, Smith V, Serago CF: Comparison of radiosurgery treatment modalities based on physical dose distribution. Int J Radiat Oncol Biol Phys 40:497–505, 1998.

CHAPTER 49

PARAGANGLIOMAS OF THE SKULL BASE

Aramis Teixeira, Ossama Al-Mefty, and Muhammad M. Husain

Glomus tumors, or *paragangliomas* (also called chemodectomas), are neoplasms originating from paraganglia tissue that belongs to the extrachromaffin cell system. These tumors are named according to their site and can appear in the head and neck as one of four types. *Carotid body* tumors arise from the carotid bifurcation and, if large, may involve the cranial nerves, especially the vagus and hypoglossal nerves. *Glomus jugulare* tumors arise from the superior vagal ganglion. *Glomus tympanicum* tumors originate from the auricular branch of the vagus, and *glomus intravaglae* tumors arise from the inferior vagal ganglion.[6,7]

In this chapter, we focus primarily on glomus jugulare tumors because of their clinical importance and cranial nerve involvement. We discuss the evaluation of these tumors, their epidemiology, the role of surgery, therapeutic management, and outcome.

LOCATION

Glomus jugulare tumors are vascular neoplasms arising from the glomus bodies in the region of the jugular bulb. With rare exceptions, they are benign, slow-growing paragangliomas. They invade locally by destroying the temporal bone, especially along preexisting pathways such as blood vessels, the eustachian tube, the jugular vein, the carotid artery, and the cranial nerves. These tumors may sometimes have a large intracranial intradural extension that compresses the brainstem and extends into the petrous bone, the clivus, and the foramen magnum.[3,18,21] They can also occur as multiples or in association with other lesions.

EPIDEMIOLOGY

Paragangliomas are not common neoplasms, accounting for only 0.03% of all neoplasms and 0.6% of head and neck tumors. Glomus jugulare tumors are relatively rare and not commonly seen in neurosurgical practice. Nonetheless, they are the most common neoplasms of the middle ear and second to vestibular schwannomas as the most common tumor involving the temporal bone.

The age at presentation ranges from the second decade or earlier to the ninth decade, although most tumors manifest in the fourth decade of life.[8,11,19,23,24] There is no clear racial

predilection, but glomus tumors seem to be more common in whites.[1] There is a marked predominance among females; women are affected three to six times more commonly than men, with a peak incidence during the fifth decade of life.[25]

Multiple paragangliomas are reported in more than 10% of cases.[3,11,13] Familial cases, most of which involve fathers and daughters, have a much higher rate of multicentricity, up to 55%.[20,23] Evidence supports an autosomal dominant inheritance pattern consistent with genomic imprinting and an association with the haplotype at chromosome band 11q23.[20] Most multicentric tumors are bilateral carotid body tumors.[20] Only a few cases of bilateral glomus jugulare tumors associated with carotid body tumors have been reported.[3,6,22,24]

DIAGNOSIS

Clinical Presentation

The clinical characteristics of a glomus jugulare tumor depend on its locally invasive behavior, its anatomic extension, the size of the tumor, and whether it secretes neuropeptide hormones. Most commonly, patients have hearing loss and pulsatile tinnitus or dizziness. Hearing loss is usually unilateral and results from invasion of the middle ear. It can be conductive if the ear canal is obstructed or sensorineural if the cochlea or labyrinth is invaded, and is often accompanied by dizziness. Pulsatile tinnitus occurs in association with a highly vascular lesion, which is seen through an otoscope as a pulsatile reddish-blue mass beneath the tympanic membrane. Occasionally, patients develop otorrhea spontaneously or after a biopsy.

Patients may also experience headache, ear pain, or neck pain. Symptoms such as hoarseness, difficulty swallowing, bronchial aspiration, aspiration pneumonia, shoulder weakness, tongue atrophy, and tongue fasciculation suggest the involvement of the lower cranial nerves. Deficits of these nerves are usually associated with large tumors. Patients with giant tumors may have facial palsy, Horner's syndrome, diplopia from invasion of the cavernous sinus, and posterior fossa symptoms such as ataxia, nystagmus, intracranial hypertension, papilledema, and occasionally paresis or plegias from brainstem compression.

Often these tumors secrete a low level of catecholamine, which is not recognized clinically but may be responsible for preoperative hypertension or wide fluctuations in blood pressure and bronchoconstriction during surgical manipulation.

Paragangliomas can also secrete serotonin and its precursor, 5-hydroxytryptamine. In rare cases, they are associated with the clinical presentation of carcinoid syndrome (bronchoconstriction, abdominal pain, explosive diarrhea, severe headache, cutaneous flushing, hypertension, hepatomegaly, and hyperglycemia).[6,15]

Classification

In 1962 Alford and Guilford were the first to classify glomus tumors in the middle ear and temporal bone based on their presenting signs and symptoms.[1] Other glomus jugulare classifications have been established mainly according to size, location, and extension. In 1984 Fisch and colleagues classified these tumors, with special emphasis on those having intracranial or intradural extensions and carotid involvement.[10] Jackson developed another classification system similar to that of Fisch and colleagues.[12] In 1994 Patel and colleagues voiced reservations about a system based on size alone and included brainstem compression and vascular encasement, because these circumstances can indicate complications and are of prognostic value.[19] None of these classification systems has complete and universal acceptance, but they have been used for many series of patients.

Laboratory Evaluation

Patients believed to have glomus tumors should undergo detailed neurologic, neuro-ophthalmologic, and neuro-otologic examinations. Audiometric and vestibular tests should be performed. An endocrinologic evaluation should be routine and should include measurements of the serum catecholamine level and the level of vanillylmandelic acid and metanephrines in the 24-hour urine collection. Cytogenetic studies should be considered in patients with multicentric tumors or familial cases.

IMAGING

With advances in radiologic studies, it has become easier to diagnose glomus tumors. High-resolution computed tomography (CT) of the temporal bone with a bone algorithm shows enlargement or destruction of the jugular foramen (Figure 49-1).

CT scans of the abdomen are helpful to identify associated adrenal lesions (carcinomas, sarcomas, etc.). Multiplanar magnetic resonance (MR) images, made both with and without contrast agent, are used to delineate the size, location, and extent of the tumor. It has a typical salt and pepper appearance (Figures 49-2 and 49-3). Although well described in the radiologic literature, the phenomenon of gadolinium enhancement of static blood in the jugular system continues to be erroneously diagnosed as glomus jugulare tumors. MR angiography with a pulse sequence has proved helpful in distinguishing between an increase in signal because of tumor tissue and that due merely to slow flow. Conventional angiography is useful to delineate the vascular anatomy and blood supply, confirm the diagnosis, and identify multicentric lesions (Figure 49-4).

Differential Diagnosis

The major differential diagnosis for glomus jugular tumors includes schwannoma of the lower cranial nerves, jugular fossa meningiomas, and lesions related to the jugular foramen and

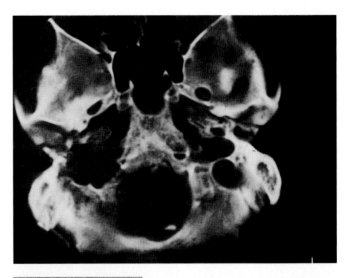

FIGURE 49-1 Axial cut computed tomography with bone windows showing enlargement and destruction of right jugular foramen by glomus tumor.

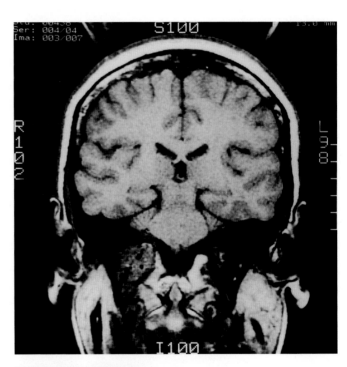

FIGURE 49-2 Coronal magnetic resonance image of right glomus jugulare.

temporal bone—cholesteatomas, chronic mastoiditis, vascular abnormalities, and primary tumors of the temporal bone such as sarcomas and carcinomas. CT, MR imaging (MRI), and angiography are complementary in defining the accurate diagnosis.[4]

TUMOR HISTOLOGY

Glomus jugulare tumors are histologically indistinguishable from carotid body tumors or any other nonchromaffin para-

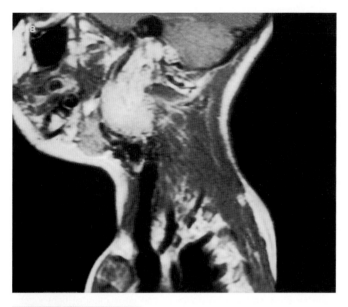

FIGURE 49-3 Sagittal magnetic resonance image of glomus vagale.

ganglioma. These tumors all show clusters (zellballen) of epithelioid (chief) cells and are invested with highly vascular stroma containing capillary-size blood vessels. Histologic criteria do not predict the clinical behavior of paragangliomas, and their malignant potential is notoriously difficult to predict. There are few if any microscopic features that allow the surgical pathologist to reliably determine whether a paraganglioma is benign or malignant. Malignancy is determined more by a clinical course of rapid, aggressive growth, usually associated with anemia, the presence of metastasis, and early death.[5,17] Low levels of neuropeptides have been reported in malignant paragangliomas (Figure 49-5).[17]

Paragangliomas usually possess secretory granules, and 4% are associated with the secretion of a wide variety of neuropeptide hormones, including adrenocorticotropic hormone (ACTH), serotonin, catecholamine, and dopamine.[8,14] The focus of reports has been on the secretion of norepinephrine.[15]

THERAPY

The introduction of computerized imaging, selective embolization, and new surgical approaches, the refinement of surgical

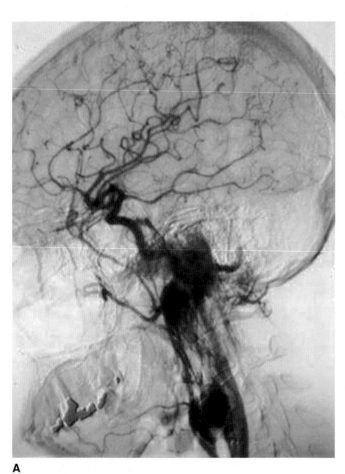

A

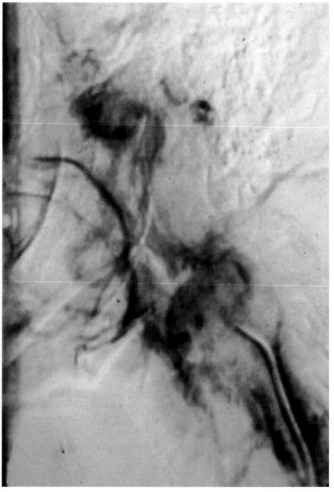

B

FIGURE 49-4 Angiography demonstrating the presence of five paragangliomas. *A,* Right carotid. *B,* Left carotid.

techniques, and increased expertise have made it possible to surgically treat glomus tympanicum and glomus jugulare tumors with good results, long-term control, or cure.[3,11,18]

Multiple paragangliomas present the greatest challenge, because the choice of appropriate treatment is not made according to a single tumor but the quality and length of the patient's life. Whether to treat, when to treat, which tumors to treat, and in which sequence with which modality (surgery or irradiation) are questions that must be addressed at the time of the first evaluation and thoroughly considered throughout the patient's follow-up. The surgeon should try to prevent multiple, bilateral cranial nerve deficits with their resulting severe morbidity and poor quality of life.[3]

Embolization

Superselective embolization techniques are used to devascularize the tumor blood supply of glomus jugulare tumors. The common feeders are from the ascending pharyngeal artery, the external carotid artery, or the vertebrobasilar system (the most common source for large tumors). Embolization decreases

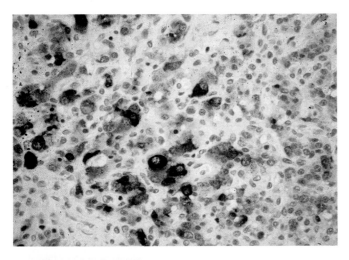

FIGURE 49-5 Immunohistochemical staining for chromogranin of a glomus jugulare tumor.

blood loss, allowing for a safer procedure and thereby increasing the degree of tumor resection (Figure 49-6). Nonetheless, there are risks involved in embolization including: cranial nerve palsy, scalp necrosis, arteriovenous shunting, and vascular accidents.

Surgery

Skull base approaches facilitate the safe removal of glomus jugulare tumors. Giant tumors remain a challenge. The main morbidity results from postoperative deficits of the lower and other cranial nerves.

The surgical approach is chosen according to the anatomic extent of the tumor and the patient's anatomy, clinical condition, and preexisting deficits. For patients with multiple paragangliomas, the surgical technique must also be modified to minimize the risk of facial nerve palsy and at least conductive hearing loss.[2] The tumor most commonly associated with a glomus jugulare tumor is an ipsilateral carotid body tumor. Because this tumor is also exposed during the approach to the glomus jugulare tumor, a unilateral carotid body tumor is best excised during the same operation.[3,11] The surgeon must also consider the role of radiosurgery for bilateral tumors.

Patients with confirmed hypersecreting tumors (a catecholamine level four times higher than normal) require preparation with an α- and β-catecholamine blocker, such as labetalol, before surgery, angiography, or embolization. β-Blockers should not be used before α-blockers. An unopposed α-agonist introduced into the setting of a β-blocker can cause severe hypertension and cardiac crisis. Lower cranial nerve deficits with associated deficits in phonation, deficits in swallowing, and pulmonary complications are the morbid deficit of large tumor that is induced by the tumor or surgical complication. Most young patients adjust in a few weeks, but older patients have longer-lasting difficulties. Vocal cord medialization may be required to improve voice and protect against aspiration.

Radiation Therapy

Radiation therapy has long been used to treat glomus tumors, particularly those that are only partially removed or have recurrence.[9] But glomus tumors are known to be radioresistant, and

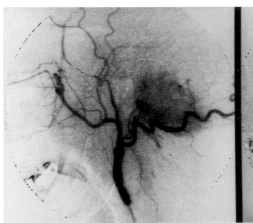
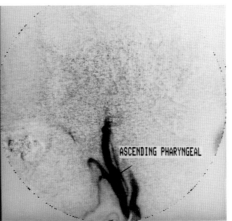

FIGURE 49-6 *A,* Pre-embolization demonstrating blood supply from the ascending pharyngeal and left occipital arteries. *B,* Postembolization.

ASCENDING PHARYNGEAL

A   B

the effect of radiation is often the induction of fibrosis, mainly along the vessels supplying the tumor. Furthermore, persistent viable tumors are often present long after the patient undergoes radiation therapy. Radiation therapy has also been associated with long-term side effects that include osteonecrosis of the temporal bone, the development of a new malignancy, and demyelination.

Early reports of stereotactic radiosurgery for glomus tumors are encouraging, and this modality may be useful in controlling symptoms.[16] Radiosurgery appears to be very effective if the target size is within the optimal size for treatment. The preliminary results of this treatment suggest a symptomatic improvement of cranial nerve function. If it is proved effective with few complications from cranial nerve deficits, radiosurgery will be a great complement to the current treatment of bilateral glomus jugulare tumors and residual lesions from the resection of giant tumors.

RECURRENCE

Glomus jugulare tumors can be cured if they are totally resected. Residual tumors are likely to grow; however, the growth rate is usually slow. Obviously, the prognosis for patients with a malignant paraganglioma is extremely poor; the majority of these patients die within a few months or up to 2 years.

References

1. Alford BR, Guilford FR: A comprehensive study of tumors of the glomus jugulare. Laryngoscope 72:765–787, 1962.
2. Al-Mefty O, Fox JL, Rifai A, Smith RR: A combined infratemporal and posterior fossa approach for the removal of giant glomus tumors and chondrosarcomas. Surg Neruol 28:423–431, 1987.
3. Al-Mefty O, Teixeira A: Complex tumors of the glomus jugulare: criteria, treatment, and outcome. J Neurosurg 97:1356–1366, 2002.
4. Arnautovic KI, Al-Mefty O: Primary jugular fossa meningiomas. J Neurosurg 97:12–20, 2002.
5. Bojrab DI, Bhansali SA, Glasscock ME III: Metastatic glomus jugulare: long-term follow-up. Otolaryngol Head Neck Surg 104:261–264, 1991.
6. Borba LA, Al-Mefty O: Paragangliomas of the skull base. Neurosurg Q 5:256–277, 1995.
7. Borba L, Al-Mefty O: Intravagel paragangliomas: report of four cases. Neurosurg 38:569–575, 1996.
8. Brown JS: Glomus jugulare tumors revisited: a ten-year statistical follow-up of 231 cases. Laryngoscope 95:284–288, 1985.
9. Cole JM, Beiler D: Long-term results of treatment for glomus jugulare and glomus vagale tumors with radiotherapy. Laryngoscope 104:1461–1465, 1994.
10. Fisch U, Fagan P, Valavanis A: The infratemporal fossa approach for the lateral skull base. Otolaryngol Clin North Am 17:513–522, 1984.
11. Green JD, Brackmann DE, Nguyen CD, et al: Surgical management of previously untreated glomus jugulare tumors. Laryngoscope 104:917–921, 1994.
12. Jackson CG: Diagnosis for treatment planning and treatment options. Laryngoscope 103 (Suppl 60):17–22, 1993.
13. Jackson CG, Glasscock ME III, McKennan KX, et al: The surgical treatment of skull-base tumors with intracranial extension. Otolaryngol Head Neck Surg 96:175–185, 1987.
14. Jackson CG, Harris PF, Glasscock ME III, et al: Diagnosis and management of paragangliomas of the skull base. Am J Surg 159:389–393, 1990.
15. Jensen NF: Glomus tumors of the head and neck: anesthetic considerations. Anesth Analg 78:112–119, 1994.
16. Jordan JA, Roland PS, McManus C, et al: Stereotactic radiosurgery for glomus jugulare tumors. Laryngoscope 110:35–38, 2000.
17. Linoilla RI, Lack EE, Steinberg SM, Keiser HR: Decreased expression of neuropeptides in malignant paragangliomas: an immunohistochemical study. Hum Pathol 19:41–50, 1988.
18. Makek M, Franklin DJ, Zhao JC, et al: Neural infiltration of glomus temporale tumors. Am J Otol 11:1–5, 1990.
19. Patel SJ, Sekhar LN, Cass SP, et al: Combined approaches for resection of extensive glomus jugulare tumors: a review of 12 cases. J Neurosurg 80:1026–1108, 1994.
20. Petropoulos AE, Luetje CM, Camarate PG, et al: Genetic analysis in the diagnosis of familial paragangliomas. Laryngoscope 110:1225–1267, 2000.
21. Sen C, Hague K, Kacchara R, et al: Jugular foramen: microscopic anatomic features and implications for neural preservation with reference to glomus tumors involving the temporal bone. Neurosurgery 48:838–848, 2001.
22. Van Baars F, van den Broek P, Cremers C, et al: Familial nonchromaffinic paragangliomas (glomus tumors): clinical aspect. Laryngoscope 91:988–966. 1981.
23. Van Der Mey AL, Frijns JH, Cornelisse CJ, et al: Does intervention improve the natural course of glomus tumors? A series of 108 patients seen in a 32-year period. Am Otol Rhino Laryngol 101:635–642, 1992.
24. Woods CI, Strasnick B, Jackson CG: Surgery for glomus tumors: the Otology Group experience. Laryngoscope 103(Suppl 60):65–70, 1993.
25. Zak FG, Lawson W: Glomus jugulare tumors. In Zak FG, Lawson W (eds): The Paraganglionic Chemoreceptor System: Physiology, Pathology, and Clinical Medicine. New York, Springer-Verlag, 1982.

CHAPTER 50

CARCINOMA OF THE PARANASAL SINUSES AND OLFACTORY NEUROBLASTOMA

Franco DeMonte, Daryl R. Fourney, Adam S. Garden, and Eduardo M. Diaz, Jr.

Sinonasal neoplasms constitute only 0.2% to 0.8% of all malignancies and 2% to 3% of all head and neck cancers.[58] The incidence rate, adjusted for age and sex, is 0.3 to 1 case per 100,000 people. The incidence increases with age beginning around the fourth decade. The median age at diagnosis is 62 years in men and 72 years in women, and the male-to-female ratio is 3:2.[76] Most patients seek treatment when they have advanced disease, which unfortunately is correlated with a less favorable outcome.[2] This problem is compounded by the proximity of the orbit, brain, and cranial nerves. The techniques of cranial base surgery can extend the anatomic margins of resection and, as part of an aggressive multimodal therapeutic approach, results in improved oncologic control of these tumors.

PATHOGENESIS

Epidemiologic studies have shown associations between a variety of environmental hazards and the development of paranasal sinus tumors. In the United States, a large case-control analysis of white males recently demonstrated a significant association between paranasal sinus tumors and cigarette smoking.[94] The risk doubles among heavy or long-term smokers, and there is a reduction in risk among long-term quitters. A significantly elevated risk of paranasal sinus carcinoma was also found among nonsmokers having a spouse who smoked. Other less pronounced associations included increased alcohol intake, high consumption of salted or smoked foods, and decreased intake of vegetables.

The association between exposure to various occupational hazards and the development of paranasal sinus tumors has been the subject of many careful epidemiologic studies (Table 50-1). In an analysis of European case-control studies, occupation was associated with 39% of all sinonasal cancers in men and 11% in women.[85] One of the earliest associations was made in nickel refining, where workers were shown to have a relative risk of developing paranasal sinus malignancy of more than 100 times that of the general population.[23] With proper management of the workplace environment, one Canadian plant achieved a zero incidence of paranasal sinus carcinoma over a 30-year period.[25] Adenocarcinoma of the ethmoid sinus is highly associated with exposure to hardwood dust. Furniture makers and wood machinists in England were shown to have

a 1000-fold increased incidence of adenocarcinoma of the ethmoid.[1,21,32] The development of paranasal sinus tumors has been linked with exposure to various other agents, including chromium compounds, radium used in watch dials, dichlorodiethyl sulfide, isopropyl oil, dust arising during the machining of shoes, textile dust, polyaromatic hydrocarbons in gas manufacture, flour dust, and asbestos.[51,77]

Asia and Africa have a relatively high incidence of paranasal sinus tumors. The Bantu of South Africa have the highest incidence in the world of carcinoma of the upper jaw, likely related to the carcinogenic effects of their homemade snuff.[33] In Japan rates are between 2 and 3.6 cases per 100,000 annually, approximately four times that of the U.S. population.[77] This is mostly due to an increased rate of squamous carcinoma of the maxillary sinus, thought to be the result of the high prevalence of chronic sinusitis and cigarette smoking among the Japanese.[27,58] Fortunately, the incidence of paranasal sinus tumors in Japan seems to be decreasing.[28] Adenocarcinoma of the paranasal sinuses is quite rare in Japan, possibly because of the extensive use of softwood rather than hardwood in the Japanese furniture industry.[27]

There is a well-known association between paranasal sinus tumors and the Epstein-Barr virus (EBV). The high incidence of sinonasal lymphoma in Uganda is due largely to cases of Burkitt's lymphoma occurring in that region.[77] Using in situ hybridization techniques, EBV RNA was found in 7 of 11 cases of sinonasal undifferentiated carcinoma in Asian patients, with no EBV RNA found in tumors of the 11 Western patients evaluated.[49]

PATHOLOGIC FEATURES

Most tumors of the nasal cavity and paranasal sinuses arise from the mucous membranes that line these air spaces, of which there are two types: respiratory mucosa and olfactory epithelium. The respiratory mucosa (schneiderian membrane) consists of pseudostratified ciliated columnar epithelium with interspersed mucus-secreting goblet cells. The surface is invaginated into numerous crypts to form the ducts of mucous glands. The respiratory mucosa gives rise to two basic types of tumors: those arising from "metaplastic" epithelium and those arising from mucous gland epithelium. The olfactory epithe-

TABLE 50-1

Occupational Hazards Associated with Paranasal Sinus Tumors

Occupational Setting	Suspected Carcinogen
Squamous Cell Carcinoma	
Nickel refining	Nickel compounds
Mustard gas manufacturing	Dichlordiethyl sulfide
Isopropyl alcohol manufacture	Isopropyl alcohol
Dial painting	Radium
Adenocarcinoma	
Woodworking	Hardwood dusts
Chrome pigment manufacture	Chromium compounds
Isopropyl alcohol manufacture	Isopropyl oil

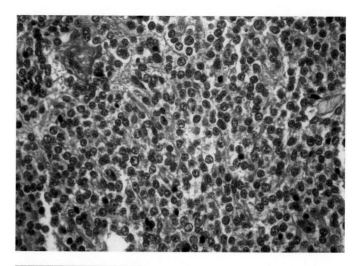

FIGURE 50-1 Photomicrograph of an olfactory neuroblastoma. Note the lobular pattern of small, uniform, round cells with prominent intercellular fibrillary material. (Courtesy of the University of Texas M. D. Anderson Cancer Center, Department of Neurosurgery, Houston, Texas.)

lium contains the nerve cell bodies and is located in the upper nasal cavity. It is nonciliated and lacks a distinct basement membrane. Olfactory neuroblastoma and neuroendocrine carcinoma are thought to originate from the olfactory epithelium.

It is often difficult to determine the exact site of origin of these neoplasms, because more than 90% are found to have invaded at least one sinus wall, and disease may extend well beyond the original sinus. The most common location is the maxillary sinus, where 55% of tumors originate. The remainder of the paranasal sinuses account for about 10% of cases, with 9% arising from the ethmoid sinus and only 1% from the sphenoid and frontal sinuses. In 35% of cases the tumor originates from within the nasal cavity.

Squamous cell carcinoma accounts for more than half of all paranasal sinus tumors in most series[58,76,89] and was the most often encountered pathology in the authors' series.[18] It most commonly arises from the maxillary antrum, with the ethmoid sinuses being the second most common site. The majority of tumors include areas of keratin formation either as sheets or as epithelial pearls. Less well-differentiated, nonkeratinizing anaplastic carcinomas make up the remainder of the lesions.

Adenocarcinoma most often occurs in the upper nasal cavity or in the ethmoid sinuses. It arises from the submucosal glands, which are direct epithelial invaginations and thus not true minor salivary glands. Adenocarcinomas may be well or poorly differentiated, and this high or low grade is related to prognosis.[35] The papillary form is the type most often seen in woodworkers and tends to have a relatively better prognosis than the other two.

Adenoid cystic carcinoma is not a common tumor. It arises from the minor salivary glands of the mucosa. This tumor occurs mainly in the lower aspect of the nasal cavity. Adenoid cystic carcinoma characteristically infiltrates diffusely, especially along perineural pathways, contributing to a high rate of recurrence and late metastasis.[60] Perineural spread is usually evident along the maxillary and mandibular divisions of the trigeminal nerve. At times, the site of secondary perineural extension may manifest itself before the diagnosis of the primary tumor. A careful evaluation usually identifies the primary tumor.[30,31] Microscopically, these tumors have a characteristic appearance as a mixture of microcystic pseudolumi-

nal spaces and tubular epithelial-lined structures with many lesions and also including solid areas.

Tumors arising from the olfactory epithelium are rare neoplasms found in the upper nasal cavity and have been described by many confusing terms, including *olfactory neurocytoma, olfactory neuroepithelioma, neuroendocrine carcinoma, esthesioneuroepithelioma, esthesioneurocytoma, neuroblastoma,* and *esthesioneuroblastoma.*[79]

In 1982 Silva and colleagues[79] divided these tumors into two types: olfactory neuroblastoma (ON) and neuroendocrine carcinoma (NEC). ON is typically composed of sheets of uniform small cells with round nuclei and scanty cytoplasm with prominent fibrillary material between the cells (Figure 50-1). Homer-Wright rosettes (a ring of neuroblastoma cells encircling a small space filled with neurofibrillary material) may be seen. Electron microscopy findings include characteristic neurosecretory (dense-core) granules. NEC is thought to arise from glandular epithelium of the exocrine glands found in the normal olfactory mucosa.[79] It thus manifests a unique admixture with glandular architecture. There is no neurofibrillary component, and the tumor is composed of solid nests of cells without rosette formation. ON is sometimes misdiagnosed, because tumors such as NEC, pituitary adenoma, melanoma, and sinonasal undifferentiated carcinoma may have a similar histopathologic appearance.[15] Careful analysis of the histopathology and electron microscopy findings and appropriate use of immunohistochemical analyses should point to the correct diagnosis (Table 50-2 and Figure 50-2).

ON and NEC should be considered separate diseases.[4,79] NEC arises from a different cell type than ON and is found more inferiorly in the nasal cavity, seldom involving the cribriform plate. Furthermore, NEC is predominantly a disease of older patients (mean age 50 years), rarely presents with regional disease, is more prone to distant metastases, has a shorter delay in the development of metastases, and causes death earlier than ON. In contrast, ON develops more superiorly in the nasal cavity and is more common in younger patients

H&E	Chromogranin	Cytokeratin

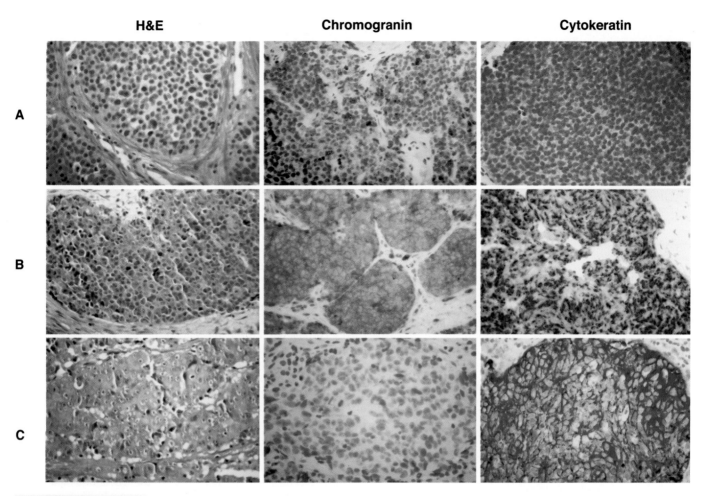

FIGURE 50-2 Tabulated photomicrographs depicting the differentiating characteristics of (A) olfactory neuroblastoma, (B) neuroendocrine carcinoma, and (C) sinonasal undifferentiated carcinoma. The stains for chromogranin are positive in both the olfactory neuroblastoma and the neuroendocrine carcinoma but negative in the sinonasal undifferentiated carcinoma. Cytokeratin staining is negative in the olfactory neuroblastoma but positive in both neuroendocrine carcinoma and sinonasal undifferentiated carcinoma. (Courtesy of the University of Texas M. D. Anderson Cancer Center, Department of Neurosurgery, Houston, Texas.)

TABLE 50-2   Immunocytological Differentiation of Olfactory Neuroblastoma

Tumor Type	Neuronal Markers*	Keratin	Pituitary Hormones	HMB-45, MART-1	CD45 (LCA)
ON	+	–	–	–	–
NEC	+	+	–	–	–
SNUC	–	+	–	–	–
Pituitary adenoma	+	+	±	–	–
Melanoma	–	–	–	+	–
Lymphoma	–	–	–	–	+

* Neuronal markers include synaptophysin and chromogranin.
NEC, Neuroendocrine carcinoma; ON, olfactory neuroblastoma; SNUC, sinonasal undifferentiated carcinoma.

(mean age 20 years). Finally, NEC has responded well to combined chemotherapy plus radiation therapy, whereas the best results with ON have been obtained with surgery and radiation therapy.[4] Grading[35] and staging[24,38] systems for these tumors have been proposed for olfactory neuroblastoma, with a recent report suggesting that the pathologic grade is the more reliable predictor of outcome (Tables 50-3 and 50-4).[56]

Sinonasal undifferentiated carcinoma (SNUC) is a rare aggressive tumor that histologically may be confused with olfactory neuroblastoma, lymphoma, or melanoma. Features of this tumor include a brisk mitotic rate, prominent cellular pleomorphism, and regions of tumor necrosis and vascular invasion. There is a high rate of early metastatic spread, and patients rarely live beyond 2 years after treatment.[34]

TABLE 50-3	Hyams Grading System for Esthesioneuroblastoma			
	Grade			
Histologic Features	1	2	3	4
Lobular architecture	Present	Present	±	±
Mitotic activity	Absent	Present	Prominent	Marked
Nuclear pleomorphism	Absent	Moderate	Prominent	Marked
Rosettes	H-W ±	H-W ±	F-W ±	Absent
Necrosis	Absent	Absent	Occasional	Common

±, Present or absent; F-W, Flexner-Wintersteiner rosette; H-W, Homer-Wright pseudorosette.
From Morita A, Ebersold MJ, Olsen KD, et al: Esthesioneuroblastoma: prognosis and management. Neurosurgery 32:706, 1993.

TABLE 50-4

Kadish and UCLA Staging Systems for Esthesioneuroblastoma

Staging After Kadish

Group A   Tumor confined to nasal cavity
Group B   Tumor extending into paranasal sinuses
Group C   Tumor spread beyond nasal cavity and paranasal cavity

UCLA Staging

T1   Tumor involving the nasal cavity or paranasal sinuses (excluding sphenoid), sparing the most superior ethmoidal cells
T2   Tumor involving the nasal cavity or paranasal sinuses (including the sphenoid) with extension to or erosion of the cribriform plate
T3   Tumor extending into the orbit or protruding into the anterior cranial fossa
T4   Tumor involving the brain

From Dulguerov P and Calcaterra T: Esthesioneuroblastoma: the UCLA experience 1070-1990. Laryngoscope 102:843–849, 1992.

Other less common malignant tumors of the nasal cavity and paranasal sinuses include mucoepidermoid carcinoma, melanoma, plasmacytoma, lymphoma, and various sarcomas. Although malignant tumors are more common overall, benign lesions such as inverting papilloma, osteoma, and paranasal fibrous tumor may occur. Other tumors involve the region by direct spread from adjacent sites, such as juvenile nasopharyngeal angiofibroma, chordoma, meningioma, nerve sheath tumors, and pituitary tumors. Metastases to the sinonasal region are rare. Renal cell carcinoma is by far the most common source of metastases to this area, followed by lung and breast cancer.[5]

Table 50-5 demonstrates the histologic distribution of paranasal sinus tumors treated at the Department of Neurosurgery at M.D. Anderson between 1992 and 2002. Because this is a neurosurgical series, there is a referral bias for advanced disease with intracranial or orbital extension, resulting in a somewhat different distribution of histologic types compared with other reports.

DIAGNOSTIC EVALUATION

The most common presenting symptom of sinonasal carcinoma is nasal airway obstruction, which is often unilateral, followed by chronic nasal discharge and epistaxis.[90] Table 50-6 summarizes the common presenting features of paranasal sinus malignancies. Signs and symptoms of maxillary sinus tumors have been grouped by regional anatomy into nasal, oral, ocular, facial, and neurologic findings.[13] Extension of the neoplasm into the nasal cavity may be seen on anterior rhinoscopy. Oral findings include unexplained pain in the maxillary teeth because of involvement of the posterior superior alveolar nerve. Further expansion may cause loosening of the teeth, malocclusion, and trismus. Fullness of the palate or alveolar ridge may manifest as ill-fitting dentures in the edentulous patient.[46] Tumor bulging into the oral cavity from an adjacent sinus may be visible. Ocular symptoms occur with upward extension into the orbit, causing unilateral tearing, diplopia, exophthalmos, epiphora, and fullness of the lids. Facial findings are most often due to involvement of the anterior antral wall. There may be facial asymmetry with cheek swelling, and in advanced cases ulceration and fistula may develop on the face. Numbness, paresthesia, and pain may be caused by involvement of the infraorbital nerve or, in more advanced disease, by posterior extension of the tumor into the pterygopalatine fossa with involvement of the maxillary division of the trigeminal nerve.[46]

Tumors of the upper nasal cavity and ethmoid may extend through the cribriform plate into the anterior cranial fossa and are associated with anosmia and headache. Carcinoma of the frontal sinus may present as acute frontal sinusitis with pain, swelling over the sinus, and evidence of bone erosion.[71] Unlike most paranasal sinus tumors, nasal obstruction, epistaxis, and nasal discharge may be absent when the tumor is located in the sphenoidal sinus. Patients with sphenoid sinus tumors most commonly experience headache, diplopia, and cranial neuropathies.[18]

Lymph node involvement or metastatic disease occurs in less than 10% of patients at presentation,[90] although the incidence varies depending on the histologic subtype, grade, and extent of the primary tumor.

Advanced disease is the most accurate predictor of poor outcome.[2] Unfortunately, the early symptomatology of malignant paranasal sinus tumors is identical to that of benign nasal and paranasal sinus disease. Combined physician–patient delay ranges from 3 to 14 months.[80] With physician's awareness

TABLE 50-5	Sinonasal Pathologies Requiring Craniofacial Surgery at The University of Texas M.D. Anderson Cancer Center (November 1992 - December 2002)

Malignant		Benign	
Squamous cell carcinoma	30	Juvenile nasopharyngeal angiofibroma	4
Adenoid cystic carcinoma	15	Schwannoma	3
Adenocarcinoma	15	Meningioma	3
Olfactory neuroblastoma	15	Inverting papilloma	3
Sinonasal undifferentiated carcinoma	6	Paranasal fibrous tumor	2
Neuroendocrine carcinoma	6	Osteoma	1
Chondrosarcoma	5	Fibrovascular polyp	1
Fibrosarcoma	5	**Total**	**17**
Osteosarcoma	5		
Metastases	5		
Mucosal melanoma	4		
Unclassified sarcoma	4		
Rhabdomyosarcoma	2		
Malignant fibrous histiocytoma	2		
Mucoepidermoid carcinoma	1		
Teratocarcinosarcoma	1		
Basosquamous carcinoma	1		
Angiosarcoma	1		
Malignant peripheral nerve sheath tumor	1		
Leiomyosarcoma	1		
Total	**125**		

TABLE 50-6	
Common Symptoms Found in 200 Patients with Malignant Tumors	
Symptoms	No. (%) of Patients
Nasal airway obstruction	89 (44.5)
Nasal discharge	78 (39)
Bloody or blood-tinged	51 (25.5)
Mucus	27 (13.5)
Facial pain	77 (38.5)
Mass in the nasal cavity	72 (36)
Exophthalmos	47 (23.5)
Swelling in cheek	43 (21.5)
Paresthesia	39 (19.5)
Epiphora	30 (15)
Diplopia	27 (13.5)
Decreased vision	21 (10.5)

From Weber AL, Stanton AC: Malignant tumors of the paranasal sinuses: radiologic, clinical and histopathologic evaluation of 200 cases. Head Neck Surg 6:761–776, 1984.

heightened, the liberal use of imaging, and early biopsy, the median patient-physician delay is reduced from 8 to 4 months, with 33% of the tumors being diagnosed at an early (T_1 or T_2) stage.

Evaluation of these patients involves a thorough examination of the head and neck, including an endoscopic evaluation of the sinonasal region. The cranial nerves must be evaluated,

and patients should have a baseline neuro-ophthalmologic review. Computed tomography (CT) and magnetic resonance imaging (MRI) are complementary studies and the radiologic methods of choice for assessing these tumors. CT is particularly useful to assess bone changes, especially erosion. Direct coronal CT images are best to assess the integrity of the anterior skull base, including the orbital roof, cribriform plate, and planum sphenoidale (Figure 50-3). The extent of tumor is best seen with MRI (Figure 50-4), which also is able to differentiate tumor from inflamed mucosa, blood, or inspissated mucus in most cases (Figure 50-5).[52] Signal voids within the tumor identified by MRI or proximity of the neoplasm to the internal carotid artery may be an indication for preoperative angiography to assess tumor vascularity and plan surgical treatment.

Management recommendations depend on the tumor histology. Flexible endoscopes permit access for biopsy to most tumors of the paranasal sinuses. In the case of deep-seated lesions, a CT-guided needle biopsy may be performed. The worth of an evaluation of the biopsy specimen by an experienced pathologist cannot be overemphasized.

TREATMENT PRINCIPLES

Tumor pathology and extent, the availability and potential success rates of adjuvant therapies, and the potential for functional impairment and esthetic deformity are all important parameters to consider when planning the best management options for a patient with a paranasal sinus tumor. In most cases, surgery and postoperative radiation therapy are recommended, but other adjuvant therapies such as radiosurgery and chemotherapy may be indicated. It is important to note that the

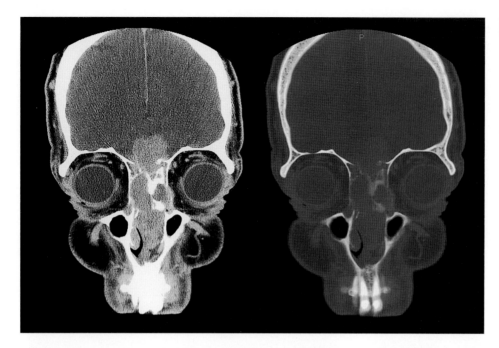

FIGURE 50-3 Coronal computed tomography scans at soft tissue and bone window levels reveal destruction of the cribriform plate by this olfactory neuroblastoma. (Courtesy of the University of Texas M. D. Anderson Cancer Center, Department of Neurosurgery, Houston, Texas.)

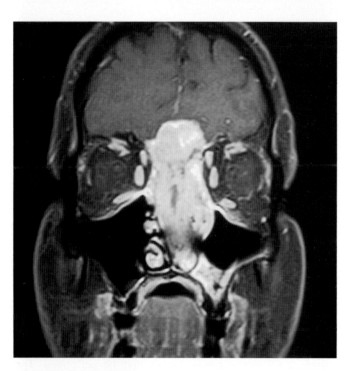

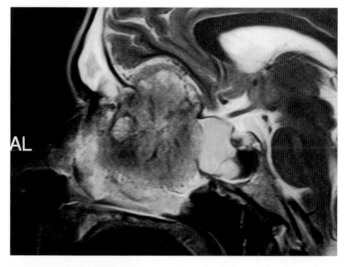

FIGURE 50-5 Sagittal T2-weighted magnetic resonance image. This sequence best differentiates between this olfactory neuroblastoma, which is of intermediate to low signal intensity, and the secretions in the frontal and sphenoid sinuses that are of high signal intensity. (Courtesy of the University of Texas M. D. Anderson Cancer Center, Department of Neurosurgery, Houston, Texas.)

FIGURE 50-4 Coronal postcontrast T1-weighted magnetic resonance image. The extensions of this olfactory neuroblastoma to the medial orbits and frontal lobe are best appreciated on magnetic resonance imaging. (Courtesy of the University of Texas M. D. Anderson Cancer Center, Department of Neurosurgery, Houston, Texas.)

management of paranasal sinus tumors is a multidisciplinary endeavor. Assistance and consultation are required from a team of specialists (Table 50-7).

Initially, consideration is given to whether a gross-total excision can be accomplished. For adenocarcinoma and adenoid cystic carcinoma, it has been our preference to begin with surgical excision and to follow with external-beam radiation therapy. If the patient has received previous radiation therapy, then induction chemotherapy may precede surgical excision for adenocarcinomas and is continued postoperatively if a response is obtained. Induction chemotherapy may also be used for squamous cell carcinoma in the context of an organ-sparing (usually orbital sparing) approach.

For patients with NEC, SNUC, and high-grade sarcoma, induction chemotherapy is recommended. This is particularly true for small cell subsets and moderately or poorly differentiated neuroendocrine cancers. If a response is obtained, then surgical excision and radiation therapy follow. In the event of a complete therapeutic response to chemotherapy, definitive local treatment with radiation therapy as a single modality or with sensitizing chemotherapy is used.

SURGICAL MANAGEMENT

The goal of surgical management is to achieve complete tumor resection with a margin of normal tissue. Early reports of the treatment of these tumors using local (piecemeal) resection such as maxillectomy combined with radiation therapy were disappointing, with an overall 5-year survival rate of less than 30%.[80] Lesions were incompletely excised because of technical difficulties in carrying out thorough *en bloc* resections.

Smith and colleagues[81] reported the first craniofacial resection for malignant disease of the ethmoid sinus involving the cribriform plate. Ketcham and colleagues[41] first reported a combined frontal craniotomy and maxillectomy to treat malignant tumors, later updating their experience with much improved survival rates.[39] Terz and colleagues further extended the limits of resection to include the middle cranial fossa,[86] so that the

TABLE 50-7
Multidisciplinary Team Members to Manage Paranasal Sinus Tumors
Neurosurgery
Head and neck surgery
Plastic surgery
Ophthalmology
Dental oncology
Diagnostic imaging
Pathology
Medical oncology
Radiation oncology

pterygoid plates and their attachments to the sphenoid bone could be removed.

Craniofacial Resection

Patients are selected for craniofacial resection because of ethmoid sinus or cribriform plate involvement by tumor or because of suspicion of dural invasion on preoperative imaging. Most purely ethmoidal tumors that extend to the skull base and invade the cribriform plate can be excised transcranially without the need for facial incisions.[6,55] A transfacial approach is needed if tumor extends to the anterior nasal cavity or laterally beyond the medial third of the maxillary sinus. In most patients, the transcranial approach is performed first followed by, if necessary, the transfacial entry into the paranasal sinuses. This sequence minimizes contact between the sinuses and the epidural space until after repair of the frontobasal dura (Figure 50-6).

Orbitectomy

Orbital exenteration was previously the standard treatment for paranasal sinus cancers that approached the eye. The periorbital membrane, like the dura, presents an interface between the sinonasal cavities and the globe that resists infiltration by tumor. This barrier allows eye-sparing protocols that may involve preoperative radiation therapy or chemotherapy.[69] A major concern with these techniques is local control. McCary and colleagues[54] reported that only 4 of 36 patients (11%) whose eyes were spared had recurrence involving the orbit. The most common tumor type, however, was olfactory neuroblastoma (13 patients), which is a relatively rare tumor in most series, making it difficult to compare results. In a clinical series with a predominance of advanced squamous cell carcinomas, there was only a 30% survival rate (10 of 34 patients) in those who had preservation of the orbital contents as compared with a 50% survival rate (28 of 55 patients) in those with resection.[40]

Another concern is a poor functional result when the eye is preserved, with some authors reporting high rates of keratitis, epiphora, diplopia, cataracts, and dysfunctional globe.[62] In the series by McCary and colleagues,[54] 14 of 31 (45%) patients with orbital preservation who underwent evaluation of function

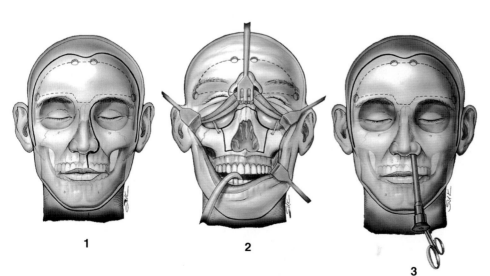

1

2

3

FIGURE 50-6 Options for transfacial approaches for resection of paranasal sinus tumors: (1) Weber-Ferguson with Lynch extension, (2) midfacial degloving, and (3) endoscopic. (Courtesy of the University of Texas M. D. Anderson Cancer Center, Department of Neurosurgery, Houston, Texas.)

in the preserved eye suffered a variety of ophthalmologic morbidities, most commonly exposure keratitis and motility disturbances. Stern and colleagues[83] reported outcome in 28 patients with squamous cell carcinoma of the maxillary sinus who underwent maxillectomy with orbital preservation. Only 3 of 18 patients (17%) who had all or part of the orbital floor resected retained significant function in the ipsilateral eye. Local recurrence occurred in eight of these patients (44%). Few eye problems occurred in the 10 patients in whom the orbital floor was preserved, especially if the eye was not included in the radiation field. Unfortunately, the local recurrence rate was higher (70%). They concluded that when the orbital floor is resected and the radiation field will include the eye, exenteration should be performed. In our experience isolated defects of the medial and lateral orbital walls do not need to be primarily reconstructed if the periorbital membrane is intact. Similarly, defects of the orbital roof, whether in isolation or in association with medial or lateral wall defects do not require reconstruction. Removal of the orbital floor (especially when more than two thirds of the bone is excised) requires primary bone and soft-tissue reconstruction, whether the defect is isolated or part of a multiwall resection.[20]

The decision of whether to spare the orbit may be made preoperatively or at the time of surgery. Transgression of the periorbita by tumor cells with invasion of the periorbital fat indicates the need for exenteration unless there is bilateral invasion or other involvement that precludes radical resection.

Reconstruction can typically be performed using the pericranial flap previously harvested and the temporalis muscle with a skin graft. At times a free rectus abdominus tissue graft is necessary. In our experience there is no significant difference between these two reconstructive methods. The free rectus transfer is preferred if there is a large defect with significant dead space or if the blood supply to the temporalis muscle is deemed tenuous.[10]

Lateral Approaches

Occasionally sinonasal tumors may require the addition of a lateral skull base exposure to achieve surgical extirpation. The most common situations in which a lateral exposure is required are for those tumors of the maxillary sinus that invade through the posterior wall and into the infratemporal fossa, those tumors with significant perineural extension along the second and third divisions of the trigeminal nerve, and tumors of the sphenoid sinus. This approach allows resection of the trigeminal nerve if it is involved by perineural tumor extension. This is generally combined with an anterior or anterolateral approach to resect the primary tumor (Figure 50-7). Reconstruction is straightforward, with subcutaneous fat being used to obliterate the opened sphenoid and maxillary sinuses. If a large resection is necessary, a free tissue transfer is used.

Complications

The incidence of complications reported in the literature is difficult to compare because of lack of uniformity in reporting. Most series report complications in 25% to 40% of patients undergoing craniofacial resection.[9,17,40,44,53,72,78,84,87] The most commonly identified complications include wound infections (especially osteomyelitis), meningitis, cerebrospinal fluid (CSF) leakage, delayed return of neurologic function, and tension pneumocephalus. The widespread use of the pericranial tissue flap for anterior skull base reconstruction has markedly reduced the incidence of infection and CSF fistula in most modern series, including our own. Our infection rate and CSF leakage rate are less

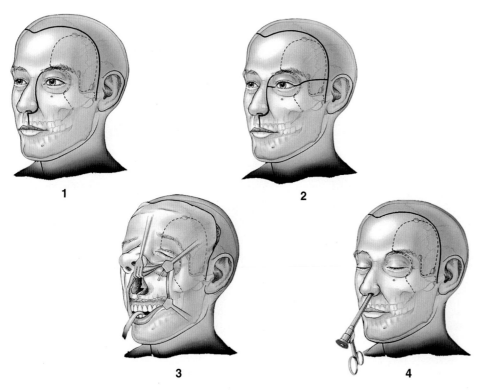

1   **2**

3   **4**

FIGURE 50-7 Options for transfacial approaches to laterally located paranasal sinus tumors include (1) Weber-Ferguson with or without Lynch extension, (2) lateral facial degloving, (3) facial translocation, and (4) endoscopic. (Courtesy of the University of Texas M. D. Anderson Cancer Center, Department of Neurosurgery, Houston, Texas.)

than 1%. Excessive frontal lobe retraction is the likely cause of delayed return of neurologic function. This complication has been totally eradicated from our series because of careful positioning of patients and operative technique that emphasizes the use and importance of the surgical microscope. Tension pneumocephalus is due to overdrainage of CSF either late in the case or in the postoperative period. Treatment consists of needle aspiration of the intracranial air delivery of 100% oxygen and diversion of the airway if needed (usually by insertion of an endotracheal tube rather than tracheotomy). An epidural blood patch may be necessary. Our overall complication rate is currently less than 5%.

RADIATION THERAPY

Radiation therapy is an important treatment modality for malignant paranasal sinus tumors. The most widely accepted view is that radiation therapy should be given after surgical resection of the tumor, especially if a complete resection is not obtained. Several studies comparing patients treated with surgery alone versus a similar group given additional postoperative radiation therapy have shown that the addition of radiation therapy improves local control.[3,29] Radiation therapy is thought to augment surgical 5-year cure rates by 10% to 15% overall.[65] Some centers routinely use preoperative radiation therapy.[11] The potential advantage of preoperative radiation is that the field size is tailored to the tumor rather than the larger operative bed. In addition, lower radiation doses are used preoperatively, potentially allowing greater safety to the optic and neural structures. Recurrence and survival benefits with preoperative irradiation are not clear, however, and there are also some concerns with wound healing.[57] Sisson and colleagues[80] found no differences in outcome or morbidity when patients who received preoperative or postoperative radiation therapy were compared.

A proposed alternative to surgical excision and postoperative radiation therapy has been radiation therapy alone with a curative intent. In a series of 48 patients with malignant paranasal sinus disease, Parsons and colleagues[68] achieved an overall 5-year survival rate of 52% with radiation therapy alone. If the 22 patients in this series with intracranial extension are considered separately, the 5-year survival rate falls to 30%. There was a 33% (16:48) incidence of unilateral blindness in this series and an 8% (4:48) incidence of bilateral blindness. Of concern is that none of the four patients who were left totally blind had orbital invasion. Similarly, not all of the patients with treatment-induced unilateral blindness had orbital invasion. Other complications of high-dose irradiation encountered in this series were CSF leakage, oral-antral fistula, acute sinusitis requiring drainage, and meningitis. For advanced, unresectable tumors, high-dose radiation therapy alone results in 5-year survival rates of 10% to 15%.[67]

At our institution, external-beam radiation therapy is usually reserved for postoperative treatment or palliation. Treatment generally consists of 60 Gy delivered to the tumor bed, with adjustments as needed to limit the dose to the optic chiasm to 54 Gy. If an orbital exenteration has not been done, it is important to construct the treatment fields to spare the lacrimal gland to avoid exposure keratitis. The cervical lymphatics are also treated in patients with advanced squamous cell or undifferentiated carcinoma of the maxillary sinus, because a high incidence of regional failure (38%) occurs when the lymphatics are not treated.[37] This strategy is applied to most histologic subtypes, although NEC and SNUC are treated with chemotherapy and irradiation. Using advanced irradiation techniques, doses ranging from 66 to 70 Gy are delivered. Based on the treatment of other head and neck tumors, irradiation and chemotherapy are often delivered at the same time.

The most common serious complication from radiation therapy is damage to the optic nerves or retina, but other significant complications may include bone necrosis, necrosis of the brain, pituitary insufficiency, and soft-tissue necrosis. Three-dimensional treatment planning has been developed to deliver higher doses of radiation to the target volume while avoiding damage to surrounding structures.[61,74] Radiosurgical techniques using Gamma Knife® or linear accelerator–based systems are proving to be helpful adjuncts for small-volume areas with residual tumor near critical structures such as the cavernous sinus or optic chiasm.[82] The precise extent to which these newer techniques reduce morbidity and diminish tumor recurrence is still to be determined.

CHEMOTHERAPY

The use of chemotherapy in paranasal sinus tumors was previously limited to the treatment of patients with systemic disease and for palliation in patients with massive recurrent tumors who had few other therapeutic options.[50] At the M.D. Anderson Cancer Center, systemic treatment with chemotherapy is considered as a potential component of primary management. Experience with chemotherapy in the setting of paranasal cancers is limited, however, and this modality has not yet gained wide acceptance as an integral component of combined modality treatment approaches. Selected patients can be treated with an induction chemotherapy format, because response rates are high, and with the achievement of a substantial tumor response, more limited surgical resection or possibly a shift from resection to definitive local treatment with radiation therapy may become feasible. Depending on the specific tumor histology, especially small cell neuroendocrine and sinonasal undifferentiated carcinomas, evidence is accumulating that chemotherapy may improve survival.

Prospective trials in squamous cell cancers of the nasopharynx and oropharynx demonstrate that local disease control and overall survival rates are superior after concomitant chemotherapy and irradiation compared with radiation therapy alone.[7,8,36,42,92,93] Data are less clear with respect to patients with primary paranasal sinus squamous cell carcinomas, because so few patients are included in large head-and-neck cancer chemotherapy studies. Although data are limited, chemotherapy has been added to combined modality treatment programs in an attempt to improve local disease control and survival, and as a component of organ preservation strategies. Early studies show promise. Choi and colleagues reported a complete response rate in excess of 90% and a 50% 5-year survival rate in 17 patients with advanced nasopharyngeal and paranasal sinus tumors involving facial bones and the skull base.[12] Split-course hyperfractionated radiation therapy and cisplatin were administered concomitantly. The University of Chicago group reported a cohort of 16 patients receiving induction chemotherapy consisting of cisplatin and infusional 5-fluorouracil (5-FU) followed by surgical resection and then postoperative concomitant irradiation and chemotherapy with

5-FU and hydroxyurea. The median total radiation dose was 60 Gy. Five patients achieved complete histologic response, and 10-year locoregional and distant control rates exceeded 90%.[47]

Intra-arterial (IA) chemotherapy is an alternative approach, developed as an organ-preservation strategy.[63,66] Paranasal sinus cancers supplied by the internal maxillary artery may be the most suitable targets for this technique. Highly selective arterial injections have greatly facilitated this therapy, resulting in concentrated drug delivery to tumor sites while lowering systemic exposures. Increasing tumor drug concentration for cisplatin is feasible, and may be critical, because a dose-response relationship seems to exist with head and neck cancers.[16,26] Lee

and colleagues reported that IA cisplatin could be administered through superselective catheterization and, when combined with systemic chemotherapy, achieved response rates of 80% (30% complete) in advanced paranasal sinus tumors.[48] Robbins and colleagues have used high-dose IA cisplatin and concomitant radiation therapy, resulting in a 96% complete response rate and 5-year survival rate of 39% in patients with head and neck squamous cell carcinomas at various primary sites.[45,75] At the M.D. Anderson Cancer Center, we are further exploring this approach with an induction chemotherapy program consisting of IA cisplatin and systemic paclitaxel and ifosfamide in patients with locally advanced maxillary sinus tumors

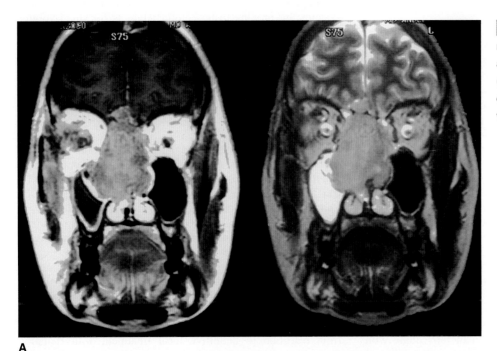

A

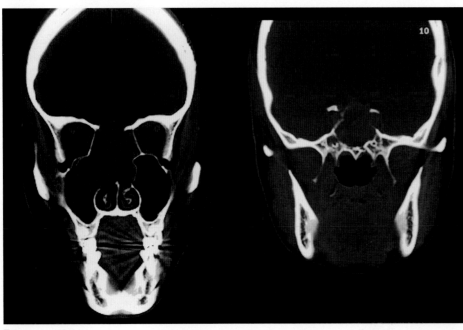

B

FIGURE 50-8 *A*, Pretreatment coronal postcontrast T1-weighted and T2-weighted magnetic resonance (MR) images. *B*, Pretreatment coronal computed tomography (CT) scans at bone window settings.

known to involve the orbit. Patients achieving a substantial chemotherapy-induced tumor response proceed to definitive local treatment with radiation therapy, and surgery is prevented.

With respect to sinonasal undifferentiated carcinoma, scattered reports of small case series suggest potential benefit from the addition of chemotherapy to combined treatment programs.[22] Righi and colleagues reported that three of six patients treated with a multimodality approach were disease free for longer than 1 year.[73] Our practice has increasingly been to use induction chemotherapy with cisplatin-based programs and then to proceed to radiation therapy, with or without surgical resection depending on the response to chemotherapy. The lit-

erature for chemotherapy for SNUC is still sparse, and no drug regimen can be identified as standard.

For patients with moderate to poorly differentiated neuroendocrine carcinoma, we have used induction chemotherapy consisting of cisplatin or carboplatin with etoposide. If a substantial remission occurs, definitive radiation therapy is the next step (Figure 50-8). If not, tumor resection is recommended followed by postoperative radiation therapy. Long-term survival has been reported with this strategy, but again, a standard chemoradiation schedule has not been defined.[64,88] These tumors are to be distinguished from olfactory neuroblastoma.[19] A subset of patients, often women in middle age, have undif-

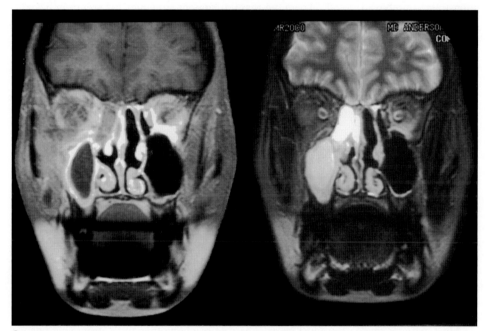

C

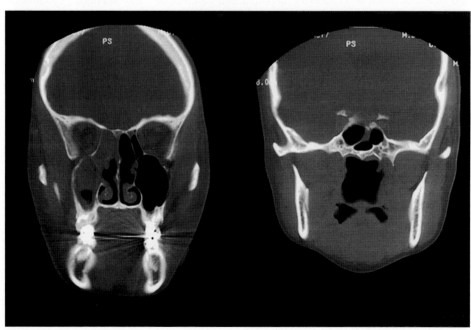

D

FIGURE 50-8 cont'd, *C,* Post-treatment coronal postcontrast T1-weighted and T2-weighted MR images. *D,* Post-treatment coronal CT scans at bone-window settings. Note complete disappearance of the tumor and the reformation of the bone of the skull base in this patient with a neuroendocrine carcinoma treated with chemotherapy and radiation therapy. (Courtesy of the University of Texas M. D. Anderson Cancer Center, Department of Neurosurgery, Houston, Texas.)

ferentiated sinonasal small-cell carcinomas.[70,91] These patients are most often treated with induction chemotherapy as described previously followed by radiation therapy. Consideration can be given to concomitant chemoradiation as in small-cell lung cancer, but there is an unpredictable risk of brain toxicity, and the more conservative sequential therapy may be preferable. Camptothecins are also highly active drugs available for treating small-cell carcinomas.

OUTCOME

Because of the variety of tumor types and the subsequent great range of biologic behavior, an analysis of outcomes is somewhat difficult. Early reports did not demonstrate a preferred treatment modality, and overall 5-year survival rates did not exceed 30%.[80] A substantial improvement in long-term disease control has been attributed to craniofacial resection of these tumors. Recent large surgical series employing craniofacial resection have reported survival rates of 47% to 70% at 5 years and 41% to 48% at 10 years[9,40,53,78,84,87] for all types of malignant tumors. Five-year survival rates are 32% to 73% for squamous cell carcinoma and 43% to 82% for adenocarcinoma.[17,53,78,87] The largest published series is that of Lund and colleagues,[53] who recently reported their 17-year experience with craniofacial resection for paranasal sinus tumors in 209 patients. The overall survival was 51% at 5 years and 41% at 10 years. For all malignant tumors, 5- and 10-year survival was 44% and 32%, respectively. Survival at 5 and 10 years for individual histologies was as follows: squamous cell carcinoma, respectively 32% and 32%; adenocarcinoma, 43% and 38%, adenoid cystic carcinoma, 51% and 36%; olfactory neuroblastoma, 62% and 47%.

McCutcheon and colleagues[55] reviewed 76 patients who underwent craniofacial (47, or 62%) or anterior transcranial (29, or 38%) resection for tumors of the paranasal sinuses at our institution between 1984 and 1993. Most patients had ethmoid sinus involvement, with adenocarcinoma (13 patients) followed by squamous cell carcinoma and olfactory neuroblastoma (11 patients each) being the most common tumor types. The mean follow-up period for the 50 patients who were still alive at the end of the study period was 34 months (range 1 month to 10.4 years). Forty-two (84%) of these patients were without evidence of disease. Calculation of survival times in only those 26 patients who died revealed that the majority (74%) had died within the first 20 months after surgery. Median survival was 20 months for squamous cell carcinoma, 26 months for adenocarcinoma, and 40 months for olfactory neu-

roblastoma. An updated review of 29 patients with olfactory neuroblastoma treated at our institution has found a 2-year and 5-year disease-free survival rate of 70% and 60%, respectively.

In the report by Lund and colleagues,[53] factors that had a significant effect on patient outcome were malignant histology, brain involvement, and orbital involvement. Pathologically positive margins and brain invasion have also been shown to be predictors of local recurrence and shorter survival.[14] Patients with malignant tumors with primary involvement of the sphenoid sinus, although accounting for only 1% to 2% of all patients with paranasal sinus tumors, are an especially difficult subgroup to manage effectively. Even in this group of patients, aggressive multimodality therapy can result in a 2-year survival rate of 44% for patients with squamous cell carcinoma.[18]

There are many treatment strategies for recurrent disease. Spread to lymph nodes, which occurs in 5% to 10% of patients during long-term follow-up review, may be managed with radical neck dissection and radiation therapy. Distant metastases to bone, lung, and liver, seen in a similar proportion of patients, may be treated with local excision or radiation therapy as well as systemic chemotherapy.[43] Intracranial metastasis is very rare.[59]

CONCLUSION

Tumors of the paranasal sinuses are best treated by a multidisciplinary approach, because they may vary significantly in terms of clinical presentation, histopathology, anatomic extent of disease, and behavior. The neurosurgeon is most likely to become involved in cases of advanced disease with infiltration of the skull base, requiring special surgical techniques to obtain clear margins while preserving cosmesis and function. Few of these advanced tumors are amenable to treatment by surgery alone, and our general recommendation is that postoperative radiation therapy with or without chemotherapy be employed in most cases. The role of chemotherapy is promising but yet to be well defined. Undifferentiated carcinomas, neuroendocrine or small cell carcinomas, and squamous carcinomas may be particularly sensitive to chemotherapy combinations, and it is expected that this modality will be integrated into multimodal regimens in the future. Despite the aggressive approach used for paranasal sinus malignancies, the overall prognosis remains less than ideal. Disease control can be achieved in the majority of patients, with some achieving long-term disease control and probable cure. Patients with recurrent tumors may be helped with additional surgery, radiation therapy, and chemotherapy.

References

1. Acheson ED, Cowdell RH, Hadfield E, et al: Nasal cancer in woodworkers in the furniture industry. Br Med J 2:587–596, 1968.
2. Alvarez I, Suarez C, Rodrigo JP, et al: Prognostic factors in paranasal sinus cancer. Am J Otolaryngol 16:109–114, 1995.
3. Anniko M, Franzen L, Lofroth PO, et al: Long-term survival of patients with paranasal sinus carcinoma. ORL J Otorhinolaryngol Relat Spec 52:187–193, 1990.
4. Austin JR, Cebrun H, Kershisnik MM, et al: Olfactory neuroblastoma and neuroendocrine carcinoma of the anterior skull base: treatment results at the M.D. Anderson Cancer Center. Skull Base Surgery 6:1–8, 1996.
5. Batsakis JG, Rice DH, Soloman AR: The pathology of head and neck tumors: squamous and mucous gland carcinomas of the nasal cavity, paranasal sinuses, and larynx. Head Neck Surg 2:497–508, 1980.

6. Blacklock JB, Weber RS, Lee YY, et al: Transcranial resection of tumors of the paranasal sinuses and nasal cavity. J Neurosurg 71:10–15, 1989.

7. Brizel DM, Albers ME, Fisher SR, et al: Hyperfractionated irradiation with or without concurrent chemotherapy for locally advanced head and neck cancer. N Engl J Med 338:1798–1804, 1998.

8. Calais G, Alfonsi M, Bardet E, et al: Randomized trial of radiation therapy versus concomitant chemotherapy and radiation therapy for advanced-stage oropharynx carcinoma. J Natl Cancer Inst 91:208–209, 1999.

9. Cantu G, Solero CL, Mariani L, et al: Anterior craniofacial resection for malignant ethmoid tumors: a series of 91 patients. Head Neck 21:185–191, 1999.

10. Chang DW, Langstein HN, Gupta A, et al: Reconstructive management of cranial base defects following tumor ablation. Plast Reconstr Surg 107:1346–1357, 2001.

11. Cheeseman AD, Lund VJ, Howard DJ: Craniofacial resection for tumors of the nasal cavity and paranasal sinuses. Head Neck Surg 8:429–435, 1986.

12. Choi KN, Rotman M, Aziz, H, et al: Concomitant infusion cisplatin and hyperfractionated radiotherapy for locally advanced nasopharyngeal and paranasal sinus tumors. Int J Radiat Oncol Biol Phys 39:823–829, 1997.

13. Choudry AP, Gorlin RJ, Mosser DG: Carcinoma of the antrum: a clinical and histopathological study. Oral Surg 13:269–281, 1960.

14. Clayman GL, DeMonte F, Jaffe DM, et al: Outcome and complications of extended cranial-base resection requiring microvascular free-flap transfer. Arch Otolaryngol Head Neck Surg 121:1253–1257, 1995.

15. Cohen ZR, Marmor E, Fuller GN, DeMonte F: Misdiagnosis of olfactory neuroblastoma. Neurosurgical Focus 12:Article 3, 2002.

16. Collins JM: Pharmacologic rationale for regional drug delivery. J Clin Oncol 2:498–504, 1984.

17. Danks RA, Kaye AH, Millar H, et al: Craniofacial resection in the management of paranasal sinus cancer. J Clin Neuroscience 1:111–117, 1994.

18. DeMonte F, Ginsberg LE, Clayman GL: Primary malignant tumors of the sphenoid sinus. Neurosurgery 46:1084–1092, 2000.

19. DeMonte F, McElroy EA, Buckner JC, Lewis JE: Chemotherapy for advanced esthesioneuroblastoma: the Mayo Clinic experience. Neurosurgery 42:1028, 1998 (comment).

20. DeMonte F, Tabrizi P, Culpepper SA, et al: Ophthalmological outcome after orbital entry during anterior and anterolateral skull base surgery. J Neurosurg 97:851–856, 2002.

21. Demers PA, Kogevinas M, Boffetta P, et al: Wood dust and sinonasal cancer: pooled reanalysis of twelve case-control studies. Am J Indust Med 28:151–166, 1995.

22. Diaz EM, Jr, Kies MS: Chemotherapy for skull base cancers in otolaryngology clinics of North America: skull base tumor. Surgery 34:1079–1085, 2001.

23. Doll R, Morgan LG, Speizer FE: Cancer of the lung and nasal sinuses in nickel workers. Br J Cancer 24:623–632, 1970.

24. Dulguerov P, Calcaterra T: Esthesioneuroblastoma: the UCLA experience 1970–1990. Laryngoscope 102:843–849, 1992.

25. Egedahl RD, Coppock E, Homik R: Mortality experience at a hydrometallurgical nickel refinery in Fort Saskatchewan, Alberta between 1954 and 1984. J Soc Occup Med 41:29–33, 1991.

26. Forastiere AA, Takasugi BJ, Baker SR, et al: High-dose cisplatin in advanced head and neck cancer. Cancer Chemother Pharmacol 19:155–158, 1987.

27. Fukuda K, Kojiro M, Hirano M, et al: Predominance of squamous cell carcinoma and rarity of adenocarcinoma of maxillary sinus among Japanese. Kurume Med J 36:1–6, 1989.

28. Fukuda K, Shabita A, Harada K: Squamous cell cancer of the maxillary sinus in Hokkaido, Japan: a case-control study. Br J Indust Med 44:263–266, 1987.

29. Gabriele P, Besozzi MC, Pisani P, et al: Carcinoma of the paranasal sinuses: results with radiotherapy alone or with a radiosurgical combination. Radiol Med (Torino) 72:210–214, 1986.

30. Ginsberg LE: Imaging of perineural tumor spread in head and neck cancer. Semin Ultrasound CT MR 20:175–186, 1999.

31. Ginsberg LE, DeMonte F, Gillenwater AM: Greater superficial petrosal nerve: anatomy and MR findings in perineural tumor spread. AJNR Am J Neuroradiol 17:389–393, 1996.

32. Gordon I, Boffetta P, Demers PA: A case study comparing a meta-analysis and a pooled analysis of studies of sinonasal cancer among wood workers. Epidemiology 9:518–524, 1998.

33. Harrison DF: The management of malignant tumors of the nasal sinuses. Otolaryngol Clin North Am 4:159–177, 1971.

34. Houston GD, Gilles E: Sinonasal undifferentiated carcinoma: a distinctive clinicopathologic entity. Adv Anat Pathol 6(6):317–323, 1999.

35. Hyams VJ, Batsakis JG, Micheals L: Tumors of the Upper Respiratory Tract and Ear, 2nd ed. Washington DC, Armed Forces Institute of Pathology, 1988.

36. Jeremic B, Shibamoto Y, Milicic B, et al: Hyperfractionated radiation therapy with or without concurrent low-dose daily cisplatin in locally advanced squamous cell carcinoma of the head and neck: a prospective randomized trial. J Clin Oncol 18:1758–1764, 2000.

37. Jiang GL, Ang KK, Peters LJ, et al: Maxillary sinus carcinomas: natural history and results of postoperative radiotherapy. Radiother Oncol 21:193–200, 1991.

38. Kadish S, Goodman M, Wang C: Olfactory neuroblastoma: a clinical analysis of 17 cases. Cancer 37:1571–1576, 1976.

39. Ketcham AS: The ethmoid sinuses: a reevaluation of surgical resection. Am J Surg 126:468–476, 1973

40. Ketcham AS, Van Buren JM: Tumors of the paranasal sinuses: a therapeutic challenge. Am J Surg 150:406–413, 1985.

41. Ketcham AS, Wilkins RH, Van Buren JM, et al: A combined intracranial facial approach to the paranasal sinuses. Am J Surg 106:698–703, 1963.

42. Kies MS, Haraf D, Rose F, et al: Concomitant infusional paclitaxel and 5-fluorouracil, oral hydroxyurea and hyperfractionated radiation for locally advanced squamous head and neck cancer. J Clin Oncol 19:1961–1969, 2001.

43. Konno A, Togawa K, Inoue S: Analysis of the results of our combined therapy for maxillary cancer. Acta Otolaryngol Suppl (Stockh) 372:1–16, 1980.

44. Kraus DH, Shah JP, Arbit E, et al: Complications of craniofacial resection for tumors involving the anterior skull base. Head Neck 16:307–312, 1994.

45. Kuma P, Wan J, Wieira F, et al: Five-year outcome analyses following treatment of stage III/IV head and neck squamous cell carcinoma using supradose intra-arterial targeted cisplatin and concurrent radiation therapy. Proc Am Soc Clin Oncol 396a, 1999.

46. Larson LG, Martensson G: Maxillary antral cancers. JAMA 219:342–345, 1972.

47. Lee MM, Vokes EE, Rosen A, et al: Multimodality therapy in advanced paranasal sinus carcinoma: superior long-term results. Cancer J Sci Am 5:219–223, 1999.

48. Lee YY, Dimery IW, Van Tassel P, et al: Superselective intra-arterial chemotherapy of advanced paranasal sinus tumors. Arch Otolaryngol Head Neck Surg 155:503–511, 1989.

49. Lopategui JR, Gaffey MJ, Frierson HF, et al: Detection of Epstein-Barr viral RNA in sinonasal undifferentiated carcinoma from Western and Asian patients. Am J Surg Pathol 18:391–398, 1994.

50. LoRusso P, Tapazoglou E, Kish JA, et al: Chemotherapy for paranasal sinus carcinoma. Cancer 62:1–5, 1988.

51. Luce D, Gerin M, Morcet JF, et al: Sinonasal cancer and occupational exposure to textile dust. Am J Indust Med 32:205–210, 1997.

52. Lund VJ, Howard DJ, Lloyd GAS, et al: Magnetic resonance imaging of paranasal sinus tumors for craniofacial resection. Head Neck 11:279–283, 1989.

53. Lund VJ, Howard DJ, Wei WI, et al: Craniofacial resection for tumors of the nasal cavity and paranasal sinuses: a 17-year experience. Head Neck 20:97–105, 1998.

54. McCary, WS, Levine PA, Cantrell RW: Preservation of the eye in the treatment of sinonasal malignant neoplasms with orbital involvement: a confirmation of the original treatise. Arch Otolaryngol Head Neck Surg 122:657–659, 1996.

55. McCutcheon IE, Blacklock JB, Weber RS, et al: Anterior transcranial (craniofacial) resection of tumors of the paranasal sinuses: surgical technique and results. Neurosurgery 38:471–479, 1996.

56. Morita A, Ebersold MJ, Olsen KD, et al: Esthesioneuroblastoma: prognosis and management. Neurosurgery 32:706–715, 1993.

57. Moss WT: Radiation therapy for tumors of the nasal cavity and paranasal sinus. In Thawley SE, Panje WR, Batsakis JG, Lindberg RD (eds): Comprehensive Management of Head and Neck Tumors, Vol 1, 2nd ed. Philadelphia, WB Saunders, 1999.

58. Muir CS, Nectroux J: Descriptive epidemiology of malignant neoplasms of nose, nasal cavities, middle ear and accessory sinuses. Clin Otolaryngol 5:195–211, 1980.

59. Murphy MA, Kaye AH, Hayes IP: Intracranial metastasis from carcinoma of the paranasal sinus. Neurosurgery 28:890–893, 1991.

60. Naficy S, Disher MJ, Esclamado RM: Adenoid cystic carcinoma of the paranasal sinuses. Am J Rhinol 13:311–314, 1999.

61. Nagata Y, Okajima K, Murata R: Three-dimensional treatment planning for maxillary sinus cancer using a CT simulator. Int J Radiat Oncol Biol Phys 30:979–983, 1994.

62. Namon AJ, Panje WR: Controversy in the management of tumors of the nasal cavity and paranasal sinuses. In Thawley SE, Panje WR, Batsakis JG, Lindberg RD (eds): Comprehensive Management of Head and Neck Tumors, Vol 1, 2nd ed. Philadelphia, WB Saunders, 1999.

63. Nishino H, Miyata M, Morita M, et al: Combined therapy with conservative surgery, radiotherapy, and regional chemotherapy for maxillary sinus carcinoma. Cancer 89:1925–1932, 2000.

64. Ordonez NG, Mackay B: Neuroendocrine tumors of the nasal cavity. Pathol Annu 28:77–111, 1993.

65. Osguthorpe JD: Sinus neoplasia. Arch Otolaryngol Head Neck Surg 120:19–25, 1994.

66. Papadimitrakopoulou VA, Hong WK: Combined-modality therapy in paranasal sinus cancer. Cancer J Sci Am 5:208–210, 1999.

67. Parsons JT, Kimsey FC, Mendenhall WM, et al: Radiation therapy for sinus malignancies. Otolaryngol Clin North Am 28:1259–1268, 1995.

68. Parsons JT, Mendenhall WM, Mancuso M, et al: Malignant tumors of the nasal cavity and ethmoid and sphenoid sinuses. Int J Radiat Oncol Biol Phys 14:11–22, 1988.

69. Perry C, Levine PA, Williamson BR, et al: Preservation of the eye in paranasal sinus cancer surgery. Arch Otolaryngol Head Neck Surg 114:632–634, 1988.

70. Raychowdhuri RN: Oat cell carcinoma and paranasal sinuses. J Laryngol Otol 79:253, 1965.

71. Rice DH, Stanley RB, Jr: Surgical therapy of tumors of the nasal cavity, ethmoid sinus, and maxillary sinus. In Thawley SE, Panje WR, Batsakis JG, Lindberg RD (eds): Comprehensive Management of Head and Neck Tumors, Vol 1, 2nd ed. Philadelphia, WB Saunders, 1999.

72. Richtsmeier WJ, Briggs RJS, Koch WM, et al: Complications and early outcome of anterior craniofacial resection. Arch Otolaryngol Head Neck Surg 118:913–917, 1992

73. Righi PD, Francis F, Aron BS, et al: Sinonasal undifferentiated carcinoma: a 10-year experience. Am J Otolaryngol 17:167–171, 1996.

74. Roa WH, Hazuka MB, Sandler HM, et al: Results of primary and adjuvant CT-based 3-dimensional radiotherapy for malignant tumors of the paranasal sinuses. Int J Radiat Oncol Biol Phys 28:857–865, 1994.

75. Robbins KT, Vicario D, Seagren S, et al: A targeted supradose cisplatin chemoradiation protocol for advanced head and neck cancer. Am J Surg 168:419–422, 1994.

76. Robin PE, Powell DJ, Stanbie JM: Carcinoma of the nasal cavity and paranasal sinuses: incidence and presentation of different histological types. Clin Otolaryngol 4:431–456, 1979.

77. Roush GC: Epidemiology of cancer of the nose and paranasal sinuses: current concepts. Head Neck Surg 2:3–11, 1979.

78. Shah JP, Kraus DH, Bilsky MH, et al: Craniofacial resection for malignant tumors involving the anterior skull base. Arch Otolaryngol Head Neck Surg 123:1312–1317, 1997.

79. Silva EG, Butler JJ, Mackay B, Goepfert H: Neuroblastomas and neuroendocrine carcinomas of the nasal cavity: a proposed new classification. Cancer 50:2388–2405, 1982.

80. Sisson GA, Sr, Toriumi DM, Atiyah RA: Paranasal sinus malignancy: a comprehensive update. Laryngoscope 99:143–150, 1989

81. Smith RR, Klopp CT, Williams JM: Surgical treatment of cancer of the frontal sinus and adjacent areas. Cancer 7:991–994, 1954.

82. Stammberger H, Anderhuber W, Walch C: Possibilities and limitations of endoscopic management of nasal and paranasal sinus malignancies. Acta Otorhinolaryngol Belg 53:199–205, 1999.

83. Stern SJ, Goepfert H, Clayman G, et al: Orbital preservation in maxillectomy. Otolaryngol Head Neck Surg 109:111–115, 1993.

84. Sundaresan N, Shah JP: Craniofacial resection for anterior skull base tumors. Head Neck Surg 10:219–224, 1988.

85. 't Mannetje A, Kogevinas M, Luce D, et al: Sinonasal cancer, occupation, and tobacco smoking in European women and men. Am J Ind Med 36:101–107, 1999.

86. Terz JJ, Alksne JF, Lawrence W: Craniofacial resection for tumors invading the pterygoid fossa. Am J Surg 118:732–740, 1969.

87. Terz JJ, Young HF, Lawrence W, Jr: Combined craniofacial resection for locally advanced carcinoma of the head and neck. II. Carcinoma of the paranasal sinuses. Am J Surg 140:618–624, 1980.

88. Thornton AF, Varvares M, McIntyre J, et al: Treatment of esthesioneuroblastoma and neuroendocrine carcinoma with combined chemotherapy and proton radiation. Proc Am Soc Clin Oncol 411a, 1998.

89. Tofano RP, Mokadam NA, Montone KT, et al: Malignant tumors of the nose and paranasal sinuses: Hospital of the University of Pennsylvania experience 1990–1997. Am J Rhinol 13:117–123, 1999.

90. Weber AL, Stanton AC: Malignant tumors of the paranasal sinuses: Radiologic, clinical, and histopathologic evaluation of 200 cases. Head Neck Surg 6:761–776, 1984.

91. Weiss MD, deFries HO, Taxy JB, et al: Primary small cell carcinoma of the paranasal sinuses. Arch Otolaryngol 109:341–343, 1983.

92. Vokes E, Kies MS, Haraf D, et al: Concomitant chemoradiotherapy as primary therapy for locoregional advanced head and neck cancer. J Clin Oncol 18:1652–1661, 2000.

93. Wendt TG, Grabenbauer GG, Rodel CM, et al: Simultaneous radiochemotherapy versus radiotherapy alone in advanced head and neck cancer: a randomized multicenter study. J Clin Oncol 16:1318–1324, 1998.

94. Zheng W, McLaughlin JK, Chow WH, et al: Risk factors for cancers of the nasal cavity and paranasal sinuses among white men in the United States. Am J Epidemiol 138:965–972, 1993.

CHAPTER 51

CRANIOPHARYNGIOMA

Tetsuo Kanno

Craniopharyngiomas are benign tumors of the central nervous system. These tumors, which arise from the squamous epithelial cell rests in Rathke's cleft, are commonly located in the suprasellar region. However, in rare cases they can occupy intrasellar or intraventricular locations. The tumors can be cystic, solid, or of a mixed type.

Craniopharyngioma accounts for 6% to 9% of all brain tumors in children and 3% of all brain tumors in adults. It is the most common suprasellar tumor in children. Age distribution of craniopharyngioma shows a bimodal pattern, with one peak at 5 to 10 years and the second at 50 to 60 years.

CLINICAL FEATURES

The classic clinical triad in children is hypothyroidism, hypogonadism, and growth retardation. Adults may have visual disturbance. Examination often reveals bitemporal hemianopia caused by chiasmal involvement. It can also cause raised intracranial pressure or hydrocephalus.

IMAGING

Plain Skull X-Ray

Sella turcica in children may show saucer-like erosion. Fleck-like calcification in the suprasellar area favors the diagnosis of craniopharyngioma.

Computed Tomography

Computed tomography (CT) scans of the head (Figure 51-1) can demonstrate solid and cystic portions of tumor. It may also demonstrate areas of calcification, which were not visible on plain x-ray studies. Cystic regions appear as hypodense or isodense areas in plain CT scans. The cyst wall and the solid parts of the tumor may show enhancement with contrast administration.

Even though differentiating it from pituitary adenoma is not very difficult, other low-density lesions like Rathke's cleft cyst, epidermoid tumor, or arachnoid cyst may closely resemble craniopharyngioma.

Magnetic Resonance Imaging

Magnetic resonance imaging (MRI) can show the relation between the tumor and its surrounding tissues such as pituitary stalk, pituitary gland, chiasm, internal carotid artery, and anterior cerebral artery (Figure 51-2). The solid part of the tumor shows slight hypointensity or isointensity on T2-weighted images and is enhanced after administration of contrast agent (gadolinium). The cystic part is often heterointense, which varies from hypointense to isointense in T1-weighted images, and it is hyperintense to cerebrospinal fluid (CSF) in T2-weighted images. Calcification and destruction of the sella is better visualized in CT scans.

TUMOR HISTOLOGY

The solid, cystic, and mixed types of craniopharyngioma occur in the ratio of 1:4:2. Macroscopically, craniopharyngioma has a clear margin and can be separated from the surrounding tissues. The cyst contains the characteristic "motor oil" fluid. The cyst can reach huge proportions, extending to the subfrontal region, sylvian fissure, and posterior fossa. The solid part often has calcification.

Histologically, two types are described, the adamantinomatous and the squamous-papillary type. Sometimes the tumor invades the hypothalamus and produces gliosis in the surrounding tissues, which makes the surgery difficult and dangerous.

SURGICAL APPROACH

The choice of surgical approach depends on the location and extent of the tumor.

Bifrontal Craniotomy with a Subfrontal Subchiasmatic Approach

A bifrontal craniotomy with a subfrontal subchiasmatic approach is used when the tumor extends anteriorly, displacing the optic chiasm posteriorly and superiorly. A more basal approach can be added to this by performing an additional orbitozygomatic osteotomy unilaterally or bilaterally, thus avoiding frontal lobe retraction.

Fronto-Temporal Craniotomy

A fronto-temporal craniotomy is used when the craniopharyngioma displaces the chiasm anteriorly and superiorly. By a transsylvian approach, the tumor is removed through the optic carotid cistern. Addition of orbitozygomatic osteotomy and

385

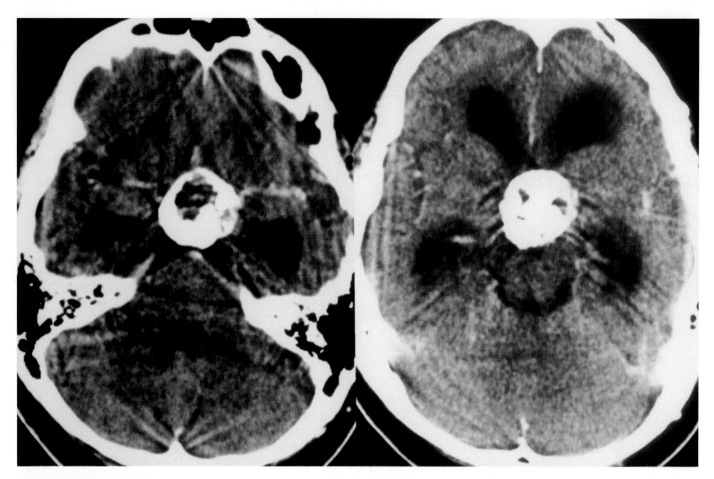

FIGURE 51-1   Computed tomography scan showing craniopharyngioma.

resection of the lesser wing of the sphenoid sinus minimizes the brain retraction.

Interhemispheric Transcallosal Approach

An interhemispheric transcallosal approach is used when the tumor occupies the third ventricle. This can be combined with a subfrontal translaminar terminalis approach.

Transsphenoidal Approach

A transsphenoidal approach is used in the rare instances of intrasellar craniopharyngiomas.

STRATEGY OF TREATMENT

The ideal treatment is total removal. This is possible in some cases of pediatric craniopharyngiomas. Total excision is often limited by the adherence of the tumor to the hypothalamus or the pituitary stalk, especially when it originates near these structures. Injury to the pituitary stalk or hypothalamus can lead to unacceptable complications, including diabetes insipidus. Leaving behind tumor remnants may lead to recurrence in the future.

The extension of tumor to adjacent regions is the other significant factor that determines treatment strategy. When the tumor extends to the posterior fossa and reaches the brainstem, attempts for total removal become hazardous. In cases where the tumor encases the perforating arteries to the brainstem or hypothalamus, total excision should be avoided. Presence of calcification need not be a significant factor influencing the strategy of total removal. However, total excision is difficult in most cases of recurrent craniopharyngiomas because of strong adhesions around the pituitary stalk and hypothalamus. Nevertheless, even in such cases it is usually possible to completely remove the tumor extensions to the posterior fossa or third ventricle. If previous surgery had involved insertion of an Ommaya tube, strong adhesions should be expected around the tube.

In cases of large multiloculated cystic lesions where total removal is precarious, insertion of an Ommaya tube, which has an extracranial reservoir, must be considered. Repeat CT and MRI scans are performed at 6 month intervals or less when the patient becomes symptomatic. If the cyst shows enlargement, the contents of the cyst are aspirated from the reservoir.

The Gamma Knife® is an adjuvant treatment modality when the excision is subtotal.[1] Local instillation of bleomycin through an Ommaya tube has been tried in pediatric craniopharyngiomas when the histology is of squamous type.[2]

RECURRENCE AND OUTCOME

The recurrence rate is almost 40% when the excision is subtotal or near total. Patients with craniopharyngioma merit a long-term and intensive follow-up. Survival rate at 5 years is 94.9%.

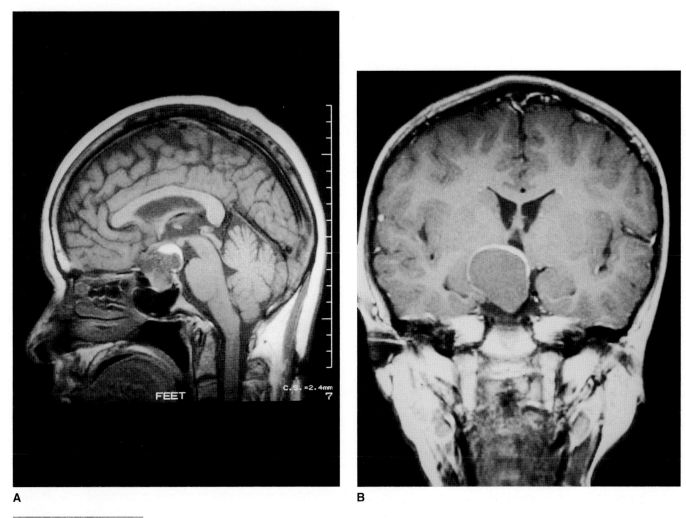

FIGURE 51-2 Magnetic resonance image showing craniopharyngioma. *A,* Sagittal view. *B,* Coronal view.

References

1. Jeffcott CR, Sugden EM, Foord T: Radiotherapy for cranio-pharyngioma in children: a national audit. Clin Oncol 15:10, 2003.

2. Mottolese C, Stan H, Hermier M, et al: Intracystic chemotherapy with bleomycin in the treatment of craniopharyngiomas. Childs Nerv Syst 17:724, 2001.

CHAPTER 52

EPIDERMOID TUMORS

Emad T. Aboud and Ali F. Krisht

Cushing said, "It's my impression that many of the cholesteatomas reported by otologists are true epidermoid tumors, which originate from aberrant epidermal rests laid down in the temporal bone during the early formation of the complicated special sense structure which it contains. Certainly all of the tumors which have a demonstrable epidermal membrane such as those encountered more often in the mastoid process and which reach a considerable size, are in all likelihood actual Cruveilhain tumor."[4]

Epidermoid tumors, the so-called pearly tumors, were first described by the French pathologist Cruveilhain in 1829. Confusion occurred when Muller (1838) proposed the term *cholesteatoma* to describe a tumor of the cranial bone containing masses of cholesterine. Other authors later found similarities with tissue formations related to chronic infections of the mastoid air cells and the middle ear compartment. In 1897 Bosteroem clarified the confusion by differentiating these infection-related epidermoid formations from the typical epidermoid tumors formed from misplaced epithelial rests during the early weeks of embryonic development. He also added that these embryonic rests can lead to either epidermoid or dermoid tumors.

The term *cholesteatoma* is generally used to refer to those inflammatory lesions appearing in the mastoid region and related to chronic middle ear infections. However, some epidermoid tumors are seen within the petrous bone. They are real epidermoid tumors even though they may overlap in their location with cholesteatomas arising from the mastoids and extending into the petrous bone.[11]

INCIDENCE

Epidermoid cysts are benign slow-growing tumors and account for 1.2% of all brain tumors. There is no sex or race predilection. Although epidermoid tumors are thought to arise from embryonic cell rests, patients become symptomatic later in life (age 20 to 40 years). By the time the tumors become symptomatic, and probably because of their slow growth rate, they have already achieved considerable size.

ORIGIN AND HISTOLOGY

Epidermoids are thought to develop as a result of the process of inclusion of ectodermal elements at the time of closure of the neural groove between the third and fifth week of embry-

onic life. Histologically, it is made up of stratified squamous epithelium with a whitish fibrous capsule containing cellular debris, including keratin and occasionally some lipid material (cholesterin) from cell membrane breakdown (Figure 52-1). The tumor is well circumscribed, and it can be smooth or lobulated. To the naked eye it has a white pearly appearance, which led Dandy to describe these tumors as the most beautiful tumors in the body (Figure 52-2A). Epidermoid tumors should be distinguished from dermoid tumors, which also result from congenital ectodermal inclusions. Dermoid inclusion cysts contain other dermal elements such as hair follicles, sebaceous glands, and sweat glands. They are mostly midline and usually accompanied by a dermal sinus. Epidermoid tumors are considered benign tumors. They rarely present with histologically malignant features.

GROWTH AND LOCATION

Epidermoid tumors tend to enlarge as epithelial cells desquamate, with the formation of keratin and cholesterol crystals. They tend to become widespread by insinuating themselves within the subarachnoid cisterns and tend to encircle cranial nerves and blood vessels.[15]

They may spread around the brainstem, and they may become very adherent to its surface. This is thought to be a result of the inflammatory process that occurs secondary to the tumor's producing cholesterol crystal, which can lead to aseptic meningitis. The most common location is the cerebellopontine angle, followed by the parasellar and suprasellar regions. They can occur anywhere within the intracranial cavity, including the middle fossa (rarely in the cavernous sinus),[5] intraventricularly,[3] intracerebrally,[8] within the brainstem,[7] or within Meckel's cave.[9]

CLINICAL PRESENTATION

The clinical picture of patients with epidermoid tumors depends on the location and the size of the mass. In general, the main presenting symptoms are related to cranial nerve deficits. Other symptoms and signs include headache, diplopia, trigeminal neuralgia, and gait ataxia.

NEUROIMAGING

Epidermoid tumors usually appear as low-density tumors on computerized tomography (CT) scans (Figure 52-3A). When

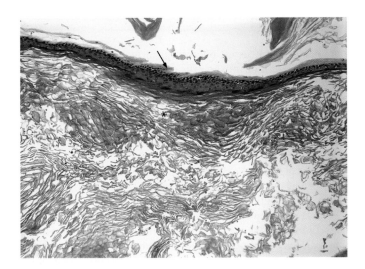

FIGURE 52-1 Histology slide shows the stratified squamous epithelium *(arrow)* surrounding the laminated keratin *(*).*

rounded, they may resemble arachnoid cysts filled with cerebrospinal fluid (CSF). On magnetic resonance imaging (MRI) they have low signal intensity on T1-weighted images (Figure 52-3B) and high signal intensity on T2-weighted images (Figure 52-3C), with no or minimal marginal enhancement seen.[10]

Calcifications are rarely seen. The mechanism of marginal enhancement, when present, is thought to be peritumoral changes in the tissues secondary to leakage of irritating cyst contents and secondary to the chemical inflammation. Handa et al suggest that, together, the inflammatory changes and compressed vessels around the tumor may account for the marginal enhancement-like picture simulating an enhancing capsule.[6] Some authors consider contrast enhancement to be very abnormal for epidermoids and suggest a malignant epithelial component.[13]

Radiologic follow-up evaluations and the confirmation of recurrence can prove difficult. This is because the tumor cavity fills with CSF and appears similar to the original tumor. Diffusion-weighted MRI has been found to be helpful in distin-

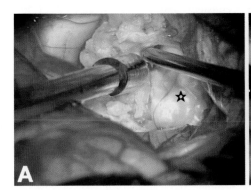
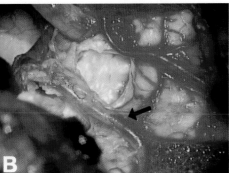

FIGURE 52-2 *A,* Intraoperative picture of epidermoid tumor *(*).* Notice its pearly white appearance. *B,* Notice the skeletonized blood vessel to which the tumor was attached *(arrow).*

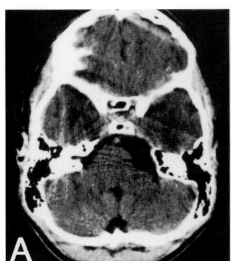
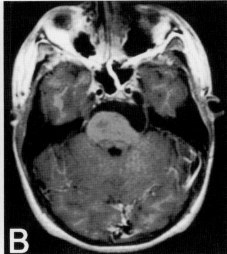
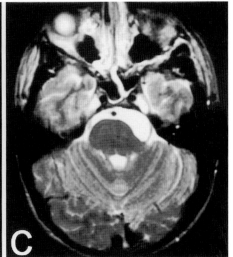

FIGURE 52-3 *A,* Computed tomography scan. Left prepontine cistern looks wide, but it was filled with an epidermoid tumor causing mass effect on the left side of the brainstem. The tumor also extends into the cerebellopontine angle. *B,* T1-weighted magnetic resonance (MR) image with gadolinium enhancement of the same tumor showing no enhancement of the hypointense tumor. *C,* T2-weighted MR image showing the same lesion with hyperintensity similar to cerebrospinal fluid.

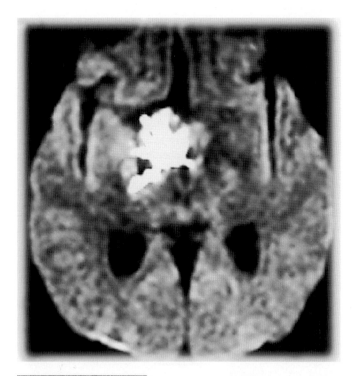

FIGURE 52-4   Diffusion-weighted magnetic resonance image shows the characteristic high signal intensity of the tumor compared with the low signal intensity of cerebrospinal fluid.

guishing between arachnoid cysts and epidermoid cysts or tumors. Although epidermoid tumors resemble CSF in T1- and T2-weighted images, they appear hyperintense on diffusion-weighted MRI, unlike CSF, which is hypointense (Figure 52-4). This is the best way to distinguish between epidermoid tumors and arachnoid cysts and help detect tumor recurrence.[12]

TREATMENT

Surgical excision using microsurgical techniques is the only treatment option of proven efficacy in the treatment of epidermoid tumors. Because it is the best option, surgery should aim at complete surgical removal with the first attempt. This is best achieved by attempting to remove the tumor capsule during the surgical excision by establishing a wide and optimal exposure that can enhance the ability to deliver the most distal portions of the tumor capsule into the surgical field.[14]

After piecemeal reduction of the mass, the capsule is teased free of adjacent neurovascular structures. In the majority of cases a plane of dissection can be established between the capsule and the underlying arachnoid (see Figure 52-2B). Occasionally, dense adhesions as a result of the inflammatory process make this task very difficult and more demanding. This should not compromise the goal of achieving radical resection, but neither should the surgeon risk injury to the adjacent neurovascular structures, especially the perforator vessels and the cranial nerves.

There is some controversy regarding the benefit related to the extent of tumor removal. Earlier, some authors believed that removing the contents with only partial removal of the capsule is enough.[1] Others consider that complete removal of the capsule is unwise and should be avoided.[2] More recent advances in microsurgical techniques and better understanding of the surgical anatomy led to better outcomes and a stronger belief that radical excision is possible in the majority of patients.[15] Because treating recurrence is much more challenging surgically, complete removal of the tumor and the capsule at the initial surgery is the only way to avoid recurrence. This is especially challenging when the capsule is the living part of the tumor.

The long-term outcome for patients with intracranial epidermoid tumors is directly related to the extent of surgical removal achieved with their first surgery. They are benign and potentially curable lesions. With successful radical surgical removal, life expectancy should not be affected.

References

1. Baumann CHH, Bucy PC: Paratrigeminal epidermoid tumors. J Neurosurg 13:455–467, 1956.
2. Berger MS, Wilson CB: Epidermoid cysts of the posterior fossa. J Neurosurg 62:214–219, 1985.
3. Bugeard R, Mahala K, Roche PH, et al: Epidermoid cysts of the lateral ventricles. Neuro-chirurgie 45:316–320, 1999.
4. Cushing, H: A large epidermal cholestiatoma of the parieto-temporal region deforming the left hemisphere without cerebral symptoms. Surg Genec Obstet 34:557–566, 1922.
5. Dufour H, Fuentes S, Metellus P, Grisoli F: Intracavernous epidermoid cysts: case report and review literature. Neuro-chirurgie. 47:55–59, 2001.
6. Handa J, Okamoto K, Nadasu Y, et al: Computed tomography of intracranial epidermoid tumors with special reference to atypical features. Acta Neurochir (Wien) 58:221–228, 1981.
7. Kachhara R, Bhattacharya RN, Radhakrishnan VV: Epidermoid cyst involving the brain stem. Acta Neurochir (Wien) 142:97–100, 2000.
8. Laconita G, Carvalho GA, Samii VP: Intracranial epidermoid tumor: a case report and review of the literature. Surg Neurol 55:218–222, 2001.
9. Miyazawa N, Yamazaki H, Wakao T, Nukui H: Epidermoid tumors of Meckel's cave: case report and review of literature. Neurosurgery 25:951–955, 1989.
10. Olson JJ, Beck DW, Crawford SC, Menezes AH: Comparative evaluation of intracranial epidermoid tumors with computed tomography and magnetic resonance imaging. Neurosurgery 21:357–361, 1987.
11. Oprador S, Lopez-Zafra JJ: Clinical features of the epidermoids of the basal cisterns of the brain. J Neurol Neurosurg Psychiat 32:450–454, 1969.
12. Samii M, Tatagiba M, Pose J, Carvalho GA: Surgical treatment of epidermoid cysts of the cerebellopontine angle. J Neurosurg 84:14–19, 1996.
13. Takeshita M, Kubo O, Tajika Y, et al: Immunohistochemical detection of carbohydrate determinant 19–9 (CA19–9) in intracranial epidermoid and dermoid cysts. Surg Neurol 40:284–288, 1993.
14. Talacchi A, Sala F, Alessandrini F, et al: Assessment and surgical management of posterior fossa epidermoid tumors: report of 28 cases. Neurosurgery 42:242–252, 1998.
15. Yazargil MG, Abernathey CD, Sarioglu AC: Microneurosurgical treatment of intracranial dermoid and epidermoid tumors. Neurosurgery 24:561–567, 1989.

SECTION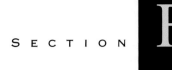

METASTASES TO
THE BRAIN

Section Editor
Raymond Sawaya

CHAPTER 53

BRAIN METASTASIS FROM NON–SMALL CELL LUNG CANCER

Adam N. Mamelak, Fredric Grannis, Robert Morgan, Jr., and Richard D. Pezner

Brain metastases from tumors arising outside the central nervous system are exceptionally common. There are an estimated 75,000 to 100,000 cases of brain metastasis each year in the United States. Approximately 30% to 60% of all brain metastases originate in a primary lung cancer. In light of the marked frequency with which this illness is encountered in general oncology practice, a thorough understanding of the principles of diagnosis and treatment is essential for all practitioners.

Lung cancers are primarily classified as either small cell or non–small cell lung cancer (NSCLC), with NSCLC representing more than 80% of cases. These two classes each have a distinct biologic activity and response to various forms of therapy and should therefore be considered as distinct entities from a clinical perspective. Only NSCLC will be considered in this chapter.

EPIDEMIOLOGIC OVERVIEW

NSCLC is the most common form of lung cancer. It is the leading cause of cancer-related deaths in the United States for both men and women and is estimated to cause 160,000 deaths per year.[10] Although the incidence of new cases of lung cancer for men appears to be at a plateau of 80 cases per 100,000 people, the incidence among women is rising, presumably because of increased smoking by women. Eight-seven percent of lung cancer cases are related to smoking, with a strong correlation between the amount of tobacco exposure and the risk of developing lung cancer. Approximately 33% of patients with NSCLC develop metastases to the brain during the course of their disease.

PATHOLOGIC OVERVIEW

NSCLC represents a heterogeneous group of tumors. Adenocarcinoma accounts for approximately 40% of cases, whereas squamous cell tumors represent approximately 30%; large cell cancer, bronchioloalveolar, and other uncommon varieties make up the remainder of cases. In addition to these general categories, some NSCLCs contain a mixture of tumor types, including small cell and neuroendocrine varieties, which can make pathologic diagnosis and selection of treatment strategies more difficult.

NON–SMALL CELL LUNG CANCER STAGING

Metastatic spread of NSCLC is very common, with bone, adrenal, and brain being the most common sites.[14] Brain metastases occur in approximately 33% of patients. Solitary metastases are noted in approximately 30% of cases. NSCLC stages are typically designated I to IV, including subsets IIA, IIB, IIIA, and IIIB. Staging is determined using standard tumor, node, and metastasis (T, N, M) criteria. The extent of staging tests performed depends on a number of factors, including the presenting symptoms, the extent of disease, and the exact tumor type. A thorough medical history and physical examination are the most important steps in the staging and subsequent work-up of a patient with suspected lung cancer. Clinical symptoms suggestive of brain metastasis include headache, seizures, or focal neurologic deficits. If a thorough medical history and physical examination demonstrate no evidence of extrapulmonary metastases, and a chest computed tomography (CT) scan suggests a localized disease process, patients are considered clinical stage I or II. Such patients do not necessarily require a full metastatic work-up. Patients with clinical evidence of either nodal or distant metastases (stages III or IV) require a full metastatic work-up, including a body CT scan, a bone scan, and typically a brain CT scan or magnetic resonance imaging (MRI) study. More recently, positron-emission tomography (PET) scans have been used to facilitate screening and assessment for disease, because this technique appears to have greater sensitivity for smaller disease burdens, and an entire body can be screened in a single study. All patients with metastases outside of the thorax are considered stage IV, including all patients harboring brain metastases regardless of the number of lesions identified.

Patients with stage IV lung cancer have very poor long-term survival or cure rates, with a 1-year actuarial survival of 10% to 20%.[15] Recent chemotherapy trials have demonstrated 1-year survival rates of up to 40%, although these patients represent a reasonably select group of patients and may not be representative of the general population of stage IV patients. Regardless, most people with brain metastases have a poor long-term prognosis, and this factor must be carefully considered when determining treatment strategies for individual patients.

SYNCHRONOUS VERSUS METACHRONOUS METASTASES FROM NON-SMALL CELL LUNG CANCER

When evaluating a patient with suspected brain metastases, consideration must be given to whether the metastases were identified at the same time that the lung tumor was identified (synchronous), or at a chronologically different time (metachronous). Some authors express pessimism regarding the treatment of NSCLC when synchronous brain metastases are present. A retrospective review of 74 patients treated at the University of Pennsylvania demonstrated that median and 5-year survivals were better in patients with metachronous brain metastases (18 months and 28.9%, respectively) than in patients with synchronous brain metastases (9.9 months and 0%, respectively). In contrast, in a series of 185 consecutive patients at Memorial Sloan-Kettering Hospital who underwent resection of brain metastases, there was no difference in 5-year survival between patients with synchronous ($n = 65$) and metachronous ($n = 120$) lesions or between T and N groups.[4] Thirteen percent survived for 5 years and seven percent lived more than 10 years. They concluded that complete resection in both the brain and the lung was the most important factor in long-term survival.

ROLE OF BRAIN IMAGING BEFORE LUNG RESECTION

Most patients with stage IV cancer are not considered surgical candidates with regard to their lung tumors. There is little debate as to the benefit of brain imaging in patients exhibiting neurologic signs or symptoms suggesting a brain metastasis. The role of such imaging in asymptomatic patients is more difficult to define. One important consideration is that the discovery of an asymptomatic brain metastasis will often direct lung cancer therapy away from curative and toward palliative

modalities. This raises the question of whether all patients with lung cancer should undergo brain imaging before surgery on the lung primary. A review of recent literature yields somewhat ambiguous results.

Several studies support the idea that routine imaging should only be performed in symptomatic patients. For example, a meta-analysis of 16 studies of potentially operable (with regard to the primary lung tumor) NSCLC patients indicated that brain metastases were found in only 3.3% (26 : 785).[7] Similar analyses corroborate these findings and indicate that routine imaging has little impact on overall survival or symptom management.

Other studies point in favor of these examinations. A review of 184 patients with NSCLC who underwent preoperative cranial CT scans identified 23 brain metastases (12.5%), of which 64% were asymptomatic.[5] At the Mayo Clinic 20.6% of asymptomatic patients with NSCLC lesions larger than 3 cm in greatest diameter had occult brain metastasis discovered by contrast-enhanced MRI. Similarly, a prospective randomized study of clinical examination versus radiographic scanning performed by the Canadian Lung Oncology Group demonstrated a statistically significant reduction in unnecessary thoracotomy and a cost saving of $823 per patient for patients who had radiographic screening. Of note, although 18-deoxyglucose PET scanning is now widely used to help stage NSCLC, it has limited use in detecting small brain metastases because of the normal uptake of glucose in the brain that leads to loss of contrast between metastasis and normal brain tissue.

The current recommendation of the National Comprehensive Cancer Network (NCCN) is that all asymptomatic patients in clinical stage IIB or higher after initial work-up of NSCLC, as well as all patients with neurologic symptoms, have cranial MRI performed before initiating definitive therapy.

ROLE OF BRAIN IMAGING IN POST-THORACOTOMY TUMOR SURVEILLANCE

It is reasonable to assume that the success of treatment of brain metastasis will be higher when such lesions are discovered at an early stage. This raises the question of whether post-thoracotomy surveillance is effective. Saitoh reported on a group of 24 patients with resection of a solitary brain metastasis after resection of the primary lung tumor. Survival was 8.3% at 5 years. Patients with an interval longer than 1 year between initial diagnosis and metastasis, a primary tumor less than 5 cm in maximal diameter, and lobectomy had better outcomes.[16] Actuarial 5-year survival was 19% in a group of patients with metachronous solitary brain metastasis. No patient with N_1 to N_2 disease survived for 2 years. Patients in a subgroup with N_0 disease and an interval of more than 14.5 months had a survival of 61%.[11] These and similar studies suggest, but do not definitively prove, that surveillance brain imaging may improve survival in patients initially seeking treatment for stage I or II disease.

TREATMENT OPTIONS FOR PATIENTS WITH BRAIN METASTASES

Because of the very poor long-term survival rates in patients with stage IV NSCLC, the management of patients with brain metastasis is largely palliative, aimed at prolonging life, improving quality of life, or diminishing neurologic symptoms. The palliative nature of this care must be taken into consideration when weighing the treatment options available.

The decision matrix for patients with identified brain metastasis depends on a large number of factors, including extent of disease within the lungs, the extent of extrathoracic systemic disease, the number of metastases identified, the location of these metastases, patient age, and functional status. Furthermore, this decision-making process must include the expected intent of any intervention and anticipated side effects and efficacy of the treatment. In an effort to clarify the decision-making process, a review of all treatment strategies as well as a basic understanding of the anticipated response of these treatments with regard to intracranial and systemic disease is useful. In evaluating the literature on this subject, one must keep in mind that the majority of publications dealing with brain metastases include multiple tumor types, although NSCLC typically represents 40% to 70% of these cases.

MEDICAL MANAGEMENT

Medical management of patients with NSCLC brain metastasis is primarily aimed at temporarily relieving symptoms attributable to the brain metastases. This falls into two broad categories: (1) reducing mass effect because of tumor burden or vasogenic edema and (2) preventing seizures. Corticosteroids are widely used to diminish the effects of vasogenic edema associated with brain metastases. When metastases induce neurologic deficits, a course of steroids is often very effective in diminishing or eliminating these symptoms until more definitive therapy is undertaken. Typical doses in the range of 8 to 32 mg of dexamethasone in divided daily doses are used. Higher doses are often employed before initiating more definitive therapy such as surgery or radiation. Steroids are often continued for several weeks or longer after treatment. In some situations patients become "steroid dependent," requiring low to moderate doses to maintain neurologic function. In these situations patients must be carefully counseled and monitored as to the negative side effects of steroid use such as demineralization of bone, significant weight gain, easy bruisability, and other signs of hypercortisolism.

Seizure is an initial symptom of brain metastasis in an estimated 20% to 45% of patients. In these patients anticonvulsants are administered and often maintained for an extended time, often for the patient's life. A wide variety of anticonvulsants are available for use, and a detailed description is beyond the scope of this chapter. Much greater controversy exists regarding the role of anticonvulsants for seizure prophylaxis. It is common practice for physicians to employ the use of anticonvulsants to prevent seizures in patients with brain metastases. Multiple retrospective studies and at least three prospective studies have attempted to determine whether anticonvulsants have a prophylactic role in preventing seizures. None of these studies have demonstrated benefit from the use of anticonvulsants.[2] In contrast, 25% to 40% of all patients on anticonvulsants will develop a toxic side effect such as rash, dizziness, or somnolence. A small percentage of patients can experience life-threatening reactions such as Stevens-Johnson syndrome. In light of the lack of proved benefit and the high chance for toxic side effects, it is our practice to not employ anticonvulsants for seizure prophylaxis.

SURGICAL MANAGEMENT

Surgical removal of brain metastases remains a significant and viable treatment option for many patients with metastatic NSCLC. Surgery is considered in two main scenarios. The first situation involves the patient with a solitary brain metastasis. Surgical resection of the solitary brain metastasis can significantly improve long-term survival, even in situations when whole-brain radiation therapy (WBRT) is withheld. A landmark study by Patchell et al demonstrated that patients with solitary brain metastases who underwent surgical resection followed by WBRT had an improved survival rate relative to patients who received WBRT alone (8 to 9 months with surgery plus WBRT vs. 3 to 4 months with WBRT alone).[13] Several other studies have confirmed these findings. When these analyses have been limited to patients with NSCLC, similar results have been demonstrated. Furthermore, in patients with an isolated brain metastasis and no other signs of systemic disease, solitary resection of a single brain metastasis followed by WBRT can significantly improve long-term survival. Approximately 10% to 20% of these patients will survive for 5 years or more. Exclusion criteria include expected survival of less than 3 months, inability to tolerate surgery, patient refusal of surgery, or evidence of leptomeningeal disease.

The option of surgery should also be entertained in situations in which a solitary lesion is causing significant mass effect, edema, or neurologic deficit, even in the face of other asymptomatic cranial metastases. In these situations the goals of surgery are to reduce mass effect, restore cerebrospinal fluid (CSF) pathways, and improve neurologic function or quality of life. Surgery can often be performed with minimal morbidity and short hospital stays.

The location of brain metastases roughly parallels the size of the various brain compartments, with two thirds being found in the supratentorial compartment and one third in the infratentorial compartment. Surgery can be considered for tumors located in the cerebral hemispheres, cerebellar hemispheres, or ventricular system. It is only rarely indicated for tumors located in the basal ganglia, thalamus, or brainstem.

Our experience with the resection of solitary brain metastasis has been quite gratifying. Using frameless or frame-based stereotaxy, the overwhelming majority of metastases can be removed through very small craniotomies with low morbidity and short inpatient stays (mean 1.75 days). In our experience of more than 85 solitary NSCLC resections there have been no deaths, one reoperation for postoperative epidural hematoma, and new permanent neurologic deficits in less than 3% of patients. Even in tumors within or directly adjacent to areas of eloquent cortex, the well-defined nature of many of these lesions will often permit aggressive surgical resection without damaging the surrounding cortex.

SURGERY FOR MULTIPLE METASTASES

Surgery plays a significantly reduced role in patients harboring multiple intracranial metastases. However, the presence of multiple lesions does not automatically exclude patients from surgery. Several studies have indicated that surgical excision of two or more metastases can result in survival outcomes similar to those seen for resection of solitary metastases. With the widespread availability of frameless stereotaxy, the removal of multiple metastases via one or more craniotomies in a single setting is technically feasible. Nonetheless, surgery for patients with multiple metastases should be approached with much greater caution than surgery for solitary metastases. In our institution, surgery for multiple NSCLC metastases is generally considered only if the systemic disease is extremely limited or absent and there is a potential for cure with surgical resection.

SYNCHRONOUS BRAIN METASTASIS AND ISOLATED THORACIC DISEASE

Surgery should play a prominent role in the patient with NSCLC harboring a solitary brain metastasis and a resectable pulmonary lesion. Several well-designed studies support this view, demonstrating a 2 to 3 year median survival in 11% to 15% of patients, and in selected cases (N_0 disease) even better results. For example, in 103 French patients undergoing both brain and lung resection for NSCLC with synchronous brain metastasis, 5-year survival was 11%.[3] They concluded that it was reasonable to complete lung resection in patients after resection of brain metastasis when there is a small primary tumor and an absence of lymph node metastasis. Similar studies conclude that surgical resection of both the brain and lung disease provides one of the only opportunities for long-term survival or cure and should therefore be considered whenever feasible.

The role of surgery can also be critical in the case of an asymptomatic brain mass identified as part of the initial staging work-up for a patient with newly documented lung cancer. Because asymptomatic intracranial meningioma and other benign neoplasms may be discovered on any screening CT or MRI scan, it would be imprudent to assume that a solitary lesion identified in a patient with lung cancer is necessarily metastatic. In this situation there may be a role for surgery to define the pathologic nature of the intracranial lesion, in addition to any therapeutic benefit derived from surgical resection. We have seen several cases in which a presumptive brain metastasis has been excised, only to discover that this lesion was a meningioma. Conversely, we have operated on several patients with presumptive meningioma that has turned out to be metastatic carcinoma. Failure to adhere to this principle may exclude some stage I or II NSCLC patients from curative surgery or, conversely, expose some patients with benign neoplasms to unnecessary radiation therapy.

WHOLE-BRAIN RADIATION THERAPY

For several decades, WBRT has been the most commonly used treatment for patients with NSCLC brain metastases. Unlike surgery, WBRT can be used for patients with multiple brain metastases or a poor Karnofsky Performance Scale (KPS) score. Treatment takes only a few minutes a day. Side effects are typically minimal or absent, particularly for patients already taking dexamethasone for symptom relief.

The combination of WBRT and corticosteroid administration will produce significant symptom relief for 47% to 52% of patients. A broad range of radiation dose schedules has been used, all with relative equivalence in symptom relief and survival. A dose schedule of 30 Gy in 10 fractions over 2 weeks has become widely used. Shorter schedules using higher doses per fraction may be appropriate for patients who have a poor KPS score or who live far from the radiation oncology facility. Although symptoms will be significantly relieved in most patients, long-term tumor control is uncommon with these dose schedules. More aggressive dose schedules have not been shown to be more effective.

NSCLC patients with brain metastases have a median survival time of 3 to 7 months, depending on ambulatory status, primary tumor control, and presence of extracranial metastases.[9] Increased age, decreased KPS score, and more extensive extracranial disease all predict a worse response to therapy. In predicting the prognosis, KPS score should be based on the patient's status after a response to steroids.[9] WBRT yielded a median survival of 28 weeks for lung cancer patients who were ambulatory, had a primary tumor that was controlled, and had no evidence of extracranial metastases.

WBRT has also been used as adjuvant postoperative treatment following resection of brain metastases. The treatment goal is to eliminate residual disease in the tumor bed and occult metastases elsewhere in the brain. In a prospective randomized study, postoperative WBRT reduced the frequency of intracranial relapse.[12] Patients treated by resection alone had a tumor bed local control failure rate of 46% and an intracranial metastasis relapse rate of 70%. In comparison, patients treated by resection and postoperative WBRT (50.4 Gy in 28 fractions) had a tumor local control failure rate of 10% and an intracranial relapse rate of 18%. There was no difference in median survival between the two arms, probably because of progression of uncontrollable extracranial disease.

The risk of radiation necrosis in the brain is less than 1% with commonly used WBRT dose schedules. Radiation-induced encephalopathy occurs in 2% to 18% of patients, although the majority of these cases develop 2 years after treatment. White matter changes can occur with radiation therapy alone, although most patients with such effects received far higher total radiation doses (>50 Gy) or daily doses (>3 Gy) than routinely used for brain metastases.

STEREOTACTIC RADIOSURGERY

Stereotactic radiosurgery (SRS) has changed the paradigm of treatment of brain metastases. SRS delivers a large dose of radiation to a small intracranial target with little radiation to the surrounding brain. Several different techniques have been used, with similar efficacy and complication rates for brain metastases. MRI is preferable to target the lesions, with MRI or CT fusion used for the highest degree of accuracy. A rigid head frame is used with most systems for targeting and to provide head immobilization with less than 1 mm of movement. Frameless mask immobilization can be used with an accuracy of less than 2 mm for alert, minimally symptomatic, cooperative patients with tumors exceeding 8 mm in diameter. Compared with rigid head frame immobilization, mask immobilization allows planning appointments to be spread out over several days at the convenience of the patient, good patient comfort for treatment, shortened treatment sessions (by treating different metastases on different days), and the opportunity for a fractionated dose schedule when indicated.

The single-fraction dose of SRS for brain metastases has ranged from 10 to 25 Gy, with most patients receiving 17 to 20 Gy. Slightly lower doses may be preferable for metastases in or adjacent to brainstem, optic chiasm, and optic nerves.

Tumor response (i.e., reduction in tumor size or cessation of tumor growth) occurs in 83% to 93% of NSCLC brain metastases treated with SRS. Local control rates for the treated lesion at 1 year are in the range of 61% to 86%. Median survival rates of 10 to 14 months were reported.[8,17] Patients with bronchogenic adenocarcinoma had slightly superior survival rates compared with patients with other NSCLC histologies, although this was not statistically significant on multivariate analysis. Patient's age, KPS score, status of primary tumor, and status of extracranial disease outweigh primary tumor site or histology as positive predictors of response to SRS.

For most SRS techniques, it is not possible to treat lesions greater than 3 to 4 cm in maximum dimension. Intensity-modulated radiation therapy (IMRT) can treat lesions up to 6 cm. However, there are limitations in treating larger lesions, including increased risk of radiation necrosis. Fractionation of the radiation into several sessions may reduce the risk of radiation brain necrosis for larger lesions.

Acute toxicity occurs in 5% to 18% of patients treated with SRS.[1] This may include headaches, nausea, vomiting, exacerbation of neurologic symptoms, and seizure. The symptoms can be controlled with corticosteroids and anticonvulsants. The risk of late symptomatic radiation necrosis is 2% to 6% in most reports. This is related to total dose and size of the target volume.[18]

STEREOTACTIC RADIOSURGERY WITHOUT WHOLE-BRAIN RADIATION THERAPY: AN EMERGING TREATMENT PARADIGM

The success of SRS for treating brain metastases has led an increasing number of physicians and patients to consider SRS alone as the initial radiotherapeutic treatment approach for selected patients with brain metastases.[19] This may be appropriate for patients with favorable prognostic factors. Because there would be no treatment of potential occult brain metastases, a higher rate of intracranial disease relapse would be expected in patients treated by SRS alone. However, close follow-up of these patients would allow appropriate WBRT or SRS intervention for subsequent brain metastases. Survival time of patients treated with SRS alone appears to be comparable with that of patients who were managed by WBRT with an SRS boost.

CHEMOTHERAPY

Chemotherapy is effective as palliative treatment of metastatic NSCLC and has been shown to prolong patients' survival and improve their overall quality of life compared with patients treated with supportive care alone. Platinum-based chemotherapeutic regimens are the most widely used for the management of systemic metastases. Response rates are moderate, with greater than 40% of patients demonstrating objective responses

to chemotherapy. Chemotherapy has, however, been thought to be of limited potential for the treatment of central nervous system metastases, because of the presence of the blood-brain barrier (BBB), which impedes the ability of chemotherapeutic agents to cross over into the central nervous system in effective concentrations. However, measurable cerebrospinal fluid (CSF) levels of multiple chemotherapeutic agents have been reported. Achievable CSF concentrations of cisplatin depend on the specific route of administration, with intra-arterial administration resulting in higher levels than intracarotid or intravenous dosing. Nonetheless, the labor-intensive and interventional nature of these procedures has generally limited their application to the research setting.

Until recently, chemotherapy has been used primarily in two situations: (1) as part of combined modality therapy with primary radiation, and (2) in the salvage setting after recurrence in patients who have previously received radiation therapy. Patients treated with systemic chemotherapy for brain metastases have had objective response rates of 14% to 35%, with symptomatic palliation noted in responding patients.[6] When stable disease is added, an overall clinical benefit has been reported in up to 52% of patients. Some studies suggest a benefit to the administration of chemotherapy in combination with radiation or after surgical resection of brain metastases. Other phase II trials of combination chemotherapy with radiation suggest improved overall response rates.

IMPLANTABLE CHEMOTHERAPEUTIC DEVICES

Implantable chemotherapy wafers containing 7.7 mg of carmustine (BCNU) per tablet have been developed and FDA approved for use in recurrent glioblastoma (Gliadel, Guilford Pharmaceuticals, Baltimore, Md.). Each eight-wafer dose delivers 61.6 mg of time-released BCNU over 4 to 6 weeks. Ongoing research studies are investigating the role of these wafers in the management of patients with metastatic carcinoma. The wafers can be implanted only into a tumor resection cavity, a fact that effectively limits this therapy to patients with solitary resectable brain metastases. The results of these trials will be necessary to define a possible role for implantable wafers in metastatic disease, but at present they do not appear to be superior to results achieved by solitary resection followed by WBRT.

SYSTEMATIC APPROACH TO THE PATIENT WITH NON-SMALL CELL LUNG CANCER BRAIN METASTASES

For the clinician treating a patient with NSCLC there are four basic clinical scenarios in which brain metastases occur. Diagnostic and treatment considerations vary considerably among these presentations.

Scenario One

Primary presentation with neurologic symptoms caused by the brain metastasis at a time when the lung cancer remains occult.

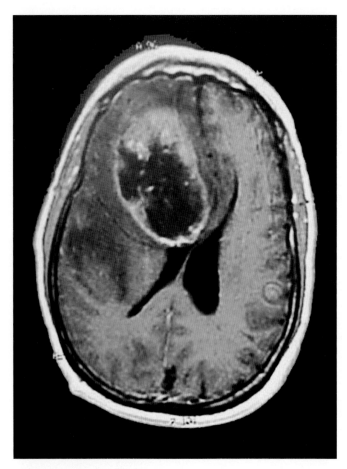

FIGURE 53-1   Large right frontal tumor causing neurological symptoms as the initial presentation of non–small cell lung cancer (NSCLC). Because of the tumor size, mass effect, and lack of a tissue diagnosis, a craniotomy was performed for tumor resection. The pathologic identification of NSCLC prompted a computed tomography scan of the chest, at which time the primary tumor was identified.

Illustrative Case

A 54-year-old male who smoked tobacco came to medical attention with altered mental status. An MRI scan revealed a right frontal lobe mass with vasogenic edema and significant mass effect (Figure 53-1). This was initially suspected to be a primary brain tumor based on appearance and the lack of a known malignancy. He underwent craniotomy and resection of a malignant tumor of the brain. The patient's neurologic symptoms resolved rapidly. Pathologic evaluation revealed NSCLC. Postoperative CT of the chest confirmed a pulmonary mass consistent with a bronchogenic carcinoma and a large pericardial effusion. Pericardial window was performed, with NSCLC cells identified in the effusion. He then received WBRT to 30 Gy in 10 sessions, radiation therapy to the lung tumor, and subsequent systemic chemotherapy.

Case Discussion

This case defines the patient with synchronous symptomatic brain metastasis in which the primary disease is occult at initial presentation. When the brain metastasis is symptomatic, the initial therapy is of necessity directed toward the brain lesion. After initiation of this therapy, consideration of treatment of the intrathoracic lung cancer is in order. Resection was performed because of the need to reduce mass effect rapidly and the lack of a tissue diagnosis. Curative treatment might be expected only in patients with no other metastases who have a resectable lung cancer. The patient must also have sufficient cardiopulmonary reserve to sustain the loss of the requisite extent of lung resection. Therefore after a potentially curative resection of the brain metastasis, a careful evaluation leading toward curative resection of the primary lung tumor or palliative treatment should be performed. Because this patient had a malignant pleural effusion, lung surgery was not performed, and palliative chemotherapy and radiation therapy were initiated.

Scenario Two

Primary presentation with pulmonary symptoms caused by the NSCLC in a patient with no symptoms of brain metastasis. The presumptive brain metastasis is discovered as part of the preoperative evaluation for lung cancer and is asymptomatic at time of discovery.

Illustrative Case

A 71-year-old white male who smoked experienced hemoptysis. The CT of the chest identified a mass in the right upper lobe of the lung and enlarged mediastinal lymph nodes in the pretracheal area. Because stage IIIA cancer was presumed, an MRI scan of the brain was performed. A lesion 2 cm in maximal diameter was found in the right frontal lobe, and a tumor 2.5 cm in maximal diameter was noted in the left insular cortex (Figure 53-2). A biopsy of the mediastinal lymph node and lung lesion demonstrated NSCLC. The patient was deemed unresectable because of the mediastinal lymph node findings. His brain lesions were not considered amenable to resection because of their location and multiplicity. He received SRS to a mean dose of 18 Gy to the two brain lesions plus WBRT to 30 Gy, along with irradiation to the lung fields. He began chemotherapy but died 8 months later from widespread metastatic disease.

Case Discussion

See the discussion for scenario three.

Scenario Three

Simultaneous presentation with pulmonary and neurologic symptoms in a patient with NSCLC and brain metastases.

Illustrative Case

A 56-year-old woman who was an ex-smoker was found to have a left lower lobe pulmonary mass 2 cm in maximal diameter. On careful questioning, the patient reported mild disequilibrium. An MRI scan of the brain revealed a solitary lesion 2.5 cm in maximal diameter in the left cerebellum. The remainder of the metastatic work-up revealed no evidence of disease. She underwent craniotomy for removal of the brain metastasis, followed by thoracotomy for resection of the lung primary. The

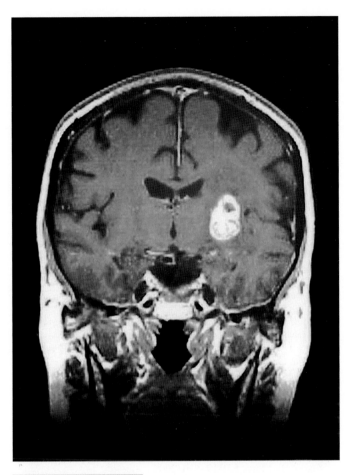

FIGURE 53-2 Metastatic non–small cell lung cancer (NSCLC) in a patient with multiple brain lesions and a synchronous primary lung lesion. Surgical resection was not considered because of the tumor's location and the multiplicity of lesions, as well as the lack of mass effect or neurologic symptoms. Stereotactic radiosurgery was employed for palliative tumor control.

pathology report revealed NSCLC. She received postoperative irradiation of the lung and brain. She remains disease free 5 years after her surgery.

Case Discussion

In both scenarios two and three, the questions that need to be addressed next in the management of the patient are whether there is a potential for long-term control of the brain tumor and whether there is a potential for long-term control of the primary lung cancer. If the answer in each case is yes, then the next steps are to determine the T and N status of the lung cancer and to determine the resectability of each neoplasm and the general medical status of the patient vis-à-vis the ability to undergo potentially curative treatment of both lesions. In scenario two, the presence of mediastinal lymph nodes rendered the chances for cure exceptionally low, and palliative treatment of the asymptomatic brain lesions with SRS and WBRT was employed. In scenario three, there was a 10% to 20% chance of long-term control or cure, so surgical resection of the brain tumor followed by WBRT was recommended.

Scenario Four

Neurologic symptoms develop during the postoperative follow-up care of a patient with NSCLC.

Illustrative Case

A 50-year-old white male developed headache and experienced a grand mal seizure 1 year after resection and radiation therapy for a right superior sulcus tumor. CT scan of the brain demonstrated a brain metastasis 3 cm in maximal diameter in the left temporal lobe. He was given anticonvulsants and steroids and offered the option of SRS or surgical resection. He opted for surgical resection. He received WBRT to 30 Gy in 10 fractions after surgery. He developed widespread metastases to the adrenal gland, bone, and lungs, and died 11 months later despite aggressive chemotherapy in a clinical trial.

Case Discussion

The group of patients with metachronous symptomatic metastases is probably the easiest to deal with. The stage is already known (stage IV), allowing a fairly accurate assessment of the possibility of recurrence at other sites. The interval between initial treatment of the primary tumor and discovery of brain metastasis also gives an indication of the chance of long-term cure. In patients who develop brain metastasis at some time after curative treatment, the first task is to complete a general evaluation to rule out local recurrence or other distant metastases. If this evaluation, including PET scan, reveals no other sites of metastasis and there is no significant comorbidity, then the next step is referral for neurosurgical and radiation oncology evaluation. The chance of cure depends on the initial stage and interval between treatment of the primary tumor and the brain metastasis and the brain metastases' size, location, and number. In contrast, if multiple systemic metastases are identified or numerous intracranial lesions defined, then greater emphasis will be directed toward short-term palliation with WBRT and, possibly, SRS or chemotherapy.

CONCLUSION

NSCLC remains one of the top killers in most of the world. Brain metastases are extremely common in patients with NSCLC. A variety of treatment options are now available for the management of the brain metastasis, including surgery, stereotactic radiosurgery, WBRT, chemotherapy, and experimental clinical trials. Although the majority of these interventions are palliative, they can have a significant impact on both the length of survival and quality of survival for patients with this devastating illness. When approaching the patient with a solitary metastasis from an NSCLC, the possibility for cure or long-term survival should always be kept in mind if there is no other evidence of metastatic disease and the primary lung lesion is amenable to surgical resection or already removed. Despite these treatment advances, smoking cessation remains the single most effective strategy for preventing deaths from NSCLC, soundly proving the adage that an ounce of prevention is worth a pound of cure.

References

1. Alexander E, Moriarty TM, Davis RB, et al: Stereotactic radiosurgery for the definitive, noninvasive treatment of brain metastases. J Natl Cancer Inst 87:34–40, 1995.
2. Batchelor T, DeAngelis LM: Medical management of cerebral metastases. Neurosurg Clin N Am 7:435–446, 1996.
3. Bonnette P, Puyo P, Gabriel C, et al: Surgical management of non-small cell lung cancer with synchronous brain metastases. Chest 119:1469–1475, 2001.
4. Burt M, Wronski M, Arbit E, et al: Resection of brain metastases from non-small-cell lung carcinoma. Results of therapy. Memorial Sloan-Kettering Cancer Center Thoracic Surgical Staff. J Thorac Cardiovasc Surg 103:399–410; discussion 410–391, 1992.
5. Ferrigno D, Buccheri, G: Cranial computed tomography as a part of the initial staging procedures for patients with non-small-cell lung cancer. Chest 106:1025–1029, 1994.
6. Franciosi V, Cocconi G, Michiara M, et al: Front-line chemotherapy with cisplatin and etoposide for patients with brain metastases from breast carcinoma, nonsmall cell lung carcinoma, or malignant melanoma: a prospective study. Cancer 85:1599–1605, 1999.
7. Hillers TK, Sauve MD, Gyatt GH: Analysis of published studies on the detection of extrathoracic metastases in patients presumed to have operable non-small cell lung cancer. Thorax 49:14–19, 1994.
8. Hoffman R, Sneed PK, McDermott MW, et al: Radiosurgery for brain metastases from primary lung carcinoma. Cancer J 7:121–131, 2001.
9. Lagerwaard FJ, Levendag PC, Nowak PJ, et al: Identification of prognostic factors in patients with brain metastases: a review of 1292 patients. Int J Radiat Oncol Biol Phys 43:795–803, 1999.
10. Landis SH, Murray T, Bolden S, et al: Cancer statistics, 1998. CA Cancer J Clin 48:6–29, 1998.
11. Mussi A, Pistolesi M, Lucchi M, et al: Resection of single brain metastasis in non-small-cell lung cancer: prognostic factors. J Thorac Cardiovasc Surg 112:146–153, 1996.
12. Patchell RA, Tibbs PA, Regine WF, et al: Postoperative radiotherapy in the treatment of single metastases to the brain: a randomized trial. JAMA 280:1485–1489, 1998.
13. Patchell RA, Tibbs PA, Walsh JW, et al: A randomized trial of surgery in the treatment of single metastases to the brain. N Engl J Med 322:494–500, 1990.
14. Quint LE, Tummala S, Brisson LJ, et al: Distribution of distant metastases from newly diagnosed non-small cell lung cancer. Ann Thorac Surg 62:246–250, 1996.
15. Riquet M, Manac'h D, Le Pimpec Barthes F, et al: Prognostic value of T and N in non small cell lung cancer three centimeters or less in diameter. Eur J Cardiothorac Surg 11:440–443; discussion 443–444, 1997.
16. Saitoh Y, Fujisawa T, Shiba M, et al: Prognostic factors in surgical treatment of solitary brain metastasis after resection of non-small-cell lung cancer. Lung Cancer 24:99–106, 1999.
17. Sanghavi SN, Miranpuri SS, Chappell R, et al: Radiosurgery for patients with brain metastases: a multi-institutional analysis, stratified by the RTOG recursive partitioning analysis method. Int J Radiat Oncol Biol Phys 51:426–434, 2001.
18. Shaw E, Scott C, Souhami L, et al: Single dose radiosurgical treatment of recurrent previously irradiated primary brain tumors and brain metastases: final report of RTOG protocol 90-05. Int J Radiation Oncol Biol Phys 47:291–298, 2000.
19. Sneed PK, Suh JH, Goetsch SJ, et al: A multi-institutional review of radiosurgery alone vs. radiosurgery with whole brain radiotherapy as the initial management of brain metastases. Int J Radiat Oncol Biol Phys 53:519–526, 2002.

CHAPTER 54

SMALL CELL LUNG CARCINOMA

Deborah T. Blumenthal, Gordon A. Watson, and Richard Wheeler

EPIDEMIOLOGY

The American Cancer Society has estimated that 173,770 new cases of lung cancer occurred in 2004 (93,110 in males and 80,660 in females), with 154,900 deaths.[2a] Lung cancers make up 14% of all cancer diagnoses.[22] Small cell lung cancer (SCLC) constitutes close to 25% (approximately 30,000 to 45,000 new cases per year in the United States) of new lung cancers.[22,41] Smoking remains the most significant risk factor for almost all cases of lung cancer. For SCLC in particular, smoking is implicated as a causative factor in up to 98% of cases.

SCLC is a cancer of epithelial origin. SCLC grows aggressively when untreated, with a shorter doubling time and higher frequency of metastases than non-SCLC. Most patients have metastatic disease at diagnosis, even in the absence of radiographically demonstrable lesions. The World Health Organization classification identifies three subtypes of SCLC: oat cell, intermediate, and combined small cell, mixed with adenocarcinoma or squamous cell carcinoma. Up to 30% of patients have combined SCLC and non-SCLC at autopsy, suggesting a common stem cell of origin that may differentiate along more than one path. Patients with the combined subtype have a better prognosis, most likely the result of more localized and resectable disease.

Patients with SCLC usually have one or more pulmonary symptoms, most commonly cough, wheezing, hemoptysis, obstructive pneumonia, or chest pain. Chest plain x-rays generally reveal a centrally located tumor with hilar and mediastinal adenopathy. Peripheral SCLC is rare. As many as 10% of patients have superior vena cava syndrome, which is not surprising given the tumor's propensity for central location and mediastinal involvement.[43] SCLC cells are submucosal but often can be identified by sputum cytology. Bronchoscopy is often sufficient to establish the diagnosis.

SCLC is associated with several paraneoplastic syndromes that are related to circulating polypeptides or antibodies. The syndrome of inappropriate antidiuretic hormone (SIADH) release may be seen in 11% of SCLC patients.[32] Cushing's syndrome is seen in 5% of SCLC patients and may portend a poorer prognosis.[45] These paraneoplastic syndromes are best treated by addressing the primary cancer. However, neurologic syndromes can persist or even progress despite successful treatment of the cancer.

Lambert-Eaton myasthenic syndrome (LEMS) is a paraneoplastic illness caused by impaired presynaptic release of acetylcholine from neurotransmitters at the neuromuscular junction. It is now known that autoantibodies to the P/Q type voltage-dependent calcium channel underly this syndrome. Although the syndrome affects less than 3% of SCLC patients, the diagnosis of LEMS is associated with SCLC in 50% to 70% of cases. Cases associated with cancer differ in terms of weight loss, male predominance, and older age at diagnosis.[16,50] About 16% of patients with SCLC produce a low titer of antineuronal antibody (anti-Hu) that can be asymptomatic and correlates with better cancer prognosis.[9,14] Less than 1% of patients with SCLC have a clinical paraneoplastic syndrome of encephalomyelitis and sensory ganglionopathy associated with this anti-Hu neuronal antibody in higher titers.[10]

STAGING

Although the conventional American Joint Committee on Cancer (AJCC) staging system for lung cancer is applicable to SCLC, a functional system of limited or extensive disease is generally employed. Limited SCLC is confined to one hemithorax (including the contralateral mediastinum) and may include ipsilateral supraclavicular node involvement. Patients with distant metastases or involvement of contralateral lymph nodes outside the mediastinum are classified as having extensive disease. Approximately one third of patients will have limited SCLC at diagnosis, with 60% to 70% having extensive disease.[1] Favorable prognostic factors include high performance status, female gender, and limited stage of disease, specifically absence of liver and brain metastases. Conversely, the metabolic abnormalities of elevated lactate dehydrogenase (LDH) and alkaline phosphatase and low sodium indicate a poor prognosis.[2] The central nervous system (CNS) is involved in up to 14% of SCLC cases at diagnosis; up to 30% of patients will develop CNS involvement during the course of their illness.[44] Bone, liver, and marrow are the most common sites of metastasis.[35]

The standard minimum evaluation should include a medical history (with careful neurologic review) and examination. Staging should include LDH and other blood tests and chest and abdominal computed tomography (CT). Bone marrow involvement without other sites of metastasis is rare; thus there is some controversy regarding the utility of bone marrow aspiration and biopsy when staging. A unilateral bone marrow examination may be appropriate in the setting of suspected limited-stage disease.

The usefulness of screening asymptomatic patients at diagnosis with brain CT or other cranial imaging is not clear. There is no evidence that asymptomatic patients whose SCLC brain metastases are diagnosed at screening have a more favorable prognosis than patients diagnosed by neurologic symptoms.[8] Median survival of patients with brain metastases as the only site of distant disease at diagnosis is similar to that observed in patients with other single sites of metastasis. There is a single report suggesting that patients with the brain as the only site of metastasis may survive as long as patients with limited-stage disease when treated aggressively.[13] However, magnetic resonance imaging (MRI) of the brain is a standard component of initial staging and is generally repeated in patients who achieve a complete response after induction chemotherapy. These patients will be candidates for prophylactic cranial irradiation (PCI). If prophylactic irradiation of the brain is planned, imaging should be performed beforehand, because discovery of metastases would indicate need for a higher dose of radiation therapy (RT).

In addition, SCLC patients with brain metastases are at increased risk for involvement of other areas of the CNS, including the leptomeninges, epidural space, or even intramedullary spinal cord.[34,37] Systemic chemotherapy has been reported to improve disease in patients with meningeal carcinomatosis.[48]

TREATMENT

SCLC differs from other lung cancers both in its aggressiveness when untreated and in its responsiveness to chemotherapy and radiation.[51] Surgery alone is not recommended, and a prospective, randomized trial for surgery following response to chemotherapy (cyclophosphamide, vincristine, and doxorubicin [CAV]) versus chemotherapy alone did not show a survival difference.[29]

Median survival time without treatment is only 6 to 12 weeks; however, median survival increases substantially with aggressive chemotherapy.[2] With current therapy, response rates are as high as 80% to 100% (50% to 70% complete responses [CR]) for patients with limited-stage disease, and 60% to 80% (up to 30% CR) for patients with extensive disease.[46] Patients with disease limited to the lung currently have a median survival time of 18 months and a 2-year survival rate of 25% when treated with chemotherapy and thoracic radiation. The median survival time for patients with extensive disease treated with chemotherapy alone is 9 to 12 months. In patients with limited disease, the 5-year survival rate is 7%, with relapses occurring 2 to 5 years after initial diagnosis. For patients with extensive-stage disease, the 5-year survival rate is only 1%. Those who have survived for 5 years without recurrence are generally considered cured. However, this is a population at risk for second malignancies.[24] These patients are at particularly high risk for a second smoking-related malignancy, usually non-SCLC (up to 4.4% per person per year, which is 10 times higher than the screening rate in smoking men). Hence aggressive counseling focused on smoking cessation is important.[25] The risk for non-neoplastic cardiovascular and pulmonary disorders is also increased as much as sixfold.[38]

Combination chemotherapy is the accepted first-line mode of treatment for SCLC. The most commonly used first-line chemotherapy agents are etoposide and cisplatin (EP). This combination seems to be superior to CAV. EP with early institution of concurrent thoracic radiation therapy is the treatment of choice for limited-stage disease.[11] Chest irradiation improves local control and survival in limited-stage disease, extending median survival time to 14 to 18 months.[39,46] Prior lung damage from cigarette smoking must be assessed during RT planning. SCLC can be so sensitive to radiation that resimulation of the treatment port is recommended once a week during a 3- to 5-week course of therapy. The standard dose to the involved thorax is 180 cGy daily or 150 cGy twice a day to a total dose of 450 cGy over 3 to 5 weeks when combined with chemotherapy. Chest radiation therapy begun concurrently with the first or, at the latest, the second cycle of chemotherapy appears to provide maximum benefit.[47]

The addition of irradiation to chemotherapy does not improve survival for patients with extensive disease. Recently published data from a Japanese phase III trial suggest an advantage to the combination of irinotecan and cisplatin over the standard EP regimen in patients with extensive disease.[36] Small trials of high-dose chemotherapy regimens with stem cell support have not led to a survival benefit and have produced a toxicity-associated mortality rate of 18%.[21] Chemotherapy for patients who have relapsed following initial treatment is beneficial in a minority. The median survival time following recurrence is only 4 months.[7] Response to treatment at relapse depends on the interval of recurrence. Recurrence less than 3 months after initial diagnosis is thought to indicate refractory disease and poor prognosis. Response rates for later recurrences are 20% to 50%. Topotecan may be a preferred second-line agent for patients initially treated with EP.[49]

BRAIN METASTASES

Brain metastases are diagnosed in up to 30% of patients with SCLC and found in 50% at autopsy.[18] Without CNS prophylactic treatment, the probability of brain metastases is 50% to 80% in SCLC 2-year survivors.[27] The prevalence of asymptomatic brain lesions at diagnosis may be as high as 15% in patients with normal neurologic findings, according to recent data using magnetic resonance imaging (MRI), which is more sensitive than CT.[19]

PROPHYLACTIC CRANIAL IRRADIATION

The high frequency of brain metastases in patients with SCLC has led to multiple evaluations of PCI. Randomized trials in the 1970s and 1980s evaluating the role of PCI for SCLC have consistently shown decreases in the rate of brain metastases but no clear improvement in survival. In a large, randomized trial of PCI (294 patients), Arriagada[3] showed a 45% incidence of brain metastases over 2 years in SCLC patients treated with 2400 cGy in eight fractions, versus a 67% recurrence rate in the nonirradiated control group. A trend toward improved survival was noted but was not statistically significant. Meta-analysis of individual data from seven randomized trials on 987 patients with SCLC in complete remission showed a reduction in relative risk of brain metastases to 0.46 with a 95% confidence interval of 0.38 to 0.57. PCI was also found, in meta-analysis, to impact overall survival (5.4% absolute survival advantage at 3 years in patients receiving PCI compared with controls:

15.3% versus 20.7%). The meta-analysis also discerned a trend toward decreased risk of brain metastases with earlier PCI following induction chemotherapy.[5]

These observations have been corroborated by other trials, which showed statistically significant results when comparing PCI after two to three cycles of chemotherapy with PCI following five to six cycles, which included patients with bone and bone marrow metastases.[31] The discrepancy between the significant reduction of brain metastases and the less significant effect on survival from PCI may be partially explained by the design of these trials. The studies defined brain involvement as an isolated first site of treatment failure but lacked the statistical power to show a difference in survival of approximately 5%, which was seen in the meta-analysis.

Radiation treatments in doses of 250 to 3750 cGy or 300 to 3000 cGy are used for patients with widespread systemic disease or more than three metastatic brain lesions. For patients with low systemic disease burden and fewer than three brain metastases, a dose of 200 to 4000 cGy or 250 to 3500 cGy is employed, with consideration of stereotactic radiosurgical boost.[20]

Complications from radiation sequelae, particularly with higher dose fractions (>300 cGy) and concurrent chemotherapy, have been cited as reasons for withholding PCI. Neurocognitive sequelae and ataxia in long-term survivors who have received PCI were most common in patients who received PCI concurrently with high-dose chemotherapy or in fractions of 400 cGy.[23] Prospective randomized trials using PCI doses of less than 3600 cGy have not shown significant neuropsychologic effects.[3,15] In a study of 283 SCLC patients from the Mayo Clinic, 17% of those who received PCI developed neurotoxicity, which increased to 37% in those who survived longer than 1.5 years. The mean time interval between PCI and neurologic sequelae was 17 months (range 2 to 63 months), with PCI doses of 2600 to 3600 cGy. Neurotoxicity was not seen in patients who did not receive prophylactic irradiation. The authors noted the possible synergistic role of lomustine, given in conjunction with radiation to the majority of their patients who received PCI, in causing toxicity.[12]

Patients with SCLC may also have significant neurocognitive deficits that are unrelated to their therapy. A study from The University of Texas M.D. Anderson Cancer Center found frontal lobe executive function, motor coordination, and verbal memory deficits in patients with SCLC to be no different between patients who underwent chemoradiation and newly diagnosed, untreated patients.[33] Causes of such deficits may include effects of heavy cigarette smoking or paraneoplastic effects.

The consensus regarding prophylactic irradiation for SCLC is that patients with limited-stage disease who have achieved a complete response following chemotherapy should have PCI. For patients with extensive disease, benefit from PCI is also likely if they have had complete response to induction chemotherapy. Brain metastases are more difficult to treat when they develop after induction or when treated as the initial metastatic site; in these cases, radiation must be used with therapeutic rather than prophylactic intent. Progression of brain metastases after radiation therapy in these cases is common,

with only 37% of patients free of tumor recurrence 1 year after a complete response to whole-brain radiation therapy (WBRT). Higher doses of radiation may produce improved response duration.[6]

Brain metastases typically occur within the first 2 years of disease diagnosis.[4] As many as 90% of brain metastases from SCLC are symptomatic. The risk of brain metastases increases with length of survival. Hence if PCI is not administered and as systemic chemotherapy and thoracic RT become more effective, we may see an increase in the frequency of subsequent brain metastases. Although the response rate of brain metastases to WBRT is 50%, patients with a complete remission nonetheless have a 50% chance of developing brain metastases within the next 2 years. Thus treatment of recognized metastases does not produce a cure.

The immediate response of symptoms from SCLC brain metastases to brain irradiation is 60% to 80%; however, the duration of this response is relatively short. The median survival time after diagnosis of brain metastases is 4 to 5 months. Although WBRT is considered standard treatment of brain metastases, there is evidence of efficacy for some chemotherapy regimens.[40,42] One study treated 14 patients with brain metastases, 4 of whom had the brain as their only metastatic site, with chemotherapy followed by WBRT with their fourth cycle. The median survival time was 34 weeks. Objective regression of brain lesions, mainly partial responses, was seen with chemotherapy. However, there also was significant toxicity caused by myelosuppression.[30]

A Mayo Clinic retrospective study of 30 patients with SCLC and the brain as the only site of metastasis at diagnosis reported a median survival of 14 months. Patients received 3600 to 4800 cGy of WBRT with cisplatin-based concomitant chemotherapy. There was a trend toward increased survival time for patients who also received thoracic radiation.[26]

Multiple metastases and additional extracranial metastases are poor prognostic factors.[17]

In summary, SCLC is an aggressively growing lung cancer that is highly sensitive to chemotherapy and radiation therapy treatments. A small percentage of patients with limited-stage disease at diagnosis have a chance of long-term survival. In patients with complete response to induction treatment, PCI seems to be of benefit. This preventive treatment is generally accepted, but there remains some controversy regarding its impact on overall survival and the deleterious effects of delayed neurocognitive sequelae from radiation in longer-term survivors.[28] It is clear that once brain metastases develop, unless as an isolated site of metastasis at diagnosis, salvage therapy will result in only short-term survival, underscoring the potential importance of preventive therapy.

Further research aimed at improving the treatment of brain metastases in SCLC should focus on changes in radiation dose and fractionation effect of preventive therapy to preserve neurocognitive status in patients who may go on to become long-term survivors. There may be utility in prophylactic chemotherapy protocols, possibly with agents that can permeate the blood-brain barrier. Targeted molecular therapies may also have a future role in the treatment and prevention of SCLC and brain metastases.

References

1. Abrams J, Doyle LA, Aisner J, et al: Staging, prognostic features, and special considerations in small cell lung cancer. Semin Oncol 15:261, 1988.

2. Albain KS, Crowley JJ, LeBlanc M, et al: Determinants of improved outcome in small-cell lung cancer: an analysis of the 2,580-patient Southwest Oncology Group data base. J Clin Oncol 8:1563–1574, 1990.

2a. American Cancer Society, Cancer Facts and Figures, 2004. ACS Publication 5008.04.

3. Arriagada R, Le Chevalier T, Borie F, et al: Prophylactic cranial irradiation for patients with small-cell lung cancer in complete remission. J Natl Cancer Inst 87:183–190, 1995.

4. Arriagada R, Le Chevalier T, Rivière A, et al: Patterns of failure after prophylactic cranial irradiation in small-cell lung cancer: analysis of 505 randomized patients. Ann Oncol 13:748–754, 2002.

5. Aupérin A, Arriagada R, Pignon J-P, et al: PCI for patients with small-cell lung cancer in complete remission. N Engl J Med 341:476–484, 1999.

6. Carmichael J, Crane JM, Bunn PA, et al: Results of therapeutic cranial irradiation in small cell lung cancer. Int J Radiat Oncol Biol Phys 14:455–459, 1988.

7. Chute JP, Chen T, Feigal E, et al: Twenty years of phase III trials for patients with extensive-stage small-cell lung cancer: perceptible progress. J Clin Oncol 17:1794–1801, 1999.

8. Crane JM, Nelson MJ, Ihde DC, et al: A comparison of computed tomography and radionuclide scanning for detection of brain metastases in small cell lung cancer. J Clin Oncol 2:1017–1024, 1984.

9. Dalmau J, Furneaux HM, Gralla RJ, et al: Detection of the anti-Hu antibody in the serum of patients with small cell lung cancer: a quantitative Western blot analysis. Ann Neurol 27:544–552, 1990.

10. Dalmau J, Graus F, Rosenblum MK, et al: Anti-Hu-associated paraneoplastic encephalomyelitis/sensory neuronopathy. A clinical study of 71 patients. Medicine 71:59–72, 1992.

11. Evans WK, Shepherd FA, Feld R, et al: VP-16 and cisplatin as first-line therapy for small-cell lung cancer. J Clin Oncol 3:1471–1477, 1985.

12. Frytak S, Shaw JN, O'Neill BP, et al: Leukoencephalopathy in small cell lung cancer patients receiving prophylactic cranial irradiation. Am J Clin Oncol 12:27–33, 1989.

13. Giannone L, Johnson DH, Hande KR, et al: Favorable prognosis of brain metastases in small cell lung cancer. Ann Intern Med 106:386–389, 1987.

14. Graus F, Dalmau J, Rene R, et al: Anti-Hu antibodies in patients with small cell lung cancer: association with complete response to therapy and improved survival. J Clin Oncol 15:2866–2872, 1997.

15. Gregor A, Cull A, Stephens RJ, et al: Prophylactic cranial irradiation is indicated following complete response to induction therapy in small-cell lung cancer: results of a multicentre randomized trial. Eur J Cancer 33:1752–1758, 1997.

16. Gutmann L, Phillips LH II, Gutmann L: Trends in the association of Lambert-Eaton myasthenic syndrome with carcinoma. Neurology 42:848–850, 1992.

17. Haie-Meder C, Pellae-Cosset B, Laplanche A, et al: Results of a randomized clinical trial comparing two radiation schedules in the palliative treatment of brain metastases. Radiother Oncol 26:111–116, 1993.

18. Hirsch FR, Paulson OB, Hansen HH, et al: Intracranial metastases in small cell carcinoma of the lung. Cancer 51:933–937, 1983.

19. Hochstenbag MM, Twijnstra A, Wilmink JT, et al: Asymptomatic brain metastases in small cell lung cancer: MR-imaging is useful at initial diagnosis. J Neuro-Oncol 48:243–248, 2000.

20. Hoffman R, Sneed PK, McDermott MW, et al: Radiosurgery for brain metastases from primary lung carcinoma. Cancer J 7:121–131, 2001.

21. Humblet Y, Symann M, Bosly A, et al: Late intensification chemotherapy with autologous bone marrow transplantation in selected small-cell carcinoma of the lung: a randomized study. J Clin Oncol 5:1864–1873, 1987.

22. Jemal A, Thomas A, Murray T, et al: Cancer statistics, 2002. CA Cancer J Clin 52:23–47, 2002.

23. Johnson BE, Becker B, Goff WB 2nd, et al: Neurologic, neuropsychologic, and computed cranial tomography scan abnormalities in 2- to 10-year survivors of small cell lung cancer. J Clin Oncol 3:1659–1667, 1985.

24. Johnson BE, Grayson J, Makuch RW, et al: Ten-year survival of patients with small-cell lung cancer treated with combination chemotherapy with or without irradiation. J Clin Oncol 8:396–401, 1990.

25. Johnson BE, Ihde DC, Matthews MJ, et al: Non-small cell lung cancer: major cause of late mortality in small cell lung cancer patients. Am J Med 80:1103, 1986.

26. Kochhar R, Frytak S, Shaw E: Survival of patients with extensive small-cell lung cancer who have only brain metastases at initial diagnosis. Am J Clin Oncol 20:125–127, 1997.

27. Komaki R, Cox JD, Whitson W: Risk of brain metastases from small cell carcinoma of the lung related to length of survival and prophylactic irradiation. Cancer Treat Rep 65:811, 1981.

28. Kristjansen PE, Hansen HH: Prophylactic cranial irradiation in small cell lung cancer: an update. Lung Cancer 12 Suppl 3:S23–S40, 1995.

29. Lad T, Piantadosi S, Thomas P, et al: A prospective randomized trial to determine the benefit of surgical resection of residual disease following response of small cell lung cancer to combination chemotherapy. Chest 106:320–323S, 1994.

30. Lee JS, Murphy WK, Glisson BS, et al: Primary chemotherapy of brain metastasis in small-cell lung cancer. J Clin Oncol 7:916–922, 1989.

31. Lee JS, Umsawasdi T, Barkley HT Jr, et al: Timing of elective brain irradiation: a critical factor for brain metastasis-free survival in small cell lung cancer. Int J Radiat Oncol Biol Phys 13:697–704, 1987.

32. List AF, Hainsworth JD, Davis BW, et al: The syndrome of inappropriate secretion of antidiuretic hormone in small cell lung cancer. J Clin Oncol 4:1191, 1986.

33. Meyers CA, Byrne KS, Komaki R, et al: Cognitive deficits in patients with small cell lung cancer before and after chemotherapy. Lung Cancer 12:231–235, 1995.

34. Murphy KC, Feld R, Evans WK, et al: Intramedullary spinal cord metastases from small cell carcinoma of the lung. J Clin Oncol 1:99, 1983.

35. Murren J, Glatstein E, Pass HI: Small cell lung cancer. In DeVita VT, Jr, Hellman S, Rosenberg SA (eds): Cancer: Principles and Practice of Oncology, 6th ed. Philadelphia, Lippincott Williams & Wilkins, 2001.

36. Noda K, Nishiwaki Y, Kawahara S, et al: Randomized phase III study of irinotecan (CPT-11) and cisplatin versus etoposide and cisplatin in extensive-disease small-cell lung cancer: Japan Clinical Oncology Group Study. Proc Am Soc Clin Oncol 19:1887, 2000 (Abstract).

37. Nugent JL, Bunn PA Jr, Matthews MJ, et al: CNS metastases in small cell bronchogenic carcinoma: increasing frequency and changing pattern with lengthening survival. Cancer 44:1885–1893, 1979.

38. Osterlind K, Hansen HH, Hansen M, et al: Mortality and morbidity in long-term surviving patients treated with chemotherapy with or without irradiation for small-cell lung cancer. J Clin Oncol 4:1044, 1986.

39. Pignon JP, Arriagada R, Ihde DC, et al: A meta-analysis of thoracic radiotherapy for small-cell lung cancer. N Engl J Med 327:1618–1642, 1992.

40. Postmus PE, Haaxma-Reiche H, Smit EF, et al: Treatment of brain metastases of small-cell lung cancer: comparing teniposide and teniposide with whole-brain radiotherapy. A phase III study of the European Organization for the Research and Treatment of Cancer. J Clin Oncol 18:3400–3408, 2000.

41. Ries LAG, Eisner MP, Kosary CL, et al (eds): SEER Cancer Statistics Review, 1973–1998, National Cancer Institute. Bethesda, Md, 2001, http://seer.cancer.gov/publications/CSR1973_1998.

42. Schiller JH, Adak S, Cella D, et al: Topotecan versus observation after cisplatin plus etoposide in extensive-stage small cell lung cancer: E7593—a phase III trial of the Eastern Cooperative Oncology Group. J Clin Oncol 19:2114–2122, 2001.

43. Sculier JP, Evans WK, Feld R, et al: Superior vena cava syndrome in small cell lung cancer. Cancer 57:847, 1986.

44. Sculier JP, Feld R, Evans WK, et al: Neurologic disorders in patients with small cell lung cancer. Cancer 60:2275, 1987.

45. Shepherd FA, Laskey J, Evans WK, et al: Cushing's syndrome associated with ectopic corticotropin production and small-cell lung cancer. J Clin Oncol 10:21, 1992.

46. Simon G, Ginsberg RJ, Ruckdeschel JC, et al: Small-cell lung cancer. Chest Surg Clin N Am 11:165–88, ix, 2001.

47. Takada M, Fukuoka M, Kawahara M, et al: Phase III study of concurrent versus sequential thoracic radiotherapy in combination with cisplatin and etoposide for limited-stage small-cell lung cancer: results of the Japan Oncology Group Study 9104. J Clin Oncol 20:3054–3060, 2002.

48. Van der Graaf WT, Haaxma-Reiche H, Burghouts JT, et al: Teniposide for meningeal carcinomatosis of small cell lung cancer. Lung Cancer 10:247–249, 1993.

49. von Pawel J, Gatzemeier U, Pujol JL, et al: Phase II comparator study of oral versus intravenous topotecan in patients with chemosensitive small-cell lung cancer. J Clin Oncol 19:1743–1749, 2001.

50. Wirtz PW, Smallegange TM, Wintzen AR, et al: Differences in clinical features between the Lambert-Eaton myasthenic syndrome with and without cancer: an analysis of 227 published cases. Clin Neurol Neurosurg 104:359–363, 2002.

51. Zelen M: Keynote address on biostatistics and data retrieval. Cancer Chemother Rep (part 3) 4:31, 1973.

CHAPTER 55

MANAGEMENT OF CENTRAL NERVOUS SYSTEM METASTASES FROM BREAST CARCINOMA

Ali Schwaiki, Vaneerat Ratanatharathorn, Laura F. Hutchins, Said El-Shihabi, and Mark E. Linskey

As many as 170,000 women are diagnosed yearly with breast cancer in the United States. This corresponds to an annual incidence of up to 120 new cases per 100,000 women per year. Cross-sectional population prevalence of breast cancer is estimated to be 100 per 100,000 women (0.1%). The annual incidence in the United States has been slowly rising for the past 3 decades. However, the annual breast cancer mortality rate over the same period has leveled off and now shows a slightly decreasing trend. The rising incidence may reflect earlier detection with more sensitive imaging techniques, whereas the declining annual mortality rate almost certainly reflects improving therapeutic results. The incidence of breast cancer increases with age, but the slope of this persisting increase declines after menopause. Early menarche, late menopause, and nulliparity increase the risk of developing breast cancer. A history of previous diagnosis of atypical lobular or ductal hyperplasia also increases this risk. A history of benign breast disease has only a marginal effect. Other known risk factors include early exposure to ionizing radiation, long-term postmenopausal estrogen replacement therapy, and alcohol consumption. One percent of breast cancer cases occurs in men.[66,135,136]

One of the most important risk factors for developing breast cancer is a family history of breast cancer. Approximately 5% to 10% of all breast cancers occurs in high-risk families, and there are several familial breast cancer syndromes, including the breast-ovarian cancer syndrome, the Li-Fraumeni syndrome, and Cowden's disease. Germ line mutations in breast cancer genes *BRCA1* and *BRCA2* are associated with a 50% to 85% lifetime risk of breast cancer, ovarian cancer, or both and are strongly implicated in the majority of cases of familial breast cancer cases.[31,83,138] In sporadic breast cancer cases molecular abnormalities have been identified in several genes, including *p53, bcl-2, c-myc,* and *c-myb* and overexpression of certain normal genes or gene products (e.g., HER-2/*neu* and cyclin D) has been noted in some cases.[36,79]

PRIMARY AND SYSTEMIC DISEASE DIAGNOSIS, TREATMENT, AND PROGNOSIS

Diagnosis

Regular systematic self-examination, physician clinical examination, and screening mammography are the cornerstones of early clinical detection and have contributed to a 25% to 30% reduction in mortality rates from breast cancer for women older than age 50. The lesion is most often discovered as a painless lump or an incidental finding on screening mammography. The American Cancer Society and the National Institutes of Health recommend annual screening mammography for all women older than 40. For high-risk patients with strong family histories or *BRCA1* or *BRCA2* mutations, mammography screening should begin at age 25 or 5 years earlier than the earliest age at which breast cancer was diagnosed in a family member, whichever is sooner.[16] More advanced cases may have skin dimpling, nipple retraction, bleeding from the nipple, reddening of the skin, ulceration, pain, fixation to the chest wall, and detection of enlarged axillary lymph nodes.

Breast cancer is bilateral in some cases. Therefore assessment of both breasts is required before a definitive therapeutic plan can be completed. Fine needle aspiration for cytology or core needle biopsy for histology is the standard technique for confirming the diagnosis. Image-guided core biopsy using ultrasound, mammography, and more recently, magnetic resonance imaging (MRI) have improved diagnostic sensitivity, especially for women with suspicious but nonpalpable lesions. The use of large-core needle biopsy techniques also increases diagnostic sensitivity and specificity compared with fine-needle aspiration techniques.[104,134,136]

Extent of systemic disease is usually assessed with the medical history, physical examination, and liver profile.

TABLE 55-1	Tumor (T), Node (N), and Metastasis (M) Classification for Breast Cancer	
Classification	Subcategory Criteria	Comment
T_1	± 2 cm	a. Without fixation fascia/muscle
T_2	>2–5 cm	b. With fixation fascia/muscle
T_3	>5 cm	
T_4	Extension to chest wall/skin	
	a. Chest wall	
	b. Skin edema/infiltration or ulceration	
	c. Both	
N_1	Mobile axillary	
	a. Not considered metastatic	
	b. Considered metastatic	
N_2	Fixed axillary	
N_3	Supraclavicular/edema of arm	
M_1	Any distant systemic metastatic involvement	

Source: American Cancer Society's anatomic staging classification for breast cancer, modified from the American Joint Committee (AJC) for Cancer Staging and End Results.

Contrast-enhanced chest, abdomen, and pelvic computed tomography (CT) scanning, as well as the nuclear medicine bone scan, further help to evaluate any suspicious finding. The role of positron-emission tomography (PET) scanning is emerging and may replace the other modalities. Central nervous system (CNS) imaging with contrast-enhanced MRI is the most sensitive means of detecting CNS involvement and has replaced CT scanning as the neuroimaging diagnostic modality of choice. However, in the absence of signs or symptoms, neuroimaging at the time of initial early breast cancer diagnosis is not felt to be cost-effective by most practitioners.[20]

Histology

Carcinoma of the breast is usually divided into ductal disease (89%), lobular disease (5%), or combined (6%), depending on the site of tumor origin within the glandular tissue of the breast. It usually takes the form of an adenocarcinoma. Both ductal and lobular carcinomas may be entirely or partly confined within the ductal basement membrane. Pure ductal carcinoma in situ (DCIS) and lobular carcinoma in situ (LCIS) have nearly 100% cure rates with local therapy alone. In the case of invasive ductal carcinoma, lymphoid infiltration within the tumor, tubular histology, or pure colloid or mucinous variants correlate with better prognosis than is seen in the more common infiltrating ductal adenocarcinoma. The significance of lobular disease lies in its tendency to be bilateral far more commonly than ductal carcinoma (bilateral disease eventually appears in approximately 20% of cases), its tendency toward multicentricity in the same breast, and its relatively poor prognosis.[72,78,85,86,113,119,136]

All lymph nodes within a surgical specimen need to be systematically checked for tumor involvement, because any presence of lymph node involvement significantly affects patient prognosis, and the strength of negative effect is proportional to the number of nodes involved. In addition to routine histologic study, all breast cancer specimens need to be carefully analyzed for their estrogen receptor status as well as the presence of the HER-2/neu gene product overexpression on the tumor cells. These data are critical in predicting likely response to either hormonal therapy or anti-HER-2/neu antibody therapy.[28,46,137]

Staging

The American Cancer Society's anatomic staging classification for breast cancer (modified from the American Joint Committee [AJC] for Cancer Staging and End Results) is outlined in Tables 55-1 and 55-2. This classification system significantly separates and stratifies patients according to expected survival using life table analysis methods. CNS involvement automatically classifies the patient as having stage IV disease; however, stage IV is a very heterogeneous class, containing patients with potentially disparate prognoses. This is being increasingly recognized for patients with isolated solid brain metastases or who have single solid brain tumors with demonstrably stable systemic disease. Both of these subcategories of stage IV patients may have a much more favorable prognosis than previously realized as long as the CNS disease is aggressively locally treated with more than just fractionated whole-brain radiation therapy (WBRT).

Local-Regional Disease

Randomized clinical trials (class I evidence by evidence-based medicine criteria) have established organ-sparing wide-excision lumpectomy followed by fractionated local radiation therapy as the preferred treatment for patients with stage I and II disease, with survival rates comparable with complete mastectomy.[53,71,128] Wide-excision lumpectomy followed by fractionated local radiation therapy can be curative in some cases. Noninvasive DCIS or LCIS can also be adequately treated with lumpectomy and radiation therapy.[52] Unfortunately, many patients thought to have stage I or II disease at the time of potentially curative surgery are subsequently found to develop distant metastases, confirming that subclinical metastatic disease may commonly go undetected.

TABLE 55-2	**Tumor (T), Node (N), and Metastasis (M) Classification Stage Grouping for Breast Cancer***		
Classification Stage	**T Classification**	**N Classification**	**M Classification**
Stage I	T_{1a}, T_{1b}	N_0, N_{1a}	M_0
Stage II	T_{1a}, T_{1b}	N_{1b}	M_0
	T_{2a}, T_{2b}	N_0, N_{1a}	M_0
	T_{2a}, T_{2b}	N_{1b}	M_0
Stage IIIa	T_{3a}, T_{3b}	N_0, N_1	M_0
	$T_{1a}, T_{1b}, T_{2a}, T_{1b}$	N_2	M_0
	T_{3a}, T_{3b}		
Stage IIIb	$T_{1a}, T_{1b}, T_{2a}, T_{2b}$	N_3	M_0
	T_{3a}, T_{3b}		
	T_{4a}, T_{4b}, T_{4c}	Any N	M_0
Stage IV	Any T	Any N	M_1

*Refer to Table 55-1 for the corresponding T, N, and M subcategory criteria.
Source: American Cancer Society's anatomic staging classification for breast cancer, modified from the American Joint Committee (AJC) for Cancer Staging and End Results.

Axillary Lymph Node Dissection

The probability of recurrence after treatment is higher for patients with histologically positive axillary lymph nodes and increases with additional positive nodes. Axillary lymph node dissection provides prognostic information but little or no therapeutic benefit and is responsible for most of the morbidity associated with breast cancer surgery.[51]

The positive predictive value of positive sentinel-node biopsy approaches 100%, and its negative predictive value exceeds 95%. Many patients without axillary nodal involvement could be potentially spared axillary lymph node dissection if a sentinel node biopsy was found to be negative. At present, until sentinel-node biopsy is further validated, axillary node dissection remains standard practice for patients with invasive breast cancer or large noninvasive tumors (>2.5 cm in maximal diameter).[62,63,77,129]

Locally Advanced and Inflammatory Breast Cancer

Current data suggest that patients with advanced stage III disease who are at least T_3 (>5 cm in maximal diameter), T_4 (extension to chest wall or skin), or N_2 (fixed or matted axillary lymphadenopathy) are best treated with preoperative chemotherapy or hormonal therapy, followed by surgery and then local-regional fractionated radiation therapy. Limited data support the addition of adjuvant chemotherapy or hormonal therapy postoperatively and after radiation therapy. Excellent local control can be achieved in 80% to 90% of women, and approximately 30% of women with stage IIIb disease (direct invasion of skin or chest wall) or inflammatory breast cancer remain free of cancer after 1 year.[24,68]

Radiation Therapy

Local-Regional Radiation Therapy

Local fractionated radiation therapy is standard treatment for patients with stage I or II disease undergoing organ-sparing lumpectomy. The treatment is directed to the entire breast to 50 Gy using conventional fractionation. There is no standard for boost treatment. Patients treated under National Surgical Adjuvant Breast and Bowel Project (NSABP) B-06 protocol did not receive any boost treatment. Fowble and colleagues recommended a 60 Gy total cumulative dose to the primary tumor site, implying a boost of 10 Gy with the electron beam.[55] This group of investigators defined a close margin to be tumor cells seen within 2 mm from the resection margin. For a focally positive margin, they recommended a total cumulative dose of 68 Gy, with 66 Gy recommended for patients with close margins.[123]

For more advanced disease (stage IIIa, IIIb, and IV) treated with mastectomy, postoperative irradiation reduces the incidence of local recurrence by 50% to 75%. This reduction in local recurrence rate does not translate into improved survival time in most randomized clinical trials (even when augmented in statistical power through meta-analysis). Host, Brennhovd, and Loeb[69] initially reported survival benefit. Unfortunately, this benefit was offset by an increased death rate due to cardiac complications, namely, myocardial infarction, which can be predicted from the use of an "en face" internal mammary port.[68] Similar problems were noted in the meta-analysis.[32,33] Other complications such as pneumonitis are rare. The brachial plexopathy risk is now close to zero with modern doses employed for microscopic disease, namely, 50 Gy with conventional fractionation. Because of the lack of survival benefit and potential complications, local fractionated radiation therapy after mastectomy is usually recommended only for women at highest risk for local or regional recurrence (i.e., primary tumor 5 cm or larger in greatest diameter, four or more positive axillary nodes, invasion of skin or pectoral fascia, and a positive surgical margin).

In two recent, long-term randomized studies of high-risk premenopausal women with breast cancer treated with modern radiation therapy and chemotherapy techniques versus chemotherapy alone, there were fewer local recurrences, and overall survival was significantly higher among women treated with combined therapy.[94,101] These results have led to renewed interest in fractionated radiation therapy in this additional high-risk group of patients. The Southwest Oncology Group

(SWOG) currently has an ongoing clinical trial examining the issue of postmastectomy radiation therapy.

Palliative Radiation Therapy

Palliative radiation therapy is widely used for relieving distressing local symptoms and circumventing or alleviating deficits as a result of uncontrolled local-regional diseases and the other systemic metastases. Among breast cancer patients, other than those with CNS metastasis, bone metastasis patients are the largest palliative group encountered in radiation oncology clinics. They are generally treated for either pain or complications related to bone metastases, such as impending or known fracture (post–internal fixation), and cord or nerve-root compression. The clinical judgments required for palliation are significantly more complex than for curative treatment and require a much higher degree of individualization.

The series of randomized trials for bone metastases from Europe and Canada reported similar palliative benefits with 8 Gy single-fraction doses as compared with higher dose fractionated regimens.[100] This led to the tendency to use low radiation dose in all bone metastasis patients. This approach is not supported by known tumor radiobiology theories or known biologic mechanisms of bone healing. External-beam radiation therapy induces bone healing in 65% to 85% of lesions irradiated, mostly by direct induction of osteogenesis. Gainor and Buchert reported that radiation doses of more than 30 Gy are detrimental to bone healing in long bones.[59] In contrast, Matsubayashi and colleagues reported that healing of spinal bone lesions was achieved with doses higher than 40 Gy, with a patient's survival of 6 months required to demonstrate that bone healing had taken place.[81]

These seemingly contradictory reports reflect different mechanisms of bone healing for different types of bone as well as the presence or absence of fractures. For fractured long bones stabilized with internal fixation devices, the mechanism of bone healing is by chondrogenesis, which is radiosensitive. If external-beam irradiation is given in this case, the chondrogenic phase of fracture healing can be impaired by doses usually used for treatment of bone metastases, such as 30 Gy in 10 fractions. This is one of the major arguments for performing prophylactic internal fixation of an impending fracture, so that bone healing will occur by direct osteogenesis and will not be impaired by irradiation. For actual fractures of long bones, rigid immobilization with internal fixation is required for healing. Survival for 6 months or longer and internal fixation are the important predictors of fracture healing. Postoperative local irradiation is necessary, because local tumor progression has been reported to cause higher failure rates for internal fixation devices. High radiation dose does not interfere with healing and is necessary because bone healing does not occur in the absence of adequate tumor cell kill. In general, we do not recommend single-fraction radiation therapy to treat patients with weight-bearing long bone fractures who have an expected survival of longer than 6 months. Likewise, we do not recommend that any patient with internal fixation receive radiation doses that might lead to inadequate tumor cell kill.

Prophylactic internal fixation should be considered for patients with involvement of weight-bearing bones at high risk for fracture. Criteria for prophylactic internal fixation are well described for weight-bearing long bone but not for spinal involvement, although spinal fractures occur far more commonly than long-bone fractures. The criteria for internal fixation include patients with lesions 2.5 cm or larger in maximal diameter in the highly stressed region of the femur (trochanteric and subtrochanteric region), those with avulsion fracture of the lesser trochanter, and those with cortical destruction of at least 50% of weight-bearing bone.[118] Percutaneous intramedullary nailing allows internal fixation even in infirm patients.

Extradural Spinal Cord Compression

Extradural spinal cord compression is a clinical emergency. MRI is the study of choice because it yields information regarding the entire spine and will identify multiple levels of compression, even those between two levels of complete block. It also delineates the extent of extraosseous component, thus limiting the chance of "geographic miss" of partial radiation therapy. All patients should be initially treated with high-dose intravenous glucocorticoids even as neuroimaging work-up is progressing. The probability of restoring neurologic function once it is impaired is inversely proportional to the lapse time from the onset of deficit to the initiation of treatment and inversely proportional to the degree of deficit. As a result, we recommend treating patients within 24 hours of the onset of acute neurologic symptoms. It is rare for a patient who has lost the ability to walk with assistance or to control bowels or bladder to regain these functions. However, patients who still have these functions when starting radiation therapy usually retain them. Surgical resection, decompression, or stabilization are now reserved for progression in partial neurologic deficit despite adequate steroid and radiation treatments or the development of spinal instability.

Systemic Therapy

Systemic therapy for breast cancer includes cytotoxic chemotherapy, hormonal therapies, and molecular therapies. These therapies are applied as an adjunct to surgery with curative intent, in conjunction with palliative radiation therapy or occasionally in isolation, for palliation in the metastatic disease setting.

Adjuvant Systemic Therapy

The benefit of adjunctive cytotoxic and hormonal systemic therapies has been documented through prospective randomized clinical trials that began in the 1950s. Hundreds of clinical trials have been conducted. The data from these trials have been reviewed and reanalyzed as an overview by the Early Breast Cancer Trialists' Collaborative Group,[40–45] and the National Cancer Institute has held consensus conferences regarding adjuvant therapy for breast cancer every 5 years beginning in 1985.[3,78a] The conclusions from these analyses stand as the foundation for our current recommendations.

The conclusions at this time regarding adjuvant therapy are as follows: Multiagent cytotoxic chemotherapy reduces the risk of recurrence of breast cancer by a proportional risk reduction. The proportional reduction decreases as age increases. Therefore older women have slightly less proportional risk reduction than younger women. Anthracycline-based chemotherapy is superior to nonanthracycline-based chemotherapy. Tamoxifen added to chemotherapy is superior to not adding tamoxifen in the hormone-receptor-positive subset of women. Tamoxifen alone has substantial benefit, particularly in postmenopausal patients, and may be used alone without chemotherapy. Four to six cycles of chemotherapy should be administered at standard doses. High-dose chemotherapy (usually with stem cell rescue) has not yet demonstrated any superiority to standard-dose chemotherapy.[38] Treatment for longer than six cycles has yet to demonstrate any additional therapeutic benefit.[103,125]

Therefore, the recommendation for adjuvant therapy is determined by the patient's risk, which depends on the lymph node status, tumor diameter, and tumor histologic grade. Other factors that contribute to prognosis in a less quantifiable way include S-phase fraction and HER-2/neu overexpression.[21,27,89,106,110,114] Estrogen receptor status is an independent predictor of both overall survival and of positive response to treatment with tamoxifen. It indicates that relapses are likely to be delayed, as compared with relapses in patients who are estrogen-receptor negative with otherwise identical prognostic features.[92] Overall, patient risk assessment as well as patient medical comorbidities and hormone-receptor status determine the recommended treatment options. At present, a shared decision-making process, with the patient taking an active role, is the most common approach. Some patients may elect a less efficacious therapy, such as tamoxifen alone, to avoid toxicity such as alopecia and cardiac dysfunction that may occur with anthracycline chemotherapy. If there were no medical comorbidities and no patient preference, our recommendation for therapy would include an anthracycline-based regimen for more than four cycles with or without tamoxifen for patients with hormone-receptor-positive tumors.

New approaches under investigation include substituting an aromatase inhibitor (e.g., anastrozole, letrozole, or exestemane) for tamoxifen and the addition of trastuzumab (Herceptin) to chemotherapy in patients who have tumors that overexpress the HER-2/neu oncoprotein. Early reports using aromatase inhibitors are exciting but too preliminary for universal implementation.[9] The use of trastuzumab in the adjuvant setting is investigational. Until benefit is demonstrated in the adjuvant setting, the risk of cardiac and unknown long-term toxicities do not allow a risk-benefit analysis, which would be needed to recommend its general use.

Metastatic Disease

Treatment for metastatic breast carcinoma (stage IV disease) is largely palliative. There are a few subgroups of patients who have a 1% to 5% chance of long-term disease-free survival. Most patients with metastatic disease, however, are destined to die of their disease. Two therapeutic approaches are used. One approach is to treat the patient aggressively with multiagent chemotherapy for the 1% to 5% chance of long-term disease-free control. The other approach is to treat the patient sequentially with single agents aimed at controlling the disease with the least amount of morbidity. There remains intense debate about the most appropriate approach. One recent study showed a survival advantage when combination treatment was used.[91] Currently, most oncologists treat these patients with the sequential single-agent approach.

The chemotherapy agents that palliate breast cancer are numerous. The most efficacious agents include the taxanes, including paclitaxel and docetaxel; the anthracyclines, including doxorubicin and epirubicin; vinorelbine; capecitabine; gemcitabine; liposomal doxorubicin; 5-fluorouracil (5-FU); mitomycin C; vinblastine; cyclophosamide; VP-16; carboplatin; and cisplatin. These agents are used initially for patients who are estrogen- and progesterone-receptor negative or have life-threatening visceral disease.[47,136] For patients with bone or soft-tissue disease only, who are hormone-receptor positive, the treatment of choice would be a hormonal agent. Hormonal therapies initially were surgical and included oophorectomy, hypophysectomy, and adrenalectomy. Pharmacologic treatments have included high-dose estrogen, androgens, and progesterones. In more recent years, the most commonly used agents fit into the category called selective estrogen-receptor modulators (SERMs). The two main agents in this group include tamoxifen and toremifene. A new class of drugs, selective estrogen-receptor down regulators (SERDs), has been developed. The first one available commercially is Faslodex.[70,93] A third class of agents that are commonly used are the aromatase inhibitors, which include anastrozle, letrozole, and exestemane. At present, the aromatase inhibitors have been found to be superior to the SERMs. They are currently the treatment of choice when a hormonal agent is chosen for treatment of metastatic disease.[18,19,90,120] The SERMs, progesterone agents, and Faslodex are available for second- and third-line therapies. As yet, there has been no demonstrated benefit from combined hormonal therapy.[47,136]

The first targeted therapy besides hormonal agents to become commercially available is trastuzumab (Herceptin). This drug is a monoclonal antibody directed toward the HER-2/neu protein. It is a member of the epidermal growth factor receptor family that has single-agent activity and is synergistic with many chemotherapy agents. Initial studies have shown it to provide a survival advantage in patients who are HER-2/neu overexpressing and who receive it with chemotherapy early in their disease course. There is cardiac toxicity associated with this agent as well as pulmonary toxicity in patients with extensive metastatic disease in the lung. Recent reports have speculated that brain metastases may occur more commonly in patients treated with trastuzumab (Herceptin).[25,131] It is currently being evaluated for the adjuvant setting. At this time, its use is approved only for metastatic disease.[105]

An important advance in treatment for metastatic disease has been the use of bisphosphonates. These agents are osteoclast inhibitors and have substantially reduced the risk of fractures, bone pain, and need for radiation therapy for painful bone lesions. The two drugs approved for this use are pamidronate and zoledronate. These are given intravenously monthly. This class of agents is currently being investigated in the adjuvant setting.[88,126]

CENTRAL NERVOUS SYSTEM METASTASES

Breast cancer can spread to the CNS in one of three ways. Solid brain tumors are the most common end point (85% to 95%), carcinomatous meningitis is next in frequency (approximately 5% to 15%), followed most rarely by intraparenchymal spread to the substance of the spinal cord (approximately 1%). Breast cancer is the second most common cause of solid brain metastases after lung cancer, accounting for 14% to 20% of the total (an even larger percentage among women). Estimates of the prevalence of symptomatic CNS metastases among patients with breast cancer range from 5.9% to 16.2%. By the time of autopsy, prevalence rates have increased to 18% to 30% of patients. CNS invasion is more likely to occur in premenopausal women with widely disseminated disease and in patients with estrogen-receptor-negative tumors. Recent reports have speculated that brain metastases may occur more commonly in patients treated with trastuzumab (Herceptin).[25,131] In approximately 20% of patients who develop CNS involvement, it is diagnosed at the time of original disease detection (synchronous disease); the other 80% are usually diagnosed after the primary disease and usually once systemic disease is also present (metachronous disease). The median time between the original diagnosis of breast cancer and diagnosis of brain metastasis is 2 to 3 years. A single brain tumor is less likely to be the only site of systemic disease (solitary metastasis) for patients with breast cancer than it is for those with lung cancer, melanoma, or renal cell carcinoma.[73,132,133]

Solid metastatic brain tumors tend to arise at the cortical-medullary junction (gray-white matter junction), where a large dense net of small capillaries is most likely to trap a hematogenous embolus of tumor cells. Their distribution within the brain is directly proportional to the regional distribution of cerebral blood flow (80% cerebral hemispheres, 15% cerebellum, and 5% brainstem). In contrast to other cancers that spread to the brain, breast cancer is more likely to produce single lesions. In one CT scan study, 56% of solid tumor brain metastases were single versus 44% of cases where lesions were multiple.[132]

Diagnosis

The majority of CNS metastases from breast cancer become symptomatic (approximately 70% to 80%). Symptoms can arise from varying combinations of tissue destruction, physical effect from tumor mass, surrounding vasogenic edema, and occasionally, intratumoral hemorrhage. In general, symptoms can be divided into those resulting from elevated intracranial pressure, those resulting from neuronal electrical irritation, and those related to local disruption of neuronal function specifically related to the anatomic location of the metastasis in question. The relative frequency of the most common signs and symptoms for solid tumor metastases are listed in Table 55-3.

TABLE 55-3

Relative Frequency of Common Signs and Symptoms among Patients with Symptomatic Solid Tumor Metastases to the Brain from Breast Carcinoma

Symptom	Frequency
Increased intracranial pressure	
Headache, nausea and vomiting	26–57%
Confusion or lethargy	22–41%
Seizure (supratentorial only)	6–21%
Signs/symptoms specific to location	
Focal weakness	18–75%
Ataxia	5–20%
Sensory symptoms	2–28%
Visual-field defect	1–21%
Aphasia	1–14%

Whereas CT scanning remains a readily obtainable and useful tool for quickly ruling out the potentially urgent or emergency clinical problems of intratumoral hemorrhage, herniation syndrome, and obstructive hydrocephalus, it should be considered obsolete for the evaluation of cancer metastasis to the CNS.[39] MRI with intravenous contrast administration is far more sensitive than CT scanning for identifying solid brain metastases, leptomeningeal or ventricular ependyma involvement (carcinomatous meningitis), or spinal cord parenchymal tumors. MRI can directly image in all three anatomic planes and provides far better tissue (as opposed to bone) resolution. Sensitivity can be increased further by using a double dose of contrast agent and by imaging in all three planes using fine-slice thickness (3 mm or less).

The presence of an enhanced brain mass on MRI in a patient with known cancer does not ensure that the lesion in question is a brain metastasis. In one prospective clinical trial studying single brain metastases in patients who had a definite tissue diagnosis of a known cancer primary obtained within 5 years of the diagnosis of the brain lesion, 11% of the brain lesions turned out not to be metastatic tumors.[95] Six percent were really primary brain tumors (usually a second malignancy), and 5% represented sites of inflammation or infection. Patients undergoing chemotherapy are particularly prone to brain abscess or areas of cerebritis. Although patients with a known cancer primary and multiple brain lesions are less likely to suffer from anything other than brain metastases than those with single lesions, it must be remembered that glioblastoma multiforme can rarely be multifocal and cerebral abscesses can also be multiple. Occasionally, a patient with a history of multiple different primary cancers will develop a new brain lesion. In this setting, tissue diagnosis is critical for establishing an accurate prognosis as well as guiding further systemic therapy, because choice of therapy differs for different cancer histologies.

When sufficient doubt exists, a tissue diagnosis via excisional open biopsy or stereotactic needle biopsy (if stereotactic radiosurgery is contemplated) is always warranted. On the other hand, the statistics are sufficiently in favor of a metastatic brain tumor in most instances such that insistence upon confirming tissue diagnosis in 100% of cases is unjustified and probably subjects many patients to unnecessary morbidity. It is our current practice to seriously entertain obtaining tissue diagnostic confirmation in (1) patients with single brain lesions and a history of freedom from disease from a histologically proven primary for more than 3 years, (2) patients with multiple lesions and a history of freedom from disease from a histologically proven primary for more than 5 years, and (3) patients with any number of lesions who are neutropenic or who have a fever, elevated white blood cell count with a left shift, elevated erythrocyte sedimentation rate, or cerebrospinal fluid (CSF) indices on lumbar puncture that indicate infection.

Natural History

The natural history for patients with cerebral metastases is very poor. Untreated, patients with *symptomatic* solid tumor brain metastases have a median survival time of approximately 1 month regardless of the histology of the primary tumor (small cell lung carcinoma excluded).[37,67,99] Corticosteroids have little, if any, direct cytotoxic effect on metastatic brain tumor cells (small cell lung carcinoma excluded) but can aid in controlling peritumoral vasogenic edema. Unfortunately, treatment with corticosteroids will increase the median life expectancy of patients with *symptomatic* solid tumor brain metastases to only approximately 2 months regardless of the histology of the primary tumor (small cell lung carcinoma excluded).[67,75,80,99,108,140] Whether or not glucocorticoids are used, the cause of death in 95% to 100% of cases will be increased intracranial pressure from progressive mass effect from both the tumor and surrounding vasogenic edema, with rapid clinical deterioration. Preterminal events include cerebral herniation with loss of consciousness. The natural history of untreated *asymptomatic* solid brain tumor metastases found on screening neuroimaging has not been well studied, and reliable life expectancy figures are not available.

The fact that 95% to 100% of patients die of their brain disease means that once a symptomatic metastatic brain tumor is diagnosed in a cancer patient, treatment of the brain tumor must move to first priority in their overall cancer treatment plan. The brain tumor is now the "rate limiting step" in their overall survival with their cancer. Extent of systemic disease, and the histology of their cancer primary (small cell lung carcinoma excluded) no longer matters in comparison. The fact that 95% to 100% of patients die of their brain disease also means that the newly diagnosed brain disease now becomes the dominant factor in the quality of the patient's remaining life span. The brain is the master organ of the rest of the body. It is intimately individual. The brain is the seat of our personality, our individual identity—our very humanity. No human organ has greater influence on our ability to maintain our independence in our daily activities or on our capacity to derive pleasure from interpersonal relationships and personal interests.

Treatment Options for Solid Brain Tumors

Throughout the 1970s, 1980s, and early 1990s, treatment options for patients were usually limited to treatment of the vasogenic edema surrounding the tumor with glucocorticoids and treatment of the solid tumor with fractionated WBRT. Surgical resection was, for the most part, restricted to cases where tissue diagnosis was in doubt, large tumors requiring immediate relief of symptomatic mass effect, and patients with tumors in the posterior fossa with (or at high risk for) obstructive hydrocephalus. Since the early 1990s abundant class 1 evidence (by evidence-based medicine criteria) has accumulated unequivocally, demonstrating that the key to maximizing both length of life *and* quality of life for patients with solid tumor brain metastases lies in maximizing local control through additional surgical intervention in qualifying patients.

Despite the overwhelming weight of evidence supporting this approach, less than 25% of patients who qualify for surgical intervention were ever referred to a surgeon for consultation. Patients with stage IV breast cancer will usually die of their cancer, and many are elderly. Given this setting, there would appear to exist a persistent and pervasive paternalistic attitude among many general practitioners, medical oncologists, and radiation oncologists that in some way they need to "protect their patient from the surgeon." With the demonstration in the late 1990s and early 2000s that stereotactic radiosurgery (SRS) can achieve results comparable to open surgical resection for both length-of-life and quality-of-life end points, one would have expected improvement in referral of appropriate patients for therapy that has a clearly proved benefit. Yet,

even today, less than one third of patients who potentially qualify are referred for surgical consultation for either surgical resection or SR intervention.

Whole-Brain Radiation Therapy

The use of fractionated WBRT improves expected patient median survival from 1 to 2 months to 4 to 6 months.[80,95,130] Further, it reduces the likelihood of dying directly as a result of CNS disease from 95% to 100% to approximately 50%.[95,130] Although this is a statistically significant improvement in both overall survival and quality of life achieved (through a reduction in CNS-related death), the magnitude of this effect is modest at best. Once it develops, the brain tumor remains the "rate limiting step" in patients' overall survival with their cancer despite WBRT. Extent of systemic disease and the histology of the cancer primary (small cell lung carcinoma excluded) still fail to matter in comparison. The fact that approximately 50% of patients still die of their brain disease despite WBRT also means that the brain disease remains the dominant factor in the quality of the patient's remaining life span. Between 1970 and the late 1990s, little changed in the recommended radiation therapy management of patients with brain metastases from breast cancer.

In the 1970s and early 1980s a series of Radiation Therapy Oncology Group (RTOG) trials failed to identify any differential benefit for total doses greater than 30 Gy or more complex fractionation schemes.[15,61] As a result, 30 Gy divided into 10 fractions became the most common dose prescription for WBRT. The rationale was that the potential CNS toxicity of the large 3-Gy fraction size was offset by the benefit of limiting the amount of the patient's remaining life span spent on treatment. This rationale was reinforced by observations that most patients were not likely to live long enough to experience the encephalopathic effects of 3 Gy fractions, because the latency of onset ranged from 6 months to 3 years (usually 1 to 2 years).[7,34,97] The number of long-term survivors when WBRT was used in isolation were too few to be of major concern.

The long-term encephalopathy effects of large-dose-per-fraction WBRT are usually seen approximately 1 to 2 years post treatment and are usually slowly progressive once they develop. DeAngelis et al reported WBRT-induced dementia of 1.9% to 5.1% with 25 to 39 Gy delivered with 3 to 6 Gy/fraction.[34] However, they included only the most severely affected patients in their report. The symptoms are usually gradual and nonspecific. Early on, patients generally manifest impairment of recent memory that progresses to severe dementia, ataxia, intermittent disorientation, somnolence, and urinary and bowel incontinence. Neuroimaging usually reveals ventricular enlargement (ex vacuo versus hydrocephalus), cerebral atrophy, and increased white matter signal intensity on T2-weighted MRI scans. Occasionally, focal "punched out" lesions in the white matter are seen. Patients rarely respond to steroid treatment or CSF shunt insertion. However, symptoms usually progress despite all treatments. Patients may become completely dependent for all care, become vegetative, or even eventually die as a result of cerebral end organ failure.

Decreasing the fraction size to less than 3 Gy per fraction probably lengthens the complication-free period and reduces the chance of radiation-induced encephalopathy as compared with a larger fraction size. This approach makes sense if patients can be expected to achieve long-term (>12 months) survival.[116] For patients with brain metastases who have a reasonable likelihood of long-term survival (>12 months), we usually recommend WBRT fraction sizes of 2 Gy to limit the chance of suffering these devastating sequelae. Breast cancer is quite radiosensitive. So there is no scientific need for large doses per fraction to overcome the breadth of the cell survival curve. Therefore for breast cancer patients with the potential for long-term survival, we generally treat to 40 Gy with 2 Gy per day, 5 days per week (4-week treatment vs. 2-week treatment with 30 Gy in 10 fractions). The key is prospectively identifying those patients with potentially longer-term survival.

It has long been known that not all patients with brain metastases have the same likelihood of survival. Gaspar and associates performed a recursive partitioning analysis (RPA) based on databases from three consecutive RTOG trials conducted between 1979 and 1993 (RTOG 79-16, 85-28, and 89-05) to group patients with brain metastases into class I, II, or III, which defined three distinctly separate survival curves.[60] Class I included patients with a Karnofsky Performance Scale (KPS) score of 70 or more, age younger than 65, with controlled primary tumors and no extracranial metastases. Class III included those with a KPS score of less than 70. Class II was a heterogeneous mix of the remaining patients not included in class I or III. The median survival of class I, II, and III patients with WBRT was 7.1, 4.2, and 2.3 months, respectively. Subsequently, the predictions for class I and class II survival were confirmed by this same group of investigators using the data from RTOG 91-04, because only patients in these two RPA classes were eligible for the trial.[60] Another way of looking at these results is to note that class II patients fare exactly as expected with WBRT, class I patients predictably fare better than expected, and class III patients fare much worse than expected. Although there may be some controversies regarding this classification and further fine-tuning is needed, the classification system is a useful new tool for assessing the results of clinical trials, choosing dose-fractionation schemes, and counseling patients regarding ultimate prognosis.

Whether WBRT is beneficial for patients with brain metastases who receive other forms of local therapy such as microsurgery or SRS has recently come into question. The answers for microsurgery seem the most clear. A prospective, randomized clinical trial of microsurgery alone versus microsurgery plus WBRT for patients with single brain metastases showed that the addition of WBRT reduced the chance of recurrence in the resection bed from 46% to 10%.[96] The risk of recurrence elsewhere in the brain was reduced from 37% to 4%.[96] This important study makes a strong argument for fractionated irradiation of a surgical resection bed after microsurgical resection. Whether this radiation therapy needs to include the whole brain or just the resection bed remains controversial. A large part of this decision must be based on the expected life span of the patient independent of CNS involvement, the physician's willingness to maintain close, regular surveillance for distant CNS metastases while they are small and asymptomatic, and the willingness of the patient to undergo additional therapy for any new distant lesions that might develop.

Because, unlike microsurgery, SRS delivers ionizing radiation and will have a "sterilizing" penumbra of at least 1 to 2 mm outside the border of the metastasis, the risk for failure of local tumor control at the site of SRS would theoretically be lower for SRS alone versus microsurgery alone. This has

led several investigators to question whether WBRT adds any benefit for patients treated primarily with SRS. This question is under active investigation.[121,122] Once again, this decision must be based on the expected life span of the patient independent of CNS involvement, the physician's willingness to maintain close, regular surveillance for the appearance of distant CNS metastases while they are small and asymptomatic, and the willingness of the patient to undergo additional therapy for any new distant lesions that might develop.

For WBRT, patient's images are obtained for simulation on a CT simulator with a thermoplastic mask for immobilization. Shaped blocks are designed, and isodose distribution is obtained. The isodose distribution should be examined cut by cut on the sagittal planes to ensure complete coverage of the whole brain and maximal sparing of eyes. Typical radiation fields are parallel opposed with custom blocking. The isodose distribution will generally show that 95% to 100% isodose lines cover the brain and there is 105% to 110% isodose on the top part of the brain. This dose gradient can be minimized by the creation of "segments" to block these high-dose areas. The segment is an additional lateral field with blocking conforming to the high-dose areas. Segments can be introduced either as additional right lateral field, left lateral field, or both. Usually, with this technique the gradient can be minimized to a maximum of 105% of the prescribed dose. The visualization and collection of such dose-volume data in correlation with the clinical data gathered in the follow-up phase of patient care will help the clinician to further understand the long-term effect of different dose fractionations of radiation therapy.

Microsurgical Resection

Open surgery for solid metastatic brain tumors has come a long way over the past 5 to 15 years. Improved microsurgical techniques, improved management of brain edema, and improvements in the safety of anesthesia have lowered 30-day surgical mortality rates to less than 5%, with 30-day neurologic morbidity rates now routinely less than 15%.[10,17,49,112,124] Improvements in frameless stereotactic tumor localization and intraoperative computerized navigation have largely eliminated the need for large scalp incisions or flaps. A simple, small, linear incision placed directly over the lesion is usually all that is required (Figure 55-1). Linear incisions (straight or s-shape) heal better than flap incisions, particularly in the setting of postoperative radiation therapy. Improvements in functional neuroimaging and intraoperative cortical mapping have enlarged our definition of the subset of patients with tumors in potentially resectable locations. More than 90% of patients can now be safely discharged home from hospital within 1 to 3 days after their surgery.

Microsurgical resection for patients with solid tumor brain metastases has always been accepted therapy for scenarios where tissue diagnosis was in doubt, where patients had large tumors requiring immediate relief of symptomatic mass effect, or for patients with tumors in the posterior fossa with (or at high risk for) obstructive hydrocephalus (Figure 55-2). For other settings the role of surgical resection remained controversial until two landmark prospective clinical trials, published in the early 1990s, studied microsurgery followed by WBRT versus WBRT alone for patients with single lesions.[95,130] Both studies confirmed the expected 4- to 6-month median survival of patients with single lesions treated with WBRT alone.

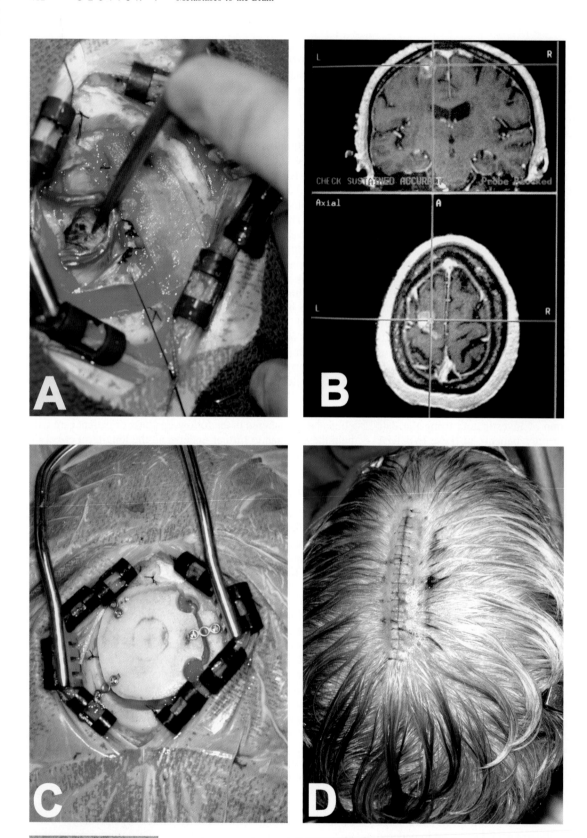

FIGURE 55-1   A woman with a small symptomatic isolated metastatic adenocarcinoma in her left posterior frontal lobe that was micro-surgically removed with the use of frameless stereotactic intraoperative neuronavigation. Preoperative functional imaging confirmed that the lesion arose in the superior frontal gyrus immediately adjacent to the primary motor strip (separated by one sulcus posteriorly). *A,* Intraoperative photograph of the resection cavity with the neuronavigation probe touching the medial wall. *B,* Coronal and axial plane magnetic resonance images revealing the position of the navigation probe where the crosshairs intersect. *C,* Intraoperative photograph of the small trephine craniotomy required when frameless stereotaxis is used to precisely localize the bone flap. *D,* Intraoperative photograph of the simple small linear incision that can be used when frameless stereotaxis precisely localizes the incision.

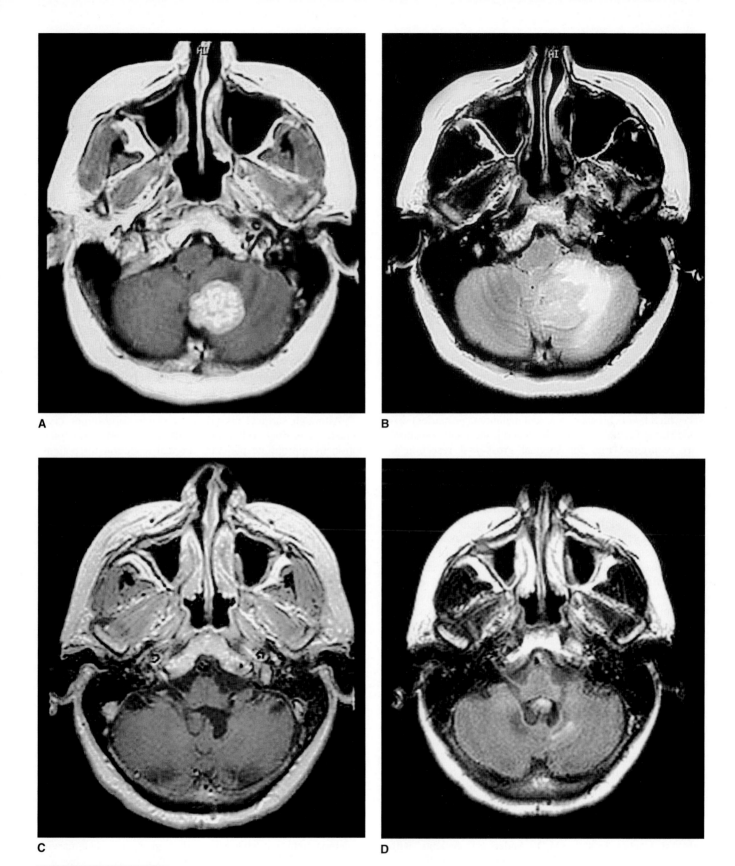

FIGURE 55-2 A 54-year-old woman with a single symptomatic cerebellar metastasis from breast cancer 3 cm in maximal diameter with compression of her fourth ventricle. Her Karnofsky Performance Scale (KPS) score was 90 and she had no evidence of disease elsewhere in her body. The lesion was microsurgically resected with intraoperative ultrasound guidance and was treated with whole-brain radiation therapy post-operatively. *A,* Preoperative T1-weighted, contrast-enhanced magnetic resonance (MR) axial image of the tumor. *B,* Preoperative fluid-attenuated inversion recovery (FLAIR) MR axial image of the tumor and surrounding vasogenic edema. *C,* T1-weighted, contrast-enhanced MR axial image obtained 16 months postoperatively revealing gross-total resection of tumor and no evidence of recurrence. *D,* FLAIR MR axial image obtained 16 months postoperatively revealing complete resolution of vasogenic edema.

More important, both studies confirmed a very significant survival advantage, adding surgical resection to the treatment strategy (median survival, 10 months). Quality of life (QOL) was also significantly improved by adding surgery. In the study by Patchell et al, "cerebral deaths" were reduced from 50% for WBRT alone to 29% when surgery was added, and the median time spent at a KPS score of 70 or greater improved from 2 months to 9.5 months.[95] In the study by Vecht et al, the median time before World Health Organization (WHO) QOL score or RTOG Neurological Functional Scale score dropped to 1 or less increased from 3.5 months to 7.5 months.[130]

Inclusion criteria for those studies were similar. Patients had to have single solid brain lesions, be older than 18 years, have had a tissue diagnosis of a primary cancer (within 5 years for Patchell et al), have a KPS score of at least 70 (or WHO QOL scale and RTOG Neurological Functional Scale of 2 or less), and their tumor in a resectable (noneloquent) location. Overall, approximately 20% to 25% of all patients with newly diagnosed solid tumor brain metastases satisfy these inclusion criteria. In both studies, favorable prognostic factors other than surgical resection included young age and absence of systemic disease. In the study by Patchell et al, a prolonged time from the diagnosis of the primary to the diagnosis of the brain metastasis (which favors breast cancer and melanoma primaries) was an additional favorable factor. In general, the local resection-cavity recurrence rate for surgical gross-total resection is approximately 10% if WBRT is added postoperatively but is 46% if WBRT is withheld, presumably due to the local persistence of microscopic disease.[96]

Given that the median time interval from diagnosis of the primary tumor until the diagnosis of a solid tumor brain metastasis in breast cancer patients is 2 to 3 years, the availability of several effective means for successful treatment of ongoing systemic disease, and the relative sensitivity of breast cancer to fractionated radiation therapy, it should be no surprise that selected surgical resection series of patients with solid brain tumor metastases from breast cancer report even better median life expectancies than those reported for brain metastases in general. The two largest modern series of surgical resection for metastatic brain tumors number 70 and 63 patients, respectively.[98,139]

In the report from Memorial Sloan-Kettering, median life expectancy in patients with metastatic brain tumors from breast cancer treated with surgical excision plus WBRT was 16.2 months from the diagnosis of the brain tumor and 14 months from the time of craniotomy (some patients had WBRT first rather than postoperatively).[139] The 1-, 2-, 3-, and 4-year postcraniotomy survival rates were 55.3%, 25.7%, 18.6%, and 7%, respectively. However, this series is confounded by the inclusion of patients who also had carcinomatous meningitis at the time of surgery. If these patients are excluded, the median life expectancy after craniotomy increases even further to 17.4 months. In the report from The University of Texas M.D. Anderson Cancer Center (M.D. Anderson), patients with metastatic brain tumors from breast cancer treated with surgical excision plus WBRT had a median life expectancy from the time of craniotomy of 16 months, and the 3- and 5-year survival rates were 22% and 17%, respectively.[98]

In the Memorial Sloan-Kettering study, significant factors predicting survival with univariate analysis included positive hormonal receptor status (positive effect) and the presence of carcinomatous meningitis (negative effect). Only the presence or absence of carcinomatous meningitis remained significant

with multivariate analysis.[139] In the M.D. Anderson study, significant factors predicting survival with univariate analysis included younger age (positive effect), higher KPS score (positive effect), and preoperative systemic disease status (both no evidence of disease vs. systemic disease, and controlled vs. active systemic disease).[98] All three remained significant on multivariate analysis. Factors not found to be statistically significant in the Sloan-Kettering study included age, lesion size, neurologic functional status, positive axillary nodes, and supratentorial versus infratentorial location. Systemic disease status was not analyzed. Factors not found to be statistically significant in the M.D. Anderson study included menopausal status, supratentorial versus infratentorial location, subtotal versus total resection, and the presence or absence of chemotherapy.

In both the Memorial Sloan-Kettering and the M.D. Anderson studies, 50% of patients with metastatic brain tumors from breast cancer died from "neurologic causes" or from "progression of neurologic disease."[98,139] This rate is higher for breast cancer than for metastatic brain disease from other primaries and may reflect the higher chance with breast cancer of eventually developing carcinomatous meningitis in addition to the shared risks of developing recurrent or new solid brain tumors.

Although surgical resection for single solid-tumor brain metastases is now well established as a preferred treatment option in appropriate patients, surgical resection for patients with multiple solid brain tumors or recurrent solid brain tumors remains controversial. Certainly, patients with multiple or recurrent solid brain tumor metastases are less likely than their single-lesion counterparts to have high functional neurologic status or controlled systemic disease, both of which are strong predictors of outcome. A large part of the controversy, however, exists because of the relative absence of good data regarding outcome in these patients.

The most often quoted paper regarding surgical resection for multiple metastatic brain tumors in a single session is that by Bindal et al.[10] They performed a retrospective case-control study of three groups of patients from the same institution treated over a similar time period, who were matched for patient sex and age, KPS score, type of primary tumor, time from primary to brain tumor diagnosis, and presence or absence of systemic disease. Group A included 30 patients who had one or more lesions left unresected. Group B included 26 patients who had all lesions resected (23, two lesions removed; 3, three lesions removed). Group C included 26 matched patients with single lesions that were removed. Breast cancer was the second most common histology in groups B and C. In this report, resection of all lesions provided similar survival benefit to removal of a single lesion (14 months median survival with the addition of WBRT), and both strategies provided results significantly superior to removal of selected lesions only (6-month median survival with the addition of WBRT). This article was the first to demonstrate that what was really important in dealing with metastatic solid brain tumors was the ability to completely and definitively address all of the CNS disease and not necessarily the total number of lesions involved. Most important, 30-day complication rates did not differ among groups (8% to 9%) despite the additional craniotomies performed, and 30-day mortality rates for the three groups were 3%, 4%, and 0%, respectively.[10] For this approach to be practically feasible, all of the lesions in question must arise in surgically accessible locations. Indeed, ideally all lesions should be accessible under the same general anesthesia administration and with the patient remaining in the same surgical position.

Even with the addition of WBRT and neuroimaging evidence of gross-total resection of the original tumor, metastatic brain tumors can recur locally at the previous resection site in up to 10% of cases.[96] Although patients with breast cancer or melanoma as the primary cancer diagnosis tend to fare worse than patients with other primary histologies, reresection of the lesion can provide additional length of life and QOL benefits in selected patients, as long as they have a good KPS score and have controlled systemic disease.[11]

Stereotactic Radiosurgery

SRS is a means of delivering an overwhelming single high dose of radiation to a precisely defined, and confined, volume of tissue, with little delivery of radiation to tissue even 2 mm from the treatment volume. The neurosurgical procedure requires a specialized radiation delivery mechanism to provide the extreme radiation concentration and steep volume edge radiation falloff. The delivery system is coupled to frame-based stereotactic targeting to provide the spatial accuracy necessary to ensure that all of the lesion is included in the therapeutic dose and that surrounding normal tissue is, for the most part, excluded. The delivery system can be a gamma unit with 201 separate cobalt-60 sources (Gamma Knife®), a rotational arc linear accelerator (LINAC), a robotic arm–mounted "point and shoot" linear accelerator (Cyberknife®), or a charged-particle cyclotron (using the Bragg peak effect). Because the radiobiology of single-fraction SRS is quite different from the radiobiology of fractionated radiation therapy, the standard radiation therapy concept of radioresistance no longer applies. Indeed, SRS works equally well for traditionally radioresistant histologies such as melanoma and renal cell carcinoma as it does for traditionally radiosensitive histologies such as breast cancer or lung cancer. SRS does not vaporize a tumor. Its goal is to take a tumor that grows and turn it into one that never can grow again. Presumed biologic end points include immediate cell death, delayed apoptosis triggered when a damaged cell tries to enter mitosis, and irreversible cellular growth arrest. Successful treatment is measured in terms of tumor control (absence of tumor growth). Although many tumors do shrink to varying degrees, and some go on to disappear on neuroimaging studies (Figure 55-3), this is not the goal of the treatment and cannot be reliably predicted preoperatively.

The Gamma Knife and LINAC are the devices most commonly used for SRS. Both provide similar targeting and delivery accuracy as well as radiation falloff for the treatment of a single isocenter. For spherical or ellipsoidal volumes with predominantly convex surfaces (such as most solid metastatic brain tumors), both provide equivalent degrees of three-dimensional targeting conformality. The only difference between the two for the treatment of most metastases is that the LINAC delivers the tumor margin dose to the 80% or 90% isodose line, whereas the Gamma Knife prescribes the margin dose to the 40% or 50% isodose line. This means that for a LINAC the maximum dose to the tumor center is 1.1 to 1.25 times the minimal margin dose, whereas for the Gamma Knife the tumor maximum dose is 2 to 2.5 times the minimal margin dose. Although this accentuated tumor "hot spot" is a theoretical advantage for the Gamma Knife and may account for the 2.84-fold relative risk for local failure after brain tumor treatment with LINAC SRS compared with Gamma Knife SRS as seen in the RTOG phase I trial of SRS for brain tumors (for equivalent tumor volumes and margin doses),[115] this has yet to be shown to translate into a clinical difference between the two techniques in outcomes after SRS for patients with brain metastasis.

For reasons related to dose-volume toxicity, SRS is limited to treatment volumes of 30 cc (<3.5 cm in diameter if spherical). It can treat lesions in any location regardless of their proximity to eloquent brain (Figure 55-4), including the deep gray matter and brainstem, and can treat multiple lesions in one sitting.[6,76] The procedure is performed without general anesthesia, and patients usually go home to full preoperative activity level within 24 hours. Minimal margin doses of 15 to 25 Gy are delivered, adjusting for the final treatment volume (usually 1.5 to 2 times the lesion volume). If SRS is to be used alone (without WBRT), larger margin doses of at least 18 Gy are necessary to maintain acceptable local control rates.[117]

Although class 1 evidence (by evidence-based medicine criteria) through a prospective randomized clinical trial is not available to assess SRS plus WBRT for patients with single brain metastases, many prospective, often multi-institutional, series (class 2 evidence) have now been published that evaluate both Gamma Knife and LINAC SRS.[4,5,8,54,82] All show a median life expectancy of 9 to 13 months, median time of 7 to 11 months spent at KPS score of 70 or greater, and the percentage of patients dying from their brain tumor reduced to 20% to 25%. All of these values are equivalent to those obtainable with open surgical resection.[95,130]

There has been no 30-day mortality directly related to SRS. Acute complications from SRS after previous WBRT include a 2% to 10% incidence of mild nausea and a 2% to 6% incidence of seizure during the first 24 hours. Subacute complications include an approximately 5% risk of focal alopecia if the scalp dose is 4.4 Gy or greater. Chronic complications include a 5% to 15% incidence of a transient new or worsened neurologic deficit, a 1% to 5% risk of a new permanent neurologic deficit, and a 1% to 6% incidence of radiation necrosis requiring surgical resection or chronic steroid dependence. The risk of radiation necrosis critically depends on the total dose of WBRT prescribed before the SRS. Local tumor control rates (absence of tumor growth) after SRS plus WBRT for single solid brain tumor metastases range from 85% to 95%. With minimum tumor margin doses of at least 18 to 20 Gy, these local control rates are maintained for SRS without WBRT.[57,84,117] However, if lower doses are used for SRS without the addition of WBRT, local recurrence rates can be between 20% and 82%.[57,102,121] Because the development of distant new brain metastases would not be affected by SRS, the incidence of distant tumor control failure in the brain due to development of a new brain tumor is, as expected, higher with SRS alone versus SRS plus WBRT.[58,102,121]

The multi-institutional study by Auchter et al[8] was specifically designed to match patients undergoing SRS plus WBRT to inclusion criteria used in the randomized prospective clinical trial of surgical resection plus WBRT performed by Patchell et al.[95] Using a comparable patient population, median survival for the SRS plus WBRT group for patients with single solid tumor brain metastases was 56 weeks (13 months), with 1- and 2-year actuarial survival rates of 53% and 30%, respectively. The median time spent at a KPS score of 70 or greater was 11 months, and 25% of deaths were attributable to the brain tumor.

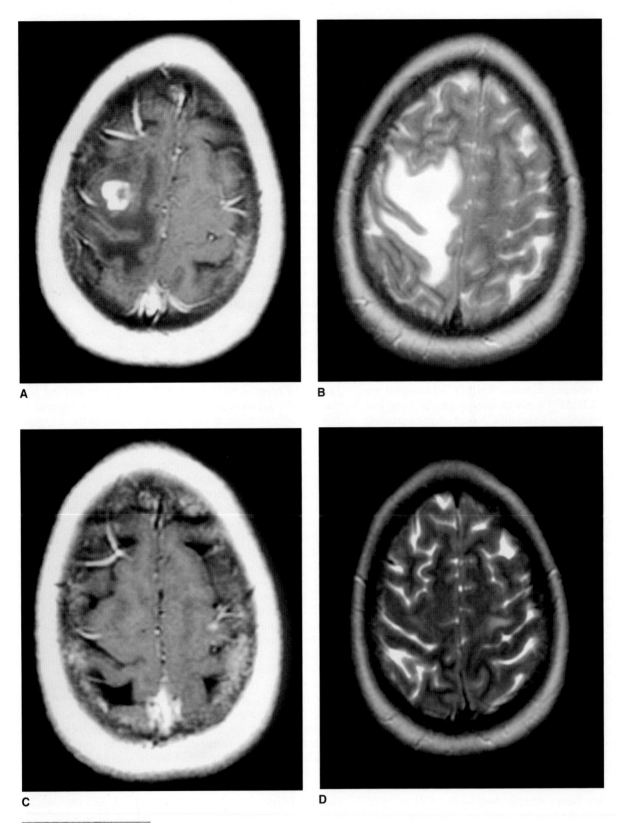

FIGURE 55-3 A 46-year-old woman with new-onset seizure and rapidly progressing new-onset left hemiparesis was found to have a single posterior right frontal lobe brain metastasis. Preoperative functional imaging confirmed that the lesion arose within a primary motor strip. She had a Karnofsky Performance Scale (KPS) score of 80 and had controlled systemic disease. She was treated with Gamma Knife stereotactic radiosurgery (16 Gy to the 50% isodose line at the tumor margin) and whole-brain radiation therapy (WBRT). *A,* Preoperative T1-weighted, contrast-enhanced magnetic resonance (MR) axial image of the tumor. *B,* Preoperative T2-weighted MR axial image of the tumor and surrounding vasogenic edema. *C,* T1-weighted, contrast-enhanced MR axial image obtained 12 months postoperatively revealing complete response. *D,* T2-weighted, contrast-enhanced MR axial image obtained 12 months postoperatively revealing complete resolution of vasogenic edema.

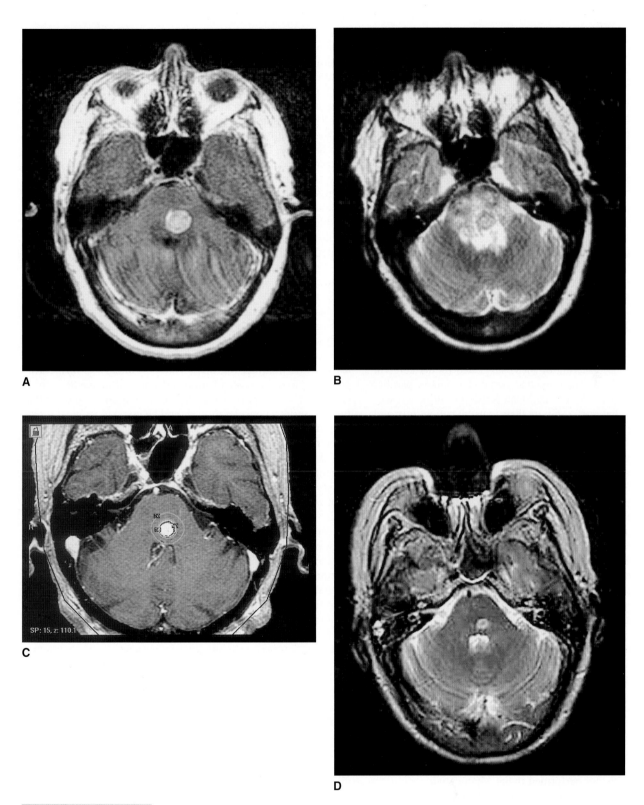

FIGURE 55-4   A 70-year-old woman with a single breast cancer brainstem metastasis within the substance of her pons. She had a Karnofsky Performance Scale (KPS) score of 60 with a right hemiparesis and sensory deficits in her right arm. Her systemic disease was responding to therapy, and she had already received whole-brain radiation therapy (WBRT). She was treated with Gamma Knife stereotactic radiosurgery (SRS) (16 Gy to the 50% isodose line at the tumor margin). Within 2 months of SRS she had improved to a KPS score of 90 (mild residual right arm paresthesias only, living and functioning independently). *A,* Preoperative T1-weighted, contrast-enhanced magnetic resonance (MR) axial image of the tumor. *B,* Preoperative T2-weighted MR axial image of the tumor and surrounding vasogenic edema. *C,* Gamma Knife SRS MR treatment plan revealing the location and distribution of the 50%, 40%, and 20% isodose lines. *D,* T2-weighted contrast-enhanced MR axial image obtained 6 months postoperatively revealing complete resolution of vasogenic edema and reduced tumor size.

Multivariate analysis revealed that baseline KPS score and absence of systemic disease were significant predictors of outcome.

There are two studies of SRS limited to patients with breast cancer brain metastases. The first, from the University of Pittsburgh, included 30 patients and 58 treated tumors (14 patients with single lesions, 15 patients with two to four lesions, and 1 patient with six lesions), and all but 4 also received WBRT either before or after their SRS.[50] The second study, from a private practice group in Miami, included 68 patients and treated approximately 544 tumors (average of 8 tumors per patient) in 110 SRS sessions.[6] Fifteen patients had single lesions, 26 had one to three lesions, 18 had four to seven lesions, and 24 had eight or more lesions. The maximum number of lesions treated in a single session was 25. Thirty-eight patients had received WBRT, but thirty patients were treated with SRS alone. The overall median survival interval from the time of SRS was 13 months (18 months from tumor diagnosis) for the Pittsburgh group and 7.8 months for the Miami group.

The Pittsburgh results[50] confirm the impression that breast cancer patients tend to do better than patients having other cancer histologies with additional local control measures (whether surgical resection or SRS) suggested by the surgical resection series.[98,139] Their median survival numbers parallel those reported by the Memorial Sloan-Kettering surgical resection plus WBRT report.[139] Given their unusual patient mix and aggressive treatment strategy, the results of the Miami group must be stratified by lesion number if they are to be comparable. Although their overall median survival time for patients with breast cancer brain metastases treated with SRS with or without WBRT was 7.8 months from SRS, the results for patients with one to three lesions treated (a group more comparable to the Pittsburgh, M.D. Anderson, and Sloan-Kettering groups) were much better. Indeed, within their length of follow-up (median 7.8 months), the Kaplan-Meier plot for this group never crossed 50% and was level at 60% by 14 months after SRS, suggesting that the median survival interval is likely to be 14 months or longer for this group.[6]

The cause of death was related to cerebral disease in 38% of deaths in the Pittsburgh report and only 9% in the Miami report.[6,50] This is in sharp contrast to the higher than expected 50% death rates from cerebral disease noted in both the M.D. Anderson and the Sloan-Kettering breast cancer brain metastasis resection plus WBRT reports.[98,139] In the Pittsburgh study, both smaller tumor volume and presence of only one brain tumor correlated with survival by univariate analysis, but only presence of a single brain tumor remained significant upon multivariate analysis.[50] Patient age, presence of systemic disease, previous WBRT, and supratentorial versus infratentorial tumor location were not found to be significant. Multifactorial statistical analysis was not performed in the Miami study.

Multiple metastatic brain tumors can be readily treated during a single SRS session. Excellent data exist for the results and efficacy of treating up to four tumors at one time. The Gamma Knife group at the University of Pittsburgh performed a prospective randomized clinical trial of WBRT plus SRS versus WBRT alone for patients with 2 to 4 solid tumor brain metastases.[76] Breast cancer was the third most common cancer histology in the study. This class 1 evidence study evaluated both local tumor control and median survival time as end points. The interim results for local tumor control were so strik-

ingly significant that the study had to be stopped for ethical reasons at the 60% accrual point (in accordance with original Institutional Review Board approved study design). One-year local control failure rates were 100% for WBRT alone versus 8% for WBRT and SRS. Although the patients' median survival rates were 7.5 months for WBRT versus 11 months for WBRT and SRS, the study was stopped before it had sufficient power for these results to reach statistical significance. Interestingly, just as noted from the surgical resection study of multiple metastatic brain tumors by Bindal et al,[10] the median survival time of patients with multiple tumors when SRS definitively addresses all tumors appears to be no different from that of patients with single lesions treated with SRS. No additional morbidity accrues with SRS for multiple lesions versus SRS for single lesions, at least as has been studied for up to four tumors treated in a single session.

For the 5% to 15% of patients with breast cancer metastatic to the brain who demonstrate tumor growth after WBRT and SRS, repeat SRS remains an option, with a chance similar to the original SRS treatment of again achieving local control.[6] The risk of radiation necrosis, however, increases slightly with each successive SRS procedure, especially if a significant total dose of fractionated radiation therapy has already been given. This risk is minimal for small volume tumors (<5 mL, corresponding to a diameter of up to 2.1 cm) but increases significantly for volumes of 10 to 30 mL. For these larger volume tumors, serious consideration should be given to surgical resection if they progress despite SRS and are in a surgically resectable location.

As previously stated, approximately 20% to 25% of all patients with newly diagnosed solid tumor brain metastases satisfy the inclusion criteria outlined in both prospective, randomized studies of surgical resection plus WBRT (single solid brain lesions, older than 18, tissue diagnosis of a primary cancer, KPS score of 70 or greater, and tumor in a resectable location). For SRS, however, location of the lesion no longer matters, and patients with up to four lesions have been proved to significantly benefit from the therapy versus WBRT alone. With these revisions accounted for, approximately 60% to 68% (two thirds) of patients with newly diagnosed metastatic brain tumors would be candidates for referral for consideration for treatment with SRS. Whether to proceed with therapy will at that time depend on the presence or absence of other systemic disease, and if systemic disease is present, whether it is controlled or potentially controllable. To benefit from the effects of SRS, a patient would have to have an expected life span (irrespective of any CNS disease) of at least 6 months, which is the maximal benefit likely to be afforded by WBRT alone (the default treatment alternative).

Chemotherapy for Brain Metastases

Systemic cytotoxic chemotherapy has not been extensively evaluated in the treatment of patients with brain metastasis. A study published in 1986 showed significant response rates in a fairly heterogeneous group of patients with brain metastases due to breast cancer.[107] Approximately 63% of these patients had received prior adjuvant chemotherapy, primarily CMF (cyclophosphamide, methotrexate, and 5-FU) or cyclophosphamide and doxorubicin. Response rates, including partial and complete responses, measured approximately 30 to 50 percent. A similar study focusing on breast cancer also demonstrated impressive results.[14] Additional studies included other primary sites and have also demonstrated responses using a variety of chemotherapy agents.[29,30,56,74,141] Recent reports in mixed patient populations have demonstrated benefit with a newer chemotherapy drug, temozolomide, which is known to obtain adequate levels in the CNS with oral administration, can be given on a chronic basis (years in some patients), and is associated with relatively low toxicity.[1,2,26]

Chemotherapy can also be delivered to extracellular fluid space in doses higher than those safely achievable with intravenous or intra-arterial administration through surgical implantation of chemotherapy-impregnated, biodegradable, sustained-release polymers at the time of tumor resection. Experimental animal evidence suggests this approach might be effective for metastatic breast cancer lesions.[48] Clinical use of this technology in patients with brain metastasis is currently under active investigation. Whether it finds a role, particularly for patients with very large brain metastases that cannot be treated with SRS, remains to be seen.

All of these studies demonstrate a proof of principle: cytotoxic chemotherapy can have an impact on CNS metastasis (Figure 55-5). The blood-brain barrier does not prevent, or even significantly inhibit, the efficacy of these agents. The studies mentioned previously have small numbers of patients, and their systemic disease burden is variable, making it difficult to draw clear guidelines for treatment recommendations. Most patients develop metastases while receiving systemic therapy. Moving to the next systemic agent does not ensure success, and the morbidity from uncontrolled CNS metastases can be devastating, causing most clinicians to proceed with WBRT. The issue becomes more pertinent for patients who, except for their CNS disease, are long-term survivors and have already been treated with WBRT but who are not candidates for SRS or microsurgery due to multiplicity of lesions (e.g., more than four lesions). Here cytotoxic chemotherapy has the potential to have the greatest effect on CNS disease.

Many research questions remain regarding the role of chemotherapy for brain metastasis. How should we stratify patients based on their systemic disease burden and prior treatments? What is the relative benefit of chemotherapy compared with WBRT? Would there be additive benefit if both modalities were used? Should they be used together or sequentially? What agents are optimal? All of these issues remain to be studied.

Treatment Approach for Patients with Solid Brain Tumors

Work in neuro-oncology over the past 12 years has clearly demonstrated that the key to improving both length of life and QOL for patients with dissemination of their cancer to the brain is achieving complete local control of the brain tumors. Equivalent degrees of local control can be achieved through open microsurgical resection or through SRS. With the addition of either of these two surgical modalities, average life span for patients with single metastatic tumors improves to 10 months or more. More important, now fewer than one in four patients will die as a direct result of their brain tumor. This means two very important things. First, because brain function has the greatest impact of any organ on functional independence, this translates into significant gains in patient QOL. Second, the type of cancer a patient has, and how well the rest of the disease

is controlled, now determines longevity. For patients with cancers that are sensitive to chemotherapy or hormonal therapy (such as breast cancer) or patients with little disease other than their brain tumor, extended survival measured in years, and even cure, now becomes possible.

Ideally, what we need to have to complete our comparative analysis of treatment options for patients with solid tumor brain metastases from breast cancer would be a prospective randomized clinical trial comparing surgical resection plus WBRT with WBRT plus SRS for patients with single brain tumors. In the mid 1990s RTOG and at least three universities opened studies for just that purpose. All went on to close due to inadequate patient accrual. Some of the poor accrual was due to reluctance of some clinicians to randomize in this setting. However, the majority was due to reluctance of patients to agree to potentially be randomized to open surgical resection once they knew that a less invasive alternative was available that was being studied as a potentially equivalent therapy. Attempts to get at this comparative issue retrospectively within single institutions have yielded conflicting results.[12,87] For now, we need to be satisfied with class 2 strength of evidence for the equivalence of the SRS alternative.

Both open surgical resection and SRS have a roughly equivalent capability of maximizing local tumor control, providing an additional length of life benefit, reducing the incidence of cerebral tumor-induced death, and of maximizing QOL for patients with single metastatic solid brain tumors. However, open surgical resection and SRS each have their own advantages and disadvantages, which are outlined in Table 55-4. Both treatment options should be available within a comprehensive, state-of-the-art, multidisciplinary neuro-oncology treatment program.

Arkansas Cancer Research Center Neuro-Oncology Program Strategy

What follows is a description of our current treatment philosophy and priority ranking in the Neuro-Oncology Program at the Arkansas Cancer Research Center. A breakdown of our case distribution for each treatment modality over the past 3.5 years according to tumor number and the tumor location relative to eloquent brain is given in Figure 55-6. All patients with breast cancer and solid brain tumor metastases receive WBRT at our institution. A single brain metastasis as the only evidence of residual disease (isolated metastasis) is extremely rare with breast cancer, as compared with the situation with non–small cell lung cancer, melanoma, or renal cell carcinoma. We reserve additional measures to maximize local control, such as surgical resection or SRS, in an effort to increase life expectancy for patients with a KPS score of 70 or greater who have controlled or "controllable" disease (defined as a reasonable chance of at least a 6-month life expectancy if the CNS disease were not present). If patients are candidates for surgical resection or SRS for this goal, care is taken to ensure that WBRT fraction size is no greater than 2 Gy, with a total dose of 40 Gy, to limit long-term cognitive side effects as well as the cumulative risk of radiation necrosis (if SRS is to be used) in these patients with longer projected life spans.

In our program, we consider open surgical resection as the clearly superior treatment choice for (1) the rare breast cancer patient with an isolated solid metastatic brain tumor (the only evidence of disease) who has the potential for cure, (2) patients

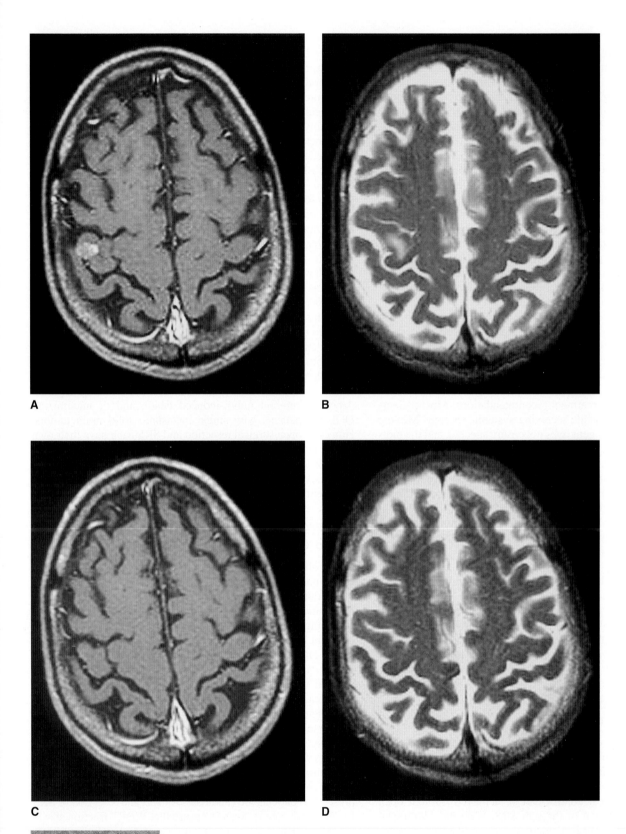

FIGURE 55-5 A 55-year-old man with a head and neck neuroendocrine (carcinoid) tumor developed multiple new brain metastases despite successful whole-brain radiation therapy (WBRT) and three separate Gamma Knife stereotactic radiosurgery (SRS) procedures over 3 years for previous metastatic lesions. He was placed on oral temozolomide chemotherapy and within 3 months demonstrated a significant response as seen by neuroimaging. *A,* Before chemotherapy, T1-weighted, contrast-enhanced magnetic resonance (MR) axial image of one of the new (not previously treated) tumors. *B,* Before chemotherapy, T2-weighted MR axial image demonstrating surrounding vasogenic edema. *C,* T1-weighted, contrast-enhanced MR axial image obtained 3 months after starting chemotherapy, demonstrating a complete tumor response. *D,* T2-weighted MR axial image obtained 3 months after starting chemotherapy, demonstrating resolution of vasogenic edema.

TABLE 55-4	Advantages and Disadvantages of Surgical Resection versus Stereotactic Radiosurgery plus WBRT for Patients with Breast Cancer Solid Brain Tumor Metastases

Advantage Surgical Resection/Disadvantage Stereotactic Radiosurgery	Relative Equivalence For Both	Advantage Stereotactic Radiosurgery/ Disadvantage Surgical Resection
Tissue diagnosis without additional procedure	Local control of disease	Can treat lesions in any location
Can treat lesions >3.5 cm in maximal diameter	Extension of life span	Can easily treat multiple lesions
Can immediately relieve symptomatic mass effect	Maximization of quality of life	One-day return to preoperative functional level
Potential for cure with an "isolated" brain metastasis	Reduction in incidence of "cerebral death"	No general anesthesia
More complete and faster relief of vasogenic edema		Minimally invasive
Faster time to improvement in baseline neurological deficit		Lower cost and less hospitalization time
No risk of radiation necrosis		No craniotomy morbidity/mortality

"Cerebral death," Death from growth of cerebral (metastatic) tumor; WBRT, Whole-brain radiation therapy.

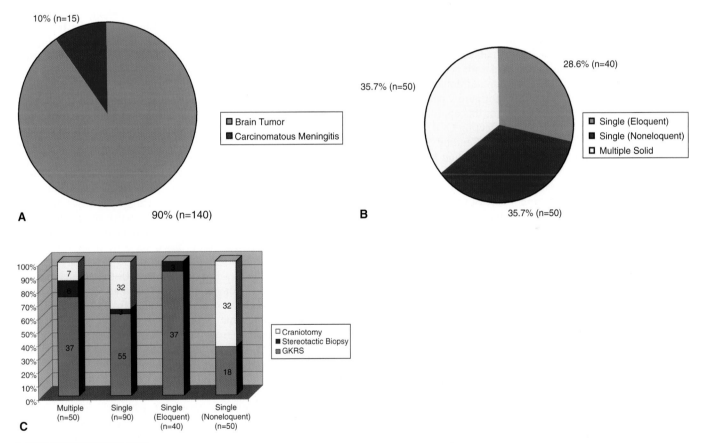

FIGURE 55-6   Case analysis for metastatic central nervous system disease referred to the multidisciplinary Neuro-Oncology Program at Arkansas Cancer Research Center from December 1993 through June 2001 (3.5 years). *A,* Pie graph demonstrating the distribution of carcinomatous meningitis relative to solid tumor disease. *B,* Pie chart demonstrating the relative distributions of patients with single solid tumors arising in eloquent brain, patients with single solid tumors arising in noneloquent brain, and patients with multiple tumors, among patients with solid tumor disease. *C,* Bar graph depicting the relative frequency of surgical intervention with diagnostic stereotactic biopsy, microsurgical resection, or Gamma Knife stereotactic radiosurgery depending on whether the patient had a single lesion located in noneloquent brain, a single lesion located in eloquent brain, or multiple lesions.

with symptomatic mass effect from tumors larger than 3.5 cm in greatest diameter, and (3) patients with obstructive hydrocephalus from their tumor or at high risk for obstructive hydrocephalus from a large posterior fossa tumor abutting the fourth ventricle. We consider open surgical resection to be the preferred option for breast cancer patients with a single solid brain tumor metastasis in a surgically resectable location who (1) have no evidence of systemic disease outside of the CNS and (2) are younger than 65. We consider SRS to be the preferred option for breast cancer patients (1) with a single solid brain tumor metastasis located in an eloquent brain location, (2) with a single solid brain tumor metastasis who have systemic disease outside of the CNS, (3) with a single solid brain tumor metastasis who pose an unacceptable medical risk for general anesthesia or open surgery, (4) who refuse recommended open surgical resection, and (5) with two to four solid metastatic tumors of appropriate size.

Patients with more than four solid metastatic brain tumors or with one to four lesions who have rapidly progressing systemic disease are candidates for systemic chemotherapy after their WBRT. The choice of agents must be determined by the extent of extracranial disease and the prior chemotherapy history. Occasionally, breast cancer patients with more than four solid metastatic brain tumors and with actively progressing systemic disease will benefit from additional intervention with either surgical resection or SRS for purely palliative QOL reasons. Targeting the correct lesion for this approach requires that the symptom or sign adversely affecting QOL be one that can accurately localize the specific offending lesion neuroanatomically. Ideally, the candidate offending lesion should be one that has been shown to have grown or increased in the amount of surrounding vasogenic edema during the clinical period in question. In this setting it is reasonable to selectively target the offending lesion while leaving the other lesions alone. If the lesion is 3.5 cm in maximal diameter or larger or is causing symptoms from obstructive hydrocephalus and is surgically accessible, we advocate an open surgical approach. If it is smaller than 3.5 cm and is not causing obstructive hydrocephalus, we advocate selective SRS as the preferred approach.

Controversies

Demonstration of longer survival possibilities with aggressive treatment of breast cancer patients who have solid tumor brain metastases, recognition that SRS (with a 2 mm penumbra) is theoretically less likely to leave behind untreated microscopic disease, and the desire to avoid the potential cognitive side effects of WBRT has led many clinicians to advocate treating with SRS and withholding WBRT.[6,57,84,117,121] This requires one to treat with SRS to minimal doses of 18 to 20 Gy to avoid an increase in local recurrence rate when WBRT is eliminated.[57,102,117] Although this strategy will predictably lead to an increase in the number of distant tumor control failures in the brain, the argument goes that imaging surveillance will pick up these failures, as well as any potential local control failures, and allow for salvage SRS if needed.[121] Although we acknowledge and support this treatment strategy for patients with radioresistant tumor histologies (e.g., renal cell carcinoma or melanoma— where WBRT is not likely to provide significant benefit in exchange for its potential cognitive toxicity), we are not yet convinced that there is enough evidence of advantage to justify this approach for radiosensitive histologies like breast cancer.

If both WBRT and SRS are to be used, the issue of which to do first is controversial. We generally perform WBRT first for several reasons. First, it may provide some tumor shrinkage, which will allow us to safely deliver a higher SRS margin dose and optimize our result. Second, it allows the 2 to 4 weeks of WBRT to be used as a "triage trial." For those patients with newly diagnosed systemic disease or progressing systemic disease being shifted to a different systemic therapy, it allows for a period of observation to assess whether the systemic disease is stabilizing before committing to SRS. For those rare breast cancer patients who develop additional brain metastases while being treated with WBRT, it allows canceling SRS if a total of more than four lesions develop, as well as inclusion of all additional lesions if the total remains four or less.

Multiple metastatic brain tumors can be readily treated during a single SRS session. Indeed, several groups have now reported treating up to 25,[6] and even 78, lesions (M. Yamamoto, Mito, Japan, personal communication, June 2001) with a single stereotactic frame placement. Many groups consider an arbitrary cutoff for the number of lesions that should be treated to be artificial and to have little scientific basis in the literature. Although we recognize the artificial and somewhat arbitrary nature of a limit of four lesions for SRS, we also recognize that in at least one study for breast cancer the number of metastases did significantly affect outcome for patients with brain metastases independently of the extent of systemic disease.[50] We will selectively consider SRS for breast cancer patients with more than four solid brain tumor metastases if they have a KPS score of 70 or greater, are younger than 65, and have CNS tumors as their only evidence of disease.

The RPA performed by Gaspar and colleagues on multiple RTOG WBRT studies to try to stratify brain metastasis patients into separate definable prognostic categories[60] has unfortunately been misapplied by many third-party payers to try to limit patients' access to potentially beneficial therapy with SRS. Despite categories not being based on SRS results data and never intended to be applied to limit access to therapy, several payers in several states limit access to SRS to patients in class 1 (KPS score of 70 or greater, younger than 65, "controlled" primary tumor, and no extracranial metastases). In fact, the only class from the RPA that predicted a median life span less than the median expected from WBRT in general (4 to 6 months) was class 3 (KPS score <70, median survival 2.3 months). This is perhaps the most appropriate class of patients to unilaterally restrict from access to additional expensive therapies associated with at least some risk of additional morbidity. Class 2 is an extremely heterogeneous group of patients (defined as an exclusionary grab bag or "catch-all"—all patients not class 1 or 3), many of whom will benefit from either open surgical resection or SRS.

The truth is that at least two studies have now shown that SRS plus WBRT provides significant survival benefit for patients across all three RTOG RPA classes.[23,111] In the retrospective 10-institution study of 502 patients with solid tumor brain metastases treated with SRS plus WBRT, the median survival times of patients across RPA classes were 16.1, 10.3, and 8.7 months, respectively,[23] as compared with median survivals of 7.1, 4.2, and 2.3 months observed in the RTOG RPA analysis.[60] Apparently, the improvement in survival afforded by SRS plus WBRT relative to WBRT alone is not restricted by RPA class-selected patients. There is also now a study demonstrating that SRS alone significantly improves survival for patients in all three RPA classes[122] compared with survival times predicted for WBRT alone.[60]

Carcinomatous Meningitis

Breast cancer is one of the most common cancer types leading to leptomeningeal involvement, along with melanoma, lymphoma, and lung cancer. The frequency of leptomeningeal disease in clinical series of breast cancer patients is 2% to 5%, with similar rates of 3% to 6% seen at autopsy. Lobular carcinoma has a predilection to spread to the subarachnoid space, as compared with ductal disease (16% versus 0.3% in one study).[35] Patients with solid tumor metastatic brain disease can develop carcinomatous meningitis, and this will occur in up to one third of symptomatic cases. Clinical symptoms of carcinomatous meningitis include symptoms from hydrocephalus and raised intracranial pressure (headache, nausea, vomiting, somnolence, memory problems, other alterations in mental status), cranial neuropathy (diplopia and auditory symptoms most common), back pain, radiculopathy, or cauda equina syndrome.

Diagnosis is made by a combination of neuroimaging and CSF sampling for cytologic analysis. Contrast-enhanced MRI of the head and total spine is the imaging tool of choice (Figure 55-7). Even MRI, however, will miss the diagnosis in 25% to 30% of patients who have a positive CSF cytology. Disease may be limited to the ventricular ependyma or the leptomeningeal surface, or may involve both. False-negative CSF cytologies are common despite obvious evidence of disease by neuroimaging. Both the quantity of CSF removed for analysis and the number of samples analyzed are important to maximize diagnostic yield. To reach a yield of more than 70% requires that a minimum of 10.5 mL of CSF be spun down for cells, with a minimum of two separate samples. To reach more than 80% diagnostic sensitivity requires a minimum of 8 mL to be spun for cells on three separate occasions.[65] If the disease is restricted to the ventricular lining as seen on neuroimaging, ventricular CSF obtained at the time of CSF reservoir placement may be necessary to confirm the diagnosis. A high suspicion of the condition and a combination of MRI and aggressive CSF sampling are required to make the correct diagnosis. Neuroimaging should be obtained before the lumbar puncture to rule out the potential for tapping below an intradural block as well as to limit any associated imaging artifact as a result of the tap.

Another confounding factor in breast cancer patients is that solid tumor brain metastases will occasionally be dural based.[109] Distinction of a dural-based solid tumor metastasis from carcinomatous meningitis with nodular disease, and even from

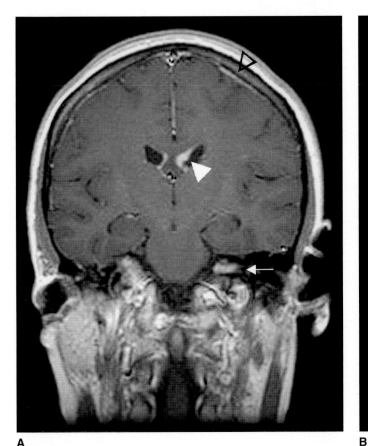

A

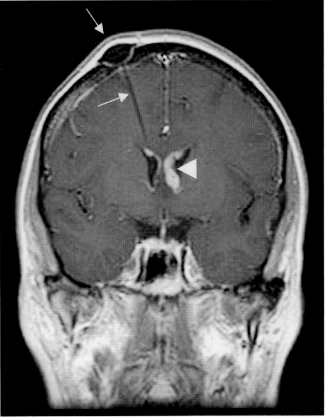

B

FIGURE 55-7 T1-weighted, contrast-enhanced coronal magnetic resonance images of a young woman with carcinomatous meningitis. *A*, Image taken at the level of the foramen of Monro and internal auditory canal demonstrating characteristic leptomeningeal convexity enhancement *(open arrow)*, ependymal enhancement of the ventricular system *(closed arrow)*, and enhancement filling the internal auditory canal *(small arrow)*. *B*, Image taken at the level of the coronal suture and the pituitary stalk demonstrating ependymal enhancement of the ventricular system *(large arrow)* and the outline of the Ommaya reservoir with ventricular catheter in the right coronal position *(small arrows)*.

an associated or incidental meningioma,[13] is extremely important, because all three portend markedly different prognoses.

Survival without treatment for patients with carcinomatous meningitis is extremely poor, with death from the leptomeningeal disease usually occurring within 1 to 2 months. Treatment includes intrathecal chemotherapy delivered via an implanted ventricular CSF reservoir. A nuclear medicine CSF flow study should be obtained after the reservoir is placed and before intrathecal treatment to rule out a block to CSF flow that might limit the drug's access to different compartments or increase drug toxicity by concentrating the drug in a smaller trapped volume of CSF. If a blockage is identified, low-dose focal fractionated irradiation to the blocked area is usually sufficient to reestablish flow.[64] Inability to reestablish free CSF flow is a very poor prognostic sign.[22,64]

Roughly equivalent results have been achieved using methotrexate alone, thiotepa alone, and methotrexate and cytosine arabinoside in combination. Most patients are treated with some form of combined intrathecal chemotherapy and fractionated radiation therapy. Fractionated radiation therapy is used for areas of nodular disease that cannot be reached by diffusion from the CSF (approximately 2 mm maximal penetration) and for clinically symptomatic areas. Cranial-spinal radiation therapy is usually avoided because of the increased risks of myelosuppression and the multifocal encephalopathy toxicity encountered when intrathecal methotrexate is combined with supratentorial fractionated radiation therapy. If the disease is primarily nodular or more than 2 mm thick diffusely, the best treatment is a combination of fractionated radiation therapy and systemic chemotherapy.

Overall response rate to treatment is approximately 65%, with median survival time in responding patients improved to 4.5 to 7.2 months. Although nonresponders tend to die of their CNS disease, approximately 50% of responders actually die from an extra-CNS cause. Complications of intrathecal chemotherapy via a ventricular CSF reservoir over time also include an approximately 20% risk of infection, wound breakdown, or catheter or reservoir failure.[35,73] Experimental treatments with intrathecal monoclonal antibodies conjugated to radioisotopes or potent cellular toxins such as ricin have not improved the grim outlook for patients with this form of CNS metastasis from breast cancer.

Parenchymal Spinal Cord Metastases

Parenchymal spinal cord solid tumor metastases are the rarest form of extension of breast carcinoma to the CNS and indeed are extremely rare for any histologic primary.[127] They must be distinguished from nodular surface accentuation of carcinomatous meningitis, which is far more common. They usually cause myelopathy and spinal cord syndromes associated with the predominant location of the lesion within the spinal cord. They are best diagnosed with contrast-enhanced MRI. Lesions arising above the level of the innervation of the diaphragm (C3, 4, and 5) are best treated conservatively with high-dose steroids and fractionated radiation therapy to avoid the disastrous QOL outcome of respirator-dependent quadriplegia. Lower lesions can be surgically explored and occasionally resected with good outcome depending on the lesion's proximity to the dorsal surface of the cord (Figure 55-8). All lesions should be treated initially with high-dose intravenous glucocorticoid therapy and fractionated radiation therapy regardless of whether resection

is possible. Good data do not exist for median survival or functional outcome in this very rare subgroup of patients, nor do good data exist comparing the outcome of surgical resection and radiation therapy to radiation therapy alone.

CONCLUSION

We are entering an exciting new era in our ability to help our patients's with CNS metastases from breast cancer. Never before have more effective means of maximizing and maintaining patients' quality of life as well as successfully achieving long-term survival for the majority of patients been available to us. The old nihilistic philosophy of simply treating patients with CNS metastases with steroids and "30 in 10" WBRT as a "no brainer" approach must now go the way of Halsted's radical mastectomy. The two keys to successfully completing this paradigm shift lie in (1) educating our colleagues that overwhelming evidence since the mid 1990s shows that the key to maximizing patient life expectancy and QOL lies in maximizing local CNS tumor control through either microsurgical resection or SRS in combination with WBRT, and (2) overcoming an apparent persistent and pervasive paternalistic attitude among many general practitioners, medical oncologists, and radiation oncologists that they need to "protect their patient from the surgeon."

Best current estimates suggest that approximately 20% to 25% of all patients with newly diagnosed solid tumor breast cancer brain metastases would qualify for referral to a neurosurgeon for consideration for microsurgical resection. Approximately 60% to 68% (two thirds) of patients with newly diagnosed metastatic brain tumors would be candidates for referral to a neurosurgeon or radiation oncologist for consideration for treatment with SRS. These two subsets of patients greatly overlap but are not identical. The majority of the remaining one third of patients do not qualify for referral because of the presence of more than four metastases. Whether future expansion of SRS indications to treat patients with more than four tumors will become scientifically validated or whether chemotherapy after WBRT might earn a significant role for this most desperate remaining subgroup of patients remains to be seen.

Of all possible primary histologies, breast cancer may be one of the most appropriate for oncologists to take an aggressive stance on once CNS metastases are identified. If local CNS tumor control can be maximized through microsurgical resection or SRS in addition to WBRT, the "rate limiting step" for the ultimate length of patients' survival becomes the patient's extent of systemic disease and the availability and effectiveness of multiple therapies for controlling that systemic disease. Given the current availability of many different effective means for successful treatment of ongoing systemic disease and the relative sensitivity of breast cancer to fractionated radiation therapy, breast cancer patients have an even greater chance of 2- to 5-year survival (or even cure) after diagnosis of a brain metastasis than their counterparts with other histologies.

Acknowledgment

The authors gratefully acknowledge Mary E. Atherton, fourth year medical student at the University of Arkansas for Medical Sciences, for her assistance with organizing and finalizing the figures for illustration and Jose Penagaricano, MD, for assistance with researching a portion of the radiation therapy section.

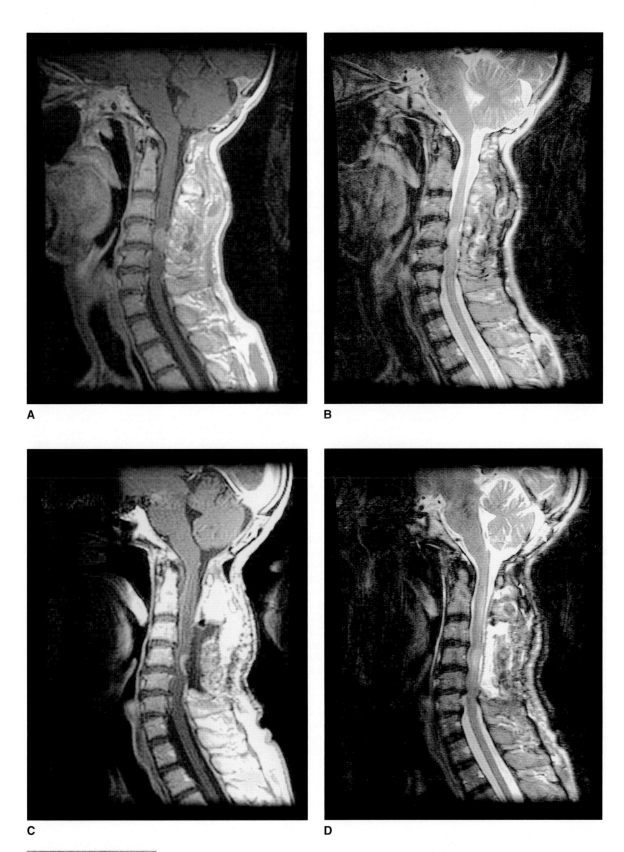

FIGURE 55-8 A 58-year-old man with a non–small cell lung cancer intraparenchymal exophytic metastasis to the spinal cord at the C4 level successfully treated with ultrasound-guided microsurgical resection followed by fractionated radiation therapy. *A*, Preoperative T1-weighted, contrast-enhanced sagittal magnetic resonance (MR) image of the tumor. *B*, Preoperative T2-weighted sagittal MR image of the tumor. *C*, T1-weighted, contrast-enhanced sagittal MR image obtained the first postoperative day revealing near-total resection. *D*, T2-weighted sagittal MR image obtained on the first postoperative day revealing near-total resection of tumor with some residual spinal cord edema.

References

1. Abrey LE, Christodoulou C: Temozolomide for treating brain metastases. Semin Onco 28:34–42, 2001.

2. Abrey LE, Olson JD, Raizer JJ, et al: A phase II trial of temozolomide for patients with recurrent or progressive brain metastases. J Neurooncol 53:259–265, 2001.

3. Adjuvant Therapy for Breast Cancer. NIH Consensus Statement 2000 November 1–3; 17:1–35, 2000.

4. Adler JR, Cox RS, Kaplan I, et al: Stereotactic radiosurgical treatment of brain metastases. J Neurosurg 76:444–449, 1992.

5. Alexander E, III, Moriarty TM, Davis RB, et al: Stereotactic radiosurgery for the definitive, noninvasive treatment of brain metastases. J Natl Cancer Inst 87:34–40, 1995.

6. Amendola BE, Wolf AL, Coy SR, et al: Gamma knife radiosurgery in the treatment of patients with single and multiple brain metastases from carcinoma of the breast. Cancer J 6:88–92, 2000.

7. Asai A, Matsutani M, Kohno T, et al: Subacute brain atrophy after radiation therapy for malignant brain tumor. Cancer 63:1962–1974, 1989.

8. Auchter RM, Lamond JP, Alexander E, et al: A multiinstitutional outcome and prognostic factor analysis of radiosurgery for resectable single brain metastasis. Int J Radiat Oncol Biol Phys 35:27–35, 1996.

9. Baum M: The ATAC (arimidex, tamoxifen, alone or in combination) adjuvant breast cancer trial in post-menopausal women. The 24th Annual San Antonio Breast Cancer Symposium, Dec 10–13, 2001.

10. Bindal RK, Sawaya R, Leavens ME, et al: Surgical treatment of multiple brain metastases. J Neurosurg 79:210–216, 1993.

11. Bindal RK, Sawaya R, Leavens ME, et al: Reoperation for recurrent metastatic brain tumors. J Neurosurg 83:600–604, 1995.

12. Bindal AK, Bindal RK, Hess KR, et al: Surgery versus radiosurgery in the treatment of brain metastasis. J Neurosurg 84:748–754, 1996.

13. Bonito D, Giarelli L, Falconieri G, et al: Association of breast cancer and meningioma. Report of 12 cases and review of the literature. Path Res Pract 189:399–404, 1993.

14. Boogerd W, Dalesio O, Bais EM, et al: Response of brain metastases from breast cancer to systemic chemotherapy. Cancer 69:972–980, 1992.

15. Borgelt B, Gelber R, Kramer S, et al: The palliation of brain metastases: final results of the first two studies by the Radiation Therapy Oncology Group. Int J Radiat Oncol Biol Phys 6:1–9, 1980.

16. Burke W, Daly M, Garber J, et al: Recommendations for follow-up care of individuals with an inherited predisposition to cancer. BRCA1 and BRCA2. Cancer Genetics Studies Consortium. JAMA 277:997–1003, 1997.

17. Burt M, Wronski M, Arbit E, et al: Resection of brain metastases from non-small-cell lung carcinoma. Results of therapy. Memorial Sloan-Kettering Cancer Center Thoracic Surgical Staff. J Thorac Cardiovasc Surg 103:399–410, 1992.

18. Buzdar AU, Jones SE, Vogel CL, et al: A phase III trial comparing anastrozole (1 and 10 milligrams), a potent and selective aromatase inhibitor, with megestrol acetate in postmenopausal women with advanced breast carcinoma. Arimidex Study Group. Cancer 79:730–739, 1997.

19. Buzdar AU, Jonat W, Howell A: Anastrozole versus megestrol acetate in the treatment of postmenopausal women with advanced breast carcinoma: results of a survival updated based on a combined analysis of data from two mature phase III trials. Arimidex Study Group. Cancer 83:1142–1152, 1998.

20. Carlson RW: Update: NCCN practice guidelines for treatment of breast cancer. Oncology 13:41–68, 1999.

21. Carter CL, Allen C, Henson DE: Relation of tumor size, lymph node status and survival in 24,740 breast cancer cases. Cancer 63:181–187, 1989.

22. Chamberlain MC, Kormanik PR: Carcinomatous meningitis secondary to breast cancer: predictors of response to combined modality therapy. J Neuroonc 35:55–64, 1997.

23. Chidel MA, Suh JH, Reddy CA, et al: Application of recursive partitioning analysis and evaluation of the use of whole brain radiation among patients treated with stereotactic radiosurgery for newly diagnosed brain metastases. Int J Radiat Oncol Biol Phys 47:993–999, 2000.

24. Chittoor SR, Swain SM: Locally advanced breast cancer: role of medical oncology. In Bland KI, Copeland EM (eds): The Breast: Comprehensive Management of Benign and Malignant Diseases, 2nd ed, Vol 1. Philadelphia, WB Saunders, 1998.

25. Chock JY, Domchek S, Burstein HJ, et al: Central nervous system metastases in women who receive trastuzumab for metastatic breast cancer. American Society of Clinical Oncology 38th Annual Meeting, May 18–21, 2002.

26. Christodoulou C, Bafaloukos D, Kosmidis P, et al: Phase II study of temozolomide in heavily pretreated cancer patients with brain metastases. Ann Oncol 12:249–254, 2001.

27. Clark G, Mathieu M, Owens M, et al: Prognostic significance of S-phase fraction in good-risk node-negative breast cancer patients. J Clin Oncol 10:428–432, 1992.

28. Clark GM: Prognostic and predictive factors. In Harris JR, Lippman ME, Morrow M, Osborne CK (eds): Diseases of the Breast, 2nd ed. Philadelphia, Lippincott Williams & Wilkins, 2000.

29. Cocconi G, Lottici R, Bisagni G, et al: Combination therapy with platinum and etoposide of brain metastases from breast carcinoma. Cancer Invest 8:327–334, 1990.

30. Colleoni M, Graiff C, Nelli P, et al: Activity of combination chemotherapy in brain metastases from breast and lung adenocarcinoma. Am J Clin Oncol 20:303–307, 1997.

31. Couch FJ, DeShano ML, Blackwood MA, et al: BRCA1 mutations in women attending clinics that evaluate the risk of breast cancer. N Engl J Med 336:1409–1415, 1997.

32. Cuzick J, Stewart H, Peto R, et al: Overview of randomized trials comparing radical mastectomy without radiotherapy against simple mastectomy with radiotherapy in breast cancer. Cancer Treat Rep 71:7–14, 1987.

33. Cuzick J, Stewart HJ, Peto R, et al: Overview of randomized trials of postoperative adjuvant radiotherapy in breast cancer. Recent Results Cancer Res 111:108–129, 1988.

34. DeAngelis LM, Delattre JY, Posner JB: Radiation-induced dementia in patients cured of brain metastases. Neurology 39: 789–796, 1989.

35. DeAngelis LM, Rogers LR, Foley KM: Leptomeningeal metastasis. In Harris JR, Lippman ME, Morrow M, Osborne CK (eds): Diseases of the Breast, 2nd ed. Philadelphia, Lippincott Williams & Wilkins, 2000.

36. DeMichele A, Weber BL: Inherited genetic factors. In Harris JR, Lippman ME, Morrow M, Osborne CK (eds): Diseases of the Breast, 2nd ed. Philadelphia, Lippincott Williams & Wilkins, 2000.

37. DiStefano A, Yong Yap Y, Hortobagyi GN, et al: The natural history of breast cancer patients with brain metastases. Cancer 44:1913–1918, 1979.

38. Davidson NE, Kennedy MJ, Armstrong DK: Dose-intensive chemotherapy. In Harris JR, Lippman ME, Morrow M, Osborne CK (eds): Diseases of the Breast, 2nd ed. Philadelphia, Lippincott Williams & Wilkins, 2000:633–644.

39. Davis PC, Hudgins PA, Peterman SB, et al: Diagnosis of cerebral metastases: double-dose delayed CT vs contrast-enhanced MR imaging. Am J Neuroradiol 12:293–300, 1991.

40. Early Breast Cancer Trialists' Collaborative Group: Effects of adjuvant tamoxifen and of cytotoxic therapy on mortality in early breast cancer. An overview of 61 randomized trials among 28,896 women. N Engl J Med 319:1681–1692, 1998.

41. Early Breast Cancer Trialists' Collaborative Group: Systemic treatment of early breast cancer by hormonal, cytotoxic, or immune therapy. Lancet 339:71–85, 1992.

42. Early Breast Cancer Trialists' Collaborative Group: Ovarian ablation in early breast cancer. Overview of the randomised trials. Lancet 348:1189–1196, 1996.

43. Early Breast Cancer Trialists' Collaborative Group: Review: ovarian ablation improves survival in women younger than 50 years with breast cancer. Am Coll Physicians Club 2:75–85, 1997.

44. Early Breast Cancer Trialists' Collaborative Group: Polychemotherapy for early breast cancer. An overview of the randomised trials. Lancet 352:930–942, 1998.

45. Early Breast Cancer Trialists' Collaborative Group: Tamoxifen for early breast cancer. An overview of the randomised trials. Lancet 351:1451–1467, 1998.

46. Elledge RM, Fuqua SAW: Estrogen and progesterone receptors. In Harris JR, Lippman ME, Morrow M, Osborne CK (eds): Diseases of the Breast, 2nd ed. Philadelphia, Lippincott Williams & Wilkins, 2000.

47. Ellis MJ, Hayes DF, Lippman ME: Treatment of metastatic breast cancer. In Harris JR, Lippman ME, Morrow M, Osborne CK (eds): Diseases of the Breast, 2nd ed. Philadelphia, Lippincott Williams & Wilkins, 2000.

48. Ewend MG, Sampath P, Williams JA, et al: Local delivery of chemotherapy prolongs survival in experimental brain metastases from breast carcinoma. Neurosurgery 43:1185–1193, 1998.

49. Ferrara M, Bizzozzero L, Talamonti G, et al: Surgical treatment of 100 single brain metastases. Analysis of the results. J Neurosurg Sci 34:303–308, 1990.

50. Firlik KS, Kondziolka D, Flickinger JC, et al: Stereotactic radiosurgery for brain metastases from breast cancer. Ann Surg Oncol 7:333–338, 2000.

51. Fisher B, Bauer M, Wickerham L, et al: Relation of number of positive axillary nodes to the prognosis of patients with primary breast cancer: an NSABP update. (With the contribution of Cruz A and other NSABP Investigators) Cancer 52:1551–1557, 1983.

52. Fisher B, Costantino J, Redmond C, et al: Lumpectomy compared with lumpectomy and radiation therapy for the treatment of intraductal breast cancer. N Engl J Med 328:1581–1586, 1993.

53. Fisher B, Anderson S, Redmond CK, et al: Reanalysis and results after 12 years of follow-up in a randomized clinical trial comparing total mastectomy with lumpectomy with or without irradiation in the treatment of breast cancer. N Engl J Med 333:1456–1461, 1995.

54. Flickinger JC, Kondziolka D, Lunsford LD, et al: A multi-institutional experience with stereotactic radiosurgery for solitary brain metastasis. Int J Radiat Oncol Biol Phys 28:797–802, 1994.

55. Fowble B, Solin L, Schultz D, et al: Ten year results of conservative surgery and irradiation for stage I and II breast cancer. Int J Radiat Oncol Biol Phys 21:269–277, 1991.

56. Franciosi V, Cocconi G, Michiara M, et al: Front-line chemotherapy with cisplatin and etoposide for patients with brain metastases from breast carcinoma, nonsmall cell lung carcinoma, or malignant melanoma: a prospective study. Cancer 85:1599–1605, 1999.

57. Fukuoka S, Seo Y, Takanashi M, et al: Radiosurgery of brain metastases with the Gamma Knife. Stereotact Func Neurosurg 66:193–200, 1996.

58. Fuller BG, Kaplan ID, Adler J, et al: Stereotaxic radiosurgery for brain metastases: the importance of adjuvant whole brain irradiation. Int J Radiat Oncol Biol Phys 23:413–418, 1992.

59. Gainor BJ, Buchert P: Fracture healing in metastatic bone disease. Clin Orthopaedic Related Res 178:297–302, 1983.

60. Gaspar L, Scott C, Rotman M, et al: Recursive partitioning analysis (RPA) of prognostic factors in three Radiation Therapy Oncology Group (RTOG) brain metastases trials. Int J Radiat Oncol Biol Phys 37:745–751, 1997.

61. Gelber RD, Larson M, Borgelt BB, et al: Equivalence of radiation schedules for the palliative treatment of brain metastases in patients with favorable prognosis. Cancer 48:1749–1753, 1981.

62. Giuliano AE, Jones RC, Brennan M, Statman R: Sentinel lymphadenectomy in breast cancer. J Clin Oncol 15:2345–2350, 1997.

63. Giuliano AE, Kirgan DM, Guenther JM, Morton DL: Lymphatic mapping and sentinel lymphadenectomy for breast cancer. Ann Surg 220:391–398, 1994.

64. Glantz MJ, Hall WA, Cole BF, et al: Diagnosis, management, and survival of patients with leptomeningeal cancer based on cerebrospinal fluid-flow status. Cancer 75:2919–2931, 1995.

65. Glantz MJ, Cole BF, Glantz LK, et al: Cerebrospinal fluid cytology in patients with cancer: minimizing false-negative results. Cancer 82:733–739, 1998.

66. Guinee VF: Epidemiology of breast cancer. In Bland KI, Copeland EM (eds): The Breast: Comprehensive Management of Benign and Malignant Diseases, 2nd ed, Vol 1. Philadelphia, WB Saunders, 1998.

67. Hazra T, Mullins GM, Lott S: Management of cerebral metastasis from bronchogenic carcinoma. Johns Hopkins Med J 130:377–383, 1972.

68. Hortobagyi GN, Singletary SE, Strom EA: Treatment of locally advanced and inflammatory breast cancer. In Harris JR, Lippman ME, Morrow M, Osborne CK (eds): Diseases of the Breast, 2nd ed. Philadelphia, Lippincott Williams & Wilkins, 2000.

69. Host H, Brennhovd IO, Loeb M: Postoperative radiotherapy in breast cancer. Long-term results from the Oslo study. Int J Radiat Oncol Biol Phys 12:727–732, 1986.

70. Howell A, Robertson J, Albano J, et al: Fulvestrant, formerly ICI 182,780, is as effective as anastrozole in postmenopausal women with advanced breast cancer progressing after prior endocrine treatment. J Clin Oncol 20:3396–3403, 2002.

71. Jacobson JA, Danforth DN, Cowan KH, et al: Ten-year results of a comparison of conservation with mastectomy in the treatment of stage I and II breast cancer. N Engl J Med 332:907–911, 1995.

72. Johnson JE, Dutt PL, Page DL: Extent and multicentricity of in situ and invasive carcinoma. In Bland KI, Copeland EM (eds): The Breast: Comprehensive Management of Benign and Malignant Diseases, 2nd ed, Vol 1. Philadelphia, WB Saunders, 1998.

73. Johnson KA, Kramer BS, Crane JM: Management of central nervous system metastases in breast cancer. In Bland KI, Copeland EM (eds): The Breast: Comprehensive Management of Benign and Malignant Diseases, 2nd ed, Vol 1. Philadelphia, WB Saunders, 1998:1389–1402.

74. Kaba SE, Kyritsis AP, Hess K, et al: TPDC-FuHu chemotherapy for the treatment of recurrent metastatic brain tumors. J Clin Oncol 15:1063–1070, 1997.

75. Kofman S, Garvin JS, Nagamani D, et al: Treatment of cerebral metastases from breast carcinoma with prednisolone. JAMA 163:1473–1476, 1957.

76. Kondziolka D, Patel A, Lunsford LD, et al: Stereotactic radiosurgery plus whole brain radiotherapy versus radiotherapy alone for patients with multiple brain metastases. Int J Radiat Oncol Biol Phys 45:427–434, 1999.

77. Krag DN, Weaver OJ, Alex JC, Fairbank JT: Surgical resection and radiolocalization of the sentinel node in breast cancer using a gamma probe. Surg Oncol 2:335–339, 1993.

78. Lagios MD, Page DL: In situ carcinomas of the breast: Ductal carcinoma in situ, Paget's disease, lobular carcinoma in situ. In Bland KI, Copeland EM (eds): The Breast: Comprehensive Management of Benign and Malignant Diseases, 2nd ed, Vol 1. Philadelphia, WB Saunders, 1998.

78a. Lippman ME (ed): Proceedings of the National Institutes of Health Consensus Development Conference on Adjuvant Chemotherapy and Endocrine Therapy for Breast Cancer. NCI Monographs, No. 1, 1986.

79. Lynch HT, Lemon SJ, Marcus JN, et al: Breast cancer genetics: heterogeneity, molecular genetics, syndrome diagnosis, and genetic counseling. In Bland KI, Copeland EM (eds): The Breast: Comprehensive Management of Benign and Malignant Diseases, 2nd ed, Vol 1. Philadelphia, WB Saunders, 1998.

80. Markesbery WR, Brooks WH, Gupta GD, et al: Treatment for patients with cerebral metastases. Arch Neurol 35:754–756, 1978.

81. Matsubayashi T, Koga H, Nishiyama Y, et al. The reparative process of metastatic bone lesions after radiotherapy. Jap J Clin Oncology 11:253–264, 1987.

82. Mehta MP, Rozental JM, Levin AB, et al: Defining the role of radiosurgery in the management of brain metastases. Int J Radiat Oncol Biol Phys 24:619–625, 1992.

83. Miki Y, Swensen J, Shattuck-Eidens D, et al: A strong candidate for the breast and ovarian cancer susceptibility gene mutations in primary breast and ovarian carcinomas. *BRCA1*. Science 266:66–71, 1994.

84. Mori Y, Kondziolka D, Flickinger JC, et al: Stereotactic radiosurgery for brain metastasis from renal cell carcinoma. Cancer 83:344–353, 1998.

85. Morrow M, Schnitt SJ: Lobular carcinoma *in situ*. In Harris JR, Lippman ME, Morrow M, Osborne CK (eds): Diseases of the Breast, 2nd ed. Philadelphia, Lippincott Williams & Wilkins, 2000.

86. Morrow M, Schnitt SJ, Harris JR: Ductal carcinoma *in situ* and microinvasive carcinoma. In Harris JR, Lippman ME, Morrow M, Osborne CK (eds): Diseases of the Breast, 2nd ed. Philadelphia, Lippincott Williams & Wilkins, 2000.

87. Muacevic A, Kreth FW, Horstmann GA, et al: Surgery and radiotherapy compared with gamma knife radiosurgery in the treatment of solitary cerebral metastases of small diameter. J Neurosurg 91:35–43, 1999.

88. Mundy GR, Guise TA, Yoneda T: Biology of bone metastases. In Harris JR, Lippman ME, Morrow M, Osborne CK (eds): Diseases of the Breast, 2nd ed. Philadelphia, Lippincott Williams & Wilkins, 2000.

89. Muss HB, Thor AD, Berry DA, et al: C-erbB-2 expression and response to adjuvant therapy in women with node-positive early breast cancer. N Engl J Med 330:1260–1266, 1994.

90. Nabholtz JM, Buzdar A, Pollak M, et al: Anastrozole is superior to tamoxifen as first-line therapy for advanced breast cancer in postmenopausal women: results of a North American multicenter randomized trial. Arimidex Study Group. J Clin Oncol 19:2578–2582, 2001.

91. O'Shaughnessy J, Miles D, Vukelja S, et al: Superior survival with capecitabine plus docetaxel combination therapy in anthracycline-pretreated patients with advanced breast cancer: phase III trial results. J Clin Oncol 20:2812–2823, 2002.

92. Osborne CK: Steroid hormone receptors in breast cancer management. Breast Cancer Res Treat 51:227–238, 1998.

93. Osborne CK, Pippen J, Jones SE, et al: Double-blind, randomized trial comparing the efficacy and tolerability of fulvestrant versus anastrozole in postmenopausal women with advanced breast cancer progressing on prior endocrine therapy: results of a North American trial. J Clin Oncol 20:3386–3395, 2002.

94. Overgaard M, Hansen PS, Overgaard J, et al: Postoperative radiotherapy in high risk pre-menopausal women with breast cancer who receive adjuvant chemotherapy. Danish Breast Cancer Cooperative Group 82b Trial. N Engl J Med 337: 949–955, 1997.

95. Patchell RA, Tibbs PA, Walsh JW, et al: A randomized trial of surgery in the treatment of single metastases to the brain. N Engl J Med 322:494–500, 1990.

96. Patchell RA, Tibbs PA, Regine WF, et al: Postoperative radiotherapy in the treatment of single metastases to the brain: a randomized trial. JAMA 280:1485–1489, 1998.

97. Pavy JJ, Denekamp J, Letschert J, et al: EORTC Late Effects Working Group. Late effects toxicity scoring: the SOMA scale. Radiother Oncol 35:11–15, 1995.

98. Pieper DR, Hess KR, Sawaya RE: Role of surgery in the treatment of brain metastases in patients with breast cancer. Ann Surg Oncol 4:481–490, 1997.

99. Posner JB: Diagnosis and treatment of metastases to the brain. Clin Bull 4:47–57, 1974.

100. Powers WE, Ratanatharathorn V: Palliation of bone metastasis. In Brady L, Perez C (eds): Principles and Practice of Radiation Oncology. Philadelphia, Lippincott-Raven, 1998.

101. Ragaz J, Jackson SM, Le M, et al: Adjuvant radiotherapy and chemotherapy in node positive pre-menopausal women with breast cancer. N Engl J Med 337:956–962, 1997.

102. Regine WF, Huhn JL, Patchell RA, et al: Risk of symptomatic brain tumor recurrence and neurologic deficit after radiosurgery alone in patients with newly diagnosed brain metastases: results and implications. Int J Radiat Oncol Biol Phys 52:333–338, 2002.

103. Rivkin S, Green S, Metch B, et al: Adjuvant CMFVP versus concurrent CMFVP and tamoxifen for postmenopausal node-positive and estrogen receptor-positive breast cancer patients: a Southwest Oncology Group Study. J Clin Oncol 12:2078–2085, 1994.

104. Robinson DS, Sundaram M: Stereotactic imaging and breast biopsy. In Bland KI, Copeland EM (eds): The Breast: Comprehensive Management of Benign and Malignant Diseases, 2nd ed, Vol 1. Philadelphia, WB Saunders, 1998.

105. Rosen N, Sepp-Lorenzino L, Lippman ME: Biological therapy. In Harris JR, Lippman ME, Morrow M, Osborne CK (eds): Diseases of the Breast, 2nd ed. Philadelphia, Lippincott Williams & Wilkins, 2000.

106. Rosen PP, Groshen S, Kinne DW, et al: Factors influencing prognosis in node-negative breast carcinoma: analysis of 767 T1N0M0/T2N0M0 patients with long-term follow-up. J Clin Oncol 11:2090–2100, 1993.

107. Rosner D, Nemoto T, Lane WW: Chemotherapy induces regression of brain metastases in breast carcinoma. Cancer 58:832–839, 1986.

108. Ruderman NB, Hall TC: Use of glucocorticoids in the palliative treatment of metastatic brain tumors. Cancer 18:298–306.

109. Rumana CS, Hess KR, Shi WM, et al: Metastatic brain tumors with dural extension. J Neurosurg 89:552–558, 1998.

110. Russo J, Frederick J, Ownby H, et al: Predictors of recurrence and survival of patients with breast cancer. Am J Clin Pathol 88:123–131, 1987.

111. Sanghavi SN, Miranpuri SS, Chappell R, et al: Radiosurgery for patients with brain metastases: a multi-institutional analysis, stratified by the RTOG recursive partitioning analysis metastases. Int J Radiat Oncol Biol Phys 51:426–434, 2001.

112. Sawaya R, Hammoud M, Schoppa D, et al: Neurosurgical outcomes in a modern series of 400 craniotomies for treatment of parenchymal tumors. Neurosurgery 42:1044–1055, 1998.

113. Schnitt SJ, Giuidi AJ: Pathology and biological markers of invasive breast cancer. In Harris JR, Lippman ME, Morrow M, Osborne CK (eds): Diseases of the Breast, 2nd ed. Philadelphia, Lippincott Williams & Wilkins, 2000.

114. Schumacher M, Schmoor C, Sauerbrei W, et al: The prognostic effect of histological tumor grade in node-negative breast cancer patients. Breast Cancer Res Treat 25:235–245, 1993.

115. Shaw E, Scott C, Souhami L, et al: Single dose radiosurgical treatment of recurrent previously irradiated primary brain tumors and brain metastases: final report of RTOG protocol 90–05. Int J Radiat Oncol Biol Phys 47:291–298, 2000.

116. Shaw EG: Radiotherapeutic management of multiple brain metastases: "3000 in 10" whole brain radiation is no longer a "no brainer." Int J Radiat Oncol Biol Phys 45:253–254, 1999.

117. Shiau CY, Sneed PK, Shu HK, et al: Radiosurgery for brain metastases: relationship of dose and pattern of enhancement to local control. Int J Radiat Oncol Biol Phys 37:375–383, 1997.

118. Sim FH, Frassica FJ, Frassica DA: Metastatic bone disease: current concepts of clinico-pathophysiology and modern surgical treatment. Ann Acad Med 21:274–279, 1992.

119. Simpson J, Wilkinson E: Malignant neoplasia of the breast: infiltrating carcinomas. In Bland KI, Copeland EM (eds): The Breast: Comprehensive Management of Benign and Malignant Diseases, 2nd ed, Vol 1. Philadelphia, WB Saunders, 1998.

120. Smith R, Sun Y, Garin A, et al: Femara® (Letrozole) showed significant improvement in efficacy over tamoxifen as first-line treatment in postmenopausal women with advanced breast cancer. 23rd Annual San Antonio Breast Cancer Symposium. December 6–9, 2000.

121. Sneed PK, Lamborn KR, Forstner JM, et al: Radiosurgery for brain metastases: is whole brain radiotherapy necessary? Int J Radiat Oncol Biol Phys 43:549–558, 1999.

122. Sneed PK, Suh JH, Goetsch SJ, et al: A multi-institutional review of radiosurgery alone vs. radiosurgery with whole brain radiotherapy as the initial management of brain metastases. Int J Radiat Oncol Biol Phys 53:519–526, 2002.

123. Solin L, Fowble B, Schultz D, et al: The significance of the pathology margins of the tumor excision on the outcome of patients treated with definitive irradiation for early stage breast cancer. Int J Radiat Oncol Biol Phys 21:279–287, 1991.

124. Sundaresan N, Galicich JH: Surgical treatment of brain metastases. Clinical and computerized tomography evaluation of the results of treatment. Cancer 55:1382–1388, 1985.

125. Tancini G, Bonadonna G, Valagussa P, et al: Adjuvant CMF in breast cancer: comparative 5-year results of 12 versus 6 cycles. J Clin Oncol 1:2–10, 1983.

126. Theriault RL: Medical treatment of bone metastases. In Harris JR, Lippman ME, Morrow M, Osborne CK (eds): Diseases of the Breast, 2nd ed. Philadelphia, Lippincott Williams & Wilkins, 2000.

127. Tognetti F, Lanzino G, Calbucci F: Metastases of the spinal cord from remote neoplasms. Study of five cases. Surg Neurol 30:220–227, 1988.

128. Veronesi U, Luini A, Galimberti V, Zurrida S: Conservation approaches for the management of stage I/II carcinoma of the breast: Milan Cancer Institute trials. World J Surg 18:70–75, 1994.

129. Veronesi U, Paganelli G, Galimberti V, et al: Sentinel-node biopsy to avoid axillary dissection in breast cancer with clinically negative lymph-nodes. Lancet 349:1864–1867, 1997.

130. Vecht CJ, Haaxma-Reiche H, Noordijk EM, et al: Treatment of single brain metastasis: radiotherapy alone or combined with neurosurgery? Ann Neurol 33:583–590, 1993.

131. Wardley A, Danson S, Clayton A, et al: High incidence of brain metastases in patients treated with trastuzumab for metastatic breast cancer at a large cancer centre. American Society of Clinical Oncology 38th Annual Meeting, May 18–21, 2002.

132. Wen PY, Black PM, Loeffler JS: Treatment of metastatic cancer. In DeVita VT, Hellman S, Rosenberg SA (eds): Cancer: Principles and Practice of Oncology, 6th ed. Philadelphia, Lippincott Williams & Wilkins, 2001.

133. Wen PY, Shafman TD: Site-specific therapy of metastatic breast cancer. In Harris JR, Lippman ME, Morrow M, Osborne CK (eds): Diseases of the Breast, 2nd ed. Philadelphia, Lippincott Williams & Wilkins, 2000.

134. Wilkinson EJ, Masood S: Cytologic needle samplings of the breast: Techniques and end results. In Bland KI, Copeland EM (eds): The Breast: Comprehensive Management of Benign and Malignant Diseases, 2nd ed, Vol 1. Philadelphia, WB Saunders, 1998.

135. Willett WC, Rockhill B, Hankinson SE, et al: Epidemiology and assessing and managing risk. In Harris JR, Lippman ME, Morrow M, Osborne CK (eds): Diseases of the Breast, 2nd ed. Philadelphia, Lippincott Williams & Wilkins, 2000.

136. Winer EP, Morrow M, Osborne CK, Harris JR: Malignant tumors of the breast. In DeVita VT, Hellman S, Rosenberg SA (eds): Cancer: Principles and Practice of Oncology. 6th ed. Philadelphia, Lippincott Williams & Wilkins, 2001.

137. Witliff JL, Pasic R, Bland, KI: Steroid and peptide hormone receptors: methods, quality control and clinical use. In Bland KI, Copeland EM (eds): The Breast: Comprehensive Management of Benign and Malignant Diseases, 2nd ed, Vol 1. Philadelphia, WB Saunders, 1998.

138. Wooster R, Bignell G, Lancaster J: Identification of the breast cancer susceptibility gene BRCA2. Nature 378:789–792, 1995.

139. Wronski M, Arbit E, McCormick B, et al: Surgical treatment of 70 patients with brain metastases from breast carcinoma. Cancer 80:1746–1754, 1997.

140. Zimm S, Wampler GL, Stablein D, et al: Intracerebral metastases in solid-tumor patients: natural history and results of treatment. Cancer 48:384–394, 1981.

141. Zulkowski K, Kath R, Semrau R, et al: Regression of brain metastases from breast carcinoma after chemotherapy with bendamustine. J Cancer Res Clin Oncol 128:111–113, 2002.

CHAPTER 56

BRAIN METASTASES FROM MALIGNANT MELANOMA

John H. Sampson, Timothy D. Shafman, James H. Carter, Jr., Allan H. Friedman, and Hilliard F. Seigler

When diagnosed at an early stage, cutaneous melanoma can be cured by wide excision. However, patients with metastatic disease beyond the first-order lymph nodes are usually incurable despite aggressive radiation therapy, chemotherapy, or immunotherapy. After metastases to the lung, metastases to the brain represent the most common manifestation of metastatic disease in these patients, and brain metastases are often the cause of death. This chapter reviews the available data on the incidence and risk factors associated with the development of brain metastases in patients with melanoma. It also reviews the clinical presentation, results of treatment, and prognosis of these patients.

DEMOGRAPHICS

Incidence of Brain Metastases

Among primary cancers, melanoma maintains the highest propensity to metastasize to the brain. The reported frequency of brain metastases in patients with melanoma varies widely and depends on the number of patients in the study, the methods used to collect the data, and the follow-up period. In our series of 6953 patients with melanoma, we primarily used clinical and radiographic criteria to establish the diagnosis of a brain metastasis and found that 10.7% of our patients had melanoma metastases to the brain.[26] This rate is similar to those reported in other clinical studies, which have found incidence rates between 8.4% and 13.3%. The rate of brain metastases in autopsy studies has varied more widely, however. In these studies, a range between 17.5% and 75% has been reported in the literature.

Overall, in our series of 6953 patients with melanoma, 99%, 87%, and 78% of patients were alive and free of brain metastases at 1, 5, and 10 years, respectively. One surprising feature is the sometimes extraordinary delay between the original diagnosis of primary melanoma and the subsequent diagnosis of brain metastases. In our series, the mean interval between the diagnosis of primary melanoma and brain metastases was 3.7 years. This is in line with other figures reported in the literature, which generally range from 2.5 to 4 years. However, in at least one case, the delay reported was 27 years.

The reported number of brain metastases at the time of diagnosis also varies widely in reported series. Again, this probably depends on the methods used to collect the data. Still, it

is surprising that the reported incidence of single metastases is quite high, with a range of between 29% and 80% reported in the literature. However, in at least one autopsy series, 90% of patients with cerebral metastases were found to have multiple metastases. Of course, this series may overestimate the number of patients with clinically relevant multiple metastases inasmuch as the use of an autopsy study induces a significant bias toward end-stage disease.

Risk Factors for Brain Metastases

A number of factors have been identified that are present more often in patients with melanoma who develop cerebral metastases than in patients who do not develop cerebral metastases. In our series, independent factors associated with the development of brain metastases included being male; a primary lesion located on a mucosal surface or in the head, neck, or trunk; deep or ulcerated lesions; acral lentiginous or nodular histologies; and lymph node or visceral metastases, especially if the visceral metastases were to the lung or more than one organ site had metastatic lesions.[26] A number of these factors have also been identified in other series. For example, all series find that males are more prevalent among those with cerebral metastases. This may reflect the fact that primary lesions that are more likely to be involved with brain metastases, such as those located in the head and neck or trunk area, are also more common in males. It also appears that primary lesions, at least in the head and neck or the trunk, or both, are also seen more commonly in patients who develop cerebral metastases. Not unexpectedly, primary lesions with a higher Clark level (level IV or V) or greater Breslow thickness (greater than 4.0 mm) and the presence of visceral metastases at the time of primary diagnosis also predispose the patient to development of cerebral metastases. Interestingly, almost all these factors have been associated with a shorter survival time from the time of diagnosis of the primary tumor. In addition, one other study has also found that tumor thickness or the age of the patient[15] influenced survival even after the diagnosis of brain metastases, but our series and others have generally shown that survival is of short duration after the diagnosis of brain metastases and relatively uninfluenced by other demographic factors. The only exceptions in our series were patients with primary lesions of the head and neck, for whom survival was significantly shorter than average even after the development of brain metastases.

BRAIN METASTASES

Symptoms and Signs

Patients with brain metastases may be asymptomatic or may have focal neurologic deficits, nonfocal symptoms or signs suggestive of increased intracranial pressure, seizures, or intracranial hemorrhage (Table 56-1). Before the widespread use of sensitive imaging studies, brain metastases from melanoma were rarely diagnosed in the absence of symptoms; however, a small percentage of patients in most series reported were asymptomatic. In most series, the most common symptoms or signs for cerebral metastases from melanoma were focal neurologic ones. This was the case in 39% of our patients. These symptoms generally reflect the anatomic region of the brain affected, and metastases to the brain are generally distributed according to its overall mass, with no particular predilection to any given site.[26] Nonfocal symptoms such as headache, nausea, or vomiting that are usually suggestive of increased intracranial pressure occurred in 36% of our patients. In our series intracerebral hemorrhage, as an initial event, occurred in only 3% of our patients. Seizures are an initial sign in 13% of our patients. The incidence of seizures as an initial symptom or sign in the literature ranges from 11% to 50% in reported series, and a number of these series seem to indicate that the risk of seizures is slightly higher than average than for brain metastases from other types of primary tumor.

Radiographic Appearance

Computed tomography (CT) scans of the brain may reveal melanoma metastases as lesions slightly hyperdense relative to normal brain on scans without contrast.[8] These scans can also betray melanoma lesions by the presence of hemorrhage or edema. Melanoma metastases also typically enhance with iodinated contrast. Typical melanoma metastases seen on magnetic resonance imaging (MRI) scans of the brain may display either melanotic or amelanotic patterns. Melanotic lesions are bright on T1-weighted images and dark on T2-weighted images, whereas amelanotic lesions are typically the reverse, although amelanotic lesions can be isointense on multiple sequences. More atypical patterns, which may be easily overlooked, include the very subtle military pattern (Figure 56-1) and periventricular patterns (Figure 56-2). In addition to the brain,

TABLE 56-1	Demographics of Patients with Brain Metastases from Melanoma	
		Number of Patients*
Presentation	Focal neurologic symptoms	274 (39%)
	Nonfocal symptoms	253 (36%)
	Seizures	91 (13%)
	Asymptomatic	49 (7%)
	Neurologic catastrophes	21 (3%)
	Behavioral changes	14 (2%)
Number of brain metastases	1	151 (39.2%)
	2	51 (13.2%)
	3	30 (7.8%)
	>3	153 (39.8%)
Maximal diameter of largest brain metastasis	1 cm	16 (17.6%)
	2 cm	19 (20.9%)
	3 cm	31 (34%)
	4 cm	20 (22%)
	5 cm	5 (5.5%)
Other metastases	Brain only	380 (54.1%)
	Brain and lung	191 (27.2%)
	Brain and bone	20 (2.9%)
	Brain and liver	17 (2.4%)
	Brain and gastrointestinal	17 (2.4%)
	Brain and 2 other organs	55 (7.8%)
	Brain and 3 other organs	20 (2.9%)
	Brain and 4 other organs	2 (0.3%)

*Totals for some variables are less than 100 because data for those categories were unavailable or not applicable. The 32 patients with brain metastases at initial diagnosis have not been excluded. Percentages are calculated based on available data.
Source: From Sampson JH, Carter JH, Jr, Friedman AH, et al: Demographics, prognosis, and therapy in 702 patients with brain metastases from malignant melanoma. J Neurosurg 88:11–20, 1998.

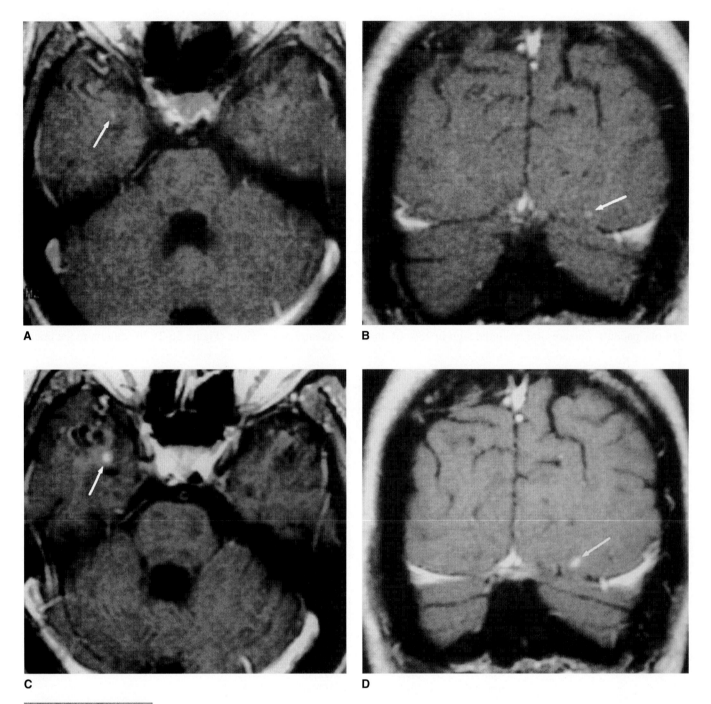

FIGURE 56-1 Military pattern of metastases. *A* and *B,* Contrast-enhanced axial T1-weighted magnetic resonance (MR) image of the inferior temporal lobes *(A)* and coronal T1-weighted MR image of the posterior occipital lobes *(B)* (750/20, one signal acquired) (both obtained on the same day) show two subtle lesions. Tiny areas of possible enhancement are seen but thought to represent artifact or vessels. The tiny hyper-intense focus in the right temporal lobe *(arrow in A)* is within an area of artifact and was thought to be artifactual or related to a vessel. The hyper-intense focus in the left occipital lobe *(arrow in B)* was seen only on coronal images and therefore was of only low suspicion and was thought probably to represent a vessel. *C* and *D,* Contrast-enhanced axial T1-weighted MR image (similar level and same parameters as *A*) *(C)* and coronal T1-weighted MR image (same level and parameters as *B*) *(D)* (both obtained 49 days later) show definite lesions *(arrow),* which appear as small enhancing nodules. (From Escott EJ: A variety of appearances of malignant melanoma in the head: a review. Radiographics 21:625–639, 2001.)

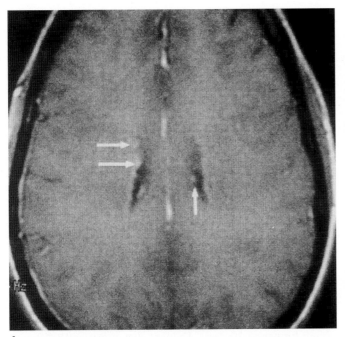

A

B

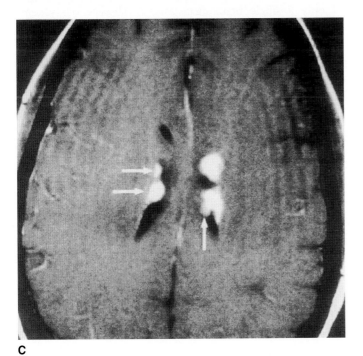

C

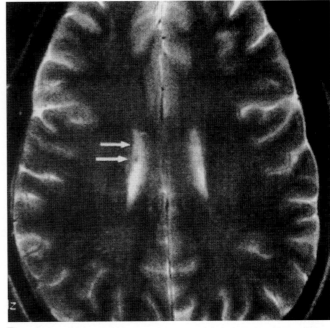

FIGURE 56-2 Periventricular pattern of metastases. *A,* Contrast-enhanced axial T1-weighted magnetic resonance (MR) image (500/24, one signal acquired) shows subtle foci of enhancement along the margins of the lateral ventricles *(arrows).* These foci could easily be mistaken for the normal vessels that are often seen in this location. *B,* Axial T2-weighted MR image (4500/95, one signal acquired) (obtained on the same day) shows the foci as subtle protrusions into the cerebrospinal fluid *(arrows),* which could still be normal vessels. *C,* Contrast-enhanced axial T1-weighted MR image (600/17, one signal acquired) of the superior aspects of the bodies of the lateral ventricles (obtained 57 days later) shows much larger subependymal nodules *(arrows).* (From Escott EJ: A variety of appearances of malignant melanoma in the head: a review. Radiographics 21:625–639, 2001.)

other structures in the head that can be involved by metastases from melanoma include the scalp, skull, temporalis muscle, nasal pharynx and mucosa, meninges, choroid plexus, internal auditory canal, and the orbit.

Prognosis

Brain metastases clearly contribute to morbidity and mortality in the majority of patients with disseminated melanoma.[1] In all reported series, when patients developed brain metastases, the metastases usually caused death.[26] Our series reported the

highest incidence of death caused by brain metastases to be 94.5%, although most series report that approximately two thirds of patients with brain metastases succumb primarily because of the brain metastases.

Survival for patients with brain metastases from malignant melanoma is alarmingly short. In our series the overall median survival time after the diagnosis of a brain metastasis was only 113 days, with only 15% of patients remaining alive at 12 months after a brain metastasis was diagnosed. These numbers are in line with other reports in the literature, which usually do not report median survival times after brain metastases much greater than 5 months. What is interesting is that in all reports a number of patients with some distinguishing characteristics were found to have survived for long periods, usually in excess of 2 or 3 years. The characteristics of these fortunate patients are discussed in more detail later.

Most series have demonstrated a survival advantage for patients with single metastases, although therapeutic selection bias in this regard may significantly skew these data.[12,30] Furthermore, not all studies have shown that the number of brain metastases correlates with survival.[15] In our series, median survival time significantly decreased with increased number of metastases ($P < .00001$, multiple pairwise comparison). Patients with a single metastasis ($N = 151$) had a median survival time of 216 days (confidence interval [CI] 168 to 267 days), whereas patients with two metastases ($N = 51$) had a median survival time of 127 days (CI 105 to 194 days), and those with greater than two metastases ($N = 183$) had a median survival time of 86 days (CI 63 to 113 days).

The extent of extracerebral disease has also been found to have a major effect on survival in most reported studies. Again, the incidence rates vary widely, but it is safe to say that 50% or more of patients with brain metastases will be found to have visceral metastases elsewhere. In our series, only 46% of patients were found to have clinical evidence of disease outside of the brain, but the incidence in the literature of clinically diagnosed extracerebral disease ranges between 45.9% and 84%, and autopsy series have shown that up to 96% of patients have associated extracerebral disease. Metastatic disease beyond the brain, however, does not appear to alter prognosis unless the lung or multiple other organ sites are involved (Figure 56-3). Unfortunately, in almost all series the lung was the most common site of extracerebral metastases.[14,23,24,26] In our series

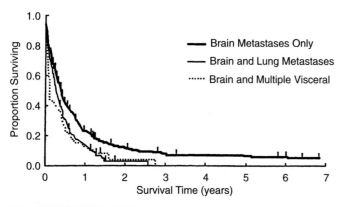

FIGURE 56-3   Graph of actuarial survival curve showing relationship between survival and visceral metastases in patients with brain metastases from malignant melanoma. Metastasis to one other organ in addition to the brain does not alter expected survival unless this organ is the lung. The median survival time for patients with isolated brain metastasis (380 patients) was 135 days. In the presence of coexistent lung metastasis (191 patients), this was significantly reduced, to 93 days ($P = .0014$). With more than one additional site of visceral metastases (77 patients), median survival time was further reduced, to 39 days ($P = .0036$). (From Sampson JH, Carter JH, Jr, Friedman AH, et al: Demographics, prognosis, and therapy in 702 patients with brain metastases from malignant melanoma. J Neurosurg 88:11–20, 1998.)

median survival time for patients with metastatic disease limited to the brain ($N = 380$) was 135 days (CI 120 to 161 days). This was significantly reduced in the presence of lung metastases ($N = 191$) to 94 days (CI 76 to 123 days, $P = .0014$) and to only 39 days (CI 24 to 131 days, $P = .0036$) in patients with more than one extracerebral site of metastatic disease. Interestingly, in at least one series, if intracerebral metastases could be well treated, they did not have a negative impact on survival time, and at least in this study, patients with well-treated extracerebral metastases had survivals that were not significantly different from patients without known extracerebral metastases.[20]

Special Patient Populations

Long-Term Survivors

Despite cerebral metastases from malignant melanoma, there exists in the literature a handful of patients, both in case reports and larger series, who have exhibited long-term survival. Most studies define long-term survival as a survival time greater than 2 or 3 years. In our series, 17 (2.4%) patients survived longer than 3 years after diagnosis of brain metastases, with one surviving for nearly 20 years. Features that consistently differentiate these patients in multiple series include the presence of only a single brain metastasis,[26,30] absence of systemic disease,[26,30] and treatment with complete surgical resection.[15,26] Of interest in this regard is that in our series and others, patients with multiple metastases who do undergo resection can have surprisingly long survival times of up to several years.

Unknown Primary

Another possibly distinct patient population comprises patients who have a brain metastasis but no evidence of primary extracerebral melanoma. This group forms a relatively large subpopulation in both our series and others. In our series, 76 of 702 patients (10.8%) had no known primary disease. However, almost all of these patients will eventually develop systemic malignant melanoma and in virtually every way conform to the expectations of patients with metastatic intracerebral lesions, thus fitting the hypothesis that most of these patients with "primary" intracerebral melanoma actually represent patients with occult systemic melanoma and cerebral metastases.

THERAPY FOR BRAIN METASTASES

Surgery for Brain Metastases

Indications and Contraindications

Surgical excision is generally indicated in patients with single metastases to the brain that can be safely and completely resected (Table 56-2). This recommendation is primarily based on two randomized trials demonstrating that surgical excision of single metastasis to the brain in addition to radiation therapy significantly reduced recurrence at the surgical site, prolonged functional independence, and increased median survival time relative to radiation therapy alone.[22,28] These data, however, were generated primarily from patients with non–small cell lung carcinoma, and only 3 of 48 of the patients in one study and 6 of 63 in the other had melanoma. This patient mix and

TABLE 56-2	Guidelines for Recommending Surgical Resection* of Brain Metastases

Indications (Strongest to Weakest)

1. Single brain metastasis accessible to safe and complete resection and no other visceral metastases present
2. Multiple brain metastases, with symptomatic or life-threatening brain metastasis accessible to safe and complete resection and no other visceral metastases present
3. Single brain metastasis accessible to safe and complete resection and one other site of visceral metastasis accessible to complete resection or responding well to systemic therapy
4. Multiple brain metastases all accessible to safe and complete resection and one other site of visceral metastasis accessible to complete resection or responding well to systemic therapy
5. Single, symptomatic, or life-threatening brain metastasis accessible to safe and complete resection and one other site of visceral metastasis present that is untreatable
6. Multiple brain metastases with symptomatic or life-threatening brain metastasis accessible to safe and complete resection and one other site of visceral metastasis present that is untreatable

Contraindications

1. Brain metastasis not accessible to safe and complete resection
2. More than one site of visceral metastasis in addition to the brain
3. Radiologic or pathologic evidence of leptomeningeal spread of tumor
4. Surgical procedure likely to be life threatening

*Could include metastases completely accessible to radiosurgery.
Source: From Sampson JH, Carter JH, Jr, Friedman AH, et al: Demographics, prognosis, and therapy in 702 patients with brain metastases from malignant melanoma. J Neurosurg 88:11–20, 1998.)

the exclusive use of CT scanning in these studies leads one to question the applicability of these data to patients with melanoma who are now imaged with much more sensitive MRI techniques. No other prospective or randomized data exist, however, to support the notion that resection of brain metastases from melanoma prolongs survival. Still, surgical therapy has generally been employed, because many retrospective studies suggest a survival benefit from surgical therapy, and these studies also suggest that surgical therapy improves quality of life by reducing patients' symptoms.[5,14,16]

Relative contraindications to surgical therapy include the presence of multiple intracerebral metastases and progressive or untreatable extracerebral metastases. Although the presence of multiple intracerebral metastases is generally considered a relative contraindication to surgery, it should be noted that Bindal et al[4] reported favorable results of surgery in a series of patients who underwent resection of multiple metastases. Because this patient series was heavily weighted toward patients with melanoma, it is of specific relevance here. They compared patients who had complete resection of all their metastases with patients who had at least one metastasis resected and with patients who had only a single metastasis that was resected. Patients in whom all multiple metastases were resected had a median survival time equivalent to patients who had a resection for a single metastasis. The median survival time in both groups was approximately 14 months. Patients with unresected metastases in this study had a comparatively low survival time of only 6 months. Similarly, in our series and others, selected patients with multiple resections[3,26] or resection of multiple metastases[4,26] have had unexpectedly long survival times.

Outcome

In almost every retrospective series, surgical therapy for melanoma brain metastases is associated with the longest

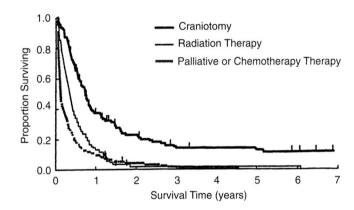

FIGURE 56-4 Graph of actuarial survival curve showing survival of patients treated with surgery, whole-brain radiation therapy, or palliative systemic chemotherapy only (P < .0001, craniotomy compared with radiation therapy; P = .0006, radiation therapy compared with palliative systemic chemotherapy). (From Sampson JH, Carter JH, Jr, Friedman AH, et al: Demographics, prognosis, and therapy in 702 patients with brain metastases from malignant melanoma. J Neurosurg 88:11–20, 1998.)

median survival time.[1,5,9,16] In our large retrospective series, 524 patients had specific therapy for their brain metastases. Of these, 205 (39.1%) were treated with systemic chemotherapy only. These patients had a median survival time of only 39 days (CI 29 to 48 days) (Figure 56-4). Treatment with radiation therapy, usually to a total dose of 3000 cGy in 10 fractions, was associated with a significantly longer median survival time of 120 days (CI 98 to 141 days) (P < .0001). Overall, patients in our series treated with surgery with or without postoperative radiation therapy had a significantly better median survival time than those who received radiation therapy or chemotherapy, however (P < .0006). Unfortunately, no randomized study dedicated to patients with melanoma brain metastases exists that compares these therapeutic approaches prospectively, and undoubtedly in our series and others a significant selection bias favoring the surgical groups existed. For example, although in our study patients selected for surgical therapy did not differ from those selected for other therapies with regard to demographics or primary lesion characteristics, they were more likely to have a single brain metastasis (P < .0001) and less likely to have other visceral metastases (P < .0001). Survival after surgical therapy for single metastasis, as reported in the literature, ranges from 4 months to 13 months, whereas survival after surgical therapy for multiple metastases, as reported in the literature, ranges from 2 months to 14 months.

Although surgical therapy has generally been shown to relieve or ameliorate neurologic symptoms in most patients,[4,26] significant complications have also been encountered. In our surgical series there was an 8.6% risk of life-threatening morbidity or mortality from the surgery. Mortality rates in other series have ranged from 0% in one small series to 15%,[4,16] and the rate of life-threatening morbidity ranges from 7.5% to 11.6%.[4,30] In addition, in our series, 22.4% of patients who underwent surgical resection did have an increase in neurologic deficit. For comparison, only 16% of our patients who underwent radiation therapy experienced an increase in neurologic deficit, and only 1.4% had life-threatening complications or died during therapy. Although these data suggest that in our series radiation therapy was less risky, these differences did not appear to be statistically significant (P = .138).

Role of Postoperative Radiation Therapy

The role of postoperative irradiation remains controversial. Although a prospective and randomized trial of postoperative radiation therapy after surgical treatment of a single metastasis to the brain has demonstrated that patients with a single metastasis to the brain who receive postoperative radiation therapy in addition to surgical resection have fewer recurrences and are less likely to die of neurologic causes, this study included only two patients with melanoma.[21] No other prospective, randomized study has addressed this question in regard to melanoma metastases to the brain specifically. Although the majority of retrospective studies demonstrate enhanced survival,[26,27] reduced rate of tumor recurrence in the brain,[12] and better rates of neurologic improvement[9,26,30] with postoperative adjuvant radiation therapy, several studies have suggested that postoperative radiation therapy may reduce survival[17,24] or have no additional benefits.[9] In our series, median survival time for patients with postoperative radiation therapy was 268 days (CI 220 to 405) and 195 days (CI 161 to 292) without radiation therapy; however, these differences were not statistically significant (P = .9998). Overall in our series, postoperative irradiation was well tolerated by most patients, and patients receiving postoperative radiation therapy were more likely to remain without neurologic deficits or to experience neurologic improvement after completion of therapy than those who did not. This must be balanced, especially in patients with completely resected single metastases, with a known risk of radiation-induced dementia at 1 year after therapy of approximately 10%.[6]

Radiation Therapy and Radiosurgery for Brain Metastases

Malignant melanoma has historically been considered a radioresistant tumor. However, experiments with melanoma cells in culture have revealed radiation survival curves and other radiobiologic parameters that overlap those of other carcinoma cell lines. In addition, clinical studies have shown that when correct dose-fractionation schemes are used, melanoma responds appropriately to radiation therapy. The results of these and other studies have led to the conclusion that, in general, melanoma should not be considered a radioresistant tumor.[11]

Treatment of brain metastasis from melanoma, as with metastasis from most other primary tumors, results in a relatively unsatisfactory outcome for nearly all patients. In an attempt to determine prognostic classes in patients with brain metastasis, a recursive partitioning analysis (RPA) was performed on patients with brain metastasis.[10] RPA is a statistical methodology designed to create a decision tree according to prognostic significance. This study included 1200 patients previously enrolled in three separate Radiation Therapy Oncology Group (RTOG) trials testing different doses, fractionation schemes, and radiation sensitizers in patients with brain metastasis. Among the factors tested were tumor histology, number of brain metastases, and interval from diagnosis of primary tumor until diagnosis of brain metastasis. The results revealed that patients younger than age 65 with a Karnofsky Performance Scale (KPS) score greater than 70 and who had controlled primary disease with no extracranial metastasis had a median survival time of 7.1 months (class I). Patients with a KPS score of less than 70 had a median survival time of 2.3 months (class III), and all others were class II, with a median survival time of 4.2 months. There were 200 patients with melanoma included in this study, accounting for 17% of the patients reviewed, and this diagnosis followed only adenocarcinoma and squamous cell histologies for the total number of patients. Histology had no prognostic value in this large group of patients, and these results suggest that patients with brain metastasis from melanoma fare no worse than those with other tumor histologies when treated with standard therapy. However, no separate data on local control, pertinent to patients with metastatic melanoma, were presented in this study.

In addition to these data, there have been a number of studies on patients with brain metastasis only from melanoma who were treated with standard whole-brain radiation therapy (WBRT). Ellerhorst et al[7] reviewed the outcome of 87 patients with brain metastasis from melanoma who were treated with WBRT (a majority received 3 Gy fractions to a total dose of 30 Gy) and found that more than half the patients were able to decrease their corticosteroid use, suggesting that the treatment was effective. The median survival time of the whole group was 4.2 months, and for patients with no extracranial metastasis it was 12 months. These results suggest that WBRT may be effective in palliation for a portion of patients with melanoma brain metastasis and that median survival rates are comparable to cohorts of patients with other types of brain metastasis. A review of similar patients treated at Duke University Medical Center has also been performed. A total of 65 patients with brain metastasis from melanoma were evaluated according to the RTOG RPA. Most patients received between 5 and 15 fractions, with between 2.5 and 4.0 Gy delivered daily. The median survival time of the whole group was 4 months, and the median survival rates according to RTOG RPA were 6.5 months, 3.5 months, and 2.5 months for classes I, II, and III, respectively. These numbers are essentially the same as those for the larger group of patients evaluated in the original RPA.[10] In summary, these studies also suggest that patients who are treated with standard WBRT for brain metastasis from melanoma have an outcome equivalent to that for patients with brain metastasis from tumors of other histologies.

Given the debate regarding dose-fractionation in melanoma, several retrospective studies have been performed to test the hypothesis that larger doses per fraction would be beneficial for patients with brain metastasis from melanoma. Vlock et al[29] reported on 46 patients treated with either high dose per fraction (HDF) (6.0 Gy each day) or low dose per fraction (LDF) (125 to 400 each day) to the whole brain. Sixty percent of patients in both groups had clinical improvement. There was no difference in median survival time (3.0 versus 2.5 months for HDF versus LDF), and 35 patients died of progressive central nervous system (CNS) disease. A separate report compares 72 patients with brain metastasis from melanoma who were treated with either 3.0 Gy per day to 30 Gy (conventional fractionation) or 5.0 to 6.0 Gy per day to 30 Gy (HDF).[31] Again, two thirds of the patients had a clinical response in both groups, and there was no difference in median survival time, 4.5 months for conventional fractionation versus 5.0 months for HDF. There was an increase in acute toxicity in the HDF arm, with 30% of these patients experiencing headache, nausea or vomiting, or other symptoms of increased intracranial pressure as compared with 12% in the conventional fractionation arm. Although there are data to support the use of larger fraction size in extracranial melanoma, it appears that standard fractionation (3.0 Gy/day to 30 Gy) is indicated for the treatment of brain metastasis from melanoma.

Recently, the use of stereotactic radiosurgery (SRS) has been reported for brain metastasis from melanoma, with impressive local control results. Mori et al[19] provided data on 60 patients who had 118 metastases treated with SRS. Fifty-one of these patients also had WBRT. The median survival time of the whole group of patients was 7 months. There were imaging-defined local control data on 72 of these tumors, and this revealed a local control rate of 90% (disappeared, 11%; shrank, 44%; and stable, 35%). Only 7 tumors recurred after SRS, although 14 tumors recurred in other sites of the brain. There were not enough patients in this study to evaluate the utility of WBRT in patients treated with SRS. In another study of 45 patients treated with SRS for 92 brain metastases from melanoma, there were image-defined local control data on 66 lesions.[18] The local control rate in this study was 82% (disappeared, 24%; shrank, 35%; and stable, 23%). Despite SRS,

12% of the tumors progressed. In 82% of patients, progressive systemic disease was the cause of death. As in the previous study, a portion of the patients also received WBRT, but the number of patients was too small to evaluate its utility. Most studies of WBRT alone do not perform imaging-based evaluation; however, death from neurologic causes is a common outcome in these patients, suggesting poorer local control than with SRS. At present, the use of SRS alone for brain metastasis is controversial and beyond the scope of this review; however, both of these studies have convincing local control rates and suggest that SRS should be considered in the therapy of patients with brain metastasis from melanoma.

Debate continues, however, with regard to the comparative efficacy of conventional surgical resection and SRS. For example, a case-control retrospective study by Bindal et al[2] reviewed the outcomes of 31 patients with brain metastases treated by radiosurgery and 62 patients treated by conventional surgery. Of particular relevance here is that 23% of the patients in each group had melanomas as a primary site of tumor. The patients were matched for histologic characteristics of the primary tumor, extent of systemic disease, preoperative KPS score, number of brain metastases, and by age and sex. This analysis suggested that surgery was superior to SRS inasmuch as patients who underwent conventional surgical treatment survived longer and had better local control, but data specific to melanoma were not presented.[2]

Systemic Therapy for Brain Metastases

Systemic treatment for melanoma that has metastasized to the brain is generally ineffective, and significant responses to systemic chemotherapy or immunotherapy have been reported only rarely. Response to systemic therapy is, in fact, so poor that most clinical studies even exclude patients with brain metastases. Chemotherapeutic options consist of dacarbazine, platinum analogs (cisplatin, carboplatin), nitrosoureas (carmustine, lomustine, semustine, and particularly, fotemustine), tamoxifen, temozolomide, and vinblastine. Potentially useful biologic agents include the interferons, interleukin 2, and thalidomide. However, even advanced therapeutic combinations that produce objective extracerebral tumor responses in the majority of patients are generally thwarted by relapse within the central nervous system. Overall, no drug combination, even when delivered directly into the internal carotid artery, produces consistent response rates of more than 30%. Direct intracerebral delivery of promising chemotherapeutic agents such as temozolomide,[13] however, may produce more encouraging results in the future. Similarly, immunization studies have recently demonstrated that systemic immune responses can be generated efficaciously against intracerebral melanoma.[25]

References

1. Amer MH, Al-Sarraf M, Baker LH, et al: Malignant melanoma and central nervous system metastases: incidence, diagnosis, treatment and survival. Cancer 42:660–668, 1978.
2. Bindal AK, Bindal RK, Hess KR, et al: Surgery versus radiosurgery in the treatment of brain metastasis. J Neurosurg 84:748–754, 1996.
3. Bindal RK, Sawaya R, Leavens ME, et al: Reoperation for recurrent metastatic brain tumors. J Neurosurg 83:600–604, 1995.
4. Bindal RK, Sawaya R, Leavens ME, et al: Surgical treatment of multiple brain metastases. J Neurosurg 79:210–216, 1993.
5. Byrne TN, Cascino TL, Posner JB: Brain metastasis from melanoma. J Neurooncol 1:313–317, 1983.

6. DeAngelis LM, Mandell LR, Thaler HT, et al: The role of post-operative radiotherapy after resection of single brain metastases. Neurosurgery 24:798–805, 1989.

7. Ellerhorst J, Strom E, Nardone E, et al: Whole brain irradiation for patients with metastatic melanoma: a review of 87 cases. Int J Radiat Oncol Biol Phys 49:93–97, 2001.

8. Escott EJ: A variety of appearances of malignant melanoma in the head: a review. Radiographics 21:625–639, 2001.

9. Fell DA, Leavens ME, McBride CM: Surgical versus nonsurgical management of metastatic melanoma of the brain. Neurosurgery 7:238–242, 1980.

10. Gaspar L, Scott C, Rotman M, et al: Recursive partitioning analysis (RPA) of prognostic factors in three Radiation Therapy Oncology Group (RTOG) brain metastases trials. Int J Radiat Oncol Biol Phys 37:745–751, 1997.

11. Geara FB, Ang KK: Radiation therapy for malignant melanoma. Surg Clin North Am 76:1383–1398, 1996.

12. Hagen NA, Cirrincione C, Thaler HT, et al: The role of radiation therapy following resection of single brain metastasis from melanoma. Neurology 40:158–160, 1990.

13. Heimberger AB, Archer GE, McLendon RE, et al: Temozolomide delivered by intracerebral microinfusion is safe and efficacious against malignant gliomas in rats. Clin Cancer Res 6:4148–4153, 2000.

14. Katz HR: The relative effectiveness of radiation therapy, corticosteroids, and surgery in the management of melanoma metastatic to the central nervous system. Int J Radiat Oncol Biol Phys 7:897–906, 1981.

15. Konstadoulakis MM, Messaris E, Zografos G, et al: Prognostic factors in malignant melanoma patients with solitary or multiple brain metastases. Is there a role for surgery? J Neurosurg Sci 44:211–218; discussion 219, 2000.

16. Madajewicz S, Karakousis C, West CR, et al: Malignant melanoma brain metastases. Review of Roswell Park Memorial Institute experience. Cancer 53:2550–2552, 1984.

17. Mendez IM, Del Maestro RF: Cerebral metastases from malignant melanoma. Can J Neurol Sci 15:119–123, 1988.

18. Mingione V, Oliveira M, Prasad D, et al: Gamma surgery for melanoma metastases in the brain. J Neurosurg 96:544–551, 2002.

19. Mori Y, Kondziolka D, Flickinger JC, et al: Stereotactic radiosurgery for cerebral metastatic melanoma: factors affecting local disease control and survival. Int J Radiat Oncol Biol Phys 42:581–589, 1998.

20. Oredsson S, Ingvar C, Stromblad LG, et al: Palliative surgery for brain metastases of malignant melanoma. Eur J Surg Oncol 16:451–456, 1990.

21. Patchell RA, Tibbs PA, Regine WF, et al: Postoperative radiotherapy in the treatment of single metastases to the brain: a randomized trial. JAMA 280:1485–1489, 1998.

22. Patchell RA, Tibbs PA, Walsh JW, et al: A randomized trial of surgery in the treatment of single metastases to the brain. N Engl J Med 322:494–500, 1990.

23. Retsas S, Gershuny AR: Central nervous system involvement in malignant melanoma. Cancer 61:1926–1934, 1988.

24. Saha S, Meyer M, Krementz ET, et al: Prognostic evaluation of intracranial metastasis in malignant melanoma. Ann Surg Oncol 1:38–44, 1994.

25. Sampson JH, Archer GE, Ashley DM, et al: Subcutaneous vaccination with irradiated, cytokine-producing tumor cells stimulates CD8+ cell-mediated immunity against tumors located in the "immunologically privileged" central nervous system. Proc Natl Acad Sci 93:10399–10404, 1996.

26. Sampson JH, Carter JH, Jr, Friedman AH, et al: Demographics, prognosis, and therapy in 702 patients with brain metastases from malignant melanoma. J Neurosurg 88:11–20, 1998.

27. Skibber JM, Soong SJ, Austin L, et al: Cranial irradiation after surgical excision of brain metastases in melanoma patients. Ann Surg Oncol 3:118–123, 1996.

28. Vecht CJ, Haaxma-Reiche H, Noordijk EM, et al: Treatment of single brain metastasis: radiotherapy alone or combined with neurosurgery? Ann Neurol 33:583–590, 1993.

29. Vlock DR, Kirkwood JM, Leutzinger C, et al: High-dose fraction radiation therapy for intracranial metastases of malignant melanoma: a comparison with low-dose fraction therapy. Cancer 49:2289–2294, 1982.

30. Zacest AC, Besser M, Stevens G, et al: Surgical management of cerebral metastases from melanoma: Outcome in 147 patients treated at a single institution over two decades. J Neurosurg 96:552–558, 2002.

31. Ziegler JC, Cooper JS: Brain metastases from malignant melanoma: Conventional vs. high-dose-per-fraction radiotherapy. Int J Radiat Oncol Biol Phys 12:1839–1842, 1986.

CHAPTER 57

BRAIN METASTASES: RENAL CELL CARCINOMA

Kevin O. Lillehei and Brian D. Kavanagh

There are approximately 31,000 new cases of renal cell carcinoma (RCC) in the United States each year. Of these, 30% to 40% will eventually become metastatic. The most common sites for metastatic dissemination are the lungs (65%), bone (40%), liver (14%), adrenals (8%), peritoneum (8%), and brain (5%). Most often, brain metastases occur at advanced stages of the disease; however, 12% of patients will have the brain as their first metastatic site, and half of these metastases will be solitary lesions.[4]

EPIDEMIOLOGY

RCC accounts for 2% of all cancers, with a male-to-female incidence ratio of nearly 2:1. The occurrence among whites and blacks in the United States appears equivalent, with a peak incidence in the sixth decade of life. Because the primary tumor is often of considerable size at the time of diagnosis, one third of patients will have synchronous metastatic disease. In the remaining two thirds of patients with disease limited to the kidney, 40% will ultimately develop metastatic disease after initial nephrectomy. The incidence of RCC is believed to be rising steadily, with an increased incidence of 38% between 1974 and 1990.[12] Of the approximately 50% to 60% of patients who have resectable disease (stage I and II, disease confined to the kidney or perinephric fat), the 5- and 10-year disease-free survival rates are 49% and 42%, respectively. The overall 5-year survival rate for patients with stage IV disease (RCC with distant metastases) is 2%, with a median survival time of 18 months.

In patients with brain metastases, 92% already carry the diagnosis of RCC, with 8% of patients having a brain mass of unknown origin. The metastatic lesions appear to be equally distributed to all parts of the brain, with no predilection for the cerebellum versus the cerebral hemispheres. The reported median survival time after diagnosis of solitary or multiple brain metastases ranges from 4 to 14 months (Table 57-1). Culine et al[4] examined factors influencing survival of patients with RCC metastatic to the brain and found that the following are associated with a worse outcome based on a univariate analysis:

1. No initial nephrectomy
2. A left-side brain metastasis
3. Temporal location

4. Presence of fever or weight loss
5. Erythrocyte sedimentation rate (ESR) greater than 50
6. Time from initial diagnosis to brain metastasis of 18 months or less.

When multivariate analysis was used, the time from initial diagnosis to the development of brain metastases remained significant, along with the presence of other extracranial sites of metastatic disease.

Approximately 50% of RCC patients with brain metastases will have a solitary brain metastasis, making these patients more amenable to local therapy (i.e., surgery or stereotactic radiosurgery).

A well-described but uncommon phenomenon associated with RCC is the occurrence of spontaneous regression, either at the primary site or in a site of metastatic disease. This curious event is seen in approximately 1% of patients, most commonly in those with lung metastases. This phenomenon supports a possible role for the immune system in modulating the course of this disease.

DIAGNOSIS

Most patients with RCC have either hematuria, flank pain, a palpable mass, or signs and symptoms of metastasis. An increasing number of patients are being diagnosed with asymptomatic renal masses as a result of computed tomography (CT), magnetic resonance imaging (MRI), or abdominal ultrasound being performed for unrelated reasons. In patients with metastatic extension to the brain, the most common symptoms are headache (24%), weakness (20%), difficulties with cognition (14%), seizures (12%), and ataxia (7%). Seven percent of patients will be found to have an asymptomatic brain lesion on screening radiographic imaging.[3] Symptoms and signs obviously vary depending on the number and size of the metastatic lesions, their location in the brain, the degree of surrounding edema, and rate of growth. Of note, with the previously described symptoms, headaches occur in less than 50% of patients. Headaches of new onset or headaches occurring in the early morning are a particularly ominous symptom and should not be ignored. These patients should undergo MRI screening in a timely manner. Unfortunately, headaches are more likely to occur in patients with a preexisting history of headaches, and the frequency and severity may not differ significantly from the

TABLE 57-1			**RTOG RPA Results versus Selected Recent Single Institution Series of Patients Treated for Brain Metastases from RCC with WBRT or SRS with or without WBRT**		
Group/Institution	N	KPS	Treatment	Median Survival	Comment
RTOG RPA class I	201	≥70	WBRT	7.1 mo	Age <65, no extracranial metastases
RTOG RPA class II	765	≥70	WBRT	4.2 mo	Age ≥65 or extracranial metastases
The University of Texas M.D. Anderson Cancer Center (Wronski, 1997)[16]	119	55% ≥70	WBRT	4.4 mo	Single metastasis significantly better than others
Daniel den Hoed Cancer Center (Lagerwaard, 1999)[10]	48	Not stated	WBRT	4.3 mo	Some patients had either no WBRT or surgery + WBRT
Institut Gustave Roussy (Culine, 1998)[4]	44	81% ≥70	WBRT	8 mo	"Average risk" patients
Institut Bergonie* (Culine, 1998)[4]	23	Not stated	WBRT	11 mo	"Average risk" patients
University of Vienna (Schoggl, 1998)[15]	23	87% ≥70	SRS	11 mo	9 patients received SRS + WBRT
Miami Neuroscience Center (Amendola, 2000)[1]	22	90% ≥ 70	SRS	8 mo	11 patients had prior WBRT
University Hospital, Tuebingen (Becker, 2002)[2]	15	Not stated	SRS	4 mo	Melanoma patients grouped with RCC patients
University of Pittsburgh (Mori, 1998)[11]	35	Median 90	SRS + WBRT	14 mo	7 patients had SRS only
Cleveland Clinic (Goyal, 2000)[9]	29	Median 80	SRS + WBRT	10 mo	13 patients had SRS only

KPS, Karnofsky Performance Scale score; RCC, renal cell carcinoma; RPA, recursive partitioning analysis; RTOG, Radiation Therapy Oncology Group; SRS, stereotactic radiosurgery; WBRT, whole-brain radiation therapy.
Source: Used as external reference data by Culine S, Bekradda M, Kramar A, et al: Prognostic factors for survival in patients with brain metastases from renal cell carcinoma. Cancer 83:2548–2553, 1998. Copyright © American Cancer Society. Reprinted by permission of Wiley-Liss, Inc., a subsidiary of John Wiley & Sons, Inc.

patient's baseline pattern (including migraine headaches with aura). A low threshold of suspicion needs to be maintained in evaluating these individuals. Of note, in patients with multiple metastatic lesions, there is often a lack of focal neurologic signs or symptoms. These patients typically exhibit either difficulties with cognition or emotional lability. The finding of papilledema is unusual and rarely exists without a multitude of additional signs and symptoms.

Brain Imaging

At the time of the initial diagnosis of RCC, and at any time thereafter, if metastatic disease is suspected, MRI scanning before and after the administration of gadolinium contrast is the test of choice. Although CT scanning with and without iodinated contrast administration is a second-best option (in patients unable to undergo MRI because of, for example, the presence of a cardiac pacemaker, ferromagnetic aneurysm clip, or severe claustrophobia), it will often miss very small metastases, particularly in the brainstem and posterior fossa. In deciding on the most appropriate therapy, the presence of these additional lesions becomes very important. Although the findings on MRI are not diagnostic of metastatic disease, the following strongly suggest the presence of a metastatic lesion[3]:

- A roughly spherical lesion with homogeneous contrast enhancement or, if greater than 2 cm in maximal diameter, a hypointense center with a regular ring of contrast enhancement. Irregularly shaped lesions with serpiginous areas of contrast enhancement are more likely to be primary gliomas of the brain.

- Lesions occurring at the gray-white matter junction of the brain. This finding is consistent with the hematogenous propagation of tumors that become trapped in a region of the brain where the arterioles suddenly narrow into a rich capillary bed.
- Enhancement of the lesions following the administration of contrast. In very small lesions the pinpoint contrast enhancement seen may be difficult to differentiate from an end-on vessel. The presence of any surrounding edema or growth of the lesion over time, however, will be helpful in ultimately differentiating between the two.

TREATMENT

Although nephrectomy has been the primary therapy for localized RCC, its benefit in patients with metastatic disease remained unsettled until recently. Prognostic factors recognized to have major influence upon survival in patients with metastatic RCC include the following[5]:

- The number of metastatic sites
- Previous chemotherapy
- Performance status
- Weight loss
- Time from diagnosis to therapy

Recently, a multi-institutional randomized study involving more than 240 patients with metastatic RCC indicated that nephrectomy followed by interferon therapy results in a significantly longer survival time among patients with metastatic RCC than does interferon therapy alone.[6] In this particular study, the absolute magnitude of the survival benefit achieved by reducing a patient's overall burden of disease via nephrectomy was modest, representing an increase in median survival from 8.1 months without surgery to 11.1 months with nephrectomy. Nevertheless, the intriguing result supports consideration of nephrectomy in selected patients with metastatic RCC and good performance status. Although nephrectomy and immunotherapy with interferon-alpha or interleukin 2 has shown promise in the treatment of metastatic disease, the use of chemotherapy has been generally disappointing. Over the past 10 years, more than 30 agents have been tested in phase II studies involving more than 200 patients. The overall response rate was less than 10%, with vinblastine being the most beneficial single agent tested. Combination therapy has been slightly more successful, with response rates not exceeding 20%. These multiagent regimens, however, were significantly more toxic. The two most successful regimens to date are weekly gemcitabine combined with continuous 5-fluorouracil (5-FU) and tamoxifen and colchicine-modulated vinblastine followed by 5-FU.

For the treatment of metastatic brain lesions secondary to RCC, chemotherapy and immunotherapy have had little impact, with surgery and radiation therapy remaining the mainstays of therapy.

Surgery

In general, surgical resection of RCC metastatic to the brain is limited to one or two lesions and, rarely, three if proximally located. The benefit of surgery lies in its ability to control local disease. In patients with multiple intracranial tumors this is not usually feasible; however, surgery in this setting may be indicated for the resection of a single large symptomatic tumor, particularly if located in the posterior fossa. Surgical resection of such a lesion, in most cases, will offer rapid relief of symptoms and have a significant benefit on a patient's quality of life. Its effect on overall survival, however, is often limited.

For solitary tumors metastatic to the brain, the benefit of surgery alone as a single long-term therapy is controversial. Patchell et al[14] conducted a randomized study in which patients with solitary brain metastases, from a variety of cancers, were randomized to receive either surgery alone or surgery in combination with whole-brain radiation therapy (WBRT). Results from the study indicated that the addition of WBRT significantly lowered the rate of tumor recurrence at the site of resection from 46% to 10%. Recurrence at sites distant to the surgical site occurred in 37% of the surgery-only cases, compared with 14% of the cases treated with surgery plus WBRT. In addition, the administration of WBRT made patients less likely to die of neurologic causes but had no effect on the overall length of survival or the length of time that patients remained functionally independent. In a separate randomized study, Patchell et al[13] compared WBRT alone with surgery plus WBRT. This latter study demonstrated that overall survival was significantly improved in the group of patients treated with surgery plus WBRT over WBRT alone (40 weeks vs. 15 weeks, respectively).

Radiation Therapy

Corticosteroids and WBRT remain an acceptable standard of care for the palliation of symptoms in patients with metastatic RCC. Approximately three quarters of patients experience a meaningful benefit after receiving a dose of radiation on the order of 30 Gy in 10 fractions.[4] Interestingly, neurologic improvement after conventionally fractionated radiation therapy does not necessarily correlate with radiographic evidence of tumor shrinkage.

During the past decade there have been numerous efforts to identify key prognostic factors that allow identifying subgroups of patients who might benefit from arguably more aggressive therapeutic interventions. One such therapy is surgery, as described previously, or stereotactic radiosurgery (SRS). SRS involves the use of multiple small beams of high-dose radiation that all converge on a single discrete area, largely sparing the remainder of the brain. Like surgery, SRS is a very focused therapy, and its use has been investigated as a treatment either alone or in combination with WBRT. Unlike surgery, however, it may take 6 to 12 months after treatment to see radiographic evidence of tumor shrinkage. Therefore in tumors that are causing significant signs and symptoms secondary to their mass effect, the use of SRS may not be the best option.

One of the most important radiation studies concerning patients with brain metastases was published by the Radiation Therapy Oncology Group (RTOG) and involved a recursive partitioning analysis (RPA) of the outcomes of 1200 patients who had been enrolled in three consecutive clinical trials between 1979 and 1993.[7] Among 21 clinical characteristics and treatment parameters examined, including tumor control at the primary site and the number of brain metastases, only the Karnofsky Performance Scale (KPS) score, patient's age, status of tumor control at the primary site, and presence or absence of extracranial metastases provided meaningful information by which patients could be grouped according to expected clinical outcome. Prognosis was universally very poor for patients with a KPS score of less than 70 (implying inability to carry on normal activity or active work and need for at least occasional assistance in self-care). This group of patients, referred to as RPA class III, demonstrated a median survival time of only 2.3 months. The most favorable subgroup of patients were those with a KPS score greater than or equal to 70, younger than age 65, and having stable systemic disease with no evidence of extracranial metastases. Median survival time for this subgroup of patients (RPA class I) was 7.1 months. For the remaining group of patients (RPA class II), median survival time fell into the intermediate level of 4.2 months. The RTOG RPA classification system has subsequently been validated in other studies and has proved to be a very useful prognostic tool for critically reviewing various treatment regimens.[8]

Table 57-1 is a compilation of selected single-institution series published since 1997 of patients with RCC metastatic to the brain treated with either WBRT, SRS, or SRS with WBRT. Included in this table are the RTOG RPA class I and class II subgroups for comparison. Studies are classified as SRS plus WBRT if more than half the patients treated received WBRT in addition to the SRS. Review of this table reveals that the best survival results are seen in patients who received the most aggressive therapy, consisting of SRS combined with WBRT. It must be pointed out, however, that in these series and in the series with SRS alone, a generally more favorable mix of patients was selected, exhibiting a higher KPS score. This selection bias may account for the modestly better median survival times seen in these series.

One drawback in the use of SRS alone (as seen with surgery alone) is the high frequency with which patients known to have one or more radiographically evident metastatic lesions in the brain eventually manifest lesions in other parts of the brain that were not evident at the time of diagnosis. This problem provides a strong argument for including WBRT in the treatment of all patients. As would be predicted, the best reported median survival time among the series quoted in Table 57-1 was achieved with what appears to be the most favorably selected patients, treated with the most aggressive therapy, with 80% of the patients receiving WBRT in addition to SRS.[11]

The optimal combination of WBRT and SRS remains a matter of ongoing investigation. The RTOG recently completed a trial in which patients with brain metastases were randomized to receive either WBRT alone or WBRT in combination with SRS given as a boost dose to selected lesions. Results from this trial will probably influence the future management of patients with brain metastases. A trial comparing surgical resection of a solitary brain metastasis with surgical resection plus WBRT has already demonstrated that patients with a single metastasis to the brain who receive WBRT after surgical resection will have fewer recurrences of cancer in the brain and are less likely to die of neurologic causes than patients treated with surgical resection alone.[14] Similar studies comparing SRS with SRS and WBRT have been initiated. An important consideration in these studies will clearly be quality of life. It remains to be seen if the therapeutic benefit obtained from WBRT, in its ability to minimize the neurologic problems associated with the emergence of new lesions, outweighs any added short-term side effects of the radiation itself.

CONCLUSION

Treatment of RCC metastatic to the brain involves a multidisciplinary team approach. Vital to the success of this approach is treatment of the primary disease with surgery or immunotherapy, treatment of the solitary brain lesion with surgery or SRS, and the addition of WBRT in confronting multiple lesions. Surgery and SRS both have a role in the local control of RCC metastatic to the brain, with large symptomatic lesions better treated with surgery and multiple small lesions better treated with SRS.

Although survival is limited following the diagnosis of RCC metastatic to the brain, with the armamentarium currently available, we do have the ability to significantly affect our patients' quality of life and, in certain instances, to even affect their overall survival.

Acknowledgment

The authors wish to acknowledge support for this work from the University of Colorado Comprehensive Cancer Center.

References

1. Amendola BE, Wolf AL, Coy SR, et al: Brain metastases in renal cell carcinoma: management with gamma knife radiosurgery. Cancer J 6:372–376, 2000.

2. Becker G, Jeremic B, Engel C, et al: Radiosurgery for brain metastases: the Tuebingen experience. Radiother Oncol 62:233–7, 2002.

3. Bender AL, Posner JB: Current treatment of brain metastases. In Maciunas RJ (ed): Advanced Techniques in Central Nervous System Metastases. Parkridge, Ill, The American Association of Neurological Surgeons, 1998.

4. Culine S, Bekradda M, Kramar A, et al: Prognostic factors for survival in patients with brain metastases from renal cell carcinoma. Cancer 83:2548–53, 1998.

5. Elson PJ, Witte RS, Trump DL: Prognostic factors for survival in patients with recurrent or metastatic renal cell carcinoma. Cancer Res 48:7310–7313, 1988.

6. Flanigan RC, Salmon SE, Blumenstein BA, et al: Nephrectomy followed by interferon alfa-2b compared with interferon alfa-2b alone for metastatic renal-cell cancer. N Engl J Med 345:1655–1659, 2001.

7. Gaspar L, Scott C, Rotman M, et al: Recursive partitioning analysis (RPA) of prognostic factors in three Radiation Therapy Oncology Group (RTOG) brain metastases trials. Int J Radiat Oncol Biol Phys 37:745–751, 1997.

8. Gaspar LE, Scott C, Murray K, et al: Validation of the RTOG recursive partitioning analysis (RPA) classification for brain metastases. Int J Radiat Oncol Biol Phys 47:1001–1006, 2000.

9. Goyal LK, Suh JH, Reddy CA, et al: The role of whole brain radiotherapy and stereotactic radiosurgery on brain metastases from renal cell carcinoma. Int J Radiat Oncol Biol Phys 47:1007–1012, 2000.

10. Lagerwaard FJ, Levendag PC, Nowak PJ, et al: Identification of prognostic factors in patients with brain metastases: a review of 1292 patients. Int J Radiat Oncol Biol Phys 43:795–803, 1999.

11. Mori Y, Kondziolka D, Flickinger JC, et al: Stereotactic radiosurgery for brain metastasis from renal cell carcinoma. Cancer 83:344–353, 1998.

12. Motzer RJ, Bander NH, Nanus DM: Renal-cell carcinoma. N Engl J Med 335:865–875, 1996.

13. Patchell RA, Tibbs PA, Walsh JW, et al: A randomized trial of surgery in the treatment of single metastases to the brain. N Engl J Med 322:494–500, 1990.

14. Patchell RA, Tibbs PA, Regine WF, et al: Postoperative radiotherapy in the treatment of single metastases to the brain: a randomized trial. JAMA 280:1485–1489, 1998.

15. Schoggl A, Kitz K, Ertl A, et al: Gamma-knife radiosurgery for brain metastases of renal cell carcinoma: results in 23 patients. Acta Neurochir (Wien) 140:549–555, 1998.

16. Wronski M, Maor MH, Davis BJ, et al: External radiation of brain metastases from renal carcinoma: a retrospective study of 119 patients from the M.D. Anderson Cancer Center. Int J Radiat Oncol Biol Phys 37:753–759, 1997.

CHAPTER 58

INTRACEREBRAL METASTATIC COLON CARCINOMA

Timothy Ryken, Thomas Carlisle, and John M. Buatti

Cancer of the colon represents a major public health problem and is of particular concern in well-developed countries. The reason behind the increased incidence in these countries is unclear but probably relates to dietary factors. The increase has attracted the attention of numerous investigators. Metastatic dissemination to the brain is less common than with other cancers, such as lung cancer or breast cancer, and therefore has not been examined as closely. The purpose of this chapter is to focus on those aspects of metastatic brain tumors unique to patients with colon cancer. As there are no large-scale randomized clinical studies available, the data reviewed are retrospective. Many of the opinions and management options discussed have had to be extrapolated from the general literature on metastatic brain tumors.

EPIDEMIOLOGY

Colon cancer ranks second in women and third in men in overall frequency but ranks fourth as the cause of mortality, giving it a slightly better prognosis than other more common cancers.[21,28] Cancers of the gastrointestinal tract accounted for more than 6% of all patients' visits to the University of Iowa for central nervous system (CNS) metastatic disease over a 10-year period, ranking fourth behind lung, breast, and skin (melanoma) as the site of primary disease (Table 58-1). The 5-year survival rate in most studies exceeds 60% from the time of primary diagnosis.[21,28] As seen in other forms of cancer, improvements in treatments and improved local control for colon cancer has resulted in an increased likelihood of metastatic disease becoming symptomatic before life-threatening disease from the primary tumor. Nonetheless, spread to the CNS continues to carry a dismal prognosis despite aggressive treatment, as discussed in the later section on specific management options.

A significant number of cases of colon cancer metastases to the brain occur in the posterior fossa. Depending on the series, this ranges from 35% to 55%, which is significantly higher than the occurrence in lung adenocarcinoma, breast adenocarcinoma, or melanoma.[1,9,13,15] This occurred in 40% of our patients in a limited review (Table 58-2) and may be related to the vascular anatomy of the colon.

The risk factors that may lead to genetic alterations in the colonic mucosa include meat intake, fecal mutagens, bile acids, altered vitamin and mineral intake, fecal pH, and a predisposition to the effects of mutagens. None of these factors has been thoroughly investigated for its impact on CNS metastatic disease.[15]

Preventive or protective factors that have been described include adjusting dietary factors, limiting tobacco and alcohol use, hormonal therapies, and nonsteroidal anti-inflammatory use.[33] The impact of cyclo-oxygenase-2 (COX-2) receptor inhibition by superselective pharmaceuticals has been an area of active investigation.[19]

PRESENTATION

Patients at particular risk for colon cancer include those who are older than age 50 and those who have polyposis, inflammatory bowel disease, multiple abdominal surgeries, or a history of pelvic irradiation.[1,13,15,34]

Despite public health and preventive medical efforts, less than 20% of people aged 50 and older are screened for colon cancer. The majority of patients are diagnosed based on symptomatic presentation. Symptoms at the time the colon cancer is diagnosed include rectal bleeding, abdominal pain, bowel obstruction, nausea and vomiting, weight loss, anemia, and fatigue. The diagnosis of colon cancer is generally made following colonoscopy.

Patients are diagnosed with CNS metastases either concurrently with their initial diagnosis (synchronous presentation) or following their initial diagnosis (metachronous presentation). The majority of patients with colon carcinoma metastases to the brain were metachronously diagnosed. A synchronous presentation occurs in only approximately 10% to 15% of cases. A patient with brain metastases generally has headache (24%), weakness (20%), behavioral or cognitive alterations (14%), seizures (12%), ataxia (7%), or no symptoms (7%).[25]

PATHOLOGY

The classic pathologic descriptions and classifications for colon cancer were published early in the nineteenth century and remain in common use today (Figure 58-1). Pathologic evaluation of the primary site of colon cancer involves various subtypes: mucinous adenocarcinoma, signet-ring adenocarcinoma, squamous cell carcinoma, small-cell carcinoma, choriocarcinoma, and medullary carcinoma. The vast majority of these are moderately differentiated adenocarcinomas. The degree of differentiation probably plays a role in the development of metastatic propagation, although it is unclear if a specific subtype has a propensity for the CNS. It does appear that invasion into the submucosa of the colon is a key factor in the development of metastatic dissemination.

Possible mechanisms of dissemination of local disease in colon cancer include local extension, lymphatic extension, hematogenous propagation, and detachment and implantation. Hematogenous propagation is the most likely route of metastasis to the brain. The relative infrequency of this occurrence is likely to be related to the vascular anatomy of the colon. Only 10% to 15% of patients have distant disease at the time of diag-

nosis, with the majority having metastatic extension to the liver. Venous drainage of the upper colon is via the hepatic portal system, accounting for this predilection. The lower colon and rectum drain to both the portal system and to the inferior vena cava, allowing widespread dissemination.[6,9]

Brown and Warrens' historical study describes an autopsy series of 70 patients with colon cancer that demonstrated an incidence of 33% liver metastases and 9% lung metastases.[6] Patients with lung metastases all had lower colon primary tumors. Given the propensity of lung carcinoma to metastasize to the brain, it seems likely that a significant number of patients with invasion of the cerebral hemispheres incur the metastasis via secondary propagation from the pulmonary circulation.

In this same series, 14% of patients had vertebral involvement. The presumed route of metastasis is via the vertebral venous plexus and may account for the cases of disease metastatic to the posterior fossa.

First described in 1965, carcinoma embryonic antigen (CEA) has become the most reliable marker for detecting active colon carcinoma. At present, the role of CEA in colon cancer metastatic to the brain is unproved. A number of other molecules are also under evaluation as potential therapeutic targets, including bcl-2 and vascular endothelial growth factor (VEGF).[24]

MANAGEMENT

As with other forms of CNS metastatic disease,[3] management options for the patient with metastatic CNS colon carcinoma center on surgery and radiation-based therapies (Figures 58-2 and 58-3). The role of chemotherapy is thought to be limited in application and cannot be recommended as a first-line therapy. Given the poor prognosis of these patients, with a median survival time of 6 to 10 months, only supportive care may be most appropriate in selected patients and should be mentioned at diagnosis. This section reviews the therapeutic options for CNS metastatic colon carcinoma, focusing on the rather limited literature available specifically on colon carcinoma.

TABLE 58-1

Distribution of Intracerebral Metastatic Lesions by Primary Pathology at the University of Iowa over a 10-year period (1992–2002)

Primary Site	Number	Percentage
Lung	568	44.0
Breast	153	11.9
Melanoma	131	10.2
Gastrointestinal	81	6.3
Unknown Primary	74	5.7
Female Genital	54	4.2
Renal	51	3.9
Testicular and Prostate	44	3.4
Oral cavity and pharynx	27	2.1
Bladder and ureteral	19	1.5
Thyroid	18	1.4
Lymphoma	14	1.1
Larynx	12	1
Other known	24	2
Total	1291	

TABLE 58-2   Clinical Data on Treatment of 10 Patients with Colon Carcinoma Metastatic to the CNS

Age/Sex	Interval to CNS Metastatic Presentation	Symptoms	Location/Number	Treatment	Survival Time (Overall/from Secondary Diagnosis)
53/F	7 mo	Headache	Left cerebellar/2	SRS	8 mo/1 mo
50/F	7 yr	Headache	Right frontal/1	Craniotomy, SRS	8 yr/12 mo
72/M	11 yr	Ataxia	Right cerebellar/1	Craniotomy, WBRT, SRS	11 yr 2 mo/2 mo
78/M	7 yr	Left hemiparesis	Right frontoparietal/1	Craniotomy, WBRT	7 yr 3 mo/3 mo
49/F	5 yr	Right hemiparesis	Left parietal/1	WBRT	5 yr 2 mo/2 mo
51/F	Synchronous	Headache, mental status changes	Right parietal/1	Craniotomy, WBRT, SRS	1 yr
52/F	2 yr	Headache	Left frontal and right frontal/2	WBRT	2 yr 4 mo/4 mo
70/M	9 yr	Right hemiparesis	Left thalamus/1	WBRT	9 yr 2 mo/2 mo
65/M	1 yr	Ataxia	Left cerebellum/1	Craniotomy, SRS	1 yr 6 mo/6 mo
78/F	4 yr	Headache	Right cerebellum/1	Craniotomy, WBRT, SRS	4 yr 9 mo/9 mo

CNS, Central nervous system; F, female; M, male; SRS, stereotactic radiosurgery; WBRT, whole-brain radiation therapy.

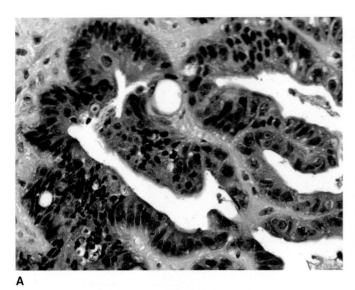

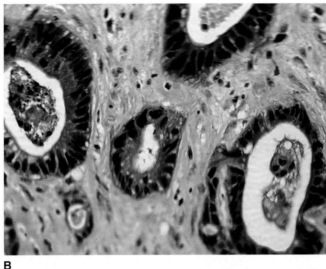

A   B

FIGURE 58-1 Representative histopathologic microphotographic images of metastatic colon carcinoma stained with hematoxylin and eosin (original magnification ×40). *A,* Note the undulating glandular pattern seen in this moderately well-differentiated colon adenocarcinoma. Interestingly, this pattern is similar to that seen in choroid plexus carcinoma. *B,* Note the rests of metastatic tumor tissue intermingled with normal parenchyma on the edge of this metastatic specimen. This microscopic invasion is the reason behind the rationale for many of the adjuvant treatment options in metastatic central nervous system disease.

Surgery

Indications for surgical intervention for metastatic CNS disease include obtaining diagnostic tissue, local control for limited CNS metastatic lesions, and symptomatic debulking of large metastatic lesions. The continued development of frameless stereotaxy (image-guided surgery) has decreased the extent of surgery required for multiple lesions and improved the ease of locating smaller lesions. Intraoperative magnetic resonance imaging and image-guided ultrasound also allow real-time feedback on extent of resection. Open surgical approaches also allow the option of intracavitary therapies available as a surgical adjunct. At present, the options include intracavitary chemotherapy and brachytherapy (Figure 58-4). Both methodologies are under active investigation in the management of metastatic intracranial disease.

The median survival time of patients with colon carcinoma treated with craniotomy has been reported to range from 8.7 to 10 months.[1,9,13,15,30,35] Wronski and Arbit describe a series of 73 patients with metastatic CNS colon carcinoma undergoing craniotomy for surgical resection. This represented 73 of 709 patients (10%) over 19 years (1974 to 1993). There were 43 women and 30 men, with a median age of 61.5 years. The interval between primary and secondary diagnosis was reported as 27.6 months. The median survival time from the time of craniotomy was 8.3 months, with a 1-year disease-free survival rate of 31.5%. Operative mortality was only 4%. The only significant factor in the multivariate analysis was the presence of a cerebellar tumor, which showed a decrease in survival time and a worse prognosis (5.1 months for infratentorial locations vs. 9.1 months for supratentorial ones, *P* < .002). This series represents the largest surgical series available for review and argues in support of surgical resection.[34]

Salvati et al published a series of 24 patients with colon cancer, all of whom had disease metastatic to the brain.[30] This series demonstrated a median survival time of 10 months. In this series, 27% had metastatic lung disease and 12% had developed liver metastases.

Farnell et al describes a series of 50 patients treated with craniotomy (1976 to 1992) who had a median survival time of 10 months and a 1-year survival rate of only 34%. The subgroup that also received whole-brain radiation therapy (WBRT) had an increased 1-year survival rate of 44%.[12] Alden et al reviewed 19 patients with an overall 6.2% survival rate at 1 year and a median survival time of 2.8 months. Only five patients were treated with a craniotomy, but they had an increased median survival time of 4.1 months.[1]

Hammoud et al[13] described experience with 100 patients with colon cancer (38 male and 62 female), of whom 24% had brain metastases at the initial diagnosis. Of these patients, 36% had multiple and 52% had supratentorial lesions. The overall median survival time was 5 months. The patients receiving only WBRT had a survival time of 3 months. Among patients in the subgroup who had undergone craniotomy, the median survival time was 9 months. The authors concluded that surgical resection is of benefit; however, limitations in the study design and patient entry criteria do not allow a definitive statement to be made.[13] Extrapolation from studies of other patients with limited intracranial metastatic disease supports this conclusion.[2,23,32]

The increased incidence of colon cancer metastases to the posterior fossa represents a potential management problem from direct brainstem compression or secondary effects of the intracerebellar mass causing hydrocephalus by obstructing the cerebrospinal fluid pathways. These patients may undergo surgery to relieve mass effect or require cerebrospinal fluid diversion. The cerebellar location has been shown to be associated with decreased survival time.[34]

In most series, surgical resection provides a significant survival advantage over radiation therapy alone. Given the current

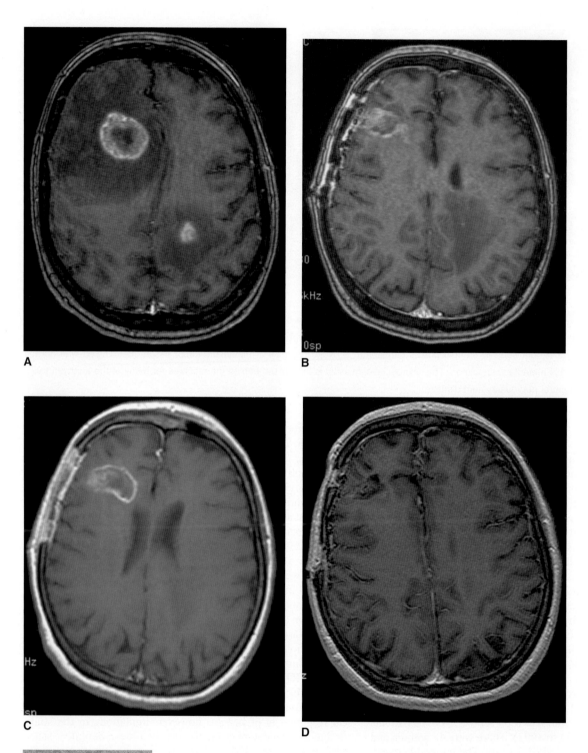

FIGURE 58-2 Comparison of treatment options in this 47-year-old woman with two metastatic lesions from colon carcinoma. For the right frontal lesion she underwent resection by craniotomy followed by stereotactic radiosurgery (SRS). For the left parietal lesion she underwent SRS alone. At her approximately 1-year follow-up evaluation, it is difficult to differentiate between the sites. *A,* Preoperative gadolinium-enhanced axial magnetic resonance image. *B,* Early postoperative view. *C,* 3 months after surgery and 2 months after SRS. *D,* 12 months after surgery and 11 months after SRS. Note the near resolution of enhancement and lack of adjacent edema.

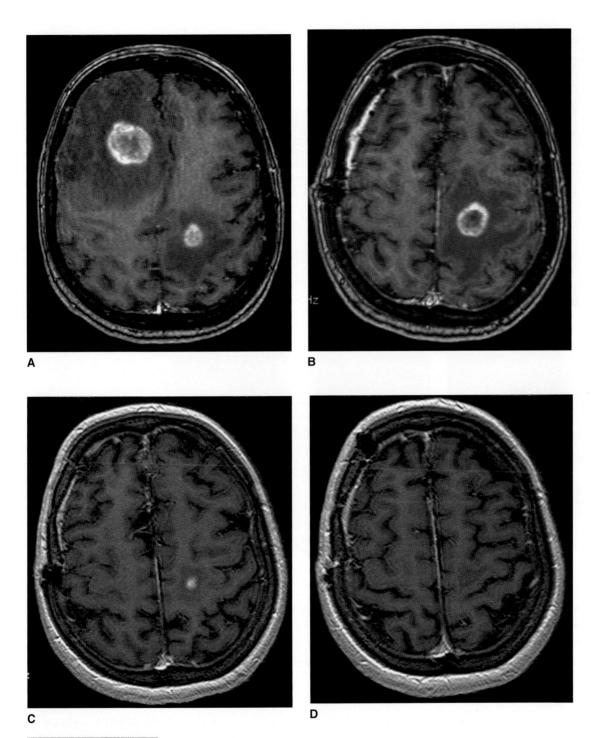

FIGURE 58-3 *A,* Gadolinium-enhanced axial magnetic resonance (MR) image focusing on the left parietal region before stereotactic radiosurgery (SRS). *B,* Image of the same patient 3 months after treatment with SRS. Note the apparent enlargement and alteration in the pattern of enhancement. In retrospect, this did not represent disease progression. *C,* MR image of the patient at 6 months after SRS. Note the clear reduction in the amount of enhancement. *D,* Nearly 1 year after SRS, the lesion has resolved.

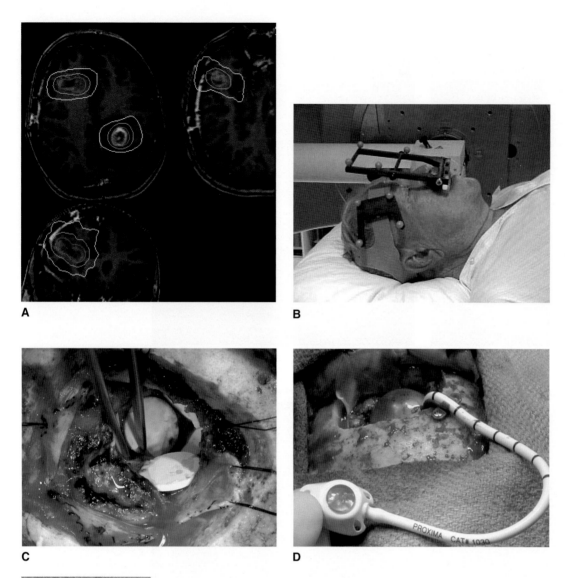

FIGURE 58-4   Modalities change for treating metastatic central nervous system lesions. *A* and *B,* Stereotactic radiosurgery has become increasingly popular as a component in the management of intracranial metastatic lesions. Techniques have been developed that completely avoid the requirement for rigid attachment of a stereotactic ring to a patient's skull. The setup for this frameless technique is shown. *C,* Implantation of a chemotherapeutic polymer in the tumor resection cavity is an option, particularly in patients who have already received external-beam radiation therapy. *D,* Systems for delivery of interstitial radiation therapy are available. Using this technique, an expandable balloon catheter is left in the surgical bed to receive a postoperative radiation dose.

data, the recommendations for surgical management should follow that for other metastatic lesions, and therefore surgical resection is generally the treatment of choice in single (or multiple) lesions of more than 2.5 cm in greatest diameter that are surgically accessible.

Radiation Therapy

WBRT remains the most widely chosen therapeutic option in the management of CNS metastases. Wronski and Arbit's report of 73 patients treated with surgical resection of colon cancer metastases included 33 patients treated with both craniotomy and WBRT (mean dose 3124 cGy).[34] This increased the median survival time from 6.8 months to 9 months but was not statistically significant. Smaller series have also been reported. Farnell

et al reported on 79 patients treated with WBRT for metastatic colon cancer who had a median survival time of only 3.6 months.[12] Hammoud et al's series of 57 patients treated with WBRT alone had a median survival time of only 3 months.[13] Other studies have reported similar results.[1,9,16,30] Overall, studies have results are consistent in implying a poor outlook for WBRT as a sole treatment modality.

By comparison, a large series of 1292 patients reported by Lagerwward et al included all types of metastatic diagnoses, with an overall median survival time of 3.4 months in patients treated with WBRT alone and 8.9 months in patients who could be treated with craniotomy and WBRT in combination.[18] In this study, only performance status, response to steroids, and extent of systemic disease correlated with improved survival. Although the pathology of the primary tumor was not significant, the number of patients with colon cancer was probably too small to influence the overall results.

The improved survival times for selected patients treated with a combination of craniotomy and radiation therapy has suggested a role of stereotactic radiosurgery as an adjuvant in the treatment of metastatic disease.[27,31] In some cases a decision has been made to treat with stereotactic radiosurgery alone, in an attempt to limit the potential toxicity from WBRT.[2,4,5,8,17,31] Techniques using both the standard stereotactic head ring (frame-based) and frameless techniques have been developed and used with success in selected cases.[7,8,29]

Chemotherapy

There is no proven benefit to the use of chemotherapy in treating colon cancer that has spread to the CNS. No convincing data exist specifically on its use to treat CNS metastases from colon carcinoma.[14,20,22,23,32] Metastatic disease from colon carcinoma is generally thought to be resistant to chemotherapy. It is believed that this is related to multiple-drug resistance gene expression and protection against antioxidants. These alterations coupled with the challenge of crossing the blood-brain barrier make the likelihood of a response to systemic chemotherapy treatment for CNS colon cancer metastases unlikely. Despite limited clinical evidence for the role of chemotherapy in patients with colon cancer and CNS metastatic disease, Ewends et al's work with the CT26 colon carcinoma line in an animal model system demonstrated the possible role of local chemotherapy in the form of polymer delivery for intracranial metastatic disease in selected patients.[11] This method is the subject of several current trials but remains of uncertain benefit in humans.

As a form of salvage therapy, various regimens have been attempted based primarily on the response of primary colon cancer and the fact that contrast-agent enhancement occurs with brain metastasis.[25] This raises the question of how to get other potentially therapeutic materials across the blood-brain barrier in the region of the metastatic lesion. The likely choice would be 5-fluorouracil (5-FU) with or without leucovorin, but it results in limited improvement in 5-year survival rates when used in patients with primary colon cancer. Promising results have also been obtained with the addition of irinotecan (CPT 11) or oxaliplatin.[10,26]

INSTITUTIONAL EXPERIENCE

To compare the available literature with our experience and provide representative cases for discussion, a series of 10 patients treated over a 2-year period were retrospectively reviewed. This group was selected because they had all been treated since the availability of stereotactic radiosurgery as a treatment modality and all had a minimum of 2-year follow-up evaluations available at the time of review. A portion of the clinical data are summarized in Table 58-2. This group included six females and four males ranging in age from 49 to 78; eight had single lesions and four had infratentorial lesions. Only one patient had been synchronously diagnosed and the rest metachronously, with a range of 7 months to 11 years between the initial diagnosis and the appearance of a CNS lesion. Patients had symptoms representative of the location as expected. The median survival time for the group from the time of the CNS metastatic presentation was 5.3 months (range 1 to 12 months). The treatments used included WBRT alone, craniotomy plus WBRT, craniotomy plus WBRT and stereotactic radiosurgery, and stereotactic radiosurgery alone. This group appears to be relatively representative of the patients described in the literature. Given the variation in treatments and the overall poor survival regardless of treatment, it is not possible to draw conclusions on treatment recommendations.

CONCLUSION

Colon cancer metastatic to the CNS represents less than 10% of all CNS metastases. Based on the relatively limited retrospective data available, it appears that it carries a prognosis at least as grim as other more common metastatic tumors, with a median survival time in the range of 3 to 10 months regardless of treatment. The metastatic process in colon cancer appears to have a predilection for the posterior fossa and produces a single lesion with some frequency. The limited response to radiation therapy and systemic chemotherapy suggests applying aggressive surgical and radiosurgical treatments in selected patients, which may improve survival and quality of life. Management decisions would benefit from prospective data collection and development of alternate treatment methodologies in the future.

References

1. Alden TD, Gianino JW, Saclarides TJ: Brain metastases from colorectal cancer. Dis Col Rect 39:541, 1996.
2. Alexander E, III, Loeffler JS: The case for radiosurgery. Clin Neurosurg 45:32, 1999.
3. Arnold SM, Patchell RA: Diagnosis and management of brain metastases. Hematol Oncol Clin North Am 15:1085, 2001.
4. Bindal AK, Bindal RK, Hess KR, et al: Surgery versus radiosurgery in the treatment of brain metastasis. [see comments.] J Neurosurg 84:748, 1996.
5. Boyd TS, Mehta MP: Stereotactic radiosurgery for brain metastases. Oncology (Huntington) 13:1397, 1999; discussion.
6. Brown C, Warren S: Visceral metastasis from carcinoma. Surg Gynecol Obstet 66:611, 1938.
7. Buatti JM, Bova FJ, Friedman WA, et al: Preliminary experience with frameless stereotactic radiotherapy. Int J Radiat Oncol Biol Phys 42(3):591, 1998.
8. Buatti JM, Meeks SL, Friedman WA, et al: Stereotactic radiosurgery: techniques and clinical applications. Surg Oncol Clin North Am 9:469, 2000.
9. Cascino TL, Leavengood JM, Kemeny N, et al: Brain metastases from colon cancer. J Neuro-oncol 1:203, 1983.
10. Cunningham D, Pyrhonen S, James RD, et al: Randomised trial of irinotecan plus supportive care versus supportive care alone after fluorouracil failure for patients with metastatic colorectal cancer. Lancet 352:1413, 1998.
11. Ewend MG, Sampath P, Williams JA, et al: Local delivery of chemotherapy prolongs survival in experimental brain metastases from breast carcinoma. Neurosurgery 43:1185, 1998.
12. Farnell GF, Buckner JC, Cascino TL, et al: Brain metastases from colorectal carcinoma. The long term survivors. [see comments.]. Cancer 78:711, 1996.

13. Hammoud MA, McCutcheon IE, Elsouki R, et al: Colorectal carcinoma and brain metastasis: distribution, treatment, and survival. Ann Surg Oncol 3:453, 1996.

14. Kaba SE, Kyritsis AP, Hess K, et al: TPDC-FuHu chemotherapy for the treatment of recurrent metastatic brain tumors. J Clin Oncol 15:1063, 1997.

15. Ko FC, Liu JM, Chen WS, et al: Risk and patterns of brain metastases in colorectal cancer: 27-year experience. Dis Colon Rect 42:1467, 1999.

16. Kohno M, Matsutani M, Sosaki T, et al: Solitary metastasis to the choroid plexus of the lateral ventricle. Report of three cases and a review of the literature. J Neurooncol 27:47, 1996.

17. Kondziolka D, Patel A, Lundsford LD, et al: Stereotactic radiosurgery plus whole brain radiotherapy versus radiotherapy alone for patients with multiple brain metastases. [see comments.]. Int J Radiat Oncol Biol Phys 45:427, 1999.

18. Lagerwaard FJ, Levendag PC: Prognostic factors in patients with brain metastases. Forum 11:27, 2001.

19. Muscat J, Stellman S, Wynder E: Nonsteroidal antiinflammatory drugs and colorectal cancer. Cancer 74:1847, 1994.

20. Newton HB: Novel chemotherapeutic agents for the treatment of brain cancer. Expert Opin Invest Drugs 9:2815, 2000.

21. Parkin D, Pisani P, and Ferlay J: Global cancer statistics. CA Cancer J Clin 49:33, 1999.

22. Patchell RA: Brain metastases. Neurol Clin 9:817, 1991.

23. Patchell RA: The treatment of brain metastases. Cancer Invest 14:169, 1996.

24. Peethambaram P, Weiss M, Loprinzi CL, et al: An evaluation of postoperative followup tests in colon cancer patients treated for cure. Oncology 54:287, 1997.

25. Posner JB: Brain metastases: 1995. A brief review. J Neurooncol 27:287, 1996.

26. Project A: Modulation of fluorouracil by leucovorin in patients with advanced colorectal cancer: evidence in terms of response rate. Advanced Colorectal Cancer Meta-Analysis Project. J Clin Oncol 10:896, 1992.

27. Regine WF, Huhn JL, Patchell RA, et al: Risk of symptomatic brain tumor recurrence and neurologic deficit after radiosurgery alone in patients with newly diagnosed brain metastases: results and implications. Int J Radiat Oncol Biol Phys 52:333, 2002. Erratum, Int J Radiat Oncol Biol Phys 53:259, 2002.

28. Ries L, et al: SEER cancer statistics review 1973–1995. In Bethesda, National Cancer Institute, 1998.

29. Ryken TC, Meeks SL, Pennington EC, et al: Initial clinical experience with frameless stereotactic radiosurgery: analysis of accuracy and feasibility. Int J Radiat Oncol Biol Phys 51:1152, 2001.

30. Salvati M, Cervoni L, Paolini S, et al: Solitary cerebral metastases from intestinal carcinoma. Acta Neurochirurgica 133:181, 1995.

31. Sanghavi SN, Miranpuri SS, Chappell R, et al: Radiosurgery for patients with brain metastases: a multi-institutional analysis, stratified by the RTOG recursive partitioning analysis method. Int J Radiat Oncol Biol Phys 51:426, 2001.

32. Sawaya R, Ligon BL, Bindal RK: Management of metastatic brain tumors. Ann Surg Oncol 1:169, 1994.

33. Winawer S, Shike M: Dietary factors in colorectal cancer and their possible effects on earlier stages of hyperproliferation and adenoma formation. J Natl Cancer Inst 84:74, 1992.

34. Wronski M, Arbit E: Resection of brain metastases from colorectal carcinoma in 73 patients. Cancer 85:1677, 1999.

35. Wronski M, Lederman G: A randomized trial to assess the efficacy of surgery in addition to radiotherapy in patients with a single cerebral metastasis. [letter; comment.] Cancer 80:1002, 1997.

CHAPTER **5 9**

GYNECOLOGIC MALIGNANCIES

Sabrina M. Walski-Easton and Walter A. Hall

The American Cancer Society estimates that there will be 1,284,900 new cases of cancer and more than 550,000 cancer-related deaths in 2002.[20] Of the estimated 647,400 cancers occurring in women, gynecologic malignancies will account for approximately 13% and contribute to 10% of cancer deaths in women.[20] Brain metastasis occurs in 20% to 40% of all solid tumor malignancies. However, the incidence of gynecologic malignancies with metastasis to the brain appears to be much lower in frequency. Ovarian cancer constitutes 2% of all brain metastases, and 0.8% of patients with ovarian cancer will develop metastatic brain disease.[22,25] Despite these low rates, the occurrence of metastatic brain lesions in gynecologic malignancies appears to have increased over the past several years.[1,14,15,17,22,25,41] This increase may be due to increased survival rates from improved treatment options and early diagnosis of widespread disease.[5,31]

The prognosis for untreated cancer metastatic to the brain is extremely poor, with a median survival time of only 1 month.[30,32] Advancements in the treatment of brain metastases, including corticosteroids and whole-brain radiation therapy (WBRT), have improved survival time to 3 to 6 months.[24,30] Studies have shown that surgical excision of a solitary lesion with subsequent WBRT extended survival time from 4 to 6 months to 10 months.[33,43] Despite these advances, only approximately 10% of patients will survive for more than 2 years.[16]

Brain metastases from gynecologic tumors are most commonly located in the cerebral hemispheres, with cerebellar lesions constituting only 8.7%.[40]

A summary of the most common gynecologic malignancies is listed in Table 59-1.[4,35] Uterine, ovarian, and cervical cancers represent the first, second, and third most common genital malignancies affecting women in the United States, respectively.[20] Of these, ovarian cancer most often metastasizes to the brain.[32]

METASTASIS

Metastatic gynecologic disease occurs in 15% to 85% of cases, depending on tumor type, primarily by direct extension, peritoneal seeding, or lymphatic dissemination. The most common sites of metastasis are liver, lung, bone, and lymph nodes.[8,35]

Central nervous system (CNS) metastases are presumed to occur via hematogenous seeding or by direct invasion from previous bone metastasis, though the latter is rare. The development of metastatic foci is thought to be related to tumor cell behavior, host immune response, and the number of tumor cells that embolize.[29] Distant metastatic disease is causally associated with poorly differentiated tumors and advanced stage disease.[8] Many patients have concurrent pulmonary and brain metastases, and pulmonary disease may be a predisposing factor for the latter.[46]

Chemotherapy has also been implicated in the development of CNS metastases,[46] by transiently weakening the blood-brain barrier and allowing tumor invasion of the brain. Because most chemotherapeutic agents do not cross the blood-brain barrier, a "sanctuary" for tumor growth may be created in the CNS in those who have undergone systemic chemotherapy.

CLINICAL PRESENTATION

Symptoms in gynecological brain metastasis are usually slowly progressive over days to weeks; are typical of intracranial mass lesions; and include headache, focal neurologic deficit, ataxia, and seizures. For patients with cerebellar metastasis, nausea, vomiting, vertigo, and hydrocephalus caused by obstruction of cerebrospinal fluid (CSF) outflow may also be present.

Occasionally, patients with gynecologic malignancies will have acute onset of neurologic symptoms attributable to hemorrhage into the tumor. In one study, ovarian cancer brain metastasis had a hemorrhage rate of 7%.[30]

Although brain metastases are rare, the development of neurologic symptoms in patients with gynecologic malignancies should be investigated promptly with contrast-enhanced magnetic resonance imaging (MRI) or computed tomography (CT).

DIAGNOSIS

Contrast-enhanced MRI or CT of the brain should be performed for all patients with new neurologic symptoms. MRI is more sensitive than CT, particularly when evaluating posterior fossa lesions. Approximately 20% of patients with a single metastasis on CT will have multiple metastases when an MRI evaluation is performed.[27] Lesions usually appear round, uniform, or occasionally ring-enhanced and are located at the gray matter–white matter junction. Stereotactic or open biopsy may be indicated to confirm an uncertain diagnosis, particularly for patients in whom brain metastasis is the first sign of recurrence or when a positive diagnosis would significantly alter treatment. CSF cytology analysis is rarely useful, unless carcinomatous meningitis is suspected.[21]

TABLE 59-1

Most Common Gynecologic Malignancies

Uterine (48%)	
Endometrial carcinoma	90%*
Adenocarcinoma	
Leiomyosarcoma	3% of uterine CA
Other	
Ovarian (29%)	
Malignant epithelial cell tumors (serous, mucinous, endometrioid, clear cell adenocarcinoma)	90%
Malignant germ cell tumors (teratoma, germinoma, endodermal sinus tumor, choriocarcinoma)	5%†
Malignant stromal cell tumors	
Other	
Cervical (16%‡)	
Squamous cell tumors	85%
Adenocarcinoma	15%
Other (clear cell tumors [DES], sarcomas, lymphomas)	
Vulvar (4–5%)	
Squamous cell tumors	90%
Other	
Vaginal (1–2%)	
Squamous cell tumors	95%
Adenocarcinoma	5%
Other (melanoma)	
Fallopian Tube (<1%)	
Adenocarcinoma	
Other (metastatic from ovary or uterine, mullerian tumors, choriocarcinomas, fibromas)	
Malignant Gestational Trophoblastic Disease (Choriocarcinoma)	
Occurs in 10% of patients with previous molar pregnancy	

*Most common genital malignancy.
†Most common ovarian tumor in women younger than age 20, accounting for 60% of ovarian cancer.
‡In United States due to pap smear screening. Most common gynecologic malignancy worldwide.
DES, Diethylstilbestrol; CA, cancer.
Source: Adapted from Beckmann CRB, Ling FW, Barzansky BM, et al: Obstetrics and Gynecology. Baltimore, Williams & Wilkins, 1995 and Robinson JB, Morris M: Cervical carcinoma metastatic to the brain. Gynecol Oncol 66:324–326, 1997.

Ovarian Cancer

Ovarian cancer is the fourth most common cancer and the second most common genital malignancy in women.[20] Fortunately, metastatic CNS disease is not a common complication. This is supported by autopsy data that indicate that ovarian cancer comprises 1% of all brain metastases and that 0.8% of patients with ovarian cancer will develop metastatic brain disease.[25] More recent reports show an increased incidence of CNS involvement ranging from 2% to 4%.[1,14,15,17,22,25,41] It has been suggested that this increased incidence is related to extended disease-free survival primarily related to early diagnosis, aggressive surgical and chemotherapeutic treatments, increased detection because of improvements in radiologic diagnosis from CT and MRI scanning, or, possibly, changes in tumor biology.[2,7,14,17,22,25,41]

Ovarian cancer is usually asymptomatic until late in the course of the disease. At the time of diagnosis, it is usually widely disseminated, with 85% of patients having extrapelvic disease. Many patients will also have active intra-abdominal disease at the time of the diagnosis of brain metastasis.[26] Second-look laparotomies with findings of recurrent intra-abdominal tumor are associated with the development of multiple brain metastases ($P = .03$). However, survival is not significantly different from those with a negative laparotomy.[26]

The median age at diagnosis of ovarian cancer for women who develop intracranial disease is 55 years. The median interval from the diagnosis of ovarian cancer to discovery of brain disease ranges from 18.1 to 23 months.[30,40] In approximately 6% of patients, brain involvement was the first indication of ovarian carcinoma.[26] Single metastatic lesions occur in 43% to 57% of patients and multiple lesions in 41% to 43%.[26,30] Median survival time is 6 to 8 months, with 23% surviving for 2 years and only 7.8% 3 years or longer.[16,26,30] There are anecdotal reports of long-term survivors.[26,42] The incidence of hemorrhage is approximately 7%.[30]

Surgery ($P = .1$) and chemotherapy ($P = .001$) were identified as independent predictors of survival in a retrospective analysis of 104 patients with ovarian brain metastases.[26] Patients with a single metastasis having surgery with or without WBRT or chemotherapy had a median survival time of 21 months versus 6 months without surgical intervention ($P = .049$). Patients who received cisplatin-based chemotherapy as part of their treatment protocol survived for 13 months versus 5 months without chemotherapy ($P = .002$). Of note, 93% of patients in this series also received WBRT.

Cervical Cancer

Cervical cancer is the most common gynecologic malignancy, worldwide, and the most common cancer in women in some parts of the world.[21,28] Widespread screening in the United States has decreased the incidence of cervical cancer, making it the third most common genital cancer in American women.[20]

Metastatic dissemination occurs mainly by direct local extension and lymphatic propagation. Vascular dissemination, the presumed mechanism for brain metastasis, occurs in 5% of tumors, is associated with anaplasia, and occurs late in the course of the disease.[35] The frequency of metastatic brain disease ranges from 0.5% to 1.2% in clinical series to 15% in autopsy data.[11] The median time from diagnosis of the primary tumor to diagnosis of brain involvement is 30 months (range 0 to 8 years).[35] The majority of brain metastases arise from squamous cell carcinomas, although adenocarcinomas, mixed tumors, and carcinoid tumors are also commonly reported primary tumors.[35] Supratentorial lesions predominate, but cerebellar and spinal epidural lesions have been reported.[10,35] Two thirds of cases had multiple lesions.[11]

Most cervical cancers are widely disseminated by the time CNS disease is identified, and multiple lesions are most common. Thus the prognosis is poor, with a median survival time of less than 3 months.[21] In these cases, WBRT for palliation is often recommended. In one review, one third of patients with brain metastases from cervical cancer who received WBRT had resolution of neurologic symptoms. However, median survival time was only 3 months.[13,21,23,38] In contrast, three patients, two with multiple metastases, who underwent craniotomy and WBRT survived for 4.1, 7.5, and 10.3 months.[19] Occasionally, there are reports of long-term survival after craniotomy and WBRT.[35,44] Given the high rate of multiple brain lesions in cervical cancer, stereotactic radiosurgery (SRS) with WBRT may be an attractive option for these patients. Chemotherapy with cisplatin may help control systemic disease, but its effect on CNS disease has not yet been demonstrated.

Brain metastasis in patients with cervical cancer carries a poor prognosis, mainly because the disease is usually widespread once CNS involvement occurs. For certain specific patients with stable systemic disease, surgery or radiation may offer improved survival.

Uterine Cancer

Endometrial cancer is the most common malignant gynecologic neoplasm,[20] the fourth most common female malignancy, and the eighth leading cause of cancer deaths in women. Of women with endometrial cancer, 0.3% to 0.9% will develop brain metastasis, and the median interval between primary diagnosis and CNS metastasis is 26 months.[12,34] Figure 59-1 illustrates a case of a 50-year-old woman with uterine cancer metastatic to the brain. The lesion was cystic and filled with proteinaceous fluid as demonstrated in the T2-weighted coronal MRI scan.

Factors conclusively associated with the development of endometrial brain metastases have not been identified. Suspected characteristics include advanced clinical stage of disease and high-grade anaplasia.[12] The fact that patients with early-stage, well-differentiated tumors have developed CNS disease may implicate intrinsic tumor biologic factors as being causative. Brain involvement was seen in 30% of patients with distant recurrent disease but in only 3% and 6% of patients with progressive or locally recurrent disease, respectively.[12]

Cerebral hemispheric metastases are most common, but cerebellar and meningeal lesions have been documented.[6,12] Uterine adenocarcinoma appears to be more common than uterine sarcoma,[46] which is a highly aggressive and lethal tumor. There are six reports of cerebral metastasis appearing before or at the time of the diagnosis of endometrial cancer.[34,39] In contrast to other gynecologic neoplasms, the CNS was the only site of detectable disease in 60% of patients in one series.[12]

Patients treated with palliative WBRT survived for approximately 3 months, but with surgical excision and radiation therapy this duration was extended to 23 to 83 months.[12,34] There is one report of a patient with synchronous presentation of brain and uterine disease who underwent craniotomy, radio-

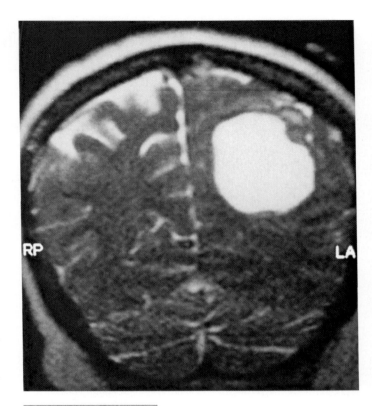

FIGURE 59-1 Magnetic resonance (MR) image of the brain showing a large posterior parietal cystic lesion in a 50-year-old woman 11 months following the diagnosis of a high-grade endometrial carcinoma. She was treated with MR-guided surgical resection and whole-brain radiation therapy (3000 cGy whole brain; 1400 cGy conformal boost). She was found to have pleural and rib metastases and was treated with systemic chemotherapy. No further brain lesions were identified on follow-up examinations.

surgery, chemotherapy, and repeat craniotomy for recurrence with no evidence of disease at 171 months.[34]

Doxorubicin, cyclophosphamide, and cisplatin appear to be the most cytotoxic chemotherapeutic agents for this disease, and overall, endometrial cancer has a good prognosis.[34] Although brain metastases have a poor prognosis, endometrial adenocarcinoma treated aggressively with surgery and radiation therapy may offer patients an extended survival time of greater than 2 years. It is unclear whether chemotherapy affects the clinical outcome in the presence of intracranial disease.[12]

Fallopian Tube Cancer

Primary tumors of the fallopian tube are extremely rare entities, accounting for less than 1% of gynecologic malignancies.[37] These tumors appear to behave in a manner similar to ovarian cancer and are classified and treated in much the same way. Some fallopian tube neoplasms may be prone to early blood-borne micrometastasis, resulting in poor long-term disease-free survival and contributing to the formation of brain metastasis.[37,47] The few cases of such brain metastases reported in the irradiation literature were treated with brain irradiation and systemic chemotherapy because of the presence of active pul-

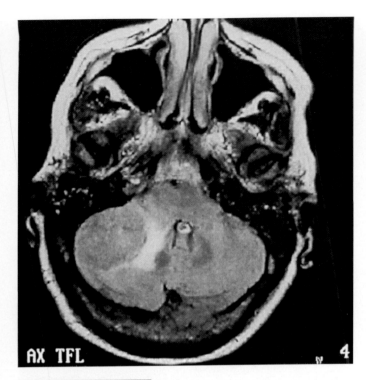

FIGURE 59-2 Magnetic resonance image illustrating a right cerebellar mass in a 53-year-old woman with a 13-year history of stage IIIc fallopian tube carcinoma metastatic to the retroperitoneum, supraclavicular lymph nodes, and thyroid. Surgical resection was performed and the pathology revealed metastatic fallopian tube carcinoma. She underwent stereotactic radiosurgery 18 months later for recurrence. Routine follow-up evaluation at 20 months showed no evidence of recurrence or new brain metastases.

monary involvement, with an approximately 1-year survival. Figure 59-2 illustrates a 53-year-old woman with a cerebellar metastasis from fallopian tube carcinoma on an axial turbo-fluid-attenuated inversion recovery (FLAIR) MRI scan.

CARCINOMATOUS MENINGITIS

Carcinomatous meningitis has been reported for most types of gynecologic malignancies. It is a rare complication associated with advanced systemic disease and a poor prognosis. MRI and high volume lumbar puncture for CSF cytologic analysis are the most useful diagnostic tests. Treatment includes radiation therapy and systemic or intrathecal chemotherapy.

SPINAL EPIDURAL METASTASIS

Spinal epidural metastasis from gynecologic neoplasms is extremely uncommon, accounting for only 3.3% of cases of spinal cord compression or cauda equina syndrome (CES).[36] Epidural metastasis occurs hematogenously through spinal epidural veins (also known as Batson's plexus) or by direct perinervous spread from the pelvis.[3]

Pain, particularly at night or persisting in recumbency, is characteristic of spinal epidural metastasis. Other symptoms include weakness, sensory disturbance, and urinary retention or urgency. Rapidly progressive lower extremity weakness or bowel and bladder involvement signifies spinal cord compression or CES and requires emergent evaluation by MRI or CT myelogram and rapid treatment. Because treatment does not prolong survival, pain control and minimization of neurologic deficit is the ultimate goal. This includes institution of high-dose steroids, surgical decompression, or radiation therapy. One complicating factor is that previous pelvic irradiation may preclude radiation therapy because of overlapping treatment fields.

TREATMENT

Data are limited on the treatment of gynecologic malignancies metastatic to the brain because of a small patient population. However, these tumors appear to behave in a manner similar to other solid malignancies. The following treatment strategies are used in the management of brain metastases.

Surgery

Patients with solitary, surgically accessible lesions, stable systemic disease, Karnofsky Performance Scale score of 70 or greater, and an expected survival time of more than 3 months are considered good candidates for surgical resection. When these criteria are not met, but the lesion is life threatening or severely symptomatic, surgery is usually considered. Two randomized series have shown a statistically significant increase in survival time for patients with a single metastasis treated with surgery time and WBRT.[33,43] Postoperative morbidity rates range from 3% to 8%, with a 30-day mortality rate of approximately 2% to 6%.[29,45] Studies have not provided convincing evidence delineating a clear role for surgery for patients with multiple metastases, as they generally have a poor prognosis.[5,18,30,32]

In univariate and multivariate analyses, evaluation of patients with ovarian cancer brain metastasis revealed surgical therapy to be an independent predictor of prolonged survival ($P = .01$).[26] Surgery combined with WBRT or chemotherapy provided a statistically significant longer median survival time for patients with ovarian cancer brain metastasis, with the longest survival reported in those with a single metastasis.[26]

Nonsurgical candidates are generally referred for palliative WBRT or SRS.

Whole-Brain Radiation Therapy

WBRT is used as adjuvant to surgery to control micrometastasis and as palliative therapy for unresectable lesions.[42] Doses range from 30 to 50 Gy divided into 1.8 to 2.0 Gy daily fractions administered over several weeks. The smaller daily fractions reduce neurotoxicity and well-known complications of radiation therapy, including radiation necrosis and radiation-induced dementia.[12] Of those patients treated with WBRT alone, 50% will have resolution of symptoms and, on average, a survival time of 3 to 6 months, with 50% of patients dying from their CNS disease. WBRT and cisplatin-based chemotherapy may offer an improved survival time over WBRT alone for gynecologic malignancies.[26]

Stereotactic Radiosurgery

At the time of diagnosis, gynecologic malignancies metastatic to the brain often show multiple lesions and advanced systemic disease, precluding surgical therapy. Consequently, SRS may be a valuable tool for treatment of this population. Some studies indicate that control rates for SRS with WBRT are equal to those obtained with surgery and WBRT,[5] but this has not been studied in gynecologic malignancies specifically.

Chemotherapy

The role of chemotherapy in the treatment of CNS disease in gynecologic malignancies is unclear. An obstacle to successful treatment with chemotherapy is the blood-brain barrier, which causes most agents to have poor CNS penetration. However, this barrier may be altered by radiation therapy, surgery, or by the tumor itself, allowing higher concentrations of chemotherapy agents to reach intracranial tumors.[9,17,21] There are reports of the objective response of ovarian cancer brain metastases to systemic carboplatin chemotherapy,[9] and cisplatin-based chemotherapy in ovarian cancer brain metastasis is associated with a statistically significant increase in patients' survival time.[26] In multivariate analysis, chemotherapy was an independent predictor of survival regardless of surgical intervention.[26]

Unfortunately, because of the recurrent nature of gynecologic malignancies, particularly ovarian cancer, and the lack of effective salvage chemotherapy, most patients will follow a course of progressive systemic disease, even when control of CNS disease is achieved. As advancements in therapeutics are made, long-term survival may become more common.

CONCLUSION

Gynecologic malignancies account for a significant number of new cancer diagnoses and cancer-related deaths in women each year. Fortunately, neurologic involvement is rare. As survival time improves for patients with gynecologic malignancies, uncommon complications such as brain metastases are increasing. The brain is the primary site of CNS involvement in most cases, but rarely there may be leptomeningeal or spinal involvement. Clinicians should be aware of signs of increased intracranial pressure, and the development of neurologic symptoms should be investigated promptly with appropriate radiologic studies. Evaluation for new or recurrent systemic disease should also be performed, as brain metastasis is commonly associated with active, widespread disease. The rarity of this disease makes the analysis of specific treatment regimens difficult; however, as we gain more experience with this entity, we have been able to achieve successful control of the CNS disease in many patients, and more cases of long-term survivors are being reported. There is often ongoing or recurrent systemic disease at the time of diagnosis of CNS metastasis, which complicates treatment options. As advancements in systemic treatment protocols continue to improve survival rates, a more aggressive approach to treating intracranial disease is warranted. An integrated team of medical, surgical, and radiation oncology specialists, together with those in neurosurgery, can offer a wide range of treatment options that take into account the patient's medical condition, systemic disease status, and neurologic performance status.

References

1. Barker GH, Orledge J, Wiltshaw E: Involvement of the central nervous system in patients with ovarian carcinoma. Br J Obstet Gynaecol 88:690–694, 1981.
2. Reference deleted in proofs.
3. Batson OV: The function of the vertebral veins and their role in the spread of metastases. Ann Surg 112:138–149, 1940.
4. Beckmann CRB, Ling FW, Barzansky BM, et al: Obstetrics and Gynecology. Baltimore, Williams & Wilkins, 1995.
5. Bindal RK, Sawaya R, Leavens ME, Lee JJ: Surgical treatment of multiple brain metastases. J Neurosurg 79:210–216, 1993.
6. Brezinka C, Fend F, Huter O, et al: Cerebral metastasis of endometrial carcinoma. Gynecol Oncol 38:278–281, 1990.
7. Bruzzone M, Campora E, Chiara S, et al: Cerebral metastasis secondary to ovarian cancer. Still an unusual event. Gynaecol Oncol 49:37–40, 1993.
8. Chang TC, Jain S, Ng KK, et al: Cerebellar metastasis from papillary serous adenocarcinoma of the ovary mimicking Meniere's disease. A case report. J Reprod Med 46:267–269, 2001.
9. Cooper KG, Kitchener HC, Parkin DE: Cerebral metastases from epithelial ovarian carcinoma treated with carboplatin. Gynecol Oncol 55:318–323, 1994.
10. Cormio G, Colamaria A, DiVagno G, et al: Surgical decompression and radiation therapy in epidural metastasis from cervical cancer. Eur J Obstet Gynecol Reprod Biol 89:59–61, 2000.
11. Cormio G, Colamaria A, Loverro G, et al: Surgical resection of a cerebral metastasis from cervical cancer: case report and review of the literature. Tumori 85:65–67, 1999.
12. Cormio G, Lissoni A, Losa G, et al: Brain metastasis from endometrial carcinoma. Gynecol Oncol 61:40–43, 1996.
13. Cormio G, Pellegrino A, Landoni F, et al: Brain metastases from cervical carcinoma. Tumori 82:394–396, 1996.
14. Dauplat J, Meiberg RK, Hacker N: Central nervous system metastases in epithelial ovarian cancer. Cancer 60:2559–2562, 1987.
15. Deutsch M, Beck D, Manor D, Brandes J: Metastatic brain tumor following negative second-look operation for ovarian carcinoma. Gynecol Oncol 27:116–120, 1987.
16. Hall WA, Djalilian HR, Nussbaum, Cho KH: Long-term survival with metastatic cancer to the brain. Med Oncol 17:279–286, 2000.
17. Hardy JR, Harvey VJ: Cerebral metastasis in patients with ovarian cancer treated with chemotherapy. Gynaecol Oncol 33:296–300, 1989.
18. Hazuka MB et al: Multiple brain metastases are associated with poor survival in patients treated with surgery and radiotherapy. J Clin Oncol 11:369–373, 1993.
19. Ikeda S, Yamada T, Katsumata N, et al: Cerebral metastasis in patients with uterine cervical cancer. Jpn J Clin Oncol 28:27–29, 1998.
20. Jemal A, Thomas A, Murray T, Thun M: Cancer statistics. Ca Cancer J Clin 52:23–47, 2002.
21. Kumar L, Tanwar RK, Singh SP: Intracranial metastases from carcinoma cervix and review of literature. Gynecol Oncol 46:391–392, 1992.
22. Larson DM, Copeland LJ, Moser, et al: Central nervous system metastases in epithelial ovarian carcinoma. Obstet Gynecol 68:746–750, 1986.

23. Lefkowitz D, Asconape J, Biller J: Intracranial metastases from carcinoma of the cervix. South Med J 76:519–521, 1983.

24. Markesbery WR, Brooks WH, Gupta GD, Young AB: Treatment for patients with cerebral metastases. Arch Neurol 35:754–756, 1978.

25. Mayer RJ, Berkowitz RS, Griffiths CT: Central nervous system involvement by ovarian carcinoma. Cancer 41:776–783, 1978.

26. McMeekin DS, Kamelle SA, Vasilev SA, et al: Ovarian cancer metastatic to the brain: what is the optimal management? J Surg Oncol 78:194–201, 2001.

27. Mintz AP, Cairncross JG: Treatment of a single brain metastasis. The role of radiation following surgical excision. JAMA 280:1527–1529, 1998.

28. National Cancer Registry: Annual report 1986. New Delhi, Indian Council of Medical Research, 1986.

29. Nielsen SL, Posner JB: Brain metastasis localized to an area of infarction. J Neurooncol 1:191–195, 1983.

30. Nussbaum ES, Djalilian HR, Cho KH, Hall WA: Brain metastases: histology, multiplicity, surgery and survival. Cancer 78:1781–1788, 1996.

31. Patchell RA: Brain metastases. Neurol Clin 9:817–824, 1991.

32. Patchell RA: Metastatic brain tumors. Neurol Clin 13:915–925, 1995.

33. Patchell RA, Tibbs RA, Walsh JW, et al: A randomised trial of surgery in the treatment of single metastases to the brain. N Engl J Med 322:494–500, 1990.

34. Petru E, Lax S, Kurschel S, Gucer G, Sutter B: Long-term survival in a patient with brain metastasis preceding the diagnosis of endometrial cancer. Report of two cases and review of the literature. J Neurosurg 94:846–848, 2001.

35. Robinson JB, Morris M: Cervical carcinoma metastatic to the brain. Gynecol Oncol 66:324–326, 1997.

36. Rome RM, Nelson JH: Compression of the spinal cord of cauda equina complicating gynecological malignancy: report of five cases and a review of the literature. Gynecol Oncol 5:273–290, 1997.

37. Ryuko K, Iwanari O, Abu-Musa A, et al: Primary clear cell adenocarcinoma of the fallopian tube with brain metastasis: a case report. Asia-Oceanic J Obstet Gynaecol 20:135–140, 1994.

38. Saphner T, Gallion HH, van Nagel JR, et al: Neurologic complications of cervical cancer. A review of 2261 cases. Cancer 64:1147–1151, 1989.

39. Sawada M, Inagaki M, Ozaki M, et al: Long-term survival after brain metastasis from endometrial cancer. Jpn J Clin Oncol 20:312–315, 1990.

40. Sood A, Kumar L, Sood R, Sandhu MS: Epithelial ovarian carcinoma metastatic to the central nervous system: a report on two cases with review of literature. Gynaecol Oncol 62:113–118, 1996.

41. Stein M, Steiner M, Klein B, et al: Involvement of the central nervous system by ovarian carcinoma. Cancer 58:2066–2069, 1986.

42. Suzuki M, Tsukagoshi S, Ohwada M, et al: A patient with brain metastasis from ovarian cancer who showed complete remission after multidisciplinary treatment. Gynecol Oncol 74:483–486, 1999.

43. Vecht CJ, Haaxma-Reiche H, Noordijk EM, et al: Treatment of single brain metastasis radiotherapy alone or combined with neurosurgery? Ann Neurol 3:583–590, 1993.

44. Vieth RG, Odom GI: Intracranial metastases. J Neurosurg 23:375–383, 1965.

45. White KT, Fleming TR, Laws E: Single metastasis to the brain. Surgical treatment in 122 consecutive patients. Mayo Clin Proc 56:424–428, 1981.

46. Wronski M, de Palma P, Arbit E: Leiomyosarcoma of the uterus metastatic to brain: a case report and a review of the literature. Gynecol Oncol 54:237–241, 1994.

47. Young JA, Kossman CR, Green MR: Adenocarcinoma of the fallopian tube: report of a case with an unusual pattern of metastasis and response to combination chemotherapy. Gynecol Oncol 17:238–240, 1984.

CHAPTER 60

MULTIDISCIPLINARY MANAGEMENT OF PATIENTS WITH BRAIN METASTASES FROM AN UNKNOWN PRIMARY TUMOR

Robert J. Bohinski, Kevin P. Redmond, Abdul-Rahman Jazieh, and Ronald E. Warnick

Cancer from an unknown primary tumor site is diagnosed when metastatic lesions are discovered and no primary site can be identified. Specifically, these patients have a histologically proved cancer in which complete medical history, comprehensive physical examination, and appropriate laboratory and diagnostic work-ups fail to detect a primary site.[4] Thus a diagnosis of cancer from an unknown primary site is not made at the time a patient seeks treatment but as a diagnosis of exclusion. Those with cancer from an unknown primary site represent between 3% and 10% of all cancer patients[16] and as a group have a median survival time of only 6 months. However, identifiable subgroups of patients with favorable clinicopathologic characteristics survive significantly longer; some may be cured by the timely administration of appropriate disease-specific therapy.[1,19,27] Much of the recent clinical effort in the management of patients with cancer from an unknown primary site has focused on identifying subgroups of patients who are candidates for specific treatment protocols and who have a more favorable prognosis than the group as a whole (Table 60-1).

Some patients with cancer from an unknown primary site are first diagnosed because of neurologic symptoms that seem to represent a distinct clinical entity. The best management of these patients, which is the subject of this chapter, constitutes a multidisciplinary effort that involves the expertise of clinicians from neurosurgery, pathology, medical oncology, and radiation oncology. Well-controlled prospective studies that specifically examine treatment algorithms for patients with brain metastases from cancer from an unknown primary site are lacking. In addition, current treatment recommendations are based on a review of retrospective studies and small populations of patients (Table 60-2). However, recent studies show that in many patients excellent control of intracranial disease is achievable, translating into increased survival time. Patients with brain metastases and an unknown primary tumor die from progression of systemic disease. However, a few have systemic disease that is limited in extent, amenable to effective systemic therapy, or both, and have significantly prolonged survival compared with the group as a whole.

Between 3% and 35% (most estimate between 5% and 12%) of all patients who are diagnosed with brain metastases have an unknown primary cancer site.[6,7,11,12,22,24,28,34,49] In most studies, an unknown primary cancer site ranks third in frequency, following the lung and breast as the two most commonly identified primary sites.[11,34,49] The broad estimated range is probably caused by the inconsistent terminology used to define this patient population. Studies that report a high incidence of an unknown primary site typically include all patients who have brain metastases as the first sign of cancer. Although many of these patients have a primary neoplasm that is identified during the course of the initial diagnostic evaluation, they do not accurately represent the subgroup with brain metastases and an *undetectable* primary tumor.

A further distinction exists between patients who have brain metastases and an undetected tumor, and those who have brain metastases as the *only* manifestation of cancer.[28,33] In the former situation, a patient may have extracerebral metastases at the time of diagnosis; in the latter situation, a patient without evidence of metastases outside of the brain represents a unique clinical situation. Brain metastases may be single, multiple, or solitary. *Single brain metastasis* refers to the detection of only one brain metastasis without any implication regarding the existence of a primary site or extracerebral metastatic disease. *Solitary brain metastasis* is specific and refers to the unique situation in which a single brain metastasis is the only known site of metastasis in the body, without implying the existence of a primary site. Given these definitions, it is important to recognize that brain metastases from an unknown primary site can be single, solitary, or multiple.

CLINICAL PRESENTATION

Patients typically are diagnosed with brain metastases from an unknown primary site during the fifth or sixth decade (see Table 60-2), timing that does not appear to differ from that of the general population of patients with brain metastases.[34,39] Most series report a slight male predominance. Neurologic symptoms

Neoplasm	Type of Treatment
Breast cancer	Palliative hormone therapy, chemotherapy
Endometrial cancer	Palliative hormone therapy
Ovarian cancer	Chemotherapy
Prostate cancer	Palliative hormone therapy
Germ cell tumors	Chemotherapy
Lymphoma	Chemotherapy
Melanoma	Local treatment
Thyroid cancer	Radioactive iodine
Head and neck squamous cell cancer	Chemotherapy, local treatment

Source: Modified from Brigden ML, Murray N: Improving survival in metastatic carcinoma of unknown origin. Postgrad Med 105:63–74, 1999. Copyright © 1999 The McGraw-Hill Companies. All rights reserved.

include headache, weakness, seizure, mental disturbances, language difficulty, gait difficulty, incoordination, nausea, emesis, and numbness; the most common complaints are headache and weakness, in 30% to 50% of patients. The most common signs are focal motor weakness and altered level of consciousness associated with increased intracranial pressure; these are followed by other focal neurologic deficits. Signs and symptoms of extracerebral metastases, if present, can provide valuable clues to the location of a primary site and to the overall tumor burden.[30,46] Clinical presentation is also similar for the small subgroup of patients who have brain metastases as the only manifestation of an undetected tumor, except that signs of cerebellar involvement may occur more often.[33]

EXTENT AND DISTRIBUTION OF METASTATIC DISEASE

Patients with brain metastases and an unknown primary site often have extracerebral metastatic disease present in lymph

T A B L E   6 O - 2   **Summary of Clinical Series: Presentation, Management, and Outcome of Patients with**

Author, Publication Year	Time of Clinical Series	No. Patients	Mean Patient Age	% Male	% Female	Most Common Symptom or Sign	Distribution of Metastases (%) Single	Multiple	Cerebellar
Ebels and vander Meulen, 1978	1966–74	19	53	63	37	NS	NS	NS	NS
Dhopesh and Yagnik, 1985	NS	26	59	65	34	Headache, motor deficit	58	42	15
Le Chevalier et al, 1985	1959–79	120	54	74	26	Elevated ICP, motor deficit	77	23	12
Eapen et al, 1988	1970–82	43	60	70	30	Elevated ICP, motor deficit	63	37	26
Merchut, 1989	1977–87	56	59	54	46	Motor deficit	57	43	30
Chee, 1990	1973–84	33	60s	61	39	Focal neurologic deficit	52	48	15
Debevec, 1990	1973–87	75	(40-59)	77	23	NS	41	59	NS
Salvati et al, 1995	1976–88	100	50s	75	25	Headache, focal signs	100	Excluded	26
van de Pol et al, 1996	1987–94	72	65	64	36	NS	NS	NS	NS
Khansur et al, 1997	1982–89	32	57	75	25	Headache, paresis	44	56	9
Nguyen et al, 1998	1977–96	39	55	54	46	Headache, weakness	49	51	33
Maesawa et al, 2000	1988–98	15	57	47	53	Focal neurologic deficit	60	30	40
Ruda et al, 2001	1987–96	33	51	85	15	Headache, paresis	67	33	15

adeno, Adenocarcinoma; GI, gastrointestinal; ICP, intracranial pressure; NS, not stated; SCC, squamous cell carcinoma; small cell, small cell lung cancer; TCC, transitional cell carcinoma; UC, undifferentiated carcinoma; UG, urogenital.

nodes, bone, liver, or lung. In one series of 15 patients referred for radiosurgical treatment of brain metastases, 10 (75%) also had synchronous metastatic disease outside of the brain (e.g., lung, lymph nodes).[28] In another study, 181 (82%) of 220 patients with brain metastases and an unknown primary tumor site had evidence of extracerebral metastases.[33] Therefore approximately 75% of patients with brain metastases and an undetected primary tumor are likely to have coexistent systemic metastases when they first seek treatment. This is important, because one of the most significant predictors of patient outcome is the extent of extracerebral tumor burden.[6,15,24] This estimate of extracerebral disease burden is comparable with the results of a series in which the primary site was known.[5] Unfortunately, most patients with initially undetectable systemic disease will develop extracerebral metastases within a few months after the diagnosis of brain metastases, whether the primary site becomes known or remains occult.[5,33]

Single brain metastases occur in 41% to 77% of patients with unknown primary tumors (see Table 60-2); this range is similar to that reported for brain metastases with a known primary site.[26,39] When the primary site remains unknown, parenchymal brain metastases may be found in the cerebral hemispheres, diencephalon, brainstem, or cerebellum.[7,22,28,33,43] A potentially significant difference between patients is that the cerebellum appears to be overrepresented as a site of brain metastasis when the primary site remains unknown versus when known. In the general population of patients with brain metastases, the cerebellum is involved in 12% to 15% of cases.[11,34] When the primary site is unknown, the cerebellum is involved (not necessarily as the only site of brain involvement) in 26% to 40% of cases (see Table 60-2). Tumors that arise in the abdomen and pelvis are known to metastasize preferentially to the posterior fossa[11]; the mechanism underlying this preference may be either retrograde venous dissemination of tumor emboli to the posterior fossa by virtue of its connections with Batson's plexus or the ability of the cerebellum to preferentially support the growth of tumor cells from certain organs.[8,9] This latter effect may be attributed to cerebellum-specific growth factors or to permissive extracellular matrix components. Therefore when the cerebellum is involved in patients who have an unknown

Brain Metastases and an Unknown Primary Site

% with Antemortem Diagnosis of Primary Site	Primary Sites Identified	Tumor Histology	Patients Alive at 6 mo (%)	Patients Alive at 12 mo (%)	Cause of Death
32	Lung (67%), kidney, parotid	NS	NS	NS	NS
67	Lung (67%), testes	NS	NS	NS	NS
44	Lung (45%), GI, melanoma, thyroid, breast, kidney	Adeno (44%), UC, SCC	52	18	NS
16	Lung (45%), melanoma, bladder, liver, prostate	Adeno (56%), SCC, UC	52	20	Brain metastasis
84	Lung (68%), GI, bladder, thyroid, melanoma, lymphoma	Adeno (46%), UC, SCC	55	13	NS
NS	NS	Adeno (47%), UC, SCC, sarcoma, TCC	NS	NS	NS
63	Lung (53%), breast, skin, esophagus, kidney, parotid	UC, adeno (21%), SCC	NS	18	Brain metastasis
64	Lung (65%), GI, melanoma, kidney, breast, UG	Adeno (65%), SCC, melanoma, UC	NS	30	NS
75	Lung (72%), breast, colon, melanoma	NS	~40	~20	Systemic disease
3	Lung (100%)	NS	40	9	NS
31	Lung (83%), GI	Adeno (79%), small cell, other, SCC	~80	56	Systemic disease
27	Lung (75%), liver	Adeno (67%), SCC, clear cell, UC	NS	~65	Systemic disease
82	Lung (78%), GI, prostate	Adeno, SCC	76	42	Systemic disease

primary tumor, consideration should be given to organs of the abdomen and pelvis as a primary source of the metastases.

RELATIONSHIP WITH SPECIFIC SYSTEMIC CANCERS

In patients with an unknown primary site and brain metastases, the lung represents the most common primary tumor site discovered antemortem, accounting for between 45% and 83% of identifiable primary sites (see Table 60-2). The lung also appears to be the most common primary site regardless of whether it becomes known early (within 2 months) or late (after 2 months) after the diagnosis of brain metastases.[33,46] In contrast, when the primary site is discovered only after autopsy, there does not appear to be a predominant organ of origin.[14,26,30] In the general population of patients with brain metastases, the lung is identified as a primary site in 50% to 70% of patients and is followed in frequency by breast cancer metastases in women.[24,34,49] By comparison, the breast appears to be underrepresented as a primary tumor site in patients in whom the site initially remains occult at diagnosis or autopsy[14,26,28,30,33,42]; in these studies, the abdominal and pelvic organs are typically the second most common primary site. This difference may be a result of the earlier diagnosis of primary breast cancer, which tends to metastasize at an advanced stage of the disease. Other primary tumor sites that become manifest include the skin and upper aerodigestive tract (e.g., melanoma, squamous cell carcinoma, adenocarcinoma), thyroid gland, hematologic system, and reproductive organs.

The high incidence of the lung as the primary site is not surprising given the high incidence of lung cancer in general, ease of detection of lung masses, and direct vascular connection between the lungs and brain that permits a convenient route for hematogenous dissemination. However, it is also possible that a lung mass may actually represent metastatic disease from another organ rather than a primary lung tumor, because most organs producing tumors that metastasize to the brain do so by first sending metastases to the lungs.[40,45] Therefore finding a lung mass on a chest x-ray should be interpreted cautiously.

DIAGNOSTIC EVALUATION

There has been significant controversy regarding how much initial diagnostic evaluation is needed for patients with cancer from an unknown primary site. However, most studies show that exhaustive diagnostic evaluations typically yield no more useful information than a screening diagnostic evaluation.[1,4,16,19,30] The goals of evaluation should be to identify patients with favorable clinical and histopathologic features for whom specific treatment is available. In these favorable patient subsets, more rigorous investigation may be justified. For example, specific treatment is available for patients with lymphoma and metastatic cancer arising from the thyroid gland, breast and prostate, and other reproductive organs.[1,4,16,19]

A thorough review of systems is a key component to the initial diagnostic evaluation and not only helps to locate the primary site of most symptomatic brain metastases but also to ascertain the general functional status of the patient, which is critical before making further treatment decisions.[30,46] In many cases, the history reveals organ-specific complaints that guide further diagnostic work-up, including a comprehensive physical examination, screening laboratory studies, and limited imaging evaluation. The physical examination evaluates all lymph node basins in the groin, axilla, head, and neck and includes palpation of the thyroid gland, digital rectal examination, and careful skin examination. This basic physical assessment should also include breast and gynecologic examinations in women and prostate and testicular examinations in men.

In a study of 72 patients with symptomatic brain metastases from undiagnosed primary sites, 41 (57%) had complaints that suggested an underlying malignancy.[46] Symptoms, including altered coughing pattern; hoarseness; and dyspnea, indicating a primary lung tumor, were most common. Twenty-two (31%) patients also had abnormalities found on physical examination that accurately predicted the primary tumor location. Other important signs and symptoms of a primary extracerebral tumor include anorexia, weight loss, abdominal pain, dysphagia, flank pain, hematuria, or new skin lesions.

The essential laboratory work-up should include a complete blood count, electrolyte panel, calcium concentration, liver function tests, amylase, lipase, stool for occult blood, and urinalysis. Tumor markers that are detectable in serum include prostate-specific antigen (PSA), cancer-associated antigen 125 (CA-125), and carcinoembryonic antigen (CEA); these markers may be nonspecifically increased in patients with cancer but generally lack sufficient sensitivity or specificity as screening tools.[4,37,42] Determination of such markers should be reserved for patients who are separable into one of several specific subgroups based on individual clinical characteristics and histopathology (Table 60-3).[4] For example, serum PSA may be

TABLE 60-3	Tumor Markers Useful in Specific Patient Subgroups	
Subgroup	Condition to Be Excluded	Appropriate Tumor Markers
Patients with mediastinal or retroperitoneal masses	Extragonadal primary germ cell tumors	α-Fetoprotein, β-Human chorionic gonadotropin
Women with adenocarcinoma in an axillary node	Breast cancer	CA-15/3, carcinoembryonic antigen
Women with ascites, with or without pelvic masses	Ovarian cancer	CA-125
Men with diffuse metastatic disease to bone or lungs	Prostate cancer	Prostate-specific antigen
Patients with single mass or multiple masses in liver	Hepatocellular cancer	α-Fetoprotein

CA-125, Cancer-associated antigen 125; CA-15/3, cancer-associated antigen 15/3.
Source: Reprinted from Brigden ML, Murray N: Improving survival in metastatic carcinoma of unknown origin. Postgrad Med 105:63–74, 1999. Copyright © 1999 The McGraw-Hill Companies. All rights reserved.

useful in men with brain metastases and diffuse metastatic disease to bone or lungs. In general, tumor markers are more valuable for following the effects of treatment than for making a specific diagnosis.

In the absence of organ-specific signs or symptoms, the initial radiographic work-up should include a chest x-ray and computed tomography (CT) scans of the chest, abdomen, and pelvis.[30,46] Although use of mammography rarely detects an occult primary site in women with brain metastases, the implications for treatment may justify its use in women, because effective treatment for breast cancer does exist. In one study that included 72 patients with brain metastases as the first sign of cancer, a chest radiograph detected abnormalities in 56 (78%) patients, 47 of whom were found to have primary lung tumors.[46] Similar findings obtained in another study found that 71% of patients with brain metastases as the first sign of cancer had abnormal chest x-ray studies. The diagnostic yield obtained from a simple chest x-ray examination is not surprising given the high prevalence of metastatic lung cancer among men and women. However, as mentioned previously, the finding of a lung mass must be interpreted cautiously, because many other tumor types that metastasize to the brain do so by first metastasizing to the lungs.[40,45]

Chest CT may disclose lung masses not shown by chest radiography. In a retrospective study of 32 patients with brain metastases as the first sign of systemic cancer, 12 (38%) with positive findings on chest CT had negative or unclear findings on chest radiography.[25] A CT of the abdomen and pelvis may identify a primary site in as many as 35% of patients in whom the history, physical examination, and chest x-ray are negative and may demonstrate additional or unsuspected disease in 65%.[29] Contrast studies of the gastrointestinal tract, nuclear medicine studies (e.g., bone scans), panendoscopy, bronchoscopy, lymph node dissections, and fine-needle biopsies should be limited to patients with organ-specific complaints or findings. Whole-body ^{18}F-fluorodeoxyglucose positron-emission tomography (FDG-PET) scanning is a newer diagnostic modality that in some cases may identify a primary site after a conventional diagnostic work-up fails to. However, its routine use in cases of cancer of an unknown primary site is not well established, and conflicting reports exist regarding its clinical utility.[18,23]

In patients with a single supratentorial lesion, the differential diagnosis must include primary central nervous system tumors and nontumor masses (e.g., brain abscesses). In a study by Voorhies et al, the probability of a metastatic lesion in patients without a known history of cancer was only 7% if their chest x-ray and intravenous pyelogram showed negative results.[48] Therefore in patients with a single supratentorial mass lesion, limiting the extent of preoperative diagnostic studies that examine the body for a primary tumor site is important. In these cases, resection or biopsy of the intracranial lesion will most efficiently establish a diagnosis and determine whether evaluation for an extracerebral tumor is necessary.

NEUROSURGICAL INTERVENTION

Treatment of brain metastases requires careful evaluation of numerous factors including location, multiplicity, tumor size, histology, overall functional status, extent of systemic disease, and response or potential response of systemic disease to treat-ment. For surgical candidates, the extent of systemic disease and the patient's overall functional status have the most important correlation with survival.[24] If a patient is determined to be an operative candidate and tissue is needed to make the diagnosis of metastatic cancer, then surgical considerations are based mainly on lesion accessibility and multiplicity.

Histopathologic analysis is critical to appropriately manage cancer from an unknown primary site. Therefore an overwhelming decision to operate occurs when the brain is the only known site of metastatic disease or when the diagnosis of brain metastasis is in doubt. A tissue diagnosis may be obtained by stereotactic biopsy or resection. If stereotactic biopsy is performed, care is taken to provide an adequate sample for both routine and specialized histopathologic evaluations; a cauterized sample is typically inadequate for specialized studies. If metastatic disease is present outside of the brain, then biopsy of a peripheral site (e.g., bronchial mass) may be considered, especially if it poses less risk to the patient than the neurologic procedure (e.g., a deep-seated brain metastasis). Another important indication for craniotomy is to treat overwhelming mass effect associated with a large brain metastasis. Because these patients often have a depressed level of consciousness secondary to elevated intracranial pressure, resection can result in significant clinical improvement even in advanced disease for which only palliative care is available.

Treatment options for brain metastases include surgical resection, stereotactic radiosurgery (SRS), and whole-brain radiation therapy (WBRT). Surgical resection combined with WBRT has proved superior to WBRT alone for patients with single brain metastases.[36,47] If surgical resection is performed, frameless stereotaxis is an important technical adjuvant for trajectory planning and tumor localization. SRS is an alternative to surgical resection for brain metastases that are small or deep seated or located in eloquent cortex. Although this is controversial, most patients who undergo surgical resection or SRS for brain metastases are also treated with WBRT.[31,35] Survival benefit has also been shown in patients who undergo surgical resection for multiple brain metastases. Bindal et al showed that the survival of patients who underwent craniotomy for multiple metastases was similar to patients who underwent surgery for single brain metastases if all lesions could be removed.[2]

HISTOPATHOLOGIC STUDIES

Evaluation of tissue obtained from the metastatic site is essential to identify patient subsets that may benefit from specific local, regional, or systemic therapies. In the absence of a clinically identifiable primary site, histopathology can provide valuable information that may (1) indicate a likely organ of origin for the metastases, (2) guide further specialized diagnostic work-up, and (3) assign the patient to a clinicopathologic subgroup that may benefit from specific treatment.[1,4,16,19] For these reasons, histopathologic studies are performed as soon as possible after completion of the screening clinical evaluation. In the absence of organ-specific signs or symptoms, biopsy or resection of the metastases and histopathologic evaluation should be performed before considering further clinical testing.[1,20,32] This strategy has proved more effective than exhaustive diagnostic testing.[1,16,19]

Routine light microscopy often suffices to confirm the diagnosis of a metastatic neoplasm and to classify most metas-

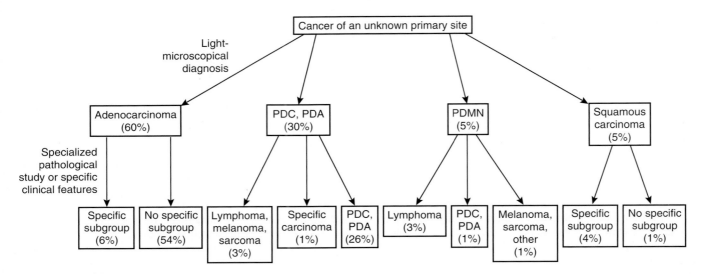

FIGURE 60-1   Distribution of various clinical and histologic subgroups of patients with cancer from an unknown primary site after optimal clinical and pathologic evaluation. PDA, Poorly differentiated adenocarcinoma; PDC, poorly differentiated carcinoma; PDMN, poorly differentiated malignant neoplasm. (Reprinted from Hainsworth JD, Greco FA: Treatment of patients with cancer of an unknown primary site. N Engl J Med 329:257–263, 1993).

tases of unknown origin into one of the following four histologic subgroups: (1) adenocarcinoma, (2) poorly differentiated carcinoma and poorly differentiated adenocarcinoma, (3) other poorly differentiated malignant neoplasm, or (4) squamous carcinoma (Figure 60-1).[19] In cases of well-differentiated metastases that retain specific cellular characteristics of the organ of origin, their source may be evident after inspection using only routine light microscopy.[21,32] For example, the presence of abundant cytoplasmic glycogen, which is characteristic of renal cell carcinoma, has been specifically referred to as "clear cell carcinoma." Melanotic or squamous cell differentiation may be obvious. For some well-differentiated adenocarcinomas, subtle glandular or microvillus architecture may also provide clues to identify the primary site. However, poor or insufficient differentiation of most metastatic adenocarcinomas and carcinomas rarely allows specific diagnosis by conventional light microscopy alone.[21,38,44] Thus evaluation of the tumor specimen usually involves specialized ancillary techniques such as immunoperoxidase staining, electron microscopy, and cytogenetic analysis. The success of these studies highly depends on the technical expertise and experience of the pathologist in dealing with cancer of an unknown primary site. Because clinical information is used to guide these studies, effective communication between the clinician and pathologist is important.

Immunoperoxidase staining is based on the detection of tissue-, organ-, or tumor-specific antigens using monoclonal or polyclonal antibodies. These antibodies can unequivocally confirm the diagnosis of important treatable subgroups such as lymphoma, melanoma, neuroendocrine tumors, and others. Many antibodies are available for this type of analysis (Table 60-4). The choice of antibody for a particular specimen is based on the results of the initial light microscopy examination and clinical information. For example, if lymphoma is suspected, then it is imperative to first perform immunohistochemistry using an antibody to common leukocyte antigen (CLA), which is highly specific for lymphoma.

Immunohistochemistry can be costly and time consuming. Therefore specific antibody tests that are based on all available clinical information should be done sequentially rather than in a shotgun approach. For example, in the case of undifferentiated adenocarcinoma, the pattern of cytokeratin-7 and cytokeratin-20 staining can often differentiate between tumors derived from the lung or breast versus those originating in the gastrointestinal tract.[38] In women, further differentiation of breast from lung primary sites may be accomplished on the basis of the staining pattern with antibodies for estrogen receptor, progesterone receptor, gross cystic disease fluid protein-15 (GCDFP-15), and thyroid transcription factor-1 (TTF-1).[3,38] Recently, TTF-1 was shown to be a highly specific marker for adenocarcinomas derived from the thyroid gland or lung.[3] To date, no breast tumor has stained positive for TTF-1. Therefore if TTF-1 staining is positive, it is reasonable to exclude the diagnosis of a treatable breast cancer and avoid diagnostic interventions designed to establish this important diagnosis. Specific antibodies are also available for melanoma (HMB-45), prostate carcinoma (PSA), and germ cell tumors (α-fetoprotein [AFP] and β-human chorionic gonadotropin [BHCG]).[44] If immunoperoxidase staining of the tumor specimen is inconclusive, electron microscopy or cytogenetic studies may be useful.[32]

PATIENTS' OUTCOME AND ADJUVANT TREATMENT OF SYSTEMIC DISEASE

The survival time for patients with brain metastases is generally poor. The median survival time of patients selected to undergo surgical resection followed by WBRT was only 8.9 months in a recent study of 1292 patients with brain metastases.[24] Although several groups have reported the outcome of patients with brain metastases from an unknown primary site,

TABLE 60-4

Immunoperoxidase Tumor Staining Useful in the Differential Diagnosis of Poorly Differentiated Neoplasms

Tumor Type	Immunoperoxidase Staining
Carcinoma	Epithelial stains (e.g., cytokeratin, EMA) +
	CLA, S-100, vimentin –
Lymphoma	CLA +, rare false –
	EMA occasionally +
	All other stains –
Mesenchymal sarcoma	Vimentin +
	Epithelial stains usually –
Rhabdomyosarcoma	Desmin +
Angiosarcoma	Factor VIII antigen +
Melanoma	HMB-45, S-100, vimentin +
	NSE often +
	Synaptophysin –
	Epithelial stains –
Neuroendocrine tumor	NSE, chromogranin, synaptophysin +
	Epithelial stains +
Germ cell tumor	HCG, AFP +
	Epithelial stains +
Prostate cancer	PSA +, rare false – and +
	Epithelial stains +
Breast cancer	ER, PR +
	Epithelial stains +
Follicular thyroid cancer	Thyroglobulin +
Medullary thyroid cancer	Calcitonin +

+, Positive result; – negative result; AFP, α-fetoprotein; CLA, common leukocyte antigen; EMA, epithelial membrane antigen; ER, estrogen receptor; HCG, human chorionic gonadotropin; NSE, neuron-specific enolase; PR, progesterone receptor; PSA, prostate-specific antigen.
Source: Reprinted from Greco AF, Hainsworth JD: Cancer of unknown primary site. In DeVita VT, Hellman S, Rosenberg SA (eds): Cancer: Principles and Practice of Oncology, 6th ed. Philadelphia, Lippincott Williams & Wilkins, 2001.

the authors derived differing conclusions based on their results. Compared with patients in whom the primary site was known when they first sought treatment, some authors report that the prognosis of patients whose primary site remained occult was worse, because appropriate treatment of the primary tumor was delayed.[26] Others argue that these latter patients had a better overall outcome because of the relative lack of significant extracranial disease.[28,30,33,43]

In two recent studies, the median survival time of patients treated for brain metastases from an unknown primary site were 13.4 and 15 months, respectively.[28,33] In these studies, the near doubling of median survival time compared with all patients with brain metastasis was most likely because of the following: one study[33] excluded patients with extracranial metastases present at the time of initial diagnosis; the other study[28] selected patients with brain metastases smaller than 3.5 cm in maximal diameter (a size suitable for radiosurgical treatment) and most of whom had a Karnofsky Performance Scale (KPS) score of 80 or more. In addition, both studies excluded patients whose primary site became known within 2 months after diagnosis of brain metastases. The authors stated that in some cases, a 2-month interval was necessary to allow urgent treatment of the brain metastases and to ensure a complete diagnostic evaluation. However, this 2-month interval naturally excluded patients with biologically aggressive tumors who would have experienced a rapidly progressive clinical course. Older studies with less stringent patient inclusion criteria demonstrate survival times similar to the brain metastasis group as a whole.[10,13,22,26,30,46]

In a 2001 study of patients with brain metastases from an unknown primary tumor, survival was comparable in those whose primary tumor became known during follow-up and in those in whom it remained occult.[41] Overall survival was not affected by disclosure of the primary site, because most patients with brain metastases were ultimately found to have lung cancer, for which effective systemic therapy is unavailable. However, a few patients received specific treatment in a timely fashion, which probably resulted in their improved survival.

In earlier studies in which surgical resection or SRS was not uniformly used to treat patients with brain metastases, the cause of death was usually progression of the intracranial disease.[10,13] By comparison, in all studies in which contemporary aggressive treatment was performed for the brain metastases, the cause of death was progression of systemic disease.[28,33,46] Even patients with brain metastases as the *only* manifestation of an undetected tumor typically die because of the development of systemic neoplastic disease.[33] Because intracranial disease can be controlled in many patients, efforts should be made to identify those for whom effective systemic treatment is available.

Several studies indicate that a small subgroup of patients with brain metastases from cancer of an unknown primary site survive for a long time without developing systemic metastatic disease or a known primary site. In these patients, the biology of the primary tumor remains an enigma. Their essential characteristics are that their KPS score was good when they sought treatment and they received definitive treatment (i.e., surgical resection or SRS) of brain metastases. In one study, 7 of 39 patients were alive 8 years after treatment of metastatic brain tumors.[33] In another study, 3 of 15 patients were alive 26 to 51 months after radiosurgical treatment of multiple brain metastases.[28] In these two studies, the other patients died because of progression or development of uncontrollable systemic disease despite effective control of disease metastatic to the brain.

After treatment of disease metastatic to the brain, patients must make decisions regarding their general oncologic state. No information available in the literature adequately addresses the subsequent care of these patients. The evolution of systemic treatment strategies for patients with cancer from an unknown primary site is largely based on clinical studies in those who had metastatic disease from an undetected primary tumor outside of the central nervous system. These patients have heterogeneous clinical presentations; therefore it is inadvisable to generalize treatment strategies and prognosis. As already mentioned, clinicopathologic characteristics can be used to subgroup patients with unknown primary tumors.[1,4,16,19] The strategy that has evolved is the identification of favorable clinicopathologic subgroups for which effective systemic treatment strategies exist. For example, the prognosis of women with adenocarcinoma found in an axillary node is significantly better than the group as a whole after modified radical mastectomy and adjunctive radiation therapy and chemotherapy.[1,19] Patients with squamous cell carcinoma in a high- or mid-cervical lymph node appear to benefit from surgical treatment and specific adjuvant therapies.[1,19] Patients with other specific tumor histologies such as melanoma, lymphoma, prostate, germ cell tumor, or sarcoma should undergo treatment according to established guidelines.

Currently, it is unclear whether empirical systemic treatment benefits patients with unfavorable epithelial tumor histologies, such as those of lung or gastrointestinal origin.[16,17] In these patients, a response rate only as high as 20% should be expected, with a median survival time ranging from 2 to 11 months. The chemotherapeutic regimen chosen is usually cisplatin-based.[16] If empirical chemotherapy is considered, the physician must decide if it is appropriate for the given situation because of the potentially toxic side effects with little gain. When presented with the low response rates and potential for harmful side effects, many patients opt only for palliative care. Aggressive chemotherapy is best suited to young, healthy patients who have good functional status.

CONCLUSION

Patients diagnosed with brain metastases from cancer from an unknown primary site rank third in terms of frequency of occurrence, preceded only by patients diagnosed with lung and breast primaries. The clinical characteristics of these patients do not differ significantly from the general group of all patients with brain metastases, except that signs and symptoms of cerebellar involvement may occur more frequently. Diagnosis is made only after a screening clinical and diagnostic evaluation fails to disclose a likely primary site. In the absence of organ-specific signs or symptoms, diagnostic studies should be minimal. Specialized histopathologic evaluation is essential to plan further diagnostic and therapeutic interventions and should be aimed at identifying treatable subgroups of patients. A primary lung tumor, which will ultimately become manifest, carries a poor prognosis. A few patients will have primary tumors discovered for which effective systemic therapy is available.

The use of surgical resection and SRS has significantly improved patients' survival time. Although patients live longer after treatment of their brain metastases, most die from the progression of systemic disease that is not amenable to effective systemic therapy. A unique situation occurs when brain metastases represent the only manifestation of an undetected tumor. Although most of these latter patients will ultimately develop a tumor outside of the brain, a few survive for several years after treatment directed only at the brain metastases. The biology of tumors that metastasize to only the brain and remain occult at their primary site and other sites for several years remains an enigma.

References

1. Abbruzzese JL, Abbruzzese MC, Lenzi R, et al: Analysis of a diagnostic strategy for patients with suspected tumors of unknown origin. J Clin Oncol 13:2094–2103, 1995.
2. Bindal RK, Sawaya R, Leavens ME, et al: Surgical treatment of multiple brain metastases. J Neurosurg 79:210–216, 1993.
3. Bohinski RJ, Bejarano PA, Balko G, et al: Determination of lung as the primary site of cerebral metastatic adenocarcinomas using monoclonal antibody to thyroid transcription factor-1. J Neurooncol 40:227–231, 1998.
4. Brigden ML, Murray N: Improving survival in metastatic carcinoma of unknown origin. Postgrad Med 105:63–74, 1999.
5. Cairncross JG, Kim JH, Posner JB: Radiation therapy for brain metastases. Ann Neurol 7:529–541, 1980.
6. Chan RC, Steinbok P: Solitary cerebral metastasis: the effect of craniotomy on the quality and the duration of survival. Neurosurgery 11:254–257, 1982.
7. Chee CP: Brain metastasis of unknown origin. Singapore Med J 31:48–50, 1990.
8. Cho KG, Hoshino T, Pitts LH, et al: Proliferative potential of brain metastases. Cancer 62:512–515, 1988.
9. Coman DR, Delong RP: The role of the vertebral venous system in the metastasis of cancer to the spinal column: experiments with tumor cell suspension in rats and rabbits. Cancer 4:610–618, 1951.
10. Debevec M: Management of patients with brain metastases of unknown origin. Neoplasma 37:601–606, 1990.
11. Delattre JY, Krol G, Thaler HT, et al: Distribution of brain metastases. Arch Neurol 45:741–744, 1988.
12. Dhopesh VP, Yagnik PM: Brain metastasis: analysis of patients without known cancer. South Med J 78:171–172, 1985.
13. Eapen L, Vachet M, Catton G, et al: Brain metastases with an unknown primary: a clinical perspective. J Neurooncol 6:31–35, 1988.
14. Ebels EJ, van der Meulen JD: Cerebral metastasis without known primary tumour: a retrospective study. Clin Neurol Neurosurg 80:195–197, 1978.
15. Gaspar L, Scott C, Rotman M, et al: Recursive partitioning analysis (RPA) of prognostic factors in three Radiation Therapy Oncology Group (RTOG) brain metastases trials. Int J Radiat Oncol Biol Phys 37:745–751, 1997.
16. Greco AF, Hainsworth JD: Cancer of unknown primary site. In DeVita VT, Hellman S, Rosenberg SA (eds): Cancer: Principles and Practice of Oncology, 6th ed. Philadelphia, Lippincott Williams & Wilkins, 2001.
17. Greco FA, Hainsworth JD: Poorly differentiated carcinoma or adenocarcinoma of unknown primary site: long-term results with cisplatin-based chemotherapy. Semin Oncol 21:77–82, 1994.
18. Greven KM, Keyes JW Jr, Williams DW III, et al: Occult primary tumors of the head and neck: lack of benefit from positron emission tomography imaging with 2-[F-18]fluoro-2-deoxy-D-glucose. Cancer 86:114–118, 1999.
19. Hainsworth JD, Greco FA: Treatment of patients with cancer of an unknown primary site. N Engl J Med 329:257–263, 1993.
20. Hammar S, Bockus D, Remington F: Metastatic tumors of unknown origin: an ultrastructural analysis of 265 cases. Ultrastruct Pathol 11:209–250, 1987.
21. Hammar SP: Metastatic adenocarcinoma of unknown primary origin. Hum Pathol 29:1393–1402, 1998.
22. Khansur T, Routh A, Hickman B: Brain metastases from unknown primary site. J Miss State Med Assoc 38:238–242, 1997.
23. Kole AC, Nieweg OE, Pruim J, et al: Detection of unknown occult primary tumors using positron emission tomography. Cancer 82:1160–1166, 1998.
24. Lagerwaard FJ, Levendag PC, Nowak PJ, et al: Identification of prognostic factors in patients with brain metastases: a review of 1292 patients. Int J Radiat Oncol Biol Phys 43:795–803, 1999.

25. Latief KH, White CS, Protopapas Z, et al: Search for a primary lung neoplasm in patients with brain metastasis: is the chest radiograph sufficient? AJR Am J Roentgenol 168:1339–1344, 1997.

26. Le Chevalier T, Smith FP, Caille P, et al: Sites of primary malignancies in patients presenting with cerebral metastases. A review of 120 cases. Cancer 56:880–882, 1985.

27. Lembersky BC, Thomas LC: Metastases of unknown primary site. Med Clin North Am 80:153–171, 1996.

28. Maesawa S, Kondziolka D, Thompson TP, et al: Brain metastases in patients with no known primary tumor. Cancer 89:1095–1101, 2000.

29. McMillan JH, Levine E, Stephens RH: Computed tomography in the evaluation of metastatic adenocarcinoma from an unknown primary site. A retrospective study. Radiology 143:143–146, 1982.

30. Merchut MP: Brain metastases from undiagnosed systemic neoplasms. Arch Intern Med 149:1076–1080, 1989.

31. Mintz AP, Cairncross JG: Treatment of a single brain metastasis: the role of radiation following surgical resection. JAMA 280:1527–1529, 1998.

32. Mrak RE: Origins of adenocarcinomas presenting as intracranial metastases. An ultrastructural study. Arch Pathol Lab Med 117:1165–1169, 1993.

33. Nguyen LN, Maor MH, Oswald MJ: Brain metastases as the only manifestation of an undetected primary tumor. Cancer 83:2181–2184, 1998.

34. Nussbaum ES, Djalilian HR, Cho KH, et al: Brain metastases. Histology, multiplicity, surgery, and survival. Cancer 78:1781–1788, 1996.

35. Patchell RA, Tibbs PA, Regine WF, et al: Postoperative radiotherapy in the treatment of single metastases to the brain: a randomized trial. JAMA 280:1485–1489, 1998.

36. Patchell RA, Tibbs PA, Walsh JW, et al: A randomized trial of surgery in the treatment of single metastases to the brain. N Engl J Med 322:494–500, 1990.

37. Pavlidis N, Kalef-Ezra J, Briassoulis E, et al: Evaluation of six tumor markers in patients with carcinoma of unknown primary. Med Pediatr Oncol 22:162–167, 1994.

38. Perry A, Parisi JE, Kurtin PJ: Metastatic adenocarcinoma to the brain: an immunohistochemical approach. Hum Pathol 28:938–943, 1997.

39. Posner JB: Neurologic Complications of Cancer. Philadelphia, FA Davis Company, 1995.

40. Raab SS, Berg LC, Swanson PE, et al: Adenocarcinoma in the lung in patients with breast cancer. A prospective analysis of the discriminatory value of immunohistology. Am J Clin Pathol 100:27–35, 1993.

41. Ruda R, Borgognone M, Benech F, et al: Brain metastases from unknown primary tumour. A prospective study. J Neurol 248:394–398, 2001.

42. Ruddon RW, Norton SE: Use of biological markers in the diagnosis of cancers of unknown primary tumor. Semin Oncol 20:251–260, 1993.

43. Salvati M, Cervoni L, Raco A: Single brain metastases from unknown primary malignancies in CT-era. J Neurooncol 23:75–80, 1995.

44. Takahashi JA, Llena JF, Hirano A: Pathology of cerebral metastases. Neurosurg Clin North Am 7:345–367, 1996.

45. Takakura K, Sano K, Hojo S, et al: Metastatic tumors of the central nervous system. Tokyo, Igaku-Shoin Ltd, 1982.

46. van de Pol M, van Aalst VC, Wilmink JT, et al: Brain metastases from an unknown primary tumour: Which diagnostic procedures are indicated? J Neurol Neurosurg Psychiatry 61:321–323, 1996.

47. Vecht CJ, Haaxma-Reiche H, Noordijk EM, et al: Treatment of single brain metastasis: radiotherapy alone or combined with neurosurgery? Ann Neurol 33:583–590, 1993.

48. Voorhies RM, Sundaresan N, Thaler HT: The single supratentorial lesion. An evaluation of preoperative diagnostic tests. J Neurosurg 53:364–368, 1980.

49. Zimm S, Wampler GL, Stablein D: Intracerebral metastases in solid-tumor patients: natural history and results of treatment. Cancer 48:384–394, 1981.

CHAPTER 61

SKULL BASE METASTASIS

Franco DeMonte, Fadi Hanbali, and Matthew T. Ballo

Metastases to the basal cranium are among the least common tumors of the skull base.[48] Patients with cranial base metastases usually have cranial neuropathies caused by invasion or compression of the cranial nerves as they exit the basal foramina. Headache or pain is not uncommon.[13,15,53] The management of tumors involving the skull base is complex because of the density of critical neurovascular structures, the proximity of these structures to the relatively contaminated spaces of the paranasal sinuses or the ear and mastoid, the varied pathologic entities encountered, and the relative lack of anatomic familiarity.[20] Table 61-1 summarizes the histologic types of tumors that may involve the cranial base.

INCIDENCE

An appreciation of the rarity of skull base metastases can be gleaned from centers that treat a large population of patients with malignancy. Hall et al noted a 0.13% incidence of cranial neuropathy resulting from osseous metastases in 7725 new patients with carcinoma of the breast evaluated at The University of Texas M.D. Anderson Cancer Center (M.D. Anderson).[30] Bitoh et al identified only 16 patients with secondary malignancies of the parasellar or cavernous sinus region over 18 years, whereas Ahmad et al found five such lesions among 2170 patients reviewed at the University of Miami.[1,11] Greenberg et al at Memorial Sloan-Kettering Cancer Center identified breast, lung, prostate, and head and neck carcinomas as the most common malignancies to metastasize to the skull base (Table 61-2).[28] Their report of 43 patients spanned 7 years.

Autopsy studies report a somewhat higher incidence of skull base metastasis. Belal reviewed 703 temporal bones from 357 patients and found a 3% incidence of temporal bone metastasis in the general population.[8] Jung et al reported metastasis to the temporal bone in approximately 24% of 249 temporal bones taken from patients with a history of malignancy.[36] Gloria-Cruz et al examined 415 temporal bones from 212 patients with primary nondisseminated malignant neoplasms and showed that 22.2% of these had cancer cells characteristic of the primary tumor.[26] The breast and lung are the most common primary sites.[8,26,51]

In a series of 877 consecutive cases of orbital neoplasms examined histopathologically at the Institute of Ophthalmology in New York, Reese noted an incidence of metastatic carcinoma of approximately 3%.[54] A similar incidence of unilateral exophthalmos was reported by Zizmor et al.[72] Breast and the lung

were the most common primary sites, followed by the genitourinary tract and the gastrointestinal (GI) tract.[22]

Paranasal sinus metastasis may become symptomatic before the primary tumor is diagnosed in 50% to 65% of cases.[5,10,64] At other times, metastasis to the paranasal sinuses is diagnosed many years after treatment of the primary tumor.[10,62] Renal cell carcinoma is by far the most common primary tumor metastasizing to the paranasal sinuses, with tumors of the lung, breast, and the remainder of the urogenital tract and the gastrointestinal tract following distantly.[4,10,50] Bernstein et al examined 82 patients with metastatic tumors of the sinonasal region. Renal cell carcinoma was the site of origin in 40 patients, lung cancer in 10 patients, breast cancer in 8 patients, testicular cancer in 6 patients, and GI malignancy in 5 patients.[10] The maxillary sinus is the most common site of metastasis, accounting for almost 50% of all metastases to the sinonasal region. The maxillary sinus is followed, in decreasing order of frequency, by the ethmoid sinus, frontal sinus, nasal cavity, and sphenoid sinus.[6,10,50] Mickel et al reported on seven patients with cancer metastatic to the sphenoid sinus, with the prostate and the lung being the most common primary sites.[44] Eight similar cases were reported by Barrs et al.[6]

Metastases to the skull base are certainly rare among skull base tumors reported in surgical series. Jackson et al, reporting on 97 patients with malignant tumors of the skull base, included metastases in a subgroup labeled *rare tumors* that represented less than 8% of the total cases.[33] Of 734 patients with cranial base tumors treated at the George Washington University Medical Center between 1993 and 1997, metastatic tumors accounted for less than 0.55% of the patients.[48]

PATHOPHYSIOLOGY

Hematogenous spread is the likely etiology of most skull base metastases. Blood-born emboli reach the basal cranium through small anastomotic arteries at the neural foramina. Tumor-derived factors can enhance invasion of the arterial walls.[33] Neural compression and osseous invasion follow. Batson's plexus of veins has also been incriminated in the dissemination of tumor emboli. With increased intra-abdominal and intrathoracic pressure, blood is shunted through the valveless vertebral, prevertebral, and epidural veins to reach the basilar plexus of veins without transiting the lungs.[7,18,33] This plexus of veins is continuous with the venous plexi of the basicranium.

TABLE 61-1   Classification of Cranial Base Tumors

Benign Tumors	Intermediate Malignant Tumors (Low Grade, Slow Growing)	Highly Malignant Tumors (Fast Growing)
Meningioma	Chordoma	Carcinoma
Schwannoma	Chondrosarcoma	Sarcoma
Hemangioma	Low-grade esthesioneuroblastoma	High-grade esthesioneuroblastoma
Paraganglioma	Adenoid cystic carcinoma	Lymphoma
Pituitary adenoma		Myeloma
Epidermoid cyst		Metastasis
Juvenile angiofibroma		
Fibrous dysplasia		
Cholesterol granuloma		

Source: From Morita A, Sekhar LN, Wright DC: Current concepts in the management of tumors of the skull base. Cancer Control 5:138–149, 1998.

TABLE 61-2   Metastases to Base of Skull: Localization

Primary Tumor	N	Site of Metastasis				
		Orbit	Parasellar	Middle Fossa	Jugular Foramen	Occipital Condyle
Breast	17	2	2	7	2	4
Lung	6	1	1	2	1	1
Prostate	5	0	2	1	1	1
Head and neck	6	0	0	2	4	0
Lymphoma	3	0	1	1	0	1
Miscellaneous	6	0	1	2	1	2
Total	43	3	7	15	9	9

Source: From Greenberg HS, et al: Metastasis to the base of the skull: clinical findings in 43 patients. Neurology 31:S30–137, 1981.

Tumors may also extend from adjacent regions such as the paranasal sinuses, external ear, and nasopharynx. Although these may not represent true metastases, they can invade or compress the cranial nerves, accounting for a significant proportion of secondary skull base neoplasms. Neural foramen invasion is a common complication of nasopharyngeal carcinoma, occurring in approximately 15% to 35% of patients.[33,53,67,69] Other pathways of tumor extension include the muscles attached to the skull base; the fibrofatty spaces between these muscles; and along the neurovascular bundles, specifically along the perineural spaces.[24,25,70]

DIAGNOSIS

The development of a cranial neuropathy in patients with known neoplasia is a strong indication of metastasis. Other malignant disorders, however, including leptomeningeal carcinomatosis, and metastasis to the brainstem and cerebellum may cause the same clinical picture but require different therapy.[28]

Most tumors metastatic to the skull base produce lytic lesions, with the exception of prostate and lung cancers, which may produce either lytic or blastic lesions.[23,33,58] Plain x-rays of the

cranial base may show evidence of bone erosion, but interpretation is often difficult, and these examinations have a low yield.[12,14]

Computed tomography (CT) scans with high spatial resolution and bone windowing are ideal for outlining subtle osseous destruction or sclerosis of the skull base (Figure 61-1). Bone window and three-dimensional CT scans are helpful in determining the surgical approach.[12,23,33,47,48] Magnetic resonance imaging (MRI) is superior to CT for defining the soft tissue component of metastases and for delineating invasion of cranial nerves, the underlying dura, leptomeninges, and brain[14,19,23,33] (Figure 61-2).

Examination of the cerebrospinal fluid (CSF) for tumor cells is essential for diagnosis and to rule out an infectious etiology for the patients' symptoms. High opening pressure and elevated protein may be present. If the spinal fluid is normal, skull base metastasis becomes the most likely cause of the multiple cranial neuropathies. In the presence of negative CSF studies and inconclusive CT and MRI, other imaging modalities may be required to establish the diagnosis in patients where a skull base metastasis is highly suspected. Radionuclide scanning is the most sensitive method of detecting skull base metastasis.[13,28,33,53] Approximately 30% to 50% of lesions seen on the bone scans are not identified on other radiographic

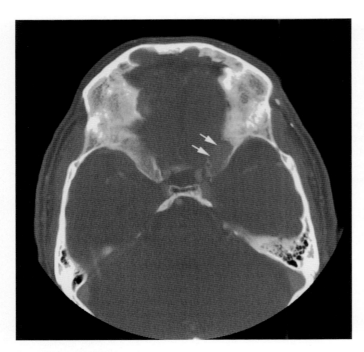

FIGURE 61-1 Axial high-resolution computed tomography scan at bone window reveals the subtle destruction of the left anterior clinoid process caused by metastatic renal cell carcinoma *(arrows).* (Used by permission of Dr. Franco DeMonte, Department of Neurosurgery, and the University of Texas M.D. Anderson Cancer Center. All rights reserved.)

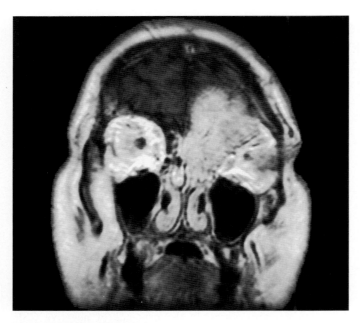

FIGURE 61-2 Coronal T1-weighted magnetic resonance image following contrast administration accurately reveals the involvement of the orbital soft tissues, the transcranial extension, and the intracerebral invasion of this metastatic renal cell carcinoma. (Used by permission of Dr. Franco DeMonte, Department of Neurosurgery, and the University of Texas M.D. Anderson Cancer Center. All rights reserved.)

studies.[39,43,52] One major drawback of bone scintigraphy is the increased activity associated with conditions such as sinusitis, mastoiditis, or temporomandibular joint arthrosis. Bone single-photon emission computed tomography (SPECT) offers a considerable advantage compared with planar bone scintigraphy, because the superimposed activity of adjacent structures is eliminated, and transaxial, coronal, and sagittal sections improve localization value in the complex anatomy of the skull base and allow better discrimination between inflammatory and malignant skull base diseases.[13,17,35,49]

Angiography is being replaced by magnetic resonance angiography (MRA) and three-dimensional CT angiography as a means of determining the major arterial and venous anatomy. Angiograms remain superior, however, in identifying the vascular anatomy and blood supply to the tumor and are necessary should tumor embolization or surgical manipulation of major vessels be indicated.[20,48]

CLINICAL FINDINGS

Cranial neuropathies secondary to a skull base metastasis may be the first sign of a distant cancer.[42,57,68] They may also be a manifestation of metastatic disease years after a cancer has been successfully treated.[29,53] Invasion of bone by metastatic tumor is the most common cause of pain, and such pain usually precedes neurologic signs and symptoms by weeks.[15,33] Several clinical syndromes associated with skull base metastases have been reported describing the entrapment of one or more cranial nerves at different sites in the skull base (Table 61-3).

Orbital Syndrome

Tumors rarely metastasize directly to the soft tissues of the orbit.[40,53] Metastases usually primarily involve the bony orbit and are most commonly of breast, lung, and prostatic tumor origin, in a decreasing order of frequency.[22,28,53,68] Greenberg reported a 2.5% incidence of orbital metastasis among 213 patients examined for eye disorders.[28] Font documented 28 patients with orbital metastasis among 235 patients with metastases to the eye, an incidence of 11.9%.[22] A progressive, dull, continuous pain in the supraorbital area is usually the first manifestation of an orbital metastasis.[28,53,68] According to Henderson, slowly increasing orbital pain is an early feature in metastatic orbital disease, not observed with other orbital neoplasms.[31] The first symptom other than pain is usually proptosis of the involved eye, accompanied by some degree of external ophthalmoplegia (Figure 61-3). Other prominent symptoms include blurred binocular vision, periorbital swelling and tenderness, palpable intraorbital mass, and decreased vision.[22,28,53] Decreased vision, visual field cuts, and papilledema rarely occur until very late in the disease course, probably because the tumors grow into the orbit from bone and do not invade the muscle cone where the optic nerve is located.[3,28] Many patients have decreased sensation along the ophthalmic division of the trigeminal nerve. Enophthalmos, rarely reported, is most typically associated with scirrhous carcinoma of the breast.[22,59]

Parasellar or Sphenocavernous Syndrome

Parasellar or sphenocavernous syndrome usually results from metastases to the bone of either the petrous apex or the sella

TABLE 61-3   Manifestations of Syndromes Involved in Skull Base Metastases

Location	Syndrome	Neural Structures	Manifestations
Anterior Skull Base	Orbital	Extraocular muscles; CNs III, IV, V$_1$, and VI	Supraorbital and orbital pain Blurred vision Proptosis No diplopia External ophthalmoplegia Enophthalmos Periorbital swelling and tenderness
Middle Skull Base	Parasellar (sphenocavernous)	CNs III, IV, V$_1$, and VI	Unilateral frontal headache No proptosis No visual loss Ocular paresis Periorbital edema Diplopia Papilledema Facial pain/numbness along CN V$_{1,2}$
	Gasserian ganglion	CN V (all branches, sensory and motor); Possible CNs III, IV, VI, VII	Numbness, parasthesias, and pain along CN V$_{2,3}$ Unilateral pterygoid and/or masseter weakness Abducens weakness
	Temporal bone	Middle ear CNs VII, VIII	Hearing loss Otalgia Periauricular swelling Facial paresis
Posterior Skull Base	Jugular foramen	CNs IX, X, XI, XII	Unilateral occipital/postauricular pain Dysphagia Hoarseness Weakness of palate, vocal cord paralysis, SCM/trapezius atrophy, tongue atrophy, Horner's syndrome
	Occipital condyle	CN XII	Occipital pain Neck stiffness/pain Dysarthria Dysphagia Ipsilateral tongue weakness

CN, Cranial nerve; SCM, sternocleidomastoid muscle.
Source: From Hanbali F, DeMonte F: Metastatic tumors of the skull base. In Sawaya R (ed): Intracranial Metastases: Current Management Strategies. Elmsford, NY, Blackwell/Futura, 2004.

turcica with secondary extension into the cavernous sinus.[67] It may less commonly result from a direct metastasis to the cavernous sinus. The parasellar syndrome is usually unilateral but may be bilateral.[46,53] It typically manifests as a unilateral frontal supraorbital headache and ocular paresis. Proptosis, if present, is minimal. Diplopia usually evolves rapidly or abruptly.[14] One or both of the oculomotor or abducens nerves are most commonly involved as they traverse the cavernous sinus. Sometimes the ophthalmic division and, rarely, the maxillary division of the trigeminal nerve is involved. Some patients complain of numbness, hypesthesia, or continuous painful dysesthesia of the face, not typical of trigeminal neuralgia.[11,12,28,53] The parasellar syndrome is relatively common in patients with systemic cancer. Roessmann et al reported 16 parasellar bony lesions (27%) in a postmortem examination of 60 consecutive cases of carcinoma; 9 were due to breast cancer.[56] Metastatic carcinoma accounted for parasellar syndrome 23 of 102 patients (25%)

described by Thomas and Yost.[67] Breast, prostate, or lung primaries were typically responsible.

Middle Fossa (Gasserian Ganglion) Syndrome

Numbness, paresthesias, and pain referred to the trigeminal nerve distribution are the typical complaints of middle fossa or Gasserian ganglion syndrome. The numbness or sensory loss usually begins close to the midline on the upper lip or chin and progresses laterally to the anterior part of the ear. Pain consists of either a dull ache in the cheek, jaw, or forehead or lightning-like pain similar to trigeminal neuralgia. Headache rarely forms part of this syndrome, being reported in 28% of the cases reported by Greenberg et al compared with 83% of patients with parasellar syndrome.[28] There is usually sensory loss in the distribution of one or more of the trigeminal divisions, with some evidence of dysfunction of the motor root as well. Obvious

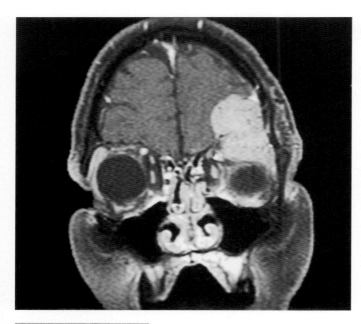

FIGURE 61-3   Coronal T1-weighted magnetic resonance image following contrast administration identifies a paraganglioma metastatic to the orbital bone. This tumor was the cause of the patient's orbital syndrome. (Used by permission of Dr. Franco DeMonte, Department of Neurosurgery, and the University of Texas M.D. Anderson Cancer Center. All rights reserved.)

weakness of the pterygoids or the masseter muscles may not be present; electromyography, however, may show evidence of denervation. Tumor spread beyond the Gasserian ganglion and over the anterior surface of the petrous ridge may compress the abducens nerve in Dorello's canal, resulting in diplopia. Tumor extension medially into the parasellar area may involve other ocular motor nerves. Spread along the posterior ridge of the petrous bone may compress or invade the facial nerve.[41] Of 15 patients with the metastatic middle fossa syndrome, 4 had isolated abducens nerve palsy, another 4 had a combination of extraocular palsies, and 3 had involvement of the facial nerve.[28]

Temporal Bone Syndrome

Conductive hearing loss is the most common manifestation of temporal bone metastasis. It is present in approximately 30% to 40% of symptomatic patients and is almost always the result of dysfunction of the eustachian tube with secondary serous otitis media.[9,26,61] Sensorineural hearing loss, if it occurs, is usually due to involvement of the cochlear fibers in the internal auditory meatus.[61] Maddox emphasized the triad of symptoms of otalgia, periauricular swelling, and facial nerve paresis as being the most suspect for malignant involvement of the temporal bone.[41] He reported an incidence of facial nerve paralysis of 34% in his series. Schuknecht et al also reported a high incidence of facial palsy.[63] Saito et al found that only 50% of patients with invasion of the facial canal manifested facial paralysis, although 100% of those who had tumors extending beyond the epineural sheath had complete paralysis.[60] Much less common findings are otorrhea, vertigo, tinnitus, or a middle ear effusion. The otic capsule may be involved, with

tumor approaching the endosteum, but the cochlea is rarely invaded, and seldom is the membranous labyrinth affected.[9,26]

Jugular Foramen Syndrome

Patients with lesions of the jugular foramen have a combination of cranial nerve palsies. The jugular foramen syndrome may include unilateral occipital or postauricular pain and progressive hoarseness or dysphagia. Signs include weakness of the palate, vocal cord paralysis, weakness and atrophy of the ipsilateral sternocleidomastoid muscle and the upper part of the trapezius, and occasionally Horner's syndrome. Papilledema has been reported as a result of compression of the sigmoid sinus or the jugular vein by the tumor. Ipsilateral weakness and atrophy of the tongue is sometimes noted, indicating extension of the tumor to the hypoglossal nerve. Metastasis to the jugular foramen is the most common cause of this syndrome.[21,27,28,53,55,66]

Occipital Condyle Syndrome

Metastasis to the area of the occipital condyle is more common than to the jugular foramen. The clinical picture is uniform. This syndrome is characterized by continuous, severe, localized, unilateral occipital pain that worsens upon neck flexion. The pain sometimes radiates toward the ipsilateral temporal area or eye and is often associated with a stiff neck. Approximately half of the patients will complain of dysarthria, dysphagia, or both, specifically related to difficulty in moving the tongue. The ipsilateral tongue is atrophic, and fasciculations may be noted.[15,53] Seven of nine patients with the occipital condyle syndrome in Greenberg's series had the typical occipital pain, four had dysarthria, and two had dysphagia; all had ipsilateral tongue weakness.[28] Carcinoma of the breast in women and prostate carcinoma in men were the most common metastatic sites of origin in the 11 patients reported by Capobianco et al.[15]

TREATMENT

The treatment of skull base metastases depends on the nature of the underlying tumor and its location. The available treatment modalities for cranial base metastases include surgical resection, irradiation, and chemotherapy. Recent technical advances in surgical therapy for primary skull base tumors occasionally make such approaches feasible in patients with a solitary metastasis.[20,33,34] Surgical patients should be critically selected based on the clinical status of the patient, the extent of primary and metastatic disease, pertinent radiographic studies, and the tumor's biologic nature. Small cell lung cancer, breast cancer, and prostate tumors are particularly sensitive to radiation and chemotherapy or hormone therapy. On the other hand, renal cell carcinoma, melanoma, and most sarcomas are relatively radioresistant, and other modalities of treatment should be considered. Only a minority of patients with skull base metastases, however, are candidates for surgical resection.

Over the past 10 years only 12 patients have undergone resection of skull base metastases at M.D. Anderson (Table 61-4). Over the same period, 439 other skull base tumor resections were performed (with an overall incidence of operations for skull base metastasis of 2.7%). Of these 12 patients, the diag-

TABLE 61-4	Patients with Metastases to the Skull Base Treated Surgically at the University of Texas M.D. Anderson Cancer Center (November 1992–August 2002)				
Pt	Pathology	Location	Reason for Operation	Adjuvant Therapy	Time to Recurrence
1	Renal cell carcinoma	Frontal and ethmoid sinuses, orbit	Progressive proptosis	None	3 mo
2	Renal cell carcinoma	Anterior clinoid	Progressive optic neuropathy	5-FU, α-interferon, fractionated stereotactic irradiation	Stable disease at 22 mo
3	Leiomyosarcoma	Orbit, frontal bone	Progressive proptosis	None	NED at 16 mo
4	Ductal carcinoma of breast	Sella	Progressive optic neuropathy, bilateral	None	Died at 2 mo
5	Melanoma	Orbit, ethmoid sinus	Progressive local recurrence following maxillectomy	None	1.5 mo
6	Follicular carcinoma of thyroid	Orbit, greater wing of sphenoid bone	Progressive proptosis	^{131}I, suppression therapy	NED at 34 mo
7	Mesenchymal chondrosarcoma	Infratemporal fossa	Massive disease, pain, temporomandibular joint dysfunction	None	8 mo
8	Renal cell carcinoma	Frontal and ethmoid sinuses, orbit	Progressive diplopia	None	5 mo
9	Paraganglioma	Frontal sinus, orbit	Progressive ptosis and diplopia	None	NED at 6 mo
10	Leiomyosarcoma	Sphenoid and ethmoid sinuses	Progressive optic neuropathy, bilateral	Intensity modulated radiation therapy	NED at 7 mo
11	Osteosarcoma	Greater sphenoid wing, orbit	Enlarging temporal mass	External-beam radiation therapy	6 mo
12	Renal cell carcinoma	Ethmoid sinus	Nasal obstruction, epistaxis	External-beam radiation therapy	NED at 1 mo

5-FU, 5-Fluorouracil; NED; no evidence of disease.
Source: From Hanbali F, DeMonte F: Metastatic tumors of the skull base. In Sawaya R (ed): Intracranial Metastases: Current Management Strategies. Elmsford, NY, Blackwell/Futura, 2004.

nosis of skull base metastasis was established preoperatively in 10. In the patients with metastatic carcinoma of the breast and thyroid, a preoperative presumptive diagnosis of meningioma had been made (Figure 61-4). Six of the 12 patients experienced local tumor recurrence, with the mean time to recurrence being a mere 4.3 months (range 1.5 to 8 months). Six patients remained free of recurrence at a mean of 14.3 months postresection (range 1 to 34 months). The local control rate has been quite poor for patients with malignant epithelial tumors such as renal cell carcinoma and melanoma. An exception is the patient with follicular carcinoma of the thyroid. These patients probably represent a more favorable group in which to consider surgical resection. Very effective postsurgical therapy is available with radioactive iodine and thyroid suppression. Another category of patients that should be considered for surgical resection are those with metastatic sarcomas, especially those of low or intermediate grade. Of the four patients with metastatic sarcomas, two remain free of local disease 7 (Figure 61-5) and 16 months, respectively, following surgery, although the patient with metastatic mesenchymal chondrosarcoma achieved local control for 8 months initially and a further 6 months following re-resection. The patient with metastatic osteosarcoma developed a local recurrence at 6 months.

The fact remains that for the majority of patients with metastatic tumors of the skull base, complete surgical resection is not feasible, and conventional fractionated radiation therapy remains the primary treatment. Although few radiation therapy series specifically address this unusual site of metastasis, it does appear as though localized radiation therapy can result in significant pain relief and improvement of neurologic deficits. Specifically, Vikram et al noted a 78% improvement of symptoms in 46 patients treated with conventional fractionated irradiation.[71] In 81% of these patients the relief was long term. Furthermore, there appeared to be an increase in the response to radiation as the duration of symptoms shortened and the dose of radiation was increased. In a second smaller series of 13 patients, Ampil reported complete or almost complete restoration of cranial nerve function in eight patients using varied radiation therapy dosage schedules and techniques.[2] Only three of the patients in this series were without documented response to the radiation therapy.

Given the generally poor overall survival of this patient population, we recommend 35 Gy in 14 fractions over 3 weeks and agree with others' findings that radiation is more effective if delivered early.[28,71] This rapid fractionation schedule is well tolerated with little risk of long-term sequelae. For patients with controlled systemic disease and a long life expectancy, we recommend a more protracted course of therapy. In these situations 50 Gy at 1.8 or 2 Gy per fraction is reasonable. As for the field of irradiation, we usually cover the radiologically visible

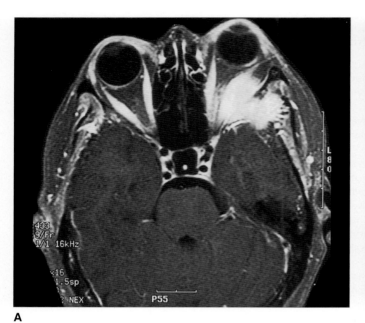

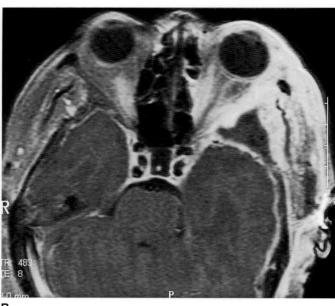

A

B

FIGURE 61-4   Preoperative (A) and postoperative (B) axial T1-weighted, fat-suppressed postcontrast magnetic resonance images reveal complete removal of this metastatic follicular carcinoma of the thyroid. The tumor involved the left greater sphenoid wing and orbit and was preoperatively diagnosed as a meningioma. (Used by permission of Dr. Franco DeMonte, Department of Neurosurgery, and the University of Texas M.D. Anderson Cancer Center. All rights reserved.)

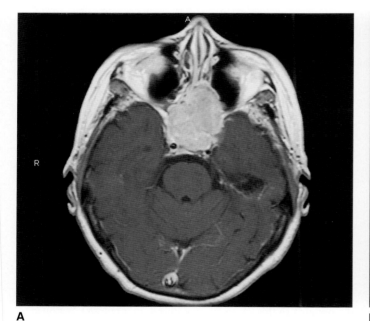

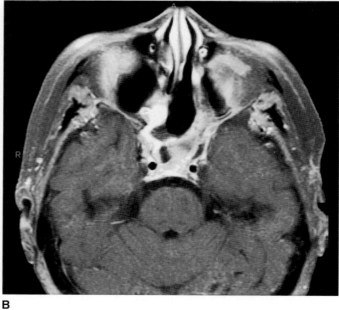

A

B

FIGURE 61-5   Preoperative (A) and postoperative (B) axial T1-weighted postcontrast magnetic resonance images depicting complete removal via a transbasal approach of this large metastatic leiomyosarcoma of the sphenoid sinus. The patient's optic neuropathy completely resolved following tumor resection. (Used by permission of Dr. Franco DeMonte, Department of Neurosurgery, and the University of Texas M.D. Anderson Cancer Center. All rights reserved.)

disease with a margin that includes at least a small portion of the clinically uninvolved skull base (Figure 61-6). Although both primary and metastatic lesions of the skull base may occur as solitary lesions, it is likely that the blood-born emboli responsible for metastatic disease result in a wider area of involvement.

In addition to conventional radiation therapy techniques, there is a growing body of literature supporting stereotactic radiosurgery or fractionated stereotactic radiation therapy for skull base tumors. These techniques are particularly attractive for patients previously irradiated for primary malignancy of the head and neck who subsequently develop a metastasis or local recurrence at the base of skull. Both represent highly conformal radiation-therapy delivery techniques where the tumor is treated to a very high dose in either a single large fraction (stereotactic radiation surgery) or in several smaller fractions (fractionated stereotactic radiation therapy). These techniques are able to deliver very high doses of radiation to the tumor but very little radiation to the surrounding previously irradiated normal tissues and critical structures (Figure 61-7). Unfortunately, because of the tight treatment, fields inherent in these techniques, there is significant potential for missing disease in the surrounding skull base. Regardless, for many patients stereotactic radiosurgery or fractionated stereotactic radiation therapy represents their only treatment option.

The effectiveness of stereotactic radiosurgery in the treatment of skull base tumors has been well documented (Table 61-5).[38,66] Iwai and Yamanaka reported a 67% tumor control and a 61% improvement of cranial neuropathies in 18 patients with

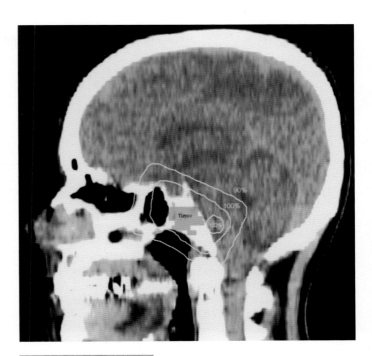

FIGURE 61-6 Parallel opposed 6 MV photon beams delivered 50 Gy in 5 weeks to this metastatic Ewing's sarcoma within the clivus with additional coverage of uninvolved skull base. Dosimetric planning revealed adequate coverage of the tumor with limited dose to surrounding structures. (Used by permission of Dr. Franco DeMonte, Department of Neurosurgery, and the University of Texas M.D. Anderson Cancer Center. All rights reserved.)

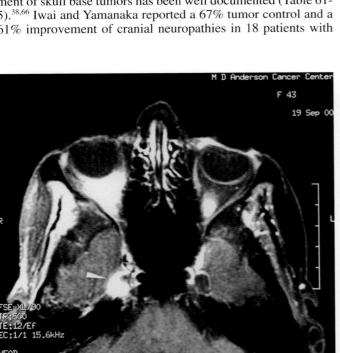

A

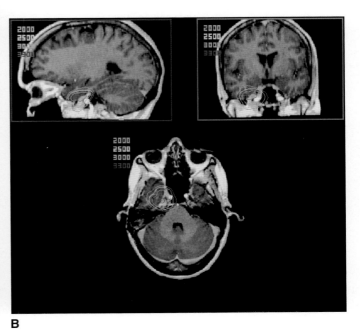

B

FIGURE 61-7 *A,* Axial T1-weighted postcontrast magnetic resonance image reveals an area of recurrence in this patient with a history of myoepithelial carcinoma. The recurrence is due to perineural tumor extension. *B,* In light of previous irradiation (60 Gy delivered using an appositional 20 MeV electron beam), fractionated stereotactic irradiation was recommended. A dose of 30 Gy was delivered in five fractions to the recurrent lesion through 12 noncoplanar, 6 MV photon beams. Two months later disease recurred along the path of the trigeminal nerve and continued back toward the brainstem. Despite an additional course of stereotactic radiosurgery, the patient died from local progression. (Used by permission of Dr. Franco DeMonte, Department of Neurosurgery, and the University of Texas M.D. Anderson Cancer Center. All rights reserved.)

TABLE 61-5	Treatment of Skull Base Metastasis with Stereotactic Radiosurgery				
Author	Number of Patients	Radiosurgery Type	Median Radiation Dose (Gy)	Median F/U (mo)	Tumor Control (%)
Iwai and Yamanaka	8	GK	16.2	10.5	67
Miller et al	32	GK	15	27.6	91
Kocher et al	13	LAC	15	22.6	77
Cmelak et al	47	LAC	20	9	69

F/U, Follow-up; GK, Gamma Knife®; LAC, linear accelerator.
Source: From Hanbali F, DeMonte F: Metastatic tumors of the skull base. In Sawaya R (ed): Intracranial Metastases: Current Management Strategies. Elmsford, NY, Blackwell/Futura, 2004.

skull base metastases, with a median follow-up of 10.5 months.[32] Miller et al treated 32 patients with malignant skull base tumors 4 cm or smaller in maximal diameter. Local control of tumor was excellent, and most patients experienced symptom relief. At a median follow-up of 2.3 years, 75% of the patients remained alive, 41% had stable disease, 28% had partial regression, 22% had complete resolution of disease, and 9% had progression.[45] Kocher and Cmelak reported similar findings (see Table 61-5).[16,37] These more conformal techniques

are a reasonable treatment modality for selected patients with skull base tumor recurrences and metastases, particularly in patients who are inoperable because of lesion location, medical contraindications, or the patient's refusal to undergo surgery. Early results suggest that radiosurgery provides good tumor control with complications comparable to standard radiation therapy. Patients with larger lesions near sensitive structures or in previously irradiated fields might benefit from fractionated stereotactic radiation techniques.

References

1. Ahmad K, Kim YH, Post MJ, Fayos JV: Involvement of the cavernous sinus region by malignant neoplasms: report of 5 cases. J Am Osteopath Assoc 87:504/91–508/95, 1987.
2. Ampil F: Palliative radiation therapy for metastases in base of skull and cranial nerves. Acta Oncologica 27:293–294, 1988.
3. Arger PH, Mishkin MM, Nenninger RH: An approach to orbital lesions. Am J Roentgenol Radium Ther Nucl Med 115:595–606, 1972.
4. Batsakis JG: The pathology of head and neck tumors: the occult primary and metastases to the head and neck, Part 10. Head Neck Surg 3:409–23, 1981.
5. Batsakis JG, McBurney TA: Metastatic neoplasms to the head and neck. Surg Gynecol Obstet 133:673–7, 1971.
6. Barrs DMMT, Whisnant JP: Metastatic tumors to the sphenoid sinus. Laryngoscope 89:1239–1243, 1979.
7. Batson OV: The function of the vertebral veins and their role in the spread of metastases. 1940 (classical article). Clin Orthop 312:4–9, 1995.
8. Belal A, Jr: Metastatic tumours of the temporal bone. A histopathological report. J Laryngol Otol 99:839–46, 1985.
9. Berlinger NT, Koutroupas S, Adams G, et al: Patterns of involvement of the temporal bone in metastatic and systemic malignancy. Laryngoscope 90:619–27, 1980.
10. Bernstein JM, Montgomery WW, Balogh K, Jr: Metastatic tumors to the maxilla, nose, and paranasal sinuses. Laryngoscope 76:621–50, 1966.
11. Bitoh S, Hasegawa H, Ohtsuki H, et al: Parasellar metastases: four autopsied cases. Surg Neurol 23:41–8, 1985.
12. Bitoh S HH, Obashi J, Maruno M: Secondary malignancies involving parasellar region: clinical manifestations, diagnosis and management in 16 patients. Medical Journal of Osaka University 36:17–27, 1985.
13. Brillman J, Valeriano J, Adatepe MH: The diagnosis of skull base metastases by radionuclide bone scan. Cancer 59:1887–91, 1987.
14. Bumpous JM, Maves MD, Gomez SM, et al: Cavernous sinus involvement in head and neck cancer. Head Neck 15:62–6, 1993.
15. Capobianco DJ, Rubino FA, Dalton JN: Occipital condyle syndrome. Headache 42:142–146, 2002.
16. Cmelak AJ, Cox RS, Adler JR, et al: Radiosurgery for skull base malignancies and nasopharyngeal carcinoma (see comments). Int J Radiat Oncol Biol Phys 37:997–1003, 1997.
17. Collier BD, Jr, Hellman RS, Krasnow AZ: Bone SPECT. Semin Nucl Med 17:247–66, 1987.
18. Delattre JY, Krol G, Thaler HT, et al: Distribution of brain metastases. Arch Neurol 45:741–4, 1988.
19. Delpassand ES, Kirkpatrick JB: Cavernous sinus syndrome as the presentation of malignant lymphoma: case report and review of the literature. Neurosurgery 23:501–4, 1988.
20. DeMonte F: Surgery of skull base tumors. Curr Opin Oncol 7:201–6, 1995.
21. DiChiro G, Fisher RL, Nelson KB: The jugular foramen. J Neurosurg 21:447–460, 1964.
22. Font RL, Ferry AP: Carcinoma metastatic to the eye and orbit III. A clinicopathologic study of 28 cases metastatic to the orbit. Cancer 38:1326–35, 1976.
23. Ginsberg LE: Neoplastic diseases affecting the central skull base: CT and MR imaging. AJR Am J Roentgenol 159:581–9, 1992.
24. Ginsberg LE, DeMonte F: Imaging of perineural tumor spread from palatal carcinoma. AJNR Am J Neuroradiol 19:1417–22, 1998.
25. Ginsberg L, DeMonte, F: Palatal adenoid cystic carcinoma presenting as perineural spread to the cavernous sinus. Skull Base Surg 8:39–43, 1998.
26. Gloria-Cruz TI, Schachern PA, Paparella MM, et al: Metastases to temporal bones from primary nonsystemic malignant neoplasms. Arch Otolaryngol Head Neck Surg 126:209–14, 2000.
27. Graus F, Slatkin NE: Papilledema in the metastatic jugular foramen syndrome. Arch Neurol 40:816–8, 1983.

28. Greenberg HS, Deck MD, Vikram B, et al: Metastasis to the base of the skull: clinical findings in 43 patients. Neurology 31:530–7, 1981.

29. Gupta SR, Zdonczyk DE, Rubino FA: Cranial neuropathy in systemic malignancy in a VA population (see comments). Neurology 40:997–9, 1990.

30. Hall SM, Buzdar AU, Blumenschein GR: Cranial nerve palsies in metastatic breast cancer due to osseous metastasis without intracranial involvement. Cancer 52:180–4, 1983.

31. Henderson J: Metastatic carcinoma. In Henderson J (ed): Orbital Tumors. New York, Decker, 1980.

32. Iwai Y, Yamanaka K: Gamma Knife radiosurgery for skull base metastasis and invasion. Stereotact Funct Neurosurg 72(Suppl 1):81–7, 1999.

33. Jackson CG, Netterville JL, Glasscock ME III, et al: Defect reconstruction and cerebrospinal fluid management in neurotologic skull base tumors with intracranial extension. Laryngoscope 102:1205–14, 1992.

34. Janecka IP, Sekhar LN: Surgical management of cranial base tumors: a report on 91 patients. Oncology (Huntingt) 3:69–74; discussion 79–80, 1989.

35. Jansen BP, Pillay M, de Bruin HG, et al: 99mTc-SPECT in the diagnosis of skull base metastasis. Neurology 48:1326–30, 1997.

36. Jung TT, Jun BH, Shea D, et al: Primary and secondary tumors of the facial nerve. A temporal bone study. Arch Otolaryngol Head Neck Surg 112:1269–73, 1986.

37. Kocher M, Voges J, Staar S, et al: Linear accelerator radiosurgery for recurrent malignant tumors of the skull base. Am J Clin Oncol 21:18–22, 1998.

38. Kondziolka D, Lunsford LD: Stereotactic radiosurgery for squamous cell carcinoma of the nasopharynx. Laryngoscope 101:519–22, 1991.

39. Krishnamurthy GT, Tubis M, Hiss J, et al: Distribution pattern of metastatic bone disease. A need for total body skeletal image. JAMA 237:2504–6, 1977.

40. Liu GT, Schatz NJ, Curtin VT, et al: Bilateral extraocular muscle metastases in Zollinger-Ellison syndrome (letter). Arch Ophthalmol 112:451–2, 1994.

41. Maddox HE: Metastatic tumors of the temporal bone. Ann Otol Rhinol Laryngol 76:149–65, 1967.

42. Massey EW, Moore J, Schold SC, Jr: Mental neuropathy from systemic cancer. Neurology 31:1277–81, 1981.

43. McNeil BJ: Rationale for the use of bone scans in selected metastatic and primary bone tumors. Semin Nucl Med 8:336–45, 1978.

44. Mickel RA, Zimmerman MC: The sphenoid sinus—a site for metastasis. Otolaryngol Head Neck Surg 102:709–16, 1990.

45. Miller RC, Foote RL, Coffey RJ, et al: The role of stereotactic radiosurgery in the treatment of malignant skull base tumors. Int J Radiat Oncol Biol Phys 39:977–81, 1997.

46. Mills RP, Insalaco SJ, Joseph A: Bilateral cavernous sinus metastasis and ophthalmoplegia. Case report. J Neurosurg 55:463–6, 1981.

47. Morita A PD: Tumors of the skull base. In Vecht C (ed): Handbook of Clinical Neurology: Neurooncology, part I. Amsterdam, Elsevier Science, 1997.

48. Morita A, Sekhar LN, Wright DC: Current concepts in the management of tumors of the skull base. Cancer Control 5:138–149, 1998.

49. Murray IP, Dixon J: The role of single photon emission computed tomography in bone scintigraphy. Skeletal Radiol 18:493–505, 1989.

50. Nahum AM BB: Malignant tumors metastatic to the paranasal sinuses: case report and review of the literature. The Laryngoscope 73:942–953, 1963.

51. Nelson EG, Hinojosa R: Histopathology of metastatic temporal bone tumors. Arch Otolaryngol Head Neck Surg 117:189–93, 1991.

52. Osmond JD, Pendergrass HP, Potsaid MS: Accuracy of 99mTC-diphosphonate bone scans and roentgenograms in the detection of prostate, breast and lung carcinoma metastases. Am J Roentgenol Radium Ther Nucl Med 125:972–77, 1975.

53. Posner J: Cancer involving cranial and peripheral nerves. In Posner J (ed): Neurologic Complications of Cancer. Philadelphia, FA Davis, 1995.

54. Reese A: Tumors of the Eye, 2nd ed. New York, Harper & Row, 1962.

55. Rivers MH, Svien, HJ, Baker HL: Diagnostic principles in the Jugular foramen syndrome. Surg Clin North Am 43:1129–1133, 1963.

56. Roessmann U, Kaufman B, Friede RL: Metastatic lesions in the sella turcica and pituitary gland. Cancer 25:478–80, 1970.

57. Rubinstein MK: Cranial mononeuropathy as the first sign of intracranial metastases. Ann Intern Med 70:49–54, 1969.

58. Ryan MW, Rassekh CH, Chaljub G: Metastatic breast carcinoma presenting as cavernous sinus syndrome. Ann Otol Rhinol Laryngol 105:666–8, 1996.

59. Sacks JG, O'Grady RB: Painful ophthalmoplegia and enophthalmos due to metastatic carcinoma: simulation of essential facial hemiatrophy. Trans Am Acad Ophthalmol Otolaryngol 75:351–4, 1971.

60. Saito H, Chinzei K, Furuta M: Pathological features of peripheral facial paralysis caused by malignant tumour. Acta Otolaryngol Suppl, 446:165–71, 1988.

61. Saldanha CB, Bennett JD, Evans JN, et al: Metastasis to the temporal bone, secondary to carcinoma of the bladder. J Laryngol Otol 103:599–601, 1989.

62. Schantz JC, Miller SH, Graham WPD: Metastatic hypernephroma to the head and neck. J Surg Oncol 8:183–90, 1976.

63. Schuknecht HF, Allam AF, Murakami Y: Pathology of secondary malignant tumors of the temporal bone. Ann Otol Rhinol Laryngol 77:5–22, 1968.

64. Sesenna E, Tullio A, Piazza P: Treatment of craniofacial metastasis of a renal adenocarcinoma: report of case and review of literature. J Oral Maxillo Surg 53:187–93, 1995.

65. Svien H, Baker HL, Rivers MH: Jugular foramen syndrome and allied syndromes. Neurology (Minneap) 13:797–809, 1963.

66. Tanaka T, Kobayashi T, Kida Y, et al: The results of gamma knife radiosurgery for malignant skull base tumors. No Shinkei Geka 24:235–9, 1996.

67. Thomas J, Waltz AG: Neurologic manifestations of nasopharyngeal carcinoma. JAMA 192:103–106, 1965.

68. Tijl J, Koornneef L, Eijpe A, et al: Metastatic tumors to the orbit—management and prognosis. Graefes Arch Clin Exp Ophthalmol 230:527–30, 1992.

69. Turgman J, Braham J, Modan B, et al: Neurological complications in patients with malignant tumors of the nasopharynx. Eur Neurol 17:149–54, 1978.

70. Vignaud J, Pharabaz C, Mourag M: Tumors of the skull base. In Portman M (ed): Rhino-otological Microsurgery of the Skull Base. Edinburgh, Churchill Livingstone, 1995.

71. Vikram B, Chu FC: Radiation therapy for metastases to the base of the skull. Radiology 130:465–8, 1979.

72. Zizmor J, Fasano CV, Smith B, et al: Roentgenographic diagnosis of unilateral exophthalmos. JAMA 197:343–6, 1966.

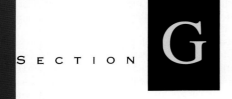

SECTION G SPINAL AXIS TUMORS

Section Editors

Andrew T. Parsa and Paul C. McCormick

CHAPTER 62

SPINAL AXIS TUMORS: INCIDENCE, CLASSIFICATION, AND DIAGNOSTIC IMAGING

Andrew T. Parsa, Tarik Tihan, and Paul C. McCormick

The consideration of spinal tumor is important in the complete differential diagnosis for any patient with myelopathy, radiculopathy, or neck or back pain. An expeditious and thorough work-up can quickly rule out a spinal tumor, and timely diagnosis can substantially improve the outcome for some patients with these lesions. Primary tumors that involve the spinal cord or nerve roots are similar to intracranial tumors in cellular type. They may arise from glial cells located within the parenchyma of the cord, Schwann cells of the nerve roots, or meningeal cells covering the cord. Primary tumors that are unique to the spine can arise from the intraspinal vascular network, the sympathetic chain, or bony elements of the vertebral column. Metastatic spinal tumors can result from dissemination of a primary systemic cancer or, more rarely, from drop metastasis of primary intracranial lesions.

PATHOLOGY AND EPIDEMIOLOGY

The location of a spinal tumor's cell of origin has an important anatomic correlate that serves to guide diagnosis and treatment. Spinal tumors are divided according to location into three major groups: intramedullary, intradural extramedullary, and extradural.[33] Intramedullary tumors are typically derived from glial or ependymal cells that are found throughout the interstitium of the cord. Intradural extramedullary lesions include meningiomas derived from meningeal cells lining the surface of the cord. Extradural lesions are typically due to metastatic disease or schwannomas derived from the cells covering the nerve roots. Occasionally, an extradural tumor extends through the intervertebral foramina, lying partially within and partially outside of the spinal canal (dumbbell or hourglass tumors).

The histologic characteristics of different types of primary and secondary spinal tumors are similar to those of intracranial tumors. Intramedullary tumors are rare, accounting for only 5% to 10% of all spinal tumors. In contrast, the benign encapsulated tumors such as meningiomas and schwannomas constitute between 55% and 65% of all primary spinal tumors. As a rule, intramedullary tumors are more common in children, and extramedullary tumors are more common in adults. The leading primary sites of metastatic tumors to the spine in order of frequency are lung, breast, and prostate[45]; however, several other systemic sites of spinal metastasis have been reported, including gastrointestinal tract, lymphoma, melanoma, kidney, sarcoma, and thyroid.[8,9,14,20,23,32,54]

Tumors of the spinal cord are much less common than intracranial tumors, with the overall prevalence approximating one spinal tumor for every four intracranial lesions.[33] When stratified for tumor type, this ratio of prevalence varies. For example, the intracranial-to-spinal ratio of astrocytomas is approximately 10:1, whereas the intracranial-to-spinal ratio of ependymomas can range from 3:1 to 20:1 depending upon the specific histologic variant. Gender prevalence is equal except in the case of meningiomas, which are more common in women, and ependymomas, which are more common in men.[37,38] Spinal tumors occur predominantly in young or middle-aged adults and are less common in childhood and old age. Although spinal tumors are more common in the thoracic region, when the lengths of the various portions of the spinal cord are taken into consideration, the distribution is relatively equal. Ependymomas may be either intramedullary or extramedullary. Ependymomas that originate at the conus (i.e., myxopapillary ependymomas) can be wholly or partially extramedullary at this site.

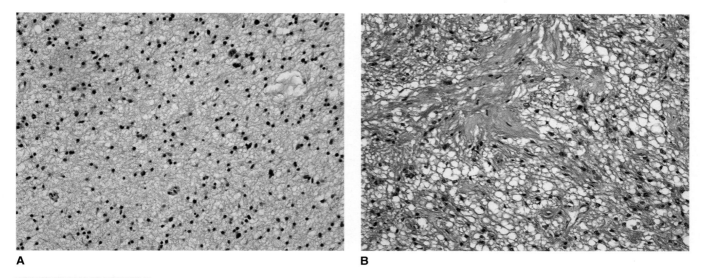

FIGURE 62-1 *A*, Histologic appearance of an infiltrating astrocytoma. The neoplasm blends imperceptibly into neuropil and focally displays a microcystic pattern composed of a small collection of myxoid substance. *B*, Typical histologic features of pilocytic astrocytoma composed of pink compact and loose areas, giving it a biphasic pattern. Rosenthal fibers can be seen in both but are more conspicuous in compact areas.

INTRAMEDULLARY TUMORS

Astrocytoma

Approximately 3% of central nervous system (CNS) astrocytomas arise within the spinal cord.[6,38] These tumors occur at any age but are most prevalent in the first 3 decades of life. They are also the most common pediatric intramedullary spinal cord tumor, accounting for approximately 90% of intramedullary tumors in patients younger than age 10 and approximately 60% of adolescent intramedullary neoplasms.[25] By approximately 30 years of age, ependymomas become slightly more common than astrocytomas and increasingly predominate in the middle decades of life.[40] After the sixth decade of life, astrocytomas and ependymomas are encountered with approximately equal frequency. Nearly 60% of spinal astrocytomas occur in the cervical and cervicothoracic segments. Thoracic, lumbosacral, or conus medullaris locations are less common. Filum terminale examples are rare. Spinal cord astrocytomas represent a heterogeneous group with respect to histology, gross characteristics, and natural history.[26] These tumors include fibrillary astrocytomas grade II-IV, pilocytic astrocytoma, and mixed gliomas. Approximately 90% of pediatric astrocytic tumors are low grade or indolent lesions such as pilocytic astrocytoma or grade II fibrillary astrocytomas.[41] Malignant astrocytomas (WHO grades III and IV) account for approximately 10% of intramedullary astrocytomas. These lesions are characterized by rapidly progressing clinical course, high incidence of cerebrospinal fluid (CSF) tumor dissemination, and poor survival.[11,51] Fibrillary astrocytomas prevail in the adult, whereas juvenile pilocytic astrocytomas are rare and usually limited to early adulthood (Figure 62-1).

Ependymoma

Ependymomas are the most common intramedullary tumor in adults. They occur throughout life but are most common in the

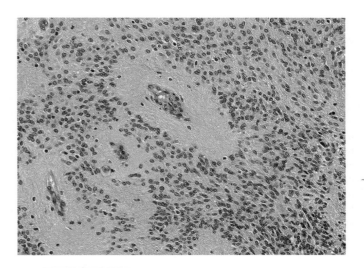

FIGURE 62-2 Histologic appearance of a classic ependymoma with perivascular pseudorosettes.

middle adult years. Although the spinal cord and filum terminale account for only 3% of the CNS by weight, nearly half of all CNS ependymomas originate within the spinal canal. The cervical region is the most common level of true intramedullary occurrence; however, 40% of intradural ependymomas arise from the filum.[40] For anatomic and surgical reasons, these lesions are generally considered to be extramedullary tumors.

A variety of histologic ependymoma subtypes may be encountered. The cellular ependymoma is the most common (Figure 62-2), but epithelial, tanycytic (fibrillar), subependymoma, myxopapillary, or mixed examples also occur. Histologic differentiation from astrocytoma may be difficult, but the presence of perivascular pseudorosettes or true rosettes establishes the diagnosis. Most spinal ependymomas are histologically benign, though necrosis and intratumoral hemorrhage

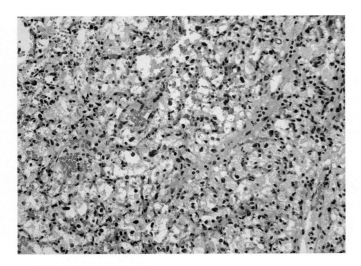

FIGURE 62-3 Hemangioblastoma showing vascular, stromal, and somewhat lipidized cells, which constitute the three cellular components of this neoplasm.

are common.[64] Although unencapsulated, these glial-derived tumors are usually well circumscribed and do not infiltrate adjacent spinal cord tissue.

Hemangioblastoma

Hemangioblastomas are benign tumors of uncertain histogenesis that are sharply circumscribed but not encapsulated. Almost all have a pial attachment and are dorsally or dorsolaterally located. They are distributed evenly throughout the spinal cord but show a cervical predominance when they occur in association with von Hippel-Lindau (VHL) disease.[13,42] Spinal hemangioblastomas account for 3% to 8% of intramedullary tumors and arise in any age group but are rare in early childhood[38] (Figure 62-3). Most patients seek treatment before age 40. Lesions are generally sporadic, but up to 25% of patients will have evidence of VHL disease. Patients with VHL disease tend to become symptomatic at an earlier age and occasionally have multiple tumors.[13,46,61,62]

Miscellaneous Intramedullary Pathology

Metastases account for approximately 2% of intramedullary tumors. This low prevalence is likely due to the small size of the spinal cord and its poor vascular accessibility to hematogenous tumor emboli.[12]

Other non-neoplastic entities can occur as intramedullary spinal lesions.[33,38] Vascular malformations, particularly cavernous angiomas, may occur in the spinal cord. Inclusion tumors and cysts are rarely intramedullary. Lipomas are the most common dysembryogenic lesion and account for approximately 1% of intramedullary masses. These are not true neoplasms but probably arise from inclusion of mesenchymal tissue within the spinal cord itself. They typically enlarge and produce symptoms in early and middle adult years through increased fat disposition in metabolically normal fat cells. Lipomas are often considered juxtamedullary, because they occupy a subpial location.

Genetic Syndromes Associated with Intramedullary Spinal Cord Tumors

Neurofibromatosis

The prevalence of certain intramedullary tumors in patients with genetic syndromes warrants consideration in formulating a differential diagnosis. There are two distinct types of neurofibromatosis (NF), each affecting cells embryologically derived from the neural crest. NF1 is a disease characterized by autosomal dominant inheritance, with almost complete penetrance and variable expressivity. Approximately 50% of cases are new mutations with a 1 in 3000 prevalence.[7,50] The NF1 gene is located on the long arm of chromosome 17 and codes for a neurofibromin guanosine triphosphatase activating protein that influences cell proliferation and differentiation. Tumors associated with the NF1 syndrome include neurofibromas, malignant nerve sheath tumors, optic nerve gliomas, rhabdomyosarcomas, pheochromocytomas, and carcinoid tumors.

NF2 also segregates by autosomal dominant inheritance, with high penetrance. The NF2 gene is located on chromosome 22q12 with approximately 50% of reported cases representing new mutations.[30] It is much less prevalent than NF1, with a rate of 1 in 40,000. The NF2 gene product encodes the protein merlin, which is a member of the ezrin-radixin-moesin protein family that links the cytoskeleton to the plasma membrane.[7] Neoplasms associated with NF2 include bilateral acoustic schwannomas, neurofibromas, ependymomas, gliomas, and meningiomas. There are two subtypes of NF2. The severe, or Wishart, form is characterized by early onset, rapid clinical progression, and multiple tumors. The mild, or Garner, form has a later onset, slower clinical progression, and fewer tumors.

In 1996 Lee and colleagues published one of the largest series of intramedullary spinal cord tumors in patients with NF.[31] Nine patients were described, including three patients with NF1, five patients with NF2, and one with "type uncertain." The predominant pathology associated with NF1 was astrocytoma (two low grade and one anaplastic), whereas ependymoma was most closely associated with NF2 (four of five patients). The reported incidence of intramedullary spinal cord tumors in the NF population was approximately 19% (9 of 48). This incidence may reflect referral patterns associated with highly specialized neurosurgical services. In 1997 Yagi and colleagues described a series of 44 patients with intramedullary spinal cord tumors, two of whom had NF1.[63] In both cases the pathology of the lesion was astrocytoma (i.e., anaplastic astrocytoma and glioblastoma). Taken together, along with selected case reports in the literature,[16] these studies support the presumption that solitary intramedullary spinal cord tumors in NF1 patients will most likely be astrocytoma. Similarly, it is reasonable to assume that an NF2 patient with an intramedullary tumor will most likely have an ependymoma. However, NF2 patients have also been described with intramedullary schwannoma.[31]

Von Hippel-Lindau Disease

VHL disease is an autosomal dominant disorder with 90% penetrance attributable to loss of a tumor-suppressor gene on chromosome 3p25-26.[15,30] Lesions associated with VHL disease include CNS hemangioblastoma, retinal angioma, renal cysts, renal cell carcinoma, pancreatic cysts, pheochromocytoma, and epididymal cystadenoma.[21,49] VHL-disease families can be grouped according to the presence or absence of pheochromo-cytomas.[42] Nearly all families with pheochromocytomas have missense mutations of the VHL gene. Hemangioblastomas are predominantly made up of endothelial cells and pericytes in a dense network of vascular channels, intermixed with lipid-laden stromal cells.[49] Using tissue microdissection, Vortmeyer and colleagues have recently demonstrated consistent loss of heterozygosity at the VHL gene locus in the stromal cells,[60] implicating these cells in the pathogenesis of hemangioblastoma.

CNS hemangioblastoma occurs in both type I (without pheochromocytoma) and type II (with pheochromocytoma) VHL-disease families. Sites of predilection are the posterior fossa (80%) and the cervical or lumbar regions of the spinal cord (20%). Specific point mutations and deletions in the VHL gene have been characterized in both sporadic and VHL-related spinal hemangioblastoma.[15,28,43,44] Hypermethylation of the VHL gene has also been implicated as a modality of inactivation.[47] Several models of how VHL inactivation results in tumor formation have been proposed.[49] The VHL tumor-suppressor protein is known to inhibit transcription elongation through interaction with the elongin protein.[57] The VHL protein also suppresses vascular endothelial growth factor (VEGF) production.[22] Loss of VHL protein function could cause VEGF up-regulation followed by angiogenesis.

EXTRAMEDULLARY TUMOR

Meningioma

Meningiomas arise from arachnoid cap cells embedded in dura near the nerve root sleeve, reflecting their predominant lateral location and meningeal attachment. Other speculated cells of origin include fibroblasts associated with the dura or pia, which may account for occasional ventral or dorsal locations of these tumors. Meningiomas occur in all age groups, but the majority arise in individuals between the fifth and seventh decades of life.[37] Between 75% and 85% occur in women, and approximately 80% are thoracic.[19,29] The upper cervical spine and foramen magnum are also common sites.[24] Here, meningiomas often occupy a ventral or ventrolateral position and may adhere to the vertebral artery near its intradural entry and initial intra-cranial course. Low cervical and lumbar meningiomas are uncommon. The majority of spinal meningiomas are entirely intradural; however, approximately 10% may be both intradural and extradural or entirely extradural. Meningiomas are generally solitary, but multiplicity can be observed in patients with neurofibromatosis. The overall prevalence of multiplicity in the spine is 1% to 2%.[10] The gross characteristics range from smooth and fibrous to the more common variegated, fleshy, and friable appearance. Microscopic calcification may occur. The dural attachment is often broader than expected, but en plaque examples are unusual. Bony involvement does not occur in the spine because of the well-defined epidural space. Psammomatous men-ingioma is the most common histologic subtype (Figure 62-4).

Peripheral Nerve Sheath Tumor: Schwannoma and Neurofibroma

Nerve sheath tumors are categorized as either schwannomas or neurofibromas. Although evidence from tissue culture, electron

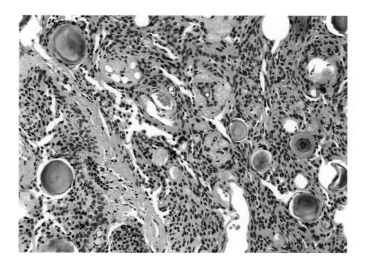

FIGURE 62-4 Meningioma with numerous psammoma-tous calcifications and whorls.

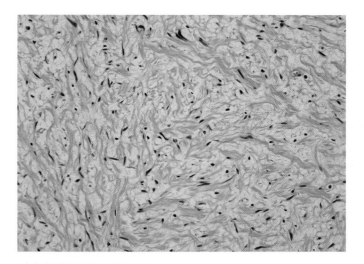

FIGURE 62-5 Neurofibroma demonstrating the typical slender wavy nuclei in a loose fibrillary and partially myxoid background.

microscopy, and immunohistochemistry supports a common Schwann cell origin of the neurofibroma and schwannoma, the morphologic heterogeneity of neurofibromas suggests participation of additional cell types, such as the perineural cell and fibroblast.[37] Neurofibromas and schwannomas merit separate consideration because of distinct demographic, histologic, and biologic characteristics. The histologic appearance of neurofibromas consists of an abundance of fibrous tissue and the conspicuous presence of nerve fibers within the tumor stroma (Figure 62-5). Grossly, the tumor produces fusiform enlargement of the involved nerve, which makes it impossible to distinguish normal from neoplastic tissue. Multiple neurofibromas establish the diagnosis of neurofibromatosis, but this syndrome is considered even in patients with solitary involvement. Schwannoma appears grossly as a smooth globoid mass, which

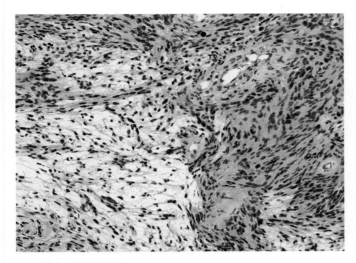

FIGURE 62-6 Typical biphasic appearance of a schwannoma with compact (Antoni A) and loose (Antoni B) areas. The compact areas also harbor palisaded structures composed of ribbons of nuclei known as Verocay bodies.

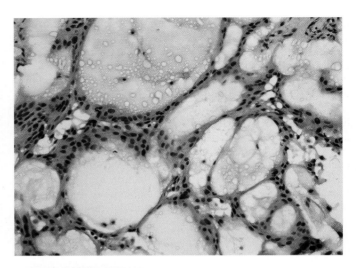

FIGURE 62-7 Characteristic appearance of myxopapillary ependymoma showing acellular myxoid center surrounded by tumor cell. Some of the loose myxoid areas also contain two center vascular cores.

does not produce enlargement of the nerve but is suspended eccentrically from it by a discrete attachment. The histologic appearance consists of elongated bipolar cells with fusiform, darkly staining nuclei arranged in compact interlacing fascicles, which tend to palisade (Antoni A pattern). A loosely arranged pattern of stellate-shape cells (Antoni B pattern) is less common (Figure 62-6).[56]

Nerve sheath tumors account for approximately 25% of intradural spinal cord tumors in adults.[37,56] Most are solitary schwannomas, which occur throughout the spinal canal. The fourth through sixth decades of life represent the peak incidence of occurrence, with men and women equally affected. The majority of nerve sheath tumors arise from a dorsal nerve root, whereas ventral root tumors are more commonly neurofibromas. Most nerve sheath tumors are entirely intradural but 10% to 15% extend through the dural root sleeve as a dumbbell tumor with both intradural and extradural components.[35,36] Approximately 10% of nerve sheath tumors are epidural or paraspinal in location. One percent of nerve sheath tumors are intramedullary and are believed to arise from the perivascular nerve sheaths that accompany penetrating spinal cord vessels. Centripetal growth of a nerve sheath tumor may also result in subpial extension. This occurs most often with plexiform neurofibromas. In these cases both intramedullary and extramedullary tumor components will be apparent. Brachial or lumbar plexus neurofibromas may extend centrally into the intradural space along multiple nerve roots. Conversely, retrograde intraspinal extension of a paraspinal schwannoma usually remains epidural.

Approximately 2.5% of intradural spinal nerve sheath tumors are malignant.[55] At least one half of these occur in patients with neurofibromatosis. Malignant nerve sheath tumors carry a poor prognosis with survival generally less than 1 year. These tumors must be distinguished from the rare cellular schwannoma, which has aggressive histologic features but is associated with a favorable prognosis.[53,55]

Filum Terminale Ependymoma

Although filum ependymomas have been classified as intramedullary lesions by virtue of the neuroectodermal derivation of the filum terminale, it is appropriate to consider them with extramedullary tumors from an anatomic and surgical perspective.[18] Approximately 40% of spinal canal ependymomas arise within the filum terminale in its proximal intradural portion.[33,37] Astrocytoma, oligodendroglioma, and paraganglioma may also originate in the filum but are rare. Filum terminale ependymomas occur throughout life but are most common in the third to fifth decades, with men slightly more commonly affected than women. Filum ependymomas and cauda equina nerve sheath tumors occur with approximately equal frequency.[37]

Lesions are typically red, sausage-shaped growths with moderate vascularity. Although unencapsulated, they are usually well circumscribed and may be covered by arachnoid. Myxopapillary ependymoma is the most common histologic type encountered in this region. The microscopic appearance consists of a papillary arrangement of cuboidal or columnar tumor cells surrounding a vascularized core of hyalinized and poorly cellular connective tissue (Figure 62-7). Nearly all filum ependymomas are histologically benign but tend to be more aggressive in younger age groups.[4]

Miscellaneous Extramedullary Pathology

Extramedullary masses may be neoplastic or non-neoplastic. Dermoids, epidermoids, lipomas, teratomas, and neurenteric cysts are inclusion lesions that result from disordered embryogenesis.[39] They may occur throughout the spinal canal but are more common in the thoracolumbar and lumbar spine. Intramedullary locations have also been reported. Associated anomalies such as cutaneous lesions, sinus tracts, occult anterior or posterior rachischisis, or split cord malformations may be present. Inclusion tumors and cysts generally occur as masses, but recurrent meningitis, tethered cord syndrome, or congenital deformities may be the predominant clinical finding.

Paragangliomas are rare tumors of neural crest origin, which may arise from the filum terminale or cauda equina.[17,27] These are benign and usually nonfunctioning tumors, which histologically resemble extra-adrenal paraganglia. They appear grossly as a well-circumscribed vascular tumor and may be clinically and radiographically indistinguishable from filum terminale ependymomas. Identification of dense-core neurosecretory granules on electron microscopy establishes the diagnosis. Complete removal can be accomplished in most cases. Cavernous malformations, hemangioblastomas, and ganglioneuromas may involve an intradural nerve root and occur as an extramedullary mass. These lesions may clinically occur as a nerve sheath tumor with early radicular symptoms.

Non-neoplastic lesions such as arachnoid cysts may occur as extramedullary masses. These are most common in the thoracic spine and are usually dorsal to the spinal cord.[3] Herniated intervertebral disks have occasionally been reported to rupture through the dura and occur as an intradural, extramedullary mass.[39]

Inflammatory pathologies such as sarcoidosis, tuberculoma, or subdural empyema rarely occur as intradural mass lesions. Although spinal carcinomatous meningitis often complicates systemic cancer, secondary metastatic mass lesions of the intradural, extramedullary compartment are rare. Malignant intracranial neoplasms that are in apposition to the subarachnoid space or ventricles are the most likely intracranial tumors to demonstrate CSF drop metastasis into the spinal subarachnoid space.[5] Systemic cancer accesses the subarachnoid space either through direct dural root sleeve penetration, or more commonly, hematogenously via the choroid plexus.

EXTRADURAL TUMOR

The majority of epidural neoplasms are metastatic, with 66% of these disseminating from the breast, prostate, hematopoietic system, or lung.[52,58] Myelography of epidural lesions can reveal a characteristic sawtooth pattern of partial to complete blockage, which in conjunction with corroborating plain films and bone scans constitutes a diagnosis of epidural metastasis. The general medical condition of the patient should influence the decision to surgically treat epidural metastasis. A scoring system employing various clinical parameters has been published in an attempt to more uniformly advise neurosurgeons.[59] The system rates patients according to six variables, including Karnofsky Performance Scale score and number of metastases. Patients who score low are unlikely to survive more than 3 months postoperatively (Table 62-1). Those who score high have a reasonable chance of surviving more than a year postoperatively. In general, the surgical approach for removal of a spinal metastasis depends on the anterior or posterior location of the tumor.

The most common spine tumors of middle-to-late adulthood are metastatic. These tumors are the result of hematogenous spread through the venous system of Batson's plexus into the vertebral elements of the spine. The vertebral body retains its red marrow longer than most other bony structures, and the microemboli of metastasis have a predilection for red marrow. As a result, the spine is the most common bony structure to acquire metastases. Metastatic tumors invade the epidural space

---

TABLE 62-1

Variables Relating to Postoperative Survival for Patients with Extradural Metastases

Karnofsky rating
Neurologic status
Number of extraspinal bony metastases
Number of metastases in the vertebral body
Presence of metastases to major organs
Primary site of cancer

---

and infiltrate the epidural fat from the surrounding bony spine. The dura can act to confine metastatic tumor to the epidural compartment, with the thoracic spine being more commonly involved than other regions.

The vertebral body and bony elements of the spine give rise to paravertebral tumor, which tends to both circumscribe the vertebral column and invade the epidural compartment. The paravertebral tumor often can be targeted for posterior percutaneous biopsy under computed tomography (CT) or fluoroscopic control, with a local anesthetic and sedation. With local anesthesia, inadvertent contact with the nerve root can be immediately detected and avoided. Because 10% of spinal metastases have no known primary tumor, biopsies can play an important role.[33,34]

DIFFERENTIAL DIAGNOSIS

Spinal tumors must be differentiated from other disorders of the spinal cord. A complete differential list is extensive and can include the following: transverse myelitis, multiple sclerosis, syringomyelia, combined system disease, syphilis, amyotrophic lateral sclerosis (ALS), anomalies of the cervical spine and base of the skull, spondylosis, adhesive arachnoiditis, radiculitis of the cauda equina, hypertrophic arthritis, ruptured intervertebral discs, and vascular anomalies.

Multiple sclerosis (MS), with a complete or incomplete transverse lesion of the cord, can usually be differentiated from spinal cord tumors by the relapsing and remitting course. The signs and symptoms of lesions in more than one anatomic location as well as evoked potential studies, cranial magnetic resonance imaging (MRI), and presence of CSF oligoclonal bands are consistent with MS. Acute transverse myelitis may occasionally enlarge the cord to simulate an intramedullary tumor.[33]

The differential diagnosis between syringomyelia and intramedullary tumors is complicated, because intramedullary cysts are commonly associated with these tumors.[2] Extramedullary tumors in the cervical region may give rise to localized pains and muscular atrophy in conjunction with a Brown-Sequard syndrome, producing a clinical picture similar to that of syringomyelia. The diagnosis of syringomyelia is likely when trophic disturbances are present.

The combination of atrophy of hand muscles and spastic weakness in the legs in ALS may suggest the diagnosis of a cervical cord tumor. Tumor is excluded by the normal sensory examination, the presence of fasciculation, or atrophy in leg muscles. Cervical spondylosis, with or without rupture of the intervertebral disks, may cause symptoms and signs of root irritation and compression of the spinal cord. Osteoarthritis can be diagnosed by findings in plain radiographs, but this is so common in asymptomatic people that MRI may be necessary to determine whether there is spondylotic myelopathy or an extramedullary tumor.

Anomalies in the cervical region or at the base of the skull, such as platybasia or Klippel-Feil syndrome, are diagnosed by the characteristic radiographic findings. Occasionally arachnoiditis may interfere with the circulation in the cord, causing signs and symptoms of a transverse lesion. With arachnoiditis, the CSF protein content is moderately elevated. Diagnosis is made by complete or partial arrest of the contrast column on myelography or by fragmentation of the material at the site of the lesion. Separation of the adhesions and removal of the thickened arachnoid by surgery have been of little benefit, with steroid therapy being equally ineffective.[33,39]

Benign tumors of the spinal cord are characterized by a slowly progressive course for many years. If a neurofibroma arises from a dorsal root, there may be years of radicular pain before the tumor is evident from other manifestations of growth. Intramedullary tumors are generally benign and slow growing; they may attain enormous size (over the course of 6 to 8 years) before they are discovered. Conversely, the sudden onset of a severe neurologic disorder, with or without pain, is usually indicative of a malignant extradural tumor, such as metastatic carcinoma or lymphoma.

RADIOGRAPHIC EVALUATION

The mainstay of radiographic diagnosis for all spinal cord tumors is MRI.[33] It provides spatial and contrast resolution of neural structures that is unattainable by any other imaging modality. Plain x-ray studies have little role in the modern diagnosis of spinal cord tumors as they do not image soft tissue adequately. However, the effects of intraspinal tumors on the vertebral elements are sometimes evident. Nerve sheath tumors can cause enlargement of the intervertebral foramina. Longstanding intramedullary lesions can produce erosion or scalloping of the posterior vertebral bodies and widening of the interpedicular interval. Myelography alone has a very limited role in the work-up of spinal cord tumors. It is seldom performed without subsequent CT. Intradural extramedullary tumors typically produce rounded filling defects of the dye column on a plain myelogram. Intramedullary lesions characteristically cause focal widening of the spinal cord shadow. CT and CT-myelography greatly enhance anatomic details over plain x-ray studies and myelography. CT provides excellent visualization of osseous structures, but soft tissue detail is inferior to MRI. For extramedullary tumors, CT-myelography provides excellent visualization of tumors arising in the region of the neural foramen. Accompanying bony changes are well demonstrated. Intramedullary tumors are more difficult to demonstrate, because they are generally confined to the cord tissue. Although widening of the cord may be seen with large lesions, subtle ones may be missed. MRI with and without intravenous contrast is the optimal initial radiographic examination for both tumor types.

OTHER DIAGNOSTIC CONSIDERATIONS

Cerebrospinal Fluid

When there is a complete subarachnoid block, the CSF is usually xanthochromic as a result of the high protein content. It may be only slightly yellow or colorless if the subarachnoid block is incomplete. The cell count is usually normal, but a slight pleocytosis is found in approximately 30% of patients. Cell counts between 25 and 100 per mm^3 are found in approximately 15% of patients' subarachnoid block secondary to spinal tumor. The CSF protein content is increased in more than 95% of patients. Values of more than 100 mg/dl are present in 60% of the patients, and values of more than 1000 mg/dl are present in 5%; these values may, in rare cases, lead to communicating hydrocephalus. The glucose content is normal unless tumor of the meninges is present. Cytologic evaluation of the CSF is useful when malignant tumors are suspected.[33]

Bone Scans

Radioisotope bone scans will show increased activity in the affected area of the spine in two thirds of patients with metastatic disease. However, this modality is actually less specific in predicting cord compression than plain spine radiographs. The utility of bone scans in differentiating malignant from nonmalignant fractures is limited as well.[1]

CONCLUSIONS

The diagnosis of spinal tumor is an important inclusion in the complete differential diagnosis for any patient with myelopathy, radiculopathy, or neck or back pain. Primary tumors that involve the spinal cord or nerve roots are similar to intracranial tumors in cellular type. Primary tumors that are unique to the spine can arise from the intraspinal vascular network, the sympathetic chain, or bony elements of the vertebral column. Metastatic spinal tumors can result from dissemination of a primary systemic cancer or, more rarely, from drop metastasis of primary intracranial lesions.

References

1. An HS, Andreshak TG, Nguyen C, et al: Can we distinguish between benign versus malignant compression fractures of the spine by magnetic resonance imaging? Spine 20:1776–82, 1995.
2. Aoki N: Syringomyelia secondary to congenital intraspinal lipoma. Surg Neurol 35:360–365, 1991.
3. Aithala GR, Sztriha L, Amirlak I, et al: Spinal arachnoid cyst with weakness in the limbs and abdominal pain. Pediatr Neurol 20:155–156, 1999.
4. Asazuma T, Toyama Y, Suzuki N, et al: Ependymomas of the spinal cord and cauda equina: an analysis of 26 cases and a review of the literature. Spinal Cord 37:753–759, 1999.

5. Barloon TJ, Yuh WT, Yang CJ, Schultz DH: Spinal subarachnoid tumor seeding from intracranial metastasis: MR findings. J Comput Assist Tomogr 11:242–244, 1987.

6. Bourgouin PM, Lesage J, Fontaine S, et al: A pattern approach to the differential diagnosis of intramedullary spinal cord lesions on MR imaging. AJR Am J Roentgenol 170:1645–1649, 1998.

7. Brill CB: Neurofibromatosis. Clinical overview. Clin Orthop 245:10–15, 1989.

8. Brown PD, Stafford SL, Schild SE, et al: Metastatic spinal cord compression in patients with colorectal cancer. J Neurooncol 44:175–180, 1999.

9. Bullard DE, Cox EB, Seigler HF: Central nervous system metastases in malignant melanoma. Neurosurgery 8:26–30, 1981.

10. Chaparro MJ, Young RF, Smith M, et al: Multiple spinal meningiomas: a case of 47 distinct lesions in the absence of neurofibromatosis or identified chromosomal abnormality. Neurosurgery 32:298–301; discussion 301–302, 1993.

11. Ciappetta P, Salvati M, Capoccia G, et al: Spinal glioblastomas: report of seven cases and review of the literature. Neurosurgery 28:302–306, 1991.

12. Connolly ES, Jr, Winfree CJ, McCormick PC, et al: Intramedullary spinal cord metastasis: report of three cases and review of the literature. Surg Neurol 46:329–337; discussion 337–338, 1996.

13. Couch V, Lindor NM, Karnes PS, Michels VV: von Hippel-Lindau disease. Mayo Clin Proc 75:265–272, 2000.

14. Dechambenoit G, Piquemal M, Giordano C, et al: Spinal cord compression resulting from Burkitt's lymphoma in children. Childs Nerv Syst 12:210–214, 1996.

15. Decker HJ, Neuhaus C, Jauch A, et al: Detection of a germline mutation and somatic homozygous loss of the von Hippel-Lindau tumor-suppressor gene in a family with a de novo mutation. A combined genetic study, including cytogenetics, PCR/SSCP, FISH, and CGH. Hum Genet 97:770–776, 1996.

16. Epstein FJ, Farmer JP, Freed D: Adult intramedullary astrocytomas of the spinal cord. J Neurosurg 77:355–359, 1992.

17. Faro SH, Turtz AR, Koenigsberg RA, et al: Paraganglioma of the cauda equina with associated intramedullary cyst: MR findings. AJNR Am J Neuroradiol 18:1588–1590, 1997.

18. Ferrante L, Mastronardi L, Celli P, et al: Intramedullary spinal cord ependymomas: a study of 45 cases with long-term follow-up. Acta Neurochir 119:74–79, 1992.

19. Gezen F, Kahraman S, Canakci Z, Beduk A: Review of 36 cases of spinal cord meningioma [In Process Citation]. Spine 25:727–731, 2000.

20. Giehl JP, Kluba T: Metastatic spine disease in renal cell carcinoma: indication and results of surgery. Anticancer Res 19:1619–1623, 1999.

21. Glavac D, Neumann HP, Wittke C, et al: Mutations in the VHL tumor suppressor gene and associated lesions in families with von Hippel-Lindau disease from central Europe. Hum Genet 98:271–280, 1996.

22. Gnarra JR, Zhou S, Merrill MJ, et al: Post-transcriptional regulation of vascular endothelial growth factor mRNA by the product of the VHL tumor suppressor gene. Proc Natl Acad Sci USA 93:10589–10594, 1996.

23. Goldstein SI, Kaufman D, Abati AD: Metastatic thyroid carcinoma presenting as distal spinal cord compression. Ann Otol Rhinol Laryngol 97:393–396, 1988.

24. Guidetti B, Spallone A: Benign extramedullary tumors of the foramen magnum. Surg Neurol 13:9–17, 1980.

25. Innocenzi G, Raco A, Cantore G, Raimondi AJ: Intramedullary astrocytomas and ependymomas in the pediatric age group: a retrospective study. Childs Nerv Syst 12:776–780, 1996.

26. Innocenzi G, Salvati M, Cervoni L, et al: Prognostic factors in intramedullary astrocytomas. Clin Neurol Neurosurg 99:1–5, 1997.

27. Kamalian N, Abbassioun K, Amirjamshidi A, Shams-Shahrabadi M: Paraganglioma of the filum terminale internum. Report of a case and review of the literature. J Neurol 235:56–59, 1987.

28. Kanno H, Kondo K, Ito S, et al: Somatic mutations of the von Hippel-Lindau tumor suppressor gene in sporadic central nervous system hemangioblastomas. Cancer Res 54:4845–4847, 1994.

29. Klekamp J, Samii M: Surgical results of spinal meningiomas. Acta Neurochir Suppl 65:77–81, 1996.

30. Kley N, Whaley J, Seizinger BR: Neurofibromatosis type 2 and von Hippel-Lindau disease: from gene cloning to function. Glia 15:297–307, 1995.

31. Lee M, Rezai AR, Freed D, Epstein FJ: Intramedullary spinal cord tumors in neurofibromatosis. Neurosurgery 38:32–37, 1996.

32. Maxwell M, Borges LF, Zervas NT: Renal cell carcinoma: a rare source of cauda equina metastasis. Case report. J Neurosurg 90:129–132, 1999.

33. McCormick P, Fetell, M, Rowland L: Spinal tumors. In Rowland L (ed): Merrit's Neurology. New York, Lippincot Williams & Wilkins, 2000.

34. McCormick PC: Anatomic principles of intradural spinal surgery. Clin Neurosurg 41:204–223, 1994.

35. McCormick PC: Surgical management of dumbbell and paraspinal tumors of the thoracic and lumbar spine. Neurosurgery 38:67–74; discussion 74–75, 1996.

36. McCormick PC: Surgical management of dumbbell tumors of the cervical spine. Neurosurgery 38:294–300, 1996.

37. McCormick PC, Post KD, Stein BM: Intradural extramedullary tumors in adults. Neurosurg Clin N Am 1:591–608, 1990.

38. McCormick PC, Stein BM: Intramedullary tumors in adults. Neurosurg Clin N Am 1:609–630, 1990.

39. McCormick PC, Stein BM: Miscellaneous intradural pathology. Neurosurg Clin N Am 1:687–699, 1990.

40. McCormick PC, Torres R, Post KD, Stein BM: Intramedullary ependymoma of the spinal cord. J Neurosurg 72:523–532, 1990.

41. Nadkarni TD, Rekate HL: Pediatric intramedullary spinal cord tumors. Critical review of the literature. Childs Nerv Syst 15:17–28, 1999.

42. Neumann HP, Lips CJ, Hsia YE, Zbar B: Von Hippel-Lindau syndrome. Brain Pathol 5:181–193, 1995.

43. Oberstrass J, Reifenberger G, Reifenberger J, et al: Mutation of the Von Hippel-Lindau tumour suppressor gene in capillary haemangioblastomas of the central nervous system. J Pathol 179:151–156, 1996.

44. Olschwang S, Richard S, Boisson C, et al: Germline mutation profile of the VHL gene in von Hippel-Lindau disease and in sporadic hemangioblastoma. Hum Mutat 12:424–430, 1998.

45. Perrin RG: Metastatic tumors of the axial spine. Curr Opin Oncol 4:525–532, 1992.

46. Pluta RM, Iuliano B, DeVroom HL, et al: Comparison of anterior and posterior surgical approaches in the treatment of ventral spinal hemangioblastomas in patients with von Hippel-Lindau disease. J Neurosurg 98:117–124, 2003.

47. Prowse AH, Webster AR, Richards FM, et al: Somatic inactivation of the VHL gene in Von Hippel-Lindau disease tumors [see comments]. Am J Hum Genet 60:765–771, 1997.

48. Rauhut F, Reinhardt V, Budach V, et al: Intramedullary pilocytic astrocytomas: a clinical and morphological study after combined surgical and photon or neutron therapy. Neurosurg Rev 12:309–313, 1989.

49. Richard S, Campello C, Taillandier L, et al: Haemangioblastoma of the central nervous system in von Hippel-Lindau disease. French VHL Study Group. J Intern Med 243:547–553, 1998.

50. Roos KL, Muckway M: Neurofibromatosis. Dermatol Clin 13:105–111, 1995.

51. Sarabia M, Millan JM, Escudero L, et al: Intracranial seeding from an intramedullary malignant astrocytoma. Surg Neurol 26:573–576, 1986.

52. Sarpel S, Sarpel G, Yu E, et al: Early diagnosis of spinal-epidural metastasis by magnetic resonance imaging Cancer 59:1112–1116, 1987.

53. Seppala MT, Haltia MJ: Spinal malignant nerve-sheath tumor or cellular schwannoma? A striking difference in prognosis. J Neurosurg 79:528–532, 1993.

54. Shapiro S, Scott J, Kaufman K: Metastatic cardiac angiosarcoma of the cervical spine. Case report. Spine 24:1156–1158, 1999.

55. Sharma BS, Banerjee AK, Kak VK: Malignant schwannoma of brachial plexus presenting as spinal cord compression. Neurochirurgia (Stuttg) 32:189–191, 1989.

56. Sharma S, Sarkar C, Mathur M, et al: Benign nerve sheath tumors: a light microscopic, electron microscopic and immunohistochemical study of 102 cases. Pathology 22:191–195, 1990.

57. Stebbins CE, Kaelin WG, Jr, Pavletich NP: Structure of the VHL-ElonginC-ElonginB complex: implications for VHL tumor suppressor function. Science 284:455–461, 1999.

58. Sundaresan N, Sachdev VP, Holland JF, et al: Surgical treatment of spinal cord compression from epidural metastasis. J Clin Oncol 13:2330–2335, 1995.

59. Tokuhashi Y, Matsuzaki H, Toriyama S, et al: Scoring system for the preoperative evaluation of metastatic spine tumor prognosis. Spine 15:1110–1113, 1990.

60. Vortmeyer AO, Gnarra JR, Emmert-Buck MR, et al: von Hippel-Lindau gene deletion detected in the stromal cell component of a cerebellar hemangioblastoma associated with von Hippel-Lindau disease. Hum Pathol 28:540–543, 1997.

61. Wanebo JE, Lonser RR, Glenn GM, Oldfield EH: The natural history of hemangioblastomas of the central nervous system in patients with von Hippel-Lindau disease. J Neurosurg 98:82–94, 2003.

62. Weil RJ, Lonser RR, DeVroom HL, et al: Surgical management of brainstem hemangioblastomas in patients with von Hippel-Lindau disease. J Neurosurg 98:95–105, 2003.

63. Yagi T, Ohata K, Haque M, Hakuba A: Intramedullary spinal cord tumour associated with neurofibromatosis type 1. Acta Neurochir 139:1055–1060, 1997.

64. Yoshii S, Shimizu K, Ido K, Nakamura T: Ependymoma of the spinal cord and the cauda equina region. J Spinal Disord 12:157–161, 1999.

CHAPTER 63

NERVE SHEATH TUMORS OF THE SPINE

James Waldron and Philip R. Weinstein

Nerve sheath tumors of the spine are relatively common entities. Except in instances of rare malignant tumors, these lesions have a favorable prognosis. They arise from the supportive tissue of the peripheral nerves that begin just beyond the Obersteiner-Redlich zone that demarcates the transition from the central nervous system (CNS) to the peripheral nervous system (PNS).[8] These tumors may be intradural and extramedullary in location, may extend with the nerve root through the neural foramen to form a transdural dumbbell tumor, or may be purely extradural.

Nerve sheath tumors consist predominantly of two benign lesions, the schwannoma and the neurofibroma, and the more rare malignant peripheral nerve sheath tumor (MPNST). The prognosis for benign nerve sheath tumors is favorable. The main therapeutic challenge for benign nerve sheath tumors is preservation of the involved nerve while attempting to achieve complete resection. MPNSTs follow an aggressive course and have a poor prognosis. Accordingly, therapy for patients with MPNSTs is typically palliative.

INCIDENCE

Nerve sheath tumors of the spine make up approximately 26% of spinal tumors, making them one of the most common spinal tumors encountered in practice.[11] They occur in equal proportion in men and women and are evenly distributed along the spine. Purely intradural lesions (57%) are much more common than dumbbell lesions (16%) and purely extradural lesions (27%).[11] They occur across a wide range of ages, typically affecting patients between the third and seventh decades.[11] Nerve sheath tumors of the spine occur sporadically and in association with neurofibromatosis 1 (NF1) and neurofibromatosis 2 (NF2). The most common variety is the sporadic schwannoma, which accounts for 83% of spinal nerve sheath tumors in one series.[16] Schwannomas also occur in association with NF2, often with a large number of lesions in a single patient.[9] Despite the low prevalence of the syndrome, NF2 accounts for 2% of all spinal schwannomas.[18] Neurofibromas are a hallmark of NF1, although most common in the periphery; they account for 15% of spinal nerve sheath tumors.[16] Approximately 30% of neurofibromas are sporadic.[16]

MOLECULAR GENETICS OF NERVE SHEATH TUMORS

Neurofibromatosis 1

Neurofibromatosis 1, also known as von Recklinghausen's disease, is an autosomal dominant disease characterized by a defect in the protein neurofibromin. Its incidence is approximately 1 in 3000 to 1 in 4000, with 50% arising from *de novo* mutations.[12] NF1 is present when two or more of the National Institutes of Health Consensus criteria are met[12] (Table 63-1). NF1 is associated with a variety of malignant conditions. In addition to the malignant degeneration of neurofibromas into MPNSTs, there is an increased incidence of astrocytomas, and myeloid leukemias.[12] The majority of spinal lesions in NF1 are asymptomatic neurofibromas, often multiple. In the NF1 population spinal tumors cause neurologic symptoms in approximately 2%.[19]

The underlying mutation of NF1 occurs on chromosome 17 in the gene coding for the protein neurofibromin. Neurofibromin is a tumor-suppressor gene that regulates the activation status of the Ras-mediated cell signaling cascade. Neurofibromin serves as a GTPase-activating protein (GAP) that associates with Ras-GTP, cleaving it into the inactive Ras-GDP form. The activated form of Ras mediates a cascade associated with cell proliferation and cell survival. Individuals with NF1 are born with a single germ line neurofibromin mutation. A second "hit" leads to tumor formation.[12]

Neurofibromatosis 2

Neurofibromatosis 2 is an autosomal dominant disorder that occurs with only 10% the frequency of NF1, with an incidence of 1 in 33,000 to 40,000.[4] NF2's hallmark is the presence of bilateral acoustic neuromas, which is pathognomonic for the disease. NF2 can also be diagnosed when a first-degree relative with NF2 and either a unilateral acoustic neuroma or two of the following are present: neurofibroma, meningioma, glioma, schwannoma, or subcapsular lenticular opacities.[1] NF2 is associated with a 90% incidence of spinal tumors (intramedullary, intradural extramedullary, dumbbell, extradural), 33% of which were symptomatic in a series of 48 patients.[13] In NF2 patients,

TABLE 63-1

NIH Consensus Criteria for Neurofibromatosis 1

Six or more café-au-lait spots (>0.5 cm in prepubertal and
  >1.5 in postpubertal)
Two or more neurofibromas or the presence of a plexiform
  neurofibroma
Axillary and intertriginous freckling
Two or more Lisch nodules (benign hamartomas of the iris)
Bony dysplasia
Optic glioma
First-degree relative with NF1

NIH, National Institutes of Health.
From Lynch TM, Gutmann DH: Neurofibromatosis 1. Neurol Clin
20:841–865, 2002.

spinal tumors are typically multiple, predominantly consisting of schwannomas and meningiomas. A review of spinal magnetic resonance (MR) images of 49 patients with NF2 revealed 22 patients with more than 201 intradural extramedullary lesions. Eighty-eight percent of the lesions were consistent with nerve sheath tumors and 12% with spinal menigiomas.[14] This series included several individuals in which the sheer number of lesions along the spine made accurate counting difficult. Despite the potentially large number of lesions, malignant change is rare.[7]

NF2 has been traced to mutations in a gene that codes for the merlin protein on chromosome 22q. The merlin protein is structurally related to a group of proteins that mediate the interaction between the cytoskeleton and the cell surface. These proteins play a role in cellular remodeling and cell growth.[1] The exact function of the merlin protein has yet to be elucidated. The severity of the phenotype can vary widely among affected families, with a more severe phenotype being associated with frameshift or nonsense mutations that result in an unstable protein. A less severe phenotype is present in families with missense mutations of the merlin gene.[15]

NERVE SHEATH TUMORS

Neurofibroma

Neurofibromas are benign lesions that arise from the connective tissue elements of peripheral nerves. They are found throughout the peripheral nervous system, involving the spinal nerve roots in 2% of cases.[10] They occur primarily in patients with NF1 but may occasionally occur sporadically. They are globular lesions surrounded by a loose capsule and contain a mixture of Schwann cells, perineural-like cells, fibroblasts, and various intermediates embedded in an extracellular matrix.[20] Unlike schwannomas, neurofibromas often ensheathe or incorporate nerve fascicles within their capsule, making their dissection surgically challenging. When present in the spine, they typically arise from the sensory nerve root. They grow at variable rates, often develop during adolescence, may progress during pregnancy, and affect nearly all adults with NF1 at

some point in their lives.[12] The plexiform neurofibroma is a diffuse form of neurofibroma that may extend across multiple nerves and invest adjacent tissue. When in the spine, they may span multiple levels of nerve roots and become intimately involved with paraspinal structures, making complete resection extremely difficult. Plexiform neurofibromas are estimated to occur in 25% to 30% of individuals with NF1.[12]

Schwannoma

The majority of schwannomas occur as solitary tumors. They may be found in any region of the peripheral nervous system. Schwannomas are the most common nerve sheath tumor of the spine[17] (Figure 63-1). In patients with spinal schwannomas 2% are attributable to NF2.[18] Spinal schwannomas typically arise from the sensory nerve root as globular well-encapsulated lesions that are discrete from neural fascicles. Their natural history consists of slow, progressive growth, with deformation of surrounding structures. In rare instances, schwannomas may appear as intramedullary lesions of the spine. It is extremely rare for schwannomas to undergo malignant transformation.

Malignant Peripheral Nerve Sheath Tumors

MPNSTs include all malignancies arising from the connective tissues of the peripheral nerves. Attempts to subdivide these tumors based on cell of origin have not yielded consistent results. They are extremely rare in the general population, with an incidence of 0.001%[2]; however, they are a major cause of mortality in individuals with NF1. These patients exhibit a lifetime risk of 8% to 13%.[3] In patients with NF1, MPNSTs are thought to arise from preexisting plexiform neurofibromas and occasionally neurofibromas. MPNSTs are aggressive lesions with a poor prognosis that exhibit progressive enlargement, infiltration of surrounding tissues, and frequent metastases.

PRESENTATION AND EVALUATION

Nerve sheath tumors of the spine may remain asymptomatic for a long time because of their slow growth and gradual deformation of surrounding tissue. When clinical symptoms begin to manifest, they are often indistinguishable from symptoms originating from mechanical or degenerative sources of radicular pain and other types of spinal tumors. Localized pain, radicular symptoms, and myelopathy are all relatively common.[8] The location of the nerve sheath tumor contributes to the specific nature of the symptoms. Purely intradural lesions are well situated to induce myelopathy and, in some instances, a Brown-Sequard syndrome may develop because of lateral compression.[8] Lesions with more peripheral involvement (i.e., dumbbell tumors and purely extradural tumors) present primarily with pain and radicular symptoms.[11] Significant differences have been noted in patients for whom the nerve sheath tumor is either sporadic or associated with NF1 and those with NF2. In a retrospective survey of 87 nerve sheath tumors treated at a single center, 75% of patients with sporadic and NF1 nerve sheath tumors reported pain, 8% noted gait ataxia, and 8% noted dysesthesia as their initial symptom. In the cohort diagnosed with NF2, pain was noted as the first symptom by only 43%, although gait ataxia was reported by 30% and a motor deficit by 17%.[11] Spinal MPNSTs most commonly cause

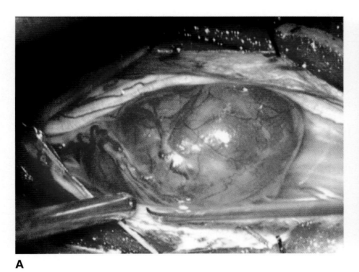 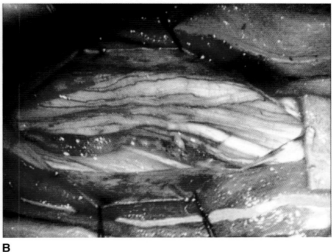

A **B**

FIGURE 63-1 Microsurgical operative photograph showing an L2 schwannoma *(A)* dissected free of surrounding cauda equina nerve roots prior to ultrasonic aspiration to shrink the mass and final dissection of the capsule before removal *(B)*. A single filament of the right L2 nerve root entered the capsule rostrally and exited from the caudal pole of the tumor. Pain was completely relieved, and a small strip of hypalgesia on the medial thigh was present postoperatively.

increased pain and progressive neurologic deficit, which may be overlooked in individuals with preexisting neurofibromas.[7]

The diagnosis of a spinal nerve sheath tumor is straightforward in a patient with known NF1 or NF2 because high suspicion leads to early use of appropriate imaging. Often the only significant challenge is determining which lesion is the source of symptoms in patients with multiple lesions. In patients with sporadic nerve sheath tumors, the diagnosis can often be missed in the standard work-up for mechanical causes of back pain and tumors of the bony spine.

Plain radiographs are rarely used in the work-up of nerve sheath tumors of the spine, although 50% may demonstrate abnormalities such as scoliosis, foraminal enlargement, and vertebral scalloping.[8] MR imaging (MRI) is the most useful test for the evaluation of nerve sheath tumors. Nerve sheath tumors are isointense on T1-weighted images and hyperintense on T2-weighted images. They are enhanced with contrast, allowing detailed resolution of the tumor border and the surrounding anatomy.[8] In the cervical region CT angiography or MR angiography (MRA) should be undertaken to elucidate the relationship between the tumor and the vertebral arteries. CT is a useful adjunct when differentiating nerve sheath tumors from bony tumors and for evaluating spinal stability during preoperative planning.[8] Current MRI technology does not allow for the consistent differentiation of MPNSTs from benign lesions.[18] Fluorodeoxyglucose positron-emission tomography (FDG-PET) scanning has shown some promise.[6]

TREATMENT AND OUTCOME

Treatment for symptomatic nerve sheath tumors of the spine consists of complete excision of the tumor mass. In addition to alleviating symptoms, complete resection decreases the rate of recurrence. A major goal during resection of spinal nerve sheath tumors is preservation of spinal nerve root function. This goal is obtainable in most cases, even when a nerve root enervating a limb is partially sacrificed during nerve sheath tumor resection. In a series of 67 patients in which a clinically relevant nerve root was resected in the cervical or lumbosacral region, 9 of 67 patients (13.4%) experienced a transient neurologic deficit lasting a maximum of 3 months, and 2 of 67 (3%) experienced a permanent neurologic deficit.[11] The ultimate goal of therapy is resolution of symptoms. Surgical resection of sporadic nerve sheath tumors and those associated with NF1 leads to alleviation of symptoms in a majority of patients,[11] although resection of nerve sheath tumors associated with NF2 leads to minimal improvement of neurologic symptoms.[11] In this same series, 10-year recurrence rates were 28.2% for the sporadic and NF1-associated nerve sheath tumors and 100% for those associated with NF2.

The prognosis for MPNSTs involving the spine is uniformly poor. Because of the locally aggressive nature of the tumor, CNS seeding typically occurs early. En bloc resection aimed at a cure is usually unobtainable because of proximity of the spinal cord.[8] Radiation assists with local control, and chemotherapy has not demonstrated any efficacy.[5] Surgery for MPNSTs should be considered a palliative option aimed at reducing symptoms.[8] Results of radiosurgery treatment are not yet available.

CONCLUSION

Spinal nerve sheath tumors are mostly benign lesions that cause radicular symptoms because of deformation of otherwise normal nerve roots or spinal cord. Surgical resection for sporadic schwannoma and neurofibroma lesions can be curative. Patients with NF1 or NF2 may have multiple lesions. Surgery for MPNSTs should be considered a palliative option aimed at reducing symptoms.

References

1. Baser ME, DG RE, Gutmann DH: Neurofibromatosis 2. Curr Opin Neurol 16:27–33, 2003.
2. Ducatman BS, Scheithauer BW, Piepgras DG, et al: Malignant peripheral nerve sheath tumors. A clinicopathologic study of 120 cases. Cancer 57:2006–2021, 1986.
3. Evans DG, Baser ME, McGaughran J, et al: Malignant peripheral nerve sheath tumours in neurofibromatosis 1. J Med Genet 39:311–314, 2002.
4. Evans DG, Huson SM, Donnai D, at al: A genetic study of type 2 neurofibromatosis in the United Kingdom. I. Prevalence, mutation rate, fitness, and confirmation of maternal transmission effect on severity. J Med Genet 29:841–846, 1992.
5. Ferner RE, Gutmann DH: International consensus statement on malignant peripheral nerve sheath tumors in neurofibromatosis. Cancer Res 62:1573–1577, 2002.
6. Ferner RE, Lucas JD, O'Doherty MJ, et al: Evaluation of (18)fluorodeoxyglucose positron emission tomography ((18)FDG PET) in the detection of malignant peripheral nerve sheath tumours arising from within plexiform neurofibromas in neurofibromatosis 1. J Neurol Neurosurg Psychiatry 68:353–357, 2000.
7. Ferner RE, O'Doherty MJ: Neurofibroma and schwannoma. Curr Opin Neurol 15:679–684, 2002.
8. Hajjar MV, Smith DA, Schmidek HH: Surgical management of tumors of the nerve sheath involving the spine. In Chapman MW (ed): Chapman's Orthopaedic Surgery. Philadelphia, Lippincott Williams & Wilkins, 2001.
9. Halliday AL, Sobel RA, Martuza RL: Benign spinal nerve sheath tumors: their occurrence sporadically and in neurofibromatosis types 1 and 2. J Neurosurg 74:248–253, 1991.
10. Huson SM, Harper PS, Compston DA: Von Recklinghausen neurofibromatosis. A clinical and population study in south-east Wales. Brain 111 (Pt 6):1355–1381, 1988.
11. Klekamp J, Samii M: Surgery of spinal nerve sheath tumors with special reference to neurofibromatosis. Neurosurgery 42:279–289; discussion 289–290, 1998.
12. Lynch TM, Gutmann DH: Neurofibromatosis 1. Neurol Clin 20:841–865, 2002.
13. Mautner VF, Lindenau M, Baser ME, et al: The neuroimaging and clinical spectrum of neurofibromatosis 2. Neurosurgery 38:880–885; discussion 885–886, 1996.
14. Patronas NJ, Courcoutsakis N, Bromley CM, et al: Intramedullary and spinal canal tumors in patients with neurofibromatosis 2: MR imaging findings and correlation with genotype. Radiology 218:434–442, 2001.
15. Ruttledge MH, Andermann AA, Phelan CM, et al: Type of mutation in the neurofibromatosis type 2 gene (NF2) frequently determines severity of disease. Am J Hum Genet 59:331–342, 1996.
16. Seppala MT, Haltia MJ, Sankila RJ, et al: Long-term outcome after removal of spinal neurofibroma. J Neurosurg 82:572–577, 1995.
17. Seppala MT, Haltia MJ, Sankila RJ, et al: Long-term outcome after removal of spinal schwannoma: a clinicopathological study of 187 cases. J Neurosurg 83:621–626, 1995.
18. Seppala MT, Sainio MA, Haltia MJ, et al: Multiple schwannomas: schwannomatosis or neurofibromatosis type 2? J Neurosurg 89:36–41, 1998.
19. Thakkar SD, Feigen U, Mautner VF: Spinal tumours in neurofibromatosis type 1: an MRI study of frequency, multiplicity and variety. Neuroradiology 41:625–629, 1999.
20. Woodruff JM: Pathology of tumors of the peripheral nerve sheath in type 1 neurofibromatosis. Am J Med Genet 89:23–30, 1999.

CHAPTER 64

SPINAL MENINGIOMAS

Aaron A. Cohen-Gadol and William E. Krauss

Meningiomas are the second-most common intradural, extramedullary spinal cord tumor, following schwannomas. Spinal meningiomas account for 25% of all primary intraspinal neoplasms and 12% of all meningiomas.[21,22] These tumors more commonly occur in women, usually from their fourth through seventh decades of life. Typically, they are well circumscribed and slow growing. They have a low propensity for recurrence after initial removal[21]; however, spinal meningiomas in younger patients are more likely to have an aggressive clinical course.[2,4,6,19] Ionizing radiation and trauma are risk factors for the later development of spinal meningiomas.[9,13]

Horsley pioneered intradural resection of benign spinal lesions when he removed a benign growth from a patient diagnosed by Gowers in 1887.[8] Later, in 1938, Cushing and Eisenhart advocated spinal meningioma surgery because "a successful operation for a spinal meningioma represents one of the most gratifying of all operative procedures."[5] Technologic advances in microsurgical techniques and neuroimaging have led to the early diagnosis and safe removal of spinal meningiomas, leading to improved surgical outcomes.

DIAGNOSIS

Definitive diagnosis of a spinal meningioma is based on histopathologic examination of tumor tissue. Before surgery, clinical, radiographic, and intraoperative findings may aid in the diagnosis of a spinal meningioma. Common symptoms are localized back pain and extremity sensory changes followed by weakness, leading to gait instability (Table 64-1).[12,14,16,23] Neurologic examination demonstrates varied patterns of a spastic myelopathy with paraparesis or tetraparesis depending on the level of the tumor. Spinal meningiomas less commonly cause radiculopathy than nerve sheath tumors.[17] Sphincter disturbances are a late manifestation seen in 15% to 40% of patients.[17] A Brown-Sequard syndrome is uncommon. Rarely, spinal meningiomas may have signs and symptoms of increased intracranial pressure such as headache and papilledema. This has been postulated to be secondary to blockage of cerebrospinal fluid (CSF) absorption, presumably because of elevated protein levels from the tumor. Venous obstruction or repeated hemorrhage are other mechanisms for increased intracranial pressure (ICP) in these patients.[1]

Mild neurologic deficits are present in 70% of patients; 30% have severe neurologic deficits.[23] The slow growth of spinal meningiomas and their variety of symptoms can cause their initial diagnosis to be delayed by several months to years.

This delay may postpone definitive treatment. Some patients may undergo inappropriate surgery, resulting in poor outcomes.[12] The natural history justifies prompt surgical resection. Most patients with untreated tumors have a progressive course of neurologic worsening and some have a rapid decline.[3,17,23] Compromise of the spinal cord vascular supply by tumor mass or edema may cause acute or subacute neurologic deterioration.

LOCATION AND SUBTYPES

Spinal meningiomas most commonly occur in the thoracic spine (80%), cervical tumors are less common (17%), and lumbar tumors are rare (3%).[3,10,11,17,20,23] However, males have equal incidence of spinal meningiomas in the cervical and thoracic spine.[17] Many cervical tumors are located anterior to the cord.[17] Presumably because of the higher concentration of arachnoid villi around the nerve root exit site, spinal meningiomas are most commonly found near the nerve root without involving the root directly. This explains their typical presentation with myelopathy, not radiculopathy. This is in contrast with schwannomas, which by definition involve a nerve root.[3,17,20,23] Up to 15% of spinal meningiomas may have extradural components.[7] Tumors that have anterior location, significant calcification, extradural extension, or en plaque features are more difficult to remove. This subset of tumors is associated with less favorable surgical outcomes.[17] Recurrent tumors pose similar risks.

The most common histologic subtype of spinal meningioma is the meningotheliomatous (syncytial) followed by the transitional variety.[10,17] Compared with their intracranial counterparts, they have more psammomatous changes and are less likely to be calcified. Malignant subtypes are rare.

PREOPERATIVE IMAGING

Plain x-rays are of limited value and may show reversal of normal spine curvatures, scoliosis, pedicle erosion, or tumor calcification.[17] Computed tomography (CT) with myelography will show classic findings of an extramedullary intradural mass. There may be a contrast block at the level of the tumor. Magnetic resonance imaging (MRI) remains the ideal imaging modality, because it accurately defines the tumor location with respect to the spinal cord. The multiplanar capabilities of MRI are essential in determining the proper surgical approach and assessing surgical risk. The typical spinal meningioma is isoin-

TABLE 64-1

Most Common Symptoms in a Large Series of Spinal Meningiomas

Symptoms	Cases (%)
Pain (focal or radicular)	72
Paresthesias	32
Cold sensations	6
Hot sensations	3
Numbness	33
Weakness	66
Sphincter dysfunction	40
Chest pain	5

tense to spinal cord on T1 and T2 sequences. It enhances uniformly with gadolinium infusion and may have a dural tail (Figure 64-1). Meningiomas may not be differentiated from schwannomas solely based on MRI findings.

SURGICAL TREATMENT AND OUTCOME

Corticosteroids are given preoperatively and continued during the immediate postoperative period. The risks of surgery include transient or permanent neurologic worsening (10%) and other medical complications, chiefly pulmonary embolism (2% to 3%).[17] Patients with multiple meningiomas or a clinical suspicion of neurofibromatosis should be evaluated by a geneticist. This may require further MRI of the brain and spinal cord seeking additional tumors. The imaging study that led to a referral for surgery may not show the symptomatic lesion in a patient harboring multiple tumors.

A safe gross-total resection of the tumor is the foremost goal of surgery. Most spinal meningiomas are benign and slow growing with a low rate of recurrence; therefore the goal of a

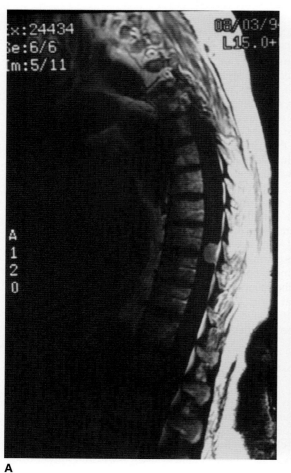

A

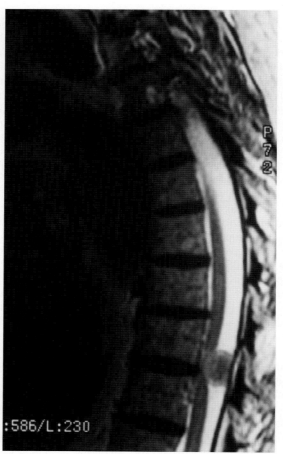

B

FIGURE 64-1   *A,* Sagittal contrast-enhanced spinal magnetic resonance (MR) image reveals a homogeneously enhancing extramedullary lesion with dural tails, consistent with a meningioma. *B,* Sagittal T2-weighted spinal MR image reveals this tumor, compressing the spinal cord.

gross-total resection may be relaxed if doing so places an elderly patient at high risk of intraoperative neurologic injury. Somatosensory or motor-evoked potentials may provide some indication of spinal cord functional status during surgery. Almost all spinal meningiomas may be resected through a posterior laminectomy, because their slow growth allows them to reach a significant size before causing neurologic symptoms. This growth pattern displaces the cord laterally, providing access to the posterior surface of the tumor via appropriate posterior bony removal. More ventrally positioned tumors may require a posterolateral approach[18] or pediculectomy to ensure safe tumor removal without cord retraction. Following tumor excision, spinal arthrodesis may be necessary if extensive bony removal has compromised spinal stability.

A midline durotomy is performed above the rostral aspect of the tumor (Figure 64-2). The surgeon uses the operating microscope for the remainder of the procedure. In most cases of anterior tumors, it is necessary to cut the dentate ligaments to allow adequate access to the tumor. On rare occasions, it may be necessary to divide a noneloquent nerve root to provide tumor access. Initially, the tumor is debulked. An ultrasonic aspirator is very helpful at this stage of the procedure. After adequate debulking, the tumor is involuted and rolled away from its interface with the spinal cord. The segment of the dura infiltrated with tumor may be resected if technically feasible; otherwise, extensive electrocautery of the involved dural

surface is performed. Cauterization of the dura instead of resection has not been associated with a higher recurrence rate.[12,23] Following the completion of tumor resection, the dura and the rest of the wound is closed in anatomic layers. Surgical treatment can have neurologic sequelae.

Postoperative neurologic improvement has been noted in 50% to 80% of patients in large series.[3,17,23] Outcomes are favorable even in the case of patients with paraplegia.[17] Features of en plaque tumors such as significant arachnoid scarring and invasion of the spinal cord parenchyma prevent complete resection. Extradural tumors can have unfavorable prognosis because of their invasiveness and their vascular nature and aggressive clinical course.[17] Predictors of poor outcome also include long duration of symptoms before diagnosis, profound neurologic deficits, subtotal tumor removal, and old age.[24]

FOLLOW-UP AND RECURRENCE

Patients undergo repeat spinal MRI 3 months after surgery. The extent of resection will be assessed at that time, and this information will be used as a baseline to compare future findings on repeat imaging (tumor recurrence versus postoperative changes). We prefer to obtain MRI scans every 1 to 2 years for the first 10 years after surgery or when the patient has new symptoms. Afterward, imaging may be performed less commonly and based on a case by case basis. In patients older than 75 years, we do not reimage the previous tumor site unless warranted by clinical change or aggressive tumor pathology.

The recurrence rate for spinal meningiomas has been reported to be 6% to 15%.[14,23] Up to 37% of patients with en plaque tumors may experience tumor recurrence.[14]

ADJUVANT THERAPIES

Radiation therapy has a limited role in the treatment of slow-growing spinal meningiomas. Even subtotally resected tumors may not change size over time.[17] Therefore the use of radiation therapy needs to be individualized and may be a more appropriate treatment for tumors with a malignant clinical course or histopathologically atypical findings. We recommend additional surgery for recurrent tumors and reserve the use of radiation therapy for tumors that show early regrowth if reoperation carries significant surgical or medical risks. Spinal metastasis of intracranial meningiomas may occur but are extremely rare. Radiation therapy has proved efficacious in the treatment of such malignant tumors.[15]

CONCLUSION

Surgical resection remains the definitive therapy for spinal meningiomas. Complete resection at the first operation offers the best opportunity for cure and is associated with excellent prognosis. Spinal meningiomas with en plaque or extradural features are infiltrative and have a high rate of recurrence. Close follow-up may be necessary to assess for early tumor regrowth. The use of radiation therapy in the treatment of spinal meningiomas is limited. Tumors with malignant features may be considered for this mode of therapy.

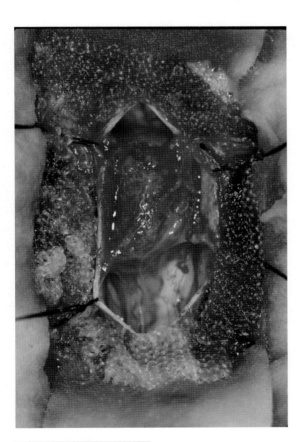

FIGURE 64-2 Intraoperative picture of a posteriorly located spinal meningioma after a durotomy (see Figure 64-1). The spinal cord is visualized anteriorly (underneath the tumor).

References

1. Arseni C, Maretsis M: Tumors of the lower spinal canal associated with increased intracranial pressure and papilledema. J Neurosurg 27:105–110, 1967.
2. Chan RC, Thopson GB: Intracranial meningiomas in childhood. Surg Neurol 21:319–322, 1984.
3. Ciapetta D, Domenicucci M, Raco A: Spinal meningiomas: prognosis and recovery factors in 22 cases with severe motor deficits. Acta Neurol Scand 77:27–30, 1988.
4. Cohen-Gadol AA, Zikel OM, Koch CA, et al: Spinal meningiomas in patients younger than 50 years of age: a 21-year experience. J Neurosurg 98:258–263, 2003.
5. Cushing H, Eisenhardt L: Meningiomas: Their Classification, Regional Behavior, Life History and Surgical Results. Springfield, Ill, Charles C. Thomas, 1938.
6. Deen Jr HG, Scheithauer BW, Ebersold MJ: Clinical and pathological study of the first two decades of life. J Neurosurg 317–322, 1982.
7. Gezen F, Kahraman S, Canakci Z, et al: Review of 36 cases of spinal cord meningiomas. Spine 25:727–731, 2000.
8. Gowers W, Horsley V: A case of the tumor of the spinal cord. Removal. Recovery. Med Chir Trans 71:377–428, 1888.
9. Harrison MJ, Wolfe DE, Tai-Shing L: Radiation-induced meningiomas: experience at the Mount Sinai Hospital and review of the literature. J Neurosurg 75:565–574, 1991.
10. Iraci G, Peserico L, Salar G: Intraspinal neurinomas and meningiomas. Int Surg 56:289–303, 1971.
11. Katz K, Reichental F, Isreali J: Surgical treatment of spinal meningiomas. Neurochirurgia 24:21–22, 1981.
12. King A, Sharr M, Gullan R, et al: Spinal meningiomas: a 20-year review. Br J Neurosurg 12:521–526, 1998.
13. Kleinschmidt-Demasters BK, Lillehei KO: Radiation-induced meningioma with a 63-year latency period. J Neurosurg 82:487–488, 1995.
14. Klekamp J, Samii M: Surgical results for spinal meningiomas. Surg Neurol 52:552–562, 1999.
15. Lee TT, Landy HJ: Spinal metastases of malignant intracranial meningioma. Surg Neurol 50:437–441, 1998.
16. Levy W, Bay J, Dohn D: Spinal cord meningiomas. J Neurosurg 57:804–812, 1982.
17. Levy WJ, Bay J, Dohn D: Spinal cord meningioma. J Neurosurg 57:804–812, 1982.
18. McCormick PC: Surgical management of dumbbell and paraspinal tumors of the thoracic and lumbar spine. Neurosurgery 38:67–75, 1996.
19. Merten DF, Gooding CA, Newton TH, et al: Meningiomas of childhood and adolescence. J Pediatr 84:696–700, 1974.
20. Rasmussen T, Kernohan J, Adson A: Pathologic classification, with surgical consideration of intraspinal tumors. Ann Surg 111:513–530, 1940.
21. Rubinstein LJ: Tumors of the Central Nervous System. Atlas of Tumor Pathology. Washington, DC, Armed Forces Institute of Pathology, 1972.
22. Slooff J, Kernohan J, MacCarty C: Primary intramedullary tumors of the spinal cord and filum terminale. Philadelphia, WB Saunders, 1964.
23. Solero CL, Fornari M, Giombini S, et al: Spinal meningiomas: review of 174 operated cases. Neurosurgery 25:153–160, 1989.
24. Souweudane MM, Benjamin V: Spinal cord meningiomas. Neurosurg Clin N Am 5:283–291, 1994.

CHAPTER 65

MYXOPAPILLARY EPENDYMOMAS

Ian F. Parney and Andrew T. Parsa

Myxopapillary ependymomas are a histopathologic variant thought to arise from primitive ependymal rests in the lumbosacral region. This chapter addresses the epidemiology, pathology, clinical presentation, imaging findings, management, and outcome for patients with myxopapillary ependymomas.

EPIDEMIOLOGY

Myxopapillary ependymomas are rare. In pathologic studies, they have constituted only 5% of intramedullary spinal cord tumors and 15% of spinal ependymomas.[14] In clinical series, they have accounted for a slightly larger percentage of spinal ependymomas (18% to 55%)[10,20,23,27] but remain relatively uncommon. They often occur in young adults, but this is not universal. Sonneland and colleagues reported that mean age at presentation was 36.4 years (range 6 to 82 years) in a series of 77 patients with myxopapillary ependymoma. In larger series, men appear to be affected more often than women (male-female ratio 1.7 to 2:1).[4,25] Predisposing conditions that increase the risk of developing a myxopapillary ependymoma have not been identified.

LOCATION, HISTOPATHOLOGY, AND MOLECULAR ABNORMALITIES

Myxopapillary ependymomas typically are intradural extramedullary lesions originating from the filum terminale within the lumbosacral thecal sac.[28] They are usually solitary and arise from the filum (65%) or filum and conus medullaris (30%)[25]; however, they can be disseminated in the spinal canal or even intracranially at presentation.[24,28] They may also involve the extradural sacrococcygeal bone or soft tissues through direct extension of an intradural tumor or as a subcutaneous mass in the sacrococcygeal region, with no clear connection to the thecal sac.[3,9,16]

Grossly, they are characteristically ovoid tumors with a delicate fibrous capsule situated within the filum terminale. Microscopically, papillae lined with cuboidal epithelium surrounding myxoid fibrovascular cores are seen.[16,25] The myxoid cores give the tumor a mucinous appearance. Pseudorosettes may be observed. Degenerative changes (microvascular hyalinization, thrombosis, hemorrhage, and hemosiderin) are com-

monly encountered. Glial fibrillary acidic protein stains are largely negative in cuboidal epithelial cells but may be positive in fibrillated ependymal cells. Neurofilament stains are negative, although S-100 and neuron-specific enolase stains are occasionally weakly positive.

Myxopapillary ependymomas do not appear to be associated with any particular risk factors or genetic syndromes. However, specific cytogenetic and molecular abnormalities have been described in myxopapillary ependymomas. These are distinct from other ependymomas. For example, myxopapillary ependymomas often have imbalanced ploidy or loss of chromosome 10q/10.[4] This distinguishes them from classic cellular spinal and intracranial ependymomas in adults, which are less likely to have chromosome 10q loss, and from childhood intracranial ependymomas, which are also more likely to have balanced ploidy.[4] Myxopapillary ependymomas have also been reported to have relative overexpression of the oncogene bcl-2 compared with other ependymoma subtypes.[18] Primary subcutaneous sacrococcygeal extradural myxopapillary ependymomas may also have a unique genetic phenotype and have been reported to have clonal telomeric fusions leading to fusion of numerous chromosomes.[19]

CLINICAL PRESENTATION

Back pain with or without a radicular component is the most common symptom and has been reported in more than 90% of patients.[21,25] Sensorimotor impairment (26% to 53%) and sphincter disturbance (20% to 36%) occur less often. Symptoms (particularly back pain) are insidious and nonspecific. A long interval between symptom onset and diagnosis is not uncommon as a result. In older pre–magnetic-resonance-imaging-era studies, a significant minority of patients underwent lumbar spinal surgery for decompression or fusion to treat pain that was subsequently attributed to the myxopapillary ependymoma.

Other presentations are uncommon. Myxopapillary ependymomas may bleed and even present with lumbar subarachnoid hemorrhage.[1] Patients with rare primary subcutaneous myxopapillary ependymomas may have a subcutaneous mass in the sacrococcygeal region.[9,16] This is often mistaken for a dermoid tumor or even for a myelomeningocele initially. Magnetic resonance imaging (MRI) usually clarifies the diagnostic considerations.

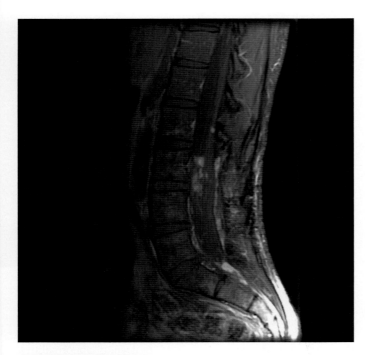

FIGURE 65-1 Sagittal postcontrast T1-weighted magnetic resonance image of the lumbar spine of a 22-year-old man with multiple enhancing intradural extramedullary masses from a myxopapillary ependymoma that was disseminated within the lumbosacral thecal sac.

IMAGING FINDINGS

MRI is the imaging test of choice. Tumors are typically intradural, extramedullary, and located in the lumbosacral region. They are typically hyperintense on T2-weighted images and enhance with gadolinium infusion. Kahan and colleagues reported that myxopapillary ependymomas were typically hyperintense on T1-weighted images and speculated that this reflected their mucinous nature[12]; however, this finding is not universal, and others have reported that myxopapillary ependymomas may be hypointense, isointense, or hyperintense on T1.[28] Typical MRI findings for a patient with a myxopapillary ependymoma are shown in Figure 65-1.

Imaging studies should include staging MRI of the entire neuraxis including brain. Computed tomography may be helpful to visualize bony anatomy for patients with osteolytic sacral involvement.[3] Myelograms typically show complete block,[25] but these studies are rarely performed in the MRI era.

MANAGEMENT

Surgery

Surgical resection is generally recommended, particularly for isolated symptomatic lesions. This allows confirmation of the histopathologic diagnosis. Gross-total resection is associated with decreased recurrence rates and better prognosis than subtotal resection[21,25,27]; however, gross total resection is achieved in only 22% to 42% of cases.[4,7,25,27] This is a lower percentage than classic cellular spinal ependymomas, which are amenable to gross-total resection in up to 97%.[7] Lower gross-total resection rates for myxopapillary ependymomas compared with other spinal ependymomas probably reflect their intimate involvement with cauda equina nerve roots and their propensity to be disseminated in the neuraxis at diagnosis.

Data on perioperative outcome are limited. Schweitzer and Batzdorf reported outcome in a series of 15 patients with cauda equina ependymomas, 10 of which were myxopapillary ependymomas. In this series, 27% had increased postoperative neurologic deficits, and 7% had regional complications.[21] Patients were symptom free or, for 75%, had only minor symptoms that did not affect activities of daily living if they had isolated pain preoperatively. This was reduced to 50% in patients with preoperative pain and neurologic deficit but intact sphincter control and was 0% if sphincter disturbance was present before surgery.

In addition to surgery for diagnosis and cytoreduction, there may be a role for spinal stabilization in select cases. As discussed previously, myxopapillary ependymomas can occasionally invade and erode bony structures in the lumbosacral region.[3] This may result in spinal instability, leading to pain and neurologic deficits that are best addressed by spinal instrumentation and fusion.[11]

Radiation

Radiation therapy's role in the management of patients with myxopapillary ependymomas is not well defined. Interpreting the literature is confounded by the fact that most published studies concerning radiation for spinal ependymomas have not clearly distinguished between myxopapillary ependymomas and classic cellular ependymomas.[10,20–22,26,27] Furthermore, most of the reported series are based on patients diagnosed and treated more than 15 years ago (in some cases more than 75 years ago).[20–22,25–27] Radiation therapy and imaging techniques have changed substantially since then, and extrapolation to the modern era is difficult.

Most authors agree that patients undergoing gross-total resection should be followed with serial imaging, deferring radiation to recurrence.[10,21,25–27] In contrast, Schild and Shaw at the Mayo Clinic have suggested that all patients with spinal ependymomas should be considered for postoperative radiation regardless of extent of resection.[20,22] However, even these authors allow that the benign natural history for low-grade tumors such as myxopapillary ependymomas may lend itself to watchful waiting after gross-total resection. For patients with subtotal resection, most authors recommend local radiation to the tumor at a dose between 45 Gy and 55 Gy.[10,20–22,27] Craniospinal irradiation is usually reserved for patients with widespread neuraxis dissemination, although Wen and colleagues proposed expanding radiation ports for spinal ependymomas to include the entire thecal sac if tumors had been resected in a piecemeal fashion.[27]

Limited data are available on early postradiation outcome. Waldron and colleagues reported that nausea was the most common side effect among spinal ependymoma patients receiving radiation and was particularly common among patients receiving craniospinal axis radiation.[26] In this series of 59 patients (16 myxopapillary ependymomas), no patients developed radiation-induced myelopathy. Similarly, no patients developed radiation-induced myelopathy in Schweitzer and Batzdorf's series of eight cauda equina region ependymoma patients receiving postoperative radiation.[21] Clover and colleagues reported that eight of nine spinal cord ependymoma patients (seven myxopapillary ependymomas) receiving postoperative radiation therapy improved neurologically following radiation.[10]

Myxopapillary ependymomas can occur in children.[6] Radiation to the neuraxis in children presents particular difficulties because of potential growth inhibition. As a result, radiation is generally used more sparingly and only when there is residual disease.[15] However, more aggressive radiation treatment, including craniospinal axis irradiation, has been reported in children with disseminated myxopapillary ependymomas.[8]

Chemotherapy

Chemotherapy is seldom employed in the treatment of patients with myxopapillary ependymomas and is reserved almost exclusively for patients with recurrent disease.[2] Case reports of etoposide, cisplatin, and tamoxifen treatment for recurrent myxopapillary ependymomas have appeared in the literature with varying degrees of success.[13,21] Slightly more data are available to support the use of etoposide in patients with recurrent classic cellular spinal ependymomas,[5] but the validity of extrapolating these data to myxopapillary ependymomas is uncertain.

OUTCOME

In general, myxopapillary ependymomas are low-grade lesions and are believed to have a good prognosis[20,25]; however, as Clover and colleagues have pointed out, many long-term survivors with myxopapillary ependymomas live with persistent or recurrent disease.[10] Patients with multiple recurrences appear to be more at risk for spinal instability or for systemic metastases, although neither of these events is common.[11,17]

In the largest published series of myxopapillary ependymomas, Sonneland and colleagues at the Mayo Clinic reported that patients with encapsulated tumors amenable to gross-total resection had a recurrence rate of 10%, and those undergoing piecemeal or subtotal resection recurred in 19%.[25] Gross-total resection was associated with a mean survival of 19 years compared with 14 years for subtotal resection. Time to recurrence ranged from 2 to 15 years. Of 77 patients, 5 (6.5%) in this series died from their disease, in all cases after a prolonged course marked by multiple recurrences. It should be noted that this series includes patients encountered during a 60-year period, from 1924 to 1983, and does not necessarily represent modern outcomes. Indeed, Schild et al reported 100% survival at 15 years for 12 myxopapillary ependymoma patients treated with surgery and radiation therapy at the Mayo Clinic after 1963.[20]

CONCLUSION

Myxopapillary ependymomas are rare tumors arising in the lumbosacral region, most commonly in young adults. They present primarily with either local back pain or radicular pain, and other neurologic deficits are less common. Gross-total resection is associated with better outcome but (in contrast to classic cellular spinal ependymomas) is often not possible. Local radiation to the tumor is generally recommended for subtotally resected tumors. Chemotherapy has a limited role in myxopapillary ependymoma management.

References

1. Argyropoulou PI, Argyropoulou MI, Tsampoulas C, et al: Myxopapillary ependymoma of the conus medullaris with subarachnoid haemorrhage: MRI in two cases. Neuroradiology 43: 489–491, 2001.
2. Balmaceda C: Chemotherapy for intramedullary spinal cord tumors. J Neurooncol 47:293–307, 2000.
3. Biagini R, Demitri S, Orsini U, et al: Osteolytic extra-axial sacral myxopapillary ependymoma. Skeletal Radiol 28:584–589, 1999.
4. Carter M, Nicholson J, Ross F, et al: Genetic abnormalities detected in ependymomas by comparative genomic hybridisation. Br J Cancer 86:929–939, 2002.
5. Chamberlain MC: Salvage chemotherapy for recurrent spinal cord ependymoma. Cancer 95:997–1002, 2002.
6. Chan HS, Becker LE, Hoffman HJ, et al: Myxopapillary ependymoma of the filum terminale and cauda equina in childhood: report of seven cases and review of the literature. Neurosurgery 14:204–210, 1984.
7. Chang UK, Choe WJ, Chung SK, et al: Surgical outcome and prognostic factors of spinal intramedullary ependymomas in adults. J Neurooncol 57:133–139, 2002.
8. Chinn DM, Donaldson SS, Dahl GV, et al: Management of children with metastatic spinal myxopapillary ependymoma using craniospinal irradiation. Med Pediatr Oncol 35:443–445, 2000.
9. Chung JY, Lee SK, Yang KH, et al: Subcutaneous sacrococcygeal myxopapillary ependymoma. AJNR Am J Neuroradiol 20: 344–346, 1999.
10. Clover LL, Hazuka MB, Kinzie JJ: Spinal cord ependymomas treated with surgery and radiation therapy. A review of 11 cases. Am J Clin Oncol 16:350–353, 1993.
11. Fourney DR, Prabhu SS, Cohen ZR, et al: Thoracolumbopelvic stabilization for the treatment of instability caused by recurrent myxopapillary ependymoma. J Spinal Disord Tech 16:108–111, 2003.
12. Kahan H, Sklar EM, Post MJ, et al: MR characteristics of histopathologic subtypes of spinal ependymoma. AJNR Am J Neuroradiol 17:143–150, 1996.
13. Madden JR, Fenton LZ, Weil M, et al: Experience with tamoxifen/etoposide in the treatment of a child with myxopapillary ependymoma. Med Pediatr Oncol 37:67–69, 2001.
14. Miller DC: Surgical pathology of intramedullary spinal cord neoplasms. J Neurooncol 47:189–194, 2000.
15. Nagib MG, O'Fallon MT: Myxopapillary ependymoma of the conus medullaris and filum terminale in the pediatric age group. Pediatr Neurosurg 26:2–7, 1997.
16. Rao IS, Kapila K, Aggarwal S, et al: Subcutaneous myxopapillary ependymoma presenting as a childhood sacrococcygeal tumor: a case report. Diagn Cytopathol 27:303–307, 2002.
17. Rickert CH, Kedziora O, Gullotta F: Ependymoma of the cauda equina. acta Neurochir (Wien) 141:781–782, 1999.
18. Rushing EJ, Brown DF, Hladik CL, et al: Correlation of bcl-2, p53, and MIB-1 expression with ependymoma grade and subtype. Mod Pathol 11:464–470, 1998.

19. Sawyer JR, Miller JP, Ellison DA: Clonal telomeric fusions and chromosome instability in a subcutaneous sacrococcygeal myxopapillary ependymoma. Cancer Genet Cytogenet 100:169–175, 1998.

20. Schild SE, Nisi K, Scheithauer BW, et al: The results of radiotherapy for ependymomas: the Mayo Clinic experience. Int J Radiat Oncol Biol Phys 42:953–958, 1998.

21. Schweitzer JS, Batzdorf U: Ependymoma of the cauda equina region: diagnosis, treatment, and outcome in 15 patients. Neurosurgery 30:202–207, 1992.

22. Shaw EG, Evans RG, Scheithauer BW, et al: Radiotherapeutic management of adult intraspinal ependymomas. Int J Radiat Oncol Biol Phys 12:323–327, 1986.

23. Shirato H, Kamada T, Hida K, et al: The role of radiotherapy in the management of spinal cord glioma. Int J Radiat Oncol Biol Phys 33:323–328, 1995.

24. Smyth MD, Pitts L, Jackler RK, et al: Metastatic spinal ependymoma presenting as a vestibular schwannoma. Case illustration. J Neurosurg 92:247, 2000.

25. Sonneland PR, Scheithauer BW, Onofrio BM: Myxopapillary ependymoma. A clinicopathologic and immunocytochemical study of 77 cases. Cancer 56:883–893, 1985.

26. Waldron JN, Laperriere NJ, Jaakkimainen L, et al: Spinal cord ependymomas: a retrospective analysis of 59 cases. Int J Radiat Oncol Biol Phys 27:223–229, 1993.

27. Wen BC, Hussey DH, Hitchon PW, et al: The role of radiation therapy in the management of ependymomas of the spinal cord. Int J Radiat Oncol Biol Phys 20:781–786, 1991.

28. Wippold FJ II, Smirniotopoulos JG, Moran CJ, et al: MR imaging of myxopapillary ependymoma: findings and value to determine extent of tumor and its relation to intraspinal structures. AJR Am J Roentgenol 165:1263–1267, 1995.

CHAPTER 66

INTRAMEDULLARY
EPENDYMOMAS

Theodore Schwartz, Andrew T. Parsa, and Paul C. McCormick

EPIDEMIOLOGY

Intramedullary ependymomas are the most common spinal cord tumor in adults, representing 34.5% of all central nervous system (CNS) ependymomas and approximately 60% of all intramedullary tumors.[10,17,23] They occur throughout life but more often in the middle adult years. Men and women are equally affected.[16] Approximately 65% will have associated syrinxes, particularly when the tumor appears in cervical locations.[19] Although the cervical cord represents only 22.5% of spinal cord tissue, approximately 68% of spinal cord tumors arise from, or extend into, the cervical cord.[15]

A variety of histologic subtypes may be encountered. The cellular ependymoma is the most common, but epithelial, tanacytic (fibrillar), malignant, subependymoma, myxopapillary, or mixed examples may occur. The myxopapillary subtype is almost exclusively observed in the filum terminale or conus and, as such, is classified as an extramedullary tumor.[23] Nearly all are histologically benign.[2,5,16–18] Although unencapsulated, these glial-derived tumors are usually well circumscribed and do not infiltrate adjacent spinal cord tissue.

CLINICAL PRESENTATION AND DIAGNOSIS

The clinical features of intramedullary ependymomas are variable. The classic central cord syndrome consisting of a dissociated suspended sensory loss with descending progression, symmetric upper extremity mixed upper and lower neuron motor weakness, and bilateral spastic lower extremities is rarely seen.[7] Early symptoms are usually nonspecific and may only subtly progress. Symptom duration before diagnosis is often in the range of 3 to 4 years, although intratumoral hemorrhage may precipitate a rapid decline.[4,16] Sensory symptoms, in particular dysesthesias, are the earliest to occur in upward of 70% of patients.[2,4,5,11,14,20] Painful aching sensations localized to the level of the tumor are rarely radicular and may also occur early in disease progression.[15]

The distribution and progression of the symptoms are related to tumor location. Upper extremity symptoms predominate with cervical neoplasms. Thoracic cord tumors produce spasticity and sensory disturbances in the lower extremities.[15] Numbness is a common complaint and typically begins distally

in the legs with proximal progression. Tumors of the lumbar enlargement often cause back and leg pain. The leg pain may be radicular in nature. Urogenital and anorectal dysfunction tend to occur early. Weakness usually occurs late in disease progression, is usually asymmetric, and indicates that the tumor has significantly thinned the surrounding spinal cord to a few millimeters.[5]

SURGICAL OBJECTIVES

The role of surgery in the management of intramedullary ependymomas has evolved significantly in recent years. Once employed for diagnosis alone, surgery now represents the most effective treatment for this benign, well-circumscribed tumor.[2,4,5,11,15,16] Because the majority of intramedullary spinal cord neoplasms are low-grade lesions, long-term tumor control or cure with preservation of neurologic function can be achieved in most patients with microsurgical removal alone.[1,4,5,11,15,16] The most important factor in determining the surgical objective is the plane between the tumor and the spinal cord. This interface can be accurately assessed only through an adequate myelotomy that extends over the entire rostral caudal extent of the tumor. Although presence of a syrinx may improve the chances of a gross-total resection, it cannot be used as an independent predictor of outcome.[19]

Ependymomas, although unencapsulated, are noninfiltrative lesions that typically display a distinct plane. Gross-total removal is the treatment of choice in these cases for optimum disease control. Intraoperative biopsy can be useful in certain circumstances but should not be used as the sole criterion dictating the surgical objective. First, interpretation of tiny biopsy fragments often is inaccurate or nondiagnostic; the fragments may consist of only peritumoral gliosis, which may be erroneously interpreted as an infiltrating astrocytoma. Second, it is difficult if not impossible to accurately assess the nature of the tumor–spinal cord interface through a tiny myelotomy. Biopsy results, however, may be particularly helpful in some circumstances; for example, identification of a histologically malignant tumor independently signals an end to the procedure, because surgery is of no benefit for malignant intramedullary neoplasms.[1,2,12] In other cases in which the tumor–spinal cord interface may not be apparent, confident histologic identification of an ependymoma reassures the surgeon that a plane must exist and that surgical removal should continue.

A

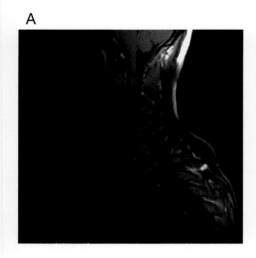

B

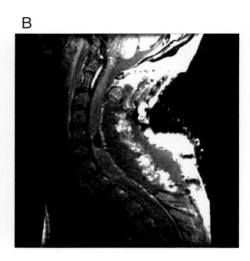

FIGURE 66-1 Preoperative *(A)* and postoperative *(B)* T1-weighted magnetic resonance image with contrast.

SURGICAL TECHNIQUE

The technique of tumor removal is determined by the surgical objective and the tumor's size and gross and histologic characteristics. If no plane is apparent between tumor and surrounding spinal cord, it is likely that an infiltrative tumor is present. Biopsy is obtained to establish a histologic diagnosis. If an infiltrating or malignant astrocytoma is identified and is consistent with the intraoperative findings, further tumor removal is not warranted. In most cases, however, a reasonably well-defined benign glial tumor will be identified. Ependymomas appear with a smooth reddish gray glistening tumor surface, which is sharply demarcated from the surrounding spinal cord. Large tumors may require internal decompression with an ultrasonic aspirator or laser.

In contrast to the ependymoma, most benign astrocytomas will present varying degrees of circumscription. Approximately one third of these patients have benign, infiltrative tumors without an identifiable tumor mass. Biopsy for diagnosis becomes the only viable surgical objective. Occasionally, an astrocytoma may be so well developed as to mimic an ependymoma. Nevertheless, astrocytomas rarely have as defined a plane as ependymomas typically do. Surgeons must rely on their own judgment and experience. Obviously, if gross tumor is easily identified, continued removal is reasonable. Changes in motor sensory evoked potentials or uncertainty of spinal cord–tumor interface should signal an end to tumor resection.

POSTOPERATIVE MANAGEMENT

Early mobilization is encouraged to prevent complications of recumbency such as deep venous thrombosis and pneumonia. Paretic patients are particularly vulnerable to thromboembolic complications. Subcutaneous heparin 5000 units twice a day is begun on the second postoperative day in these patients. Orthostatic hypotension may occasionally occur following removal of upper thoracic and cervical intramedullary neoplasms. This is usually a self-limiting problem that can be managed with liberalization of fluids and more gradual mobilization. A posterior fossa syndrome occasionally occurs following removal of a high cervical intramedullary neoplasm. This is effectively managed with steroids, although a spinal tap may be required to rule out meningitis. Complications related to wound dehiscence, infection, and cerebrospinal fluid leak are much more common in patients who have undergone prior surgery or radiation therapy.[2,15] These complications rarely resolve with conservative therapy and early reoperation is imperative to avoid exacerbation.[15]

Early and aggressive use of physical and occupational therapy will optimize functional recovery. Despite confident gross-total resection, benign intramedullary tumors present a continued risk of recurrence. Long-term clinical and radiographic follow-up is warranted in these patients. An early postoperative magnetic resonance imaging (MRI) scan—6 to 8 weeks following surgery—establishes the completeness of resection and serves as a baseline against which further studies can be compared. Serial gadolinium-enhanced MRI scans are obtained yearly, because radiographic tumor recurrence usually precedes clinical symptoms (Figure 66-1).

FUNCTIONAL OUTCOME

Most surgical series indicate that the strongest predictor of postoperative functional outcome is preoperative functional ability.[2,4,5,11,15,16] Significant improvement of a severe or long-standing preoperative neurologic deficit rarely occurs, even following technically successful surgical excision. Surgical morbidity is also greater in patients with more significant preoperative deficits. In general, most patients note sensory loss in the early postoperative period, most likely as a result of the midline myelotomy, transient edema, or vascular compromise.[5,16] These complaints are more subjective than objective in nature and can be significant even with little or no objective deficit. These deficits usually resolve within 3 months,[11] although they may not return to their preoperative baseline.[15] Additional surgical morbidity is directly related to the patient's preoperative status, the location of the tumor, and the presence of spinal cord atrophy and arachnoid scarring.[2,11,15,19] Patients with significant or long-standing deficit rarely demonstrate any significant recovery and are more likely to worsen following surgery. A shorter duration of preoperative symptoms, however, may favor improvement even in patients with a significant preoperative deficit.[11] Thoracic location has also been correlated with a decline in postoperative function,[4,11] perhaps the result of a more tenuous blood supply in this region. Appreciation of spinal cord atrophy and arachnoid scarring may indicate chronic spinal cord compression and predict poor functional outcome.[11,19] Preservation, rather than restoration, of neurologic function is the reasonable expectation for intramedullary tumor surgery. Patients who are only minimally symptomatic, therefore, derive the greatest benefit and are at the least risk of surgery for intramedullary tumors.[2,5,15,16]

ADJUVANT THERAPY

For intramedullary ependymomas, long-term outcome and risk of recurrence primarily depend on the completeness of the original resection. It has become clear that gross-total removal of benign intramedullary ependymomas more consistently provides long-term tumor control or cure than subtotal resection and radiation therapy.[4,5,11,16] Although many authors report a 100% recurrence-free survival following gross-total resection,[8,19] other authors report 5% to 10% recurrence rates.[2,9] Ependymomas are slow-growing tumors, and late recurrence can occur, even up to 12 years after surgery.[13] Nevertheless, gross-total resection is the most efficacious treatment, and most authors agree that radiation therapy is unnecessary if complete removal has been accomplished.[2,3,16,19] Subtotal resection, on the other hand, has a very high recurrence rate. Even a 99% removal can lead to tumor recurrence in up to 30% of patients despite postoperative radiation therapy, whereas a subtotal resection can lead to significant recurrence in up to 50% to 70%.[6,22] Unfortunately, these tumors are friable and often are quite adherent to the spinal cord, particularly at their polar regions, which may not allow for a microscopic total resection.

Complete removal has been reported in anywhere from 50% to 100% of intramedullary ependymomas in recent series.[2,5,16,19] The evidence to support postoperative radiation following subtotal resection is difficult to interpret, because it is largely based on studies with small patient populations, limited follow-up, and inadequate or no matched controls treated without radiation therapy. Despite these limitations, the accumulated data in these series suggests that radiation may be beneficial.[7,12,13,21] Reports of 5- and 10-year recurrence-free survivals, however, vary widely, from 60% to 100% with fractionated external-beam doses of more than 40 Gy.[7,13] At doses less than 40 Gy or at 15 years, recurrence rates approach 70% to 90%.[7,13] The presence of a dose-response curve is controversial. Doses less than 40 Gy are clearly too low,[7] but local failures have been reported with doses up to 55 Gy when risk of myelopathy becomes significant with conventional fractionation.[13,21] Craniospinal radiation is indicated only for the rare patient who has diffuse disease.[13] Although outcome is worse for this subgroup, good control rates have been reported.[13] Patients who have focal disease usually recur locally and do not manifest late dissemination.[7,13] We recommend adjuvant radiation for malignant ependymomas and the rare benign lesion that cannot be totally resected.

CONCLUSION

Intramedullary ependymomas are rare but constitute the majority of intramedullary glial neoplasms in adults. These tumors are benign, slow-growing lesions that are optimally treated with gross-total surgical resection without adjuvant therapy. Postoperative functional outcome is related to preoperative functional status; therefore early diagnosis before symptomatic progression is critical to their successful treatment. Adjuvant therapy is indicated for the rare malignant or disseminated tumor or following subtotal resection.

References

1. Cohen AR, Wisoff JH, Allen JC, Epstein FJ: Malignant astrocytomas of the spinal cord. J Neurosurg 70:50–54, 1989.
2. Cooper PR: Outcome after operative treatment of intramedullary spinal cord tumors in adults: intermediate and long-term results in 51 patients. Neurosurgery 25:855–859, 1989.
3. Cooper PR, Epstein F: Radical resection of intramedullary spinal cord tumors in adults. Recent experience in 29 patients. J Neurosurg 63:492–499, 1985.
4. Cristante L, Herrmann H-D: Surgical management of intramedullary spinal cord tumors: functional outcome and sources of morbidity. Neurosurgery 35:69–76, 1994.
5. Epstein FJ, Farmer J-P, Freed D: Adult intramedullary spinal cord ependymomas: the result of surgery in 38 patients. J Neurosurg 79:204–209, 1993.
6. Evans DGR, Huson SM, Donnai D, et al: A genetic study of type 2 neurofibromatosis in the United Kingdom: I – Prevalence, mutation rate, fitness, and confirmation of maternal transmission effect on severity. J Med Genet 29:841–846, 1992.
7. Garcia DM: Primary spinal cord tumors treated with surgery and postoperative irradiation. Int J Radiat Oncol Biol Phys 11:1933–1939, 1985.
8. Greenwood JJ: Intramedullary tumors of the spinal cord. A follow-up study after total surgical removal. J Neurosurg 20:665–668, 1963.
9. Guidetti B, Mercuri S, Vaonozzi R: Long-term results of the surgical treatment of 129 intramedullary spinal gliomas. J Neurosurg 54:323–330, 1981.
10. Helseth A, Mørk SJ: Primary intraspinal neoplasms in Norway, 1955–1986. A population-based survey of 467 patients. J Neurosurg 71:842–845, 1989.
11. Hoshimaru M, Koyama T, Hashimmoto N, Kikuchi H: Results of microsurgical treatment for intramedullary spinal cord ependymomas: analysis of 36 cases. Neurosurgery 44:264–269, 1999.
12. Kopelson G, Linggood RM: Intramedullary spinal cord astrocytoma versus glioblastoma. The prognostic importance of histologic grade. Cancer 50:732–735, 1982
13. Linstadt DE, Wara WM, Leibel SA, et al: Postoperative radiotherapy of primary spinal cord tumors. Int J Radiat Oncol Biol Phys 16:1397–1403, 1989.
14. McCormick PC, Post KD, Stein BM: Intradural extramedullary tumors in adults. Neurosurg Clin North Am 1:591–608, 1990.

15. McCormick PC, Stein BM: Intramedullary tumors in adults. Neurosurg Clin North Am 1:609–630, 1990.
16. McCormick PC, Torres R, Post KD, Stein BM: Intramedullary ependymoma of the spinal cord. J Neurosurg 72:523–533, 1990.
17. Mørk SJ, Løken AC: Ependymoma. A follow-up study of 101 cases. Cancer 40:907–915, 1977.
18. Russell DS, Rubenstein LJ: Pathology of Tumors of the Nervous System. Baltimore, Williams & Wilkins, 1989.
19. Samii M, Klekamp J: Surgical results of 100 intramedullary tumors in relation to accompanying syringomyelia. Neurosurgery 35:865–873, 1994.
20. Sandler HM, Papadopoulos SM, Thuntan AF, Ross DA: Spinal cord astrocytoma: results of therapy. Neurosurgery 30:490–493, 1999.
21. Shaw EG, Evans RG, Scheithauer BW, et al: Radiotherapeutic management of adult intraspinal ependymomas. Int J Radiat Oncol Bio Phys 12:323–327, 1986.
22. Sloof JL, Kernohan JW, McCarthy CS: Primary Intramedullary Tumors of the Spinal Cord and Filum Terminale. Philadelphia, WB Saunders, 1964.
23. Sonneland PRL, Scheithauer BW, Onofrio BM: Myxopapillary ependymoma. A clinicopathologic and immunocytochemical study of 77 cases. Cancer 56:883–893, 1985.

CHAPTER *67*

SPINAL CORD ASTROCYTOMAS: PRESENTATION, MANAGEMENT, AND OUTCOME

Ira M. Goldstein and John K. Houten

EPIDEMIOLOGY AND PATHOLOGY

Intramedullary spinal cord tumors (IMSCTs) are neoplasms that arise from the substance of the spinal cord and occur with one tenth the incidence of intracranial neoplasms—approximately 3 to 10 per 100,000 individuals.[13,28] Astrocytomas constitute 6% to 8% of all spinal cord tumors.[24] These are rare lesions that affect individuals of all ages, although they arise more commonly in the pediatric population and are seldom reported in individuals older than age 60. Astrocytomas are the most common histologic type of IMSCT encountered in the pediatric population, representing 59% of the lesions reported in a survey of the literature.[24] In adult IMSCT series, the proportion of astrocytomas varies but is generally slightly less than that of ependymomas.[13] There is a slight male predominance in the incidence of astrocytoma.[12,21]

The cervical spine is the most commonly affected region, followed closely by the thoracic spine. As IMSCTs commonly span multiple spinal levels, however, a patient may have both areas involved. Rarely, the entire spine cord may be involved. Such lesions have been termed *holocord tumors*, and are most commonly of low histologic grade.[10,24]

Spinal cord astrocytomas are categorized using the Kernohan grading scheme.[18] Though adult intracranial astrocytomas are generally high-grade tumors, adult spinal cord astrocytomas are usually low-grade lesions. High-grade lesions account for 10% to 30% of spinal cord astrocytomas in adults and 7% to 25% of spinal cord astrocytomas in children.[2,6–8,11] Juvenile pilocytic astrocytoma is a histologic subtype of low-grade astrocytoma that is generally well circumscribed from surrounding tissue and is typically associated with a better prognosis. It is common in young children but rare in adults, in whom low-grade astrocytomas are most often fibrillary.[1,19]

PRESENTATION

Patients seek treatment after symptoms have been present from months to years. As would be anticipated, more rapid symptom progression is generally seen with higher grade astrocytomas. The lack of a characteristic pattern of symptoms often leads to a delay in diagnosis; however, the ready availability of magnetic resonance imaging (MRI) has shortened the duration from symptoms to diagnosis in many cases.

Symptoms can include paravertebral pain and radicular pain.[12] The ways in which an IMSCT can cause back pain are diverse and not entirely understood. Back pain may be the result of direct pressure on the surrounding dura by the expanded spinal cord. Musculoskeletal pain may be caused by derangement of the paraspinal muscle innervation. Impingement upon or involvement of a nerve root may result in radicular pain. Radicular pain may mimic other causes: Thoracic pain may mimic angina, and lower thoracic roots may trigger pain similar to that of diverticulitis, cholelithiasis, or appendicitis.

Other common complaints relate to impingement upon the motor neurons or white matter tracts of the spinal cord. These symptoms include extremity weakness or clumsiness, gait difficulty, and abnormal sensory perception. Bowel, bladder, or sexual dysfunction are typically features of more advanced disease except in tumors of the conus medullaris, where they may be part of the initial symptoms.

Sensory disturbances besides pain may include dysesthesias, loss of pain and temperature sensation, and loss of proprioception. Centrally situated IMSCTs will destroy the crossing segmental fibers from the spinothalamic tract, resulting in impaired pain and temperature sensation. A sacral sparing may occur, given the outermost location of the lumbosacral spinothalamic fibers. Proprioceptive impairment from dorsal column impingement or invasion may cause difficulty with fine motor–control tasks, such as buttoning a shirt or typing.

Motor deficits are also a common initial complaint.[10] Tumors causing motor deficits are usually centrally located in the spinal cord. When they occur in the cervical region, the weakness in the upper extremities precedes that in the lower extremities because of the motor fiber orientation in the spinal cord. In young children, in whom verbal complaints are not articulated, pain is also identified as the most common first symptom, but gait deterioration, motor regression, torticollis, and kyphoscoliosis are also significant findings at examination.[5,6] In malignant tumors causing pain, rapid deterioration of motor function follows, resulting in significant disability within 3 to 5 months.[6,11]

HYDROCEPHALUS AND LUMBAR PUNCTURE

Hydrocephalus is occasionally present in patients with IMSCTs and is most often seen in the pediatric population.[16,25] The cause of hydrocephalus may be increased protein in the cerebrospinal fluid (CSF) or dissemination of tumor cells in the subarachnoid space. Tumors near the cervicomedullary junction may produce thickening of the leptomeninges that results in outflow obstruction from the fourth ventricle.

Lumbar puncture very rarely provides a diagnosis. Typically, CSF analysis is nonspecific, usually revealing increased protein. CSF cytology rarely yields malignant cells, even in instances where there has been frank leptomeningeal dissemination.[3]

DIAGNOSTIC IMAGING

Plain X-Ray Studies

Plain x-ray studies usually contribute little to the diagnosis of spinal cord astrocytomas in adults, though in long-standing tumors they may reveal an enlarged spinal canal with scalloping of the vertebral bodies, medial pedicle erosion, and thinning of the laminae. In children with astrocytomas, however, neuromuscular scoliosis is common. An interesting finding in many of these patients is that the apex of the curvature is on the left rather than the right as in idiopathic scoliosis.

Magnetic Resonance Imaging

MRI with and without intravenous gadolinium is the imaging technique of choice for the evaluation of spinal cord tumors. MRI is the only way to image the spinal cord substance itself and also allows for assessment of associated findings, such as edema, infarct, hemorrhage, cysts, syringomyelia, and cord atrophy. Evaluation of flow voids, nerve roots, and the relationship of tumor to avenues of safe surgical approach are invaluable in preoperative planning. In addition, cranial imaging is an important adjunct to rule out intracranial lesions or hydrocephalus.

Astrocytomas will widen the spinal cord, as is the case for other IMSCTs. In some cases, MRI with and without gadolinium may distinguish between astrocytomas and intramedullary ependymomas of the spinal cord (Figures 67-1 and 67-2). MRI signal characteristics for astrocytomas are very similar to those of ependymomas. Both lesions are isointense or hypointense with the spinal cord on T1-weighted images and hyperintense on T2-weighted images. Both astrocytoma and ependymoma enhance with contrast despite low histologic grade, although astrocytoma enhancement is usually more intense.[22] They are less often prone to hemorrhage, however, and so will rarely manifest a hemosiderin cap. An important distinction between astrocytomas and ependymomas is that astrocytomas of the cord are infiltrative and will have nondistinct margins as a result; however, the appearance of a distinct tumor margin on MRI does not always correlate with intraoperative findings.

Cysts are present in at least 50% of cases and may appear indistinguishable from solid tumor on T2-weighted studies as a consequence of a high protein content of the cyst fluid. Astrocytomas demonstrate tumor cysts much more commonly, whereas ependymomas very commonly are associated with reactive cysts. Contrast administration can help distinguish cyst from tumor, because cysts do not enhance. Astrocytomas often appear eccentric on axial views, whereas ependymomas are almost always centrally located, consistent with their assumed origin in the ependymal-lined central canal.

Computed Tomography and Myelography

Since the introduction of MRI, computed tomography (CT) with myelography is mainly relevant for patients in whom MRI is contraindicated, because it provides limited, indirect information about IMSCTs. The most significant finding on CT with myelography is widening of the spinal cord, though CT with myelography cannot reliably distinguish between an intramedullary spinal cord tumor, spinal cord swelling from non-neoplastic etiologies, and syringomyelia. In instances where MRI cannot be performed, delayed CT scanning can sometimes be used to demonstrate uptake of water-soluble contrast within the center of the spinal cord, typical of tumor associated cysts and syringomyelia.

SURGICAL GOALS AND PREOPERATIVE PATIENT SELECTION

The goals of IMSCT surgery are to obtain a tissue diagnosis and to maintain or improve neurologic function while completely resecting the tumor. Unlike other intramedullary tumors, astrocytomas may not demonstrate a clear plane of demarcation from the normal spinal cord. This may not be readily apparent on preoperative MRI. As such, the risk of subtotal resection must be weighted against the risk of neurologic impairment. Accordingly, patient selection and intraoperative technique are of great importance.

The best surgical candidates are those in whom functional independence may be prolonged by forestalling the development of severe motor deficit. Some patients with significant deficit may still benefit from surgery if sphincter function or the ability to change position in bed is preserved. Patients with few medical comorbidities generally have better postoperative courses with fewer complications. Those with complete neurologic deficits or extensive tumor dissemination are not appropriate surgical candidates.[15]

The decision to proceed to surgery in patients with very slow progressive or minor motor or sensory deficit is difficult, particularly if imaging studies suggest the presence of an infiltrating astrocytoma, which may not be removed without significant risk of neurologic deficit. One rational strategy in such cases is to follow the patient with serial neurologic assessments and MRI until there is tumor progression with functional deterioration. Some surgeons, however, take a more aggressive stance, noting that "watchful waiting" may occasionally allow a tumor in an individual with a potentially curable lesion to become unresectable. In addition, technologic advances such as the operating microscope, intraoperative ultrasound, Cavitron ultrasonic surgical aspirator, and motor- and somatosensory-evoked potential monitoring have improved the safety and effectiveness of surgery. Accordingly, patients demonstrating

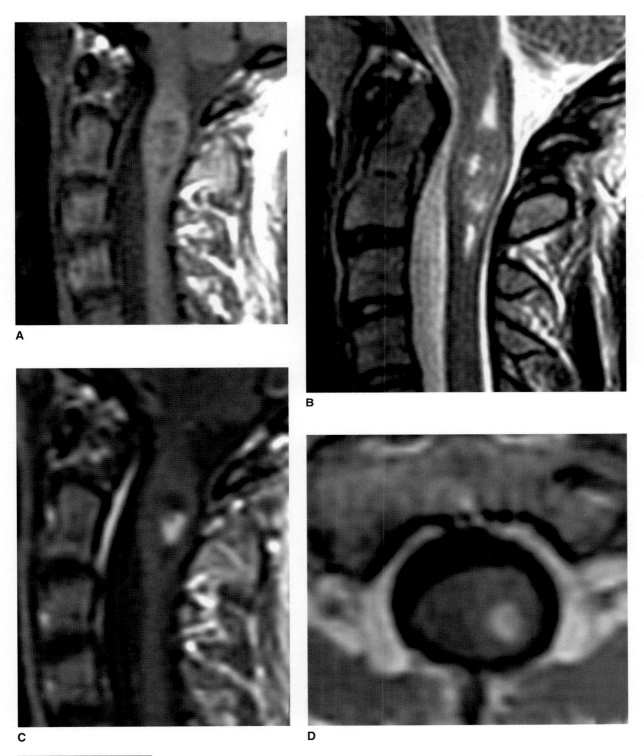

FIGURE 67-1   Magnetic resonance image of the cervical spine in a patient with an intramedullary spinal cord astrocytoma. Sagittal T1-weighted (A) and T2-weighted (B) images demonstrate widening of the spinal cord with the presence of lesion at the level of C2. The lesion is enhanced with intravenous gadolinium (C). An axial postcontrast T1-weighted image (D) shows that the tumor is eccentrically located. This is often seen with astrocytomas and strongly suggests that the lesion is not an ependymoma, because these tumors are almost always located centrally.

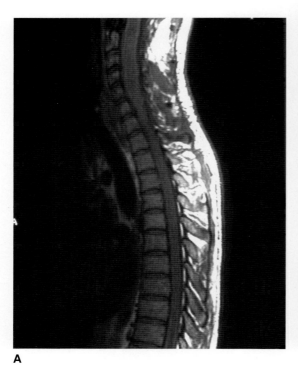
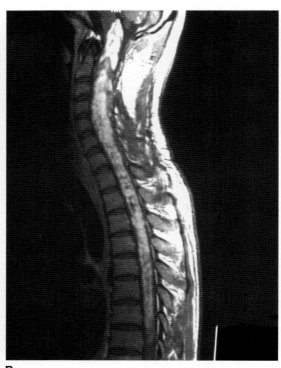

A   **B**

FIGURE 67-2   Magnetic resonance image of a holocord astrocytoma. *A,* Sagittal precontrast T1-weighted image demonstrates marked widening of the spinal cord in the cervical region and diffuse abnormality of the spinal cord with central hypointensity in the lower thoracic region. After infusion with intravenous gadolinium *(B),* the entire spinal cord is found to be enhanced.

a solitary intraspinal mass, good neurologic function, and demonstration of tumor growth are considered for early surgical intervention.

ADJUVANT THERAPY

Postoperative radiation therapy is reported to improve the recurrence rate and survival.[21,23] There is disagreement, however, on whether it should be employed if a gross-total resection is achieved, because it may complicate reoperation for recurrence.[11] It has not yet been established whether there is any role for chemotherapy in the treatment of spinal cord astrocytomas.[9]

OUTCOME

The outcome for intramedullary spinal cord astrocytoma is significantly worse than that for ependymoma, and correlates with pathologic grade.[14] Low-grade tumors (Kernohan grades I and II) may recur and result in death. Sandler reports a 5-year survival of 57% in a series of 21 patients, of whom 18 had a pathologic grade of I or II,[27] and Cooper reports a series of 11 patients with grade I or II astrocytomas, of whom 4 of died within the follow-up period, and only 4 were not neurologically worse in

functional grade.[7] In addition, we have seen tumors initially diagnosed as low-grade astrocytomas that have progressed to higher grade tumors.

Young age is a positive prognostic factor, because Sandler found that younger patients had a substantially increased time to recurrence.[27] This may be in part due to the portion of low-grade tumors in pediatric patients that are the pilocytic histologic subtype, which has the most favorable prognosis.[21]

In the immediate postoperative period, neurologic deterioration from the preoperative baseline is typically seen.[11,26] Recovery generally occurs over a period of days to months with improvement in sensory loss occurring earlier than improvements in motor deficits. Those with severe long-standing neurologic deficits, however, are unlikely to have any improvement. Preoperative neurologic function is the best prognostic indicator for functional outcome.[17,8]

The prognosis for high-grade astrocytomas is poor, with disease progression, widespread leptomeningeal dissemination, and hydrocephalus commonly observed.[4] Improvement of neurologic function after surgery is unlikely.[11] Previous reports of survival after surgery averaged 6 months in adults and 13 months in children.[4,20] The immediate cause of death is typically from pulmonary embolus and pneumonia or respiratory failure from direct tumor extension into the cervicomedullary region.

CONCLUSION

1. High-grade astrocytomas are infiltrating tumors that cannot be entirely resected.
2. The pilocytic subtype can be resected and has a favorable prognosis.
3. Functional outcome of surgery correlates well with a patient's preoperative condition.
4. The surgical objective is resection to the extent possible to allow for preservation of function.

Acknowledgments

We thank George I. Jallo, MD, and Fred J. Epstein for making the radiographic images available.

References

1. Allen JC, Aviner S, Yates AJ, et al: Treatment of high-grade spinal cord astrocytoma of childhood with "8-in-1" chemotherapy and radiotherapy: a pilot study of CCG-945. Children's Cancer Group. J Neurosurg 88:215–220, 1998.
2. Bouffet E, Pierre-Kahn A, Marchal JC, et al: Prognostic factors in pediatric spinal cord astrocytoma. Cancer 83:2391–2399, 1998.
3. Chida K, Konno H, Sahara M, et al: [Meningeal seeding of spinal cord glioblastoma multiforme without any signs of myelopathy]. Rinsho Shinkeigaku 35:1235–1240, 1995.
4. Cohen AR, Wisoff JH, Allen JC, et al: Malignant astrocytomas of the spinal cord. J Neurosurg 70:50–54, 1989.
5. Constantini S, Epstein F: Intraspinal tumors in infants and children. In Youmans J (ed): Neurological Surgery, Vol 4. Philadelphia, Saunders, 1996.
6. Constantini S, Houten J, Miller DC, et al: Intramedullary spinal cord tumors in children under the age of 3 years. J Neurosurg 85:1036–1043, 1996.
7. Cooper PR: Outcome after operative treatment of intramedullary spinal cord tumors in adults: intermediate and long-term results in 51 patients. Neurosurgery 25:855–859, 1989.
8. Cristante L, Herrmann HD: Surgical management of intramedullary spinal cord tumors: functional outcome and sources of morbidity. Neurosurgery 35:69–74; discussion 74–66, 1994.
9. Doireau V, Grill J, Zerah M, et al: Chemotherapy for unresectable and recurrent intramedullary glial tumours in children. Brain Tumours Subcommittee of the French Society of Paediatric Oncology (SFOP). Br J Cancer 81:835–840, 1999.
10. Epstein F, Epstein N: Surgical management of holocord intramedullary spinal cord astrocytomas in children. J Neurosurg 54:829–832, 1981.
11. Epstein FJ, Farmer JP, Freed D: Adult intramedullary astrocytomas of the spinal cord. J Neurosurg 77:355–359, 1992.
12. Fischer G, Brotchi J, Chignier G, et al: Clinical material. In Fischer G, Brotchi J (eds): Intramedullary Spinal Cord Tumors. Stuttgart, Germany, Thieme, 1996.
13. Fischer G, Brotchi J, Chignier G, et al: Epidemiology. In Fischer G, Brotchi J (eds): Intramedullary Spinal Cord Tumors. Stuttgart, Germany, Thieme, 1996.
14. Hardison HH, Packer RJ, Rorke LB, et al: Outcome of children with primary intramedullary spinal cord tumors. Childs Nerv Syst 3:89–92, 1987.
15. Houten JK, Cooper PR: Spinal cord astrocytomas: presentation, management and outcome. J Neurooncol 47:219–224, 2000.
16. Houten JK, Weiner HL: Pediatric intramedullary spinal cord tumors: special considerations. J Neurooncol 47:225–230, 2000.
17. Innocenzi G, Salvati M, Cervoni L, et al: Prognostic factors in intramedullary astrocytomas. Clin Neurol Neurosurg 99:1–5, 1997.
18. Kernohan J, Moabon R, Svien H: A simplified classification of the gliomas. Proc Staff Meet Mayo Clin 24:71–75, 1949.
19. McCormick PC, Stein BM: Intramedullary tumors in adults. Neurosurg Clin N Am 1:609–630, 1990.
20. Merchant TE, Nguyen D, Thompson SJ, et al: High-grade pediatric spinal cord tumors. Pediatr Neurosurg 30:1–5, 1999.
21. Minehan KJ, Shaw EG, Scheithauer BW, et al: Spinal cord astrocytoma: pathological and treatment considerations. J Neurosurg 83:590–595, 1995.
22. Osborn A: Diagnostic Neuroradiology. St. Louis, Mosby, 1994.
23. O'Sullivan C, Jenkin RD, Doherty MA, et al: Spinal cord tumors in children: long-term results of combined surgical and radiation treatment. J Neurosurg 81:507–512, 1994.
24. Reimer R, Onofrio BM: Astrocytomas of the spinal cord in children and adolescents. J Neurosurg 63:669–675, 1985.
25. Rifkinson-Mann S, Wisoff JH, Epstein F: The association of hydrocephalus with intramedullary spinal cord tumors: a series of 25 patients. Neurosurgery 27:749–754; discussion 754, 1990.
26. Samii M, Klekamp J: Surgical results of 100 intramedullary tumors in relation to accompanying syringomyelia. Neurosurgery 35:865–873; discussion 873, 1994.
27. Sandler HM, Papadopoulos SM, Thornton AF, Jr, et al: Spinal cord astrocytomas: results of therapy. Neurosurgery 30:490–493, 1992.
28. Stein BM: Surgery of intramedullary spinal cord tumors. Clin Neurosurg 26:529–542, 1979.

CHAPTER **68**

SPINAL CORD HEMANGIOBLASTOMAS

Russell R. Lonser and Edward H. Oldfield

Hemangioblastomas can be found throughout the entire central nervous system but are most commonly located in the cerebellum and spinal cord. They occur sporadically (in approximately two thirds of cases), or in association with von Hippel-Lindau (VHL) disease (in approximately one third of cases).[3] Whether they occur sporadically or in relationship to VHL disease, spinal cord hemangioblastomas are histologically identical, benign, highly vascular tumors that can be cured by complete surgical resection. Despite their benign histologic features, spinal cord hemangioblastomas may be associated with significant neurologic deficits related to their size, location, or the presence of associated edema or syrinx.[11,17] Recent insights into their natural history, as well as improvements in imaging and refinement in microsurgical removal, have enhanced the diagnosis and treatment of these tumors.

CLINICAL, RADIOGRAPHIC, AND HISTOLOGIC FEATURES

Epidemiology

Hemangioblastomas are the third most common intramedullary spinal cord tumor and represent approximately 2% to 5% of primary intramedullary spinal cord neoplasms. They are found approximately 1.5 to 2 times more often in males than females.[11,14] The average age at symptom development from spinal cord hemangioblastomas is between 33 and 35 years.

Tumor Location

Symptomatic spinal cord hemangioblastomas are found most commonly in the cervical (40% to 60%) and thoracic (40% to 50%) spinal cord and are rarely found in the lumbar spinal cord (5% to 10%) and cauda equina (less than 1%).[10,11,14] The center of the hemangioblastoma mass is most commonly found in the posterior aspect of the spinal cord (96%) in the region of the dorsal root entry zone (66%).[11] These tumors can be entirely intramedullary (30%), have intramedullary and extramedullary components (50%), or be primarily extramedullary (20%).[11]

Natural History

Understanding the natural history of spinal cord hemangioblastomas is critical for optimizing treatment and determining the efficacy of various therapies. It is especially important for VHL disease patients with central nervous system hemangioblastomas, because they may have multiple hemangioblastomas along the neuroaxis at any time and may develop new tumors over their lifetime. Recently, we examined the natural history of central nervous system (including spinal cord) hemangioblastomas in 160 consecutive patients with VHL disease.[17] Symptoms in patients with spinal cord hemangioblastomas were related to tumor size or syringomyelia-associated mass effect. As a result, symptom formation in patients with spinal cord hemangioblastomas was associated with the presence of syringomyelia and with more rapid rates of hemangioblastoma growth. The pattern of growth seen with spinal cord hemangioblastomas (and hemangioblastomas found elsewhere in the central nervous system) was variable and often marked by prolonged (several years) periods of quiescence. No reliable threshold of tumor size or threshold rate of growth could be identified that reliably predicted an association with either symptoms or a cyst. Thus neither tumor size nor rate of growth permitted an argument for early intervention when a tumor is smaller and potentially more amenable to surgery or medical therapy. Thus in the setting of VHL disease, it is probably best to reserve resection of spinal cord and other central nervous system–associated hemangioblastomas until the onset of symptoms.

Signs and Symptoms

Patients with spinal cord hemangioblastomas have a variety of signs and symptoms that are related to the spinal level of the tumor, the position of the tumor within the spinal cord (anterior versus posterior), and the presence of edema or a syrinx.[11,15,17] Consistent with their known slow, erratic growth and association with edema or syrinxes, spinal cord hemangioblastomas may have a prolonged symptomatic prodrome ranging from several months to years.[14,17]

Clinical findings associated with spinal cord hemangioblastomas include sensory changes, weakness, pain, hyperreflexia, gait difficulties, incontinence, and occasionally scoliosis (Table 68-1).[11,14] The predominance of sensory-related signs and symptoms is most likely the result of an overwhelming preponderance of posterior-located tumors (96% of spinal cord hemangioblastomas) that are often found in the dorsal root entry zone (66%).[11] Most symptom-producing spinal cord hemangioblastomas have associated syrinxes (95% of symptomatic spinal cord hemangioblastomas).[17]

TABLE 68-1

Frequency of Signs and Symptoms Associated with Spinal Cord Hemangioblastomas

Sign or Symptom	Percentage of Patients with Finding
Sensory changes	70–85%
Weakness	40–65%
Pain	15–85%
Hyperreflexia	30–60%
Gait difficulties	15–30%
Incontinence	10–15%
Scoliosis	10–15%

Source: From Roonprapunt C, Silvera VM, Setton A, et al: Surgical management of isolated hemangioblastomas of the spinal cord. Neurosurgery 49:321–327, discussion 327–328, 2001; Wanebo JE, Lonser RR, Glenn GM, et al: The natural history of central nervous system hemangioblastomas in patients with von Hippel-Lindau disease. J Neurosurg 98:82–94, 2003.

Imaging Characteristics

Postcontrast, T1-weighted magnetic resonance imaging (MRI) precisely defines these tumors and their relationship to the spinal cord (Figure 68-1).[4,6] Spinal cord hemangioblastomas are vividly enhanced on T1-weighted MRI after contrast administration. T2-weighted or fluid-attenuated inversion recovery MRI can be used to better define peritumoral edema or associated syringomyelia.

Arteriography can be used to define the vascular anatomy of large hemangioblastomas and provides a vascular "road map" during resection. However, we have found that neither preoperative selective embolization nor diagnostic arteriography are necessary for resection of spinal cord hemangioblastomas. Careful adherence to well-described microsurgical techniques[11] obviates the need for adjuvant preoperative selective embolization with its attendant risks.

Histologic Characteristics

Grossly, hemangioblastomas are bright red or red-yellow. The coloring is due to their highly vascular nature (red) and abundant lipid (yellow) content. Histologically, hemangioblastomas are benign-appearing tumors that lack mitoses and contain numerous capillaries lined by pericytes and endothelial cells. The capillaries in hemangioblastomas are surrounded by numerous bland, lipid-laden stromal cells, which have recently been shown to be the neoplastic cell of origin (Figure 68-2).[2,8,16] Common histologic patterns seen in hemangioblastomas include cyst and microcyst formation associated with vascular proliferation. These histologic components vary with hemangioblastomas of various sizes and may account for the varied natural history of these tumors.

Special Considerations

Because the occurrence of a spinal cord hemangioblastoma is significantly associated with VHL disease,[5] all patients diagnosed with a spinal cord hemangioblastoma should be screened

for it.[9] Because of the common occurrence of pheochromocytomas in VHL disease (10% to 20% of patients with VHL disease), all patients with VHL disease who are undergoing surgery should be evaluated preoperatively for the presence of a pheochromocytoma that may require priority treatment or perioperative α- and β-adrenergic blockade.[9]

TREATMENT

Surgical Resection

Indications

Microsurgical resection is the primary treatment for spinal cord hemangioblastomas. The indications for surgical resection in the setting of sporadically occurring spinal cord hemangioblastomas differ from those occurring in patients with VHL disease. In patients with sporadically occurring spinal cord hemangioblastomas, resection of the tumor is often necessary for diagnosis and can necessitate removal before symptom formation. Because spinal cord hemangioblastomas have variable patterns of growth (including long quiescent periods) and patients with VHL disease may require multiple surgeries over a lifetime, the indications for surgery in the patient with VHL are based on the presence of signs and symptoms attributable to the hemangioblastoma or its associated edema or syrinx. Thus in patients with VHL disease, asymptomatic spinal cord hemangioblastomas may be followed clinically but should be resected once they become symptomatic. Delay in removal of symptom-producing hemangioblastomas may result in progressive neurologic deficits that are not reversible. Contraindications for removal include medical instability and lack of signs and symptoms that can be attributed to the hemangioblastoma in patients with VHL disease.

Operative Results

Many patients (66%) develop new signs and symptoms or have existing ones exacerbated in the early postoperative period.[11] These neurologic changes are typically mild (do not limit function) and transient (generally lasting 2 to 6 weeks). Transient signs and symptoms found in the immediate postoperative period may include sensory disturbances (dysesthesia, pain, and numbness), motor dysfunction (mild weakness and spasticity), or bladder dysfunction.[11]

Generally, the long-term clinical outcome in patients undergoing resection of spinal cord hemangioblastomas is excellent.[11,14] More than 90% of patients will remain clinically stable or improve, although 5% to 10% of patients will be clinically worse after removal of a spinal cord hemangioblastoma. Predictors of poor outcome include significant preoperative neurologic deficits, large tumor size (greater than 500 mm^3), and anterior location (defined by the tumor mass anterior to the dentate ligament) of the hemangioblastoma.[11] Improved short- and long-term outcomes can be obtained in anterior-located spinal hemangioblastomas by direct approach rather than using posterior or posterolateral approaches.[13]

Follow-up Studies and Recurrence

The frequency of postoperative imaging studies and length of follow-up after resection of a spinal cord hemangioblastoma is

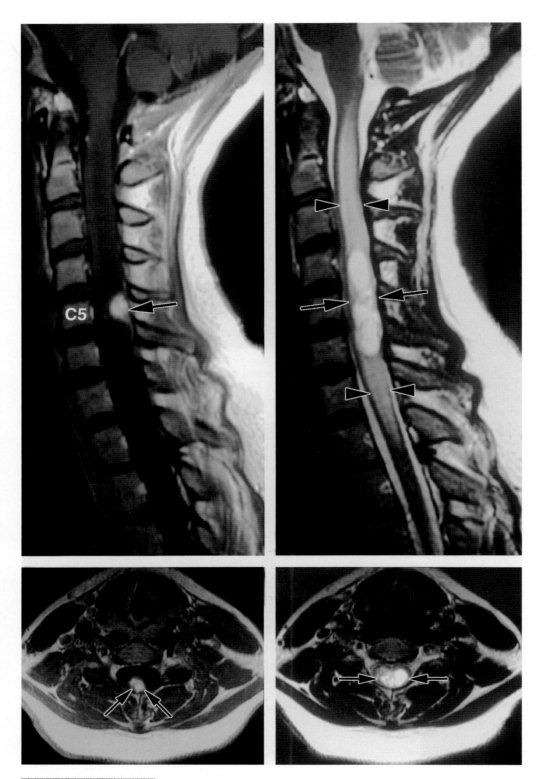

FIGURE 68-1 Magnetic resonance (MR) imaging of a 26-year-old patient with von Hippel-Lindau disease and an intramedullary hemangioblastoma at the fifth cervical level (C5). *Top left,* Postcontrast, midsagittal, T1-weighted, MR image of the cervical spinal cord demonstrating the C5 hemangioblastoma (solid enhancing area; *arrow*) with an associated syrinx (dark region in the intraspinal region). *Top right,* A midsagittal, T2-weighted, MR image clearly defines the peritumoral syrinx *(arrows)* and associated edema *(arrowheads)* of the spinal cord that extends from the cervicomedullary junction to the bottom of the first thoracic vertebrae. *Bottom left,* Postcontrast axial T1-weighted MR image of the same hemangioblastoma demonstrating the posterior location within the spinal cord of the tumor *(arrows). Bottom right,* An axial, T2-weighted, MR image demonstrates the peritumoral syrinx within the spinal cord *(arrows).*

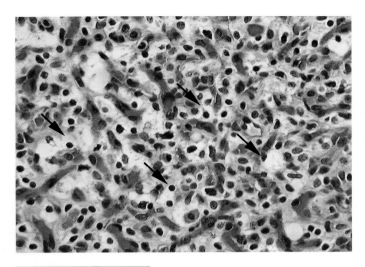

FIGURE 68-2 Hematoxylin and eosin staining of a hemangioblastoma showing the lipid-laden stromal cells *(arrows)* distributed within a capillary network (Original magnification ×40).

different between patients with sporadic and VHL-associated tumors. Generally, all patients should undergo contrast-enhanced spinal MRI 3 to 6 months after hemangioblastoma resection to confirm complete removal of the tumor. Complete resection of spinal cord hemangioblastomas should preclude recurrence and result in inactivation of an associated syrinx or edema.[11] Patients with partially resected hemangioblastomas are at significant risk for progression of tumor growth, and recurrence of symptoms that will require additional surgery.[5] Thus in patients with sporadically occurring spinal cord hemangioblastomas, follow-up after complete resection may be limited to 6 to 12 months after surgery. Because of the potential for development of new hemangioblastomas and continued growth of existing hemangioblastomas, patients with VHL disease should undergo routine serial screening of the neuraxis at 12- to 24-month intervals (with contrast-enhanced MRI) or sooner if new symptoms develop.[9]

Radiation Therapy

The role of radiation therapy in the treatment of spinal cord hemangioblastomas remains to be defined. Complete or partial craniospinal irradiation may be considered in cases of hemangioblastomatosis where surgical resection of discrete symptom-producing spinal cord hemangioblastomas is not possible. Stereotactic radiosurgery may play a role in treatment of isolated central nervous system hemangioblastomas (including spinal cord hemangioblastomas) and can avoid some of the

potential complications associated with conventional radiation-treatment paradigms.[12] Similar to the results for stereotactic radiosurgery of other central nervous system lesions, hemangioblastomas that are large (greater than 3 cm^3) or associated with cysts are less likely to respond to this therapy.[12]

Interpreting the results of radiosurgery and emerging medical therapies must be tempered by the known pattern of growth and quiescence seen in these tumors. Stability of tumor size, which is often used as a criterion for response to radiation or other medical therapies, may be misleading because of the known prolonged intervals of time in which no tumor growth may occur. Thus absence of growth may only coincide with a quiescent phase of tumor growth and may not represent a response to therapy at all.[17]

Emerging Medical Therapies

Novel medical therapies are beginning to emerge for the treatment of hemangioblastomas, particularly in the setting of VHL disease. These therapies are targeted at the known molecular abnormalities associated with loss of heterozygosity of the VHL gene (chromosome 3p25)[7] in patients with VHL disease or somatic inactivation of the VHL gene that occurs in patients with sporadic hemangioblastoma.[8] The loss of VHL gene function results in abnormal protein (pVHL) and loss of pVHL function. pVHL is a tumor-suppressor protein that is involved in oxygen-sensing homeostasis and angiogenesis. Abnormal or absent pVHL function results in enhanced expression of vascular endothelial growth factor (VEGF) through effects mediated by constitutive overproduction of hypoxia-inducible factors (HIFs).[9] Subsequently, chemotherapeutic treatment paradigms targeted at blocking HIFs and their downstream targets (such as VEGF) are promising.[1]

CONCLUSION

1. Spinal cord hemangioblastomas are histologically benign tumors that can cause significant morbidity because of their size, location, and associated edema or syrinx.
2. They are may be found sporadically or in association with VHL disease.
3. Spinal cord hemangioblastomas in these two settings (sporadic or associated with VHL disease) have different indications for surgical treatment and have variable follow-up paradigms.
4. Generally, surgical resection of these tumors is curative and should be performed at the onset of symptoms in patients with VHL disease or for diagnostic and therapeutic purposes in sporadic cases.

References

1. Aiello LP, George DJ, Cahill MT, et al: Rapid and durable recovery of visual function in a patient with von Hippel-Lindau syndrome after systemic therapy with vascular endothelial growth factor receptor inhibitor su5416. Ophthalmology 109:1745–1751, 2002.
2. Berkman RA, Merrill MJ, Reinhold WC, et al: Expression of the vascular permeability factor/vascular endothelial growth factor gene in central nervous system neoplasms. J Clin Invest 91:153–159, 1993.
3. Browne TR, Adams RD, Roberson GH: Hemangioblastoma of the spinal cord: review and report of five cases. Arch Neurol 33:435–441, 1976.
4. Chu BC, Terae S, Hida K, et al: MR findings in spinal hemangioblastoma: correlation with symptoms and with angiographic

and surgical findings. AJNR Am J Neuroradiol 22:206–217, 2001.

5. Conway JE, Chou D, Clatterbuck RE, et al: Hemangioblastomas of the central nervous system in von Hippel-Lindau syndrome and sporadic disease. Neurosurgery 48:55–63, 2001.

6. Filling-Katz MR, Choyke PL, Patronas NJ, et al: Radiologic screening for von Hippel-Lindau disease: the role of Gd-DTPA enhanced MR imaging of the CNS. J Comput Assist Tomogr 13:743–755, 1989.

7. Latif F, Tory K, Gnarra J, et al: Identification of the von Hippel-Lindau disease tumor suppressor gene. Science 260:1317–1320, 1993.

8. Lee JY, Dong SM, Park WS, et al: Loss of heterozygosity and somatic mutations of the VHL tumor suppressor gene in sporadic cerebellar hemangioblastomas. Cancer Res 58:504–508, 1998.

9. Lonser RR, Glenn GM, Walther M, et al: von Hippel-Lindau disease. Lancet 361:2059–2067, 2003.

10. Lonser RR, Wait SD, Butman JA, et al: Surgical management of lumbosacral nerve root hemangioblastomas in von Hippel-Lindau disease. J Neurosurg (Spine) 99:64–69, 2003.

11. Lonser RR, Weil RJ, Wanebo JE, et al: Surgical management of spinal cord hemangioblastomas in patients with von Hippel-Lindau disease. J Neurosurg 98:106–116, 2003.

12. Patrice SJ, Sneed PK, Flickinger JC, et al: Radiosurgery for hemangioblastoma: results of a multiinstitutional experience. Int J Radiat Oncol Biol Phys 35:493–499, 1996.

13. Pluta RM, Iuliano B, DeVroom HL, et al: Anterior versus posterior surgical approach for ventral spinal hemangioblastomas in von Hippel-Lindau disease. J Neurosurg 98:117–124, 2003.

14. Roonprapunt C, Silvera VM, Setton A, et al: Surgical management of isolated hemangioblastomas of the spinal cord. Neurosurgery 49:321–327; discussion 327–328, 2001.

15. Solomon RA, Stein BM: Unusual spinal cord enlargement related to intramedullary hemangioblastoma. J Neurosurg 68:550–553, 1988.

16. Vortmeyer AO, Gnarra JR, Emmert-Buck MR, et al: von Hippel-Lindau gene deletion detected in the stromal cell component of a cerebellar hemangioblastoma associated with von Hippel-Lindau disease. Hum Pathol 28:540–543, 1997.

17. Wanebo JE, Lonser RR, Glenn GM, et al: The natural history of central nervous system hemangioblastomas in patients with von Hippel-Lindau disease. J Neurosurg 98:82–94, 2003.

CHAPTER 69

BENIGN TUMORS OF THE SPINE

James Waldron and Christopher Ames

Benign tumors of the spinal column are rare entities that most commonly occur insidiously with progressive localized back pain. Although these lesions occur rarely, it is important for the clinician to consider benign spinal tumors in patients with localized back pain. Timely intervention can minimize the surgical challenges presented by continued growth and facilitate pain relief, neurologic improvement, and long-term cure.

INCIDENCE AND BEHAVIOR

Primary lesions of the spinal column make up a very small proportion of spine tumors, with metastatic disease accounting for the vast majority. As a subpopulation of all osseous tumors found throughout the body, spine lesions account for 10%.[15] Approximately 40% of primary bony spinal lesions are benign.[15] As is common in other tumor types, the frequency of benign and malignant lesions varies with age. In patients younger than 18 years of age, approximately 70% of primary spinal lesions are benign, whereas in those older than 18, approximately 80% are malignant.[15] Another differentiating factor between benign and malignant lesions is the location of occurrence. Eighty percent of bony malignant lesions occur in the vertebral body, compared with only 42% of benign lesions.[15]

Biologically, benign lesions grow outward from their site of origin. In addition to a pattern of bony destruction, these lesions induce reactive changes in the tissue around them, forming an osseous pseudocapsule. The degree of capsule development is related to the rate of tumor growth. Slow-growing lesions have well-defined pseudocapsules, whereas faster-growing, more aggressive lesions have a minimally developed pseudocapsule. Depending on the aggressiveness of the tumor, the lesion may remain localized within the bony structures, place pressure on the periosteum through expansion, or frankly invade the paraspinal structures.

PRESENTATION

Patients with benign bony tumors of the spine most often have a combination of back pain, weakness, and a palpable mass. The remainder are identified as incidental discoveries. The most common initial symptom is back pain. This pain is most typically localized but can also be radicular in nature. A high index of suspicion can identify many tumors before they

progress to neurologic deficits. Several differentiating features may be present (Table 69-1).

Localized pain finds its origin in the expansive pressure placed on the periosteum and the paraspinal soft tissues and, as the disease progresses, in bony destruction leading to pathologic fractures and spinal instability. Radicular pain is found with impingement on the dural sac or nerve roots caused by tumor encroachment. It occurs most commonly in the cervical and lumbar regions. In the thoracic region radiculopathy can manifest itself as dysesthesia in a dermatomal pattern. Unlike radicular pain caused by a herniated disk, pain from tumor does not improve with rest. In addition, patients may report that pain is worse at night, which is very rare with mechanical back pain.

A focal neurologic deficit is the next most common initial symptom after back pain. A contemporary retrospective series of 82 patients with spinal tumors found neurologic deficits associated with 35% of benign lesions.[15] This high frequency of neurologic symptoms in patients with benign tumors may in part reflect a substantial delay between the initial onset of symptoms and when they are brought to medical attention. Neurologic deficits can result from nerve root compression and consist of muscular weakness and diminished reflexes in the appropriate distribution or can result from direct spinal compression leading to bowel and bladder dysfunction, paraparesis, and hyperreflexia. Rare cases of aggressive benign lesions can result in permanent paralysis.

In addition to neurologic findings, physical examination may reveal a localized area of tenderness, a palpable mass, decreased range of motion, or in some instances spinal deformity. Spinal deformity can result from vertebral collapse and pain-induced muscle spasm. Vertebral collapse can lead to a kyphotic deformity, whereas muscle spasm can induce painful scoliosis and, in the case of cervical tumors, torticollis. Treatment of the lesion will most often correct a pain-induced spinal deformity.

CLINICAL EVALUATION

Initial Assessment

Once clinical suspicion of nonmechanical back pain is raised, the initial assessment should focus on ruling out metastatic disease and identifying any focal spinal lesions. In addition to careful review of the patient's medical history and risk factors,

TABLE 69-1

Typical Features of Tumor-Related Pain

Unremitting and progressive over time
Unaffected by activity and does not improve with rest
Increased when supine and at night
Well-localized and induced by direct pressure

TABLE 69-2

Laboratory Evaluation for Suspected Benign Spinal Lesions

CBC with differential
Electrolytes with Ca
ESR
Urinalysis
Serum protein and urine protein electrophoresis

CBC, Complete blood count; ESR, erythrocyte sedimentation rate.

appropriate laboratory and imaging studies should be obtained (Table 69-2).

A complete blood count (CBC) and sedimentation rate will help delineate an infectious process, whereas protein electrophoresis will help identify multiple myeloma. Additional tumor markers such as prostate-specific antigen (PSA) and vanillylmandelic acid (neuroblastoma in children) tests should be ordered when appropriate. In addition to the imaging described later to delineate the tumor, studies such as chest and abdominal computed tomography (CT) and bone scan may be used to evaluate for metastatic disease.

Relevant Imaging

Imaging allows the identification, delineation, and in some cases the diagnosis of spinal lesions. Patients should initially undergo anteroposterior and lateral radiographs followed by whole-spine survey magnetic resonance imaging (MRI) and detailed MRI series of involved regions. CT may also be useful to determine extent of bony destruction and the nature of the tissue causing spinal cord or nerve root compression. Soft tissue compression is more likely to respond to radiation therapy. Compression by fractured, retropulsed bone or hematoma is more likely to require operative decompression. Bone scan may also be useful to evaluate the extent of whole skeletal involvement. Plain anteroposterior and lateral radiographs should be the initial imaging study obtained for patients with persistent back pain or a neurologic deficit consistent with a spinal tumor. Many spinal tumors will have radiographic characteristics that will manifest on plain films and yield insight into the nature of the tumor. For tumors in the vertebral body, it is important to remember that approximately 40% to 50% of trabecular bone must be destroyed before the

lesion becomes evident. Radiographic imaging can also provide information on the presence of pathologic fractures and vertebral collapse.

Radionuclide bone scans are useful in the evaluation of back pain. By imaging areas of bone deposition, a bone scan can detect lesions not yet visible on plain radiograph and identify the multiple lesions suggestive of metastatic disease; however, it is important to note that the major drawback of a bone scan is the lack of specificity because of areas of increased uptake found in patients with osteoarthritis, fractures, and infection. Lesions caused by multiple myeloma are also not visible.

CT is appropriate to investigate lesions that have been localized to a specific spinal segment. CT provides high resolution imaging of the osseous elements allowing evaluation of the architectural integrity of the vertebral body and the posterior elements of the spine. The extent and nature of osseous change can provide clues and in some cases be diagnostic of the lesion. CT is an important part of preoperative planning and is commonly used to assist biopsy.

MRI provides unsurpassed imaging of the paraspinal soft tissues. It provides clear evidence of soft tissue extension and allows evaluation of the spinal cord and the nerve roots. MRI has supplanted CT myelography for the evaluation of the spinal cord. Occasionally, CT myelography may still be useful to assist in determining the exact relationship between extra-axial tumors and the intradural compartment if any ambiguity remains after the MRI.

Staging

Biopsy should be performed on most lesions to obtain definitive tissue diagnosis. Biopsy can take the form of CT-guided fine-needle, trocar, incisional, or excisional biopsy. The method of biopsy depends on the location, size, and likely diagnosis of the lesion.

Staging provides an important tool for the development of a treatment plan and provides perspective on prognosis. The staging system used for benign tumors of the spine is based on the skeletal tumor staging system developed by Enneking and colleagues.[5] This system divides benign tumors into three stages. Tumors are staged primarily based on radiographic information and knowledge of histology and clinical course. Stage 1 lesions are latent, either inactive or likely to heal spontaneously. They do not require intervention unless stabilization or decompression is required. Stage 2 lesions are active, demonstrate characteristics consistent with slow growth (reactive capsule), and may be mildly symptomatic. They may recur after surgical excision. Stage 3 lesions are locally aggressive, often invading neighboring tissues. They have a relatively high rate of recurrence.

TREATMENT

Treatment options available for benign primary tumors of the spine range from conservative prospective observation to surgical en bloc excision. Observation is appropriate for stage 1 lesions with a self-limiting or indolent course. For higher stage lesions, surgery is appropriate in most instances. Surgical intervention ranges from interlesional curettage to aggressive en bloc excision (spondylectomy). Given the morbidity associated with en bloc excision in the spine, it is appropriate for only a subset of the most aggressive tumors that are locally confined.

Embolization plays a therapeutic role for spinal tumors with a large vascular component. It is used preoperatively as a tool to lower surgical risk in tumors with the potential for high levels of intraoperative blood loss. Preoperative embolization may also reverse a neurologic deficit and reduce tumor size.[4] Embolization as a stand-alone therapy may have a role in some instances.[10]

Radiation therapy, in general, is used as an adjunct to surgery after incomplete resection, in instances with a large risk of recurrence, and after local recurrence. Radiation therapy has been shown to be equivalent to surgery for treatment of hemangiomas of the spine.[4] In addition, the emergence of Cyberknife® technology now allows frameless stereotactic radiosurgery of the spine. Its efficacy as a tool for the treatment of benign spinal lesions is currently under evaluation.

BENIGN PRIMARY TUMORS

Osteoid Osteoma

Osteoid osteoma is a benign lesion that most commonly occurs in children and adolescents with an average age of 16 years.[12] It occurs more often in males by a 2:1 ratio. Osteoid osteoma most commonly occurs as nonradiating back pain localized to the site of the lesion. This pain is classically relieved with the administration of aspirin or nonsteroidal anti-inflammatory drugs (NSAIDs). Additional symptoms include night pain (44%), radicular pain (44%), and neurologic deficits (18%).[12] A distinctive feature of osteoid osteoma is its association with painful scoliosis, which occurs with an incidence of approximately 63%.[12,14] This spinal deformity results from inflammation and secondary spasm of the paraspinal musculature. In almost all cases the lesion is found in the concavity of the curve near its apex.[14] In parallel fashion, paraspinal muscle spasm induced by cervical lesions may cause torticollis.

Radiographic imaging reveals a characteristic lesion, smaller than 2 cm in diameter, composed of a lucent nidus surrounded by a region of reactive sclerosis. The lesion is present in the posterior elements of the spine more than 93% of the time.[12] Because of the complex radiographic anatomy of the spine, the lesion may be difficult to visualize or missed altogether on plain radiographs. The use of radionuclide bone scan, which reveals increased uptake at the nidus of the lesion, is effective in localizing the lesion and identifying those missed on radiographic images. CT is used to fully delineate the tumor and for planning any indicated intervention. MRI findings are variable.[11]

Curative treatment consists of complete excision. Pain relief is almost immediate. Scoliosis typically resolves, although young patients in whom the scoliosis has been present for an extended period of time may require additional corrective action. Recurrence occurs in 4.5% of treated patients.[2]

Osteoblastoma

Osteoblastoma is a benign neoplastic lesion that is histologically identical to osteoid osteoma. It is differentiated from osteoid osteoma on the basis of size larger than 2 cm and by clinical course. Osteoblastoma exhibits a similar age at diagnosis (mean 18), 2:1 male predominance, and propensity for the posterior elements of the spine as osteoid osteoma.[12] Osteoblastomas are more likely to cause neurologic deficits and slightly less likely to cause scoliosis; however, osteoblastomas truly differentiate themselves in their ability to grow fairly rapidly and exhibit locally destructive and invasive behavior. Unlike osteoid osteomas, osteoblastomas invade the epidural space approximately 57% of the time, often impinging on nerve roots and in some instances causing spinal cord compression.[12] Osteoblastomas may undergo late malignant transformation.

Radiographically, osteoblastomas can appear as a benign lucent nidus surrounded by a sclerotic ring or as more aggressive expansile osseous lesions with bony destruction and invasion of soft tissue.[11] Osteoblastomas reveal increased uptake on bone scan and expansile bone remodeling surrounded by a thin sclerotic rim on CT.[11] MRI of the lesion is generally nonspecific but is effective in visualizing the effects on the spinal cord and surrounding soft tissue.[11]

Curative treatment is complete resection, which generally resolves associated pain, scoliosis, and radiculopathy. Recurrence rates of 7% for stage 2 lesions and 19% for stage 3 aggressive lesions have been reported.[2] These recurrence rates likely reflect the difficulty of obtaining complete excision for some tumors.

Osteochondroma

Osteochondroma is the most common benign primary tumor of bone; however, occurrence in the axial skeleton is fairly rare, accounting for approximately 3% of solitary lesions and a slightly higher number in patients with hereditary multiple exostosis (HME).[8] Osteochondromas are an example of dysplastic endochondral ossification and as such tend to arise in adolescent individuals during the growth that occurs during the second and third decades of life.[13] Spinal osteochondromas are more common in males and favor the posterior elements of the spine, in particular the transverse and spinous processes.[8] Spinal osteochondromas are rarely symptomatic. When clinical sequelae are present, symptoms may include localized pain, a palpable mass, and neurologic deficits secondary to compression of the spinal cord or other neurologic structures. In rare instances, spinal osteochondromas may occur in individuals who received radiation therapy earlier in life.

Spinal osteochondromas can appear as either sessile or pedunculated masses with a cartilaginous cap overlying cortex and marrow. Continuity of the cortex and marrow of the exostosis with underlying normal bone is pathognomonic for the lesion.[11] Plain radiographs provide definitive diagnosis in only 21% of cases, typically of large lesions in the cervical spine.[11] Smaller lesions may be missed altogether. CT imaging is the method of choice for visualizing continuity of cortex and marrow with underlying bone, whereas MRI provides information about the impact on surrounding soft tissues.

Treatment is necessary only for symptomatic osteochondromas. Excision serves as curative treatment in most cases, reversing neurologic deficits, with very uncommon recurrence.

Hemangioma

Vertebral hemangiomas are extremely common vascular lesions that rarely cause clinical problems. Autopsy series demonstrate an incidence of 10% to 12% in the general population.[9] Asymptomatic hemangiomas rarely progress to clinical relevance, with only 2 of 35 incidentally diagnosed hemangiomas progressing in a retrospective series from the Mayo clinic.[6] In the instances when vertebral hemangiomas become symptomatic, the typical pattern is new-onset back pain followed by the development of myelopathy and neurologic symptoms over a period of several months.[6]

Prominent vertical striations within the involved vertebrae are classically present on plain radiographs of patients with spinal hemangioma. The striations represent the presence of dilated vascular vessels surrounded by thickened trabeculae. A polka dot pattern caused by these trabeculae is often visible on CT. Symptomatic hemangiomas are often effectively treated with radiation therapy alone.[4] Lesions that require decompressive surgery often benefit from preoperative embolization.

Aneurysmal Bone Cyst

Aneurysmal bone cysts are expansile blood-filled cystic lesions with an unclear etiology. They are classified as primary when no evidence of an underlying lesion is found and as secondary when they are associated with an underlying neoplasm (giant cell tumor, osteoblastoma, chondroblastoma, osteosarcoma). Approximately 10% to 30% arise in the spine, predominantly in the posterior elements.[3] The average age of onset is younger than 20 years.[3] Clinically they cause the gradual onset of pain, a palpable mass, neurologic involvement, or axial deformity.[3] Overall, they exhibit fairly aggressive behavior. A recent series of 41 patients staged via the Enneking system demonstrated an incidence of 2% for stage 1, 20% for stage 2, and 78% for stage 3 lesions.[3]

Plain radiographs typically reveal an expansile region of remodeled bone surrounded by a thin periosteal rim, often with internal septations.[11] Although typically located in the posterior elements, expansion into the vertebral body, soft tissue, and adjacent vertebrae occurs with some frequency.[11] CT and MRI reveal the cystic nature of the lesion and characteristic fluid-fluid levels. MRI is appropriate for visualizing soft tissue and spinal cord involvement.[11]

Despite its aggressive nature, overall prognosis for aneurysmal bone cysts is generally good. Intralesional excision and embolization are similar in efficacy and rate of recurrence.[3] Radiation therapy has also been shown to be effective but should be used judiciously because of the young age of the patients. En bloc excision can be curative but because of the high associated morbidity is appropriate only for a small subset of lesions.[3]

Giant Cell Tumor

Giant cell tumors of the spine are benign lesions that often exhibit locally aggressive behavior and a high rate of recurrence. Approximately 2% to 3% of giant cell tumors of bone are located in the nonsacral vertebral spine.[7] Giant cell tumors predominantly occur in women between the ages of 20 and 30 and typically arise in the vertebral body.[7] The locally aggressive nature of these tumors combined with the sensitive nature of the local anatomy lends itself to increased morbidity and

mortality when compared with other benign lesions of the spine. Extension into paraspinal soft tissue, the posterior elements, and adjoining intervertebral disks and vertebrae is common.

Radiographically, giant cell tumors are expansile, lytic lesions. Bone scan may reveal diffuse uptake, whereas angiography reveals a diffuse vascular lesion.[11] CT and MRI reveal a heterogeneous cystic lesion with areas of hemorrhage and necrosis.[11]

Giant cell tumors carry a relatively poor prognosis because of their aggressive involvement of the sensitive structures of the spine. Treatment is aimed at achieving as complete a resection as allowed. Despite this goal, modern series of patients with giant cell tumors of the spine reveal an overall recurrence rate of 28%.[7] Because of the risk of malignant transformation, radiation therapy is generally reserved for recurrence or incomplete resection.

Eosinophilic Granuloma

Eosinophilic granuloma is a benign, self-limiting disease that occurs predominantly in young children and adolescents. Solitary eosinophilic granuloma is the most common component of the Langerhans cell histiocytosis complex that also includes the acute form of Hand-Schüller-Christian disease and the subacute form of Letterer-Siwe disease. Approximately 6% to 7% of eosinophilic granulomas involve the spine with a 2:1 male preference.[1] Patients typically have localized pain, muscle spasm, or neurologic deficit.

Radiographically, eosinophilic granulomas of the spine appear as a well-defined lytic lesion of the vertebral body. The classical presentation is of "vertebra plana," a level collapse of the involved vertebral body. It is important to remember that the "vertebra plana" finding is not pathognomic, and a biopsy is necessary to rule out malignant lesions.

Because of the self-limited nature of eosinophilic granuloma, treatment is conservative once a biopsy has confirmed the diagnosis. Surgical intervention should be undertaken only to restore spinal stability. Chemotherapy is used in the case of a systemic variant of Langerhans cell histiocytosis.

CONCLUSION

1. Despite the predominance of mechanical defects as a cause of back pain and associated neurologic deficits, benign lesions of the spine should be considered in a complete differential diagnosis.
2. The work-up should include a careful history and physical examination aimed at identifying signs indicative of lesions of the bony spine.
3. A combination of plain films, radionuclide bone scan, CT, and MRI should be used to identify and evaluate the extent of any lesions.
4. Careful staging based on radiographic, clinical, and histologic data is needed to design an optimal course of treatment.
5. In general, complete resection is curative, and even in instances of incomplete resection or recurrence, the prognosis remains favorable.

Overview of Benign Tumors of the Spine

	Incidence	Presenting Symptoms	Radiographic Appearance	Course
Osteoid Osteoma	- Children and adolescents, average age of 16 - 2:1 male-to-female ratio	- Localized nonradiating back pain - 44% night pain, 44% radicular pain, 18% neurologic deficits - 63% painful scoliosis	- <2.0 cm in diameter with a lucent nidus surrounded by reactive sclerosis - Most commonly in the posterior elements	- Excision is usually curative - Scoliosis resolves in most cases - 4.5% recurrence
Osteoblastoma	- Similar to osteoid osteoma, average age 18	- Similar to osteoid osteoma with an increased incidence of neurologic deficits and decreased incidence of scoliosis	- >2.0 cm (key differentiating factor from osteoid osteoma) - Ranges from lucent nidus with sclerotic rim to an aggressive expansile lesion with soft tissue invasion	- May grow more rapidly than osteoid osteoma and exhibit locally destructive behavior - May undergo late malignant transformation - Complete resection is curative
Osteochondroma	- Second and third decades - Male more than female - Associated with hereditary multiple exostosis and radiation therapy	- Rarely symptomatic - Localized pain, palpable mass - Rare neurologic deficits	- Sessile or pedunculated mass - Continuity of cortex and marrow is pathognomonic	- Treatment only necessary if symptomatic - Excision is curative in most cases
Hemangioma	- 10–12% incidence in the general population	- Rarely symptomatic - New onset back pain followed by the development of myelopathy and neurologic deficits over several months	- Prominent vertical striations are classic on plain radiographs - "Polka dot" pattern seen on CT secondary to traebeculae	- Treatment is necessary only if symptomatic - Radiation is sufficient in most cases - May benefit from embolization if resection required
Aneurysmal Bone Cyst	- Often associated with other neoplasms (giant cell tumor, osteoblastoma, osteosarcoma, etc) - Average age of onset <20	- Gradual but progressive onset of pain, palpable mass, neurologic deficits, and axial deformity - Often aggressive progression	- Expansile cystic region with internal septations surrounded by a thin periosteum - Frequently expands from the posterior elements into the vertebral body and soft tissues	- Good prognosis despite aggressive nature - Intralesional excision and embolization are equally effective
Giant Cell Tumor	- Female more than male - Typically occurs in 20s or 30s - Majority in sacrum	- Localized pain, neurologic deficits - Aggressive local invasion frequently causes additional symptoms	- Lytic, expansile lesion - Heterogeneous cystic lesion with areas of hemorrhage and necrosis on CT and MRI - Most frequent in the vertebral body	- Poor prognosis due to aggressive nature - Complete resection frequently limited by morbidity - 28% recurrence
Eosinophilic Granuloma	- 2:1 male-to-female ratio - Children and adolescents - Solitary granuloma is the most common expression of the Langerhans cell histiocytosis complex	- Localized pain, muscle spasms, neurologic deficits	- Well-defined lytic lesion - Typically in the vertebral body - Classic "vertebra plana"—linear collapse of the involved vertabrae	- Self-limited course - Conservative treatment once confirmed by biopsy - Surgical intervention only to restore spinal stability

CT, Computed tomography; MRI, magnetic resonance imaging.

References

1. Bertram C, Madert J, Eggers C: Eosinophilic granuloma of the cervical spine. Spine 27:1408–1413, 2002.
2. Boriani S, Capanna R, Donati D, et al: Osteoblastoma of the spine. Clin Orthop 37–45, 1992.
3. Boriani S, De Iure F, Campanacci L, et al: Aneurysmal bone cyst of the mobile spine: report on 41 cases. Spine 26:27–35, 2001.
4. Bremnes RM, Hauge HN, Sagsveen R: Radiotherapy in the treatment of symptomatic vertebral hemangiomas: technical case report. Neurosurgery 39:1054–1058, 1996.
5. Enneking WF, Spanier SS, Goodman MA: A system for the surgical staging of musculoskeletal sarcoma. Clin Orthop 106–120, 1980.
6. Fox MW, Onofrio BM: The natural history and management of symptomatic and asymptomatic vertebral hemangiomas. J Neurosurg 78:36–45, 1993.
7. Hart RA, Boriani S, Biagini R, et al: A system for surgical staging and management of spine tumors. A clinical outcome study of giant cell tumors of the spine. Spine 22:1773–1782; discussion 1783, 1997.
8. Khosla A, Martin DS, Awwad EE: The solitary intraspinal vertebral osteochondroma. An unusual cause of compressive myelopathy: features and literature review. Spine 24:77–81, 1999.
9. Lee S, Hadlow AT: Extraosseous extension of vertebral hemangioma, a rare cause of spinal cord compression. Spine 24:2111–2114, 1999.
10. Lin PP, Guzel VB, Moura MF, et al: Long-term follow-up of patients with giant cell tumor of the sacrum treated with selective arterial embolization. Cancer 95:1317–1325, 2002.
11. Murphey MD, Andrews CL, Flemming DJ, et al: From the archives of the AFIP. Primary tumors of the spine: radiologic pathologic correlation. Radiographics 16:1131–1158, 1996.
12. Raskas DS, Graziano GP, Herzenberg JE, et al: Osteoid osteoma and osteoblastoma of the spine. J Spinal Disord 5:204–211, 1992.
13. Roblot P, Alcalay M, Cazenave-Roblot F, et al: Osteochondroma of the thoracic spine. Report of a case and review of the literature. Spine 15:240–243, 1990.
14. Saifuddin A, White J, Sherazi Z, et al: Osteoid osteoma and osteoblastoma of the spine. Factors associated with the presence of scoliosis. Spine 23:47–53, 1998.
15. Weinstein JN, McLain RF: Primary tumors of the spine. Spine 12:843–851, 1987.

CHAPTER 70

MALIGNANT PRIMARY TUMORS OF THE VERTEBRAL COLUMN

Dean Chou and Ziya Gökaslan

Primary malignant tumors of the spinal column are not common; however, when they do occur, their management can be complex. Vertebral column pathologies pose particular treatment challenges not only because of their proximity to such vital structures as the spinal cord and great vessels but also because of the potential destabilization of the spinal column after surgical resection. This chapter addresses current strategies for management of primary malignant tumors of the spinal column.

CHORDOMA

Chordomas represent neoplastic changes to notochord remnants and thus occur along the spinal column axis. Between 30% and 50% of all cases of chordomas occur in the sacrococcygeal region, between 30% and 40% in the clivus, and the remainder occur throughout the rest of the axial skeleton with a slight preponderance for the cervical region. The vertebral body is usually affected. The disks are usually spared, and the posterior elements are less involved.

Symptoms are manifestations of local mass effect and bony destruction. The pain can be activity related and becomes constant. Once the tumor erodes enough bone to cause a pathologic fracture, pain occurs at rest, and night pain is common. In addition to axial pain, other signs and symptoms include radiculopathy or myelopathy from spinal root or cord compression. Rectal discomfort may also be a manifestation for anterior sacral lesions protruding on the viscera, though this happens only in approximately 20% of cases.

Chordomas affect males more than females (2:1), and they tend to be diagnosed in people between the fifth and seventh decades of life. There have been reports of children and infants who develop chordomas. The incidence in the United States is 0.08 per 100,000 people.

On imaging, the sacral chordoma (Figure 70-1) is a lytic lesion involving many segments, whereas in the axial spine usually the vertebral body is involved and not the posterior elements. Magnetic resonance imaging (MRI) is particularly useful, because the tumor is of higher signal intensity on T2-weighted imaging compared with normal surrounding soft tissue. Computed tomography (CT) scans provide vertebral-body-destruction detail and reveal calcification patterns. Radionuclide bone scans rarely show positive uptake, because these tumors are slow growing; hence there is little periosteal reaction.

Chordomas behave as malignant entities because of their local invasiveness, high recurrence rate, and potential for metastasis. Histologically, they are lobules embedded in fibrous connective tissue stroma. They may occur in many different patterns: sheets, interconnecting cords, tight clusters, or narrow strands. Nuclear pleomorphism and occasional mitotic figures are not uncommon. There can also be differentiation into conventional mesenchymal elements such as cartilage.

Surgery remains the first line of therapy, especially with new radical excision techniques coupled with reconstruction. En bloc resections of chordomas with clear margins have yielded a recurrence rate of less than 25% in the sacrococcygeal region. Because an en bloc vertebrectomy is the best chance for obtaining total resection, anterior and posterior approaches usually need to be implemented. Chordomas are highly radioresistant, and radiation therapy only has an adjuvant or palliative role.

Metastasis of chordomas occurs slowly, with some metastatic disease found as early as 1 year and some as late as 10 years after diagnosis. Regions of metastasis include lymph nodes, lung, liver, brain, or bone, and the reported incidence of metastasis varies from 5% to more than 40%.

Overall survival rates are 67% at 5 years and 40% at 10 years. The median survival is 6.3 years.[3,14]

MULTIPLE MYELOMA

Because multiple myeloma is a disease of the bone marrow, it can occur anywhere along the spinal axis. It usually involves the ribs and pelvis because of the hematopoietic nature of these areas. Initial symptoms result from tumor involvement in bone, causing pathologic fractures or compression on neural structures. There will also be constitutional symptoms given the systemic nature of the disease. Other manifestations of multiple myeloma may also be present, including renal failure or anemia. Urine and serum protein electrophoresis will demonstrate paraproteins.

Multiple myeloma is the most common primary malignancy of bone, and it specifically replaces bone marrow with cancerous plasma cells. Dyscrasias of the blood will result. The most common age of onset is in the sixth to eighth decades, and the male-to-female ratio is 1:1. The incidence is approximately 3 per 100,000, but that number rises to 50 per 100,000 in the population aged 80 or older.

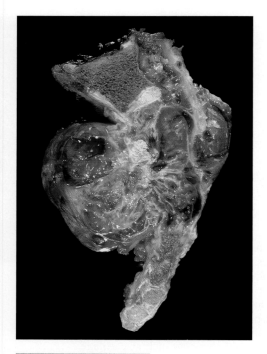

pression. Although osteosarcoma is the second most common malignant primary bone tumor after multiple myeloma, it nonetheless is rare. Its incidence is 3 per 1,000,000 people per year. The median age at diagnosis in one large study is 15 years, with symptom onset in most patients in the first 3 decades.

Visualization of this tumor is good on CT, because it is a bone-forming lesion. MRI is useful in studying not only the extent of soft tissue involvement but also the extent of the tumor's bulk. A bone scan is helpful to evaluate for multifocal disease and extent of bony metastases. The periosteal elevation and Codman's triangle—the classic radiologic findings in osteosarcoma of the long bones—are usually not present in spinal osteosarcoma. The lesions may be osteoblastic, osteoclastic, or a combination of both.

Aggressive surgical treatment is the modality that provides the best chance of extending survival. As in the appendicular tumors, neoadjuvant chemotherapy should be administered preoperatively. Wide excision or total en bloc spondylectomy with negative margins should be the goal. Postoperative radiation therapy and chemotherapy should be given to attempt cure.

Despite aggressive surgical resection, chemotherapy, and radiation therapy, outcomes for osteosarcomas remain poor. One study showed an 11% survival rate at 2-year follow-up with a mean survival of 20 months. Another study out of Northern Europe showed a 5-year survival rate of 30% and median survival from the time of diagnosis of 1.4 years.[15,9,11,17,4]

CHONDROSARCOMAS

Although chondrosarcomas occur mainly in the scapula, humerus, femur, and pelvis, approximately 4% to 8% occur in the spine. The distribution is mainly in the thoracolumbo-sacral areas, with a somewhat lower incidence in the cervical spine. As with other primary malignant spine tumors, pain is usually the chief complaint. There may also be nerve dysfunction and neurologic deficit. There may even be perception of a mass. The most common age at diagnosis is in the fifth and sixth decades, and the male-to-female ratio is 1.5:1 to 2:1.

Plain radiographs will demonstrate scalloping of the vertebral cortex or expansion or destruction of the cortex. Calcification is often present. CT scanning is useful for defining bony involvement, and MRI provides definition of soft tissue involvement. Technetium bone scanning is positive in multifocal or metastatic disease. Chondrosarcomas form hyaline cartilage and may be either primary lesions or secondary transformations of osteochondromas or endochondromas. They may also be seen in conjunction with Ollier's disease, Maffucci's syndrome, or exostoses. Higher histologic grade tumors are associated with higher recurrence rates.

Surgical resection with wide margins remains the best treatment. Total, en bloc removal should be attempted, because piecemeal removal will result in high recurrence rates. Chemotherapy has shown some benefit, and radiation therapy has a role in palliation. It has been shown that cryosurgery helps prevent local recurrence in instances in which tumor-free margins are not obtained.

In general, the histologic grade of the tumor determines the survival of the patient. In one series, median survival was 6 years, and in another study, disease-free survival at 65 months was between 63% and 71%.[18,20]

On radiographic imaging, lytic lesions will be noted on CT, and on MRI different signal patterns, ranging from normal bone marrow to focal lesions or diffuse marrow infiltration, may be seen. On T1-weighted spin-echo images, intensity is low, but there is marked enhancement after administration of gadolinium. Even in advanced stages, up to 20% of radiographs and MRI examinations may be normal.

Treatment modalities for multiple myeloma are primarily nonsurgical. Radiation therapy and chemotherapy are the mainstays of treatment. Patients are poor surgical candidates because of the diffuse nature of disease, osteopenia, anemia, neutropenia, and concomitant renal insufficiency. There are cases, however, in which surgery may be indicated if a single, isolated vertebral segment is involved. Mean survival for multiple myeloma is 49 months.[13]

OSTEOSARCOMA

Osteosarcoma is a highly malignant tumor that mainly occurs throughout the appendicular skeleton. Only approximately 3% of osteosarcomas affect the axial skeleton, involving mainly the vertebral bodies and less so the posterior elements or pedicles. Because osteosarcomas can metastasize, they may be either metastatic or primary to the spine. Moreover, they can be lesions secondary to radiation therapy, fibrous dysplasia, or Paget's disease. Reports have suggested that malignant transformation of Paget's occurs more in long bones than in the spinal column. The most common site of metastasis is the lung.

The initial symptom of osteosarcoma is pain that is localized to the area of the lesion. If the cervical spine is involved, there may be neurologic deficit or symptoms secondary to com-

EWING'S SARCOMA

Ewing's sarcoma mainly occurs in the diaphysis of the long bones; however, 8% of all Ewing's sarcoma occurs in the spine. Within the axial skeleton, the most common site is the sacrum.

Pain is the most common symptom. Neurologic deficit is common, with up to 80% of patients manifesting such signs or radiculopathy. There may also be complaint of fever, and 23% perceive a mass. Alkaline phosphatase and lactate dehydrogenase (LDH) are useful laboratory studies because their levels may be elevated. LDH is helpful as a marker of recurrent disease.

Ewing's sarcoma is a rare disease that occurs primarily in children. The average age at onset is 16.5 years. Patient's ages usually range from the first to the fourth decade. Its incidence is 3 per 1,000,000 people in the United States.

Plain x-ray examination is useful for demonstrating a lytic lesion that may have sclerotic edges. CT is useful to evaluate the extent of bony involvement, and MRI is helpful for evaluating the extent of soft tissue involvement. In addition, MRI is also helpful in defining marrow involvement. Bone scanning may be useful in the post-treatment phase of management. Histopathologically, Ewing's sarcoma is a highly malignant round cell tumor of bone, classified as a primitive neuroectodermal tumor (PNET).

Treatment modalities consist of surgery, chemotherapy, and radiation therapy. Although earlier studies have shown poor survival, with an average survival of 33 months and a 5-year survival rate of 20%, there has been significant improvement in survival of Ewing's sarcoma over the past 20 years. Wide surgical resection has also improved survival; in one study, patients receiving radical resection had a 60% 5-year survival rate versus 40% 5-year survival in patients with intralesional or incomplete resection. One study has shown that new chemotherapeutic regimens help extend 5-year survival to 64%.[12,19]

LYMPHOMA

Lymphoma may occur anywhere throughout the spine, and approximately 13% of patients with lymphoma have bony involvement. Of these patients, 15% have spinal involvement, and some may have cord compression. Patients usually have back pain, and there may be nerve dysfunction secondary to compression.

Patients usually seek treatment in the fifth to seventh decades. The incidence of lymphoma is approximately 2 to 3 per 100,000 per year, whereas non-Hodgkin's lymphoma has an incidence of approximately 10 to 20 per 100,000. Radiographic imaging demonstrates enhanced lesions on MRI, and CT may demonstrate bony involvement.

Treatment of lymphoma depends on the extent of neural compression. If there is significant compression with neurologic findings, then surgical intervention should be the procedure of choice. If there is spinal involvement without any compression or neurologic findings, then radiation therapy should be initiated. Lymphomas are very sensitive to both radiation therapy and chemotherapy, and they can be irradiated in cases in which neurologic compromise is not a factor.

Survival for non-Hodgkin's lymphoma is 40% to 60% at 5 years, whereas the 5-year survival rate for Hodgkin's lymphoma is 84% or even higher in younger people.[8,6]

SOFT TISSUE SARCOMAS

Sarcomas arise from the surrounding soft tissue of the spine. They can destroy bone, compress nerves, and cause both axial and radicular pain. They arise from the paraspinous musculature, and they are rare. One of the largest case series consists of 14 patients.

Radiographic imaging, including CT and MRI, is very important for defining both soft tissue and bony abnormalities. Radionuclide scanning should be considered for evidence of distant metastatic spread.

The types of tumor include neurofibrosarcoma, angiosarcoma, synovial sarcoma, chondrosarcoma of soft tissues, liposarcoma, leiomyosarcoma, and malignant fibrous histiocytoma. Guest et al have proposed a classification system of three classes: (1) paraspinous muscle involvement only; (2) paraspinous muscle and posterior spinous element muscle involvement; and (3) paraspinous muscle involvement, chest wall posterior element, and vertebral body involvement.

The treatment for paraspinal sarcomas includes preoperative chemotherapy before surgical resection. Aggressive en bloc surgical resection should be the goal based on location. Radiation therapy is necessary for cure, and brachytherapy may also be implemented. Postoperative chemotherapy should also be part of the treatment plan.

Because of the location of paraspinal soft tissue sarcomas, the prognosis for these tumors is probably slightly worse than for sarcomas arising in other areas. A recent Memorial Sloan-Kettering Cancer Center study looking at primary and metastatic sarcomas of the spine demonstrated that median survival after surgery was 18 months.[1,10,16]

PLASMACYTOMA

Plasmacytomas can involve such areas of the body as lymph nodes, lung, gastrointestinal tract, and spleen; however, 25% to 50% of cases involve the spine. Most of the spinal involvement is within the thoracic spine. The main symptom is pain with slow and gradual onset, and pain at night may be perceived. There may also be neural compression with subsequent symptoms—myelopathy, radiculopathy, or weakness—from mass effect of the tumor. In the population that plasmacytomas affect, more than half have radicular symptoms, and one series showed that paraplegia may not be an uncommon symptom. Because these are older patients, many are mistakenly diagnosed with rheumatoid arthritis. If plasmacytoma is suspected, a bone marrow biopsy should be performed to assess for multiple myeloma or for the presence of systemic disease. Fifty percent of patients with plasmacytoma develop multiple myeloma.

Plasmacytoma of the spine is extremely rare, with the literature consisting mainly of case reports. It is even more rare in children, with most patients being older than 50. On imaging, lytic lesions are noted, and CT and MRI are both useful for defining bony involvement and soft tissue involvement, respectively. There can be significant destruction with vertebral collapse; however, bone scans may be normal. A skeletal survey may be more useful to assess for multifocal disease. Plasmacytomas are neoplastic marrow cells that can range from mature plasma cells to tumor cells with cytologic atypia to anaplasia.

Because these lesions are radiosensitive, radiation therapy is the first choice for intervention. Surgery is indicated only when there is neurologic compromise, spinal deformity, or instability. One study showed a median survival of 47 months with a 5-year survival of 75%.[2,5,7]

CONCLUSION

Primary malignant tumors of the vertebral column are very challenging to manage, and many have poor prognoses. Multiple modalities of therapy, including surgery, radiation, and chemotherapy, are needed to properly treat these lesions. Pathologic classification, grade of tumor, and, in certain cases, extent of surgical excision can affect survival and outcome.

References

1. Bilsky MH, Boland PJ, Panageas KS, et al: Intralesional resection of primary and metastatic sarcoma involving the spine: outcome analysis of 59 patients. Neurosurgery 49:1277–1286; discussion 1286–1277, 2001.
2. Chak LY, Cox RS, Bostwick DG, et al: Solitary plasmacytoma of bone: treatment, progression, and survival. J Clin Oncol 5:1811–1815, 1987.
3. Chandawarkar RY: Sacrococcygeal chordoma: review of 50 consecutive patients. World J Surg 20:717–719, 1996.
4. Cohen ZR, Fourney DR, Marco RA, et al: Total cervical spondylectomy for primary osteogenic sarcoma. Case report and description of operative technique. J Neurosurg 97:386–392, 2002.
5. Corwin J, Lindberg RD: Solitary plasmacytoma of bone vs. extramedullary plasmacytoma and their relationship to multiple myeloma. Cancer 43:1007–1013, 1979.
6. Davidge-Pitts M, Dansey R, Bezwoda WR: Prolonged survival in follicular non Hodgkins lymphoma is predicted by achievement of complete remission with initial treatment: results of a long-term study with multivariate analysis of prognostic factors. Leuk Lymphoma 24:131–140, 1996.
7. Ellis PA, Colls BM: Solitary plasmacytoma of bone: clinical features, treatment and survival. Hematol Oncol 10:207–211, 1992.
8. Eltom MA, Jemal A, Mbulaiteye SM, et al: Trends in Kaposi's sarcoma and non-Hodgkin's lymphoma incidence in the United States from 1973 through 1998. J Natl Cancer Inst 94:1204–1210, 2002.
9. Gore L, Greffe BS, Rothenberg SS, et al: Long-term survival after intralesional resection and multi-modal therapy of thoracic spine osteosarcoma. Med Pediatr Oncol 40:400–402, 2003.
10. Guest C, Wang EH, Davis A, et al: Paraspinal soft-tissue sarcoma. Classification of 14 cases. Spine 18:1292–1297, 1993.
11. Kager L, Zoubek A, Potschger U, et al: Primary metastatic osteosarcoma: presentation and outcome of patients treated on neoadjuvant Cooperative Osteosarcoma Study Group protocols. J Clin Oncol 21:2011–2018, 2003.
12. Kennedy JG, Frelinghuysen P, Hoang BH: Ewing sarcoma: current concepts in diagnosis and treatment. Curr Opin Pediatr 15:53–57, 2003.
13. Kumar A, Loughran T, Alsina M, et al: Management of multiple myeloma: a systematic review and critical appraisal of published studies. Lancet Oncol 4:293–304, 2003.
14. McMaster ML, Goldstein AM, Bromley CM, et al: Chordoma: incidence and survival patterns in the United States, 1973–1995. Cancer Causes Control 12:1–11, 2001.
15. Meyers PA, Heller G, Healey JH, et al: Osteogenic sarcoma with clinically detectable metastasis at initial presentation. J Clin Oncol 11:449–453, 1993.
16. Nowakowski VA, Castro JR, Petti PL, et al: Charged particle radiotherapy of paraspinal tumors. Int J Radiat Oncol Biol Phys 22:295–303, 1992.
17. Ozaki T, Flege S, Liljenqvist U, et al: Osteosarcoma of the spine: experience of the Cooperative Osteosarcoma Study Group. Cancer 94:1069–1077, 2002.
18. Ruark DS, Schlehaider UK, Shah JP: Chondrosarcomas of the head and neck. World J Surg 16:1010–1015; discussion 1015–1016, 1992.
19. Stiller CA, Craft AW, Corazziari I: Survival of children with bone sarcoma in Europe since 1978: results from the EUROCARE study. Eur J Cancer 37:760–766, 2001.
20. York JE, Berk RH, Fuller GN, et al: Chondrosarcoma of the spine: 1954 to 1997. J Neurosurg 90:73–78, 1999.

CHAPTER 71

THERAPEUTIC OPTIONS FOR TREATING METASTATIC SPINE TUMORS

Mark H. Bilsky and Jeremy Wang

Therapeutic options for the treatment of metastatic spine tumors are principally external-beam radiation therapy (EBRT) and surgery. Chemotherapy, hormones, and immunotherapy play more limited roles. Regardless of the treatment modality chosen, metastatic spine tumors are treated with the intention to provide palliation. The goals of treatment are to maintain or improve the patient's neurologic and functional status, achieve mechanical stability, reduce pain, optimize local tumor control, and improve overall quality of life.[8] The indications for EBRT and surgery have evolved over the past 40 years; however, decisions are typically based on anecdotal experiences of referring physicians and institutional preferences.

Initial surgical attempts to treat metastatic tumors relied on laminectomy without instrumentation. Review of multiple series from the 1960s and early 1970s proved that laminectomy did not lead to acceptable neurologic or pain outcomes. A review of this literature showed that 55% of patients maintained ambulation, and 33% of paraparetic patients regained ambulation. In some series, more than 50% of patients were made worse with operation.* It is well recognized now that laminectomy without instrumentation does not provide adequate tumor resection of the vertebral body or epidural tumor. Iatrogenic instability was created by resecting the posterior elements in the presence of pathologic compression or burst fractures of the vertebral body. Poor preoperative assessments of systemic disease and medical comorbidities often contributed to significant postoperative complications.

As a result of suboptimal surgical outcomes and high morbidity rates, radiation therapy became the mainstay of therapy for metastatic spine disease. Neurologic and functional outcomes were as good, if not better, than with noninstrumented laminectomy. In early radiation series 80% of patients maintained ambulation, 42% of paraparetic patients improved, and less than 20% worsened neurologically over the course of radiation. Radiation therapy became the principal modality to treat metastatic spine tumors.

In the 1990s, surgeons developed more aggressive approaches to resect spine tumors, including anterior transcavitary and posterolateral approaches. The addition of anterior instrumentation and posterior segmental fixation improved neurologic and functional outcomes, with 95% of patients maintaining ambulation, 50% to 75% of paraparetic patients improving, and less than 5% of patients worsening after surgery. These improvements are likely the result of more complete tumor resections, aggressive epidural decompression, and instrumentation providing spinal stabilization. In addition, the widespread use of magnetic resonance imaging (MRI) made possible a complete assessment of the bone and epidural spinal involvement, allowing surgeons to operate before the development of significant neurologic symptoms. Extensive preoperative systemic and medical work-ups also improved surgical outcomes.†

Despite surgical advances resulting in improved outcomes, EBRT continues to play a significant role in the treatment of metastatic spine tumors and remains the primary treatment modality for most patients. The spine service at Memorial Sloan-Kettering Cancer Center (MSKCC) evaluates more than 1000 patients a year but operates on only approximately 150 tumors. In principle, EBRT is preferable to surgery, because it is less invasive and typically allows a return to systemic therapy sooner than surgery. In a radiation series reported by Maranzano and colleagues, 275 patients underwent irradiation for spinal metastases. The results of this modern radiation series are similar to surgical outcomes, with 94% of patients maintaining ambulation and 60% regaining the ability to ambulate.[38] In part, these excellent results reflect that patients with strong surgical indications, such as gross spinal instability, underwent surgery. Careful patient selection for both surgery and radiation improves palliation in the cancer population.

Surgeons, radiation oncologists, and medical oncologists often have very strong biases regarding the treatment of metastatic tumors. As noted by Maranzano and colleagues, patient selection clearly influences radiation and surgical outcomes, but therapeutic decisions are often complicated.[37] At MSKCC we use a conceptual framework to direct therapeutic assessments, known as *NOMS:* Neurologic, Oncologic, Mechanical instability, and Systemic disease and medical comorbidities. An independent assessment of each category allows the physician to decide the best single or combination of treatments for an individual patient.

---

*See references 10, 12, 13, 18, 20, 21, 24, 31, 32, 36, 39, 41, 48, 59, 61–64.

†See references 4, 5, 7, 11, 14, 17, 22, 25, 27, 29, 33, 34, 42, 43, 47, 50–52, 60.

NEUROLOGY

From a neurologic perspective (the *N* in NOMS) the overriding goals of treatment are to preserve or improve neurologic function. Resolution of myelopathy and functional radiculopathy are essential for good neurologic outcomes. The best predictor of a good neurologic outcome is neurologic function at the outset. Before the development of neurologic symptoms, patients often have nocturnal or early morning pain that can be alleviated with steroids. In a patient with known cancer, the development of biologic pain is an indication to obtain an MRI scan of the entire spinal axis. Patients with biologic pain generally have bone tumor without extensive epidural disease and have good neurologic outcomes with either radiation or surgery. Standard-fraction EBRT is strongly considered even for moderately radioresistant tumors, and surgical consideration is reserved for highly radioresistant tumors.

The development of radiculopathy and myelopathy often denotes the development of soft tissue epidural tumor. In patients with high-grade epidural spinal cord compression with or without the presence of neurologic symptoms, the treatment decision is based largely on the radiosensitivity of the tumor. For example, lymphoma and multiple myeloma are often exquisitely radiosensitive and will resolve with high-dose radiation in 2 to 3 days. Less radiosensitive tumors, such as lung and colon carcinoma, may respond but do not generally have an immediate reduction in epidural tumor compression. Thus patients treated with radiation may have ongoing compression for several weeks and show neurologic progression during or shortly following radiation. These patients are considered for operation as initial therapy (Table 71-1). Relatively radiosensitive tumors, such as breast carcinoma, with high-grade compression can often be radiated on high-dose steroids with satisfactory neurologic outcomes.

Patchell and colleagues recently reported a prospective randomized trial comparing radiation therapy with operation in patients with neurologic symptoms.[46] Out of 101 patients, 50 were randomized to surgery with postoperative radiation, and 51 received radiation alone. The patients treated all had solid tumors with high-grade spinal cord compression and neurologic deficits. Radiosensitive hematologic malignancies, such as lymphoma and multiple myeloma, were excluded from the study. Patients treated with surgery maintained ambulation significantly longer than those undergoing radiation (126 days vs. 35 days). In addition, nonambulatory patients recovered significantly more function in the operated group (9:16) compared with the irradiated group (3:16). Although these results suggest that surgery is appropriate for solid tumor metastases resulting in neurologic deficits, the survival in the operated and irradiated group was quite limited, with a median of 129 and 100 days, respectively. These relatively short survivals suggest that patients treated in this series had relatively advanced systemic disease or poor-prognosis tumors, such as colon and lung.[33] From a palliative standpoint, a patient with 3-month survival may be better served with palliative EBRT regardless of neurologic function or degree of epidural compression.

ONCOLOGY

Oncologic considerations (the *O* in NOMS) reflect how well the tumor responds to radiation therapy, surgery, or chemotherapy. The response to radiation depends on the radiosensitivity of known tumor histologies and is graded from highly sensitive to highly resistant (see Table 71-1). The highly and moderately sensitive tumors typically respond well to conventional external-beam radiation doses (e.g., 30 Gy in 10 fractions). Good responses are seen in patients with epidural tumor, including lymphoma, multiple myeloma, and breast carcinoma. Conversely, the moderately and highly radioresistant tumors do not typically respond to these conventional doses.

Until recently, higher dose radiation was not an option because of the high risk of developing radiation myelopathy. The development of systems that can deliver highly conformal doses of radiation to spinal lesions may improve our ability to treat relatively radioresistant tumors. The two iterations of three-dimensional-conformal radiation therapy currently available for spine applications are intensity-modulated radiation therapy (IMRT) and CyberKnife®. IMRT delivers a very steep dose gradient between a target volume and a nearby risk organ, such as a paraspinal tumor and spinal cord. In addition to conventional conformal techniques such as computed tomography (CT) and magnetic resonance (MR)-based three-dimensional volume rendering and conformal beam shaping using the beam's eye view, IMRT uses inverse planning techniques to generate nonuniform beam intensities that enhance the ability to deliver optimum dose distributions that may not be possible with conventional three-dimensional methods.[15,16,30,35,40,45,49,58] Of the initial eight metastatic tumors treated at our institution, all had failed prior conventional EBRT, and seven failed prior surgery. The tumors were treated to the median 100% isodose line of 20 Gy (range 20 to 30 Gy) in four or five fractions. The median dose to the spinal cord was approximately 6 Gy (range 1.5 to 5.1 Gy) in addition to the previous cord radiation. Durable pain control and recovery of functional radiculopathy was achieved in all patients. IMRT may help treat radioresistant metastatic spine tumors without operation; however, high-grade epidural compression may preclude full dose treatment to the dural margin.

TABLE 71-1
Oncologic Radiation Sensitivity

Sensitive
Myeloma
Lymphoma

Moderately Sensitive
Breast carcinoma

Moderately Resistant
Colon carcinoma
NSCLC

Highly Resistant
Thyroid carcinoma
Renal cell carcinoma
Sarcoma
Melanoma

NSCLC, Non–small cell lung carcinoma.

From an oncologic perspective, local tumor control is rarely achieved with surgery alone. Klekamp and Samii reviewed 101 metastatic tumors.[33] The recurrence rates following operation were 64% after 1 year and 96% after 4 years. Operations for highly radioresistant tumors, such as renal and thyroid cancer, often achieve local tumor control with low recurrence rates. Breast carcinoma also has a durable response to surgery. This series found that surgery did not provide long-term local tumor control for colon carcinoma, non–small cell lung carcinoma, and carcinoma of unknown primary origin. In our experience, two other tumors that may recur early following surgery are hormone refractory prostate carcinoma and melanoma.[23] Although neurologic outcomes may be improved in patients undergoing surgery for these tumor histologies, patients often do not have durable responses and may experience recurrence within 4 to 6 weeks even with aggressive tumor resection. Postoperative radiation therapy may delay recurrences, but often patients have received prior radiation either for local spine treatment or because of overlapping ports. In candidate patients, EBRT should be offered as postoperative adjuvant therapy. In tumors suspected to have aggressive tumor histologies, EBRT can be safely administered within 2 weeks of surgery.

Recently, en bloc spondylectomy has been touted for metastatic tumors.[1–3,54–57] There is little evidence that en bloc resection helps with local tumor control for metastatic tumors. En bloc tumor resection is technically demanding with a higher risk of spinal cord damage. In papers reviewing en bloc spondylectomy for metastases, there is little difference in local control between those undergoing intralesional and en bloc resection.

Systemic therapies, such as chemotherapy and hormones, are not generally used as first-line therapy for spinal metastases. With the exception of breast, prostate, and renal cell carcinoma, most metastases occur late in the course of the disease. Most patients have already failed first- and second-line systemic therapy, with progression of visceral and bone tumor. Having failed the most effective agents, these patients are unlikely to have a good response to subsequent systemic therapy. However, there are tumors that have relatively reliable responses to systemic therapy. In children these include metastatic Ewing's sarcoma, high-risk neuroblastoma, and osteogenic sarcoma. In adults, breast and prostate may respond to systemic therapy.

Bisphosphonates are a class of drugs that inhibit osteoclast activation and may have additional antineoplastic properties. Bisphosphonates such as pamidronate and zoledronate markedly reduce skeletal fractures in patients with breast carcinoma, multiple myeloma, and other osteolytic metastases.[6] In a double-blind, multicenter, parallel group trial, 372 women with stage IV breast cancer were randomized to receive either 90 mg of pamidronate or placebo intravenously every 3 to 4 weeks.[28] Over a 2-year follow-up, the proportion of patients who developed pathologic fractures or required EBRT or surgery was significantly less in the pamidronate-treated group. The median time to first skeletal event in the pamidronate-treated group was 13.9 months, and in the placebo group, 7 months. Although the drug has a high initial cost, this can be justified by the substantial quality-adjusted survival benefit.

MECHANICAL INSTABILITY

Mechanical instability (the *M* in NOMS) resulting from pathologic fractures is relatively uncommon but is often an indication for operation. Traditional concepts of instability from the trauma and degenerative literature do not directly apply to spinal tumors. Conversely, the literature regarding pathologic fractures is limited, and radiographic criteria have not been well characterized.[19,34] In our experience, patients with instability have severe pain on movement. This should be differentiated from biologic pain. Differentiating instability pain from biologic pain is essential to treatment. The vast majority of patients we see give a long history of biologic pain, which is responsive to steroids and radiation, although this depends to some degree on the radiation sensitivity of the tumor. Most patients with thoracic and lumbar compression and burst fractures have biologic pain with no evidence of movement-related pain. Movement-related pain is more often an indication for operation in candidate patients, but the level of spine involvement is important in decision making.

Atlantoaxial Spine

The atlantoaxial (AA) spine is the exception to movement-related pain representing instability. In a review of 33 patients with tumor in the AA spine who came to the neurosurgery service at MSKCC over a 6-year period, all had pain on rotation of the neck, and 11 patients had occipital neuralgia.[9,44,53] Patients with minimal fracture subluxations were treated with standard-fraction external-beam radiation (3000 cGy in 10 fractions) and immobilized in an external orthosis for the duration of the radiation and for 6 weeks post-treatment. Patients were considered unstable if they had more than 5 mm subluxation or an Effendi type 4 trauma fracture with greater than 3.5 mm subluxation and 11 degrees angulation. Of the 23 patients treated with radiation therapy (RT), 18 were successfully weaned from a hard collar and had significant pain improvement and neurologic preservation. Five required subsequent fixation, but only one had a fracture subluxation postradiation. This occurred while the patient was in rehabilitation. Two patients had fracture subluxations that met initial operative criteria, but they chose nonoperative therapy. They both required operation for persistent severe neck pain. One patient was operated on for radiographic residual metastatic osteogenic sarcoma following chemotherapy, despite an excellent pain response, and one patient underwent elective fixation.

Neutral lateral cervical spine x-ray examinations are used to evaluate fracture subluxations of the AA spine for displacement and angulation. Review of the literature and our own series confirm that patients with normal spinal alignment or minimal fracture subluxations respond to hard collar immobilization and radiation therapy. Patients who do not meet instability criteria (e.g., >5 mm subluxation) uniformly responded to nonoperative therapy, as assessed by resolution of mechanical neck pain, lack of deformity progression, and ability to be weaned from the hard collar. The tumor histology, radiosensitivity of the tumor, and extent of bone infiltration, as assessed on MRI scans, does not seem to affect response to RT or subsequent need for an operation. Osteolytic tumor often results in destruction of the C2 body, odontoid, or facet joints. Despite extensive destruction, the majority of patients with normal alignment or minimal subluxation responded to nonoperative therapy. Presumably these patients develop a fibrous union and occasionally show reossification (e.g., multiple myeloma).

Subaxial Cervical Spine

Compression and burst fractures in the subaxial cervical spine often result in severe movement-related pain. As opposed to the AA spine, radiation in an external orthosis does not typically relieve the mechanical pain. These patients often require operation. Tumor resection must often take into account the location of the vertebral artery, which is often pushed laterally and anteriorly by the tumor. Anterior reconstruction with a fibula allograft and cervical plate has been reliable. Most often anterior reconstruction is supplemented with posterior lateral mass screw-rod systems.

Thoracic Spine

In the thoracic spine, the most common symptom of instability is pain on hyperextension of the spine when the patient lies flat. This is not the equivalent of biologic pain but is true positional pain when the patient straightens the thoracic kyphosis resulting from the pathologic fracture. Radiographically, this most often results from a compression or burst fracture with the additional presence of tumor in the posterior elements. It is rare to see thoracic spine instability pain in the absence of three-column involvement. Fortunately, most compression or burst fractures in the thoracic spine are stable.

Lumbar Spine

Lumbar spine instability pain is most commonly seen with axial load on sitting or standing. Compression and burst fractures variably cause instability pain, but three-column involvement often results in movement-related pain. Mechanical radiculopathy is unique to the lumbar spine. On standing, patients develop immediate radiculopathy, resulting from a compression fracture, with tumor encasing the nerve root in the neuroforamen. Lumbar mechanical radiculopathy is a relative indication for surgery. It does not typically resolve after radiation, even with radiosensitive tumors.

SYSTEMIC DISEASE AND MEDICAL COMORBIDITIES

Decisions about treatment should be made in a multidisciplinary fashion with input from the medical oncologist and internist. The spine surgeon often meets patients late in the course of their illness and does not have a global perspective regarding the extent and pace of the disease and response to prior therapy. Evaluation of systemic disease and medical comorbidities (the *S* in NOMS) requires medical internists, who determine the need for cardiac and pulmonary evaluation and the implications of medical sequelae from prior chemotherapy and radiation. At MSKCC, most patients undergo preoperative cardiac stress and pulmonary function tests.

CASE EXAMPLES

The cases illustrated in Table 71-2 and Figures 71-1 through 71-3 illustrate several aspects of patient management.

TABLE 71-2	Case Examples: Treating Metastatic Spine Tumors

Case 1	Case 2	Case 3
Case History		
History and Physical Examination		
A 70-year-old female with a prior history of lymphoma presents with severe neck pain on movement, mild clumsy hand syndrome, and hyperactive reflexes in the upper and lower extremities.	An 80-year-old retired judge presents with a history of lung and bladder carcinoma (1983) and stage 4 prostate carcinoma (1991). Patient underwent multiple systemic therapies including androgen blockade with ketoconazole and PC-SPES. He has been on Pamidronate for one year. He presented with a 2-month history of biologic pain and 2-day history of inability to ambulate. Motor examination showed antigravity in lower extremities (ASIA C), decreased proprioception and 1200 mL residual on straight catheterization. He denies movement-related pain. Patient was loaded with Dexamethasone 100 mg followed by 24 mg every 6 hours. Within 12 hours, he was antigravity against resistance (ASIA D) in the lower extremities.	A 45-year-old with a long history of colon carcinoma and a 3-month history of biologic pain. He presented with a 3-week history of mechanical radiculopathy and left leg pain.

TABLE 71-2   **Case Examples: Treating Metastatic Spine Tumors (Continued)**

Case 1	Case 2	Case 3
Case History		
Imaging		
MRI shows a C3 pathologic burst fracture with posterior element involvement. There is spinal cord compression without cerebrospinal fluid space (see Figure 71-1A).	MRI shows multifocal osseous tumor with a T9 burst fracture without posterior element involvement (see Figure 71-2A). Circumferential high-grade epidural spinal cord compression is present (see Figure 71-2B). PET scan showed no visceral metastases, but the presence of multiple bone lesions.	MRI shows an L2 burst fracture with neuroforaminal compression on the left (see Figure 71-3A and B).
Decision Making		
Neurologic		
High-grade epidural compression with cervical myelopathy.	High-grade epidural spinal cord compression with significant neurologic symptoms.	Left L2 radiculopathy is consistent with his tumor presentation.
Oncologic		
Highly radiosensitive tumor.	Hormone refractory prostate carcinoma is relatively radioresistant; however, we have seen early failures postoperatively following surgical resection.	Colon carcinoma is considered relatively radioresistant.
Mechanical Instability		
Severe movement pain resulting from burst fracture with posterior element involvement.	The patient has no movement-related pain and a T9 burst fracture without posterior involvement. The patient was considered stable.	Mechanical component to the radiculopathy is present.
Systemic Disease and Comorbidities		
No significant medical issues and well-controlled systemic disease.	Despite no visceral disease, the patient had significant cardiac risk factors.	No significant systemic tumor or medical comorbidities.
Decision		
Operation. Despite the fact that this is a highly radiosensitive tumor and would have a rapid response to radiation, the patient is considered unstable by virtue of severe movement related pain. Operation would provide immediate spinal cord decompression, but more importantly would resolve mechanical instability issues. Operation followed by radiation: A single-staged anterior followed by posterior approach was performed. Initially the tumor was approached via an anterior transcervical approach with resection of C3 vertebral body and anterior epidural tumor and reconstruction using fibula allograft and an anterior cervical plate. The posterior operation involved a C2–C3 laminectomy with left C2–C3 facet resection and posterior lateral mass plate fixation C1 to C5 with a sublaminar wire around the posterior C1 arch to avoid fixation to the occiput (see Figure 71-1B). Because of the high radiosensitivity of the tumor, tumor was left on the left vertebral artery. Follow-up: At three year follow-up the patient remains stable without evidence of locally recurrent tumor (see Figure 71-1C).	Treatment decisions are difficult in this case. Surgery followed by radiation probably offers the best chance of durable functional recovery; however, medical co-morbidities place the patient at high risk. The patient chose EBRT over surgery. He died three weeks after radiation from systemic progression.	Operation followed by radiation is the treatment of choice as mechanical radiculopathy rarely improves even with radiosensitive tumors. Patient underwent an anterior transcavitary approach and L2 vertebral body resection. Reconstruction was performed with PEEK carbon fiber stackable cage (Johnson and Johnson, DePuy AcroMed, Inc., Raynham, MA) and an anterior plate (see Figure 71-3C). The patient had resolution of back pain and radiculopathy. He was stable for 14 months before dying from progression of systemic tumor.

EBRT, External beam radiation therapy; MRI, magnetic resonance imaging; PET, positron-emission tomography.

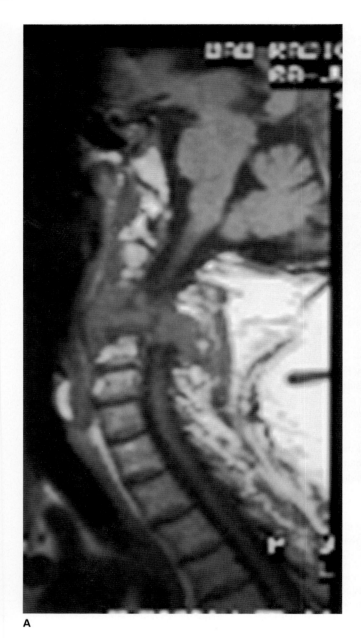

A

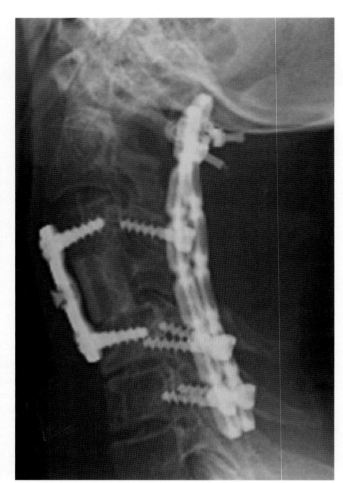

B

C

FIGURE 71-1 Magnetic resonance images of a 70-year-old female. *A,* Spinal cord compression without cerebrospinal fluid space. *B,* C2-C3 laminectomy with left C2-C3 facet resection and posterior lateral mass plate fixation C1 to C5 with a sublaminar wire around the posterior C1 arch to avoid fixation to the occiput. *C,* Three-year follow-up; the patient remains stable without evidence of locally recurrent tumor.

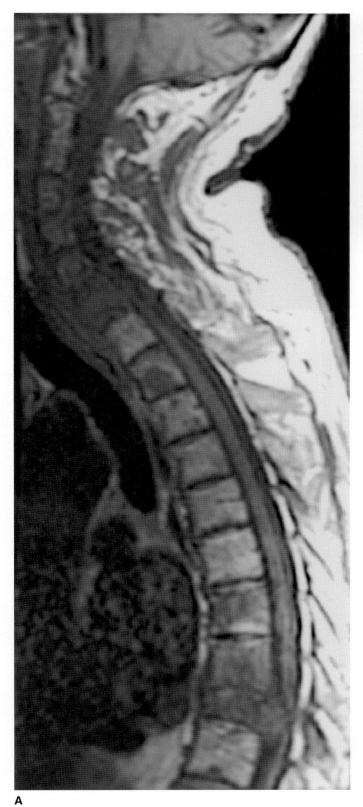

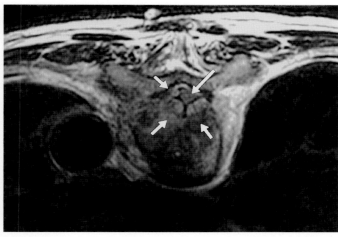

A

B

FIGURE 71-2 Magnetic resonance images of an 80-year-old male. *A,* Multifocal osseous tumor with a T9 burst fracture without posterior element involvement. *B,* Circumferential high-grade epidural spinal cord compression is present.

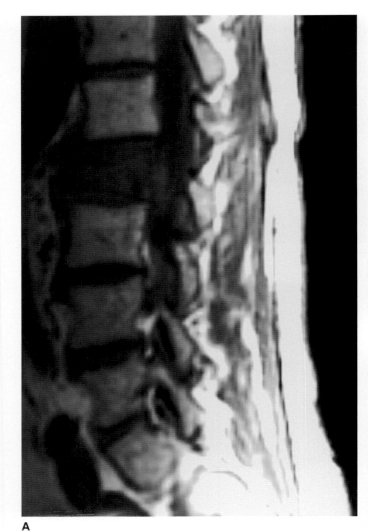

A

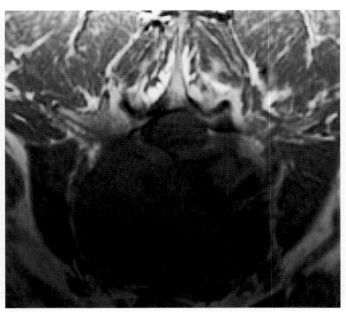

B

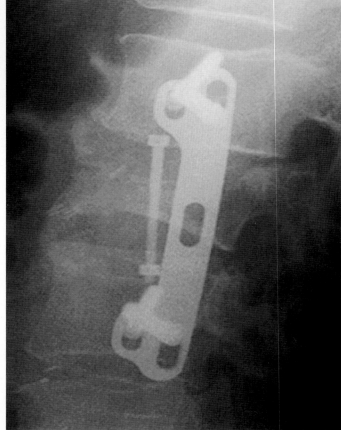

C

FIGURE 71-3 Magnetic resonance images of a 45-year-old male. *A* and *B*, L2 burst fracture with neuroforaminal compression on the left. *C*, Reconstruction was performed with PEEK carbon fiber stackable cage and an anterior plate (see Table 71-2).

References

1. Abdel-Wanis ME, Kawahara N, Murata A, et al: Thyroid cancer spinal metastases: report on 25 operations in 14 patients. Anticancer Res 22:2509–16, 2002.

2. Abe E, Kobayashi T, Murai H, et al: Total spondylectomy for primary malignant, aggressive benign, and solitary metastatic bone tumors of the thoracolumbar spine. J Spinal Disord 14:237–46, 2001.

3. Abe E, Sato K, Murai H, et al: Total spondylectomy for solitary spinal metastasis of the thoracolumbar spine: a preliminary report. Tohoku J Exp Med 190:33–49, 2000.

4. Akeyson E, McCutcheon IE: Single-stage posterior vertebrectomy and replacement combined with posterior instrumentation for spinal metastasis. J Neurosurg 85:211–220, 1996.

5. Bauer HCF, Wedin R: Survival after surgery for spinal and extremity metastases: prognostication of 241 patients. Acta Orthop Scand 66:143–146, 1995.

6. Berenson JR, Lichtenstein A, Porter L, et al: Efficacy of pamidronate in reducing skeletal events in patients with advanced multiple myeloma. N Engl J Med 334:488–493, 1996.

7. Bilsky MH, Boland P, Lis E, et al: Single-stage posterolateral transpedicle approach for spondylectomy, epidural decompression, and circumferential fusion of spinal metastases. Spine 25:2240–9, 2000.

8. Bilsky MH, Lis E, Raizer J, et al: The diagnosis and treatment of metastatic spinal tumor. Oncologist 4:459–69, 1999.

9. Bilsky MH, Shannon FJ, Shappard S, et al: Diagnosis and management of a metastatic tumor in the atlantoaxial spine. Spine 27:1062–1069, 2002.

10. Brice J, McKissock W: Surgical treatment of malignant extradural spinal tumours. Br Med J 1:1341–4, 1965.

11. Bridwell K, Jenny A, et al: Posterior segmental spinal instrumentation (PSSI) with posterolateral decompression and debulking for metastatic thoracic and lumbar spine disease: limitations and technique. Spine 13:1383–1394, 1998.

12. Cobb CA, Leavens ME, Eckles N: Indications for nonoperative treatment of spinal cord compression due to breast cancer. J Neurosurg 47: 653–658, 1977.

13. Constans JP, DeDivitiis E, Donzelli R, et al: Spinal metastases with neurological manifestations: review of 600 cases. J Neurosurg 59:111–118, 1983.

14. Cooper P, Errico T, Martin R, et al: A systematic approach to spinal reconstruction after anterior decompression for neoplastic disease of the thoracic and lumbar spine. Neurosurg 32:1–8, 1993.

15. De Neve W, Claus F, Van Houtte P, et al: [Intensity modulated radiotherapy with dynamic multileaf collimator. Technique and clinical experience]. Cancer Radiother 3:378–392, 1999.

16. De Neve W, De Wagter C, De Jaeger K, et al: Planning and delivering high doses to targets surrounding the spinal cord at the lower neck and upper mediastinal levels: static beam-segmentation technique executed with a multileaf collimator. Radiother Oncol 40:271–279, 1996.

17. DeWald RL, Bridwell KH, Chadwick P, et al: Reconstructive spinal surgery as palliation for metastatic malignancies of the spine. Spine 10:21–26, 1985.

18. Dunn, RC, Jr, Kelly WA, Wohns RNW, et al: Spinal epidural neoplasia. A 15-year review of the results of surgical therapy. J Neurosurg 52:47–51, 1980.

19. Kostuik JP, Errico TJ, Gleason TF, et al: Spinal stabilization of vertebral column tumors. Spine 13:250–6, 1988.

20. Friedman M, Kim TH, Panahon AM: Spinal cord compression in malignant lymphoma: treatment and results. Cancer 37:1485–1491, 1976.

21. Gilbert RW, Kim JH, Posner JB: Epidural spinal cord compression from metastatic tumor: diagnosis and treatment. Ann Neurol 3:40–51, 1978.

22. Gokaslan ZL, York JE, Walsh GL, et al: Transthoracic vertebrectomy for metastatic spinal tumors. J Neurosurg 89:599–609, 1998.

23. Gokaslan ZL, aladag MA, Ellerhorst JA: Melanoma metastatic to the spine: A review of 133 cases. Melanoma Res 10:78–80, 2000.

24. Hall A, Mackay N: The results of laminectomy for compression of the cord or cauda equina by extradural malignant tumour. J Bone Joint Surg (Br) 55:497–505, 1973.

25. Harrington K: Anterior decompression and stabilization of the spine as a treatment for vertebral body collapse and spinal cord compression for metastatic malignancy. Clin Orthop 233:177–197, 1988.

26. Harrington K: Anterior cord decompression and spinal stabilization for patients with metastatic lesions of the spine. J Neurosurg 61:107–117, 1984.

27. Harrington K: The use of methylmethacrylate for vertebral body replacement and anterior stabilization of pathological fracture-dislocations of the spine due to metastatic malignant disease. J Bone Joint Surg Am 63:36–46, 1981.

28. Hortobagyi GN, Theriault RL, Lipton A, et al: Long-term prevention of skeletal complications of metastatic breast cancer with pamidronate. Protocol 19 Aredia breast cancer study group. J Clin Oncol 16:2038–2044, 1998.

29. Hosono N, Yonenobu K, Fuji T, et al: Vertebral body replacement with ceramic prosthesis for metastatic spinal tumors. Spine 20: 2454–2462, 1995.

30. Hunt MA, Hsiung CY, Spirou SV, et al: Evaluation of concave dose distributions created using an inverse planning system. Int J Radiat Oncol Biol Phys 54:953–962, 2002.

31. Khan F, Glicksman A, Chu F, et al: Treatment by radiotherapy of spinal cord compression due to extradural metastases. Radiology 89:495–500, 1967.

32. Kleinman WB, Kiernan HA, Michelsen WJ: Metastatic cancer of the spinal column. Clin Orthop 136:166–172, 1978.

33. Klekamp J, Samii H: Surgical results for spinal metastases. Acta Neurochir (Wien) 140:957–967, 1998.

34. Kostuik JP: Anterior spinal cord decompression for lesions of the thoracic and lumbar spine, techniques, new methods of internal fixation results. Spine 8:512–531, 1983.

35. Leibel SA, Fuks Z, Zelefsky MJ, et al: Intensity-modulated radiotherapy. Cancer J 8:164–176, 2002.

36. Livingston KE, Perrin RG: The neurosurgical management of spinal metastases causing cord and cauda equina compression. J Neurosurg 49:839–843, 1978.

37. Maranzano E, Latini P, Beneventi S, et al: Radiotherapy without steroids in selected metastatic spinal cord compression patients. Am J Clin Oncol 19:179–183, 1996.

38. Maranzano E, Latini P: Effectiveness of radiation therapy without surgery in metastatic spinal cord compression: final results from a prospective trial. Int J Radiat Onco Biol Phys 32:959–967, 1995.

39. Marshall LF, Langfitt TW: Combined therapy for metastatic extradural tumors of the spine. Cancer 40:2067–2070, 1977.

40. Milker-Zabel S, Zabel A, Thilmann C: Clinical results of re-treatment of vertebral bone metastases by stereotactic conformal radiotherapy and intensity-modulated radiotherapy. Int J Radiat Oncol Biol Phys 55:162–167, 2003.

41. Nicholls PJ, Jarecky TW: The value of posterior decompression by laminectomy for malignant tumors of the spine. Clin Orthop 201:210–212, 1985.

42. Perrin RG, McBroom RJ: Anterior versus posterior decompression for symptomatic spinal metastasis. Can J Neurol Sci 14: 75–80, 1987.

43. Perrin RG, McBroom RJ: Spinal fixation after anterior decompression for symptomatic spinal metastasis. Neurosurgery 22: 324–327, 1998.

44. Philips E, Levine AM: Metastatic lesions of the upper cervical spine. Spine 14:1071–1077, 1989.
45. Pirzkall A, Carol M, Lohr F: Comparison of intensity-modulated radiotherapy with conventional conformal radiotherapy for complex-shaped tumors. Int J Radiat Oncol Biol Phys 48:1371–1380, 2000.
46. Regine WF, Tibbs PA, Young A, et al: Metastatic spinal cord compression: a randomized trial of direct decompressive surgical resection plus radiotherapy vs. radiotherapy alone. Int J Radiat Oncol Biol Phys 57(2 Suppl):S125, 2003.
47. Siegal T, Siegal T: Surgical decompression of anterior and posterior malignant epidural tumors compressing the spinal cord: a prospective study. Neurosurgery 17:424–432, 1985.
48. Smith R: An evaluation of surgical treatment for spinal cord compression due to metastatic carcinoma. J Neurol Neurosurg Psychiatry 28:152–158, 1965.
49. Sultanem K, Shu HK, Xia P, et al: Three-dimensional intensity-modulated radiotherapy in the treatment of nasopharyngeal carcinoma: the University of California–San Francisco experience. Int J Radiat Oncol Biol Phys 48:711–722, 2000.
50. Sundaresan N, Choi IS, Hughes JE, et al: Treatment of spinal metastases from kidney cancer by presurgical embolization and resection. J Neurosurg 73:548–554, 1990.
51. Sundaresan N, DiGiacinto GV, Krol G, et al: Spondylectomy for malignant tumors of the spine. J Clin Oncol 7:1485–1491, 1989.
52. Sundaresan N, DiGiacinto GV, Hughes JE, et al: Treatment of neoplastic spinal cord compression: results of a prospective study. Neurosurgery 29:645–650, 1991.
53. Sundaresan N, Galicich JH, Lane JM, et al: Treatment of odontoid fractures in cancer patients. J Neurosurg 54:187–192, 1981.
54. Sundaresan N, Rothman A, Manhart K, et al: Surgery for solitary metastases of the spine: rationale and results of treatment. Spine 27:1802–1806, 2002.
55. Tomita K, Kawahara N, Baba H, et al: Total en bloc spondylectomy for solitary spinal metastases. Int Orthop 18:291–8, 1994.
56. Tomita K, Kawahara N, Kobayashi T, et al: Surgical strategy for spinal metastases. Spine 26:298–306, 2001.
57. Tomita K, Toribatake Y, Kawahara N, et al: Total en bloc spondylectomy and circumspinal decompression for solitary spinal metastasis. Paraplegia 32:36–46, 1994.
58. Verhey LJ: Comparison of three-dimensional conformal radiation therapy and intensity-modulated radiation therapy systems. Semin Radiat Oncol 9:78–98, 1999.
59. Vieth R, Odom G: Extradural spinal metastases and their neurosurgical treatment. J Neurosurg 23:501–508, 1965.
60. Walsh GL, Gokaslan ZL, McCutcheon IE, et al: Anterior approaches to the thoracic spine in patients with cancer: indications and results. Ann Thorac Surg 64:1611–1618, 1997.
61. White W, Patterson R, Bergland R: The role of surgery in the treatment of spinal cord compression by metastatic neoplasm. Cancer 27:558–561, 1971.
62. Wild WO, Porter RW: Metastatic epidural tumor of the spine. Archives of Surgery 87:825–830, 1962.
63. Wright R: Malignant tumours of the spinal extradural space: results of surgical treatment. Ann Surg 157:227–231, 1963.
64. Young RF, Post EM, King GA: Treatment of spinal epidural metastases. J Neurosurg 53:741–748, 1980.

CHAPTER *72*

INTRINSIC METASTATIC SPINAL CORD TUMORS

John H. Chi and Andrew T. Parsa

Intramedullary spinal cord metastasis (ISCM) is a rare sequelae of systemic metastatic malignancy. Although historically considered to be untreatable lesions, current management paradigms have demonstrated good functional outcome and prolonged survival after aggressive treatment. Because of its overall rarity, most of the current knowledge on ISCM derives from autopsy series and small case series. Improvement in diagnostic capabilities, survival from metastatic cancer, and treatment efficacy will likely result in more patients with ISCM becoming diagnosed earlier, living longer, and requiring therapy.

DEMOGRAPHICS

ISCM affects 0.1% to 0.4% of all cancer patients.[13] True incidence may be higher but clinically silent; 2% to 4% of cancer patients will show findings of ISCM at autopsy.[1,15] Intramedullary spinal cord tumors in general are uncommon lesions in the central nervous system (CNS), and ISCM accounts for only 1% to 3% of all intrinsic spinal tumors.[7] The most common metastases to the spinal axis are extramedullary (vertebral body, epidural, or paraspinal), and only 0.8% to 3.5% of symptomatic metastases to the spine are intramedullary.[8,16] Regarding CNS metastasis as a whole, most are intracranial, with only 8.5% of CNS metastasis being ISCM.[13] The overall incidence of ISCM seems to be slowly rising as cancer patients survive longer with current chemotherapeutic and radiation therapy protocols.[5,9]

Any metastatic tumor can theoretically spread to the spinal cord (Table 72-1). Bronchogenic cancers are the most common primary source of ISCM, accounting for 54% to 85% of cases.[2,12,13] Small cell lung cancer (SCLC) accounts for 47% of these metastases and far outnumbers the other bronchogenic cancer types. Five percent of all patients with SCLC will have ISCM, whereas less than 1% of patients with non-SCLC will have ISCM.[13] Breast cancer is the second most common primary tumor and makes up 13% of ISCM.[12] Melanoma has relatively high rates of CNS metastasis with 27% to 92% of patients reported to have some form of CNS involvement, but only 9% of ISCM comes from a melanoma primary.[4] Lymphoma, renal cell carcinoma, colorectal cancer, and several others each represent 1% to 3% of ISCM.[2,16]

The presence of ISCM seems to correlate with brain metastasis and leptomeningeal disease (LMD). Of patients with ISCM, 57% will have brain metastasis, whereas 27.5% have evidence of LMD after complete work-up.[15] ISCM is an indicator of advanced systemic involvement of malignancy.

The average age of appearance of ISCM is approximately 58 years (range 38 to 78 years) and is more common in men (64%) than women (46%).[2] There is no ethnic or racial preponderance.

TUMOR LOCATION

ISCM can occur anywhere along the spinal cord. A recent review of the literature reported location of tumor in the cervical cord in 24% of patients, thoracic cord in 22%, and lumbar cord or conus in 28%.[2] Fifteen percent had multiple cord-level involvement. Individual case series have reported conflicting evidence, some stating that cervical cord metastasis is most common and others that the thoraco-lumbar cord is most susceptible.[8,12,15]

Three possible mechanisms of metastatic spread to the spinal cord have been suggested. Hematogenous dissemination probably accounts for most cases and is the commonly suggested mechanism. Spinal necroscopy shows that ISCM primarily involves the posterior horns. These areas represent spinal gray matter, which receives five times the arterial output compared with neighboring white matter and has the densest capillary bed in the spinal cord. Metastatic tumor cells bound in blood would naturally reside in areas of high blood perfusion. The higher incidence of bronchogenic cancers may be explained by the spinal cord's proximity to pulmonary veins, which provide a direct conduit for tumor cells to enter the bloodstream and circulation. Venous plexus networks throughout the vertebral column often contribute to vertebral body metastasis but probably contribute less to ISCM. In the presence of LMD, tumor cells "floating" in CSF may infiltrate the Virchow-Robin spaces of vessels, penetrating the pial layer of the spinal cord and invading spinal cord parenchyma directly. Finally, direct extension through dura or perineural spread through nerve roots may provide access for tumor bulk contiguous with neural elements into the spinal parenchyma.

Histopathologic characteristics of ISCM include (1) distinct demarcation between tumor and parenchyma, (2) hemorrhagic foci within tumor, and (3) involvement of posterior roots.[5] Histology of metastasis mirrors histology of the primary malignancy, but in 3% of ISCM, no known histopathologic tissue pattern can be discerned.[2]

TABLE 72-1

Primary Sites of Intramedullary Metastatic Spinal Cord Tumors

Site	Occurrence (%)
Bronchogenic	41–85
Breast	13
Melanoma	9
Lymphoma	5
Renal	4
Colorectal	3
Thyroid	2
Ovarian	1
Unknown	3

TABLE 72-2

Symptoms versus Physical Examination Findings in Patients with Intramedullary Metastatic Spinal Cord Tumors

Complaint	Occurrence (%)
Sensory loss	42.5
Pain	30
Weakness	30
Gait abnormality	5
Incontinence	2.5
Physical Examination	
Weakness	93
Sensory loss	78–87
Pain	52–72
Bowel or bladder dysfunction	62
Systemic symptoms	37

CLINICAL PRESENTATION

ISCM usually occurs in the setting of known malignancy and involves a rapid, progressive myelopathy occurring over several days or weeks (Table 72-2). Initial complaints commonly include sensory changes or loss (42.5%), pain (30%), weakness (30%), gait changes or abnormalities (5%), and incontinence (2.5%).[2,15] Clinical examination findings include weakness in 93% of patients, sensory changes or loss in 78% to 87%, pain in 52% to 72%, bowel or bladder dysfunction in 62%, and systemic symptoms in 37%.[2,15] Weakness and pain tend to occur earlier in a patient's clinical course, whereas sensory changes and bowel or bladder involvement seem to be later manifestations. Weakness is often lateral to one side and to a particular spinal level, whereas sensory loss is commonly referable to a specific dermatomal level. Paraplegia is present in 15% of cases.[2] The medullary pain of ISCM follows a pattern of a burning, dysesthetic, nonradicular bilateral pain.[7] Weakness and sensory changes manifest as a Brown-Sequard syndrome in 22.5% of patients, with a pseudo or partial Brown-

Sequard syndrome in another 22.5%.[15] Asymmetric physical examination findings are noted in approximately 45% of cases. The average duration of symptoms before diagnosis of ISCM averages from 28 days to 6 months, with a range from 3 days to 18 months.[2,7,15]

The mechanism for the relatively sudden development of symptoms relates to the limited reserve capacity of the spinal canal for rapid tumor growth. Direct compression of neural elements and vascular channels by tumor bulk both contribute to the onset of myelopathic signs. Tethering of the spinal cord by dentate ligaments and the filum terminale may become symptomatic when enough stretch is produced by an expanding mass. Because any mass lesion in the spinal column can cause these symptoms, distinguishing ISCM from epidural or paraspinal metastasis and compression from vertebral body metastasis becomes nearly impossible based on clinical grounds alone. The presence of a Brown-Sequard syndrome suggests ISCM but is not pathognomonic, as extramedullary tumors can also produce similar clinical findings. Radicular pain is less common in ISCM and more common in the setting of nerve root compression by extramedullary lesions or schwannomas.

In addition to ISCM and spinal column metastasis, non-neoplastic myelopathies related to malignancy or treatment of cancer can also cause progressive neurologic deterioration. Paraneoplastic necrotizing myelopathy occurs in patients with evidence of systemic cancer and can be indistinguishable from clinical symptoms of ISCM. Radiographic findings associated with paraneoplastic necrotizing myelopathy include a rostrocaudal pencil-shaped necrosis in the thoracic cord. ISCM can be distinguished from paraneoplastic necrotizing myelopathy based on the presence of serum paraneoplastic antibodies. ISCM is also more often associated with advanced metastatic disease than is paraneoplastic myelopathy. Patients receiving radiation therapy with exposure of the spinal cord are also at risk for delayed dose-related, radiation-induced myelopathy. Symptoms usually occur at least 4 months after the last dose of radiation and rarely occur in patients with less than 6000 rads if given in daily fractions of less than 200 rads/day or weekly fractions of less than 900 rads/week.[2] Obviously, the pathologic lesion of radiation-induced myelopathy must lie within the boundaries of radiation-exposed spinal cord. Compared with ISCM, both of these non-neoplastic myelopathies rarely have pain as an early or predominant symptom.

DIAGNOSTIC IMAGING AND TESTS

Historically, spinal myelography and CT myelography were the mainstay of diagnostic imaging in evaluation of spinal cord tumors. Today, magnetic resonance imaging (MRI) with gadolinium enhancement has superseded myelography in diagnostic accuracy and precision. Multiplanar T1-weighted with contrast and T2-weighted MRI sequences can demonstrate ISCM and distinguish it from extramedullary lesions.[10,11] Multiple and small lesions can also be detected on MRI, and degree of cord edema is roughly quantified.

Cerebrospinal fluid (CSF) analysis does not have a defined role in the diagnosis of ISCM. Studies have demonstrated elevated protein levels in cases of ISCM. Cytology is usually unremarkable, though in the setting of leptomeningeal dissemination white blood cell counts may be elevated. Overall, CSF analysis is uninformative, and abnormalities are grossly nonspecific.

Recently, staging of cancer patients has included full body nuclear radioisotope scans to detect potential sites of metastatic disease. These screening diagnostic scans may be helpful in detecting ISCM long before symptoms appear, but treatment strategies for asymptomatic, small ISCM are ill defined.[10]

TREATMENT

Traditionally, treatment for ISCM has consisted of dexamethasone dosing and external radiation therapy. Steroid dosing can reduce pain and provide some neurologic improvement in up to 85% of patients and is used in the acute setting as a bridge to more specific treatment.[7] Fractionated external radiation therapy is the primary treatment modality for ISCM, and general protocols use 16.3 to 45.2 Gy in 5 to 25 fractions over 2 to 4 weeks.[15] Whole-spine irradiation has been considered in the past, but the marrow toxicity involved has precluded its widespread use. Stereotactic radiosurgery has developed rapidly in the past decade and is a major treatment modality for intracranial metastatic disease. Its application in the treatment of ISCM is currently under study.[14]

Recently, several reports have advocated for surgery of ISCM in adjunct to standard therapy.[2,7] Good neurologic outcome and potential prolonged survival are purported, but the actual outcome benefit of surgical removal is still unknown. If open biopsy is required, safe excision of an intramedullary metastasis can sometimes be achieved. Surgical technique is similar to removal of primary spinal cord neoplasms, such as ependymomas, given a well-demarcated border between metastasis and spinal cord. If surgery is planned, radiation treatment should wait until after surgery, because radiation exposure can initiate scarring and obscuration of tissue planes. Some clinicians have recommended undertaking surgery for ISCM for medium to large tumors only, because a small lesion may be difficult to localize and technically more complicated to resect.[17] Currently, generous cytoreductive surgery for ISCM is a potentially safe and beneficial adjunct to standard treatment.

Chemotherapy protocols exist for most metastatic malignancies and are applied as indicated by staging. No single or combined drug strategy is unique for ISCM. Intrathecal administration of chemotherapeutic agents is possible, but the current literature supporting this adjunct is limited to anecdotal case reports.[3,6,9]

OUTCOME

In general, the presence of ISCM serves as an indicator of extensive and advanced systemic involvement of malignancy and carries a poor prognosis. Average time to death following diagnosis of ISCM is approximately 19 weeks (range 3 weeks to 27 months).[2] Death is usually secondary to systemic metastatic involvement, but the disability resulting from ISCM may predispose patients to complications such as aspiration pneumonia and pulmonary embolism from immobility. Prolonged survival correlates with aggressiveness of treatment in several small studies.[2,7,15,17] Patients receiving only steroids had average survival of 5 weeks, whereas those receiving radiation or radiation and chemotherapy had average survivals of 15 weeks and 29 weeks, respectively.[2] Prolonged functional outcomes up to 103 weeks after aggressive radiation and surgical treatment have been reported as small case series. Interestingly, melanoma demonstrates exceptionally good rates of functional survival after treatment compared with lung and breast cancer, for metastatic lesions in both intracranial and spinal disease.[2,7] Accordingly, patients with metastatic melanoma may deserve more aggressive treatment options in the setting of ISCM.

CONCLUSION

1. As patients survive longer from metastatic cancer with advancing treatment modalities, the incidence of intramedullary spinal cord metastases will steadily rise.
2. Though ISCM currently heralds poor prognosis and short survival even with maximal therapy, attempts at delineating optimal treatment strategies incorporating radiation, chemotherapeutics, and surgery are still necessary.
3. Earlier detection and newer treatment modalities with aggressive but safe cytoreductive surgery may afford extended survival with good functional status.

References

1. Amin R: Intramedullary spinal metastasis from carcinoma of the cervix. Br J Radiol 72:89–91, 1999.
2. Connolly ES, Jr., Winfree CJ, McCormick PC, et al: Intramedullary spinal cord metastasis: report of three cases and review of the literature. Surg Neurol 46:329–337; discussion 337–328, 1996.
3. Cormio G, Di Vagno G, Di Fazio F, et al: Intramedullary spinal cord metastasis from ovarian carcinoma. Gynecol Oncol 81:506–508, 2001.
4. Costigan DA, Winkelman MD: Intramedullary spinal cord metastasis. A clinicopathological study of 13 cases. J Neurosurg 62:227–233, 1985.
5. Dunne JW, Harper CG, Pamphlett R: Intramedullary spinal cord metastases: a clinical and pathological study of nine cases. Q J Med 61:1003–1020, 1986.
6. Fujimoto N, Hiraki A, Ueoka H, et al: Intramedullary spinal cord recurrence after high-dose chemotherapy and autologous peripheral blood progenitor cell transplantation for limited-disease small cell lung cancer. Lung Cancer 30:145–148, 2000.
7. Gasser TG, Pospiech J, Stolke D, et al: Spinal intramedullary metastases. Report of two cases and review of the literature. Neurosurg Rev 24:88–92, 2001.
8. Jellinger K, Kothbauer P, Sunder-Plassmann E, et al: Intramedullary spinal cord metastases. J Neurol 220:31–41, 1979.

9. Komaki R, Cox JD, Holoye PY, et al: Changes in the relative risk and sites of central nervous system metastasis with effective combined chemotherapy and radiation therapy for small cell carcinoma of the lung. Am J Clin Oncol 6:515–521, 1983.

10. Komori T, Delbeke D: Leptomeningeal carcinomatosis and intramedullary spinal cord metastases from lung cancer: detection with FDG positron emission tomography. Clin Nucl Med 26:905–907, 2001.

11. Li MH, Holtas S: MR imaging of spinal intramedullary tumors. Acta Radiol 32:505–513, 1991.

12. Okamoto H, Shinkai T, Matsuno Y, et al: Intradural parenchymal involvement in the spinal subarachnoid space associated with primary lung cancer. Cancer 72:2583–2588, 1993.

13. Potti A, Abdel-Raheem M, Levitt R, et al: Intramedullary spinal cord metastases (ISCM) and non-small cell lung carcinoma (NSCLC): clinical patterns, diagnosis and therapeutic considerations. Lung Cancer 31:319–323, 2001.

14. Ryu S, Fang Yin F, Rock J, et al: Image-guided and intensity-modulated radiosurgery for patients with spinal metastasis. Cancer 97:2013–2018, 2003.

15. Schiff D, O'Neill BP: Intramedullary spinal cord metastases: clinical features and treatment outcome. Neurology 47:906–912, 1996.

16. Schijns OE, Kurt E, Wessels P, et al: Intramedullary spinal cord metastasis as a first manifestation of a renal cell carcinoma: report of a case and review of the literature. Clin Neurol Neurosurg 102:249–254, 2000.

17. Xu QW, Bao WM, Mao RL, et al: Aggressive surgery for intramedullary tumor of cervical spinal cord. Surg Neurol 46:322–328, 1996.

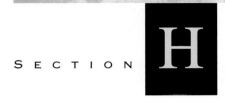
CHAPTER 73

EVALUATION AND MANAGEMENT OF BENIGN PERIPHERAL NERVE TUMORS AND MASSES

Keith Kwok, Jefferson C. Slimp, Donald E. Born, Robert Goodkin, and Michel Kliot

CLINICAL PRESENTATION

Extrapolating data from previous studies[50,69] reveals that the annual incidence rate for peripheral nerve tumors that are operated on is approximately 6 cases per 1 million people, for a total of several thousand cases in the United States. The great majority, more than 90%, of peripheral nerve tumors are benign. They can arise from any of the cellular components that make up a peripheral nerve. The 2000 World Health Organization (WHO) classification of tumors subdivides benign peripheral nerve tumors into three major types on the basis of their clinical course, histologic appearance, immunophenotypic features, and molecular or cytogenetic profile: schwannoma, neurofibroma, and perineurioma.[13,43,72] Forty-five percent of all peripheral nerve tumors occur in the head and neck region.[125] Peripheral nerve tumors arising in the limbs are relatively rare. It has been reported that these tumors account for less than 5% of all neoplasms found in the upper extremities.[76,115] The most common complaint is growth of a mass associated with neurologic symptoms such as tingling, constant burning pain, paresthesias, numbness, or weakness. The pain is often unilateral and either radicular, in the case of tumors arising from spinal nerves, or in the distribution of the involved peripheral nerve. Findings on the clinical examination include a palpable mass in the case of a superficial mass, loss of sensory or motor function in the distribution of the involved peripheral nerve, and, rarely, altered autonomic function when the mass involves either parasympathetic or sympathetic autonomic nerve fibers. Proper evaluation and management of these peripheral nerve masses involve a complete understanding of the anatomy,

pathology, clinical presentation, diagnostic studies, and medical and surgical treatments. A true team approach involving surgeons, radiologists, pathologists, oncologists, neurologists, and rehabilitation specialists is necessary to optimize treatment and clinical outcome. In addition, scientific discoveries in the fields of molecular biology and genetics, as well as advances in noninvasive imaging techniques, are all providing new opportunities for clinicians to further improve the evaluation and management of this challenging clinical problem.

DIAGNOSTIC EVALUATION

Clinical Examination

Peripheral nerve tumors are not common and are usually found incidentally during evaluation of a soft tissue mass. The most common indications are new detection or growth of a mass associated with neurologic symptoms such as tingling, pain, paresthesias, numbness, or weakness. To successfully manage these lesions, the clinical evaluation should start with a thorough clinical history and physical examination. A positive family history can help diagnose one of the genetic syndromes associated with peripheral nerve tumors, such as neurofibromatosis types 1 (NF1) and 2 (NF2). Other clinical manifestations of these genetic syndromes should be looked for, such as superficial skin masses, café-au-lait spots, axillary or inguinal freckling, Lisch nodules (melanotic pigmented hamartomas of the iris), and bone abnormalities in the case of NF1. Physical characteristics such as skin color, texture, and temperature dif-

535

ferences, as well as the presence of pain or tingling dysesthesias upon palpation (Tinel's sign), should be carefully looked for during the examination.[3] The physical examination should focus on the musculoskeletal and neurologic systems in assessing sensory, motor, reflex, and autonomic function. The cranial nerves should also be examined, because several of the genetic syndromes are associated with masses involving these nerves—for example, the optic nerve in the case of NF1 and the eighth cranial nerve complex in the case of NF2. Palpable superficial peripheral nerve masses can be mobilized most side to side in a plane orthogonal to the longitudinal axis of the nerve from which they arise. Gently palpating the mass will often give rise to a Tinel's response, in which tingling sensations radiate distally in the distribution of the involved nerve. Rapidly growing and very large, painful, and deeply located masses raise the specter of malignancy.[68] Sensory, motor, reflex, or autonomic changes allow the astute clinician, armed with a good understanding of the functional anatomy of the peripheral nervous system (PNS), to localize the peripheral nerve tumor.

Electrical Studies

Electrodiagnostic studies are extremely helpful to the clinician in localizing the mass to a particular nerve and in determining the severity or grade of nerve damage. Such information is useful both in planning for surgery and in estimating the risks of surgery for causing additional neurologic deficits. An assortment of electrophysiologic tests can be used: (1) Electromyography (EMG) assesses muscle denervation and thereby provides evidence of motor axon loss; EMG testing can differentiate between true muscle weakness and reduced use because of pain. (2) Nerve conduction studies (NCSs) assess the integrity of either sensory or motor nerve fiber pathways by measuring nerve conduction velocity and amplitude; reductions in response velocity reflect demyelination of a peripheral nerve, whereas reductions in response amplitude indicate loss of axons. (3) Somatosensory evoked potential (SSEP) responses are an evoked potential generated by repetitive activation of sensory fibers peripherally while recording from the spinal cord or brain centrally to assess the integrity of sensory pathways. These electrodiagnostic studies are all important tools, in that they may reveal subtle peripheral nerve pathology as well as aid in establishing a baseline level of function before surgical resection. These studies, as mentioned in the intraoperative monitoring section (see later discussion), are also very useful during surgery to help preserve functioning nerve fibers while resecting the tumor.

Radiologic Imaging Studies

Radiologic studies have become increasingly more important in the preoperative evaluation of peripheral nerve mass lesions. Imaging tools such as computed tomography (CT), ultrasonography, and especially magnetic resonance imaging (MRI) are widely used. CT imaging, especially following contrast administration, can visualize abnormal masses such as tumors.[98,128] Ultrasound is also capable of visualizing masses and is particularly good for distinguishing cystic from solid masses, as well as for resolving vascular structures with blood flow.[10,57,71,83] MRI is particularly useful because of its higher spatial resolution and its ability to visualize and distinguish more subtle differences in soft-tissue structures. These charac-

teristics permit MRI to visualize and distinguish the typical nerve fascicular anatomy from most mass lesions, such as tumors and cysts. Magnetic resonance neurography (MRN) techniques, employing phased-array coils in combination with particular pulse sequences and multiplanar reformation techniques, have permitted visualization of nerves and their associated mass lesions with better acuity.[46] MRN has been particularly useful in visualizing and distinguishing the fascicular structure of normal peripheral nerves from intraneural and extraneural tumors and other mass lesions, which are either enhanced following the administration of contrast agent (gadolinium) or have a more homogeneous appearance.[65] High-resolution MRN is useful preoperatively in assessing the surgical resectability of peripheral nerve tumors while preserving function (Figure 73-1).

Peripheral nerve mass lesions on MRI can be either discrete and ovoid, as is often the case for schwannomas, or more cylindrical, fusiform, or multinodular in the case of neurofibromas. Normal peripheral nerve fascicles, possibly because of the presence of endoneurial fluid within discrete fascicles, show isointense signal on T1-weighted images and slightly hyperintense signal on T2-pulse sequence images relative to the signal characteristics of adjacent normally innervated muscle tissue. Benign peripheral nerve tumors such as schwannomas and neurofibromas both show isointense to slightly hyperintense signal on T1-weighted images and hyperintense signal on T2-weighted images. These tumors can be distinguished from other types of peripheral nerve masses, such as ganglion cysts, which appear hypointense on T1-weighted images and hyperintense on T2-weighted images.[3] Most peripheral nerve tumors show enhancement on T1-weighted images following the administration of gadolinium, a contrast agent that accumulates wherever there are leaky blood vessels. One potential clinical pitfall to keep in mind is that hyperplastic lymph nodes can have very similar imaging characteristics to peripheral nerve tumors (personal unpublished observations). To date, there is no imaging study, including CT or MRI, that can separate the various classes of peripheral nerve tumor or distinguish between benign and malignant peripheral nerve tumors with confidence.[26,46,116] However, there is evidence that PET (positron-emission tomography) scanning, which uses glucose analogues such as ^{18}F-fluorodeoxyglucose to visualize metabolic activity, shows higher metabolism in malignant tumors.[35] A small study using gallium scanning has also shown specific signal characteristics in neurogenic sarcomas or malignant schwannomas.[70]

CELLULAR ANATOMY OF PERIPHERAL NERVES

Normal Anatomy

The pathology of peripheral nerve tumors can best be understood by studying the normal anatomy and cellular elements that make up a peripheral nerve (Figure 73-2), the cells from which the different types of intrinsic peripheral nerve tumors arise. In contrast, extrinsic tumors arise either from adjacent tissues with local spread or, in the case of metastatic tumors, from cells at a distance.

Peripheral nerves are part of the PNS. These axonal pathways connect the brain and spinal cord with sensory, motor, and

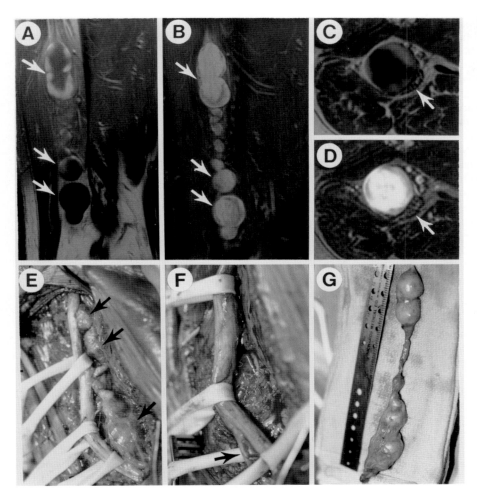

FIGURE 73-1 Magnetic resonance neurography (MRN) used to assess the resectability of a peripheral nerve tumor. MRN images of a 69-year-old-female patient with a right sciatic nerve neurofibroma in the lower thigh. *A,* Coronal fat-suppressed T1 spin echo (SE) image after administration of gadolinium showing heterogeneous enhancement of a multilobulated and cystic mass lesion *(white arrows)* in the posterior thigh. *B,* Coronal short tau inversion recovery (STIR) fast spin echo (FSE) image showing high signal within the multilobulated lesion *(white arrows)*. *C,* Axial T1 SE image after administration of gadolinium. *D,* Axial T2 FSE image showing discrete demarcation of the fascicular structure of the sciatic nerve *(white arrow)* along the posteromedial circumference of the tumor. *E,* Intraoperative photograph showing Penrose loops elevating the sciatic nerve from the multilobulated neurofibroma *(black arrows)*. *F,* Intraoperative photograph after removal of the neurofibroma. Note the splitting of the distal sciatic nerve into common peroneal and tibial *(black arrow)* nerve branches. *G,* Photograph of resected neurofibroma oriented as shown in *A* and *B*. (From Kuntz C, Blake L, Britz G, et al: Magnetic resonance neurography of peripheral nerve lesions in the lower extremity. Neurosurgery 39:750–757, 1996.)

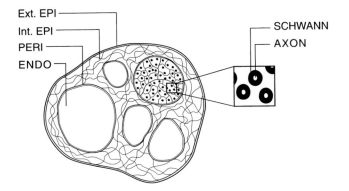

FIGURE 73-2 Schematic diagram of a cross section of a peripheral nerve showing cellular components. Individual axons are encased by Schwann cells *(inset)* within the endoneurium (ENDO). The endoneurium is in turn encircled by a connective tissue layer, the perineurium (PERI), composed of perineural cells, which divides the nerve into fascicles. Nerve fascicles are embedded in a layer of connective tissue called the internal epineurium (Int. EPI), which is surrounded by the external epineurium (Ext. EPI). (Reproduced with permission from Grossman RG, Loftus CM (eds): Principles of Neurosurgery, 2nd ed. Philadelphia, Lippincott-Raven, 1999.)

autonomic end organs. Peripheral nerves contain neural and non-neural components, which can be segregated into three functional-structural parts: (1) the action potential conducting axons; (2) the insulating ensheathing Schwann cells; and (3) a surrounding extracellular connective tissue matrix whose cells (e.g., fibroblasts, macrophages, endothelial cells, and mast cells) and molecules (e.g., proteins, glycoproteins, and proteoglycans) provide necessary nutrients, structural integrity, and an environment that can promote remyelination and the regeneration of axons following injury. Nerve fibers are ensheathed by Schwann cells, either individually in the case of myelinated fibers or in groups in the case of unmyelinated fibers. Myelinated and unmyelinated nerve fibers are embedded within a connective tissue compartment called the *endoneurium*. A compact layer called the *perineurium,* composed of concentrically arranged elongated perineural cells, encircles the endoneurium, thereby creating nerve fascicles. Characteristic features of perineural cells include abundant micropinocytotic vesicles and electron-dense cytoplasm. The perineurium partitions nerve fibers into fascicles and serves as a selective diffusion barrier. These perineural cells are believed to arise from fibroblasts despite their having a pericellular basal lamina, a characteristic of Schwann cells but not fibroblasts. Peripheral nerve fascicles surrounded by perineurium are embedded within a connective tissue layer, the internal epineurium, which in turn is surrounded by several layers of concentrically arranged cells that form the external epineurium. Both types of epineural layer include variable amounts of blood vessels, fat, fibroblasts, and macrophages.

Immunocytochemical markers can differentiate the various cellular and molecular elements of peripheral nerve. For example, perineurial cells, which normally surround the nerve fascicles within a nerve, can be distinguished from Schwann cells by their immunoreactivity for epithelial membrane antigen (EMA) and lack of reactivity for S-100 protein.[126] Schwann cells, on the other hand, can be visualized using antibodies to CNP (2,3-cyclic nucleotide-3-phosphohydrolase), S-100, Leu-7, and the low-affinity receptor to nerve growth factor.[48]

Pathology

Intrinsic tumors of the PNS may arise from any of the cellular components of a peripheral nerve, which include Schwann cells, perineural cells, fibroblasts, endothelial cells, adipose cells, and neurons. Extrinsic peripheral nerve tumors can originate from cell types not normally found in peripheral nerves, such as in the case of metastatic tumors. Pathologic descriptions of the most common types of benign peripheral nerve tumors in accordance with the WHO classification are presented first in the following sections. We then describe additional tumor and nontumor mass lesions and diseases, which can also involve peripheral nerves, that are not part of the WHO classification system.

WORLD HEALTH ORGANIZATION CLASSIFICATION OF BENIGN PERIPHERAL NERVE TUMORS

According to the WHO classification, benign peripheral nerve tumors can be categorized into three major types: (1) schwan-noma (subdivided into the most common classic type and several other less common types—cellular, plexiform, and melanotic); (2) neurofibroma (subdivided into solitary and plexiform types); and (3) perineurioma (subdivided into intraneural and soft tissue or extraneural types).

Schwannoma

Pathology

The classic type of schwannoma, also called neurilemoma or neurinoma, is a benign encapsulated peripheral nerve tumor produced by the abnormal proliferation of Schwann cells within a nerve fascicle (Figure 73-3). This neoplasm can originate from cranial, peripheral, or autonomic nerves, usually distal to the oligodendrocyte–Schwann cell junction at the interface of central nervous system (CNS) and PNS. Schwannoma is usually a solitary mass but can also be multiple masses. Their gross appearance after sectioning can be a relatively homogeneous tan or gray, although cystic cavities and yellow coloration can also be found. Proliferating Schwann cells tend to displace adjacent uninvolved nerve fibers as the tumor progressively enlarges. Histologically, these tumors consist of tissue with two characteristic patterns of cellularity, called Antoni A and Antoni B. Antoni A tissue contains densely packed spindle-shaped or elongated cells. Verocay bodies, which consist of a palisading and dense cellular pattern of tumor growth in which nuclei line up in parallel rows, are often present in Antoni A tissue. Antoni B tissue consists of less densely packed cells interspersed within areas of myxoid stroma. Occasional spindle-shaped cells are present, and mitotic figures are rarely present in Antoni B tissue. S-100 protein, an acidic protein commonly found in the supporting cells of the CNS and PNS, is present in schwannomas and is particularly prominent in the Antoni A areas. Schwann cells can also be stained positively with antibodies to Leu-7 (CD 57), the low-affinity nerve growth factor receptor (NGFr), and vimentin, which is a mesenchymal intermediate filament. The classic

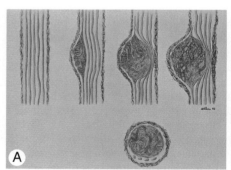
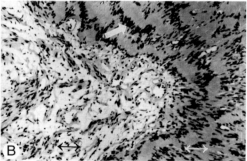

FIGURE 73-3   *A,* Schematic drawing illustrating how a growing schwannoma tumor displaces surrounding axons circumferentially away from its surface: the upper row shows tumor growth in longitudinal views of the nerve, and the lower row shows a cross section of the tumor in the nerve. (Reproduced with permission from Harkin JC, Reed RJ: Tumors of the Peripheral Nervous System. Washington, DC, Armed Forces Institute of Pathology, 1969, Plate IIIA, page 71). *B,* Hematoxylin-eosin stained section of a schwannoma demonstrating two histologic patterns of cellularity. In the right half of the section, the spindle-shaped cells are densely packed and exhibit an Antoni A histologic pattern. The nuclei of the cells have a palisading configuration in which their nuclei are aligned in rows called Verocay bodies *(white arrow).* In the left half of the section, the cells are loosely packed in an Antoni B histologic pattern *(black double arrow).* (Reproduced with permission from Grossman RG, Loftus CM (eds): Principles of Neurosurgery, 2nd ed. Philadelphia, Lippincott-Raven, 1999.)

schwannoma also stains for reticulin and collagen. However, schwannoma does not stain with antibodies to EMA. Electron microscopy (EM) shows the presence of a unique and characteristic basal lamina around Schwann cells.

There are three other less common types of schwannoma: cellular, plexiform, and melanotic variants. The cellular schwannomas are microscopically characterized by hypercellularity, hyperchromasia or dense nuclear chromatin, and the presence of up to 4 mitotic figures per 10 high power fields with no obvious tissue necrosis. They are composed predominantly of an Antoni A tissue pattern and often lack cellular palisading and Verocay bodies.[137] Ultrastructurally, cellular schwannomas are represented by well-differentiated Schwann cells. Importantly, cellular schwannomas share some of the common features often seen in soft-tissue sarcomas; for example, both types of tumors are hypercellular and hyperchromatic. Therefore cellular schwannomas can sometimes be confused with this group of malignant tumors in fine-needle aspiration specimens. One way to distinguish cellular schwannomas from malignant tumors is on the basis that cellular schwannomas show positive staining with antibody against the S-100 protein whereas soft-tissue sarcomas often show no such staining.[107] The plexiform schwannomas, also called multinodular schwannomas, are a benign encapsulated and nodular variant of schwannoma involving the small terminal nerve branches in the cutaneous and subcutaneous tissues. In plexiform schwannomas, multiple mass lesions arise and can involve one or more peripheral nerves. Histologically, these tumor nodules are separated by a loose myxomatous stroma. Both Antoni A and Antoni B tissue patterns are present in plexiform schwannomas.[27] Verocay bodies and a small number of axons are present within cutaneous plexiform schwannomas. Melanotic schwannomas are also benign encapsulated tumors. Their gross appearance after sectioning can be black, brown, or blue, and the consistency of the tissue can be either solid or spongy. Microscopically, melanotic schwannomas consist of spindle-shaped and epithelioid cells, melanin, psammoma bodies, and fat.[23-24] The spindle cells are arranged in intertwined fascicles and exhibit whorling and occasional nuclear palisading. Immunohistological sections show positive staining with antibodies to S-100 protein and vimentin but negative staining to glial fibrillary acidic protein (GFAP), actin, and keratin. Melanotic schwannomas also show two characteristic types of melanocytes: one type consists of intensely pigmented globular or fusiform-shaped cells, and the other type consists of lightly pigmented polygonal or spindle-shaped cells. The nuclei of the lighter pigmented cells are vesicular with pale chromatin and a single prominent nucleolus. Other ultrastructural features of these cells include elongated processes, a continuous basal lamina, and melanosomes.[24]

Clinical Presentation and Evaluation

Schwannomas of all types are among the most common type of peripheral nerve tumor in adults. Most patients with schwannomas are between the ages of 20 and 50, with only 10% of schwannomas found in those younger than 21 years. Both sexes are equally affected.[3,20,27,48] In the United States, the exact prevalence of benign schwannomas is unknown. However, based on a review of 3364 cases of neurogenic neoplasms of the intercostal nerves and posterior mediastinum in 1971, 141 cases (4.2%) were schwannomas. The frequency of this tumor

was ranked third, following neurofibromas and ganglioneuromas.[55] Overall, schwannomas represent 35% of peripheral nerve tumors, 35% of all head and neck tumors,[125] 29% of primary spinal tumors, and 8% of intracranial tumors.[120] There is a tendency for schwannomas to arise from sensory nerves.[93,120] They may sporadically involve the eighth cranial nerve (as in acoustic schwannomas) at the cerebellopontine angle, dorsal roots arising from the spinal cord, and peripheral nerves in the extremities. Schwannomas have a predilection for the head, neck, and flexor surfaces of the upper and lower extremities. Furthermore, the radial, median, and especially the ulnar nerves in the upper extremities are affected in 20% of reported cases.[48,68] Schwannomas also constitute less than 2% of all hand tumors.[68]

Cellular schwannomas make up 10% of schwannoma cases and are the most common variant after the classic type described previously.[84] Cellular schwannomas have a peak incidence in the fourth decade, and approximately 5% occur in childhood and adolescence.[55] Their characteristic clinical features often include a pain-free paravertebral mass in the region of the retroperitoneum, pelvis, or mediastinum. Plexiform schwannomas occur in approximately 5% of patients with schwannomas[55,68] and are mostly found in young adults. Plexiform schwannomas are usually not associated with neurofibromatosis. Melanotic schwannomas are usually small (<1 cm) and dome-shape pigmented lesions.[24] They commonly affect the posterior spinal nerve roots and the sympathetic nervous system, especially in the posterior mediastinum. The upper alimentary tract, bone, and skin may also be involved.[24,68] Melanotic schwannomas have a peak incidence in the fourth decade.[136] In contrast to the other types of schwannomas, the melanotic type is not associated with NF2. More than 50% of patients with melanotic schwannomas have Carney's syndrome.[55] Carney's syndrome, a familial multitumoral syndrome, is characterized by spotty skin pigmentation (lentigines and blue nevi), myxomas (heart, skin, and breast), endocrine tumors (adrenal cortex, pituitary, testis, and thyroid), and melanotic schwannomas. Epithelioid blue nevus and psammomatous melanotic schwannoma are two rare types of skin pigment lesion seen in Carney's syndrome. The epithelioid blue nevus is a tumor that occurs mostly on the extremities and trunk and less often on the head and neck.

Clinically, patients with schwannomas are often asymptomatic or have mild sensory symptoms. Symptoms of shooting pain and paresthesias triggered by nerve palpation (Tinel's sign) are common, whereas spontaneous pain is more often a symptom of neurofibroma or a malignant peripheral nerve tumor. Upon physical examination, classic superficial schwannomas are usually detected as palpable nodules (usually smaller than 5 cm) that can be mobilized perpendicularly more so than parallel to the longitudinal orientation of the peripheral nerve from which they arise, a characteristic feature of intrinsic peripheral nerve masses. Deep tumors that are not palpable often reach a larger size than more superficial tumors before noticeable symptoms arise. On ultrasound, schwannomas usually appear as a hypoechoic solid mass lesion. On magnetic resonance (MR) images, schwannomas usually display isointense signal with muscle on T1-weighted images and hyperintense signal on T2-weighted images, as well as enhancement following the administration of gadolinium contrast agent.[48,71] Heterogeneous enhancement may appear if the schwannoma contains cystic components.[77] Peripheral nerve fascicles adjacent to the tumor are often displaced by the schwannoma and can sometimes be visualized using high-resolution MRN techniques.[46,48,65]

Treatment and Prognosis

Symptomatic or growing schwannomas are treated by complete surgical excision whenever possible (see later discussion of surgical resection). If the tumor cannot be easily separated from the surrounding nerve fibers, the diagnosis of a neurofibroma or malignant tumor should be considered. With the aid of intraoperative electrophysiologic monitoring, nonfunctional tumor tissue should be removed while attempting to spare intact functioning nerve fibers. Complete resection of a schwannoma, often as a single mass, is usually curative, with recurrences occurring only rarely. In addition, more than 90% of these patients show minimal if any loss of sensory or motor function.[48,62] Overall, schwannomas have a recurrence rate of less than 5%. Incompletely resected schwannomas are capable of slow growth. Higher tumor recurrence rates have been reported for intraspinal, sacral, and intracranial schwannomas, as well as for complex and extensive plexiform schwannomas involving major nerves.[55] Melanotic schwannomas that are completely resected tend not to recur. Approximately 10% of the melanotic tumors are malignant, whereas the classic type and the other variants rarely undergo malignant transformation.[55,103] Malignant transformation of benign schwannomas, not to be confused with malignant schwannoma or neurogenic sarcoma, has been reported but is extremely rare.[68,120,138] The prognosis for patients with schwannomas undergoing malignant transformation is poor.[138]

Neurofibroma

Pathology

The WHO classification system divides neurofibromas into two types: a general type, also referred to as solitary, circumscribed, or globular, and a plexiform type (Figure 73-4). The gross appearance of both types of neurofibromas can be similar to schwannomas. In the skin and subcutaneous fat, solitary neurofibromas are well circumscribed but may not be encapsulated, as well as being firm with pale gray and translucent cut surfaces.[11,68,93] Neurofibromas developing in deeper nerves are more often of the plexiform type and may be encapsulated by their epineurium. These tumors can vary from a few millimeters to many centimeters. Histologically, neurofibromas have the following characteristic features: elongated spindle-shaped cells, wavy interlacing hyperchromatic nucleated cells that may represent a Schwann cell precursor, loosely packed tissue with myxoid stroma similar to the Antoni B pattern of schwannomas, and axons coursing through the tumor tissue. Mucoid background stains for mucopolysaccharide, such as Alcian blue, are positive.[59] Neurofibromas do not immunostain for EMA. They may have S-100 and Leu-7 immunoreactive cells, which often serve as markers for Schwann cells, but the immunostaining is usually less intense than for schwannomas. In 60% to 90% of patients with neurofibromas, the cells are CD34 positive.[27] Other cells, such as fibroblasts, mast cells, and perineural cells, dispersed between nerve fibers, are also found in neurofibromas. This diverse mixture of cell types within a neurofibroma compounds the confusion as to the actual cell of origin.[3,48] The diffuse proliferation of Schwann and other cells often results in fusiform enlargement of the involved nerve segment. Both myelinated and unmyelinated axons often run interspersed through the tumor cells.

Solitary neurofibromas are often discretely localized, small, globular or fusiform nodules growing in the cutaneous or subcutaneous tissue layer. Less often, solitary neurofibromas arise along a nerve trunk. They are well circumscribed but not encapsulated and often are pale gray, white-gray, or translucent.[9,68] Their intercellular matrix is characterized by bundles of collagen fibrils and a myxomatous extracellular matrix interspersed with nerve fibers.[4]

Plexiform neurofibromas are characterized by redundant loops of nerve fiber bundles and tumor tissue intermixed in a disorganized pattern. Grossly, these tumors are tortuous and complex enlargements involving nerves. They involve substantial cellular proliferation within the endoneurium of nerve fascicles, thereby displacing axons. Plexiform neurofibromas can affect both small cutaneous and major nerves. Ill-defined nodules are often detected when small cutaneous nerves are

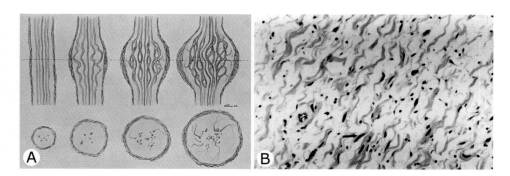

FIGURE 73-4 *A,* Schematic drawing illustrating how a growing neurofibroma tumor infiltrates the nerve and grows between the axons: the upper row shows tumor growth in longitudinal views of the nerve, and the lower row shows a cross section of the tumor in the nerve. (Reproduced with permission from Harkin JC, Reed RJ: Tumors of the Peripheral Nervous System. Washington, DC, Armed Forces Institute of Pathology, 1969, Plate IIIB, page 71). *B,* Hematoxylin-eosin stained section of a neurofibroma demonstrating spindle-shaped cells *(black arrow)* dispersed in a loose extracellular matrix rich in mucopolysaccharides. (Reproduced with permission from Grossman RG, Loftus CM (eds): Principles of Neurosurgery, 2nd ed. Philadelphia, Lippincott-Raven, 1999.)

involved. When major nerves are involved, the tumor appears as large lesions that affect long segments of a nerve, sometimes bulging and disfiguring the nerve into a convoluted mass. Furthermore, the entire extremity can be enlarged and hyperpigmented with loose overlying skin.[68] Plexiform neurofibromas are also associated with hypertrophy of underlying soft tissues and bones. Histologic sections show spindle cells, wavy collagen bundles, and increased mucinous substance. These tumors are multifocal myxoid lesions that are often described as a "bag of worms."[9] Malignant plexiform neurofibromas or malignant peripheral nerve sheath tumors may resemble fibrosarcomas.

Clinical Presentation and Evaluation

Neurofibromas are the most common benign peripheral nerve tumors in the younger age group, with most patients between the ages of 20 and 30, and both sexes are equally affected.[18,68,135–136] An epidemiologic study determined a prevalence rate of 1 lesion per 25,000 adults.[15] Neurofibromas are usually slow growing and may arise from a single large fascicle or several fascicles entering the nonfunctional tumor tissue. Ninety percent of neurofibroma patients have solitary neurofibromas.[84] However, solitary neurofibromas usually arise spontaneously and in general are not associated with neurofibromatosis, in contrast to plexiform and other less common (i.e., diffuse and multiple) types of neurofibromas, which are commonly associated with neurofibromatosis. The clinical presentation of a solitary neurofibroma is often similar to that of a schwannoma. Clinical symptoms often include spontaneous pain or dysesthesias. In contrast to schwannomas, palpation of a neurofibroma usually does not induce shooting pains or dysesthesias (i.e., a Tinel's response). Solitary neurofibromas are often small, isolated, painless nodules that mostly reside in the cutaneous or subcutaneous layer of skin and thus can cause cosmetic problems. They may be palpated under the skin. Patients with plexiform neurofibromas may have symptoms of pain, muscle weakness and atrophy, or mild sensory deficits. Cutaneous neurofibromas typically begin to appear in the prepubertal period and can develop anywhere in the body. Usually, the onset of associated symptoms begins after puberty. On ultrasound, a neurofibroma is usually a well-defined hypoechoic mass. CT scanning of neurofibromas can show low-density masses that are either homogeneously or heterogeneously enhanced, depending on the presence of cysts, and follow the trajectory of the involved peripheral nerves. MRN beautifully reveals these masses and can sometimes visualize their relation to the functional nerve fascicles of the involved peripheral nerve (see Figure 73-1). Similar to schwannomas, neurofibromas display isointense, or sometimes hypointense, signal with muscle on T1-weighted images and hyperintense signal on T2-weighted images. Furthermore, two thirds of neurofibromas have a target pattern of slightly increased central signal intensity and decreased peripheral signal intensity on T1-weighted studies and increased peripheral signal intensity and decreased central signal intensity on T2-weighted studies.[77,84] The solid tumor components show enhancement following the administration of gadolinium contrast agent.[71,117]

Treatment and Prognosis

The clinical outcome following complete resection of a solitary neurofibroma in a patient without NF1 is good or better in 80%

of cases.[3] The clinical outcome following complete resection of a solitary neurofibroma associated with NF1 is satisfactory or better in 68% of cases.[62] The clinical results following resection of a plexiform neurofibroma associated with NF1 are relatively poor because complete resection, especially of a large lesion involving a functionally important nerve, is rarely possible, whereas sparing function and recurrence is more common.[3,48,62] Therefore surgical resection of plexiform neurofibromas involving functionally important nerves is usually partial and often results in some loss of neurologic function.[76] To minimize postoperative functional deficits, surgical resection of neurofibromas, especially of the plexiform type, should be performed carefully by peripheral nerve surgeons with the aid of intraoperative electrophysiologic monitoring.[31,109–110] In contrast to neurofibromas, schwannomas can more easily be completely resected with little if any functional loss caused by displacement of the functioning axons by the proliferating Schwann cells in the tumor. High-resolution MRN images can sometimes help preoperatively in localizing and distinguishing intact and functioning nerve fascicles from tumor tissue.[65] The incidence of malignant transformation ranges from extremely rare in the case of a solitary neurofibroma to 4% in the case of a plexiform neurofibroma (see Chapter 74).[3,17–18] Plexiform neurofibromas that have undergone malignant transformation are collectively called malignant peripheral nerve sheath tumors (MPNSTs). The prognosis for benign neurofibromas following surgical resection is very good,[4] with local recurrence of neurofibromas mostly occurring in patients with neurofibromatosis.[76]

Similarities and Differences between Schwannoma and Neurofibroma

Compared with schwannomas, neurofibromas have relatively fewer Schwann cells, less reticulin, and more collagen in stained histologic sections. Both schwannomas and neurofibromas arise from supporting cells of the axon. Grossly, the most important feature that separates the two types of tumor is that axons are mixed in with tumor cells in neurofibromas, whereas axons tend to be displaced by Schwann cells in the case of schwannomas. This important difference accounts for much of the difference in clinical outcome following surgical resection of these two types of tumors. Schwannomas are histologically very homogeneous because they are composed of only Schwann cells. Neurofibromas, in contrast, have a heterogeneous cellular composition, which includes a variety of cell types in addition to Schwann cells, such as fibroblasts and mast cells. Furthermore, neurofibromas rarely but more often develop into malignant tumors than do schwannomas. Clinical symptoms of schwannomas, in contrast to neurofibromas, more often include pain and paresthesias upon palpation of the tumor (i.e., Tinel's sign).

Neurofibromatosis Syndromes and Association with Tumor Types

Neurofibromatosis disorders occur in more than 100,000 people in the United States and equally affect males and females. They are among the most common genetic disorders, and the two most common and best characterized at a molecular genetic level are types 1 and 2. Both types of neurofibromatosis are autosomal dominant disorders that can arise from either familial inheritance (~50%) or spontaneous mutation (~50%). They can affect any peripheral nerve throughout the body. Most tumors caused by neurofibromatosis are benign. Neurofibromas, especially the plexiform type, are predominantly associated with NF type 1, or von Recklinghausen's disease, whereas schwannomas of the spinal and cranial nerve roots, especially of the vestibular cranial nerve, are often associated with NF type 2.[3,51] Schwannomas can also be associated with NF1, but they are much less common than neurofibromas. The diagnostic criteria of NF1 and NF2 are based on the National Institutes of Health (NIH) Consensus Development Conference on Neurofibromatosis in 1987 (see http://consensus.nih.gov/cons/064/064_statement.htm). Although aspects of this Consensus Statement have been superceded in view of continued research, these criteria are primarily valid and valuable in the diagnostic evaluation for NF.

Neurofibromatosis 1

Molecular Genetics and Clinical Presentation.
NF1, also known as von Recklinghausen's disease or peripheral neurofibromatosis, is the most common type of neurofibromatosis and afflicts more than 85% of patients with this class of genetic phakomatoses disorder. It occurs in 1 out of every 4000 live births.[36] The NF1 gene, characterized in 1990, is located on chromosome 17 (17q11.2 locus) and codes for a protein called neurofibromin. Neurofibromin is expressed in abundance in neurons, oligodendrocytes, and nonmyelinating Schwann cells.[29] It acts through the family of Ras-GTPase activating proteins (Ras-GAP). Neurofibromin regulates cellular proliferation by inactivating Ras, thereby converting Ras-GTP to Ras-GDP. It has been postulated that neurofibromin may play two roles in the modulation of Ras-mediated activities. First, neurofibromin may inhibit the p21 Ras-mediated signaling pathway for cellular proliferation and growth. Second, it may act as a downstream modulator in the p21 Ras-mediated signaling pathway for cellular differentiation.[106] A tumor suppressor function independent of Ras-GTPase activation has also been reported. To date, more than 240 different NF1 mutations have been discovered in the large neurofibromin gene. Among patients with NF1, 30% to 50% have *de novo* mutations, representing a high spontaneous mutation rate.[3] The paternally inherited NF1 gene usually has small deletions, whereas the maternally inherited gene usually has large mutations. Clinically, a diagnosis of NF1 can be confirmed if at least two of the following clinical features are present (Figure 73-5): (1) six or more café-au-lait spots at least 5 mm in diameter in prepubertal individuals and 15 mm in postpubertal individuals (café-au-lait spots are present in 99% of NF1 patients in contrast to 10% to 20% of normal individuals); (2) two or more Lisch nodules or ocular hamartomas, which appear around puberty; (3) at least two superficial skin neurofibromas of any type, usually occurring as pea-size bumps or a single plexiform neurofibroma usually occurring as an enlarged swollen area under the skin; (4) axillary or groin freckling, which is present in 99% of NF1 patients; (5) bilateral optic nerve gliomas, which are present in 15% to 20% of NF1 patients[44]; (6) osseous abnormalities such as sphenoid dysplasia or thinning of the long bone cortex with or without pseudoarthrosis; or (7) a first-degree relative (parent, sibling, or offspring) who meets the NF1 criteria. Bone abnormalities, including abnormal curvature of the spine (scoliosis) in the lower cervical or upper thoracic regions, occur

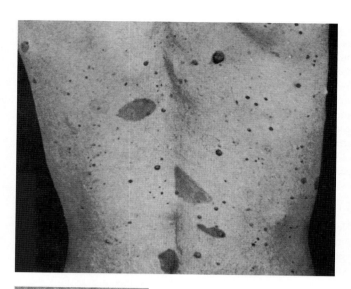

FIGURE 73-5 Photograph of the back of a patient with neurofibromatosis type 1 showing numerous skin café-au-lait spots and pigmented neurofibromas. (From Stout AP: Tumors of the peripheral nervous system. In National Research Council Committee on Pathology (eds): Atlas of Tumor Pathology, Section II, Fascicle, 6, Washington DC, Armed Forces Institute of Pathology, 1949.)

in approximately 40% of NF1 patients.[68] Occasionally, tumors may develop in the brain, on cranial nerves, or in the spinal cord. Approximately 50% of people with NF1 also have learning disabilities. Radiologically, 30% to 60% of NF1 patients show hyperintense signal on T2-weighted MR images of the brain.[33]

Treatment and Prognosis.
Patients with NF1 can have single or multiple neurofibromas. Surgical intervention for neurofibromas, particularly the plexiform type, is often difficult because of their proximity to functionally important nerves and adjacent structures, as well as their tendency to recur when incompletely resected. The surgeon, therefore, should be both strategic and cautious in deciding to operate on neurofibromas in NF1 patients. Clinical considerations that would lead the surgeon to consider surgery include disfiguring peripheral neurofibromas that can be removed in an esthetically pleasing manner; neurofibromas that are causing discomfort or functional problems that can be resected without causing significant functional deficits; and rapidly growing neurofibromas suspected of being malignant. These tumors often grow preferentially during puberty. Sometimes their growth is self-limited. The lifelong risk of malignant tumor transformation of neurofibromas in NF1 patients is approximately 4%.[11,32,103,113] Patients with NF1 have a three to five times greater risk of developing a malignancy than the general population.[44] Studies have suggested that p16 inactivation occurs during the malignant transformation of neurofibromas in NF1 patients, which may help in distinguishing neurofibromas from their malignant counterpart.[89] Thirty percent of NF1 patients ultimately die from some form of cancer in contrast to 25% in the general population.[113] Management of optic nerve glioma in patients with NF1 is challenging. Most patients with optic nerve thickening on MRI do not have significant visual symptoms. Optic glioma in NF1 patients is often stable for years, or only very slowly growing. Therefore whether

these patients require early and aggressive surgical treatment of their optic glioma remains a controversial issue.

Neurofibromatosis 2

Molecular Genetics and Clinical Presentation.
Neurofibromatosis type 2, also known as bilateral acoustic or central neurofibromatosis, is less common than NF1. NF2 occurs in 1 out of every 40,000 to 100,000 live births.[3,51] Isolated in 1993, the NF2 gene is located on chromosome 22 (22q12.2 locus) and codes for a protein called merlin, or schwannomin.[17–18,48] Merlin, or schwannomin, is expressed in fetal brain, kidney, lung, breast, and ovary. Its function is unclear but possibly involved with membrane stabilization of a cytoskeleton-associated protein and intercellular communication. The loss of merlin may lead to the elimination of intercellular contact inhibition, which could lead to tumor development.[102] In 10% of cases, NF2 patients become symptomatic before the age of 10. Fifty percent of NF2 patients become symptomatic by age 30 and 90% by age 50.[3] NF2 is characterized by schwannomas of the cranial nerve roots, particularly the vestibular portion of the eighth cranial nerve, as well as of the spinal nerve roots, mainly the sensory portion.[83,93] Schwannomas involving the cranial or spinal nerve roots usually involve multiple sites. Schwannomas rarely involve the more distal peripheral nerves in the clinical context of NF2. Clinically, NF2 is suspected when a hearing deficit is detected in patients in their teens or early twenties. An eighth nerve mass lesion can cause tinnitus and disequilibria as well as hearing loss. A diagnosis of NF2 is probable if one of the two following sets of clinical criteria is present: (1) unilateral vestibular schwannoma in a patient younger than 30 years in addition to one of the following: meningioma, glioma, schwannoma, or juvenile posterior subcapsular lenticular opacities (JPSLOs), which have a prevalence of 85% in patients with NF2,[44] or (2) multiple meningiomas in addition to unilateral vestibular schwannomas, glioma, schwannoma, or JPSLOs. A definite diagnosis of NF2 requires either (1) bilateral vestibular schwannomas or (2) first-degree relatives with NF2 in addition to unilateral vestibular schwannoma or the presence of a meningioma, glioma, schwannoma, or JPSLOs. The presence of congenital or juvenile cataracts in a person who has a first-degree relative with NF2 necessitates a detailed evaluation for NF2. Seventy-five to ninety percent of NF2 carriers develop bilateral acoustic schwannomas, and 50% develop other types of nervous system tumor.[3,83]

Treatment and Prognosis.
Surgery or radiation therapy constitutes the treatment options for vestibular schwannomas in patients with NF2. These treatments are described in detail in Chapter 43. Schwannomas of peripheral nerves in patients with NF2 are treated as described in the section on schwannomas.

Neurofibromatosis 3

NF3, also called mixed neurofibromatosis, involves both the CNS and PNS. Clinical features include a few large and pale café-au-lait spots, as well as freckling and more numerous cutaneous neurofibromas. Iris Lisch nodules do not occur in patients with NF3. Bilateral acoustic neuromas, posterior fossa and upper cervical meningiomas, and spinal or paraspinal neurofibromas are the predominant features of NF3, whereas optic gliomas have not been seen. NF3 occurs in patients between the ages of 20 and 30. Patients with NF3 often die from the effects of multiple CNS tumors.

Perineurioma

Pathology

Perineuriomas have a different pattern grossly, histologically, and ultrastructurally as compared with both neurofibromas and schwannomas (Figure 73-6). They can be found in dermal, subcutaneous, or more deeply situated tissues. In gross appearance, they are usually well circumscribed and may or may not have a hypocellular fibrous pseudocapsule. Perineuriomas are of variable size, ranging from 1 to 20 cm. These tumors comprise only perineural cells. Histologically, these cells do not stain positively with S-100 protein or Leu-7. However, they are immunoreactive to EMA, in contrast to schwannomas and neurofibromas, which, if they do stain, do so only lightly. Expression of low-affinity NGFr has also been documented in some cases of perineuriomas.[105] Perineuriomas are characterized by bland fusiform tumor cells arranged in whorls or interweaving fascicles, or they may show a storiform pattern of tumor growth in which spindle cells radiate from a central point. EM reveals an abundant collagenous stroma and the typical features of perineural cells, which include (1) an elongated nucleus with condensation of heterochromatin peripherally, (2) an incomplete and thin basal lamina, (3) the presence of multiple fine cytoplasmic processes with pinocytotic vesicles docked along the cell membrane, and (4) a wavy bipolar cytoplasm in a collagen myxoid stroma.[121] Other benign or malignant peripheral nerve tumors can also include abnormal perineural cells but not to the extent found in perineuriomas. Perineurioma has two major clinicopathologic forms: (1) intraneural and (2) soft tissue or extraneural.

Intraneural perineuriomas comprise a rare group of focal lesions arising from within peripheral nerves. Histologically, they are characterized by the proliferation of perineural cells

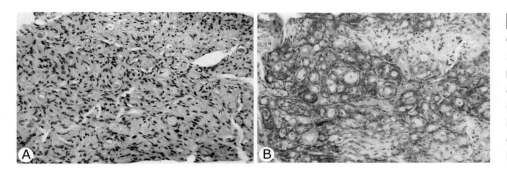

FIGURE 73-6 *A,* Hematoxylin-eosin stained section of a perineurioma. *B,* Immunohistochemical section showing positive staining of perineural cells with an antibody to epithelial membrane antigen (EMA). (From Kuntz C, Blake L, Britz G, et al: Magnetic resonance neurography of peripheral nerve lesions in the lower extremity. Neurosurgery 39:750–757, 1996.)

with a "pseudo-onion bulb" pattern around individual myelinated nerve fibers, resulting in enlargement of the involved peripheral nerve. Electron microscopy shows myelinated axons surrounded by concentric layers of cells with curved thin processes, pinocytotic vesicles, and an interrupted basal lamina. Demyelination and sometimes axonal loss occur as a result of intraneural perineurioma.[136] Other types of lesions or neoplasms, such as localized hypertrophic neuropathy and lipofibromatous hamartoma involving nerve, may be mistaken for intraneural perineuriomas because of their similar histologic patterns, including pseudo-onion bulbs. However, localized hypertrophic neuropathy can be distinguished from intraneural perineurioma by the former's positive immunostaining to S-100 protein and negative immunostaining to EMA.[103]

Soft-tissue or extraneural perineuriomas arise in the soft tissues surrounding peripheral nerves. These tumors are often small, well-circumscribed, but nonencapsulated masses. Histologically, most soft-tissue perineuriomas resemble fibroblastic tumors, which are characterized by elongated, wavy, and spindle-shaped cells with thin nuclei and elongated bipolar processes. Similar to intraneural perineurioma, they stain positively for EMA.[42] It has been reported that 30% to 40% of soft-tissue perineuriomas may be CD34 positive.[121] A distinct morphologic variant of soft-tissue perineurioma, called reticular perineurioma, has recently been characterized in the literature.[45] This particular variant is composed primarily of fusiform-shaped cells with a distinct reticular growth pattern. Both the classic type and reticular variant of soft-tissue perineuriomas are represented by bipolar cytoplasmic processes.

Clinical Presentation and Evaluation

Perineuriomas, also called storiform perineurial fibromas, are rare benign peripheral nerve tumors that occur mostly in adolescents and young adults. The chance of developing these tumors is slightly higher in females. Commonly they are a mononeuropathy, arise from soft tissues deep in the extremities, and are not associated with NF1.[3,17–18] Extraneural or soft-tissue perineuriomas, the more common form of perineuriomas, are benign tumors that are usually not associated with peripheral nerves and lie mostly within the subcutaneous and deep soft tissue of the limbs or trunk (the shoulder and back regions are common sites) of adults, especially women. They tend to occur as solitary lesions. Genetically, soft tissue perineuriomas often have part or all of chromosome 22 deleted.[42] Intraneural perineuriomas are rare benign tumors, with a little more than 50 cases reported in the literature.[53] They tend to be solitary lesions affecting major nerve trunks in the upper extremities, especially the posterior interosseous nerve.[37] Patients with intraneural perineurioma often report having muscle weakness.[136] Intraneural perineuriomas occur more often in adult males than females. Genetically, they are thought to be associated with chromosome 22 alterations. Their other names include *intraneural neurofibroma, hypertrophic interstitial neuritis, hypertrophic neurofibromatosis,* and *localized hypertrophic mononeuropathy (LHM).* In the case of intraneural perineurioma, MRI displays hyperintense signal on T2-weighted images and enhancement following gadolinium administration.[53]

Treatment and Prognosis

Complete resection of a perineurioma is curative. If resection of the tumor requires cutting functioning peripheral nerve fibers, a repair possibly with an interposition nerve graft should be considered.[47,53] Malignant transformation, recurrence, or metastasis of perineuriomas is rare but has been reported.[56]

OTHER PERIPHERAL NERVE TUMORS NOT INCLUDED IN THE WHO CLASSIFICATION SYSTEM

We have described benign peripheral nerve tumors arising primarily from Schwann cells, in the case of schwannomas and neurofibromas, and perineural cells in the case of perineuriomas. Other tumors arising from cells normally found in peripheral nerves that will be discussed include mucosal neuroma, neurothekeoma, granule cell tumor, lipoma, vascular tumors, and neuromuscular hamartoma. Peripheral nerve tumors can also originate from cells not normally found in nerves by local invasion, as in the case of desmoid tumors (i.e., from adjacent muscle tissue) or by metastatic spread in the case of primary tumors located at a distance. For example, a variety of primary tumors, such as breast and lung tumors, can metastasize to peripheral nerves and their plexi. More rarely, thyroid tumors; osteochondromas; bladder tumors; extracranial meningiomas; and malignant Ewing's tumors, which include Ewing's sarcoma, extraosseous Ewing's sarcoma, primitive neuroectodermal tumors (PNETs) or peripheral neuroepithelioma, and Askin's tumor (PNET of the chest wall), have all been found to directly involve peripheral nerves. Masses involving peripheral nerves that mimic tumors include ganglion cyst, Morton's neuroma, and traumatic neuroma. Finally, diseases that can mimic peripheral nerve tumors include inflammatory pseudotumor of the peripheral nerve, one of the Charcot-Marie-Tooth (CMT) disorders, radiation-induced neuropathy, and chronic inflammatory demyelinating polyradiculoneuropathy (CIDP). Tumors arising from neurons in the PNS include ganglioneuroma, neuroblastoma, peripheral neuroepithelioma, paraganglioma, and pheochromocytoma. They are often categorized under PNETs and tumors with nerve cell differentiation. They represent a very diverse group of tumors, often found in a pediatric population. Their clinical presentation, evaluation, and treatment are quite different from those associated with peripheral nerve tumors, and therefore this group of tumors is dealt with elsewhere in a more detailed fashion.[3,48]

Mucosal Neuroma

Mucosal neuromas are extremely rare tumors comprising a partially encapsulated aggregation or proliferation of nerve fibers, often with thickened perineurium, intertwined with one another in a plexiform pattern. This tortuous pattern of nerves is seen within a loose, endoneurium-like fibrous stroma background. Mucosal neuromas, mainly in the oral cavity, are usually associated with multiple endocrine neoplasia type 2b (MEN-2b), which consists of adrenal pheochromocytoma, medullary thyroid carcinoma, diffuse alimentary tract ganglioneuromatosis, and multiple small submucosal neuroma nodules of the upper digestive tract. It is inherited as an autosomal dominant trait, although spontaneous mutations have also been reported in many cases. The adrenal and thyroid tumors typically do not appear until after puberty, whereas the oral mucosal neuromas usually develop before puberty. The oral mucosal neuromas in

MEN-2b often occur as 2- to 7-mm yellowish-white, sessile, painless nodules in the lips, anterior tongue, and buccal commissures. Usually there are two to eight (sometimes more) neuromas, with deeper lesions having normal coloration. Similar nodules may be seen on the eyelids. The mucosal neuromas in MEN-2b are asymptomatic, self-limiting, and present no problem requiring surgical treatment. They may be surgically removed for esthetic reasons or if they are being constantly traumatized.[34,87]

Neurothekeoma

Neurothekeomas, also known as nerve sheath myxomas, are rare benign cutaneous soft-tissue tumors probably of Schwann cell origin.[12] They are commonly categorized into myxoid hypocellular and cellular types by their histology. The cellular type, occurring mostly in patients between 20 and 30 years old, is more common on the head and neck and upper extremities, whereas the myxoid hypocellular type, occurring in patients between 30 and 40 years old is more common on the trunk and lower extremities. Grossly, both types of neurothekeomas often are circumscribed masses. Microscopically, the cellular type shows higher cellularity than the myxoid type with larger spindle or epithelioid cells with vesicular nuclei. The myxoid hypocellular type shows small cytologically bland cells arranged in a loose cellular network or in loose, highly myxomatous nodules delineated by dense collagen. Myxoid tumors often show nerve sheath differentiation, whereas cellular tumors usually do not. Neurothekeoma often has spindle cells in a fascicular pattern and may contain cellular areas with little mucinous material. Mucinous lobules, if present, often have infiltrating characteristics. Cytologic atypia, mitoses, neurotropic foci, and giant cells may be present. There may be foci resembling plexiform fibrohistiocytic tumors. Cellular neurothekeomas are usually S-100 negative.[21,68] Treatment of neurothekeoma often includes surgical excision. Complete resection of the mass is usually curative. Recurrence of neurothekeoma is not very common, occurring in only 3 out of 123 reported cases, and metastasis of these tumors has not been reported.[101]

Myoblastoma

Myoblastomas, also known as granule cell tumors, are benign tumors thought to arise from Schwann cells, though the exact histogenesis has not been reported.[1,40] They occur most commonly in the skin and subcutaneous tissue as a solitary mass. On cut sections, these lesions often show a yellowish discoloration, typically have a smooth surface, and are poorly circumscribed, with infiltration into surrounding adipose tissue or muscle. Histologically, the tumor cells are large polygonal, oval, or bipolar cells with abundant fine or coarsely granular eosinophilic cytoplasm and a small pale-staining or vesicular nucleus eccentrically located in the cell. The granular cells can be stained positively with antibody to the S-100 protein. Ultrastructural studies have described the cytoplasmic granules as autophagic vacuoles containing cellular debris, including mitochondria and fragmented endoplasmic reticulum, as well as myelin. Resection of as much of the tumor while attempting to spare functioning nerve fibers or partial resection is the treatment of choice for granular cell tumor. Recurrence is seen in fewer than 7% of cases treated, even if granular cells extend beyond the surgical margins of the biopsy sample. A few reported metastasizing

granular cell tumors have appeared to be histologically benign. For this reason, tumors that recur, grow rapidly, or reach a size greater than 5 cm should be carefully followed or treated aggressively with surgery if possible. Malignant variants represent approximately 1% of all cases.[54,68,99]

Lipoma

Lipomas, also known as lipofibromatous hamartomas or neural fibrolipomas, are benign tumors arising from the proliferation of adipose or fibrous tissues. Grossly, they are well circumscribed and encapsulated and have a fusiform and yellowish appearance in the subcutaneous layer.[92] Histologically, lipomas can be intimately associated with functioning nerve fibers from which they cannot be easily separated. The median nerve is most commonly affected. Larger lipomas can envelop, infiltrate, or compress important nerves such as the brachial plexus when located in the supraclavicular fossa.[61] Overall, lipomas are the most common soft-tissue tumors in adults, occurring in 1 out of 1000 individuals.[131] They occur mostly in children or during early adulthood. Treatment includes biopsy of the tumor and decompression of the involved nerve when it becomes entrapped by surrounding structures such as the carpal tunnel. Complete resection of these tumors when involving a nerve is usually not possible without loss of neurologic function mediated by the involved nerve. Several treatment strategies therefore need to be considered. The tumors can be followed and managed conservatively if they do not grow or produce painful symptoms or loss of function. Alternatively, they can undergo biopsy, be decompressed, and be either partially resected while sparing functioning nerve fibers or fully resected with graft repair of cut and functionally important nerve fibers. The more completely the tumor is resected, the less likely it is to recur.[3,55,68] Malignant transformation has not been reported.

Vascular Tumors or Hemangioma

Hemangiomas of peripheral nerves are rare tumors arising from vascular endothelial cells. Histologically, hemangiomas show erythrocytes populated within thin-wall blood vessels within or surrounding the peripheral nerve.[18,75,94] These tumors occur mostly in younger patients. Clinical features include tenderness, pain, and the presence of a mass along with sensory or motor neurologic deficits. The surgical treatment of these tumors is similar to that of lipomas. Local recurrence sometimes occurs.

Neuromuscular Hamartoma

Neuromuscular hamartomas, also known as *benign triton tumors,* are characterized by skeletal muscle fibers mixed within bundles of disorganized nerve fascicles, containing myelinated and nonmyelinated nerve fibers. They are very rare peripheral nerve tumors, with only 20 cases reported in the literature. The exact histogenesis of these neoplastic lesions remains unclear, but they may be due to the concurrent proliferation of neuroectodermal-derived or limb-associated mesodermal tissue in a peripheral nerve fiber.[5] Grossly, these multilobulated masses are separated by fibrous septa with a hard and dark red appearance. They occur during infancy and affect both sexes equally. A majority involves major peripheral nerves, such as the sciatic or brachial plexus, causing neurologic symptoms. Cutaneous and intracranial lesions have been reported.[5,123] Complete resection often results in functional deficits. Their surgical treatment is similar to that of lipomas. Recurrence of completely resected tumors after surgery has not been reported.[81]

TUMORS ARISING FROM NEURONS

A group of tumors arises from neurons. These tumors may differ considerably in terms of their histologic appearance, state of differentiation, location, clinical presentation, and recommended treatments. Most of these tumors are benign and therefore often a surgical cure can be achieved. Those that are malignant require adjuvant therapies such as chemotherapy and radiation treatment. Although usually not included in chapters on peripheral nerve tumors, these tumors are described briefly in this chapter for the sake of being comprehensive.

Benign Tumors

Pheochromocytoma

Pheochromocytomas are rare benign tumors characterized by the abnormal proliferation of the adrenal chromaffin cells derived from the primitive neuroectoderm. As a result, a high level of catecholamine is produced. Ninety percent of these tumors are found in the adrenal medulla of the kidney. They may be associated with neurofibromatosis, von Hippel-Lindau disease, tuberous sclerosis, Sturge-Weber syndrome, and as a component of the multiple endocrine neoplasm syndrome, which is briefly described in the section on mucosal neuroma. Hypertension, whether sustained or episodic, is the most common clinical sign of pheochromocytomas. Headache, excessive truncal sweating, and palpitations are also commonly observed in these patients.[78] The diagnosis of these tumors includes assaying for serum and 24-hour urine catecholamines, as well as their metabolites such as vanillylmandelic acid (VMA) and metanephrines. Malignant transformation, by local invasion or metastasis, occurs in 10% of patients with pheochromocytomas. With nonmalignant pheochromocytomas, the 5-year survival rate is greater than 95%, and the recurrence rate after surgery is less than 10%. With malignant pheochromocytomas, the 5-year survival rate is less than 50%.[132]

Paraganglioma

Paragangliomas are rare benign tumors that originate from extra-adrenal chromaffin cells. Most paragangliomas are intra-abdominal and are especially common in the paravertebral ganglia and less common in the urinary bladder. Paragangliomas can be subclassified into carotid body tumors and chemodectomas, associated with the carotid bifurcation in the neck, or nonchromaffin paragangliomas, depending on the origin of the involved tissue.[28] The clinical presentation of these tumors mimics pheochromocytomas, their intra-adrenal counterpart. The chance of malignancy is higher with paragangliomas than with pheochromocytomas. They are also associated with a high incidence of persistent or recurrent disease after incomplete resection. It is estimated that local recurrence and metastasis develop in 5% to 10% of patients with paragangliomas.[27] The size of the tumor and the presence of metastasis are the main prognostic factors in patients with these tumors.[11]

Ganglioneuroma

Ganglioneuromas are rare benign tumors composed of a combination of Schwann and ganglion (i.e., neuronal) cells. Grossly, ganglioneuromas are usually encapsulated tumors and appear grayish-white on cut section. They represent a benign type of neuroblastic tumor, which also consists of malignant types as in neuroblastomas and ganglioneuroblastomas or differentiated neuroblastoma, which are composed of both mature and immature neurons.[19] These neuroblastic tumors are derived from primordial neural crest cells, which ultimately populate the sympathetic ganglia, adrenal medulla, and other sites. Like pheochromocytomas, ganglioneuromas along with other neuroblastic tumors are located in the adrenal medulla and sympathetic ganglia. The clinical features, diagnosis, and treatment of ganglioneuromas are similar to those of pheochromocytomas.[132] Ganglioneuromas tend to grow slowly and have no metastatic potential.

Treatment

A gross-total resection of these benign tumors should be attempted surgically whenever possible. Functionally important nerves that are involved by these tumors should be spared if possible. If it is not possible, tumor resection followed by a nerve repair with graft when necessary should be considered. In the case of pheochromocytomas, α-adrenergic receptor blocking drugs such as phenoxybenzamine or phentolamine should be administered to the patient preoperatively and as part of the treatment plan.

Malignant Tumors

Neuroblastoma

Neuroblastomas are malignant tumors derived from primitive neural crest cells. They are the most prevalent types of extracranial solid tumor in children. Neuroblastomas account for 8% to 10% of all childhood cancers. Each year approximately 525 new cases are reported in the United States.[25,140] In children, approximately 25% to 35% of neuroblastomas arise in the adrenal medulla. The other neuroblastomas can occur anywhere along the sympathetic ganglia, mostly in the paravertebral region of the posterior mediastinum and lower abdomen.[104] These tumors are characterized by rapid growth and widespread metastasis. The clinical features of neuroblastomas depend on the size and location of the tumor. For example, tumors that arise in the head and neck may be a palpable mass, and a Horner's syndrome is sometimes observed. Tumors that originate in the abdomen may cause abdominal pain and vomiting and may be palpable on physical examination. Genetically, neuroblastomas often exhibit an amplification of the N-myc oncogene. It appears that the number of N-myc copies correlates with the prognosis. Neuroblastomas may undergo spontaneous regression or, alternatively, undergo differentiation and maturation into a relatively benign ganglioneuroma. The 5-year survival rate with neuroblastomas is approximately 60%.[132]

Peripheral Neuroepithelioma

Peripheral neuroepitheliomas (i.e., of extrathoracopulmonary origin) are malignant tumors possibly originating from misplaced neuroepithelium derived from the neural crest. Histologically, sheets of small round cells in a pattern of Homer-Wright rosettes characterize peripheral neuroepitheliomas. Genetically, patients with peripheral neuroepitheliomas often can be found to have a t(11;22) translocation in common with other malignant small round-cell tumors such as Ewing's sarcomas and Askin's tumors (thoracopulmonary origin). They are rare tumors and account for less than 1% of all sarcomas. They metastasize widely, and their prognosis is poor. The 5-year survival rate with peripheral neuroepitheliomas is 10% to 35% for patients with metastasis, and 54% to 74% for patients with a localized stage of disease.[20,38]

Treatment

These malignant tumors usually require both surgical as well as adjuvant therapy such as chemotherapy and radiation treatment. Surgery is especially useful in obtaining an accurate diagnosis when treating neuroblastomas. The decision to remove peripheral neuroepithelioma is based on many factors, which include their location and relation to other important structures, as well as the patient's overall condition and prognosis.

TUMORS ARISING FROM EXTRINSIC PERIPHERAL NERVE ELEMENTS

Desmoid Tumors

Desmoid tumors, also known as *aggressive* or *deep-seated fibromatosis,* are benign fibrous tumors of mesenchymal origin usually located in muscle, particularly in the abdominal wall. When located at extra-abdominal sites such as in the neck, shoulder, or limbs, they often compress, envelop, or infiltrate peripheral nerves such as the brachial plexus, peroneal nerve, radial nerve, and sciatic nerve. Desmoid tumors are considered benign, because they do not metastasize to other parts of the body. However, they are often locally invasive to surrounding tissues, especially soft tissues such as peripheral nerves and surrounding vascular structures, and therefore they can be very difficult to treat surgically. They can also adhere to and intertwine with surrounding structures and organs. Patients often have symptoms that include a painless swelling or lump, pain or soreness caused by compressed nerves or muscles, pain and obstruction of the bowels, or limping or other difficulty using the legs, feet, arms, or hands. Treatment consists of surgical removal of the tumor along with irradiation or chemotherapy. Because desmoid tumors rarely metastasize, surgery alone often is the only treatment necessary. However, desmoid tumors have a high recurrence rate, because they are difficult to remove completely. As a result, patients with this type of tumor often require careful follow-up to manage the progressive nature of this disease. Neurologic deficits are commonly present postoperatively.[3,48,59]

Meningioma

The origin of extracranial or ectopic meningiomas has been suggested to be from the proliferation of ectopic embryonal nests of arachnoidal cells. However, these tumors may also arise from the proliferation of perineural cells of peripheral nerves because of the structural and functional similarities of perineural cells and arachnoidal cells.[66] Extracranial and extraspinal meningiomas are very rare, constituting only 2% of all meningiomas.[58,112] Previously reported locations include the orbit, parapharyngeal space, and rarely, the paranasal sinuses.[118] They are often associated with cranial nerves.[30] Primary tumor or local invasion or metastasis of an intra-axial tumor involving the peripheral nerves is extremely rare. Two cases of primary brachial plexus meningiomas and one case of secondary extension of an intra-axial lesion involving the peripheral nerves have been reported.[112] Its overall histologic appearance closely resembles an intracranial meningioma. These tumors are characterized by lobulated growth of uniform spindle cells with abundant lightly eosinophilic cytoplasm and round or oval clear nuclei with indistinct cytoplasmic borders, often arranged in concentric onion-skin-like whorls, even in the absence of psammoma bodies. The spindle tumor cells show diffuse and intense labeling for EMA and also moderate reactivity for cytokeratin and vimentin. Although locally invasive, the prognosis for these tumors is favorable if the tumor is completely removed.[39,122]

Metastatic and Other Miscellaneous Tumors

True metastatic tumors involving peripheral nerves are most commonly seen in patients with breast (24%) and pulmonary carcinoma (19%). They may also be seen in the clinical setting of lymphoma, bladder cancer, and melanoma.[61] Breast and pulmonary carcinomas often affect the brachial plexus through direct invasion and infiltration of peripheral nerves.[73] Apical pulmonary tumors, characteristic of Pancoast's syndrome, often involve the lower spinal nerve roots and trunks of the brachial plexus.[74,133] Other tumors such as pelvic tumors often infiltrate the lumbar and sacral plexus, whereas head and neck tumors often invade the cranial nerves.[6] Definitive diagnosis of these carcinomas requires multiple biopsy samples. Invasion by carcinomas can appear as a mass on CT or MRI. These tumors can cause severe neuropathic pain that often precedes weakness or sensory loss. Metastatic tumors involving the brachial plexus or other peripheral nerve elements are often approached surgically with the intent of performing a nerve decompression and neurolysis for pain relief, as opposed to attempting a more complete resection that is likely to produce significant functional deficits. Other tumors that have been associated with peripheral nerves directly include malignant PNETs, thyroid tumors, osteochondromas, and bladder tumors. PNETs typically occur in older children and young adults. The long-term survival is less than 40%. The survival rate is more optimistic for patients younger than age 1.[80]

OTHER MASSES THAT CAN MIMIC PERIPHERAL NERVE TUMORS

Ganglion Cyst

Ganglion cysts are cystic structures filled with viscous fluid and lined by fibrous hypocellular tissue. They are often a palpable mass that may produce symptoms and functional deficits in the involved peripheral nerve. They usually arise from joints or tendon sheaths and may directly or indirectly involve peripheral nerves and thereby cause neurologic symptoms and deficits. These cysts are most commonly located extraneurally, but examples of intraneural ganglion cysts developing within a peripheral nerve have also been seen. They affect the back of the hand in 60% to 70% of cases but may also involve the median and ulnar nerves at the wrist and the posterior interosseous nerve at the elbow.[124] In the lower extremity, they often involve the common peroneal nerve adjacent to the fibular head at the knee. There are at least two theories regarding their formation: (1) they directly communicate with joint spaces, with the intraneural tumors forming via articular branches to the involved joint, or (2) cystic degeneration occurs, possibly as a result of trauma.[114] Ganglion cysts often change in size and may spontaneously disappear. Ganglion cysts are best treated with total resection. Intraneural ganglion cysts are more difficult to remove than extraneural ganglion cysts because of their proximity to peripheral nerve fibers. These cysts may recur, especially in cases where total resection is not possible. An articular branch to the adjacent joint should be sought and if found should be cut to prevent cyst recurrence. A ganglion cyst can be distinguished from a peripheral nerve tumor by its unique appearance and common association with a joint capsule on MRN (Figure 73-7).[3,48,59,65,114]

Morton's Neuroma

Morton's neuromas, also known as localized interdigital neuritis, are reactive processes represented by a disorganized growth of nerve fibers. These lesions are often the result of a mechanically induced degenerative neuropathy. They are a condition characterized by a thickening of the nerve tissue caused by a swelling or tumor of the plantar digital nerves, between the metatarsal heads, most commonly the third or fourth. A burning sensation is often experienced in the ball of the foot. A fusiform enlargement of the neurovascular bundle is formed, with degeneration of the nerve and proliferation of the connective sheath layer surrounding the nerve fibers. The cause of the neuroma formation is not entirely understood but probably results from chronic and repetitive injury to the nerve in this area.[21,52] Morton's neuroma can be surgically removed by first making a small 5-cm incision between the two toes affected by the neuroma. The mass lesion is then located and removed by excising the nerve proximally. MRI reveals a low- to intermediate-signal-intensity soft-tissue mass in the intermetatarsal space.

Traumatic Neuroma

Traumatic or amputation neuromas are histologically similar to a Morton's neuroma, but they occur in a different location. They are the most common reactive process lesions associated with peripheral nerves. Traumatic neuromas arise at the severed end of a proximal peripheral nerve stump, usually 1 to 12 months after transection. They are due to severing of peripheral nerve axons with destruction of the surrounding endoneurium such that regenerating axons have no path to follow and thereby form a clump of disorganized axonal endings.[136] They can be painful, especially to direct mechanical stimuli. Histologically, they may have features in common with neurofibromas because of the presence of axons and connective tissue. The exact incidence of traumatic neuromas has not been reported, but it has been estimated that 4% of patients after digital amputations and up to 30% of patients after nerve injury develop these types of lesions.[68]

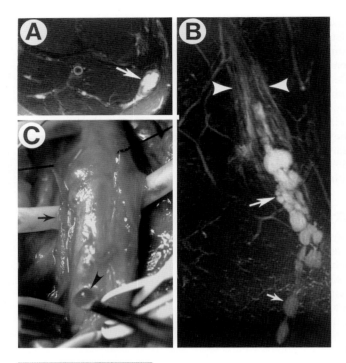

FIGURE 73-7 Magnetic resonance neurography images of a 40-year-old male patient with multiple intraneural cysts involving the left common peroneal nerve and its deep peroneal nerve branch. *A,* Axial T2-weighted fast spin echo (FSE) image showing high signal cystic lesions *(white arrow)* within the common peroneal nerve. *B,* Coronal T2-weighted FSE multiplanar reconstruction showing multiple high-signal intraneural cysts within the distal common peroneal nerve *(large white arrow)* that extend into the deep peroneal nerve branch *(small white arrow).* Note the abnormally bright nerve fascicles (between white arrowheads) splayed by the cysts. *C,* Intraoperative photograph demonstrating abnormal enlargement of the common peroneal nerve *(black arrow).* Note the extrusion of gelatinous material from a surgically ruptured cyst *(black arrowhead).* (From Kuntz C, Blake L, Britz G, et al: Magnetic resonance neurography of peripheral nerve lesions in the lower extremity. Neurosurgery 39:750–757, 1996.)

Miscellaneous Masses

Other nontumor masses that may externally or internally involve peripheral nerves include arteriovenous malformation, arteriovenous fistula, venous angiomas, traumatic pseudoaneurysms, myositis ossifans, and hyperplastic lymph nodes.[17]

OTHER DISEASES THAT CAN MIMIC PERIPHERAL NERVE TUMORS OR MASS LESIONS

Inflammatory Pseudotumor of the Peripheral Nerve

Localized or diffuse swelling of a peripheral nerve may also be due to a number of inflammatory or infectious diseases.

Inflammatory pseudotumor, also described as *nodular lymphoid hyperplasia, plasma cell granuloma,* and *fibrous xanthoma,* are all reactive and non-neoplastic processes that can mimic a peripheral nerve mass lesion. Inflammatory pseudotumors are characterized by chronic infiltration of inflammatory cells, primarily the T-cell population, as well as extensive fibrosis and collagen deposition. The etiology is unclear, but the inflammation may be triggered by various stimuli such as physical, biologic, or chemical factors. Five cases of inflammatory pseudotumor involving peripheral nerves (median nerve, facial nerve, sciatic nerve, radial nerve, and greater auricular nerve) have been reported in which the inflammatory cells penetrate the nerve fascicles.[95] The differential diagnosis often includes other non-neoplastic processes such as amyloidoma of the peripheral nerve and tuberculoid leprosy, all of which may mimic peripheral nerve tumors.[130] In general, inflammatory pseudotumor of the peripheral nerve follows a benign clinical course. This reactive process is best treated by total resection of the infiltrated fascicles while sparing functionally important nerve fibers, if possible, to minimize or avoid neurologic symptoms and functional deficits.

Amyloidoma of the Peripheral Nerve

Amyloidoma or amyloid tumor consists of a localized deposit of amyloid material, which is composed of extracellular fibrillar proteins with a β-pleated sheet secondary structure. Amyloidomas are rare and usually located in the lung and upper respiratory tract. Occasionally, these tumors have been detected in the PNS, most commonly in the trigeminal or gasserian ganglion or one of its three branches.[96,129] The etiology and pathogenesis of amyloidomas in peripheral nerves are unknown. Some studies have suggested that amyloidoma formation is due to an abnormal inflammatory response, where elevated numbers of plasma and other inflammatory cells are present surrounding the amyloid deposits. Treatment includes surgical excision of these abnormal masses.

Tuberculoid Leprosy

Leprosy, or Hansen's disease, is a severe disfiguring skin disease caused by *Mycobacterium leprae*.[85] A mild, nonprogressive form of leprosy called tuberculoid or neural leprosy is associated with type IV or cell-mediated hypersensitivity to the surface antigen of these Mycobacteria. It is characterized by nerve damage and numbness often manifested in the extremities. Grossly, the lesion appears as a macular plaque or nodular mass. Microscopically, the damaged nerve fascicles are infiltrated by mononuclear phagocytes and leukocytes organized into well-developed granulomas. At a later stage, caseous necrosis may be found in the nerve trunk. The mechanism of the nerve damage is unknown but is probably related to the cell-mediated immune response. Complications, if not treated promptly, may lead to mutilation and deformity. Standard treatment often includes a combination drug regimen of dapsone and rifampin, with or without clofazimine. Recent data have shown that multidrug therapy for leprosy may lead to the regeneration of damaged nerve fibers. However, these regenerated nerve fibers usually do not successfully reinnervate their target skin and, as a result, the cutaneous numbness continues after the treatment.

Charcot-Marie-Tooth Disorder

Charcot-Marie-Tooth (CMT) disorders, also known as hereditary motor and sensory neuropathy or peroneal muscular atrophy, represent an inherited group of neuropathies, some of whose genetic mutations have been characterized. These disorders are associated with diffusely enlarged peripheral nerves, most commonly involving the peroneal nerve. Prevalence of CMT disorder is 1 person per 2500 in the population, or approximately 125,000 patients in the United States. Patients with CMT usually have a slowly progressive degeneration of the muscles in the foot, lower leg, hand, and forearm, and a mild loss of sensation in the limbs, fingers, and toes. The first sign of CMT is generally a high-arched foot or gait disturbance. Other symptoms of the disorder may include foot bone abnormalities such as hammer toes, problems with hand function and balance, occasional lower leg and forearm muscle cramping, loss of some normal reflexes, occasional partial sight or hearing loss, and, in some patients, scoliosis (curvature of the spine). Particular genetic types of CMT include CMT-1A, which is the most common type and is inherited in an autosomal dominant pattern. The CMT-1A gene maps to chromosome 17 and is thought to code for a protein called PMP22 involved in coating peripheral nerves with myelin. Other types such as CMT-2A and CMT-2B also have an autosomal dominant inheritance pattern. CMT-3, CMT-4A, and CMT-4B refer to autosomal recessive inheritance disorders, and CMT-X has a sex-linked inheritance pattern. Full expression of CMT's clinical symptoms generally occurs by age 30.[88,127] These peripheral nerve disorders tend to be slowly progressive with no current medical treatments to reverse or slow the disease. Treatments tend to be supportive and compensatory in nature to maintain muscle strength and endurance, such as physical therapy.

Radiation-Induced Neuropathy (Plexopathy)

Peripheral nerves are relatively resistant to radiation. However, a slowly progressive neuropathy may develop locally many years after radiation therapy. It is often a diagnosis of exclusion, and therefore it is important to rule out the possibility of residual or recurrent tumor.[17-18] On MRI, the involved peripheral nerves usually have a smaller than normal diameter and increased signal on T2 and short tau inversion recovery (STIR) pulse sequences (Figure 73-8). Rarely, the involved nerves can have an enlarged appearance, though in a more uniform pattern than the irregular enlargements seen with peripheral nerve tumors and other mass lesions. Radiation-induced neuropathy or plexopathy involving the brachial plexus, often a complication following radiation therapy to the axillary and supraclavicular regions, has been most commonly reported.[8,86] The incidence of radiation-induced plexopathy is usually related to the total dose and to the dose per fraction.[97,119] The clinical features consist of a painless and slowly progressive sensory-motor disturbance, such as paresthesias and weakness, affecting especially the hand and arm, along with decreased or absent muscle stretch reflexes.[22] Shoulder discomfort is also a common symptom often seen in these patients. However, the clinician must be aware that plexopathy caused by other diseases, such as recurrent lymph node disease in the axilla, can mimic the clinical features of brachial plexopathy caused by radiation therapy. Electrodiagnostically, the most common abnormalities in patients with radiation-induced brachial neu-

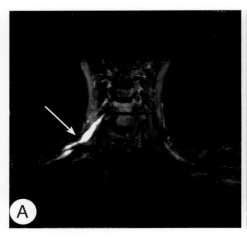 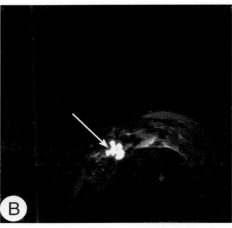

FIGURE 73-8 Coronal magnetic resonance imaging short tau inversion recovery (STIR) sequence image through the brachial plexus of a patient with a radiation-induced right brachial plexopathy following treatment for breast cancer. Abnormally increased signal involves the spinal nerves, trunks, and divisions. There was no evidence of recurrent tumor.

ropathy are signs of chronic partial muscle denervation with increased mean duration of individual motor unit potentials and decreased amplitude of compound muscle and sensory action potentials. Nerve conduction velocities are often normal.[86] Radiologically, this disorder can usually be diagnosed on MRI. However, sometimes a peripheral nerve exploration and biopsy is necessary. Treatments are supportive and include pain control and physical therapy.

Chronic Inflammatory Demyelinating Polyradiculoneuropathy

Chronic inflammatory demyelinating polyradiculoneuropathy (CIDP), also known as chronic relapsing polyneuropathy, is an immune-mediated inflammatory neuropathy. It is a rare autoimmune disorder in which there is a swelling of nerve roots and destruction of the myelin sheath over the nerves. Histologically, the damaged nerve has a well-developed onion bulb–like morphology.[7] Clinically, CIDP is characterized by slowly progressive weakness and sensory loss involving the legs and arms. Although it can occur at any age and in both sexes, CIDP is more common in young adult males. Symptoms include tingling or numbness beginning in the toes and fingers, weakness of the arms and legs, aching pain in the involved muscles, loss of deep tendon reflexes, fatigue, and abnormal sensations.[14] To diagnose CIDP, a peripheral nerve biopsy is sometimes performed. Treatment consists of a course of intravenous immunoglobulin (IV Ig), plasmapheresis, or a corticosteroid such as prednisone, which is typical for peripheral nerve disorders with an autoimmune etiology. Intermittent demyelination and remyelination, along with an onion bulb pattern, are often observed in biopsies of cutaneous nerves such as the sural nerves. Physical therapy may also be incorporated into the treatment plan to maintain and improve muscle strength, function, and mobility.

TREATMENT

Medical

Both benign and malignant peripheral nerve tumors are extremely resistant to radiation therapy, although palliation of unresectable tumors or masses may be affected with this method of treatment. In the case of malignant peripheral nerve tumors, radiation therapy may be useful in conjunction with surgery, either preoperatively, to reduce a large tumor, or postoperatively, to control residual disease (see Chapter 74). The effect of intravenous chemotherapy in the treatment of benign peripheral nerve tumors remains debatable, and we do not currently advocate or practice it. Collaborative controlled trials of 13-cis-retinoic acid (a differentiating agent) and interferon-α 2a for treatment of patients with plexiform neurofibromas are currently in progress. Furthermore, clinical studies have shown the efficacy of activin A and also a farnesyltransferase inhibitor, which blocks the normal Ras signaling pathway, in providing a new adjuvant therapeutic option for NF1 patients with neurofibromas. Similarly, quinidine or quinidine-like compounds have been shown to slow or completely halt the growth of schwannomas in NF2 patients.[64,100,139]

Surgical

The surgical treatment of benign peripheral nerve tumors or masses is aimed at obtaining a definitive diagnosis and surgically removing the lesions while preserving neurologic function whenever possible. The decision to perform a biopsy or excise peripheral nerve tumors or masses relies on clinical, radiologic, and electrodiagnostic findings. A surgical intervention is warranted if there is the need to obtain a biopsy specimen for a definitive diagnosis or if there is evidence of rapid growth of a mass, progressive neurologic symptoms with functional deficits, and intolerable pain not well controlled with medication. A team approach consisting of surgeons, electrophysiologists, and operating room staff with experience in dealing with peripheral nerve lesions is key to optimizing clinical outcome.

INTRAOPERATIVE ELECTROPHYSIOLOGIC NEUROMONITORING

Intraoperative neurophysiologic monitoring is useful in localizing functioning peripheral nerves during the dissection to expose tumors and other types of associated masses (Figure 73-9). Electrophysiologic techniques such as EMG, NCS, and SSEP tests complement patients' history, physical examination, and radiographic studies in the surgical treatment of these disorders. Intraoperative neuromonitoring techniques are employed for several important reasons: (1) to initially identify functioning nerves; (2) to distinguish functioning peripheral nerve fibers from tumor tissue and other types of mass lesions; and (3) to monitor the activity of functioning nerve fibers during the resection of mass lesions to maximize the preservation of nerve function.

Setup of the Patient Preoperatively

The recording and stimulating electrodes are often placed before or after the final positioning and draping of the patient in the operation room (see Figure 73-9). The electrodes are inserted cutaneously and percutaneously near specific nerves and muscles to monitor the electrophysiologic function of peripheral nerves either involved by or near the mass lesions. Often, additional electrodes for SSEP recording are placed over the spine and the contralateral parietal scalp to monitor sensory impulses traveling within the spinal cord and somatosensory cortex, respectively.[63] Electrophysiologic monitoring can be affected by the use of anesthetic agents. Halogenated inhalational anesthetics produce dose-related decreases in amplitude and increases in latency of SSEPs that are most marked in cortically generated components. Intravenous sedative-hypnotic drugs (droperidol, barbiturates, benzodiazepines, etomidate, propofol) produce dose-related depression of the electroencephalogram (EEG) after initial activation and dose-related depression of evoked responses to a lesser extent than do the inhalation agents. Neuromuscular blockers or paralytic agents have no significant effect on evoked potentials but confound EMG recordings. Muscle relaxation reduces artifactual signals from spontaneous muscle activity but alters muscle recordings from motor tract or nerve stimulation, making it difficult if not impossible to identify the motor fascicles.[111] Electrophysiologic recording from a limb can also be hindered by the placement of an inflatable tourniquet, a problem that can be dealt with by deflating the tourniquet intermittently to reverse accumulating tissue ischemia, which progressively attenuates nerve conduction and muscle endplate responses. Alternatively, no tourniquet is used, which is the technique preferred by us, and bleeding is controlled throughout the surgery with the use of electrocautery and hemostatic agents such as thrombin, fibrin glue, and cotton balls soaked in dilute hydrogen peroxide when necessary.

Specific Electrophysiologic Techniques and Their Intraoperative Application

Nerve Conduction Studies

Both the recording and stimulating electrodes are placed along a peripheral nerve segment, and nerve conduction responses are measured between two points. This test can record sensory, motor, or compound nerve conduction responses across the tumor or mass as it is being dissected and removed. A reduction in the amplitude of the signal waveform suggests axonal loss. Nerve conduction responses can also distinguish between functioning and nonfunctioning axons within a segment of isolated nerve.

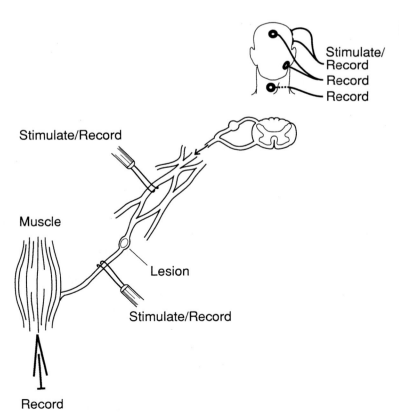

Stimulate/Record

Record
Record

Stimulate/Record

Muscle

Lesion

Stimulate/Record

Record

FIGURE 73-9 Schematic diagram illustrating the various intraoperative electrophysiologic stimulating and recording options available to the surgeon (see text for details). (From Kliot M, Slimp J: Techniques and assessment of peripheral nerve function at surgery. In Loftus C, Traynelis VC (eds): Intraoperative Monitoring Techniques in Neurosurgery. New York, McGraw Hill, 1993.)

Somatosensory Evoked Potentials

Monitoring of the sensory component of nerves included in the surgical approach may be done with SSEPs. Stimulation is conventionally to major mixed nerves such as median, ulnar, radial, tibial, or peroneal nerves, with recording at central locations such as the cervical spine, brainstem level, or scalp. In the case of tumors located very close to the spinal cord, SSEP responses, recorded either over the spine or contralateral brain (parietal scalp), to stimulation of nerve roots can be used to assess the integrity of sensory roots.

Triggered Electromyography

A peripheral nerve lesion involving motor fibers can be monitored while recording EMG activity from innervated muscles (Figure 73-10). Visible or recordable muscle contraction can be observed when motor nerves entering the proximal or distal pole of a lesion are electrically stimulated. The surface of a tumor can then be mapped delivering stimulation with a fine-tipped monopolar electrode and recording of compound motor action potentials (CMAPs) from target muscles to identify motor axons such that they can be avoided as the surgeon begins to dissect and remove the tumor. Direct electrical stimulation of the peripheral nerve lesion or mass with the use of a fine-tipped monopolar electrode permits the precise localization and mapping of the distribution of functioning nerve fibers within a mass lesion site. Direct electrical stimulation is highly advantageous in the resection of benign peripheral nerve tumors such as schwannomas, which tend to displace neighboring functional nerve fibers.

Spontaneous, Free-Running Electromyography

Continuous, free-running EMG activity on the video screen display and audio output may be used to detect the occurrence of motor unit firing. The occurrence of EMG discharges that correlate with manipulation of a nerve may indicate irritation or injury to motor fibers. Brief bursts of EMG activity may simply reflect contact and irritation of a nerve, but it may equally be an indication of injury. A sustained burst of muscle activity during tumor resection is evidence of sustained irritation or possible axonal injury.[110]

Electrophysiologic monitoring with these methods allows the surgeon to evaluate and preserve the integrity of sensory and motor axons during the resection of peripheral nerve mass lesions.

SURGICAL RESECTION OF TUMOR AND OTHER TYPES OF MASS LESIONS

In general, the main steps in resecting peripheral nerve tumors consist of (1) exposing the nerve proximal and distal to the tumor by external neurolysis; (2) directly exposing the tumor capsule, usually after incising several encircling connective tissue layers; (3) electrically mapping the tumor capsule to localize the distribution of functioning nerve fibers; (4) longitudinally (i.e., in the direction of the course of adjacent nerve fibers) cutting the tumor capsule where there are no functioning fibers in the capsule; (5) sweeping aside functioning nerve fibers that are encountered like bucket-handles; (6) entering and stimulating the tumor to identify and avoid damaging nerve fibers; (7) sending a specimen of tumor for pathologic diagnosis, with frozen sections performed to confirm a benign pathology; (8) if the tumor is thought to be malignant, closing and awaiting the final pathologic diagnosis before deciding on further treatment, as is our practice; (9) if the tumor is benign, carefully resecting while attempting to spare functioning nerve fibers using electrophysiologic motor and sensory monitoring techniques; (10) exposing the proximal and distal poles of the tumor where the entering and exiting nerve fibers are most easily identified (often useful); (11) removing tumor tissue, often using blunt dissection and suction for soft tissue or careful sharp resecting or Cavitron resection (at low power settings) of pieces for more fibrous and firm tumor tissue; and (12) sharply cutting away the residual tumor capsule that does not contain functioning nerve fibers.

Individual types of tumor may require special considerations. For example, small or medium-size schwannomas can often be circumferentially separated and excised from surrounding functioning fascicles by blunt dissection (Figure 73-11). In the end, an entering and exiting nerve fascicle that is usually nonfunctional is often found and must be cut to remove the tumor. Large schwannomas are usually best approached surgically by first performing an intratumoral debulking, thereby collapsing the tumor capsule, which facilitates the identification of functioning nerve fascicles.[3] Well-encapsulated tumors like schwannomas often are isolated from functioning nerve fascicles by (1) dissecting down upon the tumor, which usually requires incising through multiple capsular layers of connective tissue; (2) mapping the tumor capsule electrically, then making a longitudinal slit incision where there are no functioning fibers in the capsule; (3) sweeping away functioning nerve fibers like bucket handles; (4) circumferentially freeing the tumor proper and isolating nerve fascicles entering proximally and exiting distally; and finally (5) cutting them and removing the tumor. In the case where functioning nerve fibers are integrated into the capsule of the tumor, the capsule must be electrophysiologically mapped and the nonfunctional tissue cut away. In the case of tumors less easily separable from functioning nerve fibers, a combination of sharp and blunt dissection as well as using the Cavitron judiciously at low levels must be done (Figure 73-12). In some cases, the tumor cannot be separated from functioning nerve fibers, and the decision is made either to leave some tumor or to remove the tumor by sacrificing either a portion of the nerve (see Figure 73-12) or the entire nerve (Figure 73-13) and then perform a repair, usually with an interposition graft.

The surgical management of solitary neurofibromas is often comparable to that of schwannomas. However, the fascicles entering and exiting a neurofibroma are usually larger and more numerous than in schwannomas.[31,134] Key steps in resecting a solitary neurofibroma include (1) isolating and sparing important functioning fascicles infiltrating the tumor if possible; (2) resecting the tumor tissue; and (3) resecting nonfunctioning fascicles infiltrating the neurofibroma.[11,48,59–62] In the case of plexiform neurofibromas, especially those in patients with NF1, important functional nerve fibers may be intimately associated with tumor tissue.[31] In such cases, total resection of the tumor often leads to new neurologic deficits postoperatively. An alternative is to perform a subtotal resection of the tumor. Key steps involve (1) exposing the tumor and separating it from the surrounding tissues; (2) bluntly dissecting tumor nodules away from fascicles where possible; and (3) opening

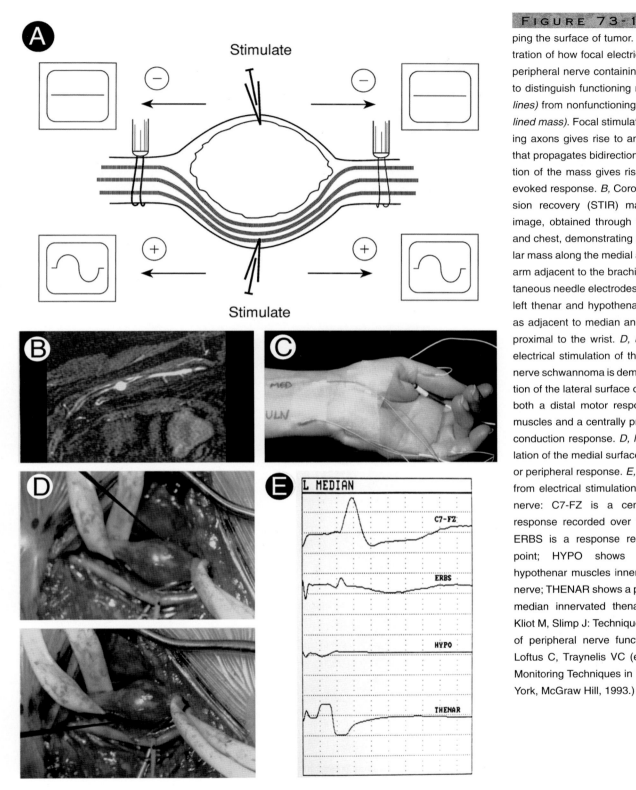

FIGURE 73-10   Needle mapping the surface of tumor. *A,* Schematic illustration of how focal electrical stimulation of a peripheral nerve containing a mass can help to distinguish functioning nerve fibers *(black lines)* from nonfunctioning tumor tissue *(outlined mass).* Focal stimulation of the functioning axons gives rise to an evoked response that propagates bidirectionally. Focal stimulation of the mass gives rise to no recordable evoked response. *B,* Coronal short tau inversion recovery (STIR) magnetic resonance image, obtained through the left upper arm and chest, demonstrating a high-signal circular mass along the medial aspect of the upper arm adjacent to the brachial artery. *C,* Percutaneous needle electrodes can be seen in the left thenar and hypothenar muscles, as well as adjacent to median and ulnar nerves just proximal to the wrist. *D, upper panel,* Focal electrical stimulation of the exposed median nerve schwannoma is demonstrated. Stimulation of the lateral surface of the tumor elicited both a distal motor response in the thenar muscles and a centrally propagating sensory conduction response. *D, lower panel,* Stimulation of the medial surface elicited no central or peripheral response. *E,* Evoked responses from electrical stimulation of the left median nerve: C7-FZ is a centrally propagating response recorded over the cervical spine; ERBS is a response recorded over Erb's point; HYPO shows no response in hypothenar muscles innervated by the ulnar nerve; THENAR shows a positive response in median innervated thenar muscles. (From Kliot M, Slimp J: Techniques and assessment of peripheral nerve function at surgery. In Loftus C, Traynelis VC (eds): Intraoperative Monitoring Techniques in Neurosurgery. New York, McGraw Hill, 1993.)

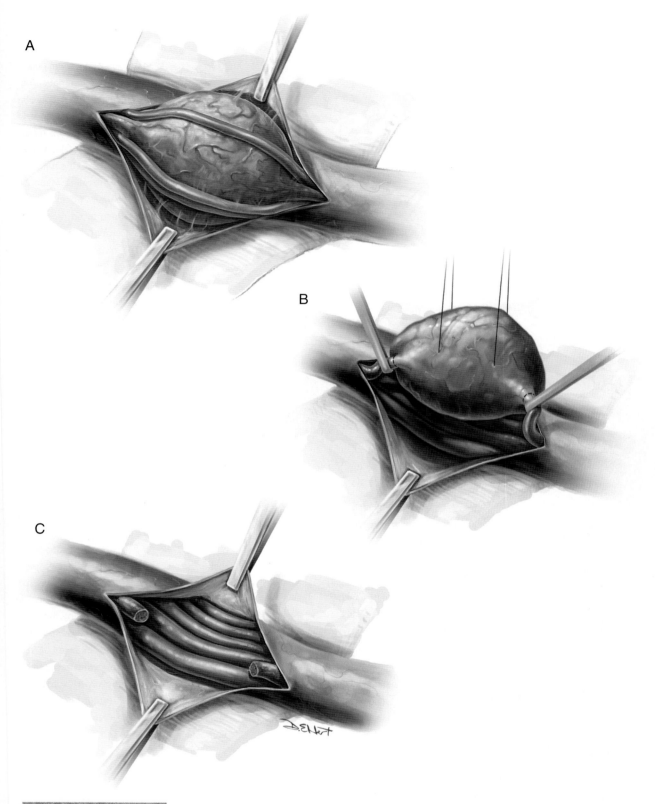

FIGURE 73-11 Schematic diagram of the surgical approach to benign neural sheath tumors. Complete resection of nerve sheath tumor that is separable from adjacent functioning nerve fibers: the steps of surgically resecting a well-circumscribed and encapsulated nerve sheath tumor are schematically illustrated. *A,* External epineurium of the nerve overlying the tumor has been longitudinally incised. An internal neurolysis is then performed to isolate and preserve functioning nerve fascicles overlying the tumor capsule; these fascicles are swept aside. *B,* Tumor is then circumferentially separated from the surrounding nerve tissue with its proximal entering and distal exiting fascicles encircled with loops. *C,* Tumor has been gross totally resected showing the cut proximal and distal fascicle, which often are nonfunctional and therefore do not require a graft repair. (Remodeled from Kline DG, Hudson AR, Kim DH: Operative steps for neural sheath tumors and lumbar sympathectomy. In Kline DG, Hudson AR, Kim DH (eds): Atlas of Peripheral Nerve Surgery. Philadelphia, WB Saunders, 2001.)

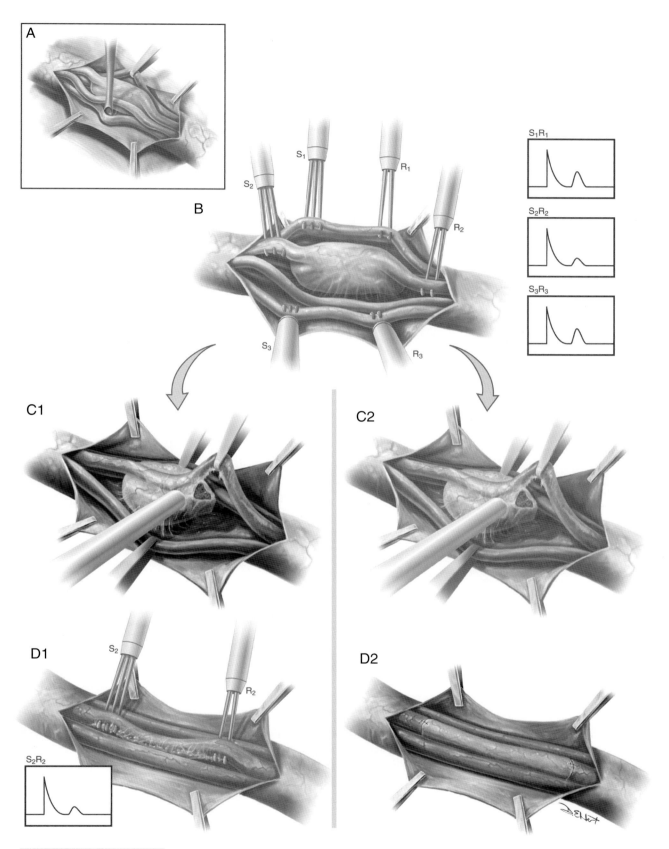

FIGURE 73-12 Schematic diagram to the surgical approach to benign neural sheath tumors. Partial resection of nerve sheath tumor partially involving functionally important nerve fibers. *A,* Longitudinal slit in the external epineurium overlying the tumor has been made and an internal neurolysis is performed to separate functioning nerve fibers from the tumor. *B,* Functioning nerve fibers entering and exiting the tumor may not be separable. *C1 and D1,* Tumor is partially removed using a Cavitron (at low power settings) to remove tumor down to the functioning nerve fibers while attempting to spare them. *C2 and D2,* Complete removal of the tumor requires sectioning of functioning nerve fibers, which are then repaired with an interposition nerve graft. (Remodeled from Kline DG, Hudson AR, Kim DH: Operative steps for neural sheath tumors and lumbar sympathectomy. In Kline DG, Hudson AR, Kim DH (eds): Atlas of Peripheral Nerve Surgery. Philadelphia, WB Saunders, 2001.)

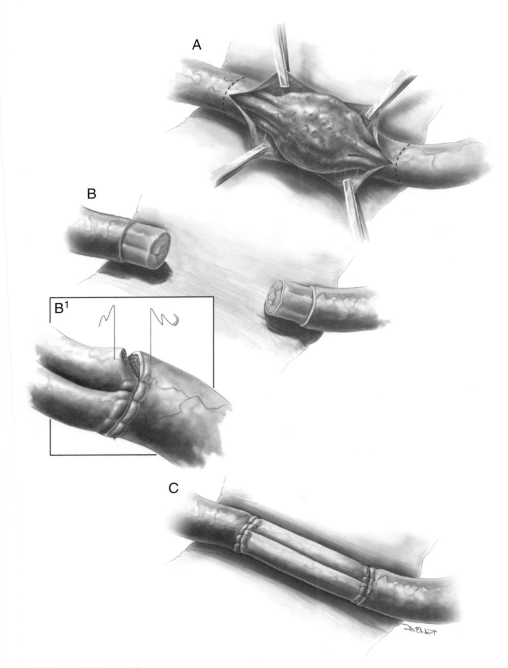

FIGURE 73-13 Schematic diagram of the surgical approach to benign neural sheath tumors. Complete resection of a nerve sheath tumor not separable from a functionally important nerve using an interposition nerve graft. *A,* Tumor has been exposed but cannot be separated from the nerve. *B,* Tumor has been completely resected, leaving the proximal and distal ends of the cut nerve stumps with an intervening gap, which is then repaired either directly (*B¹*) or with nerve grafts as shown in *C* if there is a longer gap. (Remodeled from Kline DG, Hudson AR, Kim DH: Operative steps for neural sheath tumors and lumbar sympathectomy. In Kline DG, Hudson AR, Kim DH (eds): Atlas of Peripheral Nerve Surgery. Philadelphia, WB Saunders, 2001.)

solid portions of the tumor and performing an internal debulking until functioning nerve fibers are encountered, either by eliciting neurotonic discharges in monitored muscles or by an electrical stimulation probe. Nerve grafting is sometimes necessary following the resection of a functionally important nerve. Preoperative high-resolution MRN and intraoperative electrodiagnostic monitoring enable the clinician to identify the spatial relationship between normal functioning nerve fibers and nonfunctioning tumor tissue or other types of masses (Figures 73-14, 73-15, and 73-16). This capability is especially

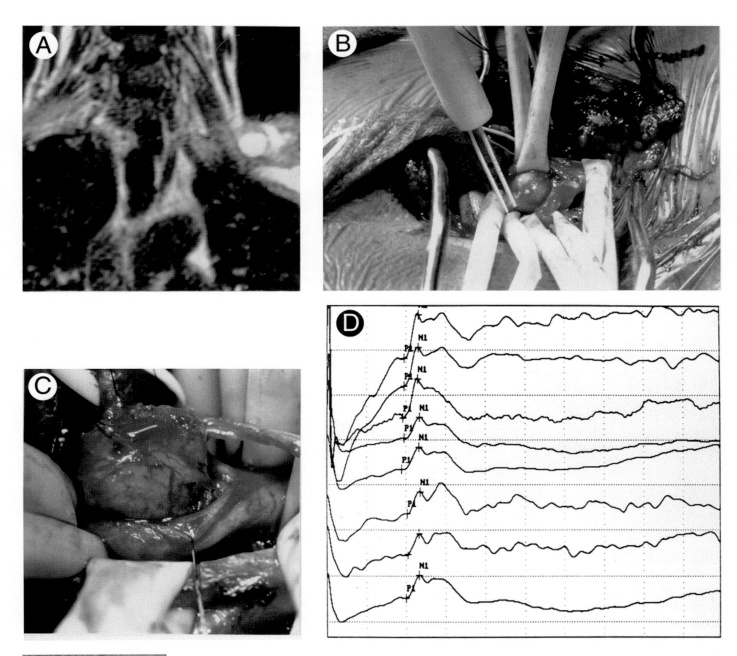

FIGURE 73-14   Monitoring during tumor resection. *A,* T1 coronal magnetic resonance image showing a gadolinium-enhanced circular mass in the left brachial plexus just above the clavicle. *B,* Surgical exposure of the mass embedded within the middle trunk of the left brachial plexus. Splayed on either side of the mass are the anterior and posterior divisions of the overlying upper trunk. Also shown is a bipolar electrode stimulating the middle trunk just distal to the mass. *C,* Surgical removal of the mass, which proved to be a schwannoma, from the middle trunk. *D,* Electrical stimulation of the median nerve distal to the tumor with central recording of the sensory evoked response over the upper cervical spine during removal of the schwannoma. (From Kliot M, Slimp J: Techniques and assessment of peripheral nerve function at surgery. In Loftus C, Traynelis VC (eds): Intraoperative Monitoring Techniques in Neurosurgery. New York, McGraw Hill, 1993.)

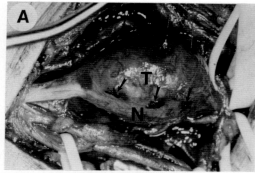

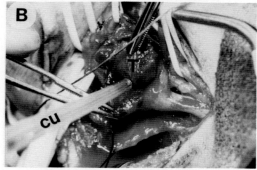

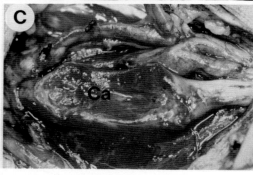

FIGURE 73-15 Intraoperative photographs demonstrating the surgical removal of an ulnar nerve neurofibroma in the distal forearm. Intraoperative stimulating and recording techniques were used to help in delineating the nonfunctional tumor (T) from the functioning ulnar nerve (N). *A,* Black arrows point to sutures placed to demarcate the tumor nerve border. *B,* Using microsurgical techniques and the Cavitron (cu) set at low power, the nonfunctional tumor is being aspirated away from the parent nerve. *C,* Residual tumor cavity (Ca) lined with functioning nerve fibers. (Reproduced with permission from Grossman RG, Loftus CM (eds): Principles of Neurosurgery, 2nd ed. Philadelphia, Lippincott-Raven, 1999.)

helpful in identifying functional nerve fibers, which may be integrated into parts of the tumor or its capsule.[65]

POSTOPERATIVE MANAGEMENT

The goals of postoperative management of patients with peripheral nerve tumor are reestablishing normal physiologic func-

tion and identifying or preventing possible systemic and neurologic complications. Neurologic and musculoskeletal examinations are performed postoperatively to evaluate any deficits, and vital signs are monitored closely. Antibiotics are administered usually at least for 24 hours postoperatively. Adequate pain medication is important both for the patient's comfort and to permit gradual and early mobilization such that an optimal functional outcome is ensured.

FOLLOW-UP PHYSICAL THERAPY AND OTHER INTERVENTIONS

Rehabilitation Interventions

Early mobilization enhances the sliding motions between nerves and the surrounding tissues, thus diminishing the development of tethering adhesions, and improves and accelerates the recovery process.[17–18] Range-of-movement exercises should be started immediately if a nerve repair has not been performed. The patient should start with gentle and slow range-of-movement exercises and gradually escalate their frequency and intensity. Such exercises should be performed several times daily. It is often useful for the patient to receive weekly physical therapy sessions for several months. Appropriate splinting to immobilize the limb for 2 weeks, followed by gradual passive then active physiotherapy, should be considered following nerve repair with or without grafts.[3] Patients are instructed in passive and active range-of-motion exercises, as well as sensory education for the involved limb to enhance or maintain neuromuscular function.[91] Strengthening exercises are supplemented postoperatively, and occupational therapy is provided as needed.[41]

Radiologic and Electrophysiologic Studies and General Follow-Up Guidelines

An initial baseline postoperative MRI study is useful either in the immediate postoperative period (first or second day after surgery) or after approximately 3 months, once the operative changes have subsided, to monitor tumor recurrence or growth of residual tumor. Electrophysiologic studies can be useful in obtaining early and objective evidence of muscle reinnervation, particularly following nerve repairs with or without grafts.[3,48] Serial clinical examinations at 3- to 6-month intervals for at least 1 to 2 years are recommended to carefully follow the recovery process of the patient. Patients should be told to contact their physician immediately should they suspect recurrence or growth of their treated tumors.

Acknowledgments

We wish to express special thanks to Janet Schukar and Paul Schwartz, in the Department of Neurological Surgery at the University of Washington Medical Center, for their wonderful photographic expertise and David Ehlert, Medical Illustrator of Health Sciences Academic Services and Facilities at the University of Washington Medical Center for creating the schematic drawings.

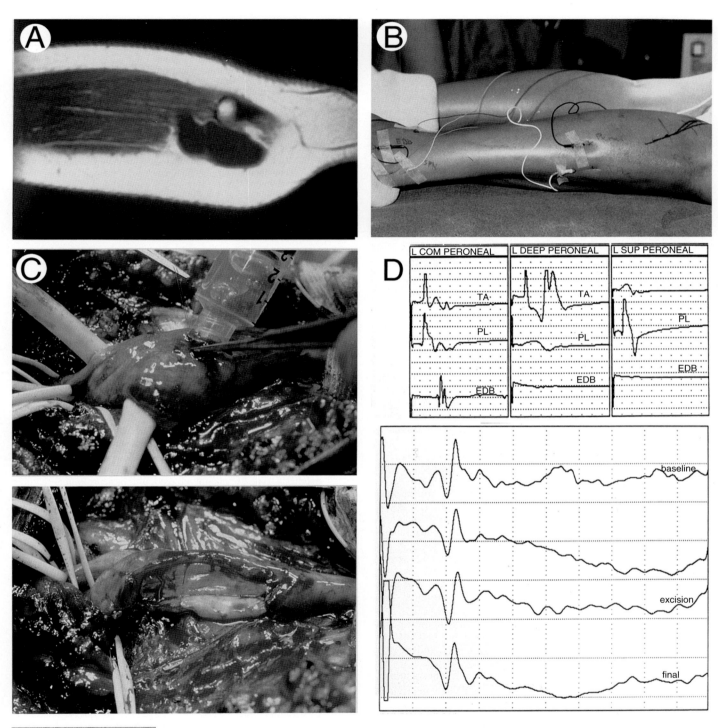

FIGURE 73-16 *A,* Sagittal T1-weighted magnetic resonance image through the right lower leg at the level of the fibular head demonstrating a large cystic structure. *B,* Percutaneous needle electrodes inserted in right superficial and deep peroneal innervated muscles of the lower leg (i.e., peroneus longus and tibialis anterior, respectively), inserted in the distal extensor digitorum brevis muscle in the foot, and adjacent to the superficial peroneal sensory branch in the foot. Note also the pen marking overlying the course of the common peroneal nerve. *C, upper panel,* Exposure of the cystic mass within the common peroneal nerve at the level of its bifurcation into superficial *(encircled by upper left loop)* and deep *(encircled by lower left loop)* branches. A small incision was made into the cyst and very viscous fluid, characteristic of a ganglion cyst, was evacuated with a syringe. The lower panel shows the common peroneal nerve after radical resection of the cyst. *D, upper panel,* Appropriate responses from distal muscles following stimulation of the common, deep, and superficial segments of the right peroneal nerve. Lower panel shows unchanging sensory conduction signals recorded across the cyst during its resection by stimulating distally the superficial sensory branch and recording proximally along the common peroneal nerve. (From Kliot M, Slimp J: Techniques and assessment of peripheral nerve function at surgery. In Loftus C, Traynelis VC (eds): Intraoperative Monitoring Techniques in Neurosurgery. New York, McGraw Hill, 1993.)

References

1. Alireza A, Connelly EM, Rowden G: An immunohistochemical investigation of S-100 protein in granular cell myoblastomas: evidence for Schwann cell derivation. Am J Clin Pathol 79:37–44, 1983.
2. Ampil FL: Radiotherapy for carcinomatous brachial plexopathy. A clinical study of 23 cases. Cancer 56:2185–2188, 1985.
3. Angelov L, Feldkamp MM, Guha A: Peripheral nerve tumors. In Kaye AH, Black PM (eds): Operative Neurosurgery. London, Churchill Livingstone, 2000.
4. Ariel I: Tumors of the peripheral nervous system. Semin Surg Oncol 4:7–12, 1988.
5. Awasthi D, Kline D, Beckman EN: Neuromuscular hamartoma (benign "triton" tumor) of the brachial plexus. J Neurosurg 75:795–797, 1991.
6. Ballantyne AJ, McCarten AB, Ibanez ML: The extension of cancer of the head and neck through peripheral nerves. Am J Surg 106:651–667, 1963.
7. Barohn RJ, Kissel JT, Warmolts JR, Mendell JR: Chronic inflammatory demyelinating polyradiculoneuropathy. Clinical characteristics, course, and recommendations for diagnostic criteria. Arch Neurol 46:878–884, 1989.
8. Barr LC, Kissin MW: Radiation-induced brachial plexus neuropathy following breast conservation and radical radiotherapy. Br J Surg 74:855–856, 1987.
9. Beggs I: Pictorial review: imaging of peripheral nerve tumors. Clinical Radiology 52:8–17, 1997.
10. Beggs I: Sonographic appearances of nerve tumors. J Clin Ultrasound 27:363–368, 1999.
11. Belzberg AJ, Campbell JN: Neoplasms of peripheral nerves. In Wilkins RH, Rengachary SS (eds): Neurosurgery. New York, McGraw-Hill, Health Professions Division, 1996.
12. Bhaskar AR, Kanvinde R: Neurothekeoma of the hand. J Hand Surg [Br] 24:631–633, 1999.
13. Biernat W: 2000 World Health Organization classification of tumors of the nervous system. Pol J Pathol 51:107–114, 2000.
14. Bouchard C, Lacroix C, Plante V, et al: Clinicopathologic findings and prognosis of chronic inflammatory demyelinating polyneuropathy. Neurology 52:498–503, 1999.
15. Bouquot JE: Common oral lesions found during a mass screening examination. J Am Dent Assoc 112:50–57, 1986.
16. Briggs RJS, Brackmann DE, Baser ME, Hitselberger WE: Comprehensive management of bilateral acoustic neuromas. Arch Otolaryngol Head Neck Surg 120:1307–1314, 1994.
17. Britz GW, Goodkin R, Kliot M: Peripheral nerve tumors: pathologic, diagnostic, and treatment considerations. In Grossman RG, Loftus CM (eds): Principles of Neurosurgery. Philadelphia, Lippincott-Raven, 1999.
18. Britz GW, Lee JC, Goodkin R, Kliot M: Peripheral nerve tumors. In Keating RF, Goodrich JT, Packer RJ (eds): Tumors of the Pediatric Central Nervous System. New York, Stuttgart Thieme, 2001.
19. Brodeur GM, Castleberry RP: Neuroblastoma. In Pizzo PA, Poplack DG (eds): Principles and Practice of Pediatric Oncology. Philadelphia, JB Lippincott, 1993.
20. Brooks D: Clinical presentation and treatment of peripheral nerve tumors. In Dyck PJ et al (eds): Peripheral Neuropathy. Philadelphia, WB Saunders, 1984.
21. Burger PC, Scheithauer BW, Vogel FS: Peripheral nerve. In Burger PC, et al (eds): Surgical Pathology of the Nervous System and Its Coverings. New York, Churchill Livingstone, 1991.
22. Burn RJ: Delayed radiation-induced damage to the brachial plexus. Clin Exp Neurol 15:221–227, 1978.
23. Carney JA: Psammomatous melanotic schwannoma. A distinctive, heritable tumor with special associations, including cardiac myxoma and the Cushing syndrome. Am J Surg Pathol 14:206–222, 1990.
24. Carney JA, Stratakis CA: Epithelioid blue nevus and psammomatous melanotic schwannoma: the unusual pigmented skin tumors of the Carney complex. Semin Diagn Pathol 15:216–224, 1998.
25. Castleberry RP: Biology and treatment of neuroblastoma. Pediatr Clin North Am 44(4):919–937, 1997.
26. Cerofolini E, Landi A, DeSantis G, et al: MR of benign peripheral nerve sheath tumors. J Comput Assist Tomgr 15:593–597, 1991.
27. Coffin CM, Dehner LP: Neurogenic tumors of soft tissue. In Coffin CM, Dehner LP, O'Shea PA (eds): Pediatric Soft Tissue Tumors: A Clinical, Pathological, and Therapeutic Approach. Baltimore, Williams & Wilkins, 1997.
28. Das Gupta TK, Chaudhuri PK: Tumors of the peripheral nerves. In Das Gupta TK, Chaudhuri PK (eds): Tumors of the Soft Tissues. Stamford, Conn, Appleton & Lange, 1998.
29. Daston MM, Scrable H, Nordlund M, et al: The protein product of the neurofibromatosis type 1 gene is expressed at highest abundance in neurons, Schwann cells, and oligodendrocytes. Neuron 8:415–428, 1992.
30. Daugaard S: Ectopic meningioma of a finger. Case report. J Neurosurg 58:778–780, 1983.
31. Donner TR, Voorhies RM, Kline DG: Neural sheath tumors of major nerves. J Neurosurg 81:362–373, 1994.
32. Ducatman BS, Scheithauer BW, Piepgras DG, et al: Malignant peripheral nerve sheath tumors. A clinicopathologic study of 120 cases. Cancer 57:2006–2021, 1986.
33. Duffner PK, Cohen ME, Seidel FG, Shucard DW: The significance of MRI abnormalities in children with neurofibromatosis. Neurology 39:373–378, 1989.
34. Dyck PJ, Carney JA, Sizemore GW, et al: Multiple endocrine neoplasia, type 2b: phenotype recognition; neurological features and their pathological basis. Ann Neurol 6:302–314, 1979.
35. Eary JF, Conrad EU: Positron emission tomography in grading soft tissue sarcomas. Semin Musculoskelet Radiol 3:135–138, 1999.
36. Eichenfield LF, Levy ML, Paller AS, et al: Guidelines of care for neurofibromatosis type I. JAAD 37:625–630, 1998.
37. Emory TS, Scheithauer BW, Hirose T, et al: Intraneural perineurioma. A clonal neoplasm associated with abnormalities of chromosome 22. Am J Clin Pathol 103:696–704, 1995.
38. Enzinger FM, Weiss SW: Soft Tissue Tumors. St Louis, Mosby, 1995.
39. Farah SE, Konrad H, Huang DT, Geist CE: Ectopic orbital meningioma: a case report and review. Ophthal Plast Reconstr Surg 15:463–466, 1999.
40. Fisher ER, Wechsler H: Granular cell myoblastoma-a misnomer: EM and histochemical evidence concerning its Schwann cell derivation and nature (granular cell schwannoma). Cancer 15:936–953, 1962.
41. Ganju A, Roosen N, Kline DG, Tiel RL: Outcomes in a consecutive series of 111 surgically treated plexal tumors: a review of the experience at the Louisiana State University Health Sciences Center. J Neurosurg 95:51–60, 2001.
42. Giannini C, Scheithauer BW, Jenkins RB, et al: Soft tissue perineurioma: evidence for an abnormality of chromosome 22, criteria for diagnosis, and review of the literature. Am J Surg Pathol 21:164–173, 1997.
43. Gonzales, M: The 2000 World Health Organization classification of tumours of the nervous system. J Clin Neurosci 8:1–3, 2001.
44. Goodrich JT: Neurofibromatosis. In Keating RF, Goodrich JT, Packer RJ (eds): Tumors of the Pediatric Central Nervous System. New York, Stuttgart Thieme, 2001.

45. Graadt van Roggen JF, McMenamin ME, Belchis DA, et al: Reticular perineurioma: a distinctive variant of soft tissue perineurioma. Am J Surg Pathol 25:485–493, 2001.

46. Grant GA, Britz GW, Goodkin R, et al: The utility of magnetic resonance imaging in evaluating peripheral nerve disorders. Muscle Nerve 25:314–331, 2002.

47. Gruen JP, Mitchell W, Kline DG: Resection and graft repair for localized hypertrophic neuropathy. Neurosurgery 43:78–83, 1998.

48. Guha A, Bilbao J, Kline DG, Hudson AR: Tumors of the peripheral nervous system. In Youmans JR (ed): Neurological Surgery: A Comprehensive Reference Guide to the Diagnosis and Management of Neurosurgical Problems. Philadelphia, Saunders, 1996.

49. Gutmann DH, Aylsworth A, Carey JC, et al: The diagnostic evaluation and multidisciplinary management of neurofibromatosis 1 and neurofibromatosis 2. JAMA 278:51–57, 1997.

50. Hajdu SI: Peripheral nerve sheath tumors: histogenesis, classification, and prognosis. Cancer 72:3549–3552, 1993.

51. Halliday A, Sobel R, Martuza R: Benign spinal nerve sheath tumors: their occurrence sporadically and in neurofibromatosis types 1 and 2. J Neurosurg 74:248–253, 1991.

52. Harkin JC, Reed RJ: Tumors of the peripheral nervous system. In Atlas of Tumor Pathology. Fascicle 3. Washington, DC, Armed Forces Institute of Pathology, 1969 (reprinted 1982).

53. Heilbrun ME, Tsuruda JS, Townsend JJ, Heilbrun MP: Intraneural perineurioma of the common peroneal nerve. J Neurosurg 94:811–815, 2001.

54. Junquera LM, de Vicente JC, Losa JL, et al: Granular-cell tumours: an immunohistochemical study. Br J Oral Maxillofac Surg 35:180–184, 1997.

55. Kao GF, Laskin WB, Olsen TG: Solitary cutaneous plexiform neurilemoma (schwannoma): a clinicopathologic, immunohistochemical, and ultrastructural study of 11 cases. Mod Pathol 2:20–26, 1989.

56. Karaki S, Mochida J, Lee YH, et al: Low-grade malignant perineurioma of the paravertebral column, transforming into a high-grade malignancy. Pathol Int 49:820–825, 1999.

57. Kaude JV: Case 51–1978: Distinguishing cystic from solid renal masses. N Engl J Med 300:985–986, 1979.

58. Kishore A, Roy D, Irvine BW: Primary extracranial meningioma of the soft palate. J Laryngol Otol 114:149–150, 2000.

59. Kline DG, Donner T, Voorhies R: Management of tumors involving peripheral nerves. In Tindall GT, Cooper PR, Barrow DK (eds): The Practice of Neurosurgery. Baltimore, Williams & Wilkins, 1996.

60. Kline DG, Hudson AR, Kim DH: Operative steps for neural sheath tumors and lumbar sympathectomy. In Kline DG, Hudson AR, Kim DH (eds): Atlas of Peripheral Nerve Surgery. Philadelphia, WB Saunders, 2001.

61. Kline DG, Hudson AR, Kim DH: Surgical management of peripheral nerve tumors. In Schmidek HH, Sweet WH (eds): Operative Neurosurgical Techniques: Indications, Methods, and Results. Philadelphia, Saunders, 2000.

62. Kline DG: Tumors involving nerves. In Kline DG, Hudson AR (eds): Nerve Injuries: Operative Results for Major Nerve Injuries, Entrapments, and Tumors. Philadelphia, WB Saunders, 1995.

63. Kliot M, Slimp J: Techniques and assessment of peripheral nerve function at surgery. In Loftus C, Traynelis VC (eds): Intraoperative Monitoring Techniques in Neurosurgery. New York, McGraw Hill, 1993.

64. Kotsuji T, Imakado S, Ichikawa E, Otsuka F: Effects of activin A on the growth of neurofibroma-derived cells from a patient with neurofibromatosis type 1. Dermatology 201:277, 2000.

65. Kuntz C, Blake L, Britz G, et al: Magnetic resonance neurography of peripheral nerve lesions in the lower extremity. Neurosurgery 39:750–757, 1996.

66. Landini G, Kitano M: Meningioma of the mandible. Cancer 69:2917–2920, 1992.

67. Laschinger JC, Cunningham JN, Jr, Cooper MM: Monitoring of somatosensory evoked potentials during surgical procedures on the thoracoabdominal aorta. I. Relationship of aortic cross-clamp duration, changes in somatosensory evoked potentials, and incidence of neurologic dysfunction. J Thorac Cardiovasc Surg 94:260–265, 1987.

68. Lee DH, Dick HM: Management of peripheral nerve tumors. In Omer GE, Spinner M, Van Beek AL (eds): Management of Peripheral Nerve Problems. Philadelphia, Saunders, 1998.

69. Legler JM, Ries LA, Smith MA, et al: Cancer surveillance series [corrected]: brain and other central nervous system cancers: recent trends in incidence and mortality. J Natl Cancer Inst 91:1382–1390, 1999.

70. Levine E, Huntrakoon M, Wetzel L: Malignant-nerve sheath neoplasms in neurofibromatosis: distinctions from benign tumors by using imaging techniques. Am J Radiol 149:1059–1064, 1987.

71. Lin J, Martel W: Cross-sectional imaging of peripheral nerve sheath tumors: characteristic signs on CT, MR imaging, and sonography. AJR Am J Roentgenol 176:75–82, 2001.

72. Lopes MBS, Vandenberg SR, Scheithauer BW: The World Health Organization classification of nervous system tumors in experimental neuro-oncology. In Levine AJ, Schmidek HH (eds): Molecular Genetics of Nervous System Tumors. New York, Wiley-Liss, 1993.

73. Ludemann W, Dorner L, Tatagiba M, Samii M: Brachial plexus palsy from nodular fasciitis with spontaneous recovery: implications for surgical management. Case illustration. J Neurosurg 94:1014, 2001.

74. Lusk MD, Kline DG, Garcia CA: Tumors of the brachial plexus. Neurosurgery 21:439–453, 1987.

75. Lusli EJ: Intrinsic hemangiomas of peripheral nerves: report of two cases and review of the literature. Arch Pathol 53:266–270, 1952.

76. MacKinnon SE, Dellon AL: Tumors of the peripheral nerve. In MacKinnon SE, Dellon AL (eds): Surgery of the Peripheral Nerve. New York, Thieme Medical Publisher, 1988.

77. Mafee MF, Coombs RJ, Shinaver CN, et al: Imaging of soft tissue sarcomas. In Das Gupta TK, Chaudhuri PK (eds): Tumors of the Soft Tissues. Stamford, Conn, Appleton & Lange, 1998.

78. Manger WM, Gifford RW, Jr: Clinical and Experimental Pheochromocytoma. Cambridge, Mass, Blackwell Science, 1996.

79. Mankin HJ: Principles of soft-tissue tumor management. In Gelberman RH (ed): Operative Nerve Repair and Reconstruction. Philadelphia, JB Lippincott, 1991.

80. Marina NM, Etcubanas E, Parham DM, et al: Peripheral primitive neuroectodermal tumor in children: a review of the St. Jude experience and controversies in diagnosis and management. Cancer 64:1952–1960, 1989.

81. Markel SF, Enzinger FM: Neuromuscular hamartoma—a benign "triton tumor" composed of mature neural and striated muscle elements. Cancer 49:140–144, 1982.

82. Martinoli C, Bianchi S, Derchi LE: Ultrasonography of peripheral nerves. Semin Ultrasound CT MR 21:205–213, 2000.

83. Martuza RL, Eldridge R: Neurofibromatosis 2 (bilateral acoustic neurofibromatosis). N Engl J Med 318:684–688, 1988.

84. Mechtler LL, Cohen ME: Primary and secondary tumors of the central nervous system. Clinical presentation and therapy of peripheral nerve tumors. In Bradley WG, Daroff RB, Fenichel GM, Marsden CD (eds): Neurology in Clinical Practice. The Neurological Disorders. Boston, Butterworth-Heinemann, 2000.

85. Miko TL, Le Maitre C, Kinfu Y: Damage and regeneration of peripheral nerves in advanced treated leprosy. Lancet 342:521, 1993.

86. Mondrup K, Olsen NK, Pfeiffer P, Rose C: Clinical and electrodiagnostic findings in breast cancer patients with radiation-induced brachial plexus neuropathy. Acta Neurol Scand 81:153–158, 1990.

87. Morrison PJ, Nevin NC: Multiple endocrine neoplasia type 2B (mucosal neuroma syndrome, Wagenmann-Froboese syndrome). J Med Genetics 33:779–782, 1996.

88. Murakami T, Garcia CA, Reiter LT, Lupski JR: Charcot-Marie-Tooth disease and related inherited neuropathies. Medicine (Baltimore) 75:233–250, 1996.

89. Nielsen GP, Stemmer-Rachamimov AO, Ino Y, et al: Malignant transformation of neurofibromas in neurofibromatosis 1 is associated with CDKN2A/p16 inactivation. Am J Pathol 155:1879–1884, 1999.

90. NIH Consensus Development Conference Statement. Neurofibromatosis. Arch Neurol 45:575–578, 1988.

91. Nori SL, Magill D: Rehabilitation. In Keating RF, Goodrich JT, Packer RJ (eds): Tumors of the Pediatric Central Nervous System. New York, Stuttgart Thieme, 2001.

92. O'Connell JX, Nielsen GP: Tumors demonstrating adipocytic differentiation. In Montgomery E, Aaron AD (eds): Clinical Pathology of Soft-Tissue Tumors. New York, Marcel Dekker, 2001.

93. Okazaki H: Neoplastic and related lesion. In Okazaki H (ed): Fundamentals of Neuropathology: Morphologic Basis of Neurologic Disorders. New York, Igaku-Shoin, 1989.

94. Patel CB, Tsai TM, Kleinert HE: Hemangioma of the median nerve: a report of two cases. J Hand Surg 11A:76–79, 1986.

95. Perez-Lopez C, Gutierrez M, Isla A: Inflammatory pseudotumor of the median nerve. Case report and review of the literature. J Neurosurg 95:124–128, 2001.

96. Pizov G, Soffer D: Amyloid tumor (amyloidoma) of a peripheral nerve. Arch Pathol Lab Med 110:969–970, 1986.

97. Powell S, Cooke J, Parsons C: Radiation-induced brachial plexus injury: follow-up of two different fractionation schedules. Radiother Oncol 18:213–218, 1990.

98. Powers KP, Norman D, Edwards MSB: Computerized tomography of peripheral nerve lesions. J Neurosurg 59:131–136, 1983.

99. Regezi JA, Batsakis JG, Courtney RM: Granular cell tumors of the head and neck. J Oral Surg 37:402–406, 1979.

100. Rosenbaum C, Kamleiter M, Grafe P, et al: Enhanced proliferation and potassium conductance of Schwann cells isolated from NF2 schwannomas can be reduced by quinidine. Neurobiol Dis 7:483–491, 2000.

101. Rosenberg AE, Dick HM, Botte MJ: Benign and malignant tumors of peripheral nerve. In Gelberman RH (ed): Operative Nerve Repair and Reconstruction. Philadelphia, JB Lippincott, 1991.

102. Rouleau G, Merel P, Lutchman M, et al: Alteration in a new gene encoding a putative membrane-organizing protein causes neurofibromatosis type 2. Nature 363:515–521, 1993.

103. Scheithauer BW, Woodruff JM, Erlandson RA: Tumors of the Peripheral Nervous System. Armed Forces Institute of Pathology, Washington DC, 1999.

104. Schofield D, Cotran RS: Diseases of infancy and childhood. In Cotran RS, Kumar V, Collins T (eds): Robbins Pathologic Basis of Disease. Philadelphia, WB Saunders, 1999.

105. Sciacco M, Scarpini E, Baron P, et al: Sural nerve immunoreactivity for nerve growth receptor in a case of localized hypertrophic neuropathy. Acta Neuropathol 83:547–553, 1992.

106. Seizinger BR: NF-1: A prevalent cause of tumorigenesis in human cancers. Nature Genet 3:97–99, 1993.

107. Seppala M, Haltia M: Spinal malignant nerve-sheath tumor or cellular schwannoma? A striking difference in prognosis. J Neurosurg 79:528–532, 1993.

108. Slavit DH, Harner SG, Harper CM, Jr: Auditory monitoring during acoustic neuroma removal. Arch Otolaryngol Head Neck Surg 117:1153–1157, 1991.

109. Slimp J, Kliot M: Electrophysiological monitoring: peripheral nerve surgery. In Andrews RJ (ed): Intraoperative Neuroprotection. Baltimore, Williams & Wilkins, 1996.

110. Slimp J: Intraoperative monitoring of nerve repairs. Hand Clinic 16:25–36, 2000.

111. Sloan TB: Anesthetic effects on electrophysiologic recordings. J Clin Neurophysiol 15:217–226, 1998.

112. Smith ER, Ott M, Wain J, et al: Massive growth of a meningioma into the brachial plexus and thoracic cavity after intraspinal and supraclavicular resection. J Neurosurg 96:107–111, 2002.

113. Sorenson S, Mulvhill J, Nielsen A: Long term follow up of von Recklinghausen neurofibromatosis. Survival and malignant neoplasms. N Engl J Med 314:1010–1015, 1986.

114. Spinner RJ, Atkinson JL, Scheithauer BW, et al: Peroneal intraneural ganglia: the importance of the articular branch. Clinical series. J Neurosurg 99:319–329, 2003.

115. Strickland JW, Steichen JB: Nerve tumors of the hand and forearm. J Hand Surg 2:285–291, 1977.

116. Stull M, Moser R, Kransdorf M, et al: Magnetic resonance appearance of peripheral nerve sheath tumors. Skeletal Radiol 20:9–14, 1991.

117. Suh JS, Abenoza P, Galloway HR, et al: Peripheral (extracranial) nerve tumors: correlation of MR imaging and histologic findings. Radiology 183:341–346, 1992.

118. Swain RE Jr, Kingdom TT, DelGaudio JM, et al: Meningiomas of the paranasal sinuses. Am J Rhinol 15:27–30, 2001.

119. Taghian AG, Powell SN: The role of radiation therapy for primary breast cancer. Surg Clin North Am 79:1091–1115, 1999.

120. Takao M, Fukuuchi Y, Koto A, et al: Localized hypertrophic mononeuropathy involving the femoral nerve. Neurology 52:389–392, 1999.

121. Theaker JM, Gatter KC, Puddle J: Epithelial membrane antigen expression by the perineurium of peripheral nerve and in peripheral nerve tumours. Histopathology 13:171–179, 1988.

122. Thompson LD, Gyure KA: Extracranial sinonasal tract meningiomas: a clinicopathologic study of 30 cases with a review of the literature. Am J Surg Pathol 24(5):640–650, 2000.

123. Tiffee JC, Barnes EL: Neuromuscular hamartomas of the head and neck. Arch Otolaryngol Head Neck Surg 124:212–216, 1998.

124. Tindall, SC: Ganglion cysts of peripheral nerves. In Wilkins R, Rengachary E (eds): Neurosurgery. Baltimore, Williams & Wilkins, 1900.

125. Torre V, Bucolo S, Galletti B, et al: Benign extracranial head and neck schwannoma: anatomical, clinical and diagnostic considerations on four cases and a review of the literature. Acta Otorhinolaryngol Ital 19:160–165, 1999.

126. Tsang WY, Chan JK, Chow LT, Tse CC: Perineurioma: an uncommon soft tissue neoplasm distinct from localized hypertrophic neuropathy and neurofibroma. Am J Surg Pathol 16:756–763, 1992.

127. Vance JM: The many faces of Charcot-Marie-Tooth disease. Arch Neurology 57:638–640, 2000.

128. Verstraete KL, Achten E, DeSchepper A, et al: Nerve sheath tumors: evaluation with CT and MR imaging. J Belg Radiol 75:311–320, 1992.

129. Vorster SJ, Lee HL, Ruggieri P: Amyloidoma of the Gasserian ganglion. Am J Neuroradiol 19:1853–1855, 1998.

130. Weiland TL, Scheithauer BW, Rock MG, Sargent JM: Inflammatory pseudotumor of nerve. Am J Surg Pathol 20:1212–1218, 1996.

131. Weiss SW, Goldblum JR: Enzinger and Weiss's Soft Tissue Tumors. St. Louis, Mosby, 2001.

132. Wilson JD, Williams RH: Williams Textbook of Endocrinology. Philadelphia, WB Saunders, 1998.

133. Wittenberg KH, Adkins MC: MR imaging of nontraumatic brachial plexopathies: frequency and spectrum of findings. Radiographics 20:1023–1032, 2000.

134. Woodhall B: Peripheral nerve tumors. Surg Clin North Am 34:1167–1172, 1954.

135. Woodruff JM: The pathology and treatment of peripheral nerve tumors and tumor-like conditions. Cancer 43:290–308, 1993.

136. Woodruff JM: Tumors of peripheral nerves and the nerve sheath. In Montgomery E, Aaron AD (eds): Clinical Pathology of Soft-Tissue Tumors. New York, Marcel Dekker, 2001.

137. Woodruff JM, Godwin TA, Erlandson RA, et al: Cellular schwannoma. A variety of schwannoma sometimes mistaken for a malignant tumor. Am J Surg Pathol 5:733–744, 1981.

138. Woodruff JM, Selig AM, Crowley K, Allen PW: Schwannoma (neurilemoma) with malignant transformation. A rare, distinctive peripheral nerve tumor. Am J Surg Pathol 18:882, 1994.

139. Yan N, Ricca C, Fletcher J, et al: Farnesyltransferase inhibitors block the neurofibromatosis type I (NF1) malignant phenotype. Cancer Res 55:3569–3575, 1995.

140. Young JLJ, Ries LG, Silverberg E, et al: Cancer incidence, survival and mortality for children younger than 15 years. Cancer 58:598, 1986.

CHAPTER **74**

MALIGNANT PERIPHERAL
NERVE TUMORS

Mubarak Al-Gahtany, Rajiv Midha, Abhijit Guha, and W. Bradley Jacobs

Peripheral nerve tumors are rare lesions that can arise anywhere on the body and as a result have a wide differential diagnosis. They commonly occur as a nonspecific mass lesion that is diagnosed as a peripheral nerve tumor at surgery. Although these tumors may initially be seen by a wide variety of surgeons, early recognition of the nature of the lesion and appropriate surgical treatment by a surgeon with expertise in peripheral nerve surgery is essential to minimize postoperative neurologic deficits. Even more rare are the malignant neoplasms of the peripheral nerves, with an incidence of 1 in 10,000 in the general population. This chapter focuses on the latter and aims to provide a classification and a management scheme for malignant peripheral nerve tumors.

NOMENCLATURE AND CLASSIFICATION

The classification scheme of malignant peripheral nerve tumors in this chapter will be based on the World Health Organization (WHO) classification.[52] As defined in the WHO system, malignant peripheral nerve sheath tumors (MPNST) are malignant tumors arising from a peripheral nerve or showing a nerve sheath differentiation, with the exception of tumors originating from epineurium or the peripheral nerve vasculature.

The MPNSTs are subclassified according to the WHO system into several variants.

Epithelioid
MPNST with divergent mesenchymal or epithelial differentiation
Melanotic
Melanotic psammomatous

In addition to their rarity, further confusion and hence uncertainty about the management of malignant peripheral nerve tumors stems from the diagnostic difficulties in differentiating these tumors from the larger group of other soft-tissue sarcomas. This has led to a large number of terms used to describe these tumors. These include *malignant schwannoma, MPNST, malignant neurilemoma,* and *neurofibrosarcoma,* all implying a known cell or structure of origin, which is an unresolved issue. The terms *neurogenic sarcoma* and *MPNST* are the most widely used. In this chapter we will use the term *MPNST* as used in the WHO classification of tumors of the nervous system.[52] Although the name MPNST implies that these tumors arise from the sheath or coverings of peripheral

nerves, this is far from certain, as are the cells of origin, which remain to be definitely defined and may be multiple in nature.

MOLECULAR BIOLOGY

The genetic aberrations, in addition to loss of the neurofibromatosis 1 (NF1) gene protein product (neurofibromin), that lead to malignant transformation of a plexiform neurofibroma to MPNST are as yet unclear. The p53 gene is a candidate, because mutations have been documented in MPNSTs and not in neurofibromas,[14] but other genetic alterations are present, and it is an area of current research. MPNSTs that arise from malignant transformation of a plexiform neurofibroma in an NF1 patient have been speculated in the past to be more aggressive as compared with *de novo* tumors,[13,17,21,36,46] a concept not supported by more recent studies.[26,51] A slightly more detailed discussion of molecular pathogenesis is discussed at the end of this chapter for its relevance to future therapy of MPNST.

PATHOLOGY

The *gross* appearance of an MPNST is that of globoid or fusiform, pseudoencapsulated tumor, which is firm to hard in consistency. It is attached to a large or medium-size nerve and is usually several centimeters in diameter at the time of diagnosis.[52] MPNSTs grow within the nerve fascicles but commonly invade through the epineurium into the adjacent soft tissues. These features explain why it is impossible to obtain gross-total resection without incurring a neurologic deficit and also explain the high recurrence rate after mere removal of the obvious lump, as is commonly done before referring these patients to tertiary care centers.

MPNSTs *microscopically* are highly cellular tumors that characteristically have a fascicular pattern, spindle-shaped nuclei, and scant cytoplasm (Figure 74-1). MPNST can be graded on a I to III scale, based on cellularity, nuclear pleomorphism, anaplasia, mitotic rate (number of mitotic figures in 10 high power fields), microvascular proliferation, and degree of necrosis and invasion.[9,10,13,50] The majority of tumors show geographic necrosis and mitotic activity. In addition, approximately 15% of cases exhibit unusual histologic features, such as epithelioid morphology and divergent differentiation.

Three immunohistochemical markers, S-100, Leu-7, and myelin basic protein, although not diagnostic by themselves

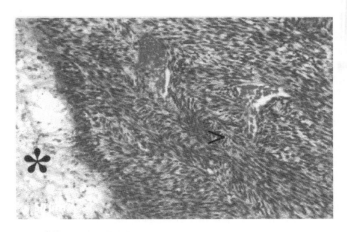

FIGURE 74-1 Histopathological appearance of a typical malignant peripheral nerve sheath tumor with adjacent plexiform neurofibroma (∗), from which it originated. The tumor (>) is hypercellular, with a fascicular pattern and spindle-shaped nuclei. On the basis of its hypercellularity and a moderate mitotic rate, it was classified grade I to II, as per the grading scheme used for soft-tissue sarcomas.

because of a significant false-positive and false-negative rate, are used to further enhance the diagnosis of neurogenic sarcoma.[17,25,53] In addition, electron microscopic examination is often found to be helpful in the pathologic diagnosis. Ultrastructural features suggestive of a neurogenic origin of the tumor recapitulate the features of normal Schwann cells, as does relative lack of ultrastructural features of other sarcomas, such as myofibrils.

In summary, the differentiation of MPNSTs from other soft-tissue sarcomas is often a diagnostic challenge, requiring a review of evidence from several sources by pathologists who are familiar with these rare tumors. This is the main reason, along with the morbidity of oncologic surgery to obtain local control, that we suggest management of these tumors in a staged and comprehensive approach, as outlined later.[3]

CLINICAL PRESENTATION

As a first step, it is crucial to obtain a thorough history (including a family history) with a focal and systemic physical examination, including an inquiry and search for the clinical findings associated with NF, because half of the cases are associated with NF1.[52] Approximately a third of neurogenic sarcomas arise *de novo,* whereas the reminder represent a sarcomatous degeneration of a preexisting plexiform neurofibroma in an NF1 or non-NF1 patient.[52] Only rarely has neurogenic sarcoma been documented to arise from conventional schwannoma, ganglioneuroblastoma or ganglioneuroma, and pheochromocytoma.[52] Hence both NF1 and NF2 can cause MPNST, although MPNST is greatly more prevalent in NF1, where there are pathologic neurofibromas, as compared with the benign schwannomas associated with NF2. The multiple dermal neurofibromas of NF1 patients should be left alone with reassurance that they do not undergo malignant transformations, which also is true for the nonsymptomatic NF2-associated benign schwan-

nomas. It is the deeper and larger plexiform neurofibromas in NF1 patients that must be clinically and radiologically followed for accelerated growth or clinical symptomatology, because they have a 3% to 5% risk of malignant conversion to an MPNST.[47] The risk of a plexiform neurofibroma converting to an MPNST in a non-NF1 patient is slightly less, with an estimated risk of less than 1%. Whether MPNSTs that occur in the setting of NF1 (50% of the cases) differ from those that arise in non-NF1 patients is not known. One would have to speculate that they do not, based on lack of any pathologic differences or similarities in their molecular pathogenesis.[22,23]

MPNST occurs as a growing mass, similar to other soft tissue sarcomas. However, this subgroup has a proportionately higher incidence of associated pain (50%) and neurologic deficits (38%) when compared with sarcoma in general.[3,24] This difference is probably related to the intimate relation of MPNSTs to the peripheral nerves and their invasive nature. Depending on the location, size, and degree of invasion, MPNSTs exhibit clinical features similar to those of benign peripheral nerve sheath tumors. These include pain or sensory deficits along the distribution of a known major nerve, mobility perpendicular to, but not along, the longitudinal axis of a known peripheral nerve, and sensory stimuli (evoked paresthesias or dysesthesias) radiating along the distribution of the nerve of origin elicited upon palpation of an MPNST. Highly invasive and large lesions may become fixed to surrounding compartments and lose their mobility. *Loss of mobility, rapid growth, and the evolution of neurologic deficits (particularly motor loss) are features that favor diagnosis of a malignant over a benign peripheral nerve tumor.* When the lesion involves the spinal canal, it may occur initially with radicular symptoms and then myelopathy as the lesion enlarges and compresses the spinal cord.

MPNSTs usually afflict adults in their third to sixth decade of life; however, the mean age is a decade younger in NF1-associated cases. The medium and large nerves are more likely to be affected than small nerves. The buttock, thigh, brachial plexus, and paraspinal regions are the most common sites. The sciatic nerve is the most commonly affected nerve.[52] No nerve, however, is immune, including, in rare examples, cranial nerves, especially the trigeminal nerve.[7,54]

In patients with NF1, a clinically symptomatic or a rapidly growing neurofibroma must be suspected to have undergone malignant transformation, an event with an incidence rate of 3% to 5%[47] of lesions. If a plexiform neurofibroma has been treated with radiation therapy and subsequently demonstrates rapid growth, malignant transformation must also be strongly considered.[1] Indeed, MPNSTs arising at the site of prior irradiation represent approximately 10% of cases.[16]

Because of the rarity of MPNSTs and a wide differential diagnosis, patients are often referred initially to other surgical disciplines and are then sent to a peripheral nerve unit after biopsy. It is recommended that, if a clinical suspicion of an MPNST is entertained or if the initial biopsy reveals a peripheral nerve tumor, the patient should be referred to a multidisciplinary peripheral nerve unit for optimal definitive management.

PREOPERATIVE TESTS

Nerve conduction and electromyography evaluations are not routinely undertaken in the management of peripheral nerve

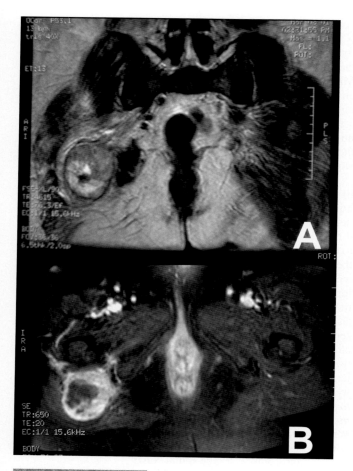

FIGURE 74-2 Coronal T2- *(A)* and T1- *(B)* weighted gadolinium-enhanced magnetic resonance images of a lesion in the right buttock growing rapidly, producing severe neuropathic pain and progressive sciatic neuropathy, in a woman with neurofibromatosis 1. The tumor, which shows regions of signal inhomogeneity and enhancement, is located deep to the gluteal muscle mass adjacent to or involving the sciatic nerve.

tumors. The importance of the history and physical examination is further stressed because of the limitation of radiologic studies to always differentiate between a peripheral nerve tumor and other soft-tissue extremity masses. In addition, computed tomography (CT) or magnetic resonance imaging (MRI) cannot distinguish between the various subtypes of peripheral nerve tumors or reliably determine whether a lesion is benign or malignant.[8,32,48,49] In general, MRI is the most useful and sensitive technique, often but not always revealing the nerve of origin (Figure 74-2). It is especially helpful in determining the relationship of the mass to adjacent anatomic structures that may be of relevance. Occasionally, remodeling of adjacent bone related to the slow progressive growth of the tumor, such as enlargement of neural foramina, can be better visualized on plain x-ray studies or CT scans, but MRI has become the investigation of choice. Ultrasound evaluation, because of its high degree of sensitivity, has an emerging role, but is still less often used.

The principal differential diagnoses of MPNST on imaging are soft tissue sarcoma, neurofibroma, and schwannoma. The rare lipomas and ganglion cysts that can mimic a peripheral nerve tumor are quite readily distinguished by their signal characteristics and association with a joint capsule, respectively, on MRI (see Chapter 73).

Whether a peripheral nerve tumor is a benign lesion or an MPNST cannot be definitely determined based on MRI or CT scan characteristics.[8,32,48,49] A positive gallium scan was reported in one small series to be specific for these tumors, but follow-up studies involving larger numbers of cases are not available.[32] Recent studies show positron-emission tomography (PET), particularly quantitative PET (high standard uptake values), appears to be a promising modality in distinguishing a region of sarcoma evolution in neurofibromas in the NF1 population.[20] Regions of nonhomogeneous enhancement on CT or MRI, suggesting intratumoral necrosis or hemorrhage, may indicate a malignant aggressive neurogenic sarcoma, but such regions are also found in (especially larger) benign schwannomas and neurofibromas and in atypical (but not malignant) schwannomas. The suggestion of a malignant tumor originating from a peripheral nerve (MPNST) or secondary involvement of a nerve from an underlying primary neoplasm (e.g., Pancoast's tumor) comes from the history and general physical examination supported by other tests, such as chest x-ray (CXR) studies and CT. Rapid growth clinically or on follow-up MRI, increasing neurologic symptoms, or preexisting NF1 with a plexiform neurofibroma should lead to consideration of an MPNST. The evaluation for metastasis, which may include baseline blood tests, including liver function tests, CXR studies, and a bone scan with or without CT scans of the chest and abdomen, is important in the management of and less so for the diagnosis of MPNST. Because a majority of MPNSTs metastasize to the lungs, similar to other soft-tissue sarcomas, a CXR study, supplemented by CT of the chest if there are any suspicious lesions, is warranted in all cases. If a suspect lesion is identified in the lung, a needle biopsy should be performed to determine if metastasis has already occurred, because this will be a major factor toward determining the aggressiveness to be used in managing the primary tumor site. Of course, the presence of metastasis will be a major negative determinant of prognosis and requires the use of adjuvant irradiation and chemotherapy from the beginning. If a metastasis is identified in the chest or is suspected elsewhere from the general physical examination, further screening for metastasis with CT or MRI of the abdomen should be undertaken.

MANAGEMENT

MPNSTs are rare tumors that remain incurable, mainly because of their high metastatic potential, and are managed by several surgical disciplines, including plastic, orthopedic, and neurosurgery, depending on local interest and expertise. The rarity of MPNSTs usually renders them to be managed according to clinical protocols used for the much more common soft-tissue sarcomas (STSs), of which MPNSTs constitute between 3% and 10%.[11,17,26,42] Whether these protocols are the most appropriate for MPNST remains uncertain; their low incidence precludes adequate data regarding their optimal management by a single center. The hypothesis that MPNSTs are not the same as other STSs both clinically and on a molecular basis is most clearly supported by the fact that 50% of all MPNSTs occur in the context of the germline cancer predisposition syndrome NF1. As previously discussed, patients with NF1 have a 3% to 5% risk of conversion of the larger proximal plexiform neurofibromas to an MPNST,[42] a risk to remember in the long-term management of these patients whose condition represents the most common cancer predisposition syndrome in humans. The molecular pathogeneses of sporadic and NF1-associated MPNSTs are probably similar and have become more clearly defined as we have deciphered the NF1 gene, its protein product (neurofibromin), and its function.[18,19,22] However, the molecular aberrations in MPNSTs are not shared by other STSs, and hence one would predict that the response of MPNST to therapies being investigated for STS may differ. In addition, the presence of germline defects in NF1 patients with MPNST may render them more susceptible to secondary tumors induced by radiation and chemotherapy, both widely used clinically in the management of STS. This potential risk, although not clinically verified because of the rarity of MPNST, has been demonstrated in mouse models of NF1.[18,19,22]

Although the foregoing discussion brings out potential differences between MPNST and STS, the reality remains that this rare tumor is ideally managed by a multidisciplinary team, with much of the management strategy borrowed from the literature dealing with STS. The management of MPNSTs that we adopt is summarized in Table 74-1. It involves local staging by means of CT or MRI, followed by biopsy and referral to a tertiary care center, then pathologic grading and metastatic survey. At that point, the case is discussed in a multidisciplinary conference leading to local treatment with wide resection (with the goal of obtaining negative margins) and possibly adjuvant radiation therapy. The patient will then be followed up at close intervals with both clinical and radiologic surveillance, looking for evidence of local recurrence or distant dissemination.[3] Before oncologic surgery, whose goals are to obtain negative tumor margins and provide the best chance for local control, a further metastatic survey including a CT or MRI scan of the chest is undertaken.

For patients with metastasis, palliative irradiation locally and to systemic metastasis combined with chemotherapy and occasionally surgery are the usual course, though with limited long-term control. Most patients, however, do not have metastasis at diagnosis, and in these cases the aim of surgery is wide oncologic resection with negative tumor margins to obtain local tumor control. Sarcomatous cells are found to spread extensively within the fascial planes,[44] resulting in high recurrence rates and ultimately systemic spread after simple excision of the tumor alone. This has led to the adoption of aggressive oncologic surgery in an attempt to maintain local control if the preoperative metastatic evaluation is negative. Historically, such surgery involved limb amputation and disarticulation; however, our center and others have found wide oncologic resections incorporating not only the tumor but also adjacent fascial and muscle planes in conjunction with neoadjuvant or adjuvant irradiation or chemotherapy to achieve the same goals without necessitating sacrifice of the limb.[38,43]

When dealing with a suspected case of MPNST, we recommend that multiple biopsies using an *open* approach should be undertaken from electrically silent areas upon electrical stimulation of the tumor (Figure 74-3). This approach is preferred over the blind needle biopsy, which sometimes leaves the patient with neuropathic pain and often does not provide an adequate and representative sample to make the diagnosis of MPNST, with the grave consequences of making an incorrect diagnosis. In the open approach, once the quick-section results are consistent with or suggestive of MPNST, the wound should be closed, without further manipulation of the tumor and without disrupting the tissue planes, to await the final expert pathologic interpretation of the diagnosis based on the permanent sections. Once the final pathology is available, the patient should be managed as outlined previously by a multidisciplinary team in a tertiary care center.

Intraoperative Evaluation and Techniques

Common intraoperative principles that are applicable to the management of all peripheral nerve tumors apply to MPNST (see Chapter 73).

The surgery should be undertaken without paralysis to allow intraoperative electrophysiologic evaluation.

The limb should be positioned and draped widely to allow anatomic accessibility and evaluation of the distal muscles that are supplied by the nerve of origin.

The surgical exposure should extend proximally and distally to allow adequate exposure of both poles of the tumor and course in a curvilinear fashion over flexor or extensor creases.

Intraoperative electrophysiologic assessment should be done that includes nerve action potentials (NAPs) and direct bipolar stimulation to identify bypassing noninvolved fascicles on the tumor capsule.

TABLE 74-1

Management Scheme for Suspected MPNST Used by the University of Toronto Multidisciplinary Sarcoma Group

Suspected MPNST
(history/examination)
↓
Local staging: CT/MRI; chest
x-ray study
↓
Referral to tertiary care center
↓
Multiple open biopsies
Definitive staging and → **Metastasis:**
pathologic grading
↓   Palliative measures:
                           • Tumor debulking
                           • Radiation therapy
                           • Chemotherapy
Multidisciplinary case conference
↓   ↓
Local wide resection including   Follow up:
fascial planes   →   Local and systemic
(Goal: negative margins)
± Preoperative or postoperative
adjuvant local radiation therapy

CT, Computed tomography; MPNST, malignant peripheral nerve sheath tumor; MRI, magnetic resonance imaging.

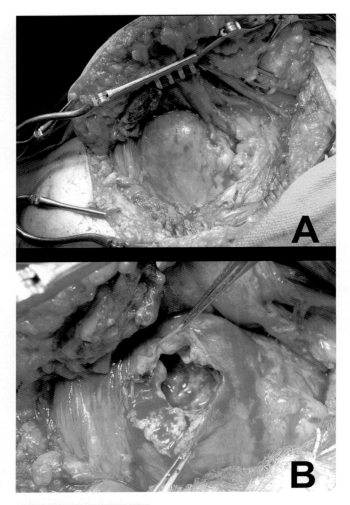

FIGURE 74-3 Operative photomicrographs showing open exposure (A) and evacuation of the internal cystic contents and intratumoral biopsy (B) of the sciatic nerve lesion illustrated in Figure 74-2. A quick-section diagnosis of neurogenic sarcoma was confirmed postoperatively and the patient was referred for definitive surgical management, as per the protocol outlined in the text and Table 74-1.

Magnification and microneurosurgical instruments are required. Ultrasonic aspiration is sometimes required to internally debulk large peripheral nerve tumors, facilitating subsequent dissection of the passing fascicles from the tumor capsule.

A quick section interpreted by an experienced pathologist should be undertaken early on to facilitate subsequent management decisions.

The proximal and distal segments of the nerve of origin are isolated, dissected from adjacent vascular and soft-tissue structures, and encircled in vessel loops. Dissection of the tumor capsule from the passing fascicles is initiated with microneurosurgical techniques. Some of the gross features of the MPNST are circumferential encasement of the whole nerve, adhesion to surrounding tissues, and areas of necrosis. The pathology in conjunction with the gross and microscopic observations will determine the extent of resection. Often it is not feasible to

reconstruct the nerve of origin of these invasive tumors after massive oncologic surgery, whose aim is to achieve tumor-free margins. However, in certain circumstances (e.g., a small tumor with tumor-free margins and a small resection gap), the nerve can be reconstructed with nerve grafting.

Because of the significant morbidity and overall poor prognosis of MPNST, one of the most crucial steps in the intraoperative management of these patients is the process of making the correct pathologic diagnosis. An STS at our center is denoted to be of neurogenic origin (an MPNST) if it fulfills one the following criteria: (1) macro or micro association with a peripheral nerve, (2) malignant transformation of a preexisting neurofibroma, or (3) immunohistochemical or ultrastructural features consistent with a peripheral nerve origin. Even with these criteria, the diagnosis is often problematic because there is significant overlap among STSs and MPNSTs in terms of association with a peripheral nerve, only a certain proportion of MPNSTs arise from a preexisting neurofibroma, and there is a lack of peripheral nerve antigenic markers in a significant proportion of MPNSTs. Therefore, in addition to the pathology assessment, the association of the sarcoma with a peripheral nerve is made on the basis of the clinical presentation (motor or sensory symptoms), preoperative gadolinium-enhanced MRI scans that demonstrate a nerve of origin and exit, and the observations of the surgeon during operation.

Management Outcome

Despite the previously mentioned management plan, the optimal management of MPNSTs remains unclear because of their small numbers and varied management schemes, which account for a lack of proper randomized prospective clinical trials with a sufficient number of patients.* The need to refer cases to tertiary care centers with proper expertise, before undertaking any major surgery or adjuvant therapy, cannot be overemphasized. Resection of only the tumor with irradiation to the tumor bed and adjacent soft tissues is inadequate, with at least a 50% incidence of early local recurrence. Systemic spread, especially with pulmonary metastasis, remains the main obstacle and the ultimate cause of death for patients with MPNSTs and other STSs. The role of additional chemotherapy after surgery and preoperative or postoperative irradiation has not proved useful in decreasing the incidence of distant metastasis or improving survival.[6,17,26,46] The arguments for preoperative irradiation is that it would allow better success in obtaining tumor-free margins and perhaps be more effective in killing the tumor cells because of the undisturbed vascularity. The arguments against preoperative irradiation are mainly related to the effects of radiation on wound healing, a serious issue because of the amount of soft-tissue removal in undertaking the *en bloc* compartmental resections. The preliminary results from a randomized multicenter study initiated by our institute suggests that no clear difference exists as to the timing of radiation therapy, and hence, in most instances, postoperative irradiation is undertaken. The usual radiation therapy protocol is 5000 to 6000 cGy applied in 25 fractions spread over 5 weeks. Because of potential of longitudinal spread, 5- to 7-cm margins on both the proximal and distal ends of the tumor are irradiated.

*References 6, 15, 17, 26–28, 30, 31, 33, 35, 40, 41, 46.

Several studies have evaluated patients with STSs and have attempted to identify clinical features or management strategies that affect patient's outcome.[5,11,24,37,42,45] In these studies large tumors, high tumor grade, surgical margins with residual tumor, and histologic subtype (specifically, neurogenic sarcomas) figure prominently as adverse prognostic features. In a study recently completed at our sarcoma center, all these features were also important prognosticators of the cohort of patients with MPNSTs.[3] Of note, the overall survival rate in our patient population was 64% at 5 years, with only an estimated 30% likely to be disease free at 5 years. This is in contrast to the 72% to 78% 5- to 12-year survival in the overall STS studies[5,24,37] and supports the suggestion that MPNSTs as a subgroup have a relatively worse prognosis.[24] Some studies have shown that patients with MPNSTs and NF have a 5-year survival rate of 16%, significantly worse than the 53% survival rate in non–NF-linked patients.[17,47] This, however, is not supported by more recent studies.[26,51]

Palliative irradiation locally and to the systemic metastases combined with chemotherapy and occasionally surgery are all undertaken, without clear-cut proved benefits. Like all STSs, MPNSTs are notoriously chemoresistant. There are some data suggesting that surgical resection of pulmonary metastasis may improve the long-term prognosis and quality of life in patients with STS (23% survival in the surgical group as compared with 2% in the nonsurgical at 3-year follow up[24]), and this has also been applied to some of our MPNST patients, with mixed results. However, the long-term success for the patients with systemic metastasis remains very guarded.

FUTURE THERAPY

The increased knowledge of the molecular pathogenesis of NF1 and non–NF1-associated MPNSTs has led to biologic therapeutics with the potential of improving the treatment of these currently incurable tumors. Similar to other syndromes associated with a germline loss of a tumor-suppressor gene, loss of neurofibromin (the gene product of the NF1 gene) occurs both in sporadic and NF1-associated plexiform neurofibromas. Neurofibromin is one of the main negative regulators of a key intracellular signal transduction pathway mediated by activation of Ras-GTP. This key pathway, which transmits mitogenic signals from a variety of growth factors, is converted to its inactive Ras-GDP bound state by neurofibromin. Absence of neurofibromin, located on chromosome 17q11.2, would result in increased levels of activated Ras-GTP, causing uncontrolled mitogenic signals to be sent to the nucleus, resulting in increased cellular proliferation.[22,23] All patients with NF1 possess a germline mutation (i.e., in all body cells) of one NF1 gene copy, with mutation or loss of the second normal allele resulting in total loss of neurofibromin and subsequent development of benign tumors such as neurofibromas, as simplistically postulated by the two-hit hypothesis of Knudson. It is likely that subsequent mutations in other genes, such as p53, are responsible for transformation of a benign neurofibroma to a malignant MPNST.[14] Understanding and subsequently rectifying these aberrant intracellular growth-promoting pathways are of interest in developing novel biologic therapeutics. One such family of agents, which has received much attention in oncology, targets the posttranslational modification of Ras, allowing for its activation, and is called *farnesyl transferase inhibitors (FTIs)*. FTIs have demonstrated efficacy in reducing growth of human MPNST in animal models, with clinical trials currently in the planning stage. Other biologic therapeutics target nonspecific aspects of tumor biology, such as tumor angiogenesis, a crucial requirement for the growth of all human solid tumors, including MPNST. Work from our laboratory on xenograft models of MPNST derived from operative specimens demonstrates marked growth reduction, with inhibition of the key angiogenic growth factor, vascular endothelial growth factor (VEGF).[4] Early clinical trials on STS with these agents, with potential application to MPNST, are promising as an adjunct to surgical and radiation therapy. These agents are the prime modalities of current treatment. It is hoped that such research will yield novel therapies with acceptable morbidity to aid in our management of MPNST in the future.

SUMMARY

MPNSTs are rare and lethal tumors that arise in the context of NF1 in nearly half of patients. Diagnosis requires a high level of initial suspicion. Rapid clinical progression, tumor growth, or heterogeneous contrast enhancement on imaging studies oblige the clinician to entertain the diagnosis of neurogenic sarcoma and embark on an appropriate management scheme. These tumors may arise *de novo* but often become manifest after sarcomatous degeneration of large plexiform neurofibromas. In contrast, their benign dermal counterparts do not pose a risk of malignant conversion. Open tumor biopsy and pathologic confirmation is required in all cases. If evidence of neurogenic sarcoma is obtained at quick-section, the incision should be closed immediately without any further attempts at tumor resection. We strongly encourage assessment of the histologic sections by an experienced pathologist and immediate referral to a multidisciplinary team consisting of surgeons, oncologists, and allied health professionals at a tertiary care center with expertise in the treatment of STSs. Definitive management will include a search for overt metastatic disease and wide oncologic resection, if indicated, coupled with radiation therapy and perhaps chemotherapy. Several prognostic factors have been identified and include tumor size, tumor grade, and the ability of the surgeon to obtain *en bloc* resection. Unfortunately, the overall prognosis for neurogenic sarcomas remains poor, with only 30% of patients disease free at 5 years.

SECONDARY MALIGNANT NON-NEURAL TUMORS

Peripheral nerves may be secondarily compressed by adjacent tumors or their metastasis to lymph nodes. Rarely, there may be direct longitudinal invasion of epineurium of the nerve by a carcinoma or sarcoma, resulting in pain or neurologic symptoms. Furthermore, there are a few reports of isolated primary neurolymphomatosis.[39] Pulmonary or breast carcinomas are the most common secondary tumors to involve the brachial plexus.[12,28–30,34] In women, breast carcinomas, either directly or by involvement of the lymphatics, should be suspected with an infraclavicular brachial plexopathy. A relatively common scenario is someone with brachial plexus pain and progressive neurologic deterioration, with a history of breast cancer and adjuvant irradiation after a long latency. The differential diagnosis of the brachial plexopathy is recurrence of the breast cancer, either as an extrinsic mass or intraneural invasion, postradiation therapy plexopathy with disruption of the extraneural and intraneural microvasculature, or a combination of both. Preoperative MRI scans are sometimes helpful in demonstrating a discrete tumor recurrence but often are not diagnostic. Another well-recognized clinical entity is Pancoast's syndrome, resulting from apical lung tumors involving the lower roots and trunks of the brachial plexus. If surgery for the lung tumor is indicated, a combined neurosurgical and thoracic surgical procedure is sometimes warranted.

Peripheral nerve (i.e., brachial plexus) surgery is warranted to make a diagnosis, if the diagnosis has not been determined, and is also warranted for treating secondary malignancies as well as intractable pain or rapidly worsening neurologic deficts that are unresponsive to radiation therapy or chemotherapy. Diagnostic indications include surgery to differentiate tumor recurrence versus radiation neuropathy, or both, as previously described.[31] In radiation plexopathy, the nerves are prone to infarction because of the already compromised microvasculature; hence they should be handled gently, and a full circumferential epineurolysis is not undertaken. This limited external neurolysis may result in good pain relief, though there may not be any return of neurologic function.[2,28,30,31,34]

References

1. Abboud HE, Dunn MJ, Newbould MJ: Post-radiation malignant peripheral nerve sheath tumour: a report of two cases. Kidney Int 38:232–239, 1990.
2. Ampil F: Radiotherapy for carcinomatous brachial plexopathy. A clinical study of 23 cases. Cancer 56:2185–2188, 1985.
3. Angelov L, Davis A, O'Sullivan B, et al: Neurogenic sarcomas: experience at the University of Toronto. Neurosurgery 43(1): 56–64; discussion 64–65, 1998.
4. Angelov L, Salhia B, Roncari L, Guha A: Inhibition of angiogenesis by blocking activation of the vascular endothelial growth factor receptor 2 leads to decreased growth of neurogenic sarcomas. Cancer Res 59:5536–5541, 1999.
5. Antman K, Corson JM, Eberlein TJ, Singer S: Prognostic factors predictive of survival and local recurrence for extremity soft tissue sarcoma. [See comments.] Archives of Surgery 127(5):548–553; discussion 553–554, 1992.
6. Basso-Ricci S: Therapy of malignant schwannomas: usefulness of an integrated radiologic. Surgical therapy. J Neurosurg Sci 33:253–257, 1989.
7. Best P: Malignant triton tumour in the cerebellopontine angle. Report of a case. Acta Neuropathol (Berl) 74:92–96, 1987.
8. Cerofolini E, Landi A, DeSantis G, et al: MR of benign peripheral nerve sheath tumors. J Comput Assist Tomog 15:593–597, 1991.
9. Chinoy RF, Ganesh B, Parikh DM, Trojanowski JQ: Malignant tumors of nerve sheath origin. J Surg Oncol Suppl 55:100–103, 1994.
10. Chinoy RF, Ganesh B, Parikh DM, Vege DS: Malignant peripheral nerve sheath tumors of the head and neck: a clinicopathological study. J Surg Oncol Suppl 55:100–103, 1994.
11. Collin C, Godbold J, Hajdu S, Brennan M: Localized extremity soft tissue sarcoma: an analysis of factors affecting survival. J Clin Oncol 5:601–612, 1987.
12. Croft PB, Wilkinson M: The incidence of carcinomatous neuromyopathy in patients with various types of carcinoma. Neurol Clin 9:857–866, 1991.
13. D'Agostino AN, Soule EH, Miller RH: Sarcomas of the peripheral nerves and somatic soft tissues associated with multiple neurofibromatosis (von Recklinghausen's disease). Cancer 16: 1015–1027, 1963.
14. Dams E, Dierick WS, Legius E: TP53 mutations are frequent in malignant NF1 tumors. Biochim Biophys Acta 1223:296–305, 1994.
15. DasGupta T: Tumors of the peripheral nerves. Clin Neurosurg 25:574–590, 1977.
16. Ducatman B, Scheithauer B: Postirradiation neurofibrosarcoma. Cancer 51:1028–1033, 1983.
17. Ducatman BS, Scheithauer BW, Piepgras DG, et al: Malignant peripheral nerve sheath tumors. A clinicopathologic study of 120 cases. Cancer 57:2006–2021, 1986.
18. Feldkamp M, Angelov L, Guha A: Neurofibromatosis type 1 peripheral nerve tumors: aberrant activation of the Ras pathway. Surg Neurol X51:211–218, 1983.
19. Feldkamp MM, Lau N, Provias JP, et al: Acute presentation of a neurogenic sarcoma in a patient with neurofibromatosis type 1: a pathological and molecular explanation. Case report. J Neurosurg 84:867–873, 1996.
20. Ferner RE, Lucas JD, O'Doherty MJ, et al: Evaluation of (18)fluorodeoxyglucose positron emission tomography ((18)FDG PET) in the detection of malignant peripheral nerve sheath tumours arising from within plexiform neurofibromas in neurofibromatosis 1. J Neurol Neurosurg Psychiatr 68:353–357, 2000.
21. Ghosh BC, Ghosh L, Huvos AG, Fortner JG: Malignant schwannoma. A clinicopathologic study. Cancer 31:184–190, 1973.
22. Guha A: The Royal College Medal in Surgery Lecture-1997: The Role of Ras Activation in Human Nervous System Tumors. Canadian J Neurol Sci 25:267–281, 1998.
23. Guha A, Lau N, Huvar I, et al: Ras-GTP Levels are elevated in human NF1 peripheral nerve tumors. Oncogene Z12:507–513, 1986.
24. Harrison LB, Leung DH, Woodruff JM, et al: Analysis of prognostic factors in 1,041 patients with localized soft tissue sarcomas of the extremities. J Clin Oncol 14:859–868, 1996.
25. Hirose T, Hasegawa T, Kudo E, et al: Malignant peripheral nerve sheath tumors: an immunohistochemical study in relation to ultrastructural features. Human Pathol 23:865–870, 1992.
26. Hruban RH, Shiu MH, Senie RT, Woodruff JM: Malignant peripheral nerve sheath tumors of the buttock and lower extremity. A study of 43 cases. Cancer 66:1253–1265, 1990.
27. Hudson A, Gentili F, Kline D: Peripheral nerve tumors. In Schmidek H, Sweet W (eds): Operative Neurosurgical Techniques. New York, Grune & Stratton, 1988.
28. Hudson A, Kline D: Peripheral nerve tumors. In Schmidek H, Sweet W (eds): Operative Neurosurgical Techniques. New York, Grune & Stratton, 1994.
29. Jaeckle KA: Nerve plexus metastases. Neurol Clin 9:857–866, 1991.
30. Kline D, Hudson A: Operative Results of Major Nerve Injuries, Entrapments and Tumors. Philadelphia, WB Saunders, 1994.
31. Lederman RJ, Wilbourn AJ: Brachial plexopathy: recurrent cancer or radiation? Neurology 34:1331–1335, 1984.
32. Levine E, Huntrakoon M, Wetzel LH: Malignant nerve-sheath neoplasms in neurofibromatosis: distinction from benign tumors by using imaging techniques. Human Pathol 18:1212–1217, 1987.
33. Louis DS, White HR, Jr: Survival in malignant schwannoma. An 18-year study. J Hand Surg American Volume 16:873–876, 1991.
34. Lusk MD, Kline DG, Garcia CA: Tumors of the brachial plexus. Neurosurgery 21:439–453, 1987.

35. Meis J, Enzinger F, Martz K: Malignant peripheral nerve sheath tumors (malignant schwannomas) in children. Am J Surg Pathol 16:694–707, 1992.

36. Nambisan RN, Rao U, Moore R, Karakousis CP: Malignant soft tissue tumors of nerve sheath origin. J Surg Oncol Suppl 25:268–272, 1984.

37. O'Sullivan B, Catton C, Bell R, et al: Outcome and prognostic factors in soft tissue sarcoma in the adult. Int J Radiat Oncol Biol Phys 27:1091–1099, 1993.

38. O'Sullivan B, Liu FF, Powell J, et al: The surgical margin in soft tissue sarcoma. J Bone Joint Surg 71:370–375, 1989.

39. Pillay PK, Hardy RW, Jr, Wilbourn AJ, et al: Solitary primary lymphoma of the sciatic nerve: case report. Neurosurgery 23:370–371, 1988.

40. Rogalski RP, Louis DS: Neurofibrosarcomas of the upper extremity. J Hand Surg American Volume 16:873–876, 1991.

41. Rosenberg A, Dick H, Botte M: Nerve tumors. In Gilberman R (ed): Operative Nerve Repair and Reconstruction. Philadelphia, JB Lippincott, 1991.

42. Russell WO, Cohen J, Enzinger F, et al: A clinical and pathological staging system for soft tissue sarcomas. Cancer 40:1562–1570, 1977.

43. Sadoski C, Suit HD, Rosenberg A, et al: Preoperative radiation, surgical margins, and local control of extremity sarcomas of soft tissues. J Surg Oncol Suppl 52:223–230, 1993.

44. Simon MA, Enneking WF: The management of soft-tissue sarcomas of the extremities. J Bone Joint Surg 58:317–327, 1976.

45. Sivaraja M, Souza K, Millis K, et al: Staging of soft-tissue sarcomas. Prognostic analysis of clinical and pathological features. J Clin Invest 98:244–250, 1996.

46. Sordillo PP, Helson L, Hajdu SI, et al: Malignant schwannoma: clinical characteristics, survival, and response to therapy. Cancer 47:2503–2509, 1981.

47. Sorensen S, Mulvhill J, Nielsen A: Longterm followup of von Recklinghausen neurofibromatosis. Survival and malignant neoplasms. N Engl J Med 314:1010–1015, 1986.

48. Stull MA, Moser RP, Jr, Kransdorf MJ, et al: Magnetic resonance appearance of peripheral nerve sheath tumors. Skeletal Radiol 20:9–14, 1991.

49. Suh JS, Abenoza P, Galloway HR, et al: Peripheral (extracranial) nerve tumors: correlation of MR imaging and histologic findings. Radiology 183:341–346, 1992.

50. Suit HD: Staging systems for sarcoma of soft tissue and sarcoma of bone. Cancer Treat Symp 23:29–36, 1984.

51. Vauthey JN, Woodruff JM, Brennan MF: Extremity malignant peripheral nerve sheath tumors (neurogenic sarcomas): a 10-year experience. Ann Surg Oncol 2:126–131, 1995.

52. WHO: Pathology and Genetics of Tumours of the Nervous System. Lyon, France, IARC press, 2000.

53. Wick MR, Swanson PE, Scheithauer BW, Manivel JC: Malignant peripheral nerve sheath tumor. An immunohistochemical study of 62 cases. Am J Clin Pathol 87:425–433, 1987.

54. Yamashiro S, Nagahiro S, Mimata C, et al: Malignant trigeminal schwannoma associated with xeroderma pigmentosum: case report. Neurol Med Chir Tokyo 34:817–820, 1994.

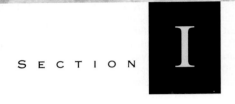
SUPRATENTORIAL LOW-GRADE GLIOMAS

Sheila K. Singh and Peter B. Dirks

Glial neoplasms in children account for up to 60% of supratentorial hemispheric tumors, with an annual incidence of five cases per million children.[14] They encompass a diverse range of pathology, including pilocytic and fibrillary astrocytomas, ependymomas, oligodendrogliomas, and gangliogliomas, as well as less common lesions unique to the pediatric age group: pleomorphic xanthoastrocytoma (PXA), dysembryoplastic neuroepithelial tumor (DNET), and desmoplastic infantile ganglioglioma (DIG). Their histologic distribution and prognostic features differ from that of adults, because the majority of these tumors in children are low grade (up to 80% of supratentorial tumors), and a strong association exists between extent of surgical resection and patient outcome.[14] Many supratentorial gliomas are also found deep, near midline structures as opposed to a more common lobar location in adults. Radiologically, pediatric low-grade gliomas also differ in that they are often enhanced with contrast, and this enhancement does not suggest that these neoplasms are malignant. Also, in contrast to adults, anatomic location favors the infratentorial compartment (posterior fossa and brainstem) in 60% to 70% of childhood gliomas, especially in the mid to latter part of the first decade of life.

In the supratentorial compartment, low-grade gliomas in children can occur in the hemisphere but also typically arise from the optic nerve, chiasm, and visual pathways, as well as deep seated in the hypothalamus, thalamus, and basal ganglia. In this chapter, we review the epidemiology, diagnosis, and management options for supratentorial low-grade gliomas in children, classified by pathologic subtype and location.

ASTROCYTOMAS

The pathologic definition of low-grade astrocytomas has been simplified by the Daumas-Duport classification,[2] which grades astrocytic tumors based on the presence of a limited number of histologic features: nuclear atypia, endothelial proliferation, and mitoses. Pilocytic astrocytomas are grade I lesions that possess none of these histologic features; they are characterized by their biphasic nature, consisting of regions of compact bipolar astrocytes alternating with microcystic regions containing eosinophilic granular bodies. Low-grade fibrillary astrocytomas typically possess one of the Daumas-Duport criteria (usually nuclear atypia) and are thus classified as grade II lesions. In a series of 1038 biopsy specimens of childhood tumors, pilocytic and grade II fibrillary astrocytomas each represented approximately one third of all gliomas (32.3% and 31.3%, respectively), with malignant gliomas occurring in a lesser number of cases (13.6%).[15] Astrocytomas are the most common childhood tumors, and although defined by cell of origin, their clinical features can be best discussed when also classified by site of tumor origin.

HEMISPHERIC ASTROCYTOMAS

Astrocytomas account for approximately 50% of hemispheric tumors in children, occurring at all ages, with a peak incidence between ages 8 and 12. There is no sex predilection, and in contrast to astrocytomas in adults, no clear genetic abnormality (such as p53 mutations) has been consistently identified in pediatric low-grade gliomas.[13] These tumors are often slow growing and may grow indolently, with an insidious onset of symptoms over a period of months or years, or may even be found incidentally. The most common clinical presentation consists of seizures and focal neurologic deficits, such as hemiparesis, hemisensory loss, or aphasia, depending on lesion location. Cortical and subcortical lesions may occur, and focal neurologic deficits often occur with deep white matter, thalamic, or basal ganglia tumors that may become quite large before symptoms manifest. In these cases, children may also have signs of long-standing raised intracranial pressure, such as papilledema. Neuroimaging typically shows a low-density lesion on noncontrast computed tomography (CT) scans that is often intensely enhanced and often cystic; magnetic resonance imaging (MRI) permits better visualization of these lesions, with a typical pattern of low T1 signal and high T2 signal, allowing tumors to be detected earlier, at less symptomatic stages.[13] Deep white matter lesions often show dense contrast enhancement on neuroimaging, but unlike in adults, this finding does not portend malignant transformation, and these tumors are often benign. An example of a lobar low-grade astrocytoma is shown in Figure 75-1.

Also in contrast to adult glial neoplasms, gross-total surgical excision provides a great prognostic advantage for childhood astrocytomas, resulting in a probable cure rate and long-term disease-free survival of greater than 80%.[12] Although gross-total resection is not always possible with deeper lesions, maximal safe surgical resection is the mainstay of therapy for hemispheric gliomas. Perioperative anticonvulsants are often used, and stereotactic guidance systems for tumors in deep or eloquent cortex, electrocorticography for identifying epileptogenic cortex adjacent to the tumor, and cortical mapping for tumors in speech and motor areas provide useful surgical adjuncts. Intraoperative use of ultrasound can also be very useful in localizing the lesion, determining location of any associated cysts, and monitoring extent of resection as the lesion is removed, because the margin is often clearly demarcated from surrounding brain. Adjuvant therapy for low-grade gliomas remains controversial, although conventional radiation remains an option for older children with recurrent or unresectable disease.[5] Small residual tumors after radical resection

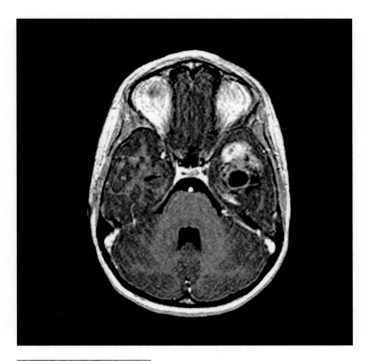

FIGURE 75-1 Axial contrast-enhanced magnetic resonance imaging demonstrates cystic and solid enhancing low-grade astrocytoma in the temporal lobe.

are often observed with serial imaging, because malignant transformation is almost unheard of in the absence of radiation treatment. Adjuvant therapy is therefore often reserved for tumor progression. Repeat surgery is also an important consideration for a local recurrence. Chemotherapy protocols typically using vincristine and carboplatin have been effective in halting disease progression in children with recurrent low-grade gliomas, especially in children with deep diencephalic tumors, but there are no universally accepted criteria for which patient gets chemotherapy and for the drug regimen.[9] Chemotherapy's main use has been in very young children to attempt to halt tumor progression in hopes of delaying radiation until a child is older. The prognosis for children with pilocytic astrocytomas is better than those with fibrillary tumors.

OPTIC PATHWAY GLIOMAS

Optic pathway gliomas represent less than 1% of all brain tumors, but because three quarters of these tumors occur in the first decade of life, they represent 4% to 6% of all brain tumors seen at major pediatric hospitals.[6] Most of these tumors occur within the first 5 years of life. They can arise anywhere from the retroorbital space, along the optic nerve, to the chiasm and hypothalamus, infiltrating these structures diffusely, and then occasionally also spreading along visual pathways posteriorly. Tumors that are confined to the optic nerve are called *optic nerve gliomas,* globular tumors involving the chiasm and hypothalamus are called *chiasmatic-hypothalamic gliomas,* and those involving multiple components of the pathway (particularly in neurofibromatosis type 1 [NF1] patients) are called *diffuse optic pathway tumors.* Collectively, these tumors are known as *optic pathway gliomas.* Although these tumors are of low-grade histology, they can have a very variable natural history based on location and patient age. Optic nerve tumors tend to be more indolent, but large chiasmatic-hypothalamic tumors when occurring in infants and very young children can be very aggressive. Despite their low-grade histology, chiasmatic tumors have a rare but recognized propensity to disseminate through cerebrospinal fluid (CSF) pathways. Optic pathway tumors are strongly associated with NF1, and the presence of an optic nerve glioma fulfills one of this disorder's six diagnostic criteria.[6]

Children with optic pathway tumors have visual loss and optic atrophy on funduscopic examination. Visual loss can be extremely difficult to detect in infants; pendular nystagmus or a squint are important clinical clues. Clinical findings reflect the anatomic pattern of tumor growth or infiltration. Optic nerve gliomas also cause proptosis and loss of extraocular movements. Large chiasmatic-hypothalamic tumors extending into the third ventricle may cause obstructive hydrocephalus resulting in macrocephaly and failure to thrive in infants. There may be appetite or sleep disturbances. Diencephalic syndrome occurring in young infants is characterized by cachexia and hyperactivity. Seizures or hemiparesis may also occur. Precocious puberty occasionally occurs, and diabetes insipidus is rare.

Diagnostic investigations include neuro-ophthalmologic and neuroendocrine assessment and MRI of the brain. Neuroimaging (Figure 75-2) typically shows fusiform enlargement of the optic nerve when this structure is involved. An optic nerve glioma can grow outside the nerve proper and encircle it

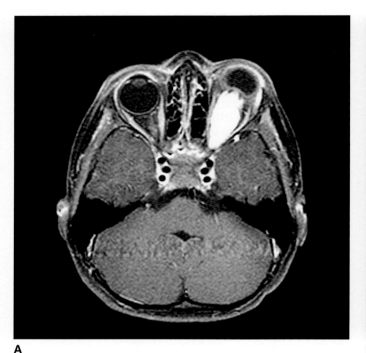

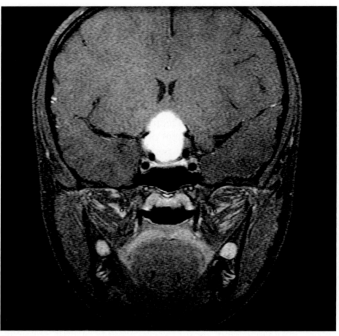

A   B

FIGURE 75-2   *A,* Axial T1 magnetic resonance imaging (MRI) with contrast agent demonstrates left optic nerve glioma in a 4-year-old boy who had proptosis and visual loss. The tumor is also encircling the nerve in the sheath. *B,* Coronal T1 image with contrast-enhanced MRI shows a chiasmatic-hypothalamic astrocytoma.

within the optic nerve sheath. Although the differential of proptosis in a child is very long, the imaging demonstration of involvement of one optic nerve or both optic nerves is usually diagnostic. For lesions in the chiasmatic-hypothalamic area, a globular mass with mixed solid and cystic lesions with intense contrast enhancement is typical. Lesions involving the chiasmatic-hypothalamic region have a wider differential. If there is a history of NF1, the diagnosis of a chiasmatic-hypothalamic glioma is certain, but if there is no history of NF1, an open biopsy is typically required to get a definitive diagnosis. Lesions such as craniopharyngiomas are usually clearly defined by imaging, and chiasmatic-hypothalamic gliomas rarely calcify, but solid masses such as germ cell tumors could be mistakenly assumed to be a chiasmatic-hypothalamic glioma in a non-NF1 patient, unless the imaging shows that the tumor infiltrates an optic nerve or optic radiations. Germ cell tumors in the suprasellar area also often occur with diabetes insipidus.

Management of these tumors remains controversial because of the variable natural history of these tumors and must in most cases be determined on an individual patient basis. Many patients do not require any treatment initially. Patients with NF1 often have optic pathway tumors that remain quiescent and require no therapy, whereas patients with rapidly growing, biologically aggressive tumors (such as infants with chiasmatic-hypothalamic tumors) may require surgery for reduction of mass effect and attempted preservation of vision.

In particular, the prognosis for patients with unilateral optic nerve tumors confined to the orbit is excellent following surgery, whereas surgery for patients with posterior tumors that infiltrate the chiasm or hypothalamus experience higher rates of morbidity and mortality. For a child with NF1 and a unilateral or bilateral optic nerve glioma, observation is usually the initial management strategy. For a non–NF1-associated unilateral optic nerve glioma, with or without involvement of the chiasm, in a patient with useful vision in the involved eye, observation is also performed initially. The role of surgery in these unilateral lesions is controversial. It has not been definitively established that optic nerve gliomas that do not involve the chiasm truly infiltrate posteriorly in time to involve the chiasm and threaten vision from the other eye. Surgery is performed mainly to manage proptosis if there is blindness in the involved eye. The nerve is sectioned anteriorly just behind the globe. The extent of posterior resection depends on whether the chiasm is involved as seen on magnetic resonance (MR) images. If the chiasm is not involved, a more aggressive surgical resection to get a clear margin is undertaken, with intradural sectioning of the nerve just anterior to the chiasm, so as to preserve von Willebrand's knee of visual fibers. Surgery has little role to play in bilateral optic nerve gliomas, but chemotherapy could be considered in a child with progressive visual loss.

In chiasmatic-hypothalamic tumors, management is also controversial. Many of these tumors can also be observed if small and associated with reasonable vision, particularly in older children. Some of these lesions do not demonstrate progressive enlargement with follow-up. If associated with NF1, observation is also initially performed. Bulky lesions in young children have a more aggressive clinical course and warrant upfront treatment. With large lesions, some groups advocate an aggressive surgical approach, and others recommend a more limited role for surgical resection. In a young child with a very large bulky chiasmatic-hypothalamic glioma, chemotherapy has recently been proposed as a first line of treatment. Surgery is held in reserve for lesions that progress on chemotherapy, and although radical debulking can be achieved, it is difficult to achieve a complete total resection. Exophytic and cystic areas can be surgically treated to debulk a progressive tumor, and relief of obstructive hydrocephalus may be achieved. A proportion of children with these tumors require CSF shunting if there has been enlargement to cause obstructive hydrocephalus at the foramen of Monro.

Radiation therapy for chiasmatic-hypothalamic tumors represents the mainstay of adjuvant therapy for older children with tumor progression, although the effectiveness is uncertain, and response is slow. Radiation treatment is becoming more focused to limit radiation to surrounding brain. Stereotactic radiosurgery has been used, or more recently fractionated stereotactic radiation has been used, and can lead to disease stabilization and regression.[4] Radiation therapy is discouraged in patients with NF1 out of concern for second malignancies and the development of moyamoya disease. Chemotherapy with vincristine and carboplatin is emerging as a very important treatment alternative for large, diffuse, or progressive optic pathway tumors, and it can result in disease stabilization or occasionally regression.[10]

INTRAVENTRICULAR ASTROCYTOMAS

Approximately 10% of all central nervous system tumors involve the ventricles. In children, supratentorial gliomas may arise from the frontal horn, septum pellucidum, third ventricle, or aqueduct; hypothalamic gliomas may extend into these regions, and anaplastic astrocytomas may invade them. An important subgroup of intraventricular astrocytic tumors, the subependymal giant cell astrocytoma (SEGA), classically occurs in children or young adults with tuberous sclerosis, a genetic disorder characterized clinically by seizures, mental retardation, adenomata sebaceum, and cortical and subependymal hamartomas, and karyotypically by mutations of genes on chromosomes 9 and 16.[19] SEGAs histologically consist of both neuronal cells and large cells resembling gemistocytic astrocytes, although few of these cells express glial fibrillary acidic protein (GFAP). These nodular tumors typically arise in the anterior third ventricle at the foramen of Monro and may therefore obstruct CSF flow, necessitating either safe surgical resection or a CSF shunting procedure (Figure 75-3). Otherwise, these tumors are typically fairly indolent and are managed with serial imaging studies to monitor growth and to look for obstructive hydrocephalus.

OLIGODENDROGLIOMAS

Although mixed oligodendroglial tumors can account for up to 30% of supratentorial low-grade gliomas, pure oligodendrogliomas are rare in children, representing only 1% to 3% of hemispheric tumors and displaying a male preponderance.[3] Histologically, these tumors are characterized by uniform sheets of cells with perinuclear halos, giving them a typical "fried-egg" appearance. Because the predominant location for these tumors is the frontal lobe, they commonly have a long history of seizures, although focal neurologic deficits and raised intracranial pressure may also occur. CT or MRI demonstrate irregular lesions that are often calcified and may be cystic with a variable pattern of contrast enhancement. These tumors are similar to childhood astrocytomas, in that they are often slow-growing lesions with a favorable prognosis (5-year survival of

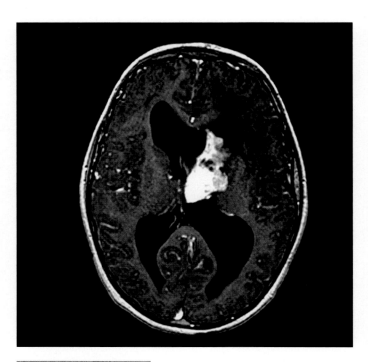

FIGURE 75-3 A 5-year-old boy with tuberous sclerosis had an enlarging ventricle caused by a large subependymal giant-cell astrocytoma in the left lateral ventricle near the foramen of Monro, as seen on magnetic resonance imaging. He underwent transcallosal debulking of the lesion and later required cerebrospinal fluid shunting.

80% to 90%) following total surgical resection alone. For cases in which only subtotal resection was achieved, the therapeutic options include expectant management or conventional radiation therapy, which is usually reserved for those children whose tumors demonstrate anaplastic features or manifest clear tumor progression.[13] Chemotherapy is also a very important consideration, because oligodendroglial tumors are known to be chemosensitive.

EPENDYMOMA

Ependymomas represent 8% to 10% of all pediatric brain tumors, but only 30% to 40% are supratentorial. They occur with a peak incidence between birth and 4 years of age, with a male preponderance.[14] They are thought to arise from ectopic ependymal cell rests within the cerebral hemispheres, adjacent to the lateral and third ventricles.[16] Histologically, ependymomas are characterized by the presence of ependymal rosettes, perivascular pseudorosettes, and blepharoblasts or basal ciliary bodies arranged around a lumen. The majority of lesions are histologically benign.[18]

Imaging shows a discrete, often calcified, heterogeneous mass lesion (Figure 75-4). Supratentorial lesions often display cystic components. Dissemination to the CSF spaces occurs in 10% to 15% of cases (more typical of infratentorial tumors), but most supratentorial ependymomas are known to frequently recur locally.[5] Therefore attempted maximal surgical excision with postoperative radiation therapy represents the standard therapy for children with this tumor. Gross-total excision is associated with a better prognosis and should be the goal of

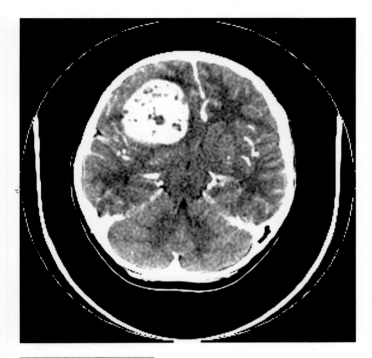

FIGURE 75-4 A contrast-enhanced computed tomography scan demonstrates a large, well-circumscribed mass in the frontal lobe. The diagnosis was ependymoma.

surgical resection. Supratentorial tumors demonstrate a more favorable 5-year survival rate of 60% compared with 10% for infratentorial tumors. Studies have shown that the combined 5-year survival rate for supratentorial and infratentorial tumors of no more than 30% with surgery alone could be improved to 40% to 50% with the addition of postoperative radiation.[11,18] Because relapse and recurrent disease are common with ependymomas and a strong association exists between postoperative residual tumor and tumor recurrence,[21] chemotherapy has also been used to attempt to improve outcomes in infants and in children. Unfortunately, no consistent evidence has yet shown that adjuvant chemotherapy improves survival.[8,17]

GANGLIOGLIOMA

This mixed neuronal-glial tumor accounts for 4% to 9% of childhood brain tumors and occurs in a predominantly supratentorial location, favoring the medial temporal lobe.[14] Thus they typically cause seizures, often complex partial in nature, and rarely manifest focal neurologic deficits. CT and MRI typically show a well-demarcated lesion of low density with common cystic regions or occasional calcification (Figure 75-5). These

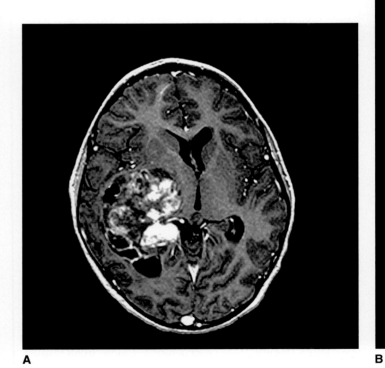

A

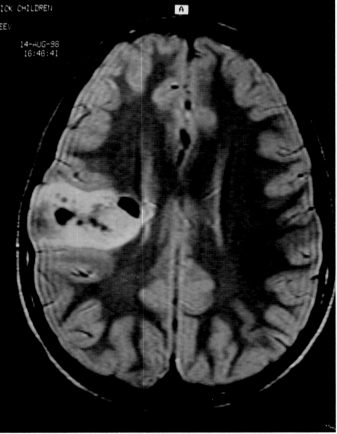

B

FIGURE 75-5 *A,* A 9-year-old girl had a hemiparesis and symptoms of raised intracranial pressure. A very large right temporal tumor was demonstrated on magnetic resonance imaging (MRI). Gross-total excision of a ganglioglioma was achieved. *B,* A 10-year-old boy had long-standing left-hand weakness and a seizure. MRI reveals a heterogeneous lesion that extends to involve the cortex. The lesion was densely calcified on computed tomography. The child's ganglioglioma was completely excised.

lesions are often indolent, superficial, and well circumscribed and are highly amenable to gross-total surgical resection, with 5-year disease-free survival rates approaching 90%. There is little need for adjuvant therapy in these relatively radioresistant tumors, and surgical re-exploration or stereotactic radiation surgery may be considered before conventional radiation therapy.

OTHER MIXED NEURONAL-GLIAL TUMORS

Desmoplastic Infantile Ganglioglioma

DIG tumors are a rare and recently described tumor of infancy that occur in a superficial cerebral location (frontal and parietal lobes). Its clinical presentation usually consists of seizures or signs of raised intracranial pressure. Radiology typically shows a massive cystic tumor with solid nodules bordering the leptomeningeal membrane (Figure 75-6). Histologically, DIG consists of a mixture of glial and neuronal cells in a fibrous stromal background. Prognosis is usually good, and recurrence rare, with total surgical resection alone.[20] Surgery can be quite hazardous because of the very large size of the tumors that occur in infants.

Pleomorphic Xanthoastrocytoma

PXA tumor, first described by Kepes et al in 1979, is characterized histologically by a mixture of large multinucleated cells with vacuolated cytoplasm, lipidized astrocytes, and ganglion cells.[7] They are usually solid and cystic tumors attached to the leptomeninges and occur superficially in the temporoparietal lobes. These tumors have a favorable long-term prognosis with surgical resection alone, and the strongest predictors of good outcome are the absence of necrosis and total surgical resection. However, tumors exhibiting necrosis do have a tendency to recur, warranting reoperation or adjuvant therapy in most cases.

Dysembryoplastic Neuroepithelial Tumor

DNET was first described by Daumas-Duport et al,[1] who described a group of pediatric patients with benign mixed neuronal-glial tumors and intractable epilepsy. DNET is typically a cortically based supratentorial tumor favoring the temporal lobes, typically with expansion of a cortical gyrus (Figure 75-7). The overlying bone can be scalloped, and the lesion can occasionally be misinterpreted as an arachnoid cyst. The lesions are not typically enhanced on CT or MRI but may be calcified. On histologic examination, these tumors show a multinodular architecture composed of glioneuronal elements, in association with cortical dysplasia. The tumor also contains loose myxoid fields containing cells resembling oligodendrocytes; indeed, DNET can be mistaken pathologically for an oligodendroglioma. These tumors respond very well to gross-total surgical resection, with very low rates of recurrence and no requirement for adjuvant therapy in most cases. Incompletely resected tumors have been shown to be very quiescent with long-term follow-up.

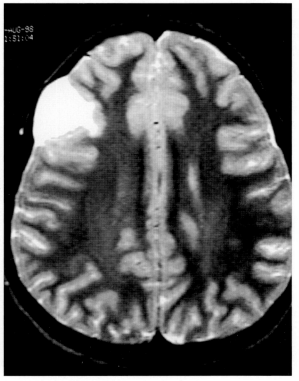

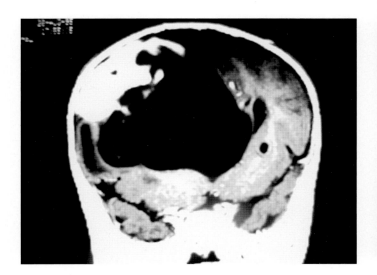

FIGURE 75-6 An infant had progressive macrocephaly and symptoms of raised intracranial pressure. Imaging revealed a very large cystic and solid mass with marked shift. The solid mass is based on the leptomeninges, and the appearance of the lesion is characteristic of desmoplastic ganglioglioma. The child is well 12 years later after a complete surgical excision without any adjuvant therapy.

FIGURE 75-7 A 12-year-old boy had a history of seizures and a right frontal lesion seen on magnetic resonance imaging. This nonenhanced lesion caused expansion of a gyrus, and there was evidence of thinning of the overlying bone. Complete surgical resection of a dysembryoplastic neuroepithelial tumor led to excellent seizure control.

References

1. Daumas-Duport C, Scheithauer BW, Chodkiewicz JP, et al: Dysembryoplastic neuroepithelial tumor: a surgically curable tumor of young patients with intractable partial seizures. Report of thirty-nine cases. Neurosurgery 23:545–556, 1988.
2. Daumas-Duport C, Scheithauer BW, O'Fallon J, et al: Grading of astrocytomas. A simple and reproducible method. Cancer 62:2152–2165, 1988.
3. Favier J, Pizzolato GP, Berney J: Oligodendroglial tumors in childhood. Childs Nerv Syst 1:33–38, 1985.
4. Gould RJ, Hilal SK, Chutorian AM: Efficacy of radiotherapy in optic gliomas. Pediatr Neurol 3:29–32, 1987.
5. Hockley AD: Tumors of the cerebral hemispheres. In Choux DRCM, Hockley AD, Walker MI (eds): Pediatric Neurosurgery. London, Churchill Livingstone, 1999.
6. Hoffman HJ: Optic pathway gliomas in children. In Albright AL, Adelson PD (eds): Principles and Practice of Pediatric Neurosurgery. New York, Thieme, 1999.
7. Kepes JJ, Rubinstein LJ, Eng LF: Pleomorphic xanthoastrocytoma: a distinctive meningocerebral glioma of young subjects with relatively favorable prognosis. A study of 12 cases. Cancer 44:1839–1852, 1979.
8. Mason WP, Goldman S, Yates AJ, et al: Survival following intensive chemotherapy with bone marrow reconstitution for children with recurrent intracranial ependymoma—a report of the Children's Cancer Group. J Neurooncol 37:135–143, 1998.
9. Packer RJ, Ater J, Allen J, et al: Carboplatin and vincristine chemotherapy for children with newly diagnosed progressive low-grade gliomas. J Neurosurg 86:747–754, 1997.
10. Packer RJ, Lange B, Ater J, et al: Carboplatin and vincristine for recurrent and newly diagnosed low-grade gliomas of childhood. J Clin Oncol 11:850–856, 1993.
11. Palma L, Celli P, Cantore G: Supratentorial ependymomas of the first two decades of life. Long-term follow-up of 20 cases (including two subependymomas). Neurosurgery 32:169–175, 1993.
12. Palma L, Guidetti B: Cystic pilocytic astrocytomas of the cerebral hemispheres. Surgical experience with 51 cases and long-term results. J Neurosurg 62:811–815, 1985.
13. Pollack I: Supratentorial hemispheric gliomas. In Albright AL, Adelson PD (eds): Principles and Practice of Pediatric Neurosurgery. New York, Thieme, 1999.
14. Pollack IF: Brain tumors in children. N Engl J Med 331:1500–1507, 1994.
15. Rorke L: Pathology of brain and spinal cord tumors. In Choux DRCM, Hockley AD, Walker MI (eds): Pediatric Neurosurgery. London, Churchill Livingstone, 1999.
16. Russell D: Pathology of Tumors of the Central Nervous System, 5th ed. Baltimore, Williams & Wilkins, 1989.
17. Siffert J, Allen JC: Chemotherapy in recurrent ependymoma. Pediatr Neurosurg 28:314–319, 1998.
18. Sutton LN, Schwartz D: Ependymomas. In Albright AL, Adelson PD (eds): Principles and Practice of Pediatric Neurosurgery. New York, Thieme, 1999.
19. Torres OA, Roach ES, Delgado MR, et al: Early diagnosis of subependymal giant cell astrocytoma in patients with tuberous sclerosis. J Child Neurol 13:173–177, 1998.
20. VandenBerg SR: Desmoplastic infantile ganglioglioma and desmoplastic cerebral astrocytoma of infancy. Brain Pathol 3:275–281, 1993.
21. Vinchon M, Soto-Ares G, Riffaud L, et al: Supratentorial ependymoma in children. Pediatr Neurosurg 34:77–87, 2001.

CHAPTER 76

OPTIC PATHWAY GLIOMAS

Cian J. O'Kelly and James T. Rutka

Optic pathway gliomas are typically low-grade astrocytomas arising from the optic nerves, the optic chiasm, or the retrochiasmal optic tracts. Although relatively rare, these tumors form a significant portion of a pediatric neuro-oncology practice, constituting 1% to 5% of all intracranial neoplasms. They typically occur in childhood and are associated with neurofibromatosis type 1 (NF1) in 20% to 30% of cases. Optic pathway gliomas exhibit tremendous variation in growth potential, ranging from quiescent, spontaneously regressing lesions to aggressive, invasive cancers.[2,5,15,16] This variability coupled with the central location of these tumors has made management controversial and challenging. This chapter attempts to clarify any controversy while providing a practical approach toward diagnosis and treatment of these tumors.

LOCATION

Optic pathway gliomas can be grouped according to location. Dodge et al classified these tumors as type I, optic nerve alone; type II, chiasm alone or with optic nerve involvement; and type III, chiasm with extension to the hypothalamus and other adjacent structures. In a large meta-analysis of 623 cases, type I accounted for 23% of cases, type II for 36%, and type III for 38%. It should be noted that in series from specialized neuro-oncology centers there is a preponderance of type III tumors, 60% to 78%, owing perhaps to a referral bias given the difficulty in managing these extensive tumors.[7,9]

The modifying effect of NF1 on location has been analyzed. Certain groups have suggested that optic glioma in the setting of NF1 is more likely to be confined to the optic nerve and less likely to exhibit a locally extensive phenotype. Others have reported no significant differences in tumor distribution between NF1 and non-NF1 patients. Bilateral optic nerve glioma is considered pathognomonic for NF1.

DIAGNOSIS

The symptoms and signs associated with optic pathway glioma are listed in Table 76-1. Not surprisingly, visual impairment is the most common initial symptom, correlating closely with the signs of impaired visual acuity and visual field deficits. Visual evoked potentials are a useful adjunct to physical examination in these patients, permitting an objective and reproducible means of evaluating the visual system in young patients. Elevated intracranial pressure, often secondary to hydrocephalus,

is responsible for headache and papilledema. The location of a particular optic glioma is predictable given its presenting features. Anterior lesions, with direct involvement of the optic nerve within the orbit, are more likely to have proptosis, strabismus, and monocular visual deficit. Posterior lesions tend to have bilateral visual field involvement, with increased incidence of nystagmus and endocrinopathy. The incidence of nystagmus and endocrinopathy is distributed differently according to age. Nystagmus is predominantly seen in patients who have progressive disease before age 4. Pituitary endocrinopathies, however, are more likely in patients older than 4 years.

The presentation of posterior optic pathway gliomas requires careful analysis because the morbidity and mortality associated with these lesions are considerably greater than are associated with their anterior counterparts. Chiasmal-hypothalamic gliomas cause relatively fewer visual complaints, with alterations in acuity and visual fields reported at 33%. Measurable endocrine dysfunction is observed in approximately half of these patients, with one third of patients exhibiting more than one type of dysfunction. The most common endocrine disorder is growth hormone deficiency followed by abnormalities in sex hormone function manifested as either precocious or delayed puberty. Abnormalities in each of the pituitary hormone systems have been reported. Accordingly, children with these posterior lesions should have a complete endocrine examination with early consultation from an endocrinologist, should abnormalities be detected. Baseline hormone levels are important to document, because treatment and progression of disease can lead to adverse alterations in endocrine function.

A diencephalic syndrome is present in 21% of patients with chiasmal-hypothalamic glioma. This syndrome includes cachexia, macrocephalus, nystagmus, and visual deficits. The child's initial symptom often is failure to thrive, with weight below the third percentile and linear growth preserved. This syndrome affects predominantly younger patients, the median age being 6 months.

The association of NF1 with optic pathway glioma deserves special consideration in the initial assessment of patients. Patients with optic glioma should be scrutinized for the clinical features of NF1. Optic glioma may present differently in the context of NF1. One study indicated increased proptosis but a lower incidence of nystagmus and signs of elevated intracranial pressure in NF1 versus non-NF1 patients, despite no significant difference in tumor location. Finally, as patients newly diagnosed with NF1 are often screened for intracranial neoplasms, asymptomatic optic pathway gliomas may be detected in this patient group. These patients need

TABLE 76-1	Symptoms and Signs at Presentation in 33 Children		
Symptom	%	Sign	%
Decreased vision	29	Decreased visual acuity	33
Headache	23	Visual field defect	33
Failure to thrive	20	Optic atrophy	21
Nausea and vomiting	14	Abnormal eye movement	21
Abnormal eye movement	14	Diencephalic syndrome	21
Symptoms of endocrine dysfunction	14	Signs of endocrine abnormalities	21
		Ataxia	12
		Papilledema	9

Source: From Rodriguez LA, Edwards MS, Levin VA: Management of hypothalamic gliomas in children: an analysis of 33 cases. Neurosurgery 26:242–247, 1990.

careful neurologic and endocrinologic assessment to ensure the identified lesions are indeed asymptomatic.

EPIDEMIOLOGY

The incidence of optic pathway glioma is generally reported at 1 per 100,000 population, with 80% to 90% occurring before the age of 20 and 60% before the age of 10. There may be a slight predilection for females versus males. The association of NF1 is variably reported in the range of 20% to 30% but may be as high as 50%. Hydrocephalus is found in 30% of patients overall but in almost 50% of those with posterior optic gliomas.

NEURO-ONCOLOGY IMAGING

Whether used for initial diagnosis, therapeutic planning, monitoring for progression, or screening for synchronous pathology of NF1, diagnostic imaging plays a crucial role in the management of optic pathway gliomas. Computed tomography (CT) has largely been supplanted by magnetic resonance imaging (MRI). Other modalities such as single-photon emission computed tomography (SPECT) and positron-emission tomography (PET) remain under investigation.

CT allows thorough evaluation of the bone structures related to the optic pathway tumor, in particular the optic canal (Figure 76-1). This is particularly useful in operative planning for these lesions. On CT, optic nerve gliomas may appear thickened or kinked. Cystic changes are common, and there may be thickening of the optic canal. These tumors may be differentiated from optic nerve meningiomas by their lack of calcification and a moderate, rather than intense, pattern of enhancement.

MRI is crucial in the diagnostic evaluation of optic pathway gliomas. It allows greater definition of the optic nerves and chiasm as well as a more accurate delineation of the intracranial extent of the lesions. As for CT, on T1 images the nerve is enlarged and kinked; it is isointense to cortex (see Figure 76-1). T2 demonstrates a hyperintense lesion again with cystic changes (Figure 76-2).

The differential diagnosis of optic nerve gliomas on the basis of neuroimaging varies with tumor location. Optic nerve

enlargement may be viewed as neoplastic versus non-neoplastic. Neoplastic enlargement of the optic nerve may be caused by glioma, meningioma, neuroma, hemangioblastoma, metastasis, or lymphoma. Non-neoplastic conditions associated with optic nerve enlargement include elevated intracranial pressure, optic neuritis, Graves disease, sarcoidosis, toxoplasmosis, central vein occlusion, and tuberculosis. Posterior optic gliomas involving the chiasm and hypothalamus must be differentiated from other sellar and suprasellar lesions, including germ cell tumors, craniopharyngiomas, and pituitary adenomas.

TUMOR HISTOLOGY

Most optic pathway gliomas are pilocytic astrocytomas. These consist of elongated cells with single elongated nuclei housing abundant chromatin. A smaller subset of cells may have the appearance of fibrillary astrocytomas. Many gliomas of the optic nerve show a propensity for leptomeningeal infiltration accompanied by resultant arachnoid hyperplasia. Most tumors stain avidly for glial fibrillary acidic protein (GFAP). Immunohistochemical markers may be useful in predicting the biologic activity of optic pathway gliomas. Optic nerve pilocytic astrocytomas with low levels of MIB-1 and p53 (labeling indices <1%) exhibit benign behavior. More aggressive pilocytic astrocytomas have elevated labeling indices for MIB-1 at 2% to 3%. Labeling indices of more than 2% for MIB-1 and p53 are predictive of a diffuse or anaplastic breed of astrocytoma.

THERAPY

The management of optic pathway gliomas is often challenging, requiring a cooperative approach between surgeons, oncologists, and rehabilitation specialists. Because many patients are initially referred to a neurosurgical clinic, the surgeon often assumes the responsibility for directing the overall management. The principal issues to address include establishment of the appropriate diagnosis, decision of when to initiate treatment, which therapeutic modalities to employ, and how to monitor for and manage recurrences.

Optic pathway gliomas are unique in that, presented with a patient demonstrating the appropriate clinical and radi-

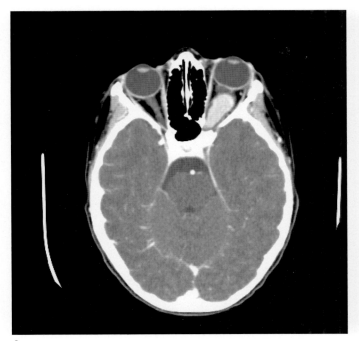

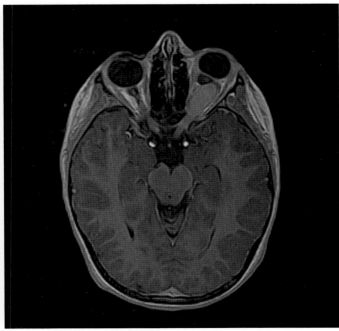

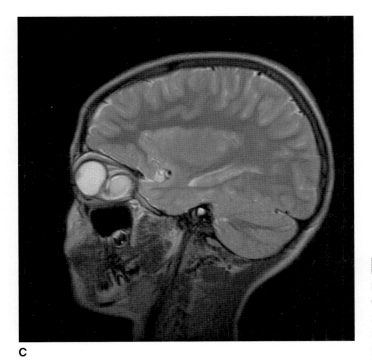

FIGURE 76-1 A 4-year-old boy who presented with a proptosis and unilateral visual loss. *A,* Axial computed tomography scan demonstrating an enlarged optic nerve. *B,* Axial T1-weighted magnetic resonance (MR) image enhanced with gadolinium shows the enlarged nerve distinct from the optic chiasm and canal. *C,* Sagittal T2-weighted MR image showing the kinked and thickened nerve.

ographic findings, the initial question is not how to confirm the diagnosis but rather whether confirmation of the diagnosis is necessary. Pediatric patients with fusiform thickening of the optic nerve, especially in the setting of NF1, do not require a biopsy to establish a diagnosis of optic glioma. An exophytic lesion confined to the optic nerve may warrant biopsy to rule out a more aggressive disease process. Posterior optic pathway tumors involving the chiasm or hypothalamus generally necessitate a formal biopsy, which may be undertaken independently or as part of a procedure to resect the bulk of the tumor.

Having established the diagnosis of optic pathway glioma, the next decision is whether to initiate treatment. The natural history of these tumors is extremely variable. Numerous groups have reported both long-term stability and even spontaneous regression of untreated lesions. This has led some authors to postulate that optic gliomas may represent benign hamartomatous lesions. However, equally many authors have described aggressive, invasive tumors with a much less favorable natural history. Despite this controversy, a policy of watchful waiting is probably indicated in a subgroup of patients. Children with

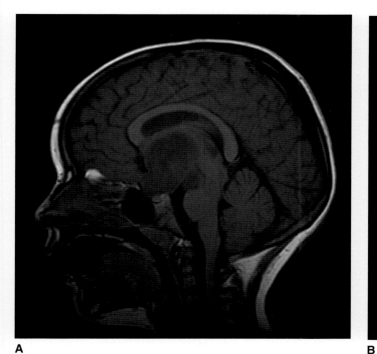

A

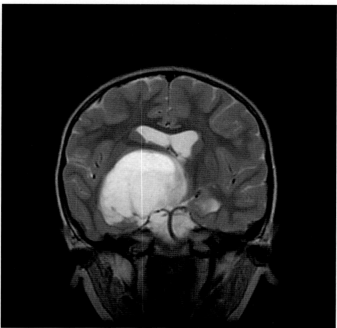

B

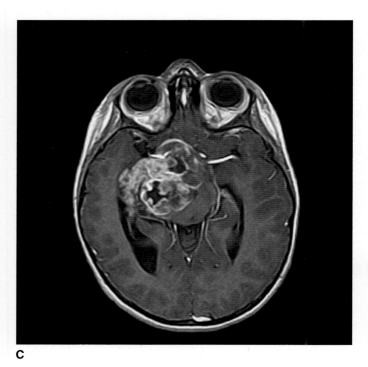

C

FIGURE 76-2   A 2-year-old girl who presented with hemiparesis and a dysconjugate gaze. *A,* Sagittal T1-weighted magnetic resonance imaging (MRI) scan demonstrating a large isointense lesion. *B,* Coronal T2-weighted MRI scan showing a hyperintense, partially cystic lesion. *C,* Diffuse enhancement seen on axial 3D MRI with gadolinium contrast.

asymptomatic or minimally symptomatic disease may be candidates for a period of careful observation. This is especially valid for younger patients unlikely to tolerate therapeutic interventions. Monitoring during this observation period should include frequent clinical visits, visual testing, endocrine assessments, and neuroimaging.

Clearly, not every patient will exhibit quiescent disease. A significant number of children will require treatment or will develop progressive disease requiring treatment. Indications for such treatment include significant visual or other neurologic

impairment, endocrinopathy or diencephalic syndrome, hydrocephalus, and radiographically progressive disease. The first decision is to determine whether surgery is required. The simplest form of surgical intervention is a biopsy. Absolute indications for surgery include the presence of hydrocephalus and decompression of neurologic structures. However, the decision to operate is often not so clear. A case-by-case assessment determines whether surgery is indicated and indicates the most appropriate operation. Symptomatology and salvageable function, patient's age and medical condition, accessibility of the tumor, as well as its proximity to vital neurologic structures, are all factors in such assessments. Regardless of the operative intervention pursued, most patients will receive some form of chemotherapy. This may be used as the primary therapy in nonoperative cases or as an adjuvant to surgical treatment.

Following these primary interventions, patients are monitored for recurrence of their optic pathway glioma. The monitoring protocol is similar to that employed for following asymptomatic lesions. Frequent clinical visits, including visual and endocrine assessments, are combined with radiologic evaluations. Recurrence may manifest as new or progressive neurologic symptoms and signs, endocrine deficit, or simply a radiographic change. Each recurrence must be carefully assessed on an individual basis. The management options include salvage surgery, radiation therapy, or experimental chemotherapy protocols. Consideration should be given to the achievable benefits versus treatment morbidity. Unfortunately, palliation may represent the most appropriate course of action in the setting of tumor recurrence.

Surgery

A variety of surgical approaches are available to the neurosurgeon managing an optic pathway glioma. Each case must be carefully evaluated to determine the most appropriate approach. The goal of the procedure often determines the approach used—for example, biopsy versus total or subtotal resection. Tumor location is also important in determining the type of procedure to pursue and the attainable goals of that particular procedure. In most cases, preservation of visual function is a priority. Monitoring of intraoperative visual evoked potentials is useful in achieving this end.

In cases where the diagnosis is uncertain but formal surgery is not indicated, a biopsy may be the most appropriate procedure. The two forms of biopsy are open and stereotactic. Open biopsy may be used for sampling of both anterior and posterior lesions. The operative approach is similar to that employed for a more formal resection in a given location. When obtaining a biopsy, it is important to sample tissue remote from vital neurologic structures. If biopsy of the optic nerve is indicated, it should be taken from a portion of the nerve in which vision has been lost. Stereotactic biopsy can be used for sampling posterior lesions. This involves placing the patient in a rigid stereotactic frame, fashioning a burr hole, and using computer generated stereotactic coordinates to guide a needle to the tumor site and aspirate a sample.

The surgical management for progressive tumors limited to the optic nerve is amputation of the nerve distal to the chiasm and enucleation of the globe. This operation should not be considered unless there is no useful vision in the affected eye or the tumor shows evidence of progression despite chemotherapy. A subfrontal approach exposing the entire optic nerve—intracranial, canal, and orbital portions—is employed. The nerve should be amputated just distal to the chiasm to avoid fibers decussating from the contralateral eye.

Posterior lesions are a more challenging undertaking than their anterior counterparts (Figure 76-3). A radical approach seeking gross-total resection is generally not feasible. The surrounding structures—the optic tracts, the thalamus and hypothalamus, the brainstem—tend to be unforgiving to such an aggressive approach. Subtotal resection is the usual objective. This may be accompanied by more specific goals such as decompression of the optic apparatus or other neuronal structures, decompression of a tumor cyst, and improvement of hydrocephalus. With regard to hydrocephalus, decompressive surgery alone may be inadequate and shunt placement required. In certain patients, ventriculoperitoneal shunt insertion is the only surgical procedure undertaken. A great variety of

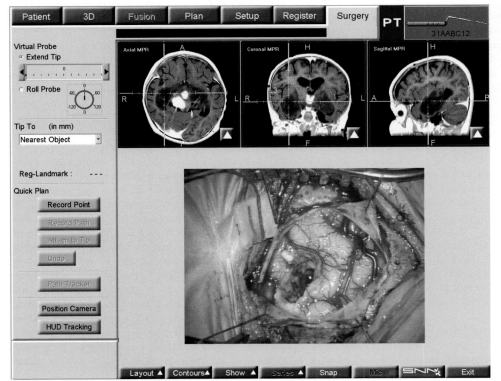

FIGURE 76-3 The surgical approach to posterior lesions is often facilitated by the use of neuronavigation. This operative photograph demonstrates an operative approach in progress, the depth of which is indicated on the navigational imaging.

approaches to tumors in this region have been described. These include subfrontal, subtemporal, transcallosal, and anterior interhemispheric. The choice of procedure will vary with the precise location of tumor and the experience or preference of the surgeon.

Chemotherapy

As for other pediatric brain tumors, chemotherapy for optic pathway gliomas is in constant evolution. A significant proportion of patients receiving treatment are enrolled in clinical trials. Chemotherapy was developed in the 1980s as an alternative to radiation therapy's significant morbidities. Although initially considered a means to delay necessary irradiation or surgical intervention, it now considered primary therapy for optic pathway glioma.

Some of the earliest experience in the literature was with the combination of actinomycin D and vincristine. This combination achieved a progression-free survival rate of 62.5% in patients with radiographic evidence of progressive optic pathway glioma. The major toxicity of vincristine is peripheral neuropathy. Similar activity was also achieved using CCNU and BCNU. Severe and delayed myelosuppression are a concern with these agents.

Recent studies have indicated that platinum-based regimens are particularly active against progressive optic pathway glioma.[1,12] A combination of platinum agent with vincristine is the most typical regimen. Carboplatin is supplanting cisplatin as the agent of choice given its decreased renal toxicity. As a single agent, carboplatin demonstrated an 83% progression-free survival rate in a phase II study. Significant toxicities experienced were thrombocytopenia and hearing loss. The use of carboplatin and vincristine has also been evaluated in children under the age of 3. These patients are a unique therapeutic challenge manifesting a more aggressive disease phenotype and yet are not candidates for radiation therapy given its deleterious cognitive effects in children at this age. A reduction in tumor volume was seen in 57%, contributing to an overall 5-year progression-free survival of 63%. In addition, neurologic improvement was demonstrated in 3 of 14 patients, whereas diencephalic syndrome responded in 4 of 6 patients.

Failure of primary chemotherapy has previously been seen as an indication for initiation of radiation therapy. However, attention has been directed toward chemotherapeutic salvage for these refractory cases. One option is to administer high-dose chemotherapy and employ bone marrow transplant or autologous stem cell transfer to salvage the patients from potentially devastating hematopoietic failure. An alternative is intraarterial administration of chemotherapeutic agents. In one pilot study, selective cannulation of both common carotid arteries and one vertebral artery was used to administer carboplatin and etoposide in combination with intravenous Cytoxan in patients who had failed intravenous carboplatin treatment. Overall, 4 of 6 patients demonstrated a response with relatively mild systemic toxicity. This mechanism of treatment has the theoretic advantage of delivering relatively high concentrations of agent to the tumor site while reducing the actual systemic dose, thereby minimizing toxicity.

Chemotherapy is enjoying an ever-expanding role in the treatment of optic pathway glioma. Currently it is first-line treatment following decompressive surgery. It is increasingly the primary treatment of choice in progressive optic pathway gliomas that are not amenable to surgical intervention (Figure 76-4). It is the only adjuvant to surgery in patients younger than age 3. Novel chemotherapy treatment strategies are also being developed as an alternative to radiation salvage for tumors resistant to conventional chemotherapy.

Radiation Therapy

Although once the mainstay of treatment, the advent of effective chemotherapy has led to a more limited role for radiation therapy in optic pathway glioma management. Radiation remains, however, an important component of the multimodal approach to the treatment of these tumors.

Overall, radiation is reserved for patients older than age 3. For patients younger than 3, the effects of radiation on neurocognitive development are considered unacceptable. Radiation is generally employed for chiasmatic or hypothalamic tumors that have not responded to chemotherapy and are either not amenable to surgical debulking or have progressed after such surgery.

External-beam irradiation is an effective means of controlling progressive optic pathway gliomas. A minimal dose of 45 to 50 Gy is delivered in fractions of 1.6 to 2 Gy. Twenty-five percent of patients exhibit a partial response, and 25% have progressive disease despite irradiation. The remaining patients achieve stable disease. Ten-year survival in these patients is in the range of 80% to 95%, with 10-year progression-free survival lower, at 69% to 75%. Visual improvement is observed in a minority of patients treated in this manner, although in most visual function is unchanged.

The toxicity of radiation therapy has limited its role in the treatment of optic pathway gliomas. The effects of radiation on neurocognitive development are well recognized. Despite the cut-off age of 3 years, cognitive problems are likely to continue to manifest in older irradiated children as learning and behavioral disorders. Other nonspecific effects of radiation include the risk of inducing a second neoplasm in the radiation field and local cutaneous irritations.

Certain toxic effects of radiation are more specific to optic pathway gliomas. Visual and endocrine disturbances are typical for these tumors. Unfortunately, although not unlike aggressive surgery, irradiation can lead to further deterioration in these systems. As many as 55% of patients irradiated for optic pathway glioma may require treatment of endocrine deficits. Patients younger than 10 years old appear to be particularly susceptible to this adverse effect. Vasculopathy also appears to be particularly prevalent following irradiation of optic pathway gliomas. Moyamoya disease, a phenomenon associated with occlusion of large intracranial arteries and subsequent development of abnormal collaterals, was observed in 5 of 28 patients irradiated for optic pathway glioma. Interestingly, this phenomenon was significantly correlated with the presence of NF1. Finally, anaplastic transformation appears to be another specific adverse reaction to irradiation of optic pathway gliomas. Anaplastic change, although the norm in adult low-grade gliomas, is extremely rare in pediatric patients. One series includes six cases of such transformation in pediatric low-grade glioma. Five of the six patients in that series had an optic pathway glioma; 5 of 30 patients with optic pathway glioma treated with surgery and radiation developed anaplastic change, whereas 0 of 25 patients treated with surgery alone developed this complication.

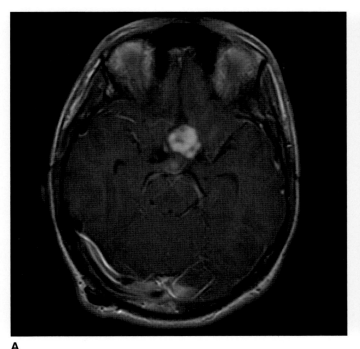
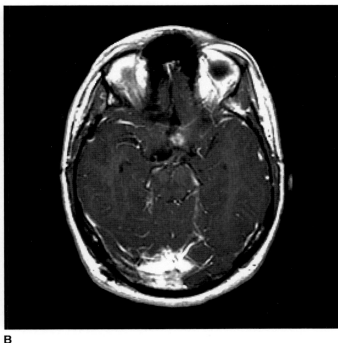

A **B**

FIGURE 76-4 This 14-year-old boy underwent a limited resection followed by adjuvant chemotherapy to achieve stable disease. *A,* Axial T1-weighted image enhanced with gadolinium immediately postoperatively. *B,* Axial T1-weighted image enhanced with gadolinium 2 years postoperatively, following chemotherapy, demonstrates shrinkage of the tumor.

Therapeutic approaches are being modified to minimize the toxic effects of radiation. Stereotactic fractionated radiation therapy shows promise in this respect. This involves giving children an anesthetic and placing them in a modified stereotactic frame. A focused dose of radiation can be given to the tumor site, limiting irradiation of surrounding structures. This should minimize toxic effects on the optic nerve and radiation-induced endocrine dysfunction. This approach also decreases irradiation of the blood vessels at the cranial base, theoretically limiting the risk of moyamoya disease. One group has reported a series of 10 patients treated in this fashion. Three patients achieved complete remission and neurologic improvement, and a further four patients had stable disease. Of note, none of the children had worsening of their vision, and only one patient experienced an endocrine deficiency. Similar to this strategy, there is a case report of the successful use of the Gamma Knife® in the management of an optic pathway glioma. Gamma Knife offers a similar targeted approach but has the convenience of the radiation being administered in a single dose, obviating the need for multiple general anesthetics.

OUTCOME

Overall outcome in optic pathway gliomas is relatively favorable. In retrospective series using combinations of surgery and radiation therapy, 10-year survival rates were in the range of 85% to 90%. Ten-year progression-free survival is lower at 65% to 75%. The impact of early use of chemotherapy on long-term survival remains to be assessed. It is clear, however, that chemotherapy can delay the use of radiation therapy or surgery, thereby improving quality of life. Of children who have a relapse, 10-year freedom from a second relapse is reported as 85%. Outcome for visual function is less encouraging. The vision in the affected eye often declines, regardless of treatment employed. The vision in the better eye often remains stable, and binocular visual acuity is also unchanged.

Numerous studies have attempted to delineate prognostic factors for optic pathway gliomas. The most consistent negative prognostic indicator is age. Children younger than 4 have poorer outcomes. This is most likely a combination of a more aggressive disease and less ability to withstand harsh therapies. Patients with anterior lesions confined to the optic nerve fare better than those with posterior lesions in terms of survival. The modifying effect of NF1 on optic pathway glioma remains the subject of some controversy. Certain studies show patients with NF1 to have improved survival, whereas others indicate that survival is impaired. Many studies show that 10-year survival rates are comparable for NF1 and non-NF1 patients. Patients without NF1 may have a shorter time to first progression despite no change in overall long-term survival. This may explain some of the discrepancies seen in the literature.

CONCLUSION

Optic pathway gliomas are fascinating tumors offering many diagnostic and therapeutic challenges to the oncology team. Overall, they offer satisfying results in terms of their response to treatment. The discovery of new forms of chemotherapy and radiation therapy offers hope for improved survival and quality of life.

References

1. Aquino VM, Fort DW, Kamen BA: Carboplatin for the treatment of children with newly diagnosed optic chiasm glioma: a phase II study. J Neurooncol 41:255–259, 1999.
2. Borit A, Richardson EP: The biological and clinical behavior of pilocytic astrocytomas of the optic pathways. Brain 105:161–187, 1982.
3. Cummings TJ, Provenzale JM, Hunter SB, et al: Gliomas of the optic nerve: histological, immunohistochemical (MIB-1 and p53), and MRI analysis. Acta Neuropathalo (Berlin) 99:563–570, 2000.
4. Debus J, Kocagoncu KO, Hoss A, et al: Fractionated stereotactic radiotherapy (FSRT) for optic glioma. Int J Radiat Oncol Biol Phys 44:243–248, 1999.
5. Dirks PB, Jay V, Becker LE, et al: Development of anaplastic changes in low-grade astrocytomas of childhood. Neurosurgery 34:68–78, 1994.
6. Grabenbauer GG, Schuchardt U, Buchfelder M, et al: Radiation therapy of optico-hypothalamic gliomas (OHG)—radiographic response, vision and late toxicity. Radiother Oncol 54:239–245, 2000.
7. Grill J, Laithier V, Rodriguez D, et al: When do children with optic pathway tumors need treatment? An oncological perspective in 106 patients treated at a single center. Eur J Pediatr 159:692–696, 2000.
8. Hollander MD, Fitzpatrick M, O'Connor SG: Optic gliomas. Radiol Clin North Am 37:59–71, 1999.
9. Jenkin D, Angyalfi S, Becker L, et al: Optic glioma in children: surveillance, resection, or irradiation? Int J Radiat Oncol Biol Phys 25:215–225, 1993.
10. Kestle JR, Hoffman HJ, Mock AR: Moyamoya phenomenon after radiation for optic glioma. J Neurosurg 79:32–35, 1993.
11. Kovalic JJ, Grigsby PW, Shepard MJ: Radiation therapy for gliomas of the optic nerve and chiasm. Int J Radiat Oncol Biol Phys 18:927–932, 1990.
12. Osztie E, Varallyay P, Doolittle ND, et al: Combined intraarterial carboplatin, intraarterial etoposide phosphate, and IV cytoxan chemotherapy for progressive optic-hypothalamic glioma in young children. Am J Neuroradiol 22:818–823, 2001.
13. Packer RJ, Sutton LN, Bilaniuk LT, et al: Treatment of chiasmatic/hypothalamic gliomas of childhood with chemotherapy: an update. Ann Neurol 23:79–85, 1988.
14. Peyster RG, Hoover ED, Hershey BL, et al: High resolution CT of lesions of the optic nerve. Am J Radiol 140:869–874, 1983.
15. Rodriguez LA, Edwards MS, Levin VA: Management of hypothalamic glioms in children: an analysis of 33 cases. Neurosurgery 26:242–247, 1990.
16. Rutka JT, Hoffman HJ, Drake JM: Suprasellar and sellar tumors in childhood and adolescence. Neurosurg Clin North Am 3:803–820, 1992.
17. Silva MM, Goldman S, Keating G: Optic pathway hypothalamic glioma in children under the three years of age: the role of chemotherapy. Ped Neurosurg 33:151–158, 2000.

CHAPTER 77

THALAMIC GLIOMAS

Mark M. Souweidane

Primary glial neoplasms of the thalamus in children possess several unique characteristics that result in challenging therapeutic decisions. The diencephalic location has significant implications negating a simple application of therapeutic strategies that have been proved effective for gliomas in other anatomic domains. Historically, the principal feature rendering this disease process as unique was the relative inaccessibility using surgical extirpation. However, recent advances in surgical technology have justified an aggressive approach toward resection for select thalamic tumors while relying on simple diagnostic sampling in others. Furthermore, an improved understanding of growth patterns, the use of high-resolution magnetic resonance imaging (MRI) and nonstructural imaging modalities, and the reliance on multimodality therapeutic schemes have all improved the potential for treatment success in children with thalamic gliomas. The central doctrine dictating a therapeutic direction relies on an individualized approach to each patient that depends primarily on the tumor growth pattern. Outcome mostly depends on this growth pattern, the histologic diagnosis, the patient age, and in patients with focal tumors, the degree of tumor resection. Although highly malignant tumors with infiltrative growth patterns remain a dismal condition, cure for well-circumscribed, low-grade gliomas is a reasonable expectation of contemporary neuro-oncologic therapy.

DEFINITION

Because the unifying feature of thalamic tumors is anatomic location, the discussion that follows is limited to only those tumors that originate within the thalamus proper. Thus other diencephalic tumors such as the hypothalamic or optic chiasmatic gliomas and tumors arising from the juxtaposed intraventricular or suprasellar compartments that affect the thalamus through direct extension will not be included.

GENERAL CHARACTERISTICS

Thalamic gliomas represent a small minority of primary neoplasms of the central nervous system (CNS). It is estimated that primary tumors of the thalamus represent approximately 1% of all intracranial neoplasms in adults[4,8,26,45] and up to 5% in children.[5,9,36] Thalamic gliomas, although occurring in all age groups, have a bimodal age distribution, with the highest incidence in children and adolescents and another peak of incidence occurring in individuals older than age 40.[5,8,16,18,22,39,45] Published series have indicated that up to 70% of patients are younger than 25 years of age[26,45] with a mean age of approximately 35 years.[19] There is no recognized gender predilection or favored lateralization. Children with the neurocutaneous syndromes neurofibromatosis type 1 (NF1) and tuberous sclerosis complex (TSC) are frequently evaluated for thalamic masses. Thalamic and basal ganglia imaging abnormalities in children with NF1 are quite common, but only approximately 10% of these children will ultimately require treatment for a diencephalic tumor, usually a hypothalamic or chiasmatic low-grade astrocytoma. Subependymal giant cell astrocytoma (SEGA) has a well-known association with TSC. Most of these tumors cause symptoms by their juxtaposition with the foramen of Monro, resulting in hydrocephalus.

DIENCEPHALIC ANATOMY

A detailed description of thalamic anatomy is beyond this chapter's scope. However, certain pertinent physiologic and anatomic details merit discussion because they have significant impact on clinical manifestations of the disease and considerations involved in surgical management. The thalamus is an ovoid collection of nuclei that accounts for the major portion of the diencephalon. The remaining three divisions of the diencephalon include the hypothalamus, the subthalamus, and the epithalamus.

The thalamus extends from the interventricular foramen anteriorly to the posterior commissure posteriorly. It is bound laterally by the posterior limb of the internal capsule and medially by the lateral and third ventricles. In the coronal plane, the superior limit is defined by the lateral ventricle, and the inferior margin approximates the hypothalamus and the rostral mesencephalon. From a surgical standpoint it is most important to note that the thalamus approximates cerebrospinal fluid (CSF)-containing structures on the dorsomedial aspect by way of the lateral ventricle and on the posterior aspect by way of the pineal and quadrigeminal cisterns. These thalamic–CSF interfaces have important implications concerning surgical approaches via natural dissection planes.

The anterior, dorsomedial, and ventrolateral nuclear groups, separated by the internal medullary lamina, serve as important relay centers for vast amounts of sensory and motor information. Topographic organization of the thalamic function is contralateral. The efferent projections distribute to a wide cortical and hypothalamic distribution, resulting in the conscious awareness of sensation and reactive emotional responses. In general, the thalamus is primarily responsible for modulating sensory input into appropriate integrated cerebral functions.

HISTOLOGY

Glial neoplasms account for approximately 90% of all primary thalamic tumors, with the vast majority being juvenile pilocytic astrocytomas (JPAs) and fibrillary astrocytomas.[4,8,15,26,45] The exact origin of the neoplastic cell has been ascribed to a rich population of subependymal glial cells and glial elements of the white matter tracts that subdivide the diencephalic nuclei.[32,38,50]

JPAs, although commonly and inadvisably grouped under the rubric of low-grade astrocytomas (World Health Organization [WHO] grade I), are biologically distinct from low-grade fibrillary astrocytomas (WHO grade II). (See Part I, Basic Principles for a detailed account of pathologic grading.) Thalamic JPA is characteristically well circumscribed with either microcystic or macrocystic features. It has been demonstrated that the incidence of a thalamic glioma having WHO grade I histology is strongly correlated to patient age, a relationship that is universal among cerebral gliomas. In the report on thalamic gliomas by Kelly, of 72 patients from whom tissue samples were obtained, 27 were diagnosed with pilocytic astrocytoma.[19] Of those 27 patients with a thalamic JPA, the average age was 16 years, with 63% of the patients being 20 years of age or younger. In a separate report that reviewed eight cases of cystic astrocytomas of the thalamus, the average age was 6 years, and no patient was older than 15 years at the time of diagnosis.[47] The identifying histologic feature of the pediatric age group with reference to thalamic gliomas is readily evident; less aggressive astrocytic tumors account for a higher percentage of gliomas in the pediatric population.

In distinction to JPA, fibrillary astrocytoma (WHO grades II to IV) exhibits a highly infiltrative capacity. Similar to the correlation that exists between JPA and the pediatric population, an association exists between malignant fibrillary astrocytoma and adults. From several studies encompassing patients of all ages, glioblastoma multiforme was responsible for roughly 45% of all thalamic tumors with confirmed pathology. This figure is comparable with the frequency of glioblastoma among all astrocytomas of the cerebral hemispheres in adults. However, high-grade astrocytomas make up a much smaller percentage of gliomas in the pediatric age group. Glioblastoma multiforme accounts for approximately 5% to 10% of pediatric brain tumors. This trend is no different for pediatric thalamic gliomas. Of 60 children with thalamic tumors reported by Bernstein et al, 41 were histologically identified, and only 5% of these were glioblastoma.[6] In agreement with a frequency of only 5%, Martinez-Lage et al confirmed only one glioblastoma in a cohort of 20 children with thalamic tumors who underwent tissue sampling.[24]

Other astrocytic thalamic tumors in children include oligodendroglioma, SEGA, and pleomorphic xanthoastrocytoma (PXA). Pilomyxoid astrocytoma, a rare variant of JPA that exhibits a more aggressive growth potential and tendency for CSF dissemination, is most often located in the suprasellar compartment but can also originate in the diencephalon. Specifically in infants, embryonal tumors include primitive neuroec-todermal tumor (PNET) and atypical teratoid-rhabdoid tumor (AT-RT). The presence of neuronal elements within the thalamic nuclear masses accounts for the rare ganglioglioma of the thalamus. Intraparenchymal ependymomas of the thalamus can also occur because of the juxtaposition of the third ventricular ependymal surface. Germ cell tumors of the thalamus have been found to represent as much as 10% of all intracranial germ cell tumors in children in some Asian populations.[20,43,51] Rare in the pediatric population, primary CNS lymphoma should be considered in the differential diagnosis in the context of acquired immunodeficiency syndrome (AIDS).

PATTERNS OF GROWTH

An appealing method for categorizing thalamic tumors into three groups is based on the tumor growth pattern as defined by radiographic imaging: focal, diffuse, and bilateral. The focal category of thalamic tumors exhibits a well-defined radiographic and histologic demarcation between tumor and surrounding brain (Figure 77-1). In distinction, the diffuse category of thalamic tumors manifests no gross or microscopic circumscription at the tumor interface (Figure 77-2). It is well established through pathologic correlation that the predominate tumor type represented in the focal category is JPA, and fibrillary astrocytoma (WHO grades II to IV) accounts for the vast majority of diffuse tumors.[2,7] Although histologically indistinguishable from the diffuse category of thalamic tumors, the bilateral thalamic glioma is defined here as a separate, third category (Figure 77-3). This distinction is due to features that uniquely affect the diagnosis, treatment, and outcome of these children. The frequency of bilateral involvement at diagnosis ranges from 2% for patients of all ages to between 11% and 33% in the pediatric population.[36] Similar to gliomatosis cerebri, this subtype of thalamic glioma is believed to have a *de novo* bilateral origin. Alternatively, secondary involvement can occur by contralateral migration via the interthalamic commissures (massa intermedia, habenular commissure, or posterior commissure) or as rostral migration of a primary mesencephalic lesion. As expected, not all histologic varieties of thalamic tumors adhere to this morphologic division, and imaging characteristics may not consistently be clearly defined. The proposed classification, however, is not meant as a substitute for histologic sampling but instead to serve as a rational basis for instituting therapy based on published outcomes and expected morbidity for thalamic tumors exhibiting these growth features.

As is true with most CNS neoplasms in children, metastatic dissemination can occur in children with thalamic tumors, albeit much less commonly. Of the 60 children with thalamic tumors reported on by Bernstein et al, 2 patients had definitive CSF dissemination into the spinal subarachnoid space.[6] The histologic variant of these tumors, however, was not identified. The rarity of this event has not typically affected the diagnostic or therapeutic recommendations for children with thalamic tumors. The recommendation for metastatic surveillance studies (MRI of the spine and CSF cytology sampling) is dictated by the histology of the primary tumor or the presence of clinical symptoms. Most practitioners would thus advocate instituting a metastatic investigation when tumors that have a high propensity for dissemination are found, such as PNET, ependymoma, germinoma, and AT-RT. One documented case

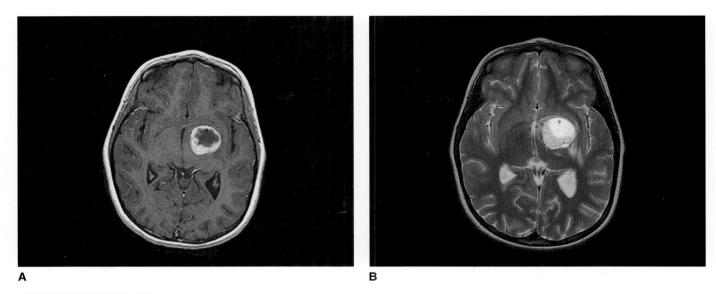

A   **B**

FIGURE 77-1   Axial magnetic resonance imaging scan of an 8-year-old girl with a right hemiparesis. The focal behavior of this tumor is demonstrated on the T1-weighted, gadolinium-enhanced sequence (A) and the T2-weighted sequence (B). Of special note is the clear delineation between the enhanced lesion and brain as well as the paucity of any signal change distant from the site of the tumor. Histological review confirmed the tumor to be a juvenile pilocytic astrocytoma (WHO grade I).

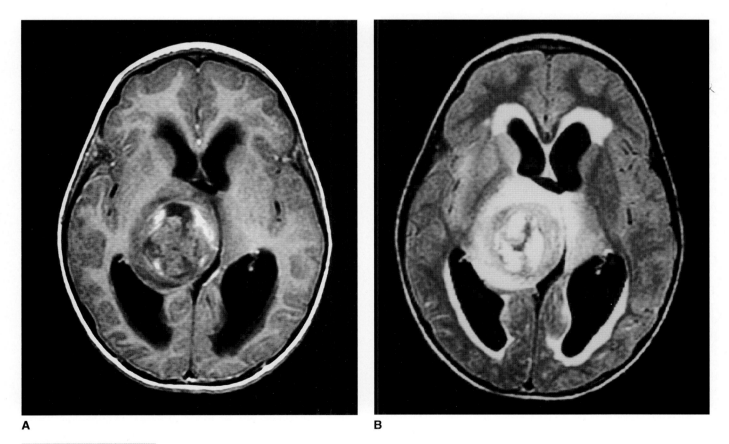

A   **B**

FIGURE 77-2   Axial magnetic resonance imaging scan of a 5-year-old boy with rapid deterioration and coma. Of note is the heterogeneous enhancement pattern, evidence of spontaneous hemorrhage, and necrotic changes seen on the contrast-enhanced T1-weighted image (A) and the diffuse hyperintensity surrounding the tumor mass on the T2-weighted sequence (B). Note the periventricular signal change indicative of transependymal fluid resorption as a result of noncommunicating hydrocephalus. A stereotactic biopsy confirmed a glioblastoma multiforme (WHO grade IV).

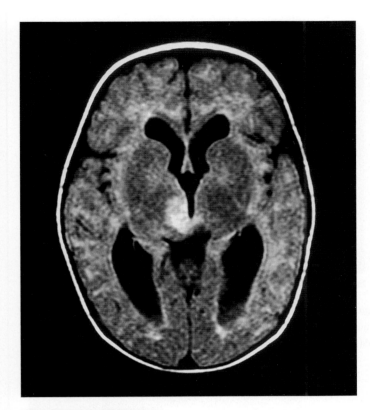

FIGURE 77-3   Early bilateral involvement of the thalamus by a presumed low-grade tumor. This axial fluid-attenuated inversion recovery (FLAIR) sequence suggests sequential bilateral involvement as evidenced by the increased signal intensity of the habenular commissure.

exists of peritoneal dissemination of a thalamic glioblastoma via a ventriculoperitoneal shunt.[23] Again, the extreme rarity of this event should not influence the routine management of patients with symptomatic hydrocephalus caused by a thalamic glioma.

CLINICAL PRESENTATION

The clinical presentation of a patient with a thalamic tumor is quite varied, but several common characteristics are found. The duration of symptoms is typically quite short, a trait not unexpected, given the compact nature of the diencephalon and the proximity of the ventricular and capsular systems. In one pediatric series, 93% of the 60 patients sought treatment with less than 1 year of symptoms, and 80% of these patients had symptoms for less than 4 months.[6] Although studies reviewing patients of all ages with thalamic tumors have similarly recognized a fairly short duration of symptoms, the average duration of symptoms is slightly more protracted in adults, with one third of patients having symptoms lasting more than 12 months.[26] This difference in symptom duration may be somewhat misleading given the differences in availability of certain imaging modalities at the time of publication.

The most common manifestation of a primary tumor within the thalamic region is a result of raised intracranial pres-

sure. This typically results from mass effect exerted by the tumor mass onto one or both of the foramina of Monro, resulting in a unilateral or biventricular noncommunicating hydrocephalus, respectively. In fact, the need to treat hydrocephalus at the time of diagnosis has been reported to be as high as 60% to 75% of children with thalamic tumors.[6,36] This set of symptoms is believed to be associated with lesions that favor the dorsomedial nuclear complex. Thus classic symptoms of elevated intracranial pressure, including headache, decreased spontaneity, and vomiting, account for the majority of symptoms. Clinical signs will somewhat depend on the age of the patient, with infants and young children manifesting most commonly with a divergent macrocrania and irritability and older children and adolescents exhibiting headache, vomiting, somnolence, and papilledema.

Physical signs referable to motor and sensory modalities primarily depend on the site of origin within the thalamus and the direction of tumor growth. The classic thalamic Dejerine-Roussy syndrome, a pain syndrome in which stimuli are vague and poorly localized, is the exception rather than the rule in patients with thalamic tumors.[4,38,45] More typically, early deficits in sensation and impairment of motor strength will accompany the signs of raised intracranial pressure. Disorders of early sensorimotor function are thought to be associated with tumors arising predominately in the ventrolateral nuclear complex because of their proximity to the internal capsule.

Interestingly, epilepsy has been described as an initial complaint or as part of the symptom complex in patients with thalamic tumors. This manifestation is reported as frequently as 30% to 40% of cases,[4,8,45] although others have found seizures to be less common.[6,17,26] The types of seizures vary from simple partial sensory seizures to complex partial epilepsy with secondary generalization.

Ocular and ophthalmologic findings are also often detected in patients with primary tumors of the thalamus. Visual field deficits resulting from compression of the optic tract or geniculate ganglia are quite common. Ocular signs most often found include a poorly reactive, myotic pupil ipsilateral to the lesion and divergent extraocular motions. An ipsilateral third nerve palsy can also occur. These findings result from tumor infiltration or compression of the optic radiations, the retrolenticular segment of the internal capsule, or the rostral mesencephalic tegmentum.

Although these lesions are in close association with the basal ganglia, involuntary movements are relatively uncommon. In series consisting of all age groups, movement disorders are present in less than 10% of cases.[21] However, in pediatric series, these presenting signs have been reported in up to 25% of children with unilateral involvement and 36% of patients with bilateral involvement.[24,36,46] These movement disorders most commonly take the form of a non-Parkinsonian tremor or focal dystonia. In rarer circumstances, hemichorea, hemiballismus, or hemiathetosis can also be found.

Language and speech disturbances, seldom an initial complaint, can sometimes be found on close examination. These deficits are typically expressive dysphasias, such as anomia and perseveration.[1,28,29] These expressive language deficits are typically limited to lesions involving the dominant thalamus.

Other less common symptoms can be predicted based on the anatomic structures involved. Inferior extension of the tumor can result in various signs and symptoms depending on the structure of involvement. Extension into the mammillothalamic fibers or the fornices can lead to alterations in cognition and memory. Involvement of the hypothalamus can potentially lead to endocrinopathies. Occasionally, sensory-motor deficits can be more exaggerated as the tumor migrates down white matter tracts and infiltrates into the midbrain and the crus cerebri.

A symptom complex recently recognized in patients harboring bithalamic involvement is characterized primarily by cognitive changes. Patients with bilateral involvement of the dorsomedial and intralaminar nuclei can exhibit personality changes, mental deterioration, memory loss, confusion, hallucination, hyperphagia, or slow mentation.[33] Because of this nonfocal and predominately cognitive symptom complex, these patients can experience a longer delay in establishing a diagnosis compared with other thalamic gliomas.

RADIOLOGIC CHARACTERISTICS

The radiologic characteristics of primary thalamic tumors, although suggestive of certain histologic subtypes, should never replace actual tissue sampling. In addition to being indicative of certain tumor histologies, the radiologic features become very important from the standpoint of dictating therapeutic options. These features are based principally on growth characteristics, because they relate to tumor infiltration and potential for surgical extirpation.

Computed tomography (CT), although serving a useful diagnostic role, has been supplanted by the higher resolution, triplanar, and spectroscopic potential of MRI. CT scanning can be quite problematic in identifying small lesions at the time of diagnosis if no cystic or necrotic areas are present. In the absence of these features, the only finding may be an area of altered density and mild asymmetry of the thalamic eminence (Figure 77-4). In the presence of mass effect on the ipsilateral or bilateral foramina of Monro, a unilateral or bilateral ventriculomegaly can be the most apparent change on a noncontrast CT scan.

With the advent of MRI, thalamic lesions are being recognized with greater specificity. An ever-expanding number of different sequences afford a very high sensitivity to mild alterations caused by regional edema or cellular density. Thus tumors of smaller dimension and lower grade histologies are being detected at an earlier point in the disease course by using MRI. Using the classification scheme outlined previously, the radiographic features are well defined for the focal, diffuse, and bilateral categories of tumors.

MRI defines the focal thalamic glioma based on the tumor-parenchymal interface, the degree of peritumoral edema, and the contrast enhancement pattern. The tumor margin on all sequences is quite distinct from the surrounding parenchymal compartment, a delineation that is better defined with longer T2-weighted sequences, and with the administration of gadolinium enhancement. In addition, homogeneous enhancement of a concentric or eccentric nodule associated with cystic changes is highly predictive of a lower grade tumor, typically JPA. Another focal thalamic tumor, the germ cell tumor, can have a frequent association with hemorrhage and multiple cystic changes.[20] Radiographic features of focal thalamic tumors have also been reported to mimic rare inflammatory or infectious processes. Thus it is stressed that neuroimaging is best used for characterizing the tumor growth patterns rather than predicting tissue histology.

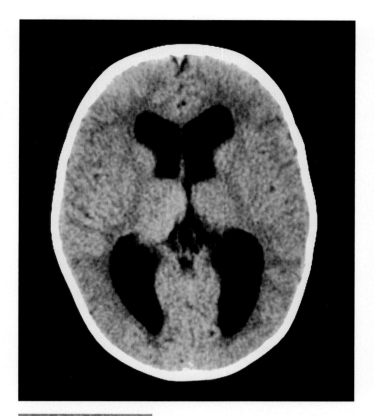

FIGURE 77-4 Axial noncontrast computed tomography (CT) examination of the brain in a 6-year-old child with symptoms of raised intracranial pressure. The right thalamic mass is recognized by the increased size relative to the contralateral side, and the increased density suggests a high cellularity and increased nuclear-to-cytoplasmic ratio. The common finding of hydrocephalus in the pediatric population is obvious on this representative CT scan.

In contrast to the focal category of thalamic tumors, the diffuse, infiltrative category of tumors does not possess many of the aforementioned features. The feature that most clearly draws the distinction between these categories is the inability to define a distinct tumor-parenchymal interface. Most fibrillary astrocytomas, whether benign or malignant, will have indistinct margins with no clear limitations. This feature is most apparent on the long T2-weighted and fluid-attenuated inversion recovery (FLAIR) sequences. With the administration of gadolinium contrast, diffuse infiltrative tumors exhibit variable enhancement patterns but in general do not show homogeneous patterns of contrast uptake. Tumor enhancement pattern is less reliable than the presence of a tumor interface for the purpose of classifying tumors into a focal or diffuse category. In the St. Jude Children's Hospital experience with 36 patients reported in 1998, 92% of the high-grade and 54% of the low-grade tumors exhibited radiographic contrast enhancement.[36] Assuming that the tissue diagnosis in that study was representative of the actual tumor, one can conclude that enhancement alone cannot definitively predict either tumor histology or prognosis. However, contrast enhancement in the appropriate context can be highly predictive of glioma grade. A ring-enhanced mass with a central area of necrosis surrounded by generous white matter infiltration and edema is usually predictive of a high-grade lesion. Thus it is the enhancement pattern in the context of other radiographic features rather than the simple presence or absence of enhancement that is more predictive of tumor grade.

The bilateral thalamic glioma is readily appreciated on standard MRI. Increased intensity using T2-weighted or FLAIR sequences serves as a very sensitive indicator for bilateral involvement. The use of MRI in establishing this diagnostic category has been critical, especially in light of the sometimes vague and nonfocal nature of the symptom complex.

In patients with NF1, unidentified bright objects (UBOs), a variant of hamartomatous or developmental lesions, can closely mimic infiltrative thalamic tumors (Figure 77-5). Similar to the low-grade fibrillary astrocytomas, these lesions exhibit thalamic enlargement, exhibit decreased intensity on T1-weighted imaging, exhibit increased signal on T2-weighted sequences, and do not enhance with the administration of contrast agents. The diagnosis is usually straightforward, however, in the context of an asymptomatic patient with NF1 who has other UBOs in predictable locations (pallidum and brachium pontis).

In addition to excellent spatial resolution and multiplanar capacity, MRI affords nonstructural or functional capabilities. Localized magnetic resonance spectroscopy (MRS) contributes toward the identification of the cellular constituents of the tissue in question by measuring metabolites in both normal and abnormal tissues. Alterations in the metabolites choline (Cho), N-acetyl aspartate (NAA), *myo*-inositol (Ins), lactate (lac), and creatinine(Cr)-phosocreatine, as well as corresponding ratios, have been shown to have a predictive value in differentiating neoplastic from normal tissue and in defining the degree of malignancy. In general, tumor tissue will typically exhibit elevated levels of Cr, Cho, and Ins, and reduced levels of NAA. It is suggested that elevated lac levels define high-grade lesions given that metabolite's association with highly concentrated areas of cell death such as in tumor necrosis. This modality has been shown to be of use in distinguishing tumors affecting the thalamus from UBOs in patients with NF1.[48] Perfusion-weighted imaging (PWI), another functional modality afforded by MRI, is purported to contribute toward the ability to assess tumor aggressiveness. Based on the principle that high-grade neoplasms possess a greater density of microvascular network than low-grade tumors, PWI can be used to measure differences in regional blood volume and thus estimate tumor grade. Limited clinical experience and some limitations have restricted the universal application of this technique. Another functional capability of MRI is diffusion-weighted imaging (DWI). This sequence has been found to assist in the differential diagnosis between necrotic tumors and thalamic abscesses.

TREATMENT

A consensus regarding the optimal therapeutic approach toward children with thalamic gliomas does not exist, as evidenced by inconsistencies in the published literature. Specifically, thalamic gliomas are typically included as a subset of patients in larger studies, with unifying features being histology, age, or location but rarely all three simultaneously. Further, these lesions are often included with other central or deep tumors surrounding the supratentorial ventricular system, such as the hypothalamic or optic nerve gliomas. Therefore attempts to summarize optimal therapeutic schemes and expected outcome for children with thalamic gliomas are limited by a paucity of dedicated reports for this specific entity. Therefore therapy is summarized later into (1) surgical options, including the treatment of hydrocephalus, obtaining accurate histologic diagnosis, and tumor resection, and (2) options for adjuvant therapy, including irradiation and chemotherapy.

SURGERY

Treatment of Hydrocephalus

The appropriate management for a patient with noncommunicating hydrocephalus secondary to a thalamic tumor includes several options. As a temporizing measure in the face of a life-threatening elevation of intracranial pressure, an emergent externalized ventricular drain is appropriate. In nonemergent situations, definitive treatment options for CSF diversion include ventriculoperitoneal shunting or endoscopic third ventriculocisternostomy. This latter procedure has the obvious advantage of avoiding implanted shunt hardware and hence complications associated with such mechanical devices. However, given the regional deformation and mass effect sur-

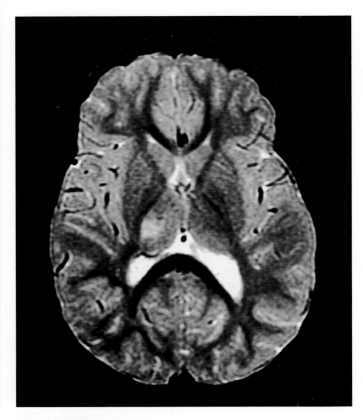

FIGURE 77-5   A T2-weighted axial image of a 5-year-old girl with known neurofibromatosis 1 depicts the common clinical scenario of a thalamic mass. The right-side lesion, indicative of either an unidentified bright object or thalamic tumor, was evaluated by magnetic resonance spectroscopy and found to have a spectral analysis inconsistent with a neoplastic process.

rounding the third ventricle, navigational capability within the third ventricle can be limited. Partial or complete tumor resection is an alternative means for reestablishing internal CSF circulatory patterns but has the obvious added morbidity of a more involved surgical procedure. Whichever mechanism is relied upon for treating hydrocephalus, one must pay particular attention to the possible risk of decompressive hemorrhage within the tumor mass secondary to deformational forces and intratumoral distortion. This latter phenomenon has been recognized in up to 20% of patients undergoing ventriculoperitoneal shunting for hydrocephalus associated with thalamic masses.[13] Therefore it is suggested that gradual release of CSF be accomplished by either using a ventriculoperitoneal shunt with a high-resistance or flow-regulated valve or using a gradual, stepwise continuum in the event of using externalized ventricular drainage.

Tissue Sampling

Although nearly 90% of all tumors involving the thalamus are of astrocytic origin, the need for tissue sampling remains essential given the variability of other pathologic processes, both neoplastic and non-neoplastic. Even within the category of astrocytomas, it remains prudent to obtain tissue samples for purposes of grading in an effort to more appropriately decide on a management scheme and to prognosticate.

Diagnostic endeavors rely on either open tissue sampling or the more minimally invasive techniques of stereotactic or endoscopic biopsy. The readily apparent advantage of open techniques for tissue sampling is the large sample size, which theoretically establishes a more representative diagnosis. In addition, partial resection also contributes to reduction of mass effect with the potential for symptom reversal depending on the individual patient. However, formal craniotomy and open tissue sampling is not without an increased relative risk versus more minimally invasive approaches. Stereotactic biopsy for lesions in and around the third ventricle is a well-established technique with little morbidity and accurate tissue sampling.[3,19,37] As an alternative to stereotactic biopsy, endoscopic transventricular biopsy affords similar benefits with respect to a minimal surgical insult. This technique has also been proved safe and effective for masses in and around the third ventricle, with a high success rate for accurate tissue sampling.[40] Even though the benefits of these minimally invasive approaches toward tissue sampling are appealing, enthusiasm is somewhat tempered by the small risk of obtaining an inaccurate diagnosis because of limited sample size and the risk of intratumoral hemorrhage. Any realistic inaccuracy in diagnosis, however, typically falls within the realm of tumor grade rather than histologic diagnosis. To reduce sampling inaccuracies in patients with thalamic gliomas, success with stereotactic biopsy using metabolic imaging with MRS and positron-emission tomography (PET) with image fusion has been reported.[27]

Surgical Resection

The surgical removal of thalamic tumors mirrors the evolution of neurosurgical techniques for other tumors of central and brainstem regions. Historically, attempts at aggressive resection of thalamic tumors met with disastrous rates of surgical morbidity and mortality. Because of those poor results, a more conservative therapeutic approach quickly evolved. Torkildsen

recommended only a palliative lateral ventriculocisternostomy in an effort to alleviate the symptoms of noncommunicating hydrocephalus from tumors in the region of the third ventricle.[44] Patients were then left to succumb to the neoplastic process at a rate dependent on tumor type. For similarly placed tumors, Ward and Spurling offered patients subtemporal decompressions followed by empiric radiation therapy.[49]

The subsequent neurosurgical era focused on the feasibility of a direct surgical approach to tumors of the thalamus. In the first of several large series, Arseni et al reported on the results of 36 patients with thalamic tumors.[4] Of the 36 patients in that series, 10 underwent surgical management, with a 30% operative mortality rate. Subsequent to that report, Greenwood described 25 patients undergoing surgery for thalamic tumors in which a radical removal was accomplished in 16.[15] Although a minority of the patients had an excellent outcome, there was a 16% mortality rate during the acute postoperative period. Justifiably, through most of the twentieth century a general philosophy remained that these deep-seated thalamic lesions were not amenable to surgery without unacceptable morbidity and mortality.

The latest era concerning surgery for thalamic tumors established a precedent of aggressive surgical management with acceptable rates of mortality and permanent morbidity. In 1984 a report from the Hospital for Sick Children in Toronto, Canada, demonstrated a 7% morbidity in a series of 44 patients harboring thalamic tumors who underwent surgical intervention.[6] In that patient cohort, 3 underwent needle biopsy, 20 had a craniotomy for biopsy, and 21 had varying degrees of resection. Since that time, numerous publications have championed the use of advanced technologies, including computer-assisted stereotactic resection, robot-assisted surgery, intraoperative electrophysiologic monitoring, intraoperative imaging, and the use of the Cavitron ultrasonic aspirator.[2,10,19,30,42] These series have quoted mortality rates ranging from 0% to 6% and permanent morbidity of less than 10%, although differences in surgical morbidity comparing resection (14%) with biopsy (6%) remain significant.[19] Thus total resection of thalamic tumors is a plausible surgical possibility (Figure 77-6). Irrespective of any benefit for long-term disease control, alleviation of symptoms through decompressive tumor resection remains a valid rationale for aggressive surgical resection of thalamic tumors in children.

In summary, contemporary neurosurgical studies have clearly proved the feasibility and safety of aggressive tumor resection for lesions situated within the thalamus. This principle is based on a thorough evaluation of the preoperative imaging, selecting an appropriate surgical route, and reliance on contemporary surgical adjuncts (Figure 77-7). Even though the technical ability for thalamic tumor removal is documented, the benefit offered to the patient can be determined on only an individual basis, based primarily on a focal growth pattern and a benign histology or by the prospect of reversing symptoms secondary to mass effect.

ADJUVANT THERAPY

Radiation Therapy

A generalization cannot be made with certainty as to the efficacy of radiation therapy (RT) for thalamic gliomas as an entity.

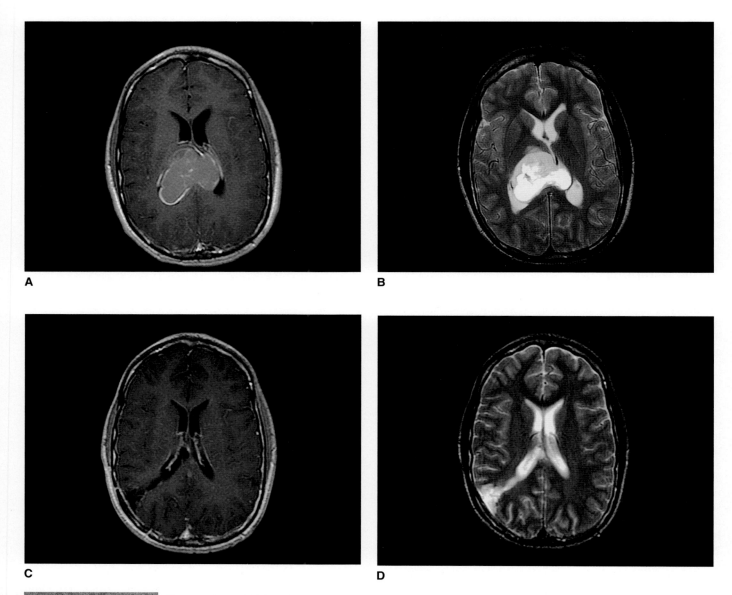

FIGURE 77-6 Preoperative axial T1-weighted image with contrast *(A)* and T2-weighted sequence *(B)* of a 17-year-old boy with headache. Given the relative focal imaging findings and the mass effect, the patient underwent a right-side, parieto-occipital-approach resection for the tumor, which was pathologically confirmed to be a World Health Organization (WHO) grade IV astrocytoma. The corresponding postoperative images *(C, D)* confirm the total tumor removal and alleviation of hydrocephalus.

However, the use of RT (50 to 60 Gy) is an important therapeutic option used in treating children with both low-grade and high-grade lesions. Response rates and disease control have been well established for children older than age 5 with low-grade diencephalic tumors that involve the optic apparatus and the hypothalamus. Several contemporary studies have documented the rationale and the benefit to using RT specifically for children with infiltrative thalamic gliomas.[6,14,16] Using RT as part of the therapeutic approach in the children, these studies indicate 5-year survival rates ranging from 20% to greater than 70%. Furthermore, most studies have also found a trend that indicates that those patients younger than 18 years of age respond better to RT than adult counterparts. Dose-escalation and hyperfractionated-schedule trials have also been under-

taken for children with thalamic gliomas.[35] Generally well tolerated, hyperfractionated RT did result in an increase in toxic side effects and in cystic changes in the radiation field. More importantly, these children enjoyed no benefit with respect to outcome, and this concept has since been abandoned.

The potential risks inherent in the use of RT in children are well recognized, including neurocognitive impairment, endocrine deficiencies, secondary neoplasms, and vascular abnormalities. These detrimental effects are directly related to the volume of irradiation and inversely related to patient age at time of irradiation. Thus, in an effort to minimize these untoward late effects, children younger than 3 to 5 years of age are typically spared irradiation. In addition, the use of highly conformal technology in an attempt to reduce these adverse effects

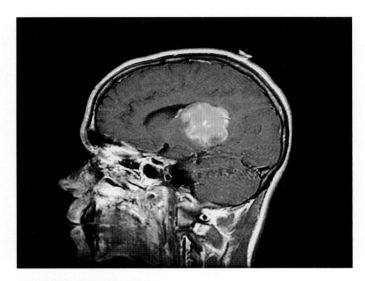

FIGURE 77-7 A preoperative sagittal magnetic resonance image with contrast administration is shown. Because of the significant tumor–cerebrospinal fluid interface within the posterior aspect of the lateral ventricle, a transventricular approach (transsplenial or parieto-occipital) for tumor removal would be appropriate. Note the fiducial on the vertex of the scalp to be used for intraoperative stereotactic registration.

is universally accepted as beneficial in children but has not been reported specifically in children with thalamic gliomas. Although this technique would predictably offer a benefit for those children with focal disease that is unresectable or recurrent, the inherent difficulty in administering a highly focused field for diffuse infiltrating tumors is self-evident.

Chemotherapy

The use of chemotherapy for the treatment of thalamic gliomas is governed primarily by the age of the child, the histologic tumor type, the previous use of other treatment modalities, and the expected toxic side effects of the regimen in question. Enthusiasm for the use of chemotherapy principally stems from documented efficacy in similar tumor types in other anatomic sites. The most thoroughly studied group of patients has been those with low-grade tumors of the diencephalon, including the thalamus and hypothalamic or optic apparatus. Combination chemotherapy using carboplatin and vincristine or a nitrosourea-based multiagent regimen are established therapies with proved control rates for low-grade gliomas in children. Using the former regimen, the Children's Cancer Study Group showed a 56% radiographic response in a group of 58 children with diencephalic tumors.[31] In that particular study, there was no difference in disease control in patients who had a complete response compared with those who had a partial response. That study revealed that a younger age was the most significant predictor of outcome. Using a similar treatment approach for children afflicted with low-grade lesions of the thalamus and mesencephalon, Hoffman et al have also shown beneficial effects.[18] Using the nitrosourea multiagent approach, Prados et al reported a radiographic response rate of 36%, with a

59% disease-stabilization rate in 42 children, 33 of whom had tumors of the hypothalamus and optic chiasmatic region.[34] Thus adequate evidence supports that low-grade astrocytomas of the diencephalon exhibit significant radiographic responses and lasting control rates with chemotherapy.

Some efficacy using chemotherapy has been documented in supratentorial malignant gliomas in children. The Children's Cancer Study Group randomized 58 children with high-grade astrocytomas to receive either surgery and RT or surgery followed by RT and multiagent chemotherapy (CCNU, vincristine, and prednisone).[41] Treatment with chemotherapy prolonged survival, and 5-year event-free survival increased from 18% to 46%. Cooperative group studies have also established modest radiographic response rates (11% to 33%) in children with high-grade gliomas using other multiagent regimens.[11] High-dose chemotherapy with autologous stem cell rescue has also been shown to benefit children with recurrent high-grade astrocytomas in the supratentorial compartment. These study results support the application of a multiagent chemotherapeutic approach for children with malignant thalamic gliomas.

OUTCOME

The outcome of children with thalamic gliomas depends on individual features that have been shown to impact the disease progression. Included in these prognostic variables are growth pattern, histology, age, and for focal tumors, extent of resection. Generally, a focal growth pattern, young age, and low-grade histology are all established positive prognostic variables. Given the current proposed categorization of thalamic gliomas into the focal, diffuse, and bilateral groups, the outcome is discussed separately for each category.

Focal Thalamic Gliomas

As referred to earlier, the focal nature of these tumors has important implications with respect to the histopathology of the tumor and the ability to accomplish a complete resection. The best outcome data for the focal thalamic glioma include 23 patients with a thalamic JPA reported by Kelly in 1989.[19] Of the 19 patients in that series who had undergone complete resection confirmed with postoperative radiographic imaging, 18 were alive and well with no evidence of recurrence at a mean follow-up period of 22 months. Similarly, in a series of 14 patients undergoing aggressive microsurgical removal of a thalamic glioma, 3 had a more than 90% resection for a JPA.[42] These children were alive with no evidence of disease at follow-up ranging from 21 months to 52 months. This experience is similar to a very large body of literature pertaining to children with pilocytic astrocytomas of other locations, more than 90% of whom are expected to enjoy a 10-year, disease-free interval.

A similar outcome is expected for patients with other low-grade glial neoplasms that exhibit a pattern of focal growth, including PXA, ganglioglioma, and SEGA. For those patients experiencing a subtotal excision or recurrent disease, radiation therapy or chemotherapy, selection of which is principally guided by the patient's age, are used with encouraging results. Outcome using these therapeutic modalities is thought to be similar to the experience in children with the more common hypothalamic or optic apparatus gliomas, namely, 10-year survival rates of greater than 70%.

Diffuse Thalamic Gliomas

The expected outcome for these children given the inability to microscopically remove the entire tumor is decidedly worse. This worse outcome is further influenced by the tendency for the low-grade tumors to eventually transform to a more malignant phenotype with time.

Within this category of infiltrative tumors, the histologic grade is the single most important parameter affecting patient outcome. Krouwer and Prados reported on prognostic variables in 57 patients with a median age of 22 years and infiltrative gliomas of the thalamus.[22] The median survival of patients with low-grade astrocytoma compared with those having anaplastic astrocytoma (WHO grade III) was 198 weeks and 54 weeks, respectively. In the 1984 Toronto series of children with thalamic gliomas, the mean survival of 20 patients with malignant gliomas was 1.1 years.[6] Of the 72 patients in Kelly's series, the mean survival times were 91, 54, and 21 weeks after stereotactic biopsy for patients with grade II, III, or IV astrocytoma, respectively.[19] In an assessment of 27 patients of all ages, Beks et al reported that every patient with a malignant tumor died within a year.[5] Steiger et al also concluded that histology of the infiltrative tumor is the primary determinant to outcome.[42] During follow-up ranging from 6 to 52 months, progression was noted in 6 of 10 patients with malignant tumors and in no patient with a low-grade tumor. Using a labeling index as an estimate of cellular kinetics, Franzini et al assessed the outcome of 70 patients with thalamic tumors.[12] Over the 3-year follow-up period in that series, patients with a low labeling index had a 20% mortality rate compared with a 100% mortality rate in patients who had a high proliferative index. Thus it can be confidently stated that histologic grade is of paramount importance in assessing outcome in children with diffuse thalamic gliomas.

Age has also been a variable affecting outcome within the category of infiltrative thalamic gliomas. Patients with thalamic tumors have been reported to have an overall 5-year survival rate of 60% for children versus 21% for adults.[16] Among the 57 patients described by Krouwer and Prados, the median survival for patients with all grades of infiltrative thalamic gliomas was 90 weeks for those younger than age 18 compared with 70 weeks for those older than age 18.[22] This association between age and outcome is most likely explained by the close correlation between low-grade histology and young age.

The importance of extent of resection for infiltrative gliomas of the thalamus is definitely less clear than for the focal thalamic tumors. Nonrepresentative biopsies, patient selection bias, and inconsistent postsurgical treatment modalities make comparisons difficult. For the low-grade fibrillary astrocytoma category, the inability to significantly impact the outcome with aggressive surgical resection, balanced by the possibility of a protracted interval without symptom progression, strongly argues against any attempt at aggressive surgical resection. Although Kelly did show some benefit in high-grade tumors treated with aggressive resection and radiation therapy (mean survival 62 weeks) compared with those patients treated with stereotactic biopsy and radiation therapy (mean survival, 22 weeks), Kelly did admit a selection bias based on preoperative radiographic imaging.[19] Steiger et al also alluded to the poor outcome in patients who successfully underwent aggressive resections of high-grade thalamic gliomas followed by radiation therapy of 60 Gy.[42] Of the 10 patients with malignant astrocytomas (WHO III and IV), all had a greater than 70% resection, with 5 of those patients having a greater than 95% resection. During the follow-up period (6 to 52 months), 6 of the 10 patients had disease progression. The experience from the Hospital for Sick Children in Toronto, Canada, a study of 60 children with thalamic gliomas, revealed that the extent of resection did not affect outcome as an independent variable.[6] Thus even in light of the ability to perform near-total and gross-total excisions of enhancing malignant fibrillary astrocytomas, recurrence is the expectation with marginal long-term benefit. This, balanced by the added morbidity of aggressive resection versus a stereotactic or endoscopic biopsy, justifies a more conservative surgical approach directed toward diagnostic sampling. Thus a logical approach toward patients with suspect fibrillary astrocytomas of the thalamus is to avoid aggressive surgical resection and instead focus on histologic subtyping. Although studies from the cooperative pediatric oncology groups have repeatedly shown a benefit with degree of resection for malignant hemispheric gliomas, the recruitment of this approach for children with infiltrative astrocytomas of the thalamus is not currently supported.

Bilateral Thalamic Gliomas

Although histologically indistinct from the fibrillary astrocytoma of varying grades found elsewhere in the cerebrum, bilateral thalamic glioma portends an overall worse outcome. This may be explained by underestimations of the degree of malignancy through inaccurate tissue sampling or by the central deep location of the tumor. The progression-free survival, overall survival, and the development of progressive disease are all statistically worse for children with bithalamic involvement than for those with unilateral thalamic disease, regardless of the histopathology. In the largest series of patients studied with bithalamic involvement, 11 of 12 children with this entity died within 2 years of diagnosis.[36] This "histology-independent" subtype of thalamic gliomas in children is very reminiscent of the clinical behavior of diffuse pontine gliomas in children.

THERAPEUTIC RECOMMENDATIONS

There is no standard of care established for children with thalamic gliomas given the variable nature of the disease. Although recommendations are made with respect to the morphologic category outlined in this chapter, each patient must be approached individually.

Focal Thalamic Gliomas

Surgery

Because of the high likelihood that a focal tumor represents a benign pathology, and most probably, a JPA, every attempt should be made to perform a total surgical removal. This goal is obviously governed by the expected morbidity of the procedure. Specifically, the anatomic position dictates the appropriate surgical goal as well as the optimal surgical route. First, only tumors that exhibit a focal pattern of growth on MRI should be considered for aggressive surgical removal. Second, the relative position of the tumor within the thalamus must be used as a guide for an optimal and safe approach. In general, the safest surgical corridor is dictated by the shortest possible route to the best defined tumor-CSF interface.

In the event of total surgical removal of a thalamic JPA, surveillance MRI is used to monitor the disease. If a subtotal resection is encountered, then an expectant approach is advisable given the proclivity of this tumor to remain static for prolonged periods and in rare situations exhibit involution. The latter phenomena are well described in the patient having NF1.

Adjuvant Therapy

In the event that the well-circumscribed tumor is not amenable to resection or if progression of residual disease is experienced, adjuvant therapy is an option. For those patients younger than 5 years of age, chemotherapy is favored in an effort to delay the use of therapeutic radiation therapy. For older children, highly conformal, three-dimensional radiation therapy is recommended.

Diffuse Thalamic Gliomas

Surgery

Because of the invasive nature of this disease, irrespective of tumor grade, aggressive surgical resection with the intent to extirpate the tumor is ill advised. Instead, stereotactic or endoscopic tumor biopsy, depending on the particular tumor and the experience of the surgeon, are recommended. Exceptions to this approach would include patients with large infiltrative tumors who may benefit from aggressive tumor removal in an effort to alleviate mass effect or re-establish CSF drainage.

Adjuvant Therapy

For the child with a pathologically confirmed, diffuse low-grade thalamic glioma, the use of adjuvant therapy is debatable.

Features that may lead to the use of adjuvant therapy include symptomatic or radiographic progression or a failure of symptom resolution with simple CSF diversion. These criteria hold more significance in the NF1 population, given the well-recognized indolent behavior of low-grade gliomas in that group of individuals. Again, the use of neoadjuvant chemotherapy is recommended for low-grade thalamic tumor if the child is younger than age 5 and has progressive disease.

RT is universally recommended for a patient older than age 5 with a high-grade thalamic glioma following pathologic confirmation. Although dependent on actual tumor distribution, use of conformal radiation schemes is advised. Most therapeutic approaches for children with malignant thalamic astrocytomas include chemotherapy. This multimodality approach, namely, radiation combined with multiagent chemotherapy, is based on the concept of reducing the total radiation exposure and creating a synergistic tumoricidal effect. For a child younger than age 5, neoadjuvant chemotherapy is recommended in an effort to delay RT.

Bilateral Thalamic Gliomas

Surgery

The extremely poor outcome for children with bilateral thalamic gliomas provides no rationale for surgical intervention beyond treatment of hydrocephalus and tissue sampling.

Adjuvant Therapy

In the patient with a confirmed bilateral thalamic glioma, tumor grade is not used when deciding on a therapeutic approach. As in the child with a confirmed unilateral malignant thalamic glioma, combined chemotherapy and RT are typically used. However, in the situation with a rapidly progressive clinical course the case is justifiably made against the added potential toxicity from chemotherapy, and instead a palliative course of RT is offered.

References

1. Ajemann GA, Ward Jr AA: Speech representation in ventrolateral thalamus. Brain 94:669–680, 1971.
2. Albright AL, Sclabassi RJ: Use of the Cavitron ultrasonic surgical aspirator and evoked potentials for the treatment of thalamic and brainstem tumors in children. Neurosurgery 17:564–568, 1985.
3. Apuzzo M, Chandrasoma P, Zelman V, et al: Computerized tomographic guidance stereotaxis in the management of lesions of the third ventricular region. Neurosurgery 15:502–508, 1984.
4. Arseni C: Tumors of the basal ganglia. Arch Neurol Psychiatry 80:18–24, 1958.
5. Beks JW, Bouma GJ, Journee HL: Tumours of the thalamic region. A retrospective study of 27 cases. Acta Neurochir (Wien) 85:125–127, 1987.
6. Bernstein M, Hoffman HJ, Halliday WC, et al: Thalamic tumors in children: long term follow-up and treatment guidelines. J Neurosurg 61:649–656, 1984.
7. Burger PC, Choen KJ, Rosenblum MK, Tihan T: Pathology of diencephalic astrocytomas. Pediatr Neurosurg 32:214–219, 2000.
8. Cheek WR, Taveras JM: Thalamic tumors. J Neurosurg 24:505–513, 1966.
9. Cuccia V, Monges J: Thalamic tumors in children. Childs Nerv Syst 13:514–521, 1997.
10. Drake JM, Joy M, Goldenberg A, Kreindler D: Computer- and robot-assisted resection of thalamic astrocytomas in children. Neurosurgery 29:27–33, 1991.
11. Finlay JL, Geyer JR, Turski PA, et al: Pre-irradiation chemotherapy in children with high-grade astrocytoma: tumor response to two cycles of the '8-drugs-in-1-day' regimen. A Childrens Cancer Group study, CCG-945. J Neurooncol 21:255–265, 1994
12. Franzini A, Leocata F, Cajola L, et al: Low-grade glial tumors in basal ganglia and thalamus: natural history and biological reappraisal. Neurosurgery 35:817–823, 1994.
13. Goel A: Preoperative shunts in thalamic tumours. Neurol India 48:347–350, 2000.
14. Greenberger JS, Cassady JR, Levene MB: Radiation therapy of thalamic, midbrain, and brain stem gliomas. Radiology 122:463–468, 1976.

15. Greenwood Jr J: Radical surgery of tumors of the thalamus and third ventricle area. Surg Neurol 1:29–33, 1973.

16. Grigsby PW, Thomas PR, Schwartz HG, Fineberg BB: Multivariate analysis of prognostic factors in pediatric and adult thalamic and brainstem tumors. Int J Radiat Oncol Biol Phys 16:649–655, 1989.

17. Hirose G, Lombroso CT, Eisenberg H: Thalamic tumors in childhood. Arch Neurol 32:740–744, 1975.

18. Hoffman HJ, Soloniuk DS, Humphreys RP, et al: Management and outcome of low-grade astrocytomas of the midline in children: a retrospective review. Neurosurgery 33:964–973, 1993.

19. Kelly PJ: Stereotactic biopsy and resection of thalamic astrocytomas. Neurosurgery 25:185–194, 1989.

20. Kim DI, Yoon PH, Ryu YH, et al: MRI of germinomas arising from the basal ganglia and thalamus. Neuroradiology 40:507–511, 1998.

21. Krauss JK, Nobbe F, Wakhloo AK, et al: Movement disorders in astrocytomas of the basal ganglia and the thalamus. J Neurol Neurosurg Psychiatry 55:1162–1167, 1992.

22. Krouwer HGJ, Prados MD: Infiltrative astrocytomas of the thalamus. J Neurosurg 82:548–557, 1995.

23. Kumar R, Jain R, Tandon V: Thalamic glioblastoma with cerebrospinal fluid dissemination in the peritoneal cavity. Pediatr Neurosurg 31:242–245, 1999.

24. Martinez-Lage JF, Perez-Espejo MA, Esteban JA, Poza M: Thalamic tumors: clinical presentation. Childs Nerv Syst 18:405–411, 2002.

25. McGirr SJ, Kelly PJ, Scheitauer BW: Stereotactic resection of juvenile pilocytic astrocytoma of the thalamus and basal ganglia. Neurosurgery 20:447–452, 1987.

26. McKissock W, Paine KWE: Primary tumors of the thalamus. Brain 81:41–63, 1958.

27. Messing-Junger AM, Floeth FW, Pauleit D, et al: Multimodal target point assessment for stereotactic biopsy in children with diffuse bithalamic astrocytomas. Childs Nerv Syst 18:445–449, 2002.

28. Nass R, Boyce L, Leventhal S, et al: Acquired aphasia in children after surgical resection of left-thalamic tumors. Dev Med Child Neurol 42:580–590, 2000.

29. Ojemann GA, Ward Jr AA: Speech representation in ventrolateral thalamus. Brain 94:669–690, 1971.

30. Ozek M, Ture U: Surgical approach to thalamic tumors. Childs Nerv Syst 18:450–456, 2002.

31. Packer RJ, Ater J, Allen J, et al: Carboplatin and vincristine chemotherapy for children with newly diagnosed progressive low-grade gliomas. J Neurosurg 86:747–754, 1997.

32. Palma L, Russo A, Mercuri S: Cystic cerebral astrocytomas in infancy and childhood. Child's Brain 10:79–91, 1983.

33. Partlow GD, del Carpio-O'Donovan R, Melanson D, Peters TM: Bilateral thalamic glioma: review of eight cases with personality change and mental deterioration. AJNR 13:1225–1230, 1992.

34. Prados MD, Edwards MS, Rabbitt J, et al: Treatment of pediatric low-grade gliomas with a nitrosurea-based multiagent chemotherapy regimen. J Neurooncol 32:235–241, 1997.

35. Prados MD, Wara WM, Edwards MSB, et al: The treatment of brain stem and thalamic gliomas with 78 Gy of hyperfractionated radiation therapy. Int J Radiation Oncology Biol Phys 32:85–91, 1995.

36. Reardon DA, Gajjar A, Sanford RA, et al: Bithalamic involvement predicts poor outcome among children with thalamic glial tumors. Pediatr Neurosurg 29:29–35, 1998.

37. Rekate HL, Ruch T, Nulsen FE, et al: Needle biopsy of tumors in the region of the third ventricle. J Neurosurg 54:338–341, 1981.

38. Smyth GE, Stern K: Tumours of the thalamus: a clinicopathological study. Brain 61:339–374, 1938.

39. Souweidane MM, Hoffman HJ: Current treatment of thalamic gliomas in children. J Neurooncol 28:157–166, 1996.

40. Souweidane MM, Sandberg DI, Bilsky MG, Gutin PH: Endoscopic biopsy for tumors of the third ventricle. Pediatr Neurosurg 33:132–137, 2000.

41. Sposto R, Ertel IJ, Jenkin RD, et al: The effectiveness of chemotherapy for treatment of high grade astrocytoma in children: results of a randomized trial. A report from the Childrens Cancer Study Group. J Neurooncol 1:165–177, 1989.

42. Steiger HJ, Götz C, Schmid-Elsaesser R, Stummer W: Thalamic astrocytomas: surgical anatomy and results of a pilot series using maximum microsurgical removal. Acta Neurochir (Wien) 142:1327–1337, 2000.

43. Tamaki N, Lin T, Shiratake K, et al: Germ cell tumors of the thalamus and the basal ganglia. Childs Nerv Syst 6:34–37, 1990.

44. Torkildsen A: Should extirpation be attempted in cases of neoplasm in or near the third ventricle of the brain? Experiences with a palliative method. J Neurosurg 5:249–275, 1948.

45. Tovi D, Schisano G, Liljeqvist B: Primary tumors of the region of the thalamus. J Neurosurg 18:730–740, 1961.

46. Villarejo F, Amaya C, Perez Diaz C, et al: Radical surgery of thalamic tumors in children. Childs Nerv Syst 10:111–114, 1994.

47. Wald SL, Fogelson MH, McLaurin RL: Cystic thalamic gliomas. Child's Brain 9:381–393, 1982.

48. Wang PY, Kaufman WE, Koth CW, et al: Thalamic involvement in neurofibromatosis type 1: evaluation with proton magnetic resonance spectroscopic imaging. Ann Neurol 47:477–484, 2000.

49. Ward A, Spurling G: The conservative treatment of third ventricle tumors. J Neurosurg 5:124–130, 1948.

50. Yasargil M: Microneurosurgery, Vol. IV A. New York, Thieme, 1994.

51. Yasue M, Tanaka H, Nakajima M, et al: Germ cell tumors of the basal ganglia and thalamus. Pediatr Neurosurg 19:121–126, 1993.

CHAPTER 78

MIDBRAIN GLIOMAS

Charles Matouk, Patrick McDonald, and James M. Drake

Midbrain gliomas constitute a distinct subgroup of brainstem tumors that arise primarily in the midbrain (diencephalon). In 1952 Kernohan and Sayre described midbrain tumors as being "in all probability the smallest tumors in the human body that led to the death of the patient."[8] Over the next 40 years, the perceived poor prognosis of all brainstem tumors was reinforced by the inexorable progression and treatment failure of the most common brainstem tumors, diffuse intrinsic pontine gliomas (DIPGs). It is only recently, in the past 15 years, with the advent of readily available computed tomography (CT) and, in particular, magnetic resonance imaging (MRI), that distinct subgroups of brainstem tumors have been identified that demonstrate a more indolent natural history and better responsiveness to therapeutic interventions. Examples include cervicomedullary and dorsal exophytic tumors, as well as the subject of this chapter, midbrain gliomas.[16]

Intrinsic midbrain tumors, like virtually all brainstem tumors, are glial in origin. They represent a heterogeneous group of lesions that can be broadly classified, based on lesion location, as tectal or tegmental. To predict lesion behavior and define an appropriate management strategy, therefore, tumor histology is often insufficient. A careful clinical evaluation and meticulous attention to imaging characteristics are the cornerstones on which treatment decisions are made. Not discussed in this chapter are tumors that arise from above (e.g., the thalamus or pineal region) or below (e.g., the pons or medulla) to encroach on the diencephalon. They demonstrate the same natural history as tumors native to their region of origin. This chapter provides a conceptual framework for the evaluation and treatment of intrinsic midbrain gliomas. Special consideration will be given to patients with neurofibromatosis type 1 (NF1) who harbor brainstem lesions, because their natural history and management strategy differ considerably from other patients. Emphasis is placed on epidemiology, diagnosis, imaging characteristics, histology, treatment, and outcome.

EPIDEMIOLOGY

Brainstem tumors constitute 20% of all pediatric brain tumors. They can arise anywhere in the brainstem; however, the majority (approximately 80%) are DIPGs that demonstrate relentless progression. Midbrain gliomas represent approximately 15% of all pediatric brainstem tumors. They are evenly distributed between the tectum and tegmentum and do not show a sex predominance.[21] Unlike their more malignant pontine counterparts, patients tend to seek treatment later in childhood;

however, midbrain tumors have been diagnosed in patients of all ages. Benign intrinsic tectal tumors, in particular, often appear after the age of 10 years.[9]

Brainstem tumors are well described in children with NF1; however, they are often difficult to distinguish from more common non-neoplastic hamartomas.[14] In one large pediatric series, 31 of 35 patients (89%) with NF1 demonstrated MRI brain abnormalities.[15] In another series of patients with NF1 and brainstem abnormalities, 11 of 25 patients had midbrain lesions.[2]

DIAGNOSIS

The clinical presentation of intrinsic midbrain gliomas is influenced by their location in the midbrain. The classical presentation of intrinsic tectal tumors is symptoms and signs of raised intracranial pressure (RICP). These tumors obstruct the aqueduct of Sylvius, resulting in acquired obstructive triventricular hydrocephalus. This produces the clinical constellation of headache, nausea and vomiting, lethargy, and altered level of consciousness. Children with long-standing hydrocephalus may also have decreased visual acuity secondary to papilledema. These symptoms may have been present for months to years. In infants and young children, physical examination may reveal macrocrania. Rarely, a disturbance of ocular movements is described as the initial presentation of a tectal mass. The most common ocular movement disorder, in this context, is Parinaud's syndrome, defined as the clinical constellation of supranuclear paresis of upward gaze, convergence-retraction nystagmus, and light-near dissociation of the pupils. It is thought to result from pressure on the tectal plate and often resolves after treatment of hydrocephalus without the institution of tumor-specific therapy.[9] Other signs include long-tract signs, ataxia, amenorrhea, and precocious puberty.[13]

In contrast, patients with tegmental tumors rarely have hydrocephalus and symptoms and signs of RICP. Clinical manifestations result from involvement (or compression) of critical midbrain structures including the cerebral peduncles and cranial nerve nuclei subserving eye movements. Their clinical prodrome is somewhat shorter in duration, ranging from weeks to months. Symptoms and signs include motor weakness, sensory disturbances, loss of coordination, and ataxia, as well as diplopia and other ocular symptoms.[17,21] Rarely they include contralateral tremor (ostensibly from involvement of the red nucleus) and parkinsonism (from probable involvement of the substantia nigra and disruption of the basal ganglia circuitry).[12]

When a midbrain glioma is suspected, a search should be undertaken for the clinical manifestations of NF1 established by the National Institutes of Health Consensus Development Conference.[10] Conversely, patients with NF1 have an increased risk of brain neoplasia. Patients with even subtle neurologic manifestations should be investigated with MRI.[13]

IMAGING CHARACTERISTICS

The widespread availability of MRI is the single most important advance in the characterization of midbrain gliomas. Unlike CT scanning, it is not hampered by bone artifact from the skull base, dental prosthetic artifacts, and poor resolution.[13] A large number of lesions can effectively be excluded based on pathognomonic imaging features, including other neoplasms (ependymoma, medulloblastoma, ganglioglioma, primitive neuroectodermal tumor), vascular malformations (arteriovenous malformation, cavernous malformation), infectious lesions (abscess, encephalitis, tuberculoma) and demyelination.[9,11] Tumors that arise in other locations and secondarily involve the diencephalon can be distinguished from intrinsic midbrain lesions more reliably with MRI. Lastly, subgroups of intrinsic midbrain gliomas can be distinguished that have an especially good prognosis (e.g., benign intrinsic tectal tumors).

Tectal gliomas may not be directly visualized on CT scans; they are betrayed only by the presence of obstructive triventricular hydrocephalus. They may also appear as a "fullness" of the tectal plate, also described as "globular" or "bulbous." Calcification is a common CT finding. MRI classically reveals a hypointense or isointense lesion on T1-weighted images and a uniformly hyperintense lesion on T2-weighted images. Imaging characteristics are variable, however, and heterogeneous signal characteristics may be present.[19] This may indicate an associated tumor cyst. Extension may occur into the basal cisterns with displacement of the thalamus and caudal brainstem. Infiltration of these adjacent structures, however, is decidedly uncommon.[9,21] Contrast enhancement is absent (or minimal) in most tectal tumors; others may demonstrate marked and homogeneous enhancement (Figure 78-1).

On CT scans, tumors of the tegmentum typically appear as hypodense or isodense lesions. Areas of increased density may represent tumoral hemorrhage or areas of calcification. MRI demonstrates tumors that are predominantly hypointense or isointense on T1-weighted images and hyperintense on T2-weighted images. Mixed signal characteristics and prominent

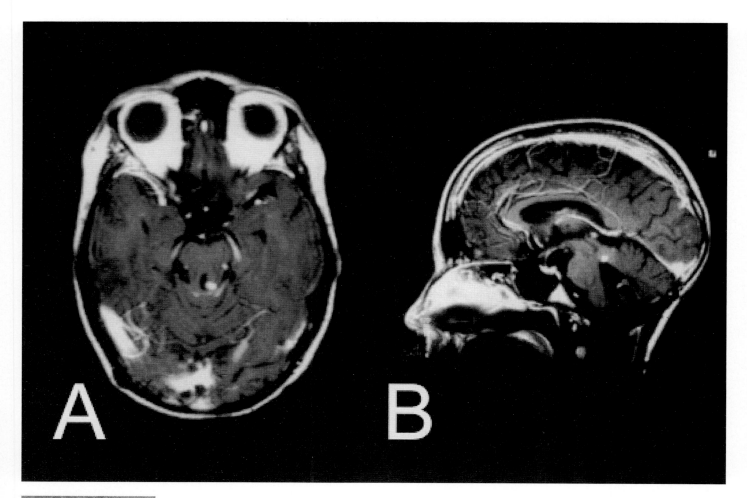

FIGURE 78-1   Axial (A) and sagittal (B) T1-weighted magnetic resonance imaging demonstrates a left-sided, focal tectal mass with marked, homogeneous contrast enhancement after the administration of gadolinium.

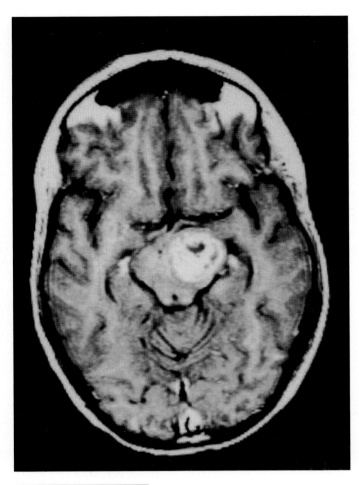

FIGURE 78-2 Axial fluid-attenuated inversion recovery (FLAIR) magnetic resonance imaging demonstrates a focal tegmental tumor of the left cerebral peduncle. Note the mixed signal characteristics and prominent enhancement after the administration of gadolinium.

cystic components are common features. Rostral and caudal extension of the tumor is also commonly seen. Contrast enhancement is typically prominent. These tumors may be *focal*, with excellent demarcation from surrounding structures, or infiltrating (*diffuse*) (Figure 78-2).[9,17,21]

In patients with NF1, distinguishing between non-neoplastic hamartomatous lesions, low-grade gliomas, and malignant tumors is not trivial. Labeled *unidentified bright objects* (UBOs), they typically appear as high signal intensity abnormalities on T2-weighted MRI in the cerebellum, brainstem, and basal ganglia. They may demonstrate mass effect and contrast enhancement.[14] They are dynamic lesions that may grow, regress, or disappear over time. It is hoped that newer techniques in neuroimaging (e.g., magnetic resonance spectroscopy and diffusion-weighted imaging) will help distinguish between UBOs and gliomas.

TUMOR HISTOLOGY

Most midbrain lesions are low-grade gliomas. Different published series report a predominance of pilocytic (WHO grade I) or fibrillary astrocytomas (WHO grade II). Some groups claim that pilocytic astrocytomas carry a better overall prognosis.[6] Other large centers have reported better outcomes for patients with fibrillary astrocytomas in the midline.[7] There is no consensus in the literature.

THERAPY

The management of intrinsic midbrain gliomas depends on their critical location in the midline and proximity to the cerebral aqueduct. For any midbrain lesion, two questions must be answered:

1. Does the patient have symptomatic hydrocephalus that requires a cerebrospinal fluid (CSF)-diversionary procedure?
2. Does the patient require any tumor-specific therapy?

Patients with midbrain gliomas may require a CSF-diversionary procedure for relief of symptomatic obstructive triventricular hydrocephalus. Ventriclo-peritoneal (VP) shunting is the standard procedure. In recent years, endoscopic third ventriculostomy (ETV) has superseded VP shunting as the treatment of choice in the management of tumoral aqueductal stenosis. The impetus for change is the high failure rate of implanted shunt systems, with nearly 50% failing in the first 2 years.[5] ETV is also a conceptually appealing alternative, because it involves the creation of a stoma in the floor of the third ventricle connecting the ventricular system directly to the subarachnoid space in the interpeduncular cistern, and bypassing the obstruction at the level of the cerebral aqueduct.[4] Recent reports indicate excellent long-term control of hydrocephalus following ETV in children with tectal plate gliomas.[22]

Tectal gliomas represent a particularly indolent form of midbrain lesion. Typically, patients have symptoms and signs of RICP and no focal neurologic deficits. MRI reveals triventricular hydrocephalus, a "bulbous" tectum that is hyperintense on T2-weighted images, and no (or minimal) contrast enhancement. Tectal tumors with these clinico-radiographic characteristics have been termed *benign intrinsic tectal tumors* and are treated by CSF-diversion alone.[3,9] No tumor-specific therapy is required. These lesions can progress, however, and require close follow-up. Our policy is to follow these children with serial MRI every 6 months in the first year and then yearly thereafter.

How are patients with tectal gliomas who have focal neurologic signs, tumor extension into the thalamus and more caudal brainstem, and contrast enhancement on MRI managed? Again, a trial of CSF-diversion alone is advocated. Many of these children show complete symptom relief and long-term lesion stability on serial MRI. Some tumors have even been observed to involute and disappear after successful ETV.[1,7] Other tumors will progress both clinically and radiographically and require a more aggressive philosophy of intervention. These lesions are subjected to biopsy, cyst drainage, or surgical debulking of any exophytic component. If biopsy only or cyst drainage is planned, the procedure may be performed by neuroendoscopy. The purpose of surgery is threefold: (1) to obtain histologic confirmation of the lesion; (2) to relieve local mass effect and possibly alleviate neurologic deficits; and (3) to reduce tumor burden. Radical excision is not the goal.[7] Adjuvant therapy is withheld unless the patient demonstrates (1) high-grade tumor histology, (2) continued tumor progression or recurrence, or (3) very large tumor size and partial resection. Adjuvant therapies are briefly discussed in the following section, "Recurrence."

The therapy of tegmental tumors has evolved considerably over the past decade. Operating within the midbrain tegmentum was once thought to carry an unacceptable risk of severe neurologic morbidity and mortality. With refinement in microneurosurgical techniques, the advent of the ultrasonic aspirator, and the use of frameless stereotaxy and image guidance, lesions of the midbrain can now be approached more safely.[7,11,21] Because these lesions typically cause progressive focal neurologic deficits, surgical intervention is often indicated. Many of these tumors have distinct tumor margins and can be completely excised. Others, for example, diffuse tegmental tumors, have indistinct margins and infiltrate adjacent neural structures. They cannot be surgically resected without unacceptable morbidity and mortality. Stereotactic or open biopsy often reveals a high-grade astrocytoma. The administration of adjuvant therapy in these cases is mandatory.

Patients with NF1 and midbrain lesions represent a special management dilemma. Whether these lesions represent true midbrain gliomas or UBOs is controversial. It appears that both demonstrate a very indolent natural history. A conservative policy of serial MRI for these patients is recommended. Many of these lesions will fluctuate over time, with the majority regressing as the patients enter adolescence and early adulthood.[2] Only in the face of relentless clinical and radiographic progression (a rare occurrence) is surgical intervention indicated.

RECURRENCE

The management of tumor recurrence is controversial and includes the following options: (1) surgery, (2) fractionated or single-dose stereotactic radiation (radiosurgery), or (3) chemotherapy.

There is reluctance to commit children with low-grade neoplasms to potentially harmful adjuvant therapies. Because prognosis is generally good and long-term survivors are expected, the harmful effects of radiation and chemotherapy are to be avoided. There is general consensus in the literature that repeated surgical resection (or debulking) is indicated for tumor recurrence and concomitant clinical progression.[7] This has produced acceptable outcomes.

Some tumors will recur (or progress) after a secondary surgical procedure, or cannot be safely reapproached. In these cases, adjuvant therapy is indicated. Fractionated stereotactic radiation therapy is given to older children. Some groups advocate the use of radiosurgery; however, its efficacy remains largely unproven.[18] The effects of ionizing radiation on the developing nervous system are not inconsequential and include intellectual and behavioral disturbances, endocrinopathies, vasculopathies (moyamoya disease, cavernous malformations), and induction of high-grade secondary malignancies. Chemotherapy, generally a combination of carboplatin and vincristine, may be given to younger children (younger than 3 years old)

in an attempt to avoid these harmful effects. Some dramatic results have been observed.[21]

OUTCOME

It can be said that the only commonality between midbrain gliomas and their more malignant counterparts, DIPG, is their brainstem location. Patients with DIPG rarely survive longer than 18 months. Patients with midbrain gliomas, in comparison, have an indolent natural history with the expectation of long-term survival.

In particular, patients with benign intrinsic tectal tumors have a particularly good outcome. One series followed six such patients for 8 months to 17 years. None demonstrated clinical or radiographic progression.[9] In another series, six of seven patients demonstrated radiographic (but not clinical) progression. Although three cases underwent biopsy, none underwent a significant surgical debulking or received adjuvant therapy. No patient experienced any tumor-related morbidity at up to 7 years of follow-up.[3] There is general agreement in the literature that outcome in these tumors is excellent.

For patients with tectal tumors that demonstrate clinical and radiographic progression, the benefit of surgery is clear, and patients rarely require adjuvant therapy. In one series, six patients with tectal gliomas and progressive clinical syndromes were treated with a minimal or major debulking procedure, two patients receiving additional postoperative radiation therapy. With a mean follow-up of 2.5 years, all patients were clinically improved from the time of diagnosis. Some lesions even demonstrated involution on serial imaging.[21]

In one recent series of tegmental tumors, aggressive surgical resection was performed in seven patients with low-grade astrocytomas of the cerebral peduncle. Patients were followed for 1 to 8.5 years, and no patient received adjuvant therapy. Only one patient had documented tumor recurrence. Three patients who had undergone subtotal resections showed spontaneous involution of the residual tumor on serial MRI.[20] Patients with diffuse tegmental tumors share the same poor prognosis as diffuse intrinsic pontine gliomas, discussed in another chapter.

CONCLUSION

Midbrain gliomas represent a distinct group of brainstem tumors in the pediatric population that demonstrate a relatively indolent course. Many of these lesions require only a CSF-diversionary procedure, while others benefit from multimodal therapy, including surgery, radiation, or chemotherapy. Deciding which tumors can be monitored and which warrant tumor-specific therapy requires careful attention to the history, physical examination, and MRI characteristics. In particular, clinical and radiographic progression mandate a more aggressive philosophy of intervention. Finally, patients with NF1 represent a unique subgroup of patients that may have midbrain lesions. These tumors are characterized by an especially benign course and can usually be followed safely with serial clinical and radiologic examinations.

References

1. Alkhani AM, Boop FA, Rutka JT: Involution of enhancing intrinsic tectal tumors after endoscopic third ventriculostomy. J Neurosurg 91:863–866, 1999.
2. Bilaniuk LT, Molloy PT, Zimmerman RA, et al: Neurofibromatosis type 1: brain stem tumors. Neuroradiology 39:642–653, 1997.
3. Bowers DC, Georgiades C, Aronson LJ, et al: Tectal gliomas: natural history of an indolent lesion in pediatric patients. Pediatr Neurosurg 32:24–29, 2000.
4. Cinalli G: Alternatives to shunting. Childs Nerv Syst 15:718–731, 1999.
5. Drake JM, Kestle JRW, Milner R, et al: Randomized trial of cerebrospinal fluid shunt valve design in pediatric hydrocephalus. Neurosurgery 43:294–305, 1998.
6. Fisher PG, Breiter SN, Carson BS, et al: A clinicopathologic reappraisal of brain stem tumor classification. Cancer 89:1569–1576, 2000.
7. Hoffman HJ, Soloniuk DS, Humphreys RP, et al: Management and outcome of low-grade astrocytomas of the midline in children: a retrospective review. Neurosurgery 33:964–971, 1993.
8. Kernohan JW, Sayre GS: Tumors of the Central Nervous System. Atlas of Tumor Pathology, Section X, Fascicle 35. Washington DC: Armed Forces Institute of Pathology, 1952.
9. May PL, Blaser SI, Hoffman HJ, et al: Benign intrinsic tectal "tumors" in children. J Neurosurg 74:867–871, 1991.
10. NIH Consensus Development Conference: Neurofibromatosis conference statement. Arch Neurol 45:575–578, 1988.
11. Pendl G, Vorkapic P, Koniyama M: Microsurgery of midbrain lesions. Neurosurgery 26:641–648, 1990.
12. Pohle T, Krauss JK: Parkinsonism in children resulting from mesencephalic tumors. Mov Dis 14:842–846, 1999.
13. Raffel C, Hudgins R, Edwards MSB: Symptomatic hydrocephalus: initial findings in brain stem gliomas not detected on computed tomographic scans. Pediatrics 82:733–737, 1988.
14. Raininko R, Thelin L, Eeg-Olofsson O: Atypical focal non-neoplastic brain changes in neurofibromatosis type I: mass effect and contrast enhancement. Neuroradiology 43:586–590, 2001.
15. Raininko R, Thelin L, Eeg-Olofsson O: Non-neoplastic brain abnormalities on MRI in children and adolescents with neurofibromatosis type 1. Neuropediatrics 32:225–230, 2001.
16. Reddy AT, Mapstone TB: Brain stem tumors. In Bernstein M, Berger MS (eds): Neuro-Oncology: The Essentials. New York, Thieme Medical Publishers, 2000.
17. Robertson PL, Muraszko KM, Brungberg JA, et al: Pediatric midbrain tumors: a benign subgroup of brainstem gliomas. Pediatr Neurosurg 22:65–73, 1995.
18. Somaza SC, Kondziolka D, Lunsford LD, et al: Early outcomes after stereotactic radiosurgery for growing pilocytic astrocytomas in children. Pediatr Neurosurg 25:109–115, 1996.
19. Sun B, Wang CC, Wang J: MRI characteristics of midbrain tumors. Neuroradiology 41:158–162, 1999.
20. Tomita T, Cortes RF: Astrocytomas of the cerebral peduncle in children: surgical experience in seven patient. Childs Nerv Syst 18:225–230, 2002.
21. Vandertop WP, Hoffman HJ, Drake JM, et al: Focal midbrain tumors in children. Neurosurg 31:185–194, 1992.
22. Wellons JC, Tubbs RS, Banks JT, et al: Long-term control of hydrocephalus via endoscopic third ventriculostomy in children with tectal plate gliomas. Neurosurgery 51:63–68, 2002.

CHAPTER 79

SUPRATENTORIAL HIGH-GRADE GLIOMAS

Ian F. Pollack

Most primary supratentorial hemispheric tumors in children are gliomas,[38] as in adults. However, in contrast to the situation in adults, high-grade gliomas are substantially less common than low-grade lesions. Although pediatric high-grade gliomas are comparable histologically to their adult counterparts, they exhibit a number of distinct properties. First, cooperative group studies have demonstrated a substantial improvement in survival with the use of chemotherapy as an adjuvant to surgery and irradiation for children with high-grade gliomas,[15] which contrasts with the modest benefits of chemotherapy for adults with these tumors. Second, such studies have indicated a strong correlation between resection extent and outcome in childhood high-grade gliomas, an association that remains controversial in adults, which may reflect age-related features in the growth properties of a subset of pediatric malignant gliomas that renders them amenable to extensive resection.[9,15,57] Third, recent molecular and biologic studies have shown notable differences between childhood and adult malignant gliomas and have called attention to the existence of prognostically distinct subsets of tumors in both age groups.[6,43,52,53] This chapter reviews the clinical presentation, epidemiology, diagnostic evaluation, pathology, treatment, and outcome of pediatric high-grade gliomas and discusses how novel therapies are being incorporated into patient management.

DIAGNOSIS

Cerebral hemispheric tumors characteristically cause seizures; focal neurologic deficits, such as hemiparesis, hemisensory deficits, or aphasia, depending on the site of the lesion; and symptoms of increased intracranial pressure.[3,9,12,37] In contrast to low-grade gliomas, which often manifest with an insidious onset of symptoms over a period of months or with a long history of seizures, the mode of symptom progression in high-grade lesions is generally more rapid. Seizures are the initial symptom in approximately 30% of children, less than with low-grade lesions. In contrast, signs of increased intracranial pressure and focal neurologic deficits are more common in high-grade gliomas. A sudden neurologic deterioration occurs in 5% to 10% of children, which in most cases reflects intratumoral hemorrhage. Apart from these stroke-like events, severe symptoms and signs appear anecdotally to be less common among children diagnosed in the magnetic resonance imaging (MRI) era than in historical reports, reflecting the earlier detection of these tumors at a less symptomatic stage.

EPIDEMIOLOGY

High-grade gliomas compose approximately 20% of hemispheric gliomas in children[38] and occur at an incidence of approximately 2 cases per million children per year. However, the exact frequency of these tumors has not been precisely defined, because previous estimates may have been confounded by the inclusion of various low-grade glioma variants, such as pleomorphic xanthoastrocytoma and aggressive-appearing pilocytic tumors,[28,36] which were sometimes mistaken for high-grade gliomas in earlier reports.[5] Current estimates, based on North American cooperative group and cancer registry data, are that approximately 100 children with high-grade supratentorial gliomas are diagnosed annually.

Although a definite environmental or genetic "cause" for most gliomas is unknown, a subgroup of affected children do have an underlying genetic syndrome, such as neurofibromatosis type 1 (NF1) or Turcot's syndrome, that predisposes them to develop central nervous system tumors. NF1 is caused by a mutation in the neurofibromin gene on chromosome 17q11.2, which encodes a protein with GTPase-activating properties that functions in signal transduction.[46] Although the most characteristic intracranial neoplasms in affected patients are optic-hypothalamic gliomas, a small percentage of patients develop lesions in the cerebral hemispheres. These are generally low-grade gliomas; however, high-grade lesions have also been observed.[46]

Patients with Turcot's syndrome exhibit colonic polyposis in association with intracranial neoplasms. This disorder results from mutations in either the *APC* gene or in DNA mismatch repair genes.[21] Affected patients generally have malignant gliomas or primitive neuroectodermal tumors (PNETs). A number of less common syndromes have also been linked anecdotally with glial neoplasms, but a molecular basis for these associations remains to be defined.

IMAGING

Computed tomography (CT) or MRI is usually the only diagnostic study needed to establish the presence of a supratentorial hemispheric tumor. High-grade gliomas typically exhibit irregular or ringlike enhancement on CT and MRI, with a surrounding area of low density on CT, low intensity on T1-weighted MRI, and high intensity on T2-weighted MRI that represents infiltrating tumor and edema. Because these lesions grow more rapidly than low-grade gliomas, they often produce substantially greater local mass effect. It is sometimes difficult to distinguish high-grade gliomas from other malignant hemispheric tumors, such as ependymomas and PNETs; however, certain features of the latter neoplasms (e.g., calcification in ependymomas) can help the clinician make an educated guess as to the identity of the tumor preoperatively. Pleomorphic xanthoastrocytomas, a subset of which are classified as high-grade gliomas histologically, characteristically arise at or close to the cortical surface in association with an underlying cyst. Enhancement of the solid tumor component is typically seen.

Other diagnostic studies are rarely needed preoperatively. Lumbar puncture should specifically be avoided because of the risk of herniation and death. Angiography is indicated only for tumors that have unusual vascularity or cause hemorrhage, specifically if concern is raised that the lesion may be a vascular malformation. Neuraxis imaging is needed only if there is strong clinical indication of the presence of disseminated disease (which is rare at the time of diagnosis) or if another diagnosis, such as primitive neuroectodermal tumor, is being considered strongly, and is best reserved for the postoperative period after a histologic diagnosis has been obtained. If indicated, it can then be combined with imaging of the head to provide an assessment of the extent of postoperative residual disease.

TUMOR HISTOLOGY

Supratentorial high-grade astrocytomas are generally subdivided into two major groups, specifically, anaplastic astrocytoma (AA; grade III) and glioblastoma multiforme (GBM; grade IV).[11,25] In recent World Health Organization classification guidelines,[25] AAs are characterized as astrocytomas with focal or diffuse hypercellularity, pleomorphism, nuclear atypia, and mitotic activity, whereas GBMs exhibit these features in addition to vascular proliferation or necrosis.

In addition to the more common high-grade gliomas, such as AA and GBM, other tumors that are classified as high-grade gliomas histologically include anaplastic oligodendroglial neoplasms and anaplastic variants of pleomorphic xanthoastrocytoma, ganglioglioma, and pilocytic astrocytoma. Oligodendroglial tumors are characterized by having spherical cells with hyperchromatic nuclei and a well-defined plasma membrane, which produces a "fried egg" appearance. Lesions that exhibit a major astrocytic component, either diffusely mixed with oligodendroglial cells or separated into distinct regions, are classified as oligoastrocytomas. Anaplastic (grade III) oligodendrogliomas and oligoastrocytomas exhibit features of anaplasia with mitoses, necrosis, and vascular proliferation that, in some cases, may be difficult to distinguish from GBM.

Pleomorphic xanthoastrocytomas arise most commonly in the temporal or parietal lobes, are often associated with a cyst, and are generally classified as low-grade, rather than high-grade, gliomas, despite their characteristic nuclear atypia, pleomorphism, and multinucleation. Abundant lipid-rich cells and pronounced reticulin reactivity, particularly in the regions of leptomeningeal invasion, are also typical. However, approximately 20% of these lesions exhibit malignant transformation with pronounced mitosis, necrosis, and endothelial prolifera-

tion[25,28,36] and are classified as high-grade (grade III or IV) gliomas. Similarly, a small subset of gangliogliomas and juvenile pilocytic astrocytomas exhibit evidence of mitosis, necrosis, and endothelial proliferation. Although these lesions are recognized as grade III (anaplastic) gliomas in contemporary histologic classification schemes,[25] the issue of whether to include such tumors in therapeutic studies with other high-grade gliomas remains controversial, because their behavior is generally more indolent than that of AAs.[15]

MOLECULAR PATHOGENESIS

Institutional studies by our group and others[6,40,45,48,52,53] have suggested that pediatric malignant gliomas may differ on a molecular and biologic basis from primary adult high-grade gliomas[22,27] and that appropriately selected tumor markers might provide a basis for refining outcome predictions for patients with these lesions. However, the small size of these institutional cohorts as well as the association between marker status and histology precluded determining whether these markers could provide data that had independent prognostic utility.

Children's Cancer Group (CCG) study B975 was therefore initiated to more conclusively evaluate the association between biologic and molecular genetic features and outcome in pediatric high-grade gliomas. This study incorporated the multi-institutional cohort of CCG-945, the largest clinical study of pediatric high-grade gliomas to date. The analysis approaches were based upon a combination of microdissection-based topographic genotyping with loss of heterozygosity and sequence analysis for genes of interest and immunohistochemical techniques.

Tumor specimens were obtained for 179 of the 231 children enrolled on this study, making this the largest collection of microdissected glioma specimens accrued from a consistently treated patient cohort and by far the largest group of childhood malignant glioma specimens ever assembled. Although this study remains in progress, its results to date indicate some notable differences in comparison with results in previous adult cohorts. In particular, there was a strong association between proliferation index (as assessed by labeling of the Ki-67 antigen using the MIB-1 antibody) and outcome, which was independent of the effect of tumor histology ($P = .004$), notwithstanding the association between histology and proliferation labeling ($P = .002$) and between histology and outcome ($P = .01$).[44] An independent association between proliferation index and outcome was also apparent after adjusting for the extent of resection, age, and sex, in addition to histology, in multivariate regression modeling ($P < .005$). An association between MIB-1 labeling index and outcome was evident among tumors classified as AA ($P = .02$) and those classified as GBM ($P = .046$).[44]

A second marker studied in this cohort was alteration in the p53 pathway, as determined both by direct mutational genotyping and p53 immunohistochemistry. To date, the status of TP53 mutations in exons 5 to 8 has been assessed in 121 tumors and p53 immunohistochemistry completed in 115. Forty tumors (33.1%) had mutations of TP53 within exons 5 to 8, and 41 had p53 overexpression. Children with tumors that had p53 overexpression or TP53 mutations exhibited a substantially worse progression-free survival than those with tumors that lacked these features.[43] Five-year progression-free survival was 44%

± 6% in the 74 children whose tumors had low levels of p53 expression versus 17% ± 6% in 41 children with p53 over-expression ($P = .0001$).

In contrast to reports involving adult high-grade gliomas, this analysis also demonstrated that p53 mutations and over-expression were significantly more common in grade IV than grade III tumors. Whereas overexpression was detected in 58% of glioblastomas, this finding was present in only 26% of AAs and only 21% of other grade III gliomas ($P < .002$). Despite the strong association between p53 alterations and histology, p53 overexpression was independently associated with outcome after stratifying for histology ($P = .005$).[43] An additional observation of this study was that p53 status was strongly associated with patient age. Children younger than 3 years had a significantly lower frequency of TP53 mutations than older children,[42] which suggests that the tumors in such patients may have arisen by a molecular pathway distinct from that in older patients. A trend toward more favorable outcomes among young children than older children with malignant gliomas has been noted by other groups,[13] which may reflect a greater sensitivity of the postoperative residual disease to adjuvant therapy associated with a normal p53 pathway.

The importance of these observations is not that they support reduction of therapy based on "favorable" marker status, but rather that they indicate prognosis in children with malignant gliomas may be significantly influenced by molecular and biologic factors, independent of clinical and histologic features, and that such factors may help to refine prognostic assessments that will facilitate the prospective evaluation of novel therapeutic strategies for these tumors.

In addition to proliferation and p53 status, a variety of other markers are currently being examined for their potential association with outcome in children with malignant gliomas, based on their known association with disease progression in adults with high-grade gliomas. These include EGFR amplification, a hallmark of primary glioblastomas in adults that appears to be less common in childhood gliomas[6,52]; PTEN deletions, which have been associated with an unfavorable outcome in an initial institutional pilot study[48]; and alterations of cell cycle–control genes, such as CDKN2A, p14[ARF], and CDK4.[22] In contrast to the potentially adverse prognostic effects of the previously discussed factors, studies involving adult high-grade gliomas indicate that deletions of chromosomes 1p and 19q may identify a subgroup of tumors with oligodendroglial features that have a generally favorable prognosis.[23] Evidence of such a potential association has not been confirmed in childhood malignant gliomas,[40] although further evaluation of the utility of this marker in oligodendroglial tumors is required. The fact that anaplastic oligodendroglial tumors from adults that have 1p deletions are now commonly treated with chemotherapy as an initial approach with deferral of irradiation is of particular interest in view of the cognitive risks of irradiation in young children. If a chemotherapy-responsive pediatric subgroup could also be reliably identified prospectively, this would offer the potential for improvement in functional outcome if irradiation could be safely deferred.[13,29]

SURGICAL TREATMENT

In general, surgical intervention forms the initial step in the treatment plan by providing tissue to establish the histologic diagnosis and by achieving cytoreduction, if this is safely feasible. Corticosteroids are generally administered upon admission in children with large tumors, or preoperatively in patients with smaller lesions, at a dose of 1 to 6 mg every 6 hours (for dexamethasone), depending on the size of the child. This medication is continued intraoperatively and then tapered during a period of 3 to 7 days if significant tumor debulking has been achieved. Because children with hemispheric tumors may be at risk for seizures during the perioperative period, anticonvulsants are generally administered preoperatively and continued for at least 1 week postoperatively.

The appropriate surgical strategy for a supratentorial high-grade glioma is influenced by the growth characteristics of the tumor as depicted by CT or, preferably, MRI. Ideally, for reasonably well-circumscribed lesions, an extensive resection should be the operative goal, if this can be achieved without inordinate risk, because resection extent has been associated with long-term outcome.[57]

Conversely, for some infiltrative, poorly circumscribed high-grade gliomas that cross the midline or extensively invade the deep nuclei and other critical brain regions, radical resection may not be feasible without unacceptable morbidity. In such instances, a percutaneous CT- or MRI-guided stereotactic biopsy may be preferable to an open operation with limited tumor removal as a means to safely establish the histologic diagnosis in preparation for adjuvant therapy. However, a number of adjuncts have become available during the past several years that facilitate extensive removal of lesions previously thought to be unresectable, or resectable only with substantial morbidity, thereby potentially increasing the percentage of tumors amenable to resection.

Frame-based or frameless stereotactic guidance systems provide three-dimensional localization of the tumor, which permits the surgeon to plan an operative approach that minimizes manipulation of functionally critical brain while providing optimal access to the tumor. Ultrasound is also useful for providing real-time feedback on the location of the lesion, which prevents problems with intraoperative brain movements that limit the accuracy of stereotactic techniques after the tumor resection has been initiated. Intraoperative MRI holds promise for further improving the accuracy of surgical navigation, assuming issues of cost and convenience can be resolved.

A variety of techniques have also been developed for functional localization of critical brain areas adjacent to or overlying the tumor. For superficial lesions, these adjuncts enable the surgeon to resect as much tumor as possible without damaging vital surrounding structures and, for deep lesions, allow the surgeon to choose a trajectory to the tumor that avoids traversing important loci. Cortical stimulation techniques are useful for identifying speech and motor areas in patients with tumors in proximity to these sites.[4] These techniques can be applied either extraoperatively, using grid or strip electrodes that have been implanted at a preliminary procedure, or intraoperatively, at the time of the planned tumor resection. Intraoperative somatosensory evoked potential recordings are also helpful for delineating the primary sensory cortex and central sulcus; however, in contrast to direct-stimulation techniques, this approach is not useful for mapping subcortical pathways. Functional MRI offers an alternative approach for localizing critical cortical and subcortical areas before beginning a tumor resection. Finally, for patients with intractable seizures in association with cerebral cortical tumors, electrocorticography is useful for determining whether the seizures originate from the area of the lesion and for identifying epileptogenic cortex adjacent to or distant from the tumor to optimize the chances for postoperative seizure control.[4]

ADJUVANT RADIATION THERAPY AND CHEMOTHERAPY

High-grade gliomas in children have conventionally been treated with maximal resection followed by radiation therapy to the tumor bed and a margin of surrounding brain, with a dosage of 5000 to 6000 cGy in 180 to 200 cGy/day fractions. Cooperative group studies have demonstrated that the administration of chemotherapy in addition to irradiation improves the chances for long-term survival, although to date the optimal treatment regimen remains uncertain. In the CCG-943 study, children who were randomly assigned to receive radiation therapy followed by CCNU (lomustine), vincristine, and prednisone (pCV) had a 5-year event-free survival of 46% versus 18% for patients treated with radiation therapy alone.[50] In a subsequent study (CCG-945), a more complex eight-drug regimen failed to further improve survival,[15] reflecting the low dose intensity of several components of the "8-in-1" regimen. This realization formed the impetus for subsequent studies that have administered more intensive submyeloablative regimens in a neoadjuvant (preirradiation) format and myeloablative regimens in both preirradiation and postirradiation settings.[2,20]

The Pediatric Oncology Group (POG) 9135 study compared the use of neoadjuvant cisplatin-BCNU versus cyclophosphamide-vincristine in patients with newly diagnosed high-grade gliomas. The cisplatin-BCNU arm was associated with a 20% 5-year event-free survival versus less than 5% for cyclophosphamide-vincristine ($P < .05$). Although encouraging results with cisplatin-BCNU were also reported in adult patients with high-grade gliomas,[19] a more recent phase III study noted no advantage in the use of neoadjuvant cisplatin-BCNU followed by radiation therapy versus radiation therapy with adjuvant BCNU. Subsequently, the CCG 9933 study compared three alkylating agents (carboplatin, ifosfamide, and cyclophosphamide), each administered with etoposide before irradiation, for patients with postoperative residual disease. Preliminary results suggested an unacceptably high rate of disease progression with a progression-free survival of only 15% at 24 months.[2] Similarly, the POG 9431 study compared neoadjuvant procarbazine and topotecan and noted insufficient activity of either agent to warrant further study.[10]

Although pilot studies of extremely high–dose chemotherapy have noted promising rates of long-term disease control, these approaches were also associated with significant rates of morbidity and mortality, which has limited their broad application for these tumors[20] and called into question whether strategies that incorporate intensification of chemotherapy improve overall outcome in terms of not only survival but also quality of life, in comparison with the results obtained with the pCV regimen from CCG-943 and -945. Unfortunately, direct comparisons between studies have until recently been hampered by the fact that inclusion criteria for many historical studies were based on institutional histologic review, whereas more recent studies have used central review based on con-

temporary World Health Organization guidelines. The importance of this distinction is highlighted by the fact that a central review of the initial histology in both the CCG-943 and -945 studies in the context of the recently published World Health Organization criteria[25] indicated that more than 30% of tumors did not fit current definitions of high-grade glioma and that the 5-year survival of review-confirmed tumors was approximately 20%,[5] substantially lower than previous reports[50] but similar to the results obtained with the nitrosourea-containing arm of the centrally reviewed POG-9135 study. Accordingly, to facilitate more reliable comparisons between study results, ongoing treatment protocols are relying almost exclusively on central review for study eligibility. In addition, planned comparisons with historical "controls" (e.g., the large randomized 945 study cohort) will be strictly limited to the subset of cases in which blinded central review of the original histologic material has been performed and has confirmed the presence of a high-grade glioma.

PROGNOSTIC FACTORS

Both the CCG-943 and -945 studies have called attention to a striking association between resection extent and outcome.[15,50,57] In the CCG-945 study, 3-year event-free survival was 54% for patients undergoing more than 90% tumor resection versus only 17% for patients undergoing biopsy.[57] It is, of course, impossible to exclude the possibility that certain tumors with more favorable biologic characteristics were inherently more amenable to extensive resection. Thus the more favorable outcome in such patients may in part have been an expression of these biologic characteristics, rather than being solely attributable to the more aggressive surgical intervention. In a similar context, the report of Campbell et al[9] noted a 5-year progression-free survival of 100% for the small subgroup of children who underwent a gross-total resection of all enhanced tumor. Such lesions typically were extremely well circumscribed both by imaging and at operation, suggesting that they constituted a biologically distinct group.

A second factor that has been associated with outcome in childhood malignant gliomas is tumor histology: Patients with GBM fare worse than those with AA,[15,50] with 5-year event-free survivals in the range of 10% to 15% and 25% to 30%, respectively. Several studies have also noted that high-grade gliomas other than AA or GBM have a more favorable outcome than predominantly astrocytic malignant gliomas.[15] This may in part result from a greater sensitivity of anaplastic oligodendroglial tumors to conventional chemotherapeutic agents, such as the combination of procarbazine, CCNU, and vincristine.[8]

As noted earlier, a number of molecular and biologic factors have been associated with outcome, specifically p53 expression status and proliferation index.[43,44] It is anticipated that additional markers will be identified during the next decade that will further refine the prognostic stratification of these tumors. However, it is important to reiterate that no marker to date has identified a "good-risk" group of pediatric malignant gliomas, and even among the subgroups with favorable marker profiles, more than 60% of patients eventually die from tumor progression, despite the best available conventional therapy. These results provide the impetus for the evaluation of a variety of novel therapeutic strategies for these challenging tumors.

RECURRENCE

The predominant site of disease progression for supratentorial malignant gliomas is at the primary site, which may be amenable to treatment by additional local therapy, such as surgical resection or stereotactic radiosurgery, or experimental chemotherapy. Despite aggressive therapy, the prognosis for long-term survival in such children is poor (albeit not hopeless), reflecting the failure of therapies to date to substantially slow the course of tumor growth in most patients. High-dose chemotherapy does appear to achieve a long-term survival rate of approximately 20% in children with localized recurrences,[20] substantially better than the results obtained with conventional doses of cytotoxic agents. Unfortunately, cerebrospinal fluid dissemination of tumor is detected in as many as one third of children with recurrent high-grade gliomas,[18] which drastically decreases the chances for achieving disease control. Improvements in the outcome of affected patients will likely depend on identifying and implementing novel therapeutic approaches that target the molecular pathways that are aberrantly activated in these tumors, employing new approaches to achieve improved local drug delivery, or initiating a host immune response to facilitate recognition and rejection of the tumor.

ONGOING STUDIES AND NOVEL THERAPIES

Although there are data to support the use of adjuvant chemotherapy in the treatment of children with high-grade glioma,[50] the appropriate agent upon which to build a more effective therapeutic platform remains unsettled. Although nitrosoureas have been a component of most active regimens for both children and adults with high-grade gliomas, their efficacy is modest, at best,[55] and the evaluation of new therapeutic approaches is warranted. At present, there are a wealth of novel agents and strategies being examined in children with newly diagnosed and, particularly, recurrent high-grade gliomas. Adequate discussion of the many single- and limited-institution pilot studies that are in progress is beyond the scope of this chapter. This presentation will therefore focus on the broader strategic initiatives that are ongoing or planned within the major pediatric cooperative groups in North America, specifically the Children's Oncology Group (COG; formed from the merger of the CCG and the POG) and the Pediatric Brain Tumor Consortium (PBTC).

One broad hypothesis that is being tested is that administration of active chemotherapeutic agents both in conjunction with and following radiation therapy will improve outcome in comparison with historical controls (e.g., the centrally reviewed cohort from the CCG-945 study treated with postirradiation CCNU and vincristine). The first pilot study that will evaluate this strategy (ACNS0126) will administer temozolomide during and after radiation therapy. This imidazotetrazine produces site-specific alkylation at the O^6 position of guanine that leads to cross-linking of DNA strands and has demonstrated

activity against malignant gliomas in adults.[35] A pediatric phase I trial in the United Kingdom observed responses in 7 of 16 children with malignant gliomas.[14] Similar results were obtained in a CCG phase I study.[32] The rationale for administering temozolomide both during and after irradiation is based upon preclinical and pilot clinical data that the combination of temozolomide with radiation therapy can potentiate the antitumor effects of each modality.[51] Temozolomide will first be administered on a daily basis during radiation therapy and then on a more conventional schedule (5 consecutive days per 28-day cycle) after irradiation; this approach has been well tolerated with promising activity against malignant gliomas in adults, with a 1-year survival rate of 71%.[51]

A second pilot study in this sequence may combine temozolomide with an antiangiogenic agent, such as SU5416, or a growth factor pathway inhibitor, such as STI571, each of which is currently undergoing phase I evaluation in the limited-institution PBTC protocols (PBTC-002 and PBTC-006, respectively) while the initial temozolomide study (ACNS0126) is in progress. These approaches are based on the hypothesis that interference with the signaling pathways that control glioma growth and angiogenesis will enhance the effects of conventional cytotoxic therapies. The combination strategy with an antiangiogenic agent will directly target the hypervascular phenotype of malignant gliomas.[31] Because antiangiogenic drugs inhibit the growth of endothelial cells, they provide a potential mechanism for blocking the enlargement of tumors that may be resistant to conventional chemotherapeutic agents.[34] Their prolonged administration has resulted in eradication of experimental tumors, suggesting the applicability of these agents in maintenance regimens. Similarly, the addition of agents with activity against the dysregulated growth factor–mediated signaling pathways that directly contribute to the proliferation of neoplastic astrocytes may potentiate the efficacy of conventional cytotoxic modalities. Based on the observation that childhood high-grade glioma cells commonly exhibit overexpression of the epidermal growth factor receptor (EGFR),[6] which may provide tumors with a growth advantage under conditions of mitogen limitation,[16] a pilot study (PBTC-007) is in progress to identify the maximal tolerated dose and activity of one EGFR inhibitor (ZD1839) in the PBTC.[1] Glioma cells also commonly exhibit overexpression of both platelet-derived growth factor (PDGF) and its receptors,[30,33] and a second pilot study (PBTC-006) is evaluating the safety and activity of a PDGF receptor (PDGF-R) inhibitor (STI571), based on promising preclinical data.[24] A third signal transduction-targeted study involving a farnesyltransferase inhibitor of Ras activity is also planned (PBTC-003), following from preclinical data that this approach has potential therapeutic activity against gliomas.[39] The results from the previously discussed pilot studies for children with recurrent disease will then be applied to build upon the results obtained with temozolomide alone in newly diagnosed patients.

An alternative strategy for enhancing the activity of temozolomide involves combining this agent with another cytotoxic agent. In the COG ADVL-0011 study, CCNU is being administered in a dose escalation design with temozolomide to determine the maximal tolerated dose and activity of this combination. This study is being conducted in parallel with the previously discussed studies and will provide a comparison of the relative efficacies of these strategies that may help in the design of subsequent therapeutic approaches. To ensure consistency of histologic inclusion criteria between studies, central review will be mandated, which will facilitate comparisons for each study group with the results obtained in the centrally reviewed CCG-945 historical cohort.

While the previously discussed studies are in progress for newly diagnosed patients, a third broad hypothesis will be tested in children with progressive disease, specifically, that intensification of chemotherapy improves outcome in patients with minimal residual disease after re-resection. This study (ACNS0231) will compare the efficacy of a single course of maximal intensity chemotherapy with carboplatin, thiotepa, and etoposide with three courses of moderately intensive therapy with thiotepa and carboplatin, administered at a higher total dose but lower dose per individual course than the other regimen. Both regimens will be supported by stem cell transplantation. This phase III study will resolve the long-standing controversy regarding the influence of chemotherapy dose intensity on outcome by providing an objective comparison of toxicity and efficacy between the two regimens and will potentially provide a platform upon which to add additional cytostatic agents in the post-transplant phase.

A fourth therapeutic paradigm that is being explored for children with supratentorial high-grade gliomas involves applications of local therapies, which builds upon single-institution pilot studies and promising results in adults with malignant gliomas. These approaches include convection-enhanced delivery of immunotoxins into the tumor bed,[26] administration of interstitial chemotherapy (i.e., Gliadel)[7] in conjunction with O^6-benzylguanine to potentially reverse alkyltransferase-mediated drug resistance,[56] and tumor-targeted immunotherapy using cytokine gene transduction-based and dendritic cell-based vaccine strategies.[47] It is anticipated that one or more of these approaches will be translated to the PBTC setting within the next year.

REHABILITATION

There is no systematic rehabilitation strategy that is pursued in children with high-grade gliomas. For lesions in noneloquent cortex, gross-total resection can often be performed with minimal neurologic morbidity. Lesions in higher risk locations are associated with a correspondingly higher frequency of serious neurologic deficits. Rehabilitative strategies are targeted to address the relevant deficits, if any, that are encountered. Given the remarkable ability of children to recover from neurologic injuries, such rehabilitative interventions yield results that are often impressive and gratifying.

OUTCOME AND QUALITY OF LIFE

As noted earlier, the overall frequency of long-term survival in children with supratentorial high-grade gliomas remains suboptimal, with less than 30% of patients in most series achieving long-term progression-free survival. Accordingly, the published literature has focused predominantly on strategies to improve survival, rather than quality of life issues. A number of factors can clearly influence functional status in affected children. Apart from the acute neurologic morbidity produced by the tumor and its resection, preirradiation or postirradiation chemotherapy carries risks of hematologic and nonhematologic toxicity that largely depend on the therapeutic regimen being employed. Whereas low-intensity regimens have generally been well tolerated,[15,50] high-dose myeloablative and submyeloablative strategies have been associated with significant morbidity and potential mortality rates in the 10% range,[20] a level high enough to enter into risk-benefit considerations for use of this therapy. Radiation therapy carries risks of more delayed sequelae for children with central nervous system tumors, although these risks are difficult to quantify for gliomas, because most of the literature on cognitive morbidity after irradiation has been based on follow-up of patients who have received whole-brain radiation therapy,[49] whereas supratentorial high-grade gliomas are generally treated with much more limited irradiation fields. Moreover, even among children with high-grade gliomas, the volume of normal brain that is irradiated can vary widely, and for large tumors, such fields can encompass a substantial percentage of the brain, which is a major concern in young patients, who are particularly vulnerable to the neurotoxic effects of irradiation. Accordingly, a number of recent studies have attempted to delay or avoid irradiation in children younger than 3 by first administering an extended course of intensive chemotherapy.[13,17,29] The use of three-dimensional conformal radiation therapy treatment planning and delivery also holds promise as a strategy for minimizing the volume of normal brain irradiated in those patients who do undergo radiation therapy.[54] However, it remains to be determined whether these approaches can translate into meaningful improvements in quality of life. A larger goal is to identify strategies to improve not only the accuracy of delivery but also the efficacy of irradiation, and thereby increase the percentage of patients who become long-term survivors.

Acknowledgment

This work was supported in part by NIH grant 1R01 NS37704.

References

1. Archer GE, Heimberger AB, McLendon RE, et al: The EGFR-specific tyrosine kinase inhibitor, ZD1839 (IRESSA™) is efficacious following oral administration against EGFR-overexpressing intracranial tumors. Neuro-oncol 2:247, 2000.

2. Arenson E, Ater J, Bank J, et al: A randomized phase II trial of high dose alkylating agents plus VP-16 in children with high grade astrocytoma. J Pediatr Hematol Oncol 21:325, 1999.

3. Artico M, Cervoni L, Celli P, et al: Supratentorial glioblastoma in children: a series of 27 surgically treated cases. Childs Nerv Syst 9:7–9, 1993.

4. Berger MS, Ojemann GA, Lettich E: Neurophysiological monitoring during astrocytoma surgery. Neurosurg Clin North Am 1:65–80, 1990.

5. Boyett J, Yates A, Gilles F, et al: When is a high-grade astrocytoma (HGA) not a HGA? Results of a central review of 226 cases of anaplastic astrocytoma (AA), glioblastoma multiforme (GBM), and other-HGA (OTH-HGA) by five neuropathologists. Proc Am Soc Clin Oncol 17:526a, 1998.

6. Bredel M, Pollack IF, Hamilton RL, James CD: Epidermal growth factor receptor (EGFR) expression in high-grade non-

brainstem gliomas of childhood. Clin Cancer Res 5:1786–1792, 1999.

7. Brem H, Piantadosi S, Burger P, et al: Placebo-controlled trial of safety and efficacy of intraoperative controlled delivery by biodegradable polymers of chemotherapy for recurrent gliomas. Lancet 345:1008–1012, 1995.

8. Cairncross JG, Macdonald DR, Ramsay DA: Aggressive oligodendroglioma: a chemosensitive tumor. Neurosurgery 31:78–82, 1992.

9. Campbell JW, Pollack IF, Martinez AJ, Shultz BL: High-grade astrocytomas in children: radiologically complete resection is associated with an excellent long-term prognosis. Neurosurgery 38:258–264, 1996.

10. Chintagumpala M, Burger P, McCluggage C, et al: DNA mismatch repair and O6-alkylguanine-DNA alkyltransferase (AGT) analysis and response to procarbazine in malignant glioma in children—a Pediatric Oncology Group (POG) study. Med Ped Oncol 33:159, 1999.

11. Daumas-Duport C, Scheithauer B, O'Fallon J, et al: Grading of astrocytomas: a simple and reproducible grading method. Cancer 62:2152–2165, 1988.

12. Dropcho E, Wisoff J, Walker R, et al: Supratentorial malignant gliomas in childhood: a review of fifty cases. Ann Neurol 22:355–364, 1978.

13. Duffner PK, Horowitz ME, Krischer JP, et al: Postoperative chemotherapy and delayed radiation in children less than three years of age with malignant brain tumors. N Engl J Med 328:1725–1731, 1993.

14. Estlin EJ, Lashford L, Ablett S, et al: Phase I study of temozolomide in paediatric patients with advanced cancer. United Kingdom Children's Cancer Study Group. Br J Cancer 78:652–661, 1998.

15. Finlay JL, Boyett JM, Yates AJ, et al: Randomized phase III trial in childhood high-grade astrocytoma comparing vincristine, lomustine, and prednisone with the eight-drugs-in-1-day regimen. Children's Cancer Group. J Clin Oncol 13:112–123, 1995.

16. Frederick L, Wang X-Y, Eley G, James CD: Diversity and frequency of epidermal growth factor receptor mutations in human glioblastomas. Cancer Res 60:1383–1387, 2000.

17. Geyer JR, Finlay JL, Boyett JM, et al: Survival of infants with malignant astrocytomas: a report from the Children's Cancer Group. Cancer 75:1045–1050, 1995.

18. Grabb PA, Albright AL, Pang D: Dissemination of supratentorial malignant gliomas via the cerebrospinal fluid in children. Neurosurgery 30:64–71, 1992.

19. Grossman SA, Wharam M, Sheidler V, et al: Phase II study of continuous infusion carmustine and cisplatin followed by cranial irradiation in adults with newly diagnosed high-grade astrocytoma. J Clin Oncol 15:2596–603, 1997.

20. Grovas AC, Boyett JM, Lindsley K, et al: Regimen-related toxicity of myeloablative chemotherapy with BCNU, thiotepa, and etoposide followed by autologous stem cell rescue for children with newly diagnosed glioblastoma multiforme: report from the Children's Cancer Group. Med Pediatr Oncol 33:83–87, 1999.

21. Hamilton SR, Lui B, Parsons RE, et al: The molecular basis of Turcot's syndrome. N Engl J Med 332:839–847, 1995.

22. Ichimura K, Bolin MB, Goike HM, et al: Deregulation of the p14^{ARF}/MDM2/p53 pathway is a prerequisite for human astrocytic gliomas with G$_1$-S transition control gene abnormalities. Cancer Res 60:417–424, 2000.

23. Ino Y, Zlatescu MC, Sasaki H, et al: Long survival and therapeutic responses in patients with histologically disparate high-grade gliomas demonstrating chromosome 1p loss. J Neurosurg 92:983–990, 2000.

24. Kilic T, Alberta JA, Zdunek PR, et al: Intracranial inhibition of platelet-derived growth factor-mediated glioblastoma cell growth by an orally active kinase inhibitor of the 2-phenylaminopyrimidine class. Cancer Res 60:143–150, 2000.

25. Kleihues P, Burger PC, Scheithauer BW, et al: World Health Organization Histological Typing of Tumours of the Central Nervous System, 2nd ed. New York, Springer-Verlag, 1993.

26. Laske DW, Youle RJ, Oldfield EH: Tumor regression with regional distribution of targetted toxin TF-CRM107 in patients with malignant brain tumors. Nature Med 3:1362–1368, 1997.

27. Louis DN: A molecular genetic model of astrocytoma histopathology. Brain Pathol 7:755–764, 1997.

28. Macauley RJ, Jay V, Hoffman HJ, et al: Increased mitotic activity as a negative prognostic indicator in pleomorphic xanthoastrocytoma. J Neurosurg 79:761–767, 1993.

29. Mason WP, Grovas A, Halpern S, et al: Intensive chemotherapy and bone marrow rescue for young children with newly diagnosed malignant brain tumors. J Clin Oncol 16:1–13, 1998.

30. Maxwell M, Naber SP, Wolfe HJ, et al: Coexpression of platelet-derived growth factor (PDGF) and PDGF-receptor genes by primary human astrocytomas may contribute to their development and maintenance. J Clin Invest 86:131–140, 1990.

31. Millauer B, Shawver LK, Plate KH, et al: Glioblastoma growth inhibited in vivo by a dominant-negative Flk-1 mutant. Nature 367:576–579, 1994.

32. Nicholson HS, Krailo M, Ames MM, et al: Phase I study of temozolomide in children and adolescents with recurrent solid tumors: a report from the Children's Cancer Group. J Clin Oncol 16:3037–3043, 1998.

33. Nister M, Claesson-Welch L, Eriksson A, et al: Differential expression of platelet-derived growth factor receptors in human malignant glioma cell lines. J Biol Chem 266:16755–16763, 1991.

34. O'Reilly MS, Holmgren L, Chen C, Folkman J: Angiostatin induces and sustains dormancy of human primary tumors in mice. Nat Med 2:689–692, 1996.

35. O'Reilly SM, Newlands ES, Glaser MG, et al: A new oral cytotoxic chemotherapeutic agent with promising activity against primary brain tumours. Eur J Cancer 7:940–942, 1993.

36. Papahill PA, Ramsay DA, Del Maestro RF: Pleomorphic xanthoastrocytoma: case report and analysis of the literature concerning the efficacy of resection and the significance of necrosis. Neurosurgery 38:822–829, 1996.

37. Phuphanich S, Edwards MSB, Levin VA, et al: Supratentorial malignant gliomas of childhood: results of treatment with radiation therapy and chemotherapy. J Neurosurg 60:495–499, 1984.

38. Pollack IF: Brain tumors in children. N Engl J Med 331:1500–1507, 1994.

39. Pollack IF, Bredel M, Erff M, et al: Inhibition of Ras and related G-proteins as a novel therapeutic strategy for blocking malignant glioma growth. II. In vivo results in a nude mouse model. Neurosurgery 45:1208–1214, 1999.

40. Pollack IF, Campbell JW, Hamilton RL, et al: Proliferation index as a predictor of prognosis in malignant gliomas of childhood. Cancer 79:849–856, 1997.

41. Pollack IF, Finkelstein SD, Burnham J, et al: Association between chromosome 1p and 19q loss and outcome in pediatric malignant gliomas: results from the CCG-945 cohort. Pediatr Neurosurg 39:114–121, 2003.

42. Pollack IF, Finkelstein SD, Burnham J, et al: Age and TP53 mutation frequency in childhood gliomas. Results in a multi-institutional cohort. Cancer Res 61:7404–7407, 2001.

43. Pollack IF, Finkelstein SD, Woods J, et al: Expression of p53 and prognosis in childhood malignant gliomas. N Engl J Med 346:420–427, 2002.

44. Pollack IF, Hamilton RL, Burnham J, et al: The impact of proliferation index on outcome in childhood malignant gliomas: Results in a multi-institutional cohort. Neurosurgery 50:1238–1244; discussion 1244–1245, 2002.

45. Pollack IF, Hamilton RL, Finkelstein SD, et al: The relationship between TP53 mutations and overexpression of p53 and prognosis in malignant gliomas of childhood. Cancer Res 57:304–309, 1997.

46. Pollack IF, Mulvihill JJ: Special issues in the management of gliomas in children with neurofibromatosis 1. J Neuro-oncol 28:257–268, 1996.

47. Pollack IF, Okada H, Chambers WH: Exploiting immune mechanisms in the treatment of central nervous system cancer. Sem Pediatr Neurol 7:131–143, 2000.

48. Raffel C, Frederick L, O'Fallon JR, et al: Analysis of oncogene and tumor suppressor gene alterations in pediatric malignant astrocytomas reveals reduced survival for patients with PTEN mutations. Clin Canc Res 5:4085–4090, 1999.

49. Silber JH, Radcliffe J, Peckham V, et al: Whole-brain irradiation and decline in intelligence: the influence of dose and age on IQ score. J Clin Oncol 10:1390–1396, 1992.

50. Sposto R, Ertel IJ, Jenkin RDT, et al: The effectiveness of chemotherapy for treatment of high grade astrocytoma in children: results of a randomized trial. J Neurooncol 7:165–177, 1989.

51. Stupp R, Ostermann S, Kraljevic A, et al: Promising survival with concomitant and adjuvant temozolomide [TMZ] for newly diagnosed glioblastoma multiforme [GBM]. Proc Am Soc Clin Oncol 19:163a, 2000.

52. Sung T, Miller DC, Hayes RL, et al: Preferential inactivation of the p53 tumor suppressor pathway and lack of EGFR amplification distinguish de novo high grade pediatric astrocytomas from de novo adult astrocytomas. Brain Pathol 10:249–259, 2000.

53. Sure U, Ruedi D, Tachibana O, et al: Determination of p53 mutations, EGFR overexpression, and loss of p16 expression in pediatric glioblastomas. J Neuropathol Exp Neurol 56:782–789, 1997.

54. Tarbell NJ, Loeffler JS: Recent trends in the radiotherapy of pediatric gliomas. J Neurooncol 28:233–244, 1996.

55. Thomas D, Brada M, Stenning S: Randomized trial of procarbazine, lomustine, and vincristine in the adjuvant treatment of high-grade astrocytoma: a Medical Research Council Trial. J Clin Oncol 19:509–518, 2001.

56. Wedge SR, Newlands ES: O6-benzylguanine enhances the sensitivity of a glioma xenograft with low O6- alkylguanine-DNA alkyltransferase activity to temozolomide and BCNU. Br J Cancer 73:1049–1052, 1996.

57. Wisoff JH, Boyett JM, Berger MS, et al: Current neurosurgical management and the impact of the extent of resection in the treatment of malignant gliomas of childhood: a report of the Children's Cancer Group trial no. CCG-945. J Neurosurg 89:52–59, 1998.

CHAPTER 80

LHERMITTE-DUCLOS DISEASE

Raafat Yahya, Todd Mainprize, Cynthia Hawkins, Juan M. Bilbao, and James T. Rutka

Lhermitte-Duclos disease is a rare condition that involves the cerebellum producing mass effect. Since its description in 1920 by Lhermitte and Duclos,[24] the disease has acquired several names, including diffuse ganglioneuroma of the cerebellar cortex,[19] gangliocytoma myelinicum diffusum of the cerebellar cortex,[9] hypertrophy (benign) of the cerebellum,[10,12] hamartoma of the cerebellum,[19] granule cell hypertrophy of the cerebellum, dysplastic gangliocytoma of the cerebellum,[23,30,35] and granulo-molecular hypertrophy of the cerebellum,[11,39] reflecting the controversy regarding the etiology and the nature of the disease. It is now most commonly referred to as Lhermitte-Duclos disease (LDD). The diagnosis of the disease is based on a characteristic appearance on pathologic examination that includes hypertrophy of the granule cell layer containing abnormal granule cells, loss of the Purkinje cell layer, widening of the molecular layer that contains hypertrophied axons, and decreased density of the subcortical white matter.[1,15,23] The etiology of the disease is still unknown, though several factors favor a developmental cause.[1,38] Surgery is the only effective treatment of the disease and significant improvement in outcome following surgical treatment of these patients has been observed.

ETIOLOGY

The etiology of LDD has been the subject of some controversy, and several theories have been put forward to explain its pathogenesis. Lhermitte and Duclos in their initial description[24] explained that the lesion is the result of two processes, one developmental and the other cancerous, arising from precursors of Purkinje cells. Duncan and Snodgrass[12] proposed that the tumor cells are actually hypertrophied granular cell layer neurons, a suggestion also supported by Pritchell and King[35] based not only on the preservation of the normal anatomy of the granule cell layer neurons and their axonal orientation but also on ultrastructural analyses that revealed features of these cells shared with the granule cell layer neurons. Further molecular analysis in patients with LDD showed that neurofilament expression in neurons of the dysplastic cerebellum is similar to that in normal cerebellar control neurons,[48] providing further support to the theory that the underlying process is non-neoplastic. Further evidence in favor of LDD being a congenital lesion came from a report by Ambler et al[1] of LDD in two members of the same family, a mother and son, who had the disease. They suggested that the disease is likely due to a congenital lesion that is transmitted in an autosomal dominant

fashion and proposed that a likely target is a growth controlling agent or its target metabolic machinery. They were also the first to associate the disease with the other phakomatoses, Sturge-Weber, tuberous sclerosis, and neurofibromatosis.

CLINICAL PRESENTATION

Patients with LDD usually seek treatment in the third to fourth decades of life. However, the disease has been reported in infants and in patients in their sixth decade. The clinical features are those of a slowly growing posterior fossa mass or increased intracranial pressure caused by obstructive hydrocephalus with ataxia, headache, nausea, vomiting, and visual disturbances. Isolated case reports of the disease causing orthostatic hypotension,[40] tinnitus,[25] double vision,[41] and subarachnoid hemorrhage[44] can be found in the literature. The duration of symptoms ranges from several weeks to many years. Acute deterioration, though not common in recent reports, was reported initially, including the first two patients diagnosed with this condition. On the other hand, the disease has also been reported as a coincidental finding at autopsy in a patient who died of unrelated conditions.[17]

RADIOLOGIC FEATURES

Before the late 1970s, radiologic studies used to investigate patients with LDD included cerebral angiography and ventriculography. The findings were those of a posterior fossa mass with obstructive hydrocephalus. Reports of computed tomography (CT) findings in patients with LDD started to appear in the early 1980s and included evidence of a hypodense mass lesion in the posterior fossa that does not enhance with contrast and compresses the fourth ventricle, producing obstructive hydrocephalus. Calcifications have been described within the lesion. Reports of the use of magnetic resonance imaging (MRI) in patients with LDD started to appear in the literature in the late 1980s.[6,36,41,43] Since then, the number of patients diagnosed with LDD has approached the number of cases reported in the pre-MRI era.

MRI is the preferred study in the diagnosis of patients with LDD. The cerebellar mass in these patients is usually unilateral and nonenhancing after contrast injection, implying an intact blood-brain barrier (Figure 80-1). Bilateral cerebellar involvement had been reported in a smaller percentage of patients, and

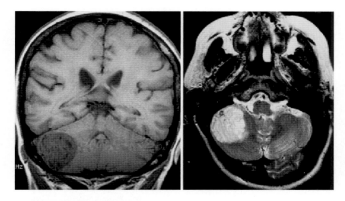

FIGURE 80-1 Typical magnetic resonance appearance of Lhermitte-Duclos disease in the cerebellum. *Left,* T1-weighted image showing discrete lesion with no significant mass effect, coronal cut. *Right,* T2-weighted axial image showing expanded and thickened folia. (Reproduced with permission from Koch R, Scholz M, Nelen MR, et al: Lhermitte-Duclos disease as a component of Cowden's syndrome. Case report and review of the literature. J Neurosurg 90:776–779, 1999.)

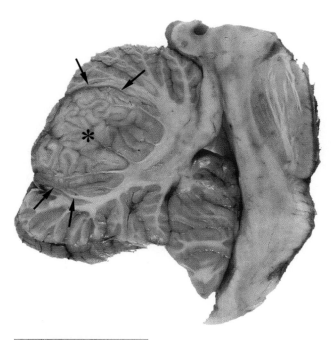

FIGURE 80-2 Midline sagittal view of the brainstem and cerebellum from a patient with Lhermitte-Duclos disease. The *asterisk* represents the center of the lesion, and the *arrows* mark the margins.

contrast enhancement with gadolinium was also observed by several authors.[2,13,33] The mass is hypointense on T1- and hyperintense on T2-weighted images. The enlarged folia characteristic of the disease appear as large parallel striations on the surface of the mass most clearly seen on short Tau inversion recovery (STIR) T1-relaxation images. This appearance occurs as a result of alternating signal from the isointense cortical layer and the hyperintense underlying white matter layer, and is referred to as the "tiger strip" structure. This finding is characteristic enough that it has been suggested to be sufficient to diagnose the disease.[6,8,16,28]

MRI also has a higher sensitivity for detecting other abnormalities that might not be well visualized on CT scanning. Syringomyelia has been reported in association with LDD on preoperative MRI.[27,41,47] Sabin was the first to report on the preoperative diagnosis of patients with LDD based on magnetic resonance (MR) images in 1988. Several other investigators since have also been able to achieve the same results. There is still, however, no established radiologic criteria for the preoperative diagnosis of LDD. The results of positron-emission tomography (PET) scanning in patients with LDD have also been reported, as well as increased cerebral blood flow through the lesion.[31,32]

PATHOLOGY

The gross appearance of the cerebellum is pathognomonic for patients with LDD.[1,7,23] The folia are enlarged and usually soft (Figure 80-2). The preservation of their architectural pattern is a constant finding. Grayish discoloration of the cerebellar surface has also been described. The mass blends into the normal cerebellar tissue, and it can be difficult to delineate its exact boundaries. The occipital bone has been reported to be thinned, indicating the prolonged preclinical course of the disease.

Microscopic examination of the cerebellum reveals a bilayer organization consisting of a molecular layer widened by an increased number of heavily myelinated axons that arise from enlarged neurons, which expand the internal granular cell layer (Figure 80-3).[1,4,23,30,35] The Purkinje cell layer is deficient. The appearance of the internal granular layer depends on the degree of involvement with the disease and ranges from a few large neurons among normal-appearing granular cells to complete replacement of the whole cellular population by large, irregular neurons that are bigger than the normal granular neurons but smaller than the Purkinje cells (Figure 80-4). Many of these cells are binucleated, and their nuclei contain two nucleoli. Their cytoplasm, contrary to normal granular neurons, is abundant and has been described as containing cytoplasmic inclusions that are periodic acid-Schiff (PAS) stain-positive. They give rise to axons that, like the normal granular neurons, are perpendicular to the pial surface. Neurons have also been described in the molecular layer. The white matter of the affected folia is significantly reduced.

Early, as well as more recent, reports described immunohistochemical[18,42,48] and electron microscopic[5,14,18,26,37] features of the cells in the internal granular layer that are characteristic of neurons, raising the suspicion that these cells are actually dysplastic granule cell layer neurons that are hypertrophied and misplaced. Mitoses and necrosis are not features of LDD. Neovascularization has been described in areas of increased neuronal density, and calcifications, when present, usually occur at the periphery of the lesion along the small capillary type vessels that are abundant in the thickened molecular layer. The gradual transition between normal and abnormal tissue is evident on microscopic examination as well and correlates with the

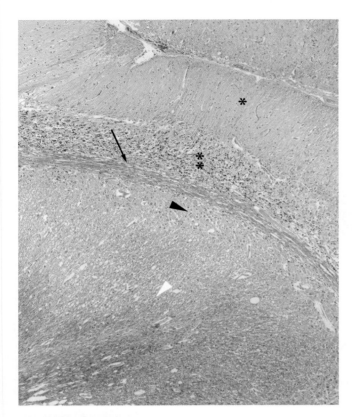

FIGURE 80-3 Microscopic appearance of the cerebellum in Lhermitte-Duclos disease (hematoxylin and eosin/luxol fast blue ×40). The *arrowhead* points to the internal granular cell layer, which has been completely replaced by large irregular neurons and beneath which is a widened molecular layer containing heavily myelinated axons. The white matter layer is reduced *(arrow)* and the internal granular layer above it *(double asterisk)* shows only a few large neurons amongst normal-appearing granular cells. The associated molecular layer *(asterisk)* is relatively preserved, with only a few large myelinated axons.

grossly indistinguishable borders of the mass, an important factor that limits total resection.

GENETICS

As mentioned earlier, Ambler was the first to suggest that LDD is due to an inherited genetic mutation. He suggested that the disease is likely transmitted in an autosomal dominant fashion. Cowden's disease is an autosomal dominant hamartomatous condition that mainly affects the skin and mucous membranes as well as other organs. The association between LDD and Cowden's disease was first reported in 1991 by Padberg.[34] Padberg reported on two unrelated patients who had Cowden's disease as well as LDD and suggested that the rarity of the two conditions makes their occurrence in the two patients very unlikely and thus concluded that the two conditions might be related. Shortly after their report, a third case with both conditions was reported.[21] Several reports followed thereafter of 33 patients with clinical manifestations of LDD who also had

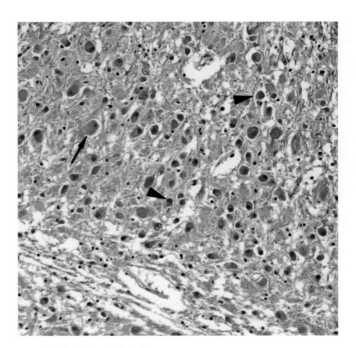

FIGURE 80-4 High-power microscopic view of the granular cell layer, which has been replaced by large irregular neurons (hematoxylin and eosin/luxol fast blue ×100).

Cowden's disease. Many of these cases are patients who were already diagnosed with LDD and were found to have manifestations of Cowden's disease on retrospective review. Recently, the diagnosis of Cowden's disease has been defined by the International Cowden consortium and is based on major and minor clinical criteria. In the presence of LDD the diagnosis of Cowden's disease is established if one other major criterion or three minor criteria are met.

The genetic lesion in Cowden's disease is a mutation in the PTEN gene, which has been localized to chromosome 10q23.[29] This gene has been found to be mutated in a large number of human cancers, including brain, kidney, breast, prostate, and skin. Accordingly, the association between CD and LDD is very important, and patients with LDD should undergo extensive clinical investigation to rule out Cowden's disease. PTEN has also been associated with several of the characteristic features of patients with LDD. Kwon et al[22] reported on an animal model of LDD, which they established by inactivating PTEN using the Cre-1oxP knockout mouse technology. They found that genetically engineered mice with an inactivated PTEN gene exhibited loss of neuronal stromal growth control with a markedly enlarged cerebellar internal granular layer and molecular layer. The Purkinje cell layer was atrophic and disorganized. The molecular layer also contained small neurons that expressed gamma-aminobutyric acid (GABA)-A receptor alpha 6, a protein expressed only in mature granule cells after migration along glial processes from the subpial space where they form the internal granular layer. This finding provides further support to the hypothesis that the basic defective mechanism in LDD is that of neuronal migration. Backman et al reported on similar findings upon examination of the brains of mice who had the embryologically lethal PTEN deletion.[3]

TREATMENT

Surgery is the definitive treatment of patients with LDD. The natural history of the disease, however, is not clear. The first patient diagnosed with LDD did not undergo surgery and died of the secondary cause of increased intracranial pressure. The pathology was revealed on postmortem examination of the brain. Christensen is credited for the first successful resection of an LDD lesion in 1937. The 34-year-old patient underwent surgery for a posterior fossa mass; no distinct tumor was found, and the patient had part of the cerebellum removed. Before 1955 only three patients were reported to have had successful treatment of LDD. Significant improvement in the outcome of patients with LDD can be noticed following the literature since then. This is due not only to the significant improvement in the surgical and anesthetic techniques that allow safe resection of tumor and better control of the intracranial pressure especially in the perioperative period, but also due to the better understanding of the disease and the ability to suspect its presence on preoperative imaging studies.

The goal of surgery is to perform a gross-total removal of the mass with relief of posterior fossa pressure and reconstitution of the normal cerebrospinal fluid (CSF) pathways. The need for preoperative ventricular drainage is dictated by the patient's condition and is required in patients who acutely decompensate. The suboccipital approach is the most commonly used route for resection of the mass; however, other posterior fossa approaches can also be used depending on the location of the mass. The extent of the surgical resection might be the most important part of the surgical planning. The tumor might not be clearly evident grossly, and the margins of the mass not clear as it meets with normal cerebellum. Recent advances in the radiologic evaluation of patients with LDD, particularly the advent of MRI and recent reports about the characteristic appearance of LDD on these imaging studies, facilitate the diagnosis preoperatively. This aids the subsequent neurosurgical approach and preoperative planning of the extent of the resection.

Another treatment option for patients with LDD was reported by Tuli et al.[45] They treated a 54-year-old female with LDD by a decompressive-type surgery with suboccipital craniectomy and removal of C1 posterior arch followed by augmentation duraplasty using autologous fascia lata graft. The patient's clinical symptoms improved and follow-up MRI revealed resolution of the hydrocephalus.

Radiation therapy has no role in patients with LDD. Two patients with LDD are reported to have received radiation therapy. Heitkamp[20] reported one who received radiation therapy for a posterior fossa mass that was thought to be a low-grade astrocytoma. She underwent suboccipital craniectomy, and the pathologic examination of the posterior fossa tumor revealed findings characteristic of LDD. The other patient, reported by Marano et al,[26] was a 13-year-old who underwent biopsy and treatment with radiation therapy. The child had worsening disease while on treatment but did well after undergoing a subtotal resection. Recurrent symptoms appeared 1 year later, and the child underwent radical resection for recurrent disease. Several other cases of disease progression and recurrence of symptoms have been reported.[36,44,46] Despite the slowly progressive nature of the disease, continued follow-up and surveillance with MRI is important for the early detection of disease progression and the institution of the appropriate treatment.

CONCLUSION

LDD is a fascinating disorder of uncertain origin that involves the cerebellum of patients causing mass effect and obstruction of CSF pathways. The presence of cases of LDD in patients with Cowden's disease suggests a role for the PTEN gene in the molecular pathogenesis of inherited forms of LDD. The diagnosis of LDD is suspected on preoperative imaging studies such as MRI, and timely surgical removal of the mass lesion is effective in limiting the emergent features of the disease. Further molecular genetic studies should be performed on sporadic cases of LDD to determine whether these are associated with mutations in the PTEN gene, so that these patients can be screened for Cowden-associated cancers.

References

1. Ambler M, Pogacar S, Sidman R: Lhermitte-Duclos disease (granule cell hypertrophy of the cerebellum) pathological analysis of the first familial cases. J Neuropathol Exp Neurol 28:622–647, 1969.
2. Awwad EE, Levy E, Martin DS, Merenda GO: Atypical MR appearance of Lhermitte-Duclos disease with contrast enhancement. AJNR Am J Neuroradiol 16:1719–1720, 1995.
3. Backman SA, Stambolic V, Suzuki A, et al: Deletion of PTEN in mouse brain causes seizures, ataxia and defects in soma size resembling Lhermitte-Duclos disease. Nat Genet 29:396–403, 2001.
4. Barone F, Noubari BA, Torrisi A, et al: Lhermitte duclos disease and Cowden disease: clinical, pathological and neuroimaging study of a case. J Neurosurg Sci 44:234–237, 2000.
5. Beuche W, Wickboldt J, Friede RL: Lhermitte-Duclos disease—its minimal lesions in electron microscope data and CT findings. Clin Neuropathol 2:163–170, 1983.
6. Carter JE, Merren MD, Swann KW: Preoperative diagnosis of Lhermitte-Duclos disease by magnetic resonance imaging. Case report. J Neurosurg 70:135–137, 1989.
7. Chen KS, Hung PC, Wang HS, et al: Medulloblastoma or cerebellar dysplastic gangliocytoma (Lhermitte-Duclos disease)? Pediatr Neurol 27:404–406, 2002.
8. Choudhury AR: Pre-operative magnetic resonance imaging in Lhermitte-Duclos disease. Br J Neurosurg 4:225–229, 1990.
9. Courville CB: Gangliocytoma myelinicum diffusum of the cerebellar cortex. Bull Los Angeles Neurol Soc 23:72, 1958.
10. Dastur HM, Pandya SK, Deshpande DH: Diffusecerebellar hypertrophy Lhermitte-Duclos disease. Neurol India 23:53–56, 1975.
11. Di Lorenzo N, Lunardi P, Fortuna A: Granulomolecular hypertrophy of the cerebellum (Lhermitte-Duclos disease). Case report. J Neurosurg 60:644–646, 1984.
12. Duncan D, Snodgrass SR: Diffuse hypertrophy of the cerebellar cortex (myelinated neurocytoma). Arch Neurol Psychiatr 50:677–684, 1943.
13. Ellis PK: Case report: Lhermitte-Duclos disease: enhancement following gadolinium-DPTA. Clin Radiol 51:222–224, 1996.
14. Ferrer I, Marti E, Guionnet N, et al: Studies with the Golgi method in central gangliogliomas and dysplastic gangliocytoma

of the cerebellum (Lhermitte-Duclos disease). Histol Histopathol 5:329–336, 1990.

15. Gessaga EC: Lhermitte-Duclos disease (diffuse hypertrophy of the cerebellum). Report of two cases. Neurosurg Rev 3:151–158, 1980.

16. Grand S, Pasquier B, Le Bas JF, Chirossel JP: Case report: magnetic resonance imaging in Lhermitte-Duclos disease. Br J Radiol 67:902–905, 1994.

17. Gyori S, Molnar P: Lhermitte-Duclos disease. Case report and review of the literature. Morphol Igazsagugyi Orv Sz 29:55–60, 1989.

18. Hair LS, Symmans F, Powers JM, Carmel P: Immunohistochemistry and proliferative activity in Lhermitte-Duclos disease. Acta Neuropathol (Berl) 84:570–573, 1992.

19. Hallervorden J: Uberdie Hamartome (Ganglioneurome) des Kleinhirns. Deutsch Z Nervenheilk 179:531–563, 1959.

20. Heitkamp JW, Rose JE: Neck pain following migration of a ventriculocervical shunt. Surg Neurol 19:285–287, 1983.

21. King MA, Coyne TJ, Spearritt DJ, Boyle RS: Lhermitte-Duclos disease and Cowden disease: a third case. Ann Neurol 32:112–113, 1992.

22. Kwon CH, Zhu X, Zhang J, et al: PTEN regulates neuronal soma size: a mouse model of Lhermitte-Duclos disease. Nat Genet 29:404–411, 2001.

23. Leech RW, Christoferson LA, Gilbertson RL: Dysplastic gangliocytoma (Lhermitte-Duclos disease) of the cerebellum. J Neurosurg 47:609–612, 1977.

24. Lhermitte J, Duclos P: Surun ganglioneurome di.us du: cortex du cervelet. Bull Assoc Fr Etud Cancer 9:99–107, 1920.

25. Lobo CJ, Mehan R, Murugasu E, Laitt RD: Tinnitus as the presenting symptom in a case of Lhermitte-Duclos disease. J Laryngol Otol 113:464–465, 1999.

26. Marano SR, Johnson PC, Spetzler RF: Recurrent Lhermitte-Duclos disease in a child. Case report. J Neurosurg 69:599–603, 1988.

27. Marcus CD, Galeon M, Peruzzi P, et al: Lhermitte-Duclos disease associated with syringomyelia. Neuroradiology 38:529–531, 1996.

28. Meltzer CC, Smirniotopoulos JG, Jones RV: The striated cerebellum: an MR imaging sign in Lhermitte-Duclos disease (dysplastic gangliocytoma). Radiology 194:699–703, 1995.

29. Nelen MR, Padberg GW, Peeters EA, et al: Localization of the gene for Cowden disease to chromosome 10q22–23. Nat Genet 13:114–116, 1996.

30. Nowak DA, Trost H-A, Porr A, Stolzle A, Lumenta CB: Dysplastic gangliocytoma of the cerebellum (Lhermitte-Duclos disease). Clin Neurol Neurosurg 103:105–110, 2001.

31. Ogasawara K, Beppu T, Yasuda S, et al: Blood flow and oxygen metabolism in a case of Lhermitte-Duclos disease: results of positron emission tomography. J Neurooncol 55:59–61, 2001.

32. Ogasawara K, Yasuda S, Beppu T, et al: Brain PET and technetium-99m-ECD SPECT imaging in Lhermitte-Duclos disease. Neuroradiology 43:993–996, 2001.

33. Ortiz O, Bloomfield S, Schochet S: Vascular contrast enhancement in Lhermitte-Duclos disease: case report. Neuroradiology 37:545–548, 1995.

34. Padberg GW, Schot JD, Vielvoye GJ, et al: Lhermitte-Duclos disease and Cowden disease: a single phakomatosis. Ann Neurol 29:517–523, 1991.

35. Pritchett PS, King TI: Dysplastic gangliocytoma of the cerebellum—an ultrastructural study. Acta Neuropathol 42:1–5, 1978.

36. Reeder RF, Saunders RL, Roberts DW, et al: Magnetic resonance imaging in the diagnosis and treatment of Lhermitte-Duclos disease (dysplastic gangliocytoma of the cerebellum). Neurosurgery 23:240–245, 1988.

37. Reznik M, Schoenen J: Lhermitte-Duclos disease. Acta Neuropathol (Berl) 59(2):88–94, 1983.

38. Roski RA, Roessmann U, Spetzler RF, et al: Clinical and pathological study of dysplastic gangliocytoma. Case report. J Neurosurg 55:318–321, 1981.

39. Rousseaux M, Combelles G, Krivosi KY, Christiaens JL: Lhermitte-Duclos disease. Granulomolecular hypertrophy of the cerebellum. Neurochirurgie 33:232–235, 1987.

40. Ruchoux MM, Gray F, Gherardi R, et al: Orthostatic hypotension from a cerebellar gangliocytoma (Lhermitte-Duclos disease). Case report. J Neurosurg 65:245–248, 1986.

41. Sabin HI, Lidov HG, Kendall BE, Symon L: Lhermitte-Duclos disease (dysplastic gangliocytoma): a case report with CT and MRI. Acta Neurochir (Wien) 93:149–153, 1988.

42. Shiurba RA, Gessaga EC, Eng LF, et al: Lhermitte-Duclos disease. An immunohistochemical study of the cerebellar cortex. Acta Neuropathol (Berl) 75:474–480, 1988.

43. Smith RR, Grossman RI, Goldberg HI, et al: MR imaging of Lhermitte-Duclos disease: a case report. AJNR Am J Neuroradiol 10:187–189, 1989.

44. Stapleton SR, Wilkins PR, Bell BA: Recurrent dysplastic cerebellar gangliocytoma (Lhermitte-Duclos disease) presenting with subarachnoid haemorrhage. Br J Neurosurg 6:153–156, 1992.

45. Tuli S, Provias JP, Bernstein M: Lhermitte-Duclos disease: literature review and novel treatment strategy. Can J Neurol Sci 24:155–160, 1997.

46. Williams DW, III, Elster AD, Ginsberg LE, Stanton C: Recurrent Lhermitte-Duclos disease: report of two cases and association with Cowden's disease. AJNR Am J Neuroradiol 13:287–290, 1992.

47. Wolansky LJ, Malantic GP, Heary R, et al: Preoperative MRI diagnosis of Lhermitte-Duclos disease: case report with associated enlarged vessel and syrinx. Surg Neurol 45:470–475; discussion 475–476, 1996.

48. Yachnis AT, Trojanowski JQ, Memmo M, Schlaepfer WW: Expression of neurofilament proteins in the hypertrophic granule cells of Lhermitte-Duclos disease: an explanation for the mass effect and the myelination of parallel fibers in the disease state. J Neuropathol Exp Neurol 47:206–216, 1988.

CHAPTER 81

CEREBELLAR ASTROCYTOMAS

Cornelia S. von Koch, John H. Chi, and Nalin Gupta

Cerebellar astrocytomas represent 12% to 17% of all pediatric brain tumors and 20% to 35% of tumors in the posterior fossa of children.[51] Four histologic grades have been defined, and in general, a higher grade is associated with worse outcome. Eighty percent of pediatric cerebellar astrocytomas are pilocytic (World Health Organization [WHO] grade I) and are considered histologically benign.[33] Higher grade tumors, fibrillary astrocytomas (WHO grade II), make up 15% of the total, whereas anaplastic astrocytomas (WHO grade III) and glioblastoma multiforme (GBM, WHO grade IV) are each less than 5% of the total.[51] Complete surgical resection is the treatment of choice for cerebellar astrocytomas, and outcome depends on extent of resection, tumor invasion, and histologic grade. Complete resection of pilocytic astrocytoma usually results in cure. The treatment of residual tumor and tumor recurrence remains controversial, and no clear roles for radiation and chemotherapy have been defined. Molecular studies are beginning to define genetic features, especially in tumors of higher grade.

LOCATION

Infratentorial tumors constitute 50% to 60% of all intracranial tumors in childhood and include cerebellar astrocytoma (20% to 35%), medulloblastoma or primitive neuroectodermal tumor (PNET) (30% to 35%), brainstem glioma (25%), ependymoma (10%), and other miscellaneous types (5%).[36] Cerebellar astrocytomas are usually thought to arise in the cerebellar hemispheres, but a large percentage also are found in the vermis. In one study of 97 patients, 41% of tumors were found in the midline, 33% in the left, and 26% in the right cerebellar hemisphere, respectively.[47] The majority of midline tumors were solid, whereas hemispheric tumors were mostly cystic. Brainstem involvement occurs in 10% to 40% of tumors, with most of these tumors being of the solid type,[26,47] whereas the cerebellar peduncles are affected in 34%.[23,35] Older patients have a higher incidence of hemispheric tumors compared with younger patients.

DIAGNOSIS

Children with cerebellar astrocytomas commonly present in the first decade of life (mean 6.8 years, range 6 months to 17 years) with symptoms often having been present for several months.[42,51] Typical symptoms include headaches, vomiting, gait disturbance, visual disturbance, diplopia, decreased level of consciousness, and neck pain or stiffness (Table 81-1).[1,47] Headaches are worse with recumbency; they often begin frontally and migrate to the occiput. Constant occipital headache and neck pain with hyperextension is an ominous sign of tonsillar herniation into the foramen magnum. Respiratory depression, preceded by cluster or ataxic breathing, may follow shortly.[45] Vomiting is the result of increased intracranial pressure and is usually not accompanied by nausea in the absence of tumor infiltration of the area postrema. This differs from ependymomas and other lesions arising from the fourth ventricle itself.

Signs elicited during physical examination are similar to those of many posterior fossa masses and include ataxia, dysmetria, hydrocephalus, papilledema, cranial nerve palsies, nystagmus, and rarely, weakness from involvement of descending motor pathways (see Table 81-1).[1,47] Lesions of the cerebellar hemisphere produce ataxia and dysmetria in the ipsilateral limbs, whereas midline lesions produce truncal and gait ataxia.[3] Obstructive hydrocephalus from tumor compressing the fourth ventricle and its outflow tracts results in dilation of the proximal ventricular system, namely the lateral and third ventricles. This pattern is readily detected on computed tomography (CT) or magnetic resonance imaging (MRI). A more indolent course is seen with slow-growing low-grade tumors (WHO grade I), with symptoms persisting for as long as several years. High-grade tumors (WHO III or IV) progress rapidly with symptoms lasting only days to weeks.

EPIDEMIOLOGY

Spontaneous Cerebellar Astrocytoma

In children, astrocytomas constitute approximately 35% to 47% of all primary brain tumors.[18,44] They can arise within the optic pathway (5%), hypothalamus (10%), cerebellum (15% to 25%), cerebral hemisphere (12%), spine (10% to 12%), or brainstem (12%).[36] Cerebellar astrocytomas represent 12% to 17% of the central nervous system (CNS) tumors in children[15] and 25% to 35% of pediatric tumors of the posterior fossa.[13] The incidence of cerebellar astrocytomas is highest between ages 4 and 10 years, with a median age at diagnosis of 6 years.[51] Therefore pilocytic astrocytomas are often termed *juvenile* pilocytic astrocytomas (JPAs). Gender does not play a role in prognosis or survival, and males and females are equally affected.[44,55] No geographic or ethnic propensity has been found for the occurrence of cerebellar astrocytomas.[18,44]

TABLE 81-1

Signs and Symptoms of Cerebellar Astrocytoma

Symptoms	%
Headache	82–86
Vomiting	66–85
Gait disturbance	64
Visual disturbance	12
Diplopia	11–31
Decreased level of consciousness	7–22
Neck pain/stiffness	5–23
Signs	
Cerebellar signs/ataxia	74–79
Hydrocephalus	85
Papilledema	78–88
Dysmetria	39
Cranial nerve palsies	39
Nystagmus	8–40
Pyramidal signs	3–6

Source: Data from Abdollahzadeh M, Hoffman HJ, Blazer SI, et al: Benign cerebellar astrocytoma in childhood: Experience at the Hospital for Sick Children 1980–1992. Childs Nerv Syst 10:380–383, 1994; and from Sgouros S, Fineron PW, Hockley AD: Cerebellar astrocytoma of childhood: Long-term follow-up. Childs Nerv Syst 11:89–96, 1997.

The incidence of pediatric brain tumors was recently believed to be rising, based on studies from the United States and Europe.[18,21] However, this trend has now been attributed to increased surveillance and reporting during the preceding 2 decades.[44,48] Prior cranial radiation therapy is a risk factor for developing malignant cerebellar astrocytomas.[51] Environmental factors, such as parents' smoking or residential proximity to electromagnetic field sources, have not been linked to pediatric brain tumors, although a parent's occupation in the chemical or electrical industry might be associated with an increased risk of astroglial tumors in offspring.[19,43] Conversely, prenatal vitamin supplementation in mothers may confer a slight protective effect.[40]

Neurofibromatosis Type 1

Neurofibromatosis type 1 (NF1) is genetic disorder inherited in an autosomal dominant manner and is associated with an increased risk of intracranial tumors, with 15% to 20% of patients developing low-grade intracranial tumors. In patients with NF1, pilocytic astrocytomas arise in the optic nerve, hypothalamus, and cerebellum. Five percent of NF1 patients will develop pilocytic cerebellar astrocytomas.[31] The growth of intracranial tumors is the main cause of death among NF1 patients.

The NF1 gene is located on chromosome 17q and encodes a GTPase activating protein, termed neurofibromin, involved in regulating the ras-p21 signaling pathway. Mutations in the NF1 gene lead to the manifestations of the disease. The exact reason that loss of neurofibromin expression, or expression of defective neurofibromin, leads to the formation of astrocytomas is unknown. NF1-associated CNS tumors, such as spontaneous pilocytic astrocytomas, rarely demonstrate alterations in other known oncogenic genes, such as p53, EGFR, PDGF, and p21.[22] In general, NF1-associated cerebellar astrocytomas resemble spontaneous pilocytic astrocytomas and are benign.[56]

DIAGNOSTIC IMAGING

Computed Tomography and Magnetic Resonance Imaging

CT and MRI are the preferred techniques for the diagnosis of cerebellar astrocytomas. CT is readily available, fast, and less expensive than MRI, but bone artifact limits visualization of the posterior fossa. MRI is the preoperative imaging technique of choice because of its accurate anatomic localization, superior resolution with no bone artifact and increased tissue distinction, and multiplanar capability. The disadvantages include increased study time and the requirement of general anesthesia in younger children and infants. Both CT and MRI adequately demonstrate the degree of hydrocephalus present. In patients with altered mental status, a rapid CT scan should be performed first to evaluate for hydrocephalus.

The classic radiologic appearance of a pilocytic cerebellar astrocytoma, observed in 30% to 60% of cases, is a large cyst with a solid mural nodule located in one of the cerebellar hemispheres.[42] On CT, the cyst is hypodense to brain and hyperdense to cerebral spinal fluid (CSF) because of its high protein content. On MRI, the cyst appears hypointense to brain on T1-weighted images (T1-WI) and hyperintense to brain but hypointense to CSF on T2-weighted images (T2-WI) (Figure 81-1). The mural nodule is hypodense to isodense to brain on CT and hyperintense to brain on T1-WI. The mural nodule enhances uniformly following contrast administration on both CT and MRI, whereas the cyst is not affected by the contrast agent. The cyst wall, however, may demonstrate contrast enhancement if neoplastic cells are present. On occasion, the compressed glial reactive tissue surrounding a cyst may also show limited enhancement. The proper treatment of the cyst wall remains controversial, and neurosurgeons often advocate resection, or at least biopsy, of the cyst wall if enhancement is seen. Other pilocytic cerebellar astrocytomas have multiple mural nodules, a single large nodule filling in a portion of the cyst, or an irregular cyst contour.

Cerebellar astrocytomas are solid lesions in 17% to 56% of cases, with 90% originating from or involving the vermis.[42] CT reveals a lesion hypodense to isodense to brain, and MRI demonstrates a mass hyperintense to brain. Uniform enhancement of the solid tumor is commonly seen on CT and MRI, although patchy enhancement and small intratumoral cysts may be present. Often, cerebellar astrocytomas show both cystic and solid features and may have a ringlike enhancement pattern with varying degrees of cyst formation. Calcifications are present in 10% to 17% of tumors and hemorrhage in only 4.5%.[3] Edema may be evident in some cases but does not predict malignancy or poor prognosis.

Magnetic Resonance Spectroscopy

On CT and MRI it remains difficult to distinguish cerebellar astrocytomas from other CNS tumors affecting the cerebellum

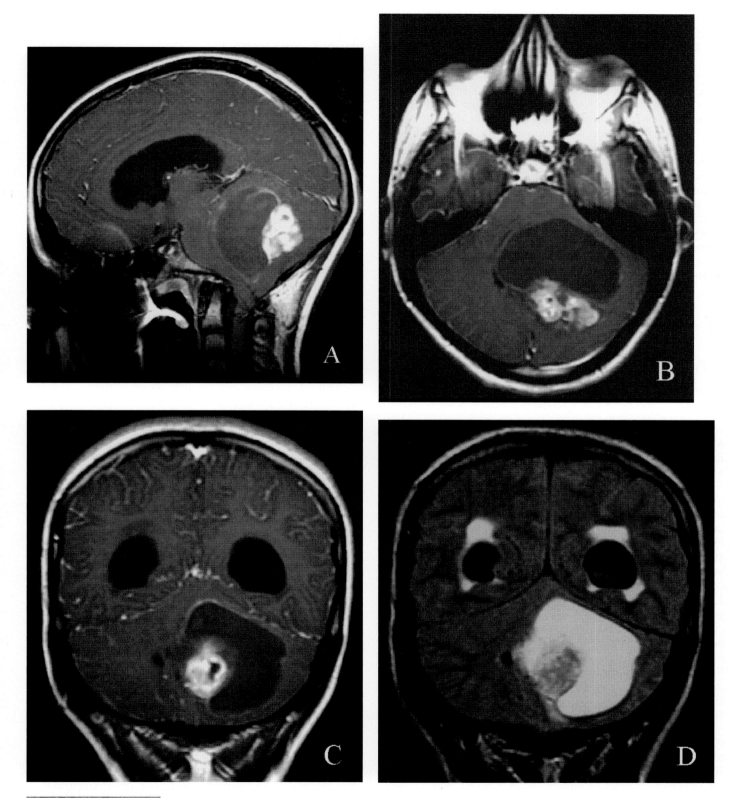

FIGURE 81-1 Preoperative magnetic resonance (MR) images of a typical pediatric pilocytic cerebellar astrocytoma. Sagittal *(A)*, axial *(B)*, and coronal *(C)* T1-weighted images with gadolinium contrast agent demonstrate a cystic hemispheric lesion with an enhanced mural nodule. On histologic examination, the cyst wall was found to contain tumor. *D,* Coronal fluid-attenuated inversion recovery (FLAIR) MR image shows the cystic nature of the cerebellar lesion and periventricular transependymal flow of the lateral ventricles secondary to hydrocephalus.

of children, such as PNET and ependymoma. Therefore histologic examination is necessary to establish a definitive diagnosis. Recently, magnetic resonance spectroscopy (MRS) has been used to distinguish pediatric cerebellar tumors based on differential levels of tumor metabolites and macromolecules. Pilocytic astrocytomas demonstrate increased choline/N-acetyl-aspartate (Cho/NAA) ratios and elevated lactate levels when compared with normal brain but similar to many other tumor types.[25,59] In one study, low-grade astrocytomas had higher NAA/Cho ratios than PNET but lower ratios than ependymoma, whereas creatine-to-Cho ratios were highest for ependymoma and lowest for PNET.[25,59] Other metabolites differentially detected in PNET and astrocytoma in vitro include glutamate, glycine, taurine, and myoinositol. Elevated lactate levels in pilocytic astrocytoma carry no indication of malignancy and may reflect aberrant glucose utilization in these tumors.[59] At present, MRS cannot replace tissue diagnosis, but it may be a useful adjuvant to MRI for the diagnosis of cerebellar astrocytomas.

TUMOR HISTOLOGY

WHO Grading and Genetics

According to the recent WHO classification of CNS tumors, cerebellar astrocytomas are grouped into four grades. WHO grade I corresponds to the pilocytic cerebellar astrocytoma and accounts for approximately 70% to 80% of pediatric cases.[51] Most pilocytic astrocytomas demonstrate normal cytogenetic findings,[6] although abnormalities in chromosomes 1, 7, 8, and 11[61,62] have been described.

Diffuse cerebellar astrocytomas are considered WHO grade II and represent 15% of childhood cases.[51] In contrast to pilocytic astrocytomas, p53 mutations are commonly reported and may represent an early event in malignant progression.[60] Other aberrations include allelic losses on chromosomes 10p, 19, and 22q.[2,57] Grade II tumors are found to have higher mitotic indices, higher percentages of cells in S phase, and more vascular endothelial growth factor (VEGF) expression than grade I tumors.[42] Experimental evidence suggests that grade I and grade II cerebellar astrocytomas develop from different precursor cells.[31] PEN5, a recently identified oligodendroglial antibody epitope, is positive in grade I tumors but not in grade II tumors. Also, NF1-related cerebellar astrocytomas demonstrate PEN5 immunoreactivity, indicating that both spontaneous grade I and NF1-related grade I cerebellar astrocytomas come from the same precursor cells, which are different from grade II tumors.

Cerebellar grade III (anaplastic astrocytoma) and IV (GBM) tumors are not common in childhood and are identical to their counterparts in adults in histology and prognosis. Grade III or IV tumors commonly show gains of chromosomes 7 and 10, structural changes of chromosomes 1, 9, 17, and 22, and loss of alleles on chromosome 17.[5] p53 Mutation and overexpression is common in both grade III and IV tumors. Epidermal growth factor receptor (EGFR) gene amplification, seen in up to 30% of adult tumors, is rare in pediatric high-grade astrocytomas.[52] PTEN mutations were found in 20% to 30% of grade IV tumors, 5.9% of grade III tumors, and 0% of grade II tumors.[41]

Gross Pathology

Cerebellar astrocytomas may be cystic, solid, or mixed. Pilocytic astrocytomas are mostly cystic, containing yellow-brown fluid and a mural nodule. The cyst wall can contain neoplastic cells or non-neoplastic glial tissue.[51] However, less than 50% of pilocytic astrocytomas manifest this classic histology. Pilocytic astrocytomas are found throughout the neuraxis, including the optic pathway, hypothalamus, and cerebral hemisphere, although most are located in the cerebellum. Diffuse subtypes are mostly solid tumors composed of somewhat circumscribed neoplastic cells without cysts. However, it is common for cerebellar astrocytomas to demonstrate a mixed histology with both cystic and solid components of the tumor.

Histopathology

Pilocytic astrocytomas are astrocytic tumors of low cellularity and rare mitotic figures. Dense areas of bipolar cells with Rosenthal fibers are intermixed with loose areas of cells with microcysts and granules. Rosenthal fibers represent elongated eosinophilic cellular inclusions. Occasional microvascular proliferation, pleomorphism, and meningeal invasion is seen and does not represent malignancy or poor prognosis.[51] In up to 50% of cases, local leptomeningeal invasion is apparent, but it has no prognostic significance.[8]

Diffuse cerebellar astrocytomas are divided into three histologic subtypes. Fibrillary astrocytoma is the most common subtype and shows a compact, uniform arrangement of fibrillary astrocytes with varying degrees of cellular atypia on a background of loosely structured tumor matrix.[51] Protoplasmic astrocytomas demonstrate low cellularity and extensive mucoid degeneration with numerous microcysts.[28] Gemistocytic astrocytomas contain tumor cells with large, slightly eosinophilic cytoplasm with nuclei displaced to the periphery.[28] Diffuse astrocytomas resemble low-grade astrocytomas of the cerebral hemispheres with poorly circumscribed borders and invasion of the surrounding parenchyma. These tumors generally occur in older children and young adults and can undergo malignant transformation.[8]

TREATMENT

Natural History

Cerebellar astrocytomas, if left untreated, tend to grow and cause progressive signs and symptoms related to hydrocephalus and cerebellar and brainstem dysfunction. The tempo of progression primarily depends on the exact location of the tumor and its grade. Ultimately, patients die from increasing mass effect and brain herniation.

Preoperative Management and Cerebrospinal Fluid Diversion

Preoperative management depends on the clinical presentation of the patient. An asymptomatic, incidentally discovered lesion can be observed with surgical intervention planned electively. More commonly, however, patients have signs of increased intracranial pressure and cerebellar dysfunction, warranting urgent intervention. High-dose dexamethasone can relieve headache, nausea, and vomiting within a day and allow for several days of relief before undertaking a surgical procedure. An initial loading dose of 4 to 10 mg given intravenously followed by 4 mg/day for patients younger than age 2, 6 to 8 mg/day for those age 2 to 6, and 12 mg/day for those older than age 6. Teenagers of adult weight may take 16 mg/day. The daily dose is divided every 6 hours and may be administered intravenously or orally.[45] In a patient who is stuporous and lethargic, with cardiorespiratory instability, relief of elevated intracranial pressure is of utmost importance and should be performed immediately. A temporary external ventricular drain should be placed in the intensive care unit or the operating room. In less urgent situations, an endoscopic third ventriculocisternostomy (ETV) can also be considered. In this procedure, a passage for CSF egress is created between the third ventricle and the basal cisterns, thereby bypassing the obstruction at the level of the fourth ventricle. This procedure, although not always successful, can avoid permanent shunt placement. Permanent shunt placement usually involves placement of a ventriculoperitoneal (VP) shunt, diverting the CSF into the peritoneal cavity. This procedure carries the risk of upward herniation and subdural hematoma from overshunting while also rendering the patient shunt-dependent for life with all of its associated complications. The risk of upward herniation is estimated at 3% and causes lethargy and obtundation 12 to 24 hours after shunt placement, with the potential for compression of the posterior cerebral arteries at the tentorium, resulting in occipital-lobe ischemia or stroke.[51]

In a stable and alert patient with hydrocephalus from a posterior fossa mass, most neurosurgeons would first resect the tumor and later determine if CSF diversion is necessary. Tumor removal alone may be sufficient to open the fourth ventricle and its outflow tracts. Permanent postoperative CSF diversion following complete tumor removal is required in 10% to 40% of cases.[27]

Surgery

Gross-total resection (GTR) is the treatment of choice for cerebellar astrocytomas and is achieved in 60% to 80% of operative cases[9] (Figure 81-2). GTR is accomplished when all visible tumor is removed during surgery and when both the surgeon's report and postoperative neuroimaging are concordant. MRI with the contrast agent gadolinium is recommended within 24 to 48 hours after resection to assess the extent of tumor removal. Postoperative changes, including edema and gliosis, appear by 3 to 5 days after surgery and can interfere with the identification of residual tumor.[3] In 10% to 15% of cases, the surgeon's and radiologist's reports are in disagreement as to whether GTR was achieved[14]; some tumor tissue visible to the surgeon may not be detected on postoperative imaging and vice versa. The clear presence of residual tumor is managed by reoperation to achieve GTR.

Classic cystic tumors with a mural nodule may require only removal of the nodule to achieve complete resection, depending on the composition of the cyst wall. A nonenhancing cyst wall does not require resection. Contrast enhancement of the cyst wall on MRI is believed to represent neoplastic tissue, and complete removal of all enhancing portions is considered essential to prevent recurrence. Recently, it has become more apparent that enhancement of the cyst wall in some cases

represents vascularized reactive gliosis that does not require resection.[51] It is difficult to distinguish these two processes, and intraoperative biopsy of the cyst wall may be beneficial, although sampling error and poor pathologic visualization on frozen section are to be kept in mind. Surgeons may choose conservative management of the enhancing cyst wall, if the wall enhancement is thin (indicating gliosis rather than tumor), biopsies are unremarkable, and the gross appearance is benign.[51]

Subtotal resection (STR) is recommended when GTR would result in unacceptable morbidity and neurologic dysfunction, usually in the setting of brainstem invasion, involvement of the floor of the fourth ventricle, leptomeningeal spread, and metastasis. Management of incompletely resected tumors remains controversial and depends on clinical circumstances. Interestingly, some low-grade astrocytomas may spontaneously regress or involute. Therefore a period of observation for residual disease that is unresectable may be indicated before reoperation is undertaken.

The role of radiation therapy after resection of cerebellar astrocytomas is unclear. Postoperative irradiation after STR of any grade improves local control and recurrence rates, but survival rates seem to be unaffected.[24] Radiation doses range from 30 to 54 Gy over 3 to 6 weeks, and some evidence suggests that doses greater than 53 Gy are necessary to see beneficial effects.[24] However, the detrimental effects on the developing nervous system preclude its use in infants younger than age 3, and current trends favor delaying radiation therapy as long as possible to allow full cognitive development. The risks of radiation therapy include decreased cognitive function[12] and an increased risk of malignant transformation.[24] Chemotherapy is rarely used for residual disease and is further discussed in the next section.

RECURRENCE

Follow-up Neuroimaging

Postoperative surveillance imaging in children with low-grade cerebellar astrocytomas depends on tumor histology and the extent of initial resection. No consistent imaging schedule is used, but large centers tend to obtain MRI scans at 3 and 6 months, then annually for 3 to 4 years. Routine imaging after GTR for a typical JPA can be stopped 3 to 5 years following resection if there is no evidence of recurrence. However, a small number of benign cerebellar astrocytomas can recur late, sometimes decades after GTR, and therefore clinical changes warrant reimaging. Completely resected grade II cerebellar astrocytomas of the diffuse or fibrillary subtype demonstrate a recurrence rate and prognosis similar to those of grade I lesions. These tumors can be followed with an imaging frequency similar to that for grade I lesions; however, most clinicians tend to follow grade II lesions more closely and for longer times, even when GTR was achieved.

STR commonly occurs with tumors of higher histologic grades and warrants more frequent examinations and neuroimaging to detect tumor progression or recurrence early. Tumor recurrence usually occurs locally at the primary site. For high-grade cerebellar astrocytomas, the entire craniospinal axis should be imaged with MRI to assess for tumor dissemination into the CSF, ideally before initial tumor removal.

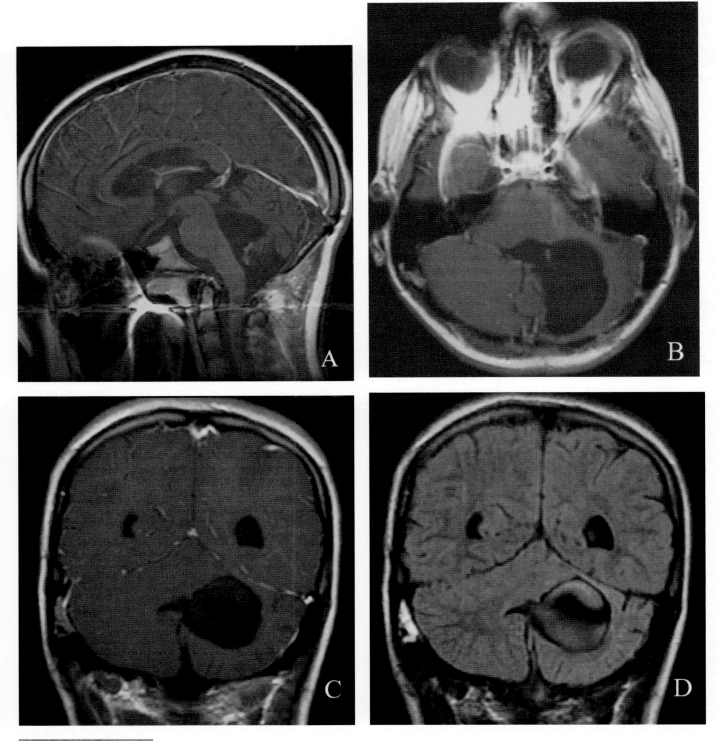

FIGURE 81-2 Magnetic resonance (MR) images made 2.5 months after resection of the pilocytic cerebellar astrocytoma shown in Figure 81-1. Sagittal *(A)*, axial *(B)*, and coronal *(C)* T1-weighted MR images with gadolinium contrast show a resection cavity in the left cerebellar hemisphere. Consistent with gross-total resection, no focus of clear residual enhancement is seen. *D,* Coronal fluid-attenuated inversion recovery (FLAIR) MR image reveals resolution of transependymal flow and reduction in size of the lateral ventricles, suggesting the resolution of hydrocephalus. No permanent cerebrospinal fluid diversion was necessary.

Treatment of Recurrence

Management of recurrence remains the most challenging aspect of treating cerebellar astrocytomas. Treatment options include a combination of reoperation, radiation therapy, and chemotherapy. Recurrence after GTR is rare, can occur several years to decades from the initial operation, and should be treated with reoperation. Few of these patients require further adjuvant therapy. For recurrence following STR, reoperation with the goal of GTR is the preferred first step. Often, however, GTR was not possible at the time of diagnosis because of brainstem or vermian involvement. It is mainly for this reason that, at reoperation, only 30% of recurrences result in GTR, whereas 70% of patients continue to have residual tumor.[14]

Eighty-eight percent of all patients whose tumor recurs have undergone STR, whereas 20% to 50% had brainstem invasion.[35] Following STR, 30% to 40% of patients have a recurrence within 3 years (mean 54 months), whereas more than 60% recur by 5 to 6 years.[14] Tumors with diffuse or fibrillary histology are more prone to recurrence, but this association is not consistent. Of all recurrent tumors, 65% are pilocytic, 31% are diffuse or fibrillary, 48% are cystic, and 52% solid.[18,47] Recurrences are commonly found in the midline or vermis. A clear predictor of disease progression is volume of residual disease.[49] Unfortunately, the relationship between STR, brainstem invasion, residual tumor volume, and histology confound each other in almost all other series.

Radiation and Chemotherapy for Recurrence

Recurrence of low-grade cerebellar astrocytomas after GTR is rare, and even after STR only 4 of 12 patients in one small study demonstrated recurrence within a mean follow-up time of 5 years.[46] For pilocytic astrocytomas, a European study found that 7% recurred after GTR, and 27% recurred after STR.[16] Spontaneous regression of residual pilocytic astrocytoma occurred more often than growth of residual tumor.[16] It is unclear why some tumors do not progress. Those tumors that do recur may remain quiescent for many years. Waller et al[58] reported progression-free survival (PFS) of 74% at 10 years, but only 41% at 20 years. The utility of radiation therapy for STR of cerebellar astrocytomas is unclear. In one study, radiation therapy decreased the frequency of disease progression but had no effect on overall survival.[9] Although experience with Gamma Knife® radiosurgery is even more limited, it is being evaluated for the treatment of small-volume residual or recurrent astrocytomas. In one recent study of nine children treated with radiosurgery, five had decreased tumor size and four had no further growth at a mean follow-up period of 19 months.[50] However, none of those astrocytomas were located in the cerebellum, and the follow-up time was short.

Chemotherapy has a limited role in the treatment of benign cerebellar astrocytoma but has been used in rare instances of multifocal disease, leptomeningeal spread, and malignant transformation.[10,54] Combination chemotherapy has been used in the adjuvant management of inoperable low-grade astrocytomas. Commonly used regimens are carboplatin with vincristine[34] and 6-thioguanine, procarbazine, CCNU, and vincristine.[39] Both regimens have been associated with complete and partial responses in a subgroup of tumors. Cyclophosphamide has been applied in the treatment of cerebellar astrocytoma with leptomeningeal spread.[32] No study has yet shown a clear benefit in recurrence or survival with chemotherapy for residual or recurrent cerebellar astrocytomas.

REHABILITATION

Surgical resection may lead to both non-neurologic and neurologic complications. Fortunately, the majority of these adverse effects are either transient or treatable, making the overall morbidity for surgical treatment of cerebellar astrocytomas quite low. Radiation therapy may result in cognitive impairment, especially in children younger than 3 years. Side effects of chemotherapy can be severe, including myeloid suppression with associated infections, but are usually transient. In patients with pilocytic astrocytomas, the functional outcome was favorable in 82% of patients, and 18% had moderate to severe disabilities.[16]

Neurologic Complications

Worsening of cerebellar dysfunction, such as limb or truncal ataxia and dysmetria, can follow retraction injury or cerebellar swelling, and function improves several weeks to months after surgery.[13] Permanent deficits can occur with significant injury to the vermis, resulting in disabling truncal ataxia and injury to the restiform body, producing ipsilateral limb ataxia. In up to 30% of postoperative patients, new neurologic deficits are found; they include cranial nerve VI and VII dysfunction, nystagmus, bulbar signs, pseudobulbar syndrome, long-tract motor signs, and transient mutism.[13] Impaired initiation of chewing, voiding, and eye opening may occur after injury to areas of the cerebellum responsible for repetitive motor movement memory. Patients with these deficits commonly have tumor involvement of the floor of the fourth ventricle, brainstem, and cerebellar peduncles. Removal of large hemispheric tumors can transiently impair cranial nerve VI function, resulting in diplopia. Half the patients with new deficits are thought to recover their function eventually.[38,51]

Cerebellar mutism can occur after the resection of large midline posterior fossa tumors. The patient is usually able to speak immediately after surgery, but within 24 to 94 hours becomes mute although alert with intact comprehension and normal cranial-nerve and motor function.[38] In the largest series to date, the incidence was 8.5% for all posterior fossa tumors and 12% for vermian tumors but did vary with histology.[11] Patients with malignant tumors, often involving the brainstem, fourth ventricle, and vermis, developed mutism more often (20%) than those with less invasive tumors (1%).[17] Recovery of speech occurs between 2 weeks to 2 months and starts as profoundly dysarthric and abnormal speech, with isolated words and phrases, and progressing to full sentences. Most patients recover fluent speech within 4 months of surgery, with an average duration of mutism lasting 6 weeks.[17,38] However, 20% of patients remain dysarthric. All patients have normal speech preoperatively and it is impossible to predict which child will develop cerebellar mutism.[38] A small radiologic review identified bilateral edema in the brachium pontis as the only factor significantly associated with mutism.[38]

Neuropsychologic changes can be found after surgical resection of posterior fossa tumors. One study described visual-spatial dysfunction in 37%, expressive language problems in 37%, verbal memory decline in 33%, and difficulty with affect control in 15% to 56%.[30] Irritability, impulsiveness, and disinhibition were the most common changes in affect and increased in parallel with greater involvement of the vermis. It is uncertain how often and to what extent these neuropsychologic changes are reversible, and long-term studies are needed. Postoperative radiation therapy is highly associated with lower IQ during childhood and affects younger children more than older ones.[20]

Non-neurologic Complications

Pseudomeningocele, the formation of a CSF collection outside the confines of the subarachnoid space, is reported in 12% to 24% of patients postoperatively.[1] It occurs 1 to 2 weeks after the initial surgery and occurs as a fluctuant, occasionally tense mass under the incision. The formation of a pseudomeningocele may indicate the presence of untreated hydrocephalus, a CSF fistula, or a wound infection. Most pseudomeningoceles resolve within days to weeks without intervention. Wound breakdown and hydrocephalus are indications for CSF diversion or shunting and antibiotic treatment if meningitis or other infection is suspected. Percutaneous needle aspiration for cell count and culture is not recommended, because risk of infection rises with skin puncture, although it may provide temporary relief of pain from skin tension or prevent wound dehiscence.

Hydrocephalus can develop from obstruction of any level along the CSF pathway from residual tumor, blood clot, swelling, or inflammation. Asymptomatic and stable hydrocephalus requires no immediate intervention, and the patient can be followed for 6 to 8 weeks before permanent shunt placement is considered. Acute hydrocephalus, persistent pseudomeningocele, and CSF leak warrant CSF diversion with either VP shunt placement or ETV and are required in 10% to 26% of patients following posterior fossa surgery.[51] The risk of extraneural metastasis from shunting in children with cerebellar astrocytomas is virtually nonexistent.[4]

Wound infections are not common (2% to 5%) in the absence of a pseudomeningocele and poor nutrition, and meningitis is seen in 3% to 8% of patients.[1] Aseptic meningitis is not unusual after posterior fossa surgery in children. Patients have increasing headache 4 to 7 days following surgery, accompanied by fever, nuchal rigidity, and CSF pleocytosis.[45] Organisms are not isolated, and symptoms seem to correspond with steroid taper. No treatment is necessary, though bacterial meningitis must be excluded.

OUTCOME

Prognostic Factors

Brainstem invasion, irrespective of tumor histology, carries a poor prognosis, with only 40% of patients alive at 5 years after diagnosis. In contrast, without brainstem involvement, 84% were alive at 5 years.[9,47] The effect of histology on PFS and outcome has been controversial. One study found pilocytic cerebellar astrocytoma to have 5-, 10-, and 20-year survival rates of 85%, 81%, and 79%, respectively, whereas diffuse subtypes had dramatically reduced survival rates of 7% at 5, 10, and 20 years each.[23] Unfortunately, the mean age of patients in both groups differed greatly (14 years for the pilocytic and 51 years for the diffuse astrocytomas), making a meaningful comparison difficult. Moreover, diffuse tumors in this study had a more malignant histology, which suggests that higher grade

lesions might have been included inappropriately. More recent series have reported 78% survival with 89% PFS for pilocytic histology and 44% survival with 52% PFS for diffuse subtypes at 5 years.[47] A European group[16] reported 5, 10, and 25 year survival rates for pilocytic astrocytomas of 90%, 89%, and 85%, respectively. Diffuse or fibrillary histology has been reported as the most important determinant for residual tumor volume, which in turn is the only predictor of tumor recurrence at any site after multivariate analysis in one study.[49]

Cystic tumors, compared with solid tumors, have greater 5-year PFS rates, and that is thought to be a result of the more complete resection of cystic tumors. After controlling for extent of tumor removal, most series do not demonstrate a survival advantage based on tumor morphology.[47,49] Tumor location, such as a hemispheric versus a vermian or midline site, does not affect prognosis,[49] even though complete resection is more often achieved with a hemispheric location than in the midline.

Clinical characteristics such as gender and age at diagnosis do not influence survival.[49] A short interval of symptoms may reflect more rapid tumor growth and, therefore, a higher tumor grade. Tumors with a long duration of symptoms are often large. Patients with neurofibromatosis can have malignant histology, but the majority of NF1 patients with cerebellar astrocytomas appear to have a quiescent course.[49]

Gross-Total and Subtotal Resection

The prognosis for patients with grade I tumors and GTR is excellent, with 5- and 10-year PFS of 80% to 100% in nearly all studies. Even a 30-year PFS is not unusual. Patients with grade II tumors after total resection have 5-year survival rates of 50% to 80%. Patients with grade III and IV lesions continue to have poor survival rates, despite GTR, at 2 years. GTR is reported in 53% of patients with tumors of a pilocytic histology and a hemispheric location but in only 19% of those with tumors not of a pilocytic histology.[9] Recurrence after GTR occurs in less than 5% of grade I cases, though recurrences have been reported as long as 45 years after initial resection.[7]

In general, STR is associated with future tumor recurrence and poorer outcome.[35] Approximately 75% of patients will have recurrence during the follow-up period, although some remain stable clinically and radiographically for several years.[29] The 5-year survival rate varies from 29% to 80%, and 10-year survival ranges from 0% to 70%,[9,47] with these variations attributable to inconsistent study design. STR is more commonly reported with solid midline tumors, usually of grade II or higher. In one prospective study, only 50% of patients with STR and no brainstem involvement demonstrated progression of disease at a follow-up interval of 8 years.[53] Interestingly, 1.5% of residual tumors spontaneously regressed without further treatment.[53] The biologic reason behind tumor quiescence or regression is unknown. STR with recurrence carries a 25% PFS at 5 years from the time of recurrence, and reoperation tends to lower subsequent recurrence rates but does not affect overall survival.[47] The extent of resection and infiltration of the brainstem influenced survival in children with grade I and grade II cerebellar astrocytoma.[16,47,49]

Malignant Transformation and Metastasis

Malignant transformation of pilocytic astrocytomas occurs rarely.[3] Several case reports describe malignant degeneration in pilocytic cerebellar astrocytomas at recurrence several years from initial resection.[3] Standard indices of aggressive histology, such as necrosis, vascular proliferation, and mitoses, do not indicate malignancy in pilocytic astrocytomas, although increased perivascular cellularity may serve as a marker of future anaplastic change.[29]

Leptomeningeal dissemination of low-grade astrocytomas occurs rarely and is associated mainly with hypothalamic tumor location.[37] Spinal metastases are the most common and were found in 3 of 72 patients.[37] Of patients with diffuse cerebellar astrocytoma, 7% had spinal metastases.[23] Long-term outcome is not known, but there is anecdotal evidence that leptomeningeal dissemination indicates impending malignant degeneration.[29] Aggressive resection of isolated metastasis, combined with irradiation and chemotherapy, may result in PFS.[37,54] CSF sampling is not helpful in detecting early leptomeningeal dissemination.[37]

CONCLUSION

Cerebellar astrocytomas of childhood commonly present during the first decade of life with cerebellar dysfunction, hydrocephalus, and at times cranial nerve palsies. Pilocytic astrocytomas (grade I) represent the predominant subtype; therefore, among pediatric brain tumors, cerebellar astrocytomas have the most favorable prognosis. Complete tumor resection is the treatment of choice and correlates with outcome, regardless of tumor histology. Cures can be achieved with grade I tumors; however, tumors of higher grade are often invasive, and only STR can be performed. Patients with grade III or IV tumors still have a poor outcome. Perioperative steroid administration and CSF diversion are often indicated. Surgical complications from tumor removal include worsening of cerebellar dysfunction, cranial-nerve dysfunction, mutism, pseudomeningocele, hydrocephalus, and wound infection and need to be discussed with the family before an operation is undertaken. Full recovery from most complications can be expected after weeks to months of recovery.

Treatment of tumor recurrence is controversial, and no clear regimen for adjuvant radiation or chemotherapy has been established. Grade I tumors rarely recur, whereas higher grade tumors and those with STR or brainstem invasion represent the majority of recurrent cerebellar astrocytomas. If feasible, re-resection should be attempted, and if not successful, radiation therapy is the preferred treatment. Radiation therapy in the setting of recurrence has not been shown to confer benefit on overall survival but may increase PFS. Chemotherapy is reserved for tumors with leptomeningeal spread, those that fail adjuvant radiation therapy, or for very young patients with tumors that are not amenable to resection. In general, PFS and overall outcome depend on extent of resection, brainstem involvement, and histologic subtype.

References

1. Abdollahzadeh M, Hoffman HJ, Blazer SI, et al: Benign cerebellar astrocytoma in childhood: experience at the Hospital for Sick Children 1980–1992. Childs Nerv Syst 10:380–383, 1994.
2. Bello MJ, de Campos JM, Kusak ME, et al: Molecular analysis of genomic abnormalities in human gliomas. Cancer Genet Cytogenet 73:122–129, 1994.
3. Berger MS: Cerebellar astrocytoma. In Becker DP, Dunsker SB, Friedman WA, et al (eds): Tumors, Vol 4, 4th ed. Philadelphia, Saunders, 1996.
4. Berger MS, Baumeister B, Geyer JR, et al: The risks of metastases from shunting in children with primary central nervous system tumors. J Neurosurg 74:872–877, 1991.
5. Biegel JA: Genetics of pediatric central nervous system tumors. J Pediatr Hematol Oncol 19:492–501, 1997.
6. Bigner SH, McLendon RE, Fuchs H, et al: Chromosomal characteristics of childhood brain tumors. Cancer Genet Cytogenet 97:125–134, 1997.
7. Boch AL, Cacciola F, Mokhtari K, et al: Benign recurrence of a cerebellar pilocytic astrocytoma 45 years after gross total resection. Acta Neurochir 142:341–346, 2000.
8. Burger PC, Scheitauer BW, Paulus W, et al: Pilocytic astrocytoma. In Cavenee PKW (ed): Tumors of the Nervous System: Pathology & Genetics. Lyon, France, IARC Press, 2000.
9. Campbell JW, Pollack IF: Cerebellar astrocytomas in children. J Neurooncol 28:223–231, 1996.
10. Castello MA, Schiavetti A, Varrasso G, et al: Chemotherapy in low-grade astrocytoma management. Childs Nerv Syst 14:6–9, 1998.
11. Catsman-Berrevoets CE, Van Dongen HR, Mulder PG, et al: Tumour type and size are high risk factors for the syndrome of "cerebellar" mutism and subsequent dysarthria. J Neurol Neurosurg Psychiatry 67:755–757, 1999.
12. Chadderton RD, West CG, Schuller S, et al: Radiotherapy in the treatment of low-grade astrocytomas. II. The physical and cognitive sequelae. Childs Nerv Syst 11:443–448, 1995.
13. Cochrane DD, Gustavsson B, Poskitt KP, et al: The surgical and natural morbidity of aggressive resection for posterior fossa tumors in childhood. Pediatr Neurosurg 20:19–29, 1994.
14. Dirven CM, Mooij JJ, Molenaar WM: Cerebellar pilocytic astrocytoma: a treatment protocol based upon analysis of 73 cases and a review of the literature. Childs Nerv Syst 13:17–23, 1997.
15. Dohrmann GJ FJ, Flannery JT: Astrocytomas in childhood: a population-based study. Surg Neurol 23:64–68, 1985.
16. Due-Tonnessen BJ HE, Scheie D, Skullerud K, et al: Long-term outcome after resection of benign cerebellar astrocytomas in children and young adults (0–19 years): report of 110 consecutive cases. Pediatr Neurosurg 37:71–80, 2002.
17. Ersahin Y, Mutluer S, Cagli S, et al: Cerebellar mutism: report of seven cases and review of the literature. Neurosurgery 38:60–65; discussion 66, 1996.
18. Gjerris F, Agerlin N, Borgesen SE, et al: Epidemiology and prognosis in children treated for intracranial tumours in Denmark 1960–1984. Childs Nerv Syst 14:302–311, 1998.
19. Gold EB, Leviton A, Lopez R, et al: Parental smoking and risk of childhood brain tumors. Am J Epidemiol 137:620–628, 1993.
20. Grill J, Renaux VK, Bulteau C, et al: Long-term intellectual outcome in children with posterior fossa tumors according to radiation doses and volumes. Int J Radiat Oncol Biol Phys 45:137–145, 1999.
21. Gurney JG, Davis S, Severson RK, et al: Trends in cancer incidence among children in the U.S. Cancer 78:532–541, 1996.
22. Gutmann DH, Donahoe J, Brown T, et al: Loss of neurofibromatosis 1 (NF1) gene expression in NF1-associated pilocytic astrocytomas. Neuropathol Appl Neurobiol 26:361–367, 2000.

23. Hayostek CJ, Shaw EG, Scheithauer B, et al: Astrocytomas of the cerebellum. A comparative clinicopathologic study of pilocytic and diffuse astrocytomas. Cancer 72:856–869, 1993.

24. Herfarth KK, Gutwein S, Debus J: Postoperative radiotherapy of astrocytomas. Semin Surg Oncol 20:13–23, 2001.

25. Hwang JH, Egnaczyk GF, Ballard E, et al: Proton MR spectroscopic characteristics of pediatric pilocytic astrocytomas. AJNR Am J Neuroradiol 19:535–540, 1998.

26. Ilgren EB, Stiller CA: Cerebellar astrocytomas. Part I. Macroscopic and microscopic features. Clin Neuropathol 6:185–200, 1987.

27. Imielinski BL, Kloc W, Wasilewski W, et al: Posterior fossa tumors in children—indications for ventricular drainage and for V-P shunting. Childs Nerv Syst 14:227–229, 1998.

28. Kaye AH, Walker DG: Low grade astrocytomas: controversies in management. J Clin Neurosci 7:475–483, 2000.

29. Krieger MD, Gonzalez-Gomez I, Levy ML, et al: Recurrence patterns and anaplastic change in a long-term study of pilocytic astrocytomas. Pediatr Neurosurg 27:1–11, 1997.

30. Levisohn L, Cronin-Golomb A, Schmahmann JD: Neuropsychological consequences of cerebellar tumour resection in children: cerebellar cognitive affective syndrome in a paediatric population. Brain 123:1041–1050, 2000.

31. Li J, Perry A, James CD, et al: Cancer-related gene expression profiles in NF1-associated pilocytic astrocytomas. Neurology 56:885–890, 2001.

32. McCowage G, Tien R, McLendon R, et al: Successful treatment of childhood pilocytic astrocytomas metastatic to the leptomeninges with high-dose cyclophosphamide. Med Pediatr Oncol 27:32–39, 1996.

33. Morreale VM, Ebersold MJ, Quast LM, et al: Cerebellar astrocytoma: experience with 54 cases surgically treated at the Mayo Clinic, Rochester, Minnesota, from 1978 to 1990. J Neurosurg 87:257–261, 1997.

34. Packer RJ, Lange B, Ater J, et al: Carboplatin and vincristine for recurrent and newly diagnosed low-grade gliomas of childhood. J Clin Oncol 11:850–856, 1993.

35. Pencalet P, Maixner W, Sainte-Rose C, et al: Benign cerebellar astrocytomas in children. J Neurosurg 90:265–273, 1999.

36. Pollack IF: Pediatric brain tumors. Semin Surg Oncol 16:73–90, 1999.

37. Pollack IF, Hurtt M, Pang D, et al: Dissemination of low grade intracranial astrocytomas in children. Cancer 73:2869–2878, 1994.

38. Pollack IF, Polinko P, Albright AL, et al: Mutism and pseudobulbar symptoms after resection of posterior fossa tumors in children: incidence and pathophysiology. Neurosurgery 37:885–893, 1995.

39. Prados MD, Edwards MS, Rabbitt J, et al: Treatment of pediatric low-grade gliomas with a nitrosourea-based multiagent chemotherapy regimen. J Neurooncol 32:235–241, 1997.

40. Preston-Martin S, Pogoda JM, Mueller BA, et al: Prenatal vitamin supplementation and pediatric brain tumors: huge international variation in use and possible reduction in risk. Childs Nerv Syst 14:551–557, 1998.

41. Raffel C, Frederick L, O'Fallon JR, et al: Analysis of oncogene and tumor suppressor gene alterations in pediatric malignant astrocytomas reveals reduced survival for patients with PTEN mutations. Clin Cancer Res 5:4085–4090, 1999.

42. Reddy ATM, Timothy B: Cerebellar astrocytoma. In McLone DG (ed): Pediatric Neurosurgery: Surgery of the Developing Nervous System, Vol 4, 4th ed. New York, Saunders, 2000.

43. Rickert CH: Epidemiological features of brain tumors in the first 3 years of life. Childs Nerv Syst 14:547–550, 1998.

44. Rickert CH, Paulus W: Epidemiology of central nervous system tumors in childhood and adolescence based on the new WHO classification. Childs Nerv Syst 17:503–511, 2001.

45. Rosenfeld JV: Cerebellar astrocytoma in children. In Kaye AH, Black PM (eds): Operative Neurosurgery, Vol 2, 1st ed. New York, Churchill Livingstone, 2000.

46. Schneider JH, Jr, Raffel C, McComb JG: Benign cerebellar astrocytomas of childhood. Neurosurgery 30:58–62; discussion 62–53, 1992.

47. Sgouros S, Fineron PW, Hockley AD: Cerebellar astrocytoma of childhood: long-term follow-up. Childs Nerv Syst 11:89–96, 1995.

48. Smith MA, Freidlin B, Ries LA, et al: Trends in reported incidence of primary malignant brain tumors in children in the United States. J Natl Cancer Inst 90:1269–1277, 1998.

49. Smoots DW, Geyer JR, Lieberman DM, et al: Predicting disease progression in childhood cerebellar astrocytoma. Childs Nerv Syst 14:636–648, 1998.

50. Somaza SC, Kondziolka D, Lunsford LD, et al: Early outcomes after stereotactic radiosurgery for growing pilocytic astrocytomas in children. Pediatr Neurosurg 25:109–115, 1996.

51. Steinbok P, Mutat A: Cerebellar astrocytoma. In Albright AL, Pollack IF, Adelson PD (eds): Principles and Practice of Pediatric Neurosurgery. New York, Thieme, 1999.

52. Sung T, Miller DC, Hayes RL, et al: Preferential inactivation of the p53 tumor suppressor pathway and lack of EGFR amplification distinguish de novo high grade pediatric astrocytomas from de novo adult astrocytomas. Brain Pathol 10:249–259, 2000.

53. Sutton LN, Cnaan A, Klatt L, et al: Postoperative surveillance imaging in children with cerebellar astrocytomas. J Neurosurg 84:721–725, 1996.

54. Tamura M, Zama A, Kurihara H, et al: Management of recurrent pilocytic astrocytoma with leptomeningeal dissemination in childhood. Childs Nerv Syst 14:617–622, 1998.

55. Viano JC, Herrera EJ, Suarez JC: Cerebellar astrocytomas: a 24-year experience. Childs Nerv Syst 17:607–610; discussion 611, 2001.

56. Vinchon M, Soto-Ares G, Ruchoux MM, et al: Cerebellar gliomas in children with NF1: pathology and surgery. Childs Nerv Syst 16:417–420, 2000.

57. von Deimling A, Nagel J, Bender B, et al: Deletion mapping of chromosome 19 in human gliomas. Int J Cancer 57:676–680, 1994.

58. Wallner KE, Gonzales MF, Edwards MSB, et al: Treatment results of juvenile pilocytic astrocytoma. J Neurosurg 69:171–176, 1988.

59. Wang Z, Sutton LN, Cnaan A, et al: Proton MR spectroscopy of pediatric cerebellar tumors. AJNR Am J Neuroradiol 16:1821–1833, 1995.

60. Watanabe K, Peraud A, Gratas C, et al: p53 and PTEN gene mutations in gemistocytic astrocytomas. Acta Neuropathol (Berl) 95:559–564, 1998.

61. Wernicke C, Thiel G, Lozanova T, et al: Numerical aberrations of chromosomes 1, 2, and 7 in astrocytomas studied by interphase cytogenetics. Genes Chromosomes Cancer 19:6–13, 1997.

62. Zattara-Cannoni H, Gambarelli D, Lena G, et al: Are juvenile pilocytic astrocytomas benign tumors? A cytogenetic study in 24 cases. Cancer Genet Cytogenet 104:157–160, 1998.

CHAPTER 82

BRAINSTEM GLIOMAS

Bruce Kaufman

Primary brainstem tumors have rightfully been considered difficult to treat.[34] They have been described as having a progressive neurologic deterioration, followed by a "slow, miserable" death within 18 months of diagnosis. In the 1960s Matson considered all brainstem gliomas (BSGs) to be inoperable and survival after diagnosis unlikely past 1 year.[27] Treatment seemed to be of little help, with radiation typically showing a transient effectiveness, at best, but was rarely curative.

More recently, approximately 6% to 20% of these patients have been observed to have long-term survival.[15,18,33,35] Improved surgical techniques, allowing direct access to some brainstem tumors, have been suggested as one factor in these improved outcomes.[9,35,36] Other factors suggested to correlate with outcome include tumor focality,[8,46] tumor growth pattern,[10,11,35,36,39,44] tumor imaging characteristics,[8,21,30,35] and tumor location.[3,28,35,39]

Brainstem tumors seem to have two broad categories, based on differing signs, findings, and often outcomes. They can be grouped as *diffuse pontine* lesions versus all others, or as *cystic or focal* versus diffuse pontine enlargement.[20] Based primarily on their imaging characteristics, four categories have also been defined, to include *focal, dorsally exophytic, cervicomedullary,* and *diffuse intrinsic.*[9,11,16]

This chapter reviews the signs and symptoms, evaluation, treatment, and outcome differences for this somewhat differing group of tumors.

EPIDEMIOLOGY AND PRESENTATION

Brainstem tumors account for approximately 10% to 20% of all pediatric central nervous system tumors.[16,29,40] The great majority of these tumors are gliomas. More than 75% of the patients with BSGs will seek treatment before age 20, with a peak of incidence at 5 to 8 years of age and a smaller peak at 36 to 45 years of age.[20,41]

Patients with these tumors on average have symptoms for less than 6 months before diagnosis, but many will have less than 2 months of symptoms. This is likely the result of a functionally densely packed anatomic region being affected and the rather noticeable effects when any of these functions are affected. The most commonly reported symptoms include headache with vomiting (80%) and a change in gait (85%) resulting from cerebellar involvement or weakness, which are present in nearly 70% of patients.[20,26] When the tumor affects the pons, cranial nerve dysfunction will be seen in approximately two thirds of patients. Diplopia or a head tilt, facial weakness, or gagging and difficulties with swallowing are the most common.[26] If the tumor involves or extends into the cerebellopontine angle, then trigeminal and auditory functions may be affected. The combination of cranial nerve dysfunction with long-tract signs has been considered highly suggestive of a BSG.

The frequency of specific symptoms is very dependent on the location of the tumor within the brainstem.[13,21,41] The more common diffuse pontine lesion will usually have a shorter duration of symptoms and more severe symptoms than the nondiffuse tumors, although the latter can yield identical findings.

The diffuse pontine tumors occur at a mean age of approximately 6 years, with a short symptom duration before diagnosis averaging only 6 weeks. Multiple cranial nerve abnormalities are present in nearly all the patients, usually affecting ocular motility and facial function. Ataxia and long-tract signs were each present in 70%. All three are found in 35% of patients with diffuse BSG.

Patients with localized BSG tend to be older, with a mean age at diagnosis of 10 years. They have a much longer average duration of symptoms before diagnosis of 65 weeks. The cranial nerves are uncommonly involved (15%), but ataxia (55%) and long-tract signs (40%) are still common. This group of patients will have more headache, nausea, and vomiting because of a higher incidence of obstructive hydrocephalus. Patients with exophytic BSG may have torticollis and unilateral abducens palsy.

As a group, the reported survivals vary widely, from none at 3 years after diagnosis to up to 50% at 5 years after diagnosis.[1,19,25] Early on, this led to multiple attempts to separate these patients into categories based on risk of progression and death. Ultimately, the most consistent grouping has been based on tumor location and magnetic resonance imaging (MRI) characteristics. Tumors outside the pons and those that were exophytic were noted to do much better.[12,28,44]

A less consistent prognostic factor is the duration of symptoms. In some reports a short duration of symptoms was associated with a worse outcome, but in other studies this was not a discerning factor.[13,32,37,41] Multiple cranial nerve involvement is usually associated with a worse outcome.[32,1] The imaging characteristic of focal contrast enhancement seems to be associated with a better prognosis, but in one study patients with nonenhanced tumors did better.[8,22,32] The patient age, sex, and the actual pathology have not been considered to be of any consistent prognostic significance.[22,41]

Patients with neurofibromatosis type 1 (NF1) often will be found on imaging to have lesions of the brainstem.[34] In general, these lesions will behave in a benign fashion, and only 20% will require treatment. Although these lesions may represent a different pathology, when biopsies are performed they look like typical astrocytomas.

IMAGING

The evaluation of brainstem tumors has evolved concurrent with the evolution in techniques of imaging. Indirect observation of these tumors was achieved using pneumoencephalography and cisternography. Computed tomography (CT) allowed for direct imaging. However, CT is limited by the beam-hardening artifacts in the posterior fossa and the nature of these tumors, which have a density similar to brain tissue and inconsistent patterns of enhancement.

MRI gives exquisite definition of normal and abnormal tissue in the brainstem and adjacent structures (Figure 82-1).[3,13,50] The evaluation and, frankly, the diagnosis of these tumors now relies on the use of MRI. A number of series have described the MRI characteristics of various brainstem tumors.

T2-weighted images provide the most sensitive visualization of tumor extent.[3] T2 imaging in the sagittal plane is especially useful in defining the anatomy and tumor of brainstem lesions. This sequence also seems to correlate best with the extent of pathology, at least in postmortem studies.[26] T2-weighted images are very sensitive to blood and blood products and thus are useful in evaluating the differential diagnosis of brainstem lesions.

MRI spectroscopy has offered hope for in vivo assessment and grading of BSGs. Unfortunately, there is a "sampling error" similar to that obtained with small biopsies. Difficulties with volume averaging occur, because the voxel of measurement can contain areas of tumor, necrosis, and invaded normal tissue.

These tumors can be classified based on imaging by their location and appearance. The most common form of BSG is the diffuse pontine type, occurring 50% to 85% of the time.[16,20,41] Focal gliomas involving the brainstem are reported from 5% to 25% and include those with a cystic component.[16,20] Ten to twenty percent of these tumors show an exophytic growth pattern, extending dorsally into the fourth ventricle, laterally into the cerebellopontine angle, or into the cervicomedullary junction (Figure 82-2).[13,16] Approximately 5% to 10% of the tumors are restricted to the cervicomedullary junction.[16]

The focal, dorsally exophytic, and cervicomedullary tumors constitute the group of nondiffuse BSGs. As a group, only half tend to be enhanced on MRI with gadolinium contrast, but the enhancement is usually uniform and bright.[13,21,50] A third may not be enhanced at all. Three quarters will have a focal pattern of growth, and a small number (perhaps as many as 10% of the nondiffuse tumors) will be located within the pons.[13]

Midbrain tumors encountered before the use of MRI were often misdiagnosed as "aqueductal stenosis," because small tumor would be missed by CT. More than 80% of these tumors would cause obstructive hydrocephalus at the level of the aqueduct.[28,39,50] MRI shows that these tumors are distributed nearly

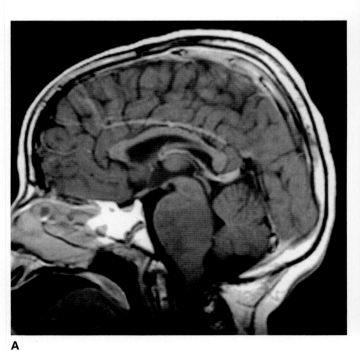

A

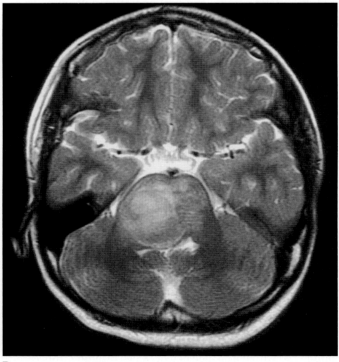

B

FIGURE 82-1 Diffuse pontine glioma. *A,* Magnetic resonance (MR), sagittal T1-weighted image with gadolinium—the pons is noted to be diffusely enlarged in all directions, obliterating the anterior cerebrospinal fluid spaces and displacing the fourth ventricle but not causing hydrocephalus; there is variable signal through the tumor but no significant enhancement. *B,* MR, axial T2-weighted image—the tumor has diffusely expanded the pons and seems to have highlighted the decussating pontine fibers.

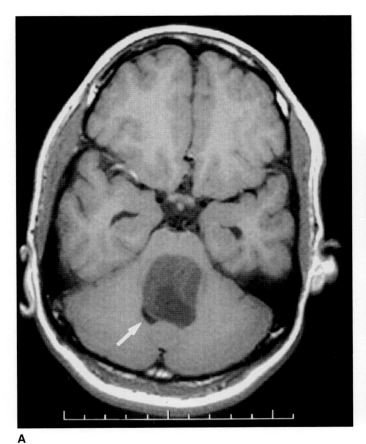

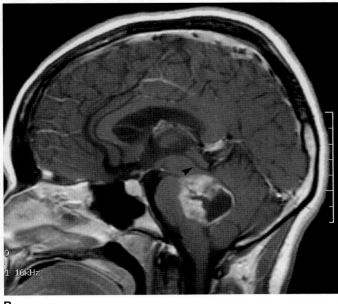

A

B

FIGURE 82-2 Dorsally exophytic brainstem glioma. *A,* Magnetic resonance (MR), axial T1-weighted image—the tumor extends dorsally and displaces the fourth ventricle posteriorly and to the right *(arrow).* The tumor is hypointense with areas suggesting more solid tumor and is well demarcated from the brainstem. *B,* MR, sagittal T1-weighted image with gadolinium—the periphery of the tumor is irregularly enhanced, with no enhancement seen in the center of the mass. Note the aqueduct displaced dorsally and superiorly *(arrowhead),* confirming the lesion is intrinsic to the brainstem.

equally among the tectum, tegmentum, and immediately adjacent areas.[13,39,50] On T1-weighted images approximately 60% are isointense, 24% are hypointense, and 18% have a mixed intensity. They all seem to be hyperintense on T2-weighted images. They are typically slow to grow, with a resulting benign clinical course.

Medullary tumors tend to be either focal or exophytic. They are hypointense on T1 images and hyperintense on T2 images. They are usually enhanced with gadolinium contrast. The few medullary tumors that are diffuse behave much like the diffuse pontine tumors, with more rapid progression and death.[21,50]

Diffuse pontine tumors, the most common BSG, enlarge the pons in the anterior-posterior and lateral dimensions.[13,14,50] With CT imaging, approximately one third are isodense, and another third are hypodense to the brainstem tissue. These tumors will show irregular and infrequent CT contrast enhancement, particularly when compared with focal and exophytic tumors in the same region.[41,50]

MRI of diffuse pontine tumors will show the enlargement of the pons, obliteration of the prepontine cistern, and even the tumor enveloping the basilar or vertebral arteries (Figure 82-3).[13,50] Although arising within the pons, there can be exten-

sion through the cerebellar peduncles into the cerebellum, extension up into the midbrain, or down into the medulla. The initial growth pattern seems to be infiltrative, with limited destruction of the involved neural structures and relatively few symptoms considering the size and extent of the mass. These tumors are hypointense on T1 and hyperintense on T2 images.[13,14,50] Gadolinium enhancement is variable and often limited, with 60% showing no enhancement. Some lesions will have mild, irregular enhancement or even ring enhancement. MRI is usually able to define leptomeningeal spread when present, seen as contrast enhancement coating the surface of the brain and spinal cord—so called *sugar coating.* Such spread is rare at diagnosis, but eventually 5% to 25% of BSG patients will show some subarachnoid spread.[50]

With the diffuse pontine tumors, the extent of MRI contrast enhancement does not correlate with the patient's prognosis or survival. In many patients, the tumor will show an increase in contrast enhancement immediately preceding a clinical decline and death. Whether this is due to rapid tumor growth or increased tumor necrosis is unknown.[30,31]

Central necrosis in diffuse tumors has been defined on both CT and MRI. CT shows a hypodense area with a rim of

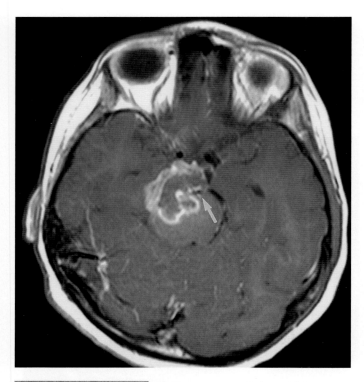

FIGURE 82-3 Diffuse pontine glioma with anterior extension. Magnetic resonance (MR), axial T1-weighted image with gadolinium—the tumor tissue is irregularly enhanced and extends anteriorly, starting to surround the basilar artery *(arrow)*.

contrast enhancement. MRI will have a low T1 signal within a lower T1 signal area, with the region showing bright signal on T2 images and a rim of enhancement. Such necrosis is seen in 20% of patients before any treatment, and the incidence of necrosis increases with time—regardless of the treatment.[31]

MRI has been quite useful with NF1 patients.[49] Many of them will have a benign enlargement of the brainstem that can resemble a typical BSG. In NF1, the degree of brainstem enlargement is less than with glioma, and the enlargement is not limited to the pons. Magnetic resonance (MR) spectroscopy may have a distinct role in this differentiation, because the presumably non-neoplastic tissue in NF1 will have a preserved N-acetylaspartate (NA) peak compared with the typical neoplastic tissue.

Imaging advances, in particular the various MRI techniques, are able to specifically define the extent and involvement of these tumors, limiting the differential diagnostic possibilities.[2,13,22,42,49] Imaging has effectively replaced biopsy of the diffuse pontine lesions, but lesions other than glioma do occur in this region.[32,48]

Primitive neuroectodermal tumors (PNETs) involving the brainstem tend to be distinct by appearance and on imaging from BSGs. PNET occurs in a somewhat younger child (<3 years old) compared with the average of 6 years old for gliomas, but there is considerable overlap in the age ranges. The PNET is typically very well circumscribed. The focal pontine lesion has a low T1 and high T2 signal with no enhancement. Often there is subarachnoid spread of tumor at the time of diagnosis, rather than later as may happen with BSGs. PNET patients may

have hydrocephalus, whereas patients with BSG typically develop hydrocephalus late in the course of the disease.

Brainstem encephalitis can have a spectrum of clinical symptoms and findings similar to those of a BSG. Encephalitis is typically preceded by a viral illness, and the CT and MRI scans are usually normal. The clinical course is rather benign and short, with resolution of symptoms within weeks. Multiple sclerosis, although often considered in the context of a solitary, demarcated brainstem lesion, is a rare occurrence in infants and children.

Vascular diseases of the brainstem that might be confused with a glioma include cavernous malformations and small arteriovenous malformations. These lesions will usually have some degree of hemosiderin, hemorrhage, or calcification that is not seen in the typical BSG. Tuberculomas can mimic the symptoms and signs seen with BSG, and infratentorial tuberculomas are more common in children. Imaging combined with skin testing should easily delineate this lesion. Parasitic cysts, such as cysticercosis, have involvement of the brain in up to 60% of affected patients but are more common in the cerebral hemispheres or within the fourth ventricle than within the brainstem. Imaging showing multiple lesions combined with serologic testing usually gives the diagnosis, but a solitary cystic glioma can mimic a typical cysticercosis cyst.

HISTOLOGY

The relatively low frequency of biopsy and the paucity of tissue obtained for examination (see surgical section) has limited the microscopic analysis of these tumors. The diffuse pontine gliomas have shown a distribution of low- to high-grade tumors. In one series of 71 biopsies of diffuse lesions, grade I astrocytomas accounted for 14%, grade II for 75%, grade III for 10%, and grade IV for 1%.[41] Unfortunately, there has been no consistent correlation between biopsy grading and the clinical outcome in this group of tumors.

Biopsy of the nondiffuse tumors reflects a predilection toward lower grade lesions. These astrocytomas have a pilocytic appearance, perhaps resulting from their being "squeezed in" among the brainstem fiber bundles.[8,10,21,26] They will have prominent cytoplasmic intermediate filaments and cell processes. In one report, two thirds were classified as low-grade astrocytomas or gangliogliomas, and another 10% to 15% were grade II lesions.[13] Again, there is some limitation in these statistics because of failure to biopsy as many as 25% of the patients.

There have been very limited molecular biologic studies of diffuse BSGs, particularly recently as they have infrequent biopsies or resections.[38] However, they seem to resemble adult glioblastoma multiforme more than a typical pediatric astrocytoma. They can have loss of heterozygosity on chromosomes 17p and 10, and p53 mutations are seen. Unfortunately, there has been no significant work reported on using markers of proliferation to predict tumor behavior.

The role of biopsy in brainstem tumors has been recognized as rather limited in utility. In early series, open biopsy resulted in new deficits in one third of the patients, and 30% of the biopsies were deemed nondiagnostic.[19,25] With the introduction of stereotactically guided biopsies, samples could be safely obtained but were quite small. There was the concern of significant sampling error leading to an incorrect diagnosis or prognosis.[34]

Concurrent with the use of stereotactic biopsy was the realization that there was little correlation between the pathologic findings in diffuse pontine lesions and the patient's clinical course.[41] In a large series from Montreal, before 1994, 70% of the diffuse lesions had biopsies. After 1994 this dropped to 35%, and the biopsy was often replaced with an open operation for selected lesions. Even nondiffuse lesions had biopsies less often because of more aggressive attempts at debulking or resection. Interestingly, the clinical behavior of adult BSGs seems to correlate with the biopsy pathology, where this is clearly not true in the pediatric population.

THERAPY

The discrepancies between diffuse and nondiffuse BSG tumors require that the tumor type be considered when evaluating treatments. Unfortunately, many of the reports on BSG treatments contain a mixture of pathologies. There is one report of the "natural" history of untreated diffuse BSG patients.[3,22] On average, these patients became bedridden by 1.5 months after diagnosis and then survived for a few weeks or up to 8 months longer. Among this group of 12 patients, however, there was one long-term survivor. Even with treatment, the diffuse lesions show a rather dismal median survival time (from diagnosis to death) of 9 months.[13] Spontaneous regressions have been reported, although they are extremely rare, and there continue to be occasional long-term survivors treated with radiation therapy.[23]

The results of treatment for the nondiffuse BSG group are much better. For example, tectal lesions can be stable for years after the treatment of the obstructive hydrocephalus, and dorsally exophytic tumors treated with significant surgical resection can be tumor progression free for years.[9,13,21,28,39] Even with subsequent disease progression, surgical debulking may be possible, and standard radiation therapy is usually used. More than 90% will have stable disease at 3- to 4-year follow-up.

Surgery

The indications for surgical intervention with BSGs are rather limited. The diffuse and infiltrative lesions cannot be resected, and as mentioned there is rarely a need for a biopsy.[26] A biopsy can be done safely if needed. Stereotactically guided needle biopsies can be performed, even on pontine lesions. The approach can be transcerebellar for the more laterally placed lesions, or transfrontal through the cerebral peduncle for the midline lesions. If more than one sample is to be obtained, an obturator tube should be passed just short of the target, allowing a biopsy needle to be placed repeatedly in the tumor without multiple passes through normal brain tissue.

When hydrocephalus is present, appropriate treatment should be considered. Patients with midbrain and tectal tumors usually have symptomatic hydrocephalus.[13,28] They respond quite well to cerebrospinal fluid (CSF) diversion, whether treated with a shunt or third ventriculostomy. The benign course of these lesions rarely requires any other surgery.

In other patients with BSGs, approximately 10% will initially have hydrocephalus.[2] Many others will develop hydrocephalus during the course of their disease. Whether to treat the hydrocephalus in the late stages of the disease depends on the patient's condition and should be discussed with patient and family. It is sometimes difficult to distinguish between a clinical change because of progressive brainstem disease or to the hydrocephalus.

Tumors of the midbrain, medulla, and cerebellar peduncle that are focal or exophytic should be considered for open debulking and resection.[9,12,21,36,44] They are commonly low-grade astrocytomas that respond well to such resection.* In many cases, the tumor remains stable after debulking. If the tumor progresses, repeat resection can be considered in addition to adjunctive radiation therapy.[35,36]

Even focal tumors beneath the floor of the fourth ventricle have been approached for subtotal resection, using microevoked potentials and cranial nerve nuclei mapping to define the relatively safe areas through which to enter the pons.[43] Such resection is still very limited by the regional anatomy and cannot be considered routine.

Radiation

Standard external-beam radiation therapy has been a mainstay treatment for BSG. Conventional doses of 55 Gy in fractions of 1.7 Gy/day have been used for the entire group of brainstem tumors, with 3- to 5-year survival reported from 7% to 35%.[16,25] However, the results with the diffuse pontine gliomas are significantly less impressive, with a median survival of only 264 days for rare long-term survivors.[22]

The poor survival with diffuse pontine gliomas treated with standard radiation therapy led to trials using hyperfractionated radiation therapy. It was hoped that the higher total doses delivered with hyperfractionated treatments would maintain a minimum of normal tissue injury while increasing the effectiveness against the tumor. A large number of studies were undertaken with similar findings.[26] Despite doses of up to 78 Gy, there was no significant improvement in survival compared with historical controls.[18,24,31,33,37] In addition, such therapy is very labor intensive and may not be feasible with children who require sedation for every therapy session.

Brachytherapy is usually not an option with BSG because of the risk of injury to the small brainstem, although it has been tried.[7] There has been no clear survival advantage with this treatment. Stereotactic radiosurgery has also been of limited utility because of the typical geometry of the lesions and their diffuse nature. Radiosurgery has been used successfully for select focal lesions.

Most patients will have some response to radiation therapy, with a maximal response seen several weeks after the completion of therapy.[26,37,50] Approximately two thirds of patients will remain in remission for 6 to 60 weeks, averaging only 27 weeks.[22] MRI shows there is a measurable decrease in the area of T2 hyperintensity. Unfortunately, there does not seem to be any correlation of response to pathology or survival.

The current standard of care for diffuse BSG includes standard radiation therapy and no longer includes hyperfractionated treatments. Nondiffuse tumors are usually treated with observation or surgery before any radiation, but if required by tumor recurrence or growth, they are treated initially with standard radiation therapy and radiation surgery in select cases. In BSGs in general, radiation does have palliative effects but cannot be considered to be curative.

---

*See references 2, 5, 9, 12, 19, 21, 35, 36, 44, 45.

Chemotherapy

A variety of chemotherapy agents have been used singly or in combination to treat BSG. The poor response of diffuse BSG to radiation therapy has led to trials with agents such as cisplatin, carboplatin, nitrosourea compounds, cyclophosphamide, and ifosfamide.[26,34] Response has been very limited, with no consistent beneficial effect.

A number of relatively small trials have attempted to use chemotherapy in conjunction with radiation therapy. Tamoxifen in high doses and for longer duration combined with standard radiation therapy had no effect on survival or outcome.[6] Combining chemotherapy with hyperfractionated radiation therapy actually resulted in patients doing worse than historical controls.[17,47] High-dose chemotherapy following radiation therapy has been tried, with no change in the survival and a significant number of patients unable to complete the chemotherapy protocol because of major toxicities.[4]

CONCLUSION

BSGs will come to attention because of the symptoms they cause. When the tumor affects the pons or medulla, those symptoms are typically related to cranial nerve dysfunction, long-tract signs, or ataxia. Midbrain lesions will usually cause symptoms related to the typical obstructive hydrocephalus. The most effective radiographic evaluation uses MRI.

Diffuse pontine gliomas have stereotypical imaging findings, allowing the diagnosis to be made on MRI alone. They do not require a biopsy when the typical clinical findings and radiographic findings exist. For unusual tumors, a stereotactic or open biopsy can be used. Treatment remains limited to conformal external radiation therapy. Given the dismal prognosis despite all therapy attempts, a number of pilot studies are under way attempting to find a more effective treatment. Even so, there are rare long-term survivors, raising hope that some effective treatment can be found.

Tectal tumors will usually cause symptoms referable to obstructive hydrocephalus. Although many of these patients will have an initial CT scan, imaging with MR will be required to make a diagnosis. Typical lesions of the tectum and tegmentum will not require biopsy. Treatment begins with the diversionary treatment of the hydrocephalus and careful observation of the tumor with serial imaging. Adjunctive therapy is reserved for progressive lesions and can include attempts at open debulking, standard radiation therapy, and occasionally stereotactic radiosurgery.

Focal or exophytic tumors will cause symptoms specific to their location in the brainstem. Again, MRI is the diagnostic test of choice defining the lesion location and extent. Hydrocephalus, if present, is treated with diversion. The focal lesion should be considered for surgical debulking and resection, taking into consideration the location and accessibility within the brainstem. Residual or surgically inaccessible tumors may be followed with serial imaging, but recurrence or tumor progression will be treated with standard radiation therapy.

References

1. Albright AL, Guthkelch AN, Packer RJ, et al: Prognostic factors in pediatric brainstem gliomas. J Neurosurg 65:751–755, 1986.
2. Albright AL, Packer RJ, Zimmerman RA, et al: Magnetic resonance scans should replace biopsies for the diagnosis of diffuse brain stem gliomas: a report from the Children's Cancer Group. Neurosurgery 33:1026–1030, 1993.
3. Barkovich AJ, Krischer J, Kun LE, et al: Brainstem glioma: a classification system based on magnetic resonance imaging. Pediatr Neurosurg 16:73–83, 1990.
4. Bouffet E, Raquin M, Doz F, et al: Radiotherapy followed by high dose busulfan and thiotepa: A prospective assessment of high dose chemotherapy in children with diffuse pontine gliomas. Cancer 88:685–692, 2000.
5. Bricolo A, Turazzi S, Cristofori L, et al: Direct surgery of brainstem tumors. Acta Neur S53:148–158, 1991.
6. Broniscer A, da Costa Leite C, Lanchote VL, et al: Radiation therapy and high-dose tamoxifen in the treatment of patients with diffuse brainstem gliomas: results of a Brazilian cooperative study. J Clin Oncol 18:1246–1253, 2000.
7. Chuba PJ, Zamarano L, Hamre M, et al: Permanent I-125 brain stem implants in children. Childs Nerv Syst 14:570–577, 1998.
8. Edwards MSB, Wara WM, Ciricillo SF, et al: Focal brainstem astrocytomas causing symptoms of involvement of the facial nerve nucleus: long term survival in six pediatric cases. J Neurosurg 80:20–25, 1994.
9. Epstein F, Wisoff JH: Intrinsic brainstem tumors in childhood: surgical indications. J Neurooncol 6:309–317, 1998.
10. Epstein FJ, Farmer J-P: Brainstem glioma growth patterns. J Neurosurg 78:408–412, 1993.
11. Epstein FJ, Wisoff JH: Surgical management of brainstem tumors of childhood and adolescence. Neurosurg Clin North Am 1:111–121, 1990.
12. Epstein F, McCleary EL: Intrinsic brain-stem tumors of childhood: surgical indications. J Neurosurg 64:11–15, 1986.
13. Farmer J-P, Montes JL, Freeman CR, et al: Brainstem gliomas: a 10-year institutional review. Pediatr Neurosurg 34:206–214, 2001.
14. Fischbein NJ, Prados MD, Wara W, et al: Radiologic classification of brain stem tumors: correlation of magnetic resonance imaging appearance with clinical outcome. Pediatr Neurosurg 24:9–23, 1996.
15. Freeman CR, Bourgouin PM, Sanford RA, et al: Long term survivors of childhood brainstem gliomas treated with hyperfractionated radiotherapy: clinical characteristics and treatment related toxicities. Cancer 77:555–562, 1996.
16. Freeman CR, Farmer J-P: Pediatric brain stem gliomas: a review. Int J Radiat Oncol Biol Phys 40:265–271, 1998.
17. Freeman CR, Kepner J, Kun LE, et al: A detrimental effect of a combined chemotherapy-radiotherapy approach in children with diffuse intrinsic brain stem gliomas? Int J Radiat Oncol Biol Phys 47:561–564, 2000.
18. Freeman CR, Krischer JP, Sanford RA, et al: Final results of a study of escalating doses of hyperfractionated radiotherapy in brain stem tumors in children: a Pediatric Oncology Group study. Int J Radiat Oncol Biol Phys 27:197–206, 1993.
19. Halperin EC, Wehn SM, Scott JW, et al: Selection of a management strategy for pediatric brainstem tumors. Med Clin North Am 17:116–125, 1989.

20. Kansal S, Jindal A, Mahapatra AK: Brain stem glioma—A study of 111 patients. Indian J Cancer 36:99–108, 1999.
21. Khatib ZA, Jenkins JJ, Fairclough DL, et al: Predominance of pilocytic histology in dorsally exophytic brainstem tumors. Pediatr Neurosurg 20:2–10, 1994.
22. Langmoen IA, Lundar T, Storm-Mathisen I, et al: Management of pediatric pontine gliomas. Childs Nerv Syst 7:13–15, 1991.
23. Lenard HG, Engelbrecht V, Janssen G, et al: Complete remission of a diffuse pontine glioma. Neuropediatrics 29:328–330, 1998.
24. Lewis J, Lucraft H, Gholkar A: UKCCSG study of accelerated radiotherapy for pediatric brainstem glimoas. Int J Radiat Oncol Biol Phys 38:925–929, 1997.
25. Littman P, Jarrett P, Bilaniuk LT, et al: Pediatric brainstem gliomas. Cancer 45:2787–2792, 1980.
26. Maria BL, Rehder K, Eskin TA, et al: Brainstem glioma: I. Pathology, clinical features, and therapy. J Child Neurol 8:112–128, 1993.
27. Matson DD: Neurosurgery of Infancy and Childhood, 2nd ed. Springfield, Thomas, 1969.
28. May PL, Blaser SI, Hoffman HJ, et al: Benign intrinsic tectal tumors in children. J Neurosurg 74:867–871, 1991.
29. Mehta V, Chapman A, McNeely PD, et al: Latency between symptom onset and diagnosis of pediatric brain tumors: an Eastern Canadian geographic study. Neurosurgery 51:365–373, 2002.
30. Moghrabi A, Kerby T, Tien RD, et al: Prognostic value of contrast-enhanced magnetic resonance imaging in brainstem gliomas. Pediatr Neurosurg 23:293–298, 1995.
31. Nelson MD, Jr, Soni D, Baram TZ: Necrosis in pontine gliomas: radiation induced or natural history? Radiology 191:279–282, 1994.
32. Nishio S, Takeshita I, Fujii K, et al: Brain stem glioma: the role of a biopsy. Br J Neurosurg 5:265–273, 1991.
33. Packer RJ, Boyett JM, Zimmerman RA, et al: Outcome of children with brainstem gliomas after treatment with 7800 cGy of hyperfractionated radiotherapy. Cancer 74:1827–1834, 1994.
34. Packer RJ, Nicholson HS, Johnson DL, et al: Dilemmas in the management of childhood brain tumors: brainstem gliomas. Pediatr Neurosurg 17:37–43, 1991.
35. Pierre-Kahn A, Hirsch J-F, Vinchon M, et al: Surgical management of brainstem tumors in children: results and statistical analysis of 75 cases. J Neurosurg 79:845–852, 1993.
36. Pollack IF, Hoffman HJ, Humphreys RP, et al: The long term outcome after surgical treatment of dorsally exophytic brainstem gliomas. J Neurosurg 78:859–863, 1993.
37. Prados MD, Wara WM, Edwards MSB, et al: The treatment of brainstem and thalamic gliomas with 78 Gy of hyperfractionated radiation therapy. Int J Radiat Oncol Biol Phys 32:85–91, 1995.
38. Raffel C: Molecular biology of pediatric gliomas. J Neurooncology 28:121–128, 1996.
39. Robertson P, Muraszko KM, Brunberg JA, et al: Pediatric midbrain tumors: a benign subgroup of brainstem gliomas. Pediatr Neurosurg 22:65–73, 1995.
40. Rubin G, Michowitz S, Horev G, et al: Pediatric brain stem gliomas: an update. Childs Nerv Syst 14:167–173, 1998.
41. Selvapandian S, Rajshekhar V, Chandy MJ: Brainstem glioma: comparative study of clinico-radiological presentation, pathology and outcome in children and adults. Acta Neurochir (Wein) 141:721–727, 1999.
42. Steck J, Friedman WA: Stereotactic biopsy of brainstem mass lesions. Surg Neurol 43:563–568, 1995.
43. Strauss C, Romstock J, Fahlbusch R: Pericollicular approaches to the rhomboid fossa. Part II. Neurophysiological basis. J Neurosurg 91:768–775, 1999.
44. Stroink AR, Hoffman HJ, Hendrick EB, et al: Diagnosis and management of pediatric brain-stem gliomas. J Neurosurg 65:745–750, 1986.
45. Tomita T, McLone DG: Medulloblastoma in childhood: results of radical resection and low dose radiation therapy. J Neurosurg 64:238–242, 1986.
46. Vandertop WP, Hoffman HJ, Drake JM, et al: Focal midbrain tumors in children. Neurosurgery 31:186–194, 1992.
47. Walter AW, Gajjar A, Ochs JS, et al: Carboplatin and etoposide with hyperfractionated radiotherapy in children with newly diagnosed diffuse pontine gliomas: a phase I/II study. Med Pediatr Oncol 30:28–33, 1998.
48. Zagzag D, Miller DC, Knopp E, et al: Primitive neuroectodermal tumors of the brainstem: investigation of seven cases. Pediatrics 106:1045–1053, 2000.
49. Zimmerman RA: Neuroimaging of pediatric brainstem diseases other than brainstem glioma. Pediatr Neurosurg 25:83–92, 1996a.
50. Zimmerman RA: Neuroimaging of primary brainstem gliomas: diagnosis and course. Pediatr Neurosurg 25:45–53, 1996b.

CHAPTER 83

DORSALLY EXOPHYTIC BRAINSTEM GLIOMAS

Prithvi Narayan and Timothy B. Mapstone

For the first half of the twentieth century, brainstem gliomas were considered uniformly malignant with an extremely poor prognosis. These tumors were considered to be a single entity, and their location was thought to preclude surgery as a therapeutic option. However, reports of successful resections in a subset of patients harboring these tumors emerged and shed some light on their heterogeneity.[4,19,25] In 1980 Hoffman et al reported on a clinically and pathologically distinct group of benign brainstem gliomas, the dorsally exophytic glioma, that was amenable to surgical resection.[14] In 1986 classification schemes for brainstem gliomas were developed based on clinical and computed tomography (CT) findings. Epstein et al defined subcategories of diffuse, focal, and cervicomedullary tumors and described their histologic and clinical correlations.[11] Stroink et al described a five-category classification scheme based on the CT appearance of these tumors.[32] Albright classified these tumors simply as focal or diffuse.[2] The advent of magnetic resonance imaging (MRI) further refined the imaging characteristics of these neoplasms and established that tumor extent was the main prognostic factor.[5,32] Based on these classification schemes, five subsets of brainstem gliomas covering the spectrum of prognosis and intervention are currently recognized: diffuse intrinsic pontine glioma, cervicomedullary tumors, dorsally exophytic tumors, tectal tumors, and focal tumors. Among these, the dorsally exophytic tumors are amenable to surgical resection and carry a good long-term prognosis despite incomplete resection or recurrence.

EPIDEMIOLOGY

Brainstem gliomas are predominantly a childhood neoplasm. They account for approximately 6% to 20% of all pediatric brain tumors and 20% to 30% of all pediatric posterior fossa tumors.[1,2,17,18,23,26,28,30,35] They are rare in adults, accounting for 1% of all brain tumors.[2] There appears to be no gender or race predilection. The age of occurrence ranges from a few months to the late teenage years with a peak prevalence from 6 to 10 years of age.[2,6,19,22] These tumors are not associated with any heritable syndromes. The majority of them are diffuse pontine gliomas. Dorsally exophytic brainstem tumors comprised approximately 20% of all brainstem gliomas. In Pollack et al's series, 19% of all brainstem gliomas treated between 1974 and 1990 were of the dorsally exophytic type.[9] All 18 patients in this study ranged in age from 1 month to 14 years at the time of diagnosis.

SIGNS AND SYMPTOMS

Patients with dorsally exophytic tumors often have signs and symptoms of increased intracranial pressure caused by obstruction of cerebrospinal fluid (CSF) pathways. Headache, vomiting, and ataxia are common in older children. Papilledema and torticollis may be evident on physical examination, reflecting increased intracranial pressure. Children younger than 3 years may have intractable vomiting and failure to thrive.[32,33] These children typically undergo extensive medical work-up before diagnosis of the tumor. Cranial nerve deficits may be seen in approximately 50% of patients.[26] Cranial nerve findings are usually isolated instead of multiple, with the abducens or facial nerves commonly affected. The onset of symptoms is usually insidious, reflecting the slow-growing nature of these tumors. In one series of 18 patients, examination revealed torticollis in 6 patients, papilledema in 13, ataxia in 12, nystagmus in 6, and cranial nerve deficits in 7.[9] Long-tract signs are usually absent, which differentiates these tumors from the diffuse gliomas. In general, patients have signs and symptoms that indicate minimal brainstem dysfunction.

DIAGNOSIS

The different subtypes of brainstem gliomas can be differentiated based on a combination of clinical history and imaging characteristics. The dorsally exophytic tumors are usually hypodense on CT scans and are brightly enhanced with contrast administration. Hydrocephalus is common, and calcification is usually absent. Although classification schemes have been developed based on CT findings,[33] the imaging is suboptimal secondary to bony artifacts in the posterior fossa.

MRI is the study of choice in evaluating patients with suspected brainstem gliomas. A number of favorable prognostic factors have been identified based on MRI. These include tumor focality, growth pattern, enhancement characteristics, and location.[12] The classic dorsally exophytic brainstem glioma is almost entirely extra-axial. It is typically large, arises from the floor of the fourth ventricle, and often fills it. Cyst formation with a mural nodule may be present, similar to low-grade astrocytomas in other locations. On MRI, these tumors are hypointense on T1-weighted images and hyperintense on T2-weighted studies and are sharply demarcated from the surrounding structures. The size of the tumor is typically the same on the different imaging sequences, suggesting a benign histology. Enhancement with contrast administration is uniform and bright, suggestive of a pilocytic astrocytoma. Because of the difference in prognosis, it is important to distinguish the dorsally exophytic gliomas from those that are exophytic in the lateral and ventral directions. The latter grow by rupturing the pia-arachnoid and are usually high-grade lesions.[1]

Brainstem evoked potentials have little role in the diagnosis of these tumors. They may be useful for postoperative evaluation to rule out brainstem dysfunction, but their role has not been established. Khatib et al postoperatively tested seven patients with dorsally exophytic gliomas using brainstem auditory evoked responses (BAERs). The patients demonstrated essentially normal central auditory conduction, reflecting little disturbance of brainstem function.[16] Cytologic analysis of CSF has little role in the diagnosis of brainstem gliomas except in cases where an infectious cause is suspected.

PATHOLOGY

Dorsally exophytic gliomas are generally low-grade astrocytomas. In Pollack et al's series of 18 patients, 16 were classified as grade I or II (low-grade) astrocytomas, 1 as grade III (anaplastic) astrocytoma, and 1 as a ganglioglioma.[23] The predominant histologic type was pilocytic astrocytoma. Grossly, they are soft, gray, and discrete. Microscopically, they are characterized by a biphasic pattern of compacted bipolar cells with Rosenthal fibers and loosely arranged multipolar cells with microcysts and granular bodies.[7] Khatib et al reported on the MRI and clinicohistologic characterization of dorsally exophytic tumors. Out of 51 patients in their series, 12 were diagnosed with dorsally exophytic gliomas emanating from the pons, pontomedullary junction, or medulla. Of 12 patients, 11 had classic juvenile pilocytic astrocytomas.[16]

The genesis of pilocytic astrocytomas is unclear. In contrast to diffuse astrocytomas, the TP53 gene does not seem to play a role.[7] Although it is the most common neoplasm in the setting of neurofibromatosis type 1 (NF1), the role of the tumor-suppressor gene NF1 in the genesis of these tumors has not been established.[7] Also, dorsally exophytic brainstem gliomas are usually sporadic and unusual in the setting of NF1.

TREATMENT

Surgery is the treatment of choice for dorsally exophytic tumors. Radiation and chemotherapy are usually reserved for progressive disease or recurrences. The goal of surgery is radical but safe excision. Although stereotactic biopsies may provide tissue for diagnosis, the location and histology of these tumors warrant an attempt at resection.

Hydrocephalus

As previously mentioned, hydrocephalus is present in most cases. Before the last decade, placement of a shunt before tumor resection was performed routinely in the management of hydrocephalus associated with posterior fossa tumors. This approach is currently used uncommonly, because only approximately 20% of patients need a shunt after tumor removal, and the attendant risks of an internal shunt can be avoided.

Today, the hydrocephalus is treated primarily with an external ventricular drain (EVD) placed just before craniotomy. This approach provides brain relaxation during tumor resection and minimizes the risk of acute postoperative hydrocephalus. Sometimes administering preoperative corticosteroids is all that is needed, and the EVD may be placed at the time of tumor resection. The placement of an EVD prophylactically before resection of these tumors when no hydrocephalus is present is controversial. Although there are no data to support its use, proponents argue that EVDs add a measure of safety and avoid the risk of transient postoperative hydrocephalus secondary to swelling.[3]

EVDs can be placed via the standard frontal or occipital approach. Drainage is continued postoperatively for a few days to clear any blood and debris and is slowly weaned. A ventriculoperitoneal shunt (VPS) is inserted if the patient does not tolerate occlusion. An alternative to internal shunting is endoscopic third ventriculostomy. This may preclude placement of an internal shunt and its attendant risks. Prophylactic third ventriculostomies before tumor resection are not indicated, because only a minority of patients require permanent CSF diversion after tumor resection.

Tumor

The goals of surgery for dorsally exophytic gliomas are safe excision and restoration of CSF pathways. Preoperative corticosteroids are typically administered to reduce peritumoral edema and decrease intracranial pressure. The timing of surgery depends on the neurologic condition of the patient. If neurologic status is deteriorating rapidly or if there is intratumoral hemorrhage and the patient is moribund, a craniotomy may need to be performed emergently. If the hydrocephalus is profound and the patient is lethargic, it is reasonable to place an EVD while the patient is in the intensive care unit to reduce the intracranial pressure and then proceed to the craniotomy when the neurologic status is stable. In general, if the patient is alert and awake, the craniotomy is usually performed within 48 to 72 hours of presentation.

The posterior fossa craniotomy is performed with the patient prone. Although a sitting position may be used, it is difficult to place infants and young children in this position. In addition, the sitting position carries the risks of air embolism and subdural hematomas or pneumoencephalus secondary to uncontrolled escape of CSF through the aqueduct of Sylvius. The prone position provides a comfortable view for the surgeon looking down into the field and avoids arm fatigue associated with the sitting position. For children with thin skulls, the head and face are placed on a well-padded horseshoe head holder. Otherwise, the head is secured with a three-pin head holder. Overflexion of the neck should be avoided to ensure adequate venous return.

Traditionally, a suboccipital craniectomy has been preferred for posterior fossa explorations. Recently, however, there has been a trend toward performing a craniotomy. This provides a more anatomic closure of the wound with reduction of dead space and decreases the risk of a postoperative pseudomeningocele. A midline approach is used, and the vermis is usually split to gain access to the tumor. Extensive splitting of the vermis is associated with the risks of cerebellar mutism and pseudobulbar syndrome.[9,34] Alternatively, the cerebellomedullary fissure approach, described by Piatt, may be used to gain access to the tumor while sparing the sectioning of the vermis and possibly lowering the risk of neurologic complications.[15] Extensive mobilization of the tumor should be avoided. A biopsy is performed for frozen section. The tumor is then removed with internal debulking using an ultrasonic aspirator or a combination of suction and bipolar cautery. Usually there is an area of attachment to the brainstem ventrally, which precludes complete resection. In Pollack et al's series, no definite tumor-brainstem interface was discerned, resulting in subtotal resections.[23] The floor of the fourth ventricle should be identified before debulking the ventral portions of the tumor. The tumor is then resected flush with the floor of the fourth ventricle, with care taken not to pursue it into the brainstem. Intraoperative ultrasound may be useful in guiding the extent of resection. Some surgeons use intraoperative brainstem mapping.[20,31] However, the efficacy of this remains unproved.

Exquisite hemostasis should be obtained and the dura closed in a watertight fashion. Dural graft or substitutes may be necessary to obtain a good closure. The bone flap is secured in place with plates or sutures and the wound is closed in layers. To facilitate muscle closure, the head can be slightly extended at this point. It is important to obtain an MRI scan of the brain with contrast within 24 to 48 hours after craniotomy to assess the extent of tumor resection and to aid in planning adjunctive treatment. This may include reoperation if adequate cytoreduction was not obtained. After 72 hours, postsurgical changes may confound the accurate assessment of residual tumor.

Complications

With modern surgical and anesthetic techniques, surgical mortality from resection of dorsally exophytic tumors is approaching zero. Cranial nerve dysfunction such as abducens and facial palsy is usually secondary to manipulation of the floor of the fourth ventricle.

Postoperative mutism, initially described by Hirsch et al in 1979, is a rare transient complication associated with posterior fossa surgery.[13] A spontaneous recovery of normal speech is the rule, but neuropsychologic deficits may persist.[27] The posterior fossa syndrome is a relatively common complication first described by Wisoff and Epstein.[34] In addition to cerebellar mutism, the syndrome is characterized by ataxia, emotional lability, and pseudobulbar palsy with or without hemiparesis developing within 72 hours after the operation. The pathogenesis is controversial, but the anatomic sites implicated are the dentato-rubro-thalamic tract and the vermis.[8,24] The cerebellar mutism is itself self-limited with complete resolution of symptoms in the majority of cases, but the remaining neurologic complications may be irreversible.[10,29]

Aseptic meningitis manifesting as postoperative headaches, photophobia, and nuchal rigidity is secondary to blood in the subarachnoid space. Careful attention to hemostasis and prevention of the entry of blood into the ventricular system can minimize this rare complication.

RECURRENCE AND OUTCOME

Most patients with dorsally exophytic tumors treated with radical surgery have long disease-free or progression-free survival despite subtotal resections. The histology is typically low grade. Residual tumor may be followed with serial MRI scans at 3- to 6-month intervals. Disease progression is seen in 25% to 30% of patients.[23] Progression is usually at the primary site and is amenable to radiation therapy, chemotherapy, or repeat surgery. If the patient is asymptomatic, continued observation often is sufficient, because these tumors may become quiescent after a brief growth spurt. Standard limited field radiation doses of 54 Gy are generally used. The role of focused radiation such as Gamma Knife® and hyperfractionated radiation has not been established in the case of exophytic tumors.

Since the first description of this subset of brainstem tumors by Hoffman, a number of studies have documented their benign nature. In Pollack et al's report, all 18 patients underwent aggressive debulking, but only subtotal resections resulted.[23] One patient died because of a shunt malfunction. Fifteen patients were observed without further intervention, and two patients received postoperative radiation because of a high-grade lesion or widespread infiltration of the brainstem surface. Seventeen patients were alive at the conclusion of the study, with a follow-up ranging from 33 to 212 months. The two patients who received postoperative radiation therapy had no evidence of residual disease on follow-up imaging at 61 and 135 months after surgery. Of the 15 patients who were observed, there was complete regression of residual tumor in 3 children, stable disease in 8, and progressive disease in 4. The progression was detected by imaging at 12 to 84 months after the initial surgery. These recurrences were managed by either repeat resections or radiation therapy with long-term disease control. Of note, the histology of the tumor from the patients with progressive disease showed no significant change from that obtained at the initial resection. There was no evidence of malignant degeneration in any of the specimens.

In another series reported by Khatib et al, 12 of 51 patients with brainstem tumors were diagnosed with dorsally exophytic brainstem gliomas.[16] Six patients had near-total or gross-total resection and six had subtotal resections. The histology in 11 of the 12 patients was classic juvenile pilocytic astrocytomas, and 1 was a low-grade astrocytoma. For 10 of the 12 patients no postoperative treatment was instituted. Two patients received either chemotherapy or radiation of 55 Gy following subtotal resection. Of the 10 patients followed postoperatively without adjunctive treatment, 3 showed progression of disease. Each of these 3 patients was subsequently treated with radiation therapy encompassing the tumor volume. One patient who was treated with chemotherapy died of acute myelogenous leukemia. Neuroimaging before death showed no evidence of tumor. Of the 11 surviving patients, 7 with subtotal or gross-total resections and no subsequent treatment remained progression free with a median follow-up of 28 months or more (range 17 or more to 60 months or more). One patient had no residual tumor, and the remaining 6 had either stable disease or continued diminution of MRI abnormalities. The three patients treated with radiation therapy following tumor progression were free of progression for 16 months or more. The overall and progression-free survival at 2 years was 100% and 67%, respectively.

One of the main concerns of radiation treatment in children is the long-term neurocognitive and neuroendocrine sequelae. To minimize the long-term effects of radiation, the use of chemotherapy to obviate or delay radiation seems an attractive option. The Children's Cancer Study Group in 1989 evaluated the efficacy of carboplatin and vincristine in the treatment of children with progressive, recurrent, or newly diagnosed low-grade gliomas.[21] Of the 78 patients enrolled in the study, 12 patients had dorsally exophytic brainstem gliomas. One patient died of sepsis after 11 months of treatment. In general, the treatment was well tolerated with acceptable toxicity. Complete radiographic responses were noted in 50% of the patients with the dorsally exophytic tumors. Only 3 patients had developed progressive disease at 2 years. For the study as a whole, the progression-free survival was 75% ± 6% at 2 years, and 68% ± 7% at 3 years. Studies are ongoing to determine the optimal chemotherapeutic regimen for progressive low-grade gliomas.

CONCLUSION

Dorsally exophytic gliomas account for approximately 20% of all brainstem tumors. They occur insidiously, causing failure to thrive in infants and signs and symptoms of increased intracranial pressure in older children. Safe surgical resection is the treatment of choice with adjuvant therapy reserved for patients with high-grade lesions or for those with progression or recurrence. Long-term survivors are common even with incomplete resections. Most of these children are able to resume normal activities, and the quality of survival is satisfactory.[14] Radiation therapy following surgery is the major cause of morbidity in these patients. The optimal adjuvant chemotherapy in the treatment of these tumors has not been established.

References

1. Abbott R: Brain stem gliomas. In McLone DG (ed): Surgery of the Developing Nervous System, 4th ed. Philadelphia, WB Saunders, 2001.
2. Albright AL: Brain stem gliomas. In Youmans JR (ed): Neurological Surgery, ed 4. Philadelphia, WB Saunders, 1996.
3. Albright AL: Medulloblastomas. In Albright AL, Pollac IF, Adelson PD (eds): Principles and Practice of Pediatric Neurosurgery. New York, Thieme, 1999.
4. Baker GS: Physiologic abnormalities encountered after removal of brain tumors from the floor of the fourth ventricle. J Neurosurg 23:245, 1964.
5. Barkovich AJ, Krischer J, Kun LE, et al: Brain stem gliomas: a classification system based on magnetic resonance imaging. Pediatr Neurosurg 16:73, 1990.
6. Berger M, Edwards M, LaMaster D, et al: Pediatric brain stem tumors: radiographic, pathological, and clinical correlations. Neurosurgery 12:298, 1983.
7. Burger PC, Scheithauer BW, Paulus W, et al: Pilocytic astrocytoma. In Kleihues P, Cavenee WK (eds): Tumours of the Nervous System. Lyon, France, IARC Press, 2000.
8. Dailey AT, McKhann GM, Berger MS: The pathophysiology of oral pharyngeal apraxia and mutism following posterior fossa tumor resection in children. J Neurosurg 83:467–475, 1995.
9. Dietz D, Mickle J: Cerebellar mutism after posterior fossa surgery. Pediatr Neurosurg 16:25, 1991.
10. Doxey D, Bruce D, Sklar F, et al: Posterior fossa syndrome: identifiable risk factors and irreversible complications. Pediatr Neurosurg 31:131–136, 1999.
11. Epstein F, McCleary EL: Intrinsic brain-stem tumors of childhood: Surgical indications. J Neurosurg 64:11, 1986.
12. Farmer JP, Montes JL, Freeman CR, et al: Brain stem gliomas: a 10-year institutional review. Pediatr Neurosurg 34:206, 2001.
13. Hirsch JF, Renier D, Czernikow P, et al: Medulloblastoma in childhood: survival and functional results. Acta Neurochir (Wien) 48:1, 1979.
14. Hoffman HJ, Becker L, Craven MA: A clinically and pathologically distinct group of benign brain stem gliomas. Neurosurgery 7:243, 1980.
15. Kellogg JX, Piatt JH, Jr: Resection of fourth ventricle tumors without splitting the vermis: the cerebellomedullary fissure approach. Pediatr Neurosurg 28:28–33, 1997.
16. Khatib ZA, Heideman RL, Kovnar EH, et al: Predominance of pilocytic histology in dorsally exophytic brain stem tumors. Pediatr Neurosurg 20:2, 1994.
17. Lassiter KRL, Alexander E, Jr, Davis CH: Surgical treatment of brain stem gliomas. J Neurosurg 34:719, 1971.
18. Lee B, Kneeland J, Walker R, et al: MR imaging of brainstem tumors. AJNR Am J Neuroradiol 9:159, 1985.
19. Littman P, Jarrett P, Bilaniuk LT, et al: Pediatric brainstem tumors. Cancer 45:2787, 1980.
20. Morota N, Deletis V, Epstein F, et al: Brain stem mapping: neurophysiological localization of motor nuclei on the floor of the fourth ventricle. Neurosurgery 37:922, 1995.
21. Packer RJ, Alter J, Allen J, et al: Carboplatin and vincristine chemotherapy for children with newly diagnosed progressive low-grade gliomas. J Neurosurg 86:747, 1997.
22. Pierre-Kahn A, Hirsch J, Vinchon M, et al: Surgical management of brain-stem tumors in children: results and statistical analysis of 75 cases. J Neurosurg 79:845, 1993.
23. Pollack IF, Hoffman HJ, Humphreys RP, et al: The long-term outcome after surgical treatment of dorsally exophytic brain-stem gliomas. J Neurosurg 78:859, 1993.
24. Pollack IF, Polinko P, Albright AL, et al: Mutism and pseudobulbar symptoms after resection of posterior fossa tumors in children: incidence and pathophysiology. Neurosurgery 37:885–893, 1995.
25. Pool JL: Gliomas in the region of the brain stem. J Neurosurg 29:164, 1968.
26. Reddy AT, Mapstone TB: Brain stem tumors. In Bernstein M, Berger MS (eds): Neuro-Oncology. New York, Thieme, 2000.
27. Rekate HL, Grubb RL, Adam DM, et al: Muteness of cerebellar origin. Arch Neurol 42:697, 1985.
28. Schoenberg B, Schoenberg DG, Christine B, et al: The epidemiology of primary intracranial neoplasms of childhood: a population study. Mayo Clin Proc 51:51, 1976.
29. Siffert J, Poussaint TY, Goumnerova LC, et al: Neurological dysfunction associated with postoperative cerebellar mutism. J Neurooncol 48:75–81, 2000.
30. Stiller C: Population based survival rates for childhood cancer in Britain 1980–1991. BMJ 309:1612, 1994.
31. Strauss C, Romstock J, Nimsky C, et al: Intraoperative identification of motor areas of the rhomboid fossa using direct stimulation. J Neurosurg 79:393, 1993.
32. Stroink AR, Hoffman HJ, Hendrick EB, et al: Diagnosis and management of pediatric brain-stem gliomas. J Neurosurg 65:745, 1986.
33. Stroink AR, Hoffman HJ, Hendrick EB, et al: Transependymal benign dorsally exophytic brain stem gliomas in childhood: diagnosis and treatment recommendations. Neurosurgery 20:439, 1987.
34. Wisoff J, Epstein F: Pseudobulbar palsy after posterior fossa operation in children. Neurosurgery 15:707, 1984.
35. Yates A, Becker L, Sachs L: Brain tumor in childhood. Childs Brain 5:31, 1979.

CHAPTER 84

CERVICOMEDULLARY GLIOMAS

Eve C. Tsai and James T. Rutka

Whereas the term *brainstem gliomas* can be applied to all intra-axial glial tumors involving the brainstem,[19] cervicomedullary gliomas describe a subset of brainstem gliomas with distinctive pathologic, therapeutic, and prognostic features. Cervicomedullary gliomas typically infiltrate regions of the upper cervical spinal cord caudally and the medulla rostrally,[21] rarely extending above the pontomedullary junction. Although in the past brainstem gliomas have been associated with a dismal prognosis,[5] cervicomedullary tumors have been shown to have a good prognosis, especially when compared with the diffuse pontine subset of brainstem tumors.[25] In this chapter, we will review the features unique to cervicomedullary gliomas with respect to diagnosis, management, and outcome.

EPIDEMIOLOGY

Although brainstem gliomas can occur at any age, most occur in children.[14] Brainstem gliomas can be grouped into three main categories—midbrain (tectal and focal), pontine (diffuse intrinsic, dorsally exophytic, and focal), and cervicomedullary[24]—and are estimated to constitute 10% of all pediatric neoplasms.[14] Cervicomedullary tumors, as a group, are relatively uncommon lesions and constitute approximately 6% of all pediatric brain tumors.[11] Although there are reports of peak occurrences of brainstem gliomas in the latter half of the first decade of life with a second peak occurring in the fourth decade,[14] cervicomedullary tumors show no age or gender predilection.[25]

SIGNS AND SYMPTOMS

Children with cervicomedullary tumors often develop symptoms and signs that can occur for several months or years before discovery of the tumor.[25] Signs and symptoms generally fall into one of three major syndromes: medullary dysfunction, spinal cord dysfunction,[24] and hydrocephalus.[25] Medullary dysfunction can lead to symptoms attributable to cranial nerve dysfunction such as facial nerve palsy or weakness,[25] dysphonia, dysarthria, dysphagia, palatal deviation, and recurrent aspiration.[21] Children may also complain of facial pain[19] and torticollis.[9] Severe neck pain may be a child's only complaint.[7,21] The respiratory centers in the medulla may also be affected, causing apnea, or irregular nocturnal breathing patterns[19]; pulmonary edema; and hiccups.[25]

Symptoms associated with the spinal cord dysfunction syndrome include motor or sensory dysfunction. The motor dysfunction can occur insidiously[21] in the upper or lower extremities and can include atrophy, hypotonia,[25] spasticity, hemiparesis, quadriparesis,[5] and hypoactive reflexes.[9] Muscle disuse may lead to contractures[25] and atrophy.[9] Sensory findings can also involve both the upper or lower extremities and can include paresthesias, dysesthesias,[21] and neuropathic pain.[13]

Patients can also have symptoms associated with increased intracranial pressure and hydrocephalus such as headache, nystagmus, and vomiting.[25] Nausea and vomiting has also been reported to occur unassociated with increased intracranial pressure.[19] Other findings that have been reported in children in association with cervicomedullary tumors include failure to thrive in infants and young children,[19] clumsiness, syncope, weight gain, ataxia,[25] and scoliosis.[12] Cervicomedullary tumors have been reported to simulate neuromuscular disorders and cause proximal upper extremity weakness (hypoactive upper extremity reflexes, proximal greater than distal weakness), atrophy, prominent scapular winging, and no sensory deficits or upper motor neuron signs.[9] Although electromyography (EMG) findings can be consistent with a chronic denervating disorder involving the upper cervical anterior horn cells or their axons,[9] use of imaging can assure the correct diagnosis.

NEUROIMAGING FEATURES

When imaging cervicomedullary tumors, technically satisfactory neurodiagnostic studies[5] must be obtained. Computerized tomography (CT) imaging can demonstrate associated hydrocephalus; however, the majority of patients with cervicomedullary tumors do not have associated hydrocephalus.[25] On CT, some cervicomedullary tumors can appear hypodense to white matter[25] and can be enhanced with the addition of contrast[19] (Figure 84-1). More often, however, the tumor is isodense to white matter and can be reported as negative.[25] The artifacts created by bone of the posterior fossa around the foramen magnum prevent CT imaging from adequately determining the complete extent of the lesion.[21]

Use of magnetic resonance imaging (MRI) is clearly the imaging modality of choice, because it allows a clear depiction of tumor and permits an analysis of the rostral-caudal extent of the tumor extension.[21] On MRI, the majority of cervicomedullary tumors are hypointense to white matter on T1-

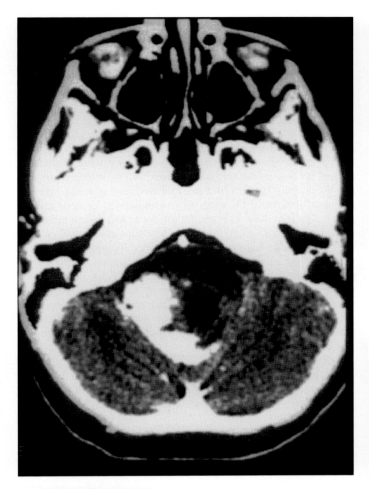

FIGURE 84-1 Contrast-enhanced axial computed tomography scan of 10-year-old boy with progressive dysphonia, sleep apnea, and difficulty swallowing. An enhanced tumor is seen arising from the cervicomedullary junction.

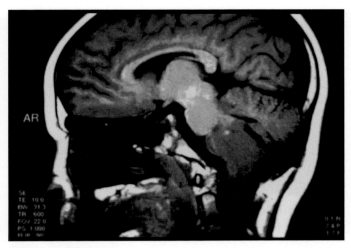

FIGURE 84-2 T1-weighted sagittal magnetic resonance image demonstrating extent of lesion within the high cervical spinal cord and the medulla. Note how the lesion does not extend into the pons.

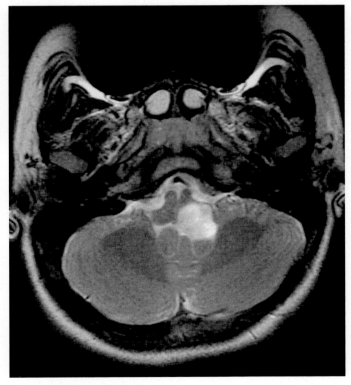

FIGURE 84-3 Axial T2-weighted image of small lesion arising from the lower medulla on the left side. The lesion appears quite discrete by magnetic resonance imaging.

weighted images[5] but can contain hyperintense foci[25] (Figure 84-2). On T2-weighted and proton density images, the lesions are often hyperintense to white matter[5,25] (Figure 84-3) but can also contain mixed areas of hyperintensity and hypointensity with fluid levels and linear septations.[25] The majority of tumors are enhanced with gadolinium,[5] and this enhancement is usually homogeneous but can also be heterogeneous (Figure 84-4). Although most tumors are solid,[25] cysts containing blood products[25] or nodules may also appear.[5] Mural nodules that are enhancing but have cyst walls that do not enhance are reported to be amenable to radical resection and carry a good prognosis. Cyst walls that are enhancing may indicate a malignant glioma for which only short-term palliation may be obtained with surgical intervention.[7]

Imaging may not reflect the surgical findings. Although the imaging studies may show a diffuse appearance of the tumor, intraoperatively a tissue-tumor plane can often be found.[19]

Although some report that the combination of MRI and clinical presentation will suggest the diagnosis of malignancy,[7] there are no presurgical tests that can definitively make a pathologic diagnosis of a cervicomedullary brainstem tumor.[25]

PATHOLOGY

Several tumor types have been reported to occur in the cervicomedullary region: however, the most common are astrocytomas, medulloblastomas, and ependymoma.[11] Other tumor types found in the cervicomedullary region of the pediatric pop-

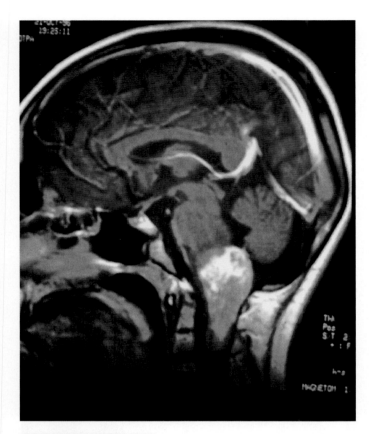

FIGURE 84-4   Gadolinium-enhanced sagittal magnetic resonance image showing extensive cervicomedullary tumor. Here, the contrast enhancement is diffuse throughout the cervicomedullary junction.

ulation include schwannoma,[12] neurofibroma,[4] angioreticuloma[2] and lipoma,[2] hemangioendothelioma,[3] meningioma,[11] neurolemmoma,[11] ganglioglioma,[24] and oliogastrocytoma.[24] For the purposes of this chapter, however, we will focus on the pathophysiology of intrinsic cervicomedullary gliomas.

Cervicomedullary gliomas occur at the cervicomedullary junction and extend rostrally and dorsally into the medulla and caudally into the spinal cord. Caudal expansion into the spinal cord may be to the level of first cervical vertebra alone or can extend as far as the fourth thoracic vertebra with a mean maximum tumor diameter of 4.4 cm.[25] Epstein et al[8] have proposed a hypothesis that describes cervicomedullary glioma growth patterns. In the spinal cord, there are no transversely oriented anatomic structures, other than crossing spinothalamic fibers that can affect growth at the spinal level. Thus intra-axial spinal tumors will expand longitudinally and cylindrically within the cord. This pattern was found to be uniform and irrespective of histologic grade.

Within the brainstem, however, the ependyma lining the fourth ventricle forms less of a barrier compared with the pia. In addition, the transverse structures of the cervicomedullary zones of decussations may act as barriers to tumor growth. At the cervicomedullary junction, anatomic barriers include the pyramidal decussation crossing from side to side, the internal arcuate fibers and medial lemniscus, and the efferent fibers from the inferior olivary complex that stream from a ventro-

medial position toward the inferior cerebellar peduncle located posterolaterally. Although some of these structures may be more of a barrier than others, in combination they could hinder axial growth in accordance with the principles of Scherer[22] and act in conjunction with the enveloping pia to direct the overall growth of a benign astrocytoma. Thus a tumor that originates within the spinal cord and below the cervicomedullary barrier would be limited in growth by the circumferential pia and the transverse fibers of the medulla. The tumor would then be directed toward the obex, the area of least resistance. The cervicomedullary barrier may be displaced rostrally but is not penetrated because of the transverse fibers. With continued growth, the lesion may rupture into the fourth ventricle at the level of the obex because of the relatively weak barrier. Epstein and his group also found the tumors that are focal and do not penetrate a barrier are more likely benign. They stipulate, however, that even high-grade lesions may be contained by a given barrier in the early stages of the disease. With expansion of the cervicomedullary tumor, cranial motor nuclei XII can be displaced either around the tumor on the floor of the fourth ventricle, or cranial motor nuclei XII and VII may remain in their original anatomic position.[16] Others suggest that as advanced tumor extends into the fourth ventricle,[1] it pushes cranial nerve motor nuclei upward.

Approximately 10% to 20%[6,24] of cervicomedullary gliomas are high grade and include anaplastic oligoastrocytoma,[24] anaplastic ganglioglioma,[19] anaplastic astrocytoma,[6,24] and glioblastoma.[6] More commonly, however, in several published surgical series, low-grade glioma is found.[5,19,24,25] Often the majority of these are pilocytic astrocytoma[10,24,25] (WHO grade I) and less commonly fibrillary astrocytoma,[10,24] gangliogliomas,[24] oligoastrocytoma,[24] and desmoplastic tumor of infancy.[25]

In the Young Poussaint et al series[25] of 11 patients, 1 had a tumor of predominant fibroblastic cell type. Infrequent glial fibrillary acidic protein (GFAP)-positive astrocytes were scattered within the dense fibroblastic (desmoplastic) proliferation. This tumor was ultimately classified as a desmoplastic tumor of infancy or "gliofibroma"; however, pilocytic astrocytomas have been reported to initiate a desmoplastic response at the surface of the brainstem in their more exophytic portions.[10]

In 8 of their 11 patients, an astrocytic tumor most consistent with a pilocytic astrocytoma (WHO grade I) was demonstrated. These tumors had loosely arranged bipolar cells with predominantly bipolar astrocytes expressing glial fibrillary acidic protein, no detectable mitoses, and a low proliferative index (MIB-1). Rosenthal fibers, brightly eosinophilic cylindrical structures, were found in all eight of these tumors, and eosinophilic granular bodies were found in six. Two of their patients had tumors where the distinction between pilocytic and fibrillary astrocytoma could not be made, and one of these tumors was associated with an abundant extracellular mucinous matrix. The differentiation between fibrillary and pilocytic astrocytomas may be significant in that fibrillary astrocytomas, when compared with pilocytic astrocytomas, have been found to more likely occur in the pons and are more infiltrative, often expanding ventrally to encircle the basilar artery. Thus although fibrillary astrocytomas may be low grade initially, they may progress to a more malignant tumor with time and have features such as vascular proliferation and necrosis (WHO grade IV). Some report that diffusely infiltrating tumors may be more likely to be fibrillary astrocytomas and hold a poorer prognostic response than circumscribed or dorsally exophytic tumors,[6,10] which more likely may be pilocytic astrocytomas and have a more favorable outcome.

Definitive pathologic diagnosis can be difficult. There have been reports of malignant transformation or biopsy sampling errors. Epstein et al report one case where a biopsy showing low-grade glioma was subsequently found to be anaplastic ganglioglioma after radiation therapy at reoperation.[19] Some tumors can contain entrapped neurons, which may make distinction of astrocytoma from the much less common ganglioglioma difficult.[10] It has also been postulated that patients with minimal neurologic deficits and symptoms lasting more than 4 months may have the topographic variant of the dysembryoplastic neuroepithelial tumor.[24]

MANAGEMENT OF CERVICOMEDULLARY TUMORS

In the past, intrinsic brainstem tumors as a group were treated with irradiation and adjunctive chemotherapy with relatively little success.[5] With MRI allowing better differentiation among the different groups of brainstem tumors, the cervicomedullary tumor group has been found to significantly benefit from surgery.[5–7,23,25] Although adults with cervicomedullary tumors have been treated successfully with observation or radiation,[14] surgery is recommended in children.[7,17] If the patient has hydrocephalus, we prefer to treat with preoperative steroids followed by tumor excision. Many children improve and stabilize with high-dose steroids before definitive resection. Shunting procedures have several disadvantages, including shunt malfunction or infection, subdural hematomas with rapid decompression of the ventricles, or upward herniation of the posterior fossa contents with brainstem compression and hemorrhage into the tumor.[21]

Surgical options for the tumor itself include biopsy or resection. MRI or CT-guided biopsy is advocated if the clinical or radiologic features are atypical, because the differential diagnosis can include other lesions such as inflammatory granuloma, pyogenic abscess, and other tumors.[18,20] If the clinical and imaging findings are in keeping with a cervicomedullary glioma, the role for biopsy is less clear. Epstein et al[5,6] suggest that if the biopsy discloses a malignant neoplasm, a poor prognosis will be obvious.

Although biopsy has been recommended by some, others recommend maximal tumor resection for the management of typical cervicomedullary gliomas.[5–7,17,18] Factors determined from retrospective analyses to be important for assessing the potential benefits of surgery include duration of the illness, the evolution of the disease, and the severity of neurologic deficits in conjunction with the MRI, the preoperative neurologic status, the size and location of the tumor within the brainstem, the presence or absence of associated edema, and the pathologic diagnosis.[5–8,24,25] A patient with symptoms lasting 4 months or longer and minimal neurologic deficits almost invariably has an indolent lesion, which is associated with a longer progression-free survival despite incomplete surgical resection.[24] The preoperative clinical status influences surgical outcome in that patients who were severely disabled did poorly postoperatively.[7] Patients with malignant tumors were also found to do poorly, although those with benign or low-grade neoplasms were found to have the potential for neurologic

recovery and long-term survival.[7,24] The goal of surgery is to reduce tumor burden. The amount of neoplastic tissue removed has been variable, ranging from 50% to more than 90%.[7] Reports of surgical resection suggest that a gross-total resection is achievable in 31% of patients, and approximately 50% of patients obtain less than 90% resection.[24]

Surgical management of patients with cervicomedullary tumors requires thorough neuroanesthetic and monitoring consideration. Atropine is useful in blunting deleterious vagal responses that often occur after laryngoscopy and administration of a neuromuscular blocking agent. Intravenous lidocaine can suppress coughing and prevents any precipitous rise in intracranial pressure during intubation.[21] Use of a nasotracheal tube allows full cervical flexion without concern for kinking and obstruction of the airway.[21] Careful intraoperative monitoring is essential and usually includes a Foley catheter, arterial and central venous lines, body temperature, and electrocardiographic monitoring.[21] The patient is often given a hyperosmotic agent such as mannitol to decrease intracranial pressure and allow improved tumor access.[21] Although patients can be positioned in a sitting position for surgery, pitfalls such as risk of air embolism, frontal pneumocephalus, systemic hypotension, and surgeon fatigue prompt our use of a prone position with gentle neck flexion.[21] Although children younger than 2.5 years of age are placed in a padded horseshoe head holder, older patients may be placed in headrests with pin fixation.[21] Somatosensory, motor, and brainstem-evoked-potential monitoring is often used to aid the surgeon in differentiating normal brain from tumor,[21] because the electrical activity becomes relatively disordered as the interface between tumor and normal neural tissue is approached.[7]

The rostral spinal cord and the lower medulla are exposed using a midline skin incision from the inion to the cervical or thoracic region, depending on the caudal extent of the tumor as indicated by sagittal MRI. The bony exposure is with a small suboccipital craniectomy and laminectomy or osteoplastic laminotomy if more than two laminae are to be removed.[24] If the tumor cannot be easily visualized, ultrasound may be of assistance. Intraoperative ultrasound can be used to help identify the rostral and caudal poles of the tumor before opening the dura and the retraction of the cerebellar tonsils laterally.[21]

After dural opening, a midline myelotomy is then performed in the spinal cord centered over the middle of the tumor rather than the poles to avoid injuring adjacent intact tissue[6,21] (Figure 84-5). Because cervicomedullary tumors can cause displacement of motor nuclei of cranial nerve XII around the tumor on the floor of the fourth ventricle or leave cranial motor nuclei of XII and VII in their original anatomic position, myelotomy should be placed only up to the cervicomedullary junction and tumor beneath the fourth ventricular floor resected by undermining it through the myelotomy.[16] In most cases, a gross-total excision of the cervical component with a subtotal removal of the medullary component can be obtained[6] (Figure 84-6). A less aggressive tumor resection in the medulla is called for because of the increased hazard of gray versus white matter injury. Cysts found in the medullary component of the tumor and cyst drainage are thought to be important because the cysts may contribute to the symptomatology.[6,21] Ultrasound may be of use in identifying cysts that may otherwise be overlooked.[6]

Tumor removal has been described using several techniques that include removing the tumor piecemeal or with mechanical, ultrasonic aspiration; bipolar coagulation and

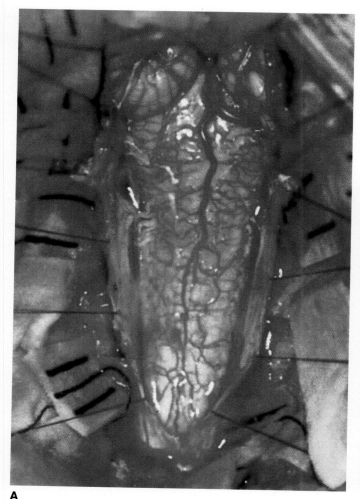

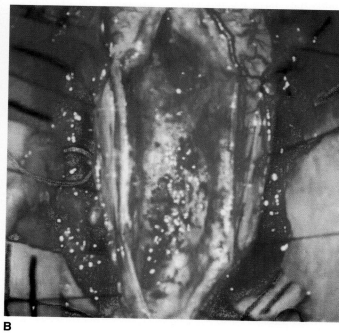

A

B

FIGURE 84-5 *A,* Preoperative exposure of lesions seen in Figure 84-4. Note expanded, swollen cervicomedullary junction. *B,* Following midline myelotomy, the tumor has been debulked, leaving behind the intramedullary component rostrally. In this case, the diagnosis was ganglioglioma.

cutting; and laser.[2,6,21] Although the Cavitron ultrasonic aspirator can be used, many prefer the laser.[6,21] The Cavitron hand piece can restrict the visibility, and the laser can be very valuable in removing small foci of firm and fibrous tumor adherent to normal spinal cord. Laser char, however, can necessitate frequent interruption of the dissection to gently remove the thin layer of blackened tissue and adequately visualize the residual neoplasm.[5] Postoperatively, patients should be followed carefully with serial neurologic and neuroimaging assessments.[17]

Adjuvant therapy can be considered either together with the initial surgery or if there is disease progression. These options can include surgery with radiation and surgery with chemotherapy and radiation.[25] Although the gross-total removal of a spinal ependymoma without the routine use of adjuvant therapy has been suggested as the treatment of choice,[17] because of the relative rarity of cervicomedullary gliomas, there is no consensus regarding the use of adjuvant treatment.[17] Incompletely resected low-grade astrocytoma can be associated with long and neurologically improved postoperative survival, and given the risks of cognitive impairment and the development of second neo-

plasms, radiation treatment may be restricted to the treatment of high-grade tumors, recurrences, and metastatic spread of tumor through the cerebrospinal fluid pathways.[17] Although there is presently no clear evidence for the role of chemotherapy in the treatment of these tumors, it has been suggested that intensive chemotherapy and radiation be used in patients with high-grade tumors.[17] There has been reported response in a patient with a pilocytic astrocytoma treated with biopsy, ranimustine, and radiation. Follow-up MRI with gadolinium contrast in this patient performed 5 years post-treatment showed no enhanced lesion and clinical improvement with respect to motor weakness and truncal ataxia.[17] Another patient with high-grade pilocytic astrocytoma, however, also treated with biopsy, radiation, and chemotherapy had tumor progression and died at 6 months. Chemotherapeutic regimens using carboplatin and vincristine have also been used for treatment of young children to avoid the neurotoxic effects of radiation. Following this chemotherapeutic regimen, radiation therapy has been used with subsequent tumor progression, resulting in interval tumor resolution with stable clinical findings.[25] Chemotherapy for gangliogliomas and

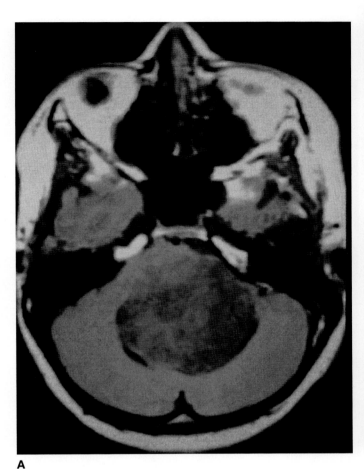

A

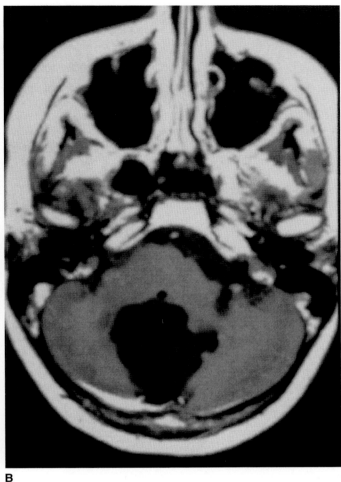

B

FIGURE 84-6   Preoperative *(A)* and postoperative *(B)* images showing gross-total resection of a cervicomedullary tumor. The diagnosis here was low-grade astrocytoma.

oligoastrocytomas of the cervicomedullary region include carboplatin and MOPP (mustargen, Oncovin, procarbazine, and prednisone),[19] respectively.

Severe neuropathic pain can also be associated with cervicomedullary tumors. There is a report of a 12-year-old patient with a partially resected glioblastoma multiforme cervicomedullary tumor who developed neuropathic pain. This pain was successfully palliated using ketamine, benzodiazepines, and morphine,[13] which allowed transferring the patient home.

OUTCOMES

The histologic subtype may be the most significant predictor of prognosis after treatment in cervicomedullary tumors.[10] Bricola reports in his series of children and adults with cervicomedullary tumors that 6 of 12 patients (one ependymoma, five benign astrocytomas) made excellent neurologic recoveries, although the remainder (four malignant gliomas, one angioreticuloma, and one lipoma) showed no appreciable improvement.[2] In Epstein's series,[7] there were 24 patients with cervicomedullary gliomas. Sixteen had grade I or II astrocytomas, and four had gangliogliomas. All 16 patients were alive

and neurologically improved 6 to 60 months postoperatively. All four patients with grade III or IV astrocytomas died 9 to 12 months postoperatively from tumor progression.

Although radical surgery offers the possibility of long-term clinical remission,[25] there are significant complications. Reported postoperative deficits can include severe quadriparesis, respiratory difficulties resulting in ventilatory dependency, and swallowing difficulties that require gastrostomy.[5,19] Mortality from meningitis and sepsis, tumor progression,[7] aspiration pneumonia,[5] aspiration with pulmonary insufficiency,[23] and apnea and respiratory arrest[25] has been reported. The immediate postoperative course has been related to the preoperative neurologic status, because patients who are severely disabled before surgery recover very slowly, whereas those who are less impaired improve more quickly.[5] Given the increased risk of respiratory and airway compromise in these patients, recommendations have been made for tracheostomy or prolonged intubation for up to 7 days postoperatively.[23] Long-term postoperative complications include cervical kyphosis in three out of nine patients after suboccipital craniotomy and cervical laminectomy requiring surgical fusion in two[25] (Figure 84-7).

The therapeutic series are too small to make definite conclusions regarding the various treatment strategies. In the

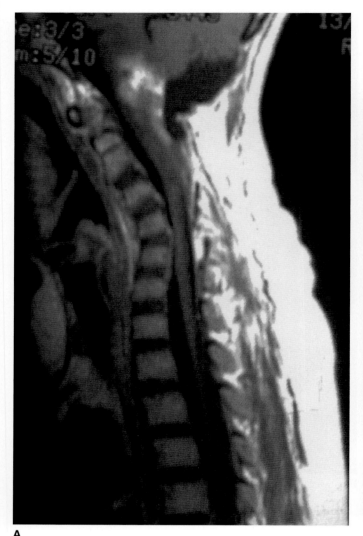

A

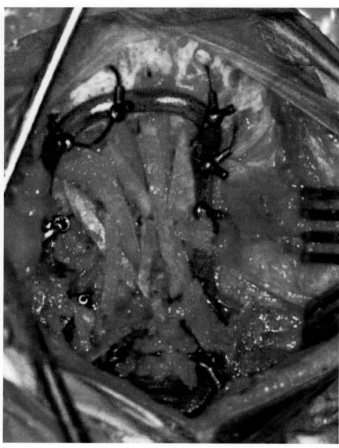

B

FIGURE 84-7   *A,* Postoperative sagittal image taken from the same case as depicted in Figure 84-4. Note radical resection of tumor but the development of cervical kyphosis. *B,* Occipital-cervical instability necessitated a fusion procedure using an occipital to C3 fusion construct with a Luque rectangle, sublaminar and suboccipital wires, and bone grafting.

Young Poussaint et al series,[25] patients underwent surgery alone, surgery with radiation, and surgery with chemotherapy and radiation. In their six patients who had surgery alone, subtotal resection was performed in four, biopsy only in one, and biopsy followed 1 month later by subtotal resection for tumor in one. Of these patients, four had stable residual disease, and two had no visible tumor. All are alive with a mean follow-up of 3.9 years (range 0.2 to 11 years). In four patients who underwent surgery followed by radiation, three underwent subtotal resection and one underwent biopsy. Progression of the disease occurred in three and the fourth died of respiratory arrest with stable residual tumor. With radiation treatment and mean follow-up of 8.2 years (range 4.3 to 10 years) of the remaining three patients, two have stable residual tumor, and one has no tumor. One patient had subtotal resection with increasing tumor enhancement found 1 month later. Because of the young age of the patient (1 year), the patient was initially treated with carboplatin and vincristine. Although decreased

tumor enhancement was initially observed, 1.5 years later the patient developed a metastatic nodule in the brain consistent with cerebrospinal fluid seeding. When the original tumor was found to increase in enhancement 2 months later, the patient underwent radiation therapy. At 2-year follow-up review, the patient was reported to have had interval tumor resolution with stable clinical findings.

With respect to tumor progression, the majority were related to local tumor growth rather than metastatic disease.[19,25] Robertson et al[19] report that 4-year actuarial progression-free survival rates and total survival rates were 70% and 100%, respectively, in patients after first surgery for a newly diagnosed tumor. Progression-free and total survival rates were poorer, 41% and 62%, respectively, in patients who had received prior radiation therapy for their tumor. Median follow-up in this series was 4 years.[19] In the three patients with newly diagnosed tumors with progression, treatment consisted of repeated resection with adjuvant radiation therapy. The histopathology of low-grade astrocytoma in two and anaplastic astrocytoma in the other was not found to have changed. In three of six patients who had progressed after prior radiation treatment and surgery, one was stable after a second resection, and two died. From this study, it was concluded that patients with prior radiation treatment or severe preoperative deficits of bulbar function (swallowing, speaking, breathing) and ambulation had the highest morbidity. Neurologic deterioration with significant disability has also been reported to occur as late as 1 to 3 years following radiation therapy.[5]

Others, however, find no correlation with radiation therapy or preoperative symptomatology. Weiner et al[24] report that no statistical correlation was found between 5-year progression-free survival, total survival, or neurologic outcome and age, gender, radiographic tumor appearance, prior surgery, radiation therapy, chemotherapy, preoperative symptomatology (spinal cord versus medullary), extent of resection, or postoperative adjuvant therapy.

CONCLUSION

Cervicomedullary gliomas are a unique, relatively rare category of brainstem gliomas that may be amenable to treatment and have a good prognosis. They occur more often in children than adults and can cause clinical syndromes associated with medullary or spinal cord dysfunction or hydrocephalus. Although these tumors can sometimes be visualized by CT, MRI is the imaging modality of choice, because it allows determination of their rostral and caudal extent. Unlike pontine brainstem tumors, cervicomedullary tumors are less likely to infiltrate the pons and are more commonly associated with low-grade astrocytoma. They are usually treated with surgical resection and with adjuvant radiation or chemotherapy if there is tumor progression. Although significant complications such as ventilator dependency can occur with surgical treatment, the majority of patients are reported to survive postoperatively without tumor progression.

References

1. Bricolo A, Turazzi S: Surgery for gliomas and other mass lesions. In Symon L (ed): Advances and Technical Standards in Neurosurgery, Vol 22. New York, Springer Wien, 1995.
2. Bricolo A, Turazzi S, Cristofori L, et al: Direct surgery for brainstem tumours. Acta Neurochir Suppl (Wien) 53:148–158, 1991.
3. Chen TC, Gonzalez-Gomez I, Gilles FH, et al: Pediatric intracranial hemangioendotheliomas: case report. Neurosurgery 40:410–414, 1997.
4. Clarke DB, Farmer JP, Montes JL, et al: Newborn apnea caused by a neurofibroma at the craniocervical junction. Can J Neurol Sci 21:64–66, 1994.
5. Epstein F, McCleary EL: Intrinsic brain-stem tumors of childhood: surgical indications. J Neurosurg 64:11–15, 1986.
6. Epstein F, Wisoff J: Intra-axial tumors of the cervicomedullary junction. J Neurosurg 67:483–487, 1987.
7. Epstein F, Wisoff JH: Intrinsic brainstem tumors in childhood: surgical indications. J Neurooncol 6:309–317, 1988.
8. Epstein FJ, Farmer JP: Brain-stem glioma growth patterns. J Neurosurg 78:408–412, 1993.
9. Felice KJ, DiMario FJ: Cervicomedullary astrocytoma simulating a neuromuscular disorder. Pediatr Neurol 20:78–80, 1999.
10. Fisher PG, Breiter SN, Carson BS, et al: A clinicopathologic reappraisal of brain stem tumor classification. Identification of pilocystic astrocytoma and fibrillary astrocytoma as distinct entities. Cancer 89:1569–1576, 2000.
11. Gilles FH, Leviton A, Hedley-Whyte ET, et al: Childhood brain tumors that occupy more than one compartment at presentation. Multiple compartment tumors. J Neurooncol 14:45–56, 1992.
12. Kaufman BA, Kaufman B, Rekate HL: Cervicomedullary junction tumor diagnosed by nuclear magnetic resonance scanning: case report. Neurosurgery 15:878–880, 1984.
13. Klepstad P, Borchgrevink P, Hval B, et al: Long-term treatment with ketamine in a 12-year-old girl with severe neuropathic pain caused by a cervical spinal tumor. J Pediatr Hematol Oncol 23:616–619, 2001.
14. Landolfi JC, Thaler HT, DeAngelis LM: Adult brainstem gliomas. Neurology 51:1136–1139, 1998.
15. Morioka T, Fujii K, Mitani M, et al: Intraoperative localization of a cervicomedullary glioma from the killed end potential: illustrative case. Neurosurgery 26:1038–1041, 1990.
16. Morota N, Deletis V, Lee M, et al: Functional anatomic relationship between brain-stem tumors and cranial motor nuclei. Neurosurgery 39:787–793; discussion 793–784, 1996.
17. Nishio S, Morioka T, Fujii K, et al: Spinal cord gliomas: management and outcome with reference to adjuvant therapy. J Clin Neurosci 7:20–23, 2000.
18. Rajshekhar V, Chandy MJ: Computerized tomography-guided stereotactic surgery for brainstem masses: a risk-benefit analysis in 71 patients. J Neurosurg 82:976–981, 1995.
19. Robertson PL, Allen JC, Abbott IR, et al: Cervicomedullary tumors in children: a distinct subset of brainstem gliomas. Neurology 44:1798–1803, 1994.
20. Rubin G, Michowitz S, Horev G, et al: Pediatric brain stem gliomas: an update. Childs Nerv Syst 14:167–173, 1998.
21. Rutka JT, Hoffman HJ, Duncan JA: Astrocytomas of the posterior fossa. In Cohen AR: Surgical Disorders of the Fourth Ventricle. Cambridge, Mass, Blackwell Science, 1996.
22. Scherer HJ: Structural development in gliomas. Am J Cancer 34:333–351, 1938.
23. Squires LA, Constantini S, Miller DC, et al: Diffuse infiltrating astrocytoma of the cervicomedullary region: clinicopathologic entity. Pediatr Neurosurg 27:153–159, 1997.
24. Weiner HL, Freed D, Woo HH, et al: Intra-axial tumors of the cervicomedullary junction: surgical results and long-term outcome. Pediatr Neurosurg 27:12–18, 1997.
25. Young Poussaint T, Yousuf N, Barnes PD, et al: Cervicomedullary astrocytomas of childhood: clinical and imaging follow-up. Pediatr Radiol 29:662–668, 1999.

CHAPTER 85

DESMOPLASTIC INFANTILE GANGLIOGLIOMA

Concezio Di Rocco, Gianpiero Tamburrini, Ceasare Colosimo, and Felice Giangaspero

The term *desmoplastic infantile ganglioglioma* (DIG) was coined by VandenBerg et al in 1987.[17] In their first report the authors referred to a rare, distinct clinicopathologic entity, the main features of which were (1) divergent astrocytic and ganglionic differentiation, (2) prominent desmoplastic stroma, (3) voluminous tumor size, (4) evidence of a cystic component, (5) occurrence within the first 18 months of life, and (6) good prognosis. Over the past 15 years this restricted definition has been the subject of much debate. The similarities with the superficial cerebral astrocytoma described by Taratuto et al in 1984[14] and with the pleomorphic xanthoastrocytoma first reported by Kepes et al in 1979[3] led to the identification of a group of massive superficial pediatric brain tumors, the desmoplastic neuroepithelial tumors, which probably have a common origin, though a different histologic differentiation. Indeed, the presence of ganglion cells, which once was considered the most distinctive histologic feature of DIG, is currently accepted as a common finding in superficial cerebral astrocytomas and in pleomorphic xanthoastrocytomas.[10]

INCIDENCE, AGE, LOCATION

Since the description in 1987, approximately 50 cases of DIGs have been described in the literature, with an incidence in autopsy series of 0.4% out of 6500 brain tumors.[5] Males are affected more commonly than females.[1,5,17,18] Diagnosis typically is obtained in the first 2 years of life, with most patients aged younger than 18 months.[2,5,9,17] This early age of onset has led to the speculation that DIGs are true prenatal or congenital neoplasms. However, several cases not occurring in infants but rather in patients with ages ranging from 5 to 19 years have been recently reported, arguing against this theory.[1,5]

DIGs are exclusively supratentorial tumors, for the most part hemispheric in location and without side prevalence. Involvement of multiple lobes is common, with a predilection for the frontal and/or parietal regions; temporal, and at times, occipital lobe extent have been described.[5,8,9]

CLINICAL MANIFESTATIONS

Despite the benign biologic behavior of DIGs, most patients have a brief clinical history with a median duration of symptoms of 3 to 6 months.[1,5,9] Rapid head growth is the presenting symptom in approximately 60% of cases, often accompanied by a bulging anterior fontanel, sunset sign, and cranial bulge overlying the tumor.[1] In children older than 1 year, the duration of symptoms is usually longer (6 to 9 months), and symptoms of intracranial hypertension are more commonly combined with focal neurologic deficits (hemiparesis: 40%).[5,13] In contrast to dysembryoplastic neuroepithelial tumors, seizures (most often partial) outline the clinical onset in only 20% of patients. Consciousness disturbances are also relatively rare, suggesting the very slow growth of these tumors.[1,5,13]

NEURO-ONCOLOGY IMAGING

Most DIGs are huge frontal or parietal mass lesions in which the vast majority of the mass effect is the result of the presence of intratumoral cysts; less often extratumoral cysts may develop and contribute to the macrocrania.[2] Almost invariably DIGS have solid superficial mass or plaque, of variable size, that appears slightly hyperdense on unenhanced computed tomography (CT), hypointense on T1-weighted images (WI), and distinctly hypointense on T2-WI. The presence of septations within the cystic mass, originating from the superficial solid tumor, represents a common feature. These septations show the same CT density and magnetic resonance (MR) signal intensity of the solid superficial mass. The solid superficial mass or plaque, the walls of the intratumoral cysts, and the cystic septations exhibit strong contrast enhancement after iodinated or paramagnetic intravenous injection.[4,6,13,15,16] The CT density and especially the hypointensity on T2-WI are the result of the abundant fibrous tissue and collagen, whereas the intense contrast enhancement results from the rich vascularity.[15,16] These imaging features are quite pathognomonic of DIGs (Figure 85-1). Differential diagnoses on the basis of CT and MRI scans include all the forms of contrast-enhanced superficial tumors encountered in the pediatric age group; however the most commonly encountered gangliogliomas and pleomorphic xanthoastrocytomas (PXAs) are almost invariably hyperintense on T2-WI. Moreover, PXAs are usually found in older children.[2,4] Similarly, dysembryoplastic neuroectodermal tumors (DNTs) are commonly discovered later in life and are easily differentiated from DIGs because DNTs are smaller and do not enhance.[4,6]

Atypical forms of DIGs were recently described: atypical locations (suprasellar), cerebrospinal fluid (CSF) seeding with

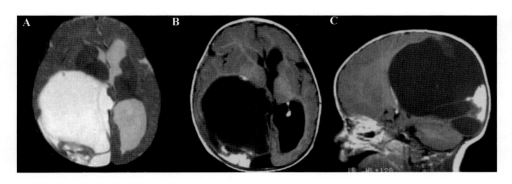

FIGURE 85-1 An 18-month-old child with desmoplastic infantile ganglioglioma. The magnetic resonance imaging examination shows the lesion's typical features, such as the hyperintense signal of the cystic component *(A)* and the hyperintensity and contrast enhancement of the solid portion of the tumor in T1-weighted image after contrast administration *(B and C).*

multiple leptomeningeal implants, and almost completely solid tumors with small cystic portions.[11] Obviously, in such instances a definitive preoperative diagnosis may be unreliable.

TUMOR HISTOLOGY

Macroscopically, these tumors are usually very large with uniloculated or multiloculated cysts filled with clear or xanthochromic fluid. The superficial portion is primarily extracerebral, involving leptomeninges and superficial cortex, and is commonly attached to the dura.[17,18] Histologically, the desmoplasia is characterized by deposition of dense collagen in combination with neuroepithelial and fibroblastic elements. The neuroepithelial component shows a variable proportion of astrocytes and neuronal cells. The neoplastic astrocytes are moderately pleomorphic, ranging from elongated to polygonal cells, most showing intense immunoreactivity for glial fibrillary acidic protein (GFAP). The leptomeningeal part consists of spindle-shaped, elongated astrocytes intermixed with collagen and reticulin fibers surrounding tumor cells (Figure 85-2). The neuronal elements range from atypical ganglioid cells to small polygonal cell types.[7,12] Immunohistochemical detection of synaptophysin or neurofilaments facilitate identification of the neuronal cell population. In addition, there is usually a population of more primitive cells. Such an undifferentiated cell component may predominate in some areas; in such areas, mitoses and small foci of necrosis can be observed. There is a sharp demarcation between the cortical surface and the desmoplastic tumor, although Virchow-Robin spaces in the underlying cortex are often filled with tumor cells. Mitotic activity is scarce and when present limited to the undifferentiated small cell population. The Ki-67 labeling index may range from less than 0.5% to 15%. In general, the histologic features that define a poor prognosis in common infiltrating astrocytomas such as necrosis, vascular proliferation, mitoses, and high Ki-67 labeling index do not have the same negative implications in DIGs.[12]

Molecular genetic studies have demonstrated that, in contrast to diffuse astrocytomas, DIGs do not display any allelic loss on chromosomes 17p and 10 and do not carry TP53 gene mutations. Despite the ambiguous histology, the prognosis of DIGs is good, corresponding to WHO grade I tumors.[12,18]

TREATMENT AND PROGNOSIS

Surgery is the treatment of choice. Typical intraoperative features of DIGs are a remarkably firm texture (resulting from

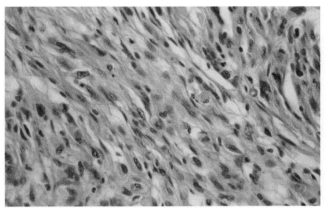

A

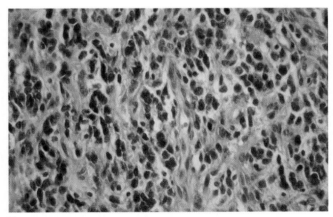

B

FIGURE 85-2 *A,* The bulk of the lesion is composed of spindle astrocytes with a marked desmoplastic component. *B,* In some areas the tumor contains aggregates of poorly differentiated cells.

desmoplasia), contact with the surface of the hemisphere, and the almost invariably present cystic component.[2,5]

Complete tumor removal can, however, be achieved only in selected cases. In a review of the literature, Duffner et al[1] could find only a 35% rate of gross-total resection. Many reasons may contribute to this relatively low rate of success. (1) A definite cleavage of the tumor from the surrounding brain can only occasionally be recognized. (2) A large percentage of these tumors are densely adherent to the tentorium, basal dura, or superior sagittal sinus or infiltrate eloquent central nervous system (CNS) structures (i.e., cerebral peduncle or hypothalamus). (3) As for every infant brain tumor, blood loss is a major intraoperative problem; the sheer size and diffuse vascularization of DIGs specifically contribute to increased hemodynamic risks.[1,2,5]

Few reports have commented on the use of adjuvant treatments—too few cases to permit definite conclusions. Duffner et al[1] reported on four patients treated with adjuvant chemotherapy (the Pediatric Oncology Group protocol of cyclophosphamide, vincristine, cisplatin, and etoposide administered to one patient aged 12 months; one aged 18 months; two aged 24 months). One patient had undergone a gross-total resection, and the remaining three patients had debulking procedures only. Among those infants with measurable residual disease, one had a complete response, one had a partial response, and one remained stable, with a follow-up of 32 to 60 months.

In a review paper, VandenBerg[18] reports on an 8.7-year median follow-up of 14 cases of DIGs from different institutions. Treatment modality was known in 90% of the cases: 31% had a near-total resection and no further treatment, 38% surgery and radiation therapy, 23% surgery and chemotherapy, and 8% surgery and both chemotherapy and radiation therapy. There were no deaths in any of these groups. Only one patient, initially receiving a gross-total tumor resection without adjuvant therapy, had a documented recurrence of the lesion 2 years after surgery; he went on to have a repeat surgical procedure, described as complete, and radiation therapy. No sign of tumor regrowth was later documented (at follow-up of 8 years).

The conclusion from the available literature is that no complementary treatment is needed in the case of complete tumor resection. When tumor recurrence or residual tumor is demonstrated, a second operation should be considered the treatment of choice. Chemotherapy is a reasonable further option in infants with progressive disease after surgery and when no further tumor removal can be performed (e.g., infiltration of eloquent CNS structures). Radiation therapy is advised as a last resort in children older than 5 years of age and unresponsive to chemotherapy. The very young age of the patients and the usually large volume of the involved brain make the risks of radiation neurotoxicity too high. Despite the occasional reports of fatal cases, DIGs have a generally good prognosis, and recurrence-free intervals range from 6 months to 14 years.

References

1. Duffner PK, Burger PC, Cohen ME, et al: Desmoplastic infantile gangliogliomas: an approach to therapy. Neurosurgery 34:583–589, 1994.
2. Ildan F, Tuna M, Gocer IA, et al: Intracerebral ganglioglioma: clinical and radiological study of eleven surgically treated cases with follow-up. Neurosurg Rev 24:114–118, 2001.
3. Kepes JJ, Rubinstein LJ, Eng LF: Pleomorphic xanthoastrocytoma: a distinct meningocerebral glioma of young subjects with relatively favorable prognosis. A study of 12 cases. Cancer 44:1839–1852, 1979.
4. Koeller KK, Henry JM: From the archives of the AFIP: superficial gliomas: radiologic-pathologic correlation. Radiographics 21:1533–1556, 2001.
5. Mallucci C, Lellouch-Tubiana A, Salazar C, et al: The management of desmoplastic neuroepithelial tumours in childhood. Childs Nerv Syst 16:8–14, 2000.
6. Martin DS, Levy B, Awwad EE, Pittman T: Desmoplastic infantile ganglioglioma: CT and MR features. AJNR 12:1195–1197, 1991.
7. Moreno A, de Felipe J, Garcia Sola R, et al: Neuronal and mixed neuronal glial tumors associated to epilepsy. A heterogeneous and related group of tumours. Histol Histopathol 16:613–622, 2001.
8. Paulus W, Schlote W, Perentes E, et al: Desmoplastic supratentorial neuroepithelial tumours of infancy. Histopathology 21:43–49, 1992.
9. Rothman S, Sharon N, Shiffer J, et al: Desmoplastic infantile ganglioglioma. Acta Oncol 36:655–657, 1997.
10. Rushing EJ, Rorke LB, Sutton L: Problems in the nosology of desmoplastic tumors of childhood. Pediatr Neurosurg 19:57–62, 1993.
11. Setty SN, Miller DC, Camras L, et al: Desmoplastic infantile astrocytoma with metastases at presentation. Mod Pathol 10:945–951, 1997.
12. Shao L, Tihan T, Burger PC: Desmoplastic infantile ganglioglioma: a clinical and pathological review of eight cases. J Neuropath Exp Neurol 61:466, 2002.
13. Sperner J, Gottschalk J, Neumann K, et al: Clinical, radiological and histological findings in desmoplastic infantile ganglioglioma. Childs Nerv Syst 10:458–463, 1994.
14. Taratuto AL, VandenBerg SR, Rorke LB: Desmoplastic infantile astrocytoma and ganglioglioma. In Kleihues P and Cavanee WK: Pathology and Genetics of Tumours of the Nervous System. Lyon, France, IARC Press, 2002.
15. Tenreiro-Picon OR, Kamath SV, Knorr JR, et al: Desmoplastic infantile ganglioglioma: CT and MRI features. Pediatr Radiol 25:540–543, 1995.
16. Tseng JH, Tseng MY, Kuo MF, et al: Chronological changes on magnetic resonance images in a case of desmoplastic infantile ganglioglioma. Pediatr Neurosurg 36:29–32, 2002.
17. VandenBerg SR, May EE, Rubinstein LJ, et al: Desmoplastic supratentorial neuroepithelial tumors of infancy with divergent differentiation potential ("desmoplastic infantile gangliogliomas"). Report of 11 cases of a distinctive embryonal tumor with favorable prognosis. J Neurosurg 66:58–71, 1987.
18. Vandenberg SR: Desmoplastic infantile ganglioglioma and desmoplastic cerebral astrocytoma of infancy. Brain Pathol 3:275–281, 1993.

CHAPTER 86

PLEOMORPHIC XANTHOASTROCYTOMA

Ganesh Rao and John R.W. Kestle

Since its original description in 1979,[18] pleomorphic xanthoas-trocytoma (PXA) has been regarded as a distinct astrocytic tumor with a favorable outcome.[19] In general, this is a rare tumor that classically occurs as a cystic mass in the temporal lobe. PXA often arises in adolescents and young adults and is amenable to surgical resection with good disease control, although it may harbor the potential for malignant transformation. In this chapter, we discuss specific characteristics of this tumor type, including diagnostic and therapeutic considerations.

LOCATION AND DIAGNOSIS

PXA typically occurs in the supratentorial compartment and, most commonly, in the temporal lobe.[3,4,8,13,15,23,25,31,33–35] This tumor has been reported in the cerebellum, pineal region, spinal cord, and even the retina.[6,10,12,21,22,26,32,37,41] PXA has also been reported in association with oligodendrogliomas and gangli-ogliomas.[6,20,22,29,30] Given the tumor's predilection for involving the superficial temporal lobe, it commonly causes seizures, and nearly 80% of patients will have epilepsy.[2,5,28] Although its occurrence is uncommon, PXA should be considered in the differential diagnosis when a patient has a cystic mass in the temporal lobe.

EPIDEMIOLOGY

PXA is a rare tumor, and although epidemiologic estimates are speculative at best, PXA likely represents approximately 0.5% of gliomas.[3] PXA most commonly occurs in adolescents and young adults, although it has been reported in patients as young as 2 years and as old as 82 years of age.[28,29]

IMAGING

PXA has a characteristic appearance on neuroimaging modalities such as computed tomography (CT) and magnetic resonance imaging (MRI). Typically, it appears as a superficial, cystic mass in the temporal lobe.[28] On noncontrast CT scan, PXA is usually hypodense and cystic in appearance, and calcifications are unusual.[27,40] MRI with contrast is the study of choice for this type of tumor (Figure 86-1). PXAs will appear hypointense or isoin-tense to normal brain.[34] A peripheral, mural nodule may be

present that is avidly contrast enhanced.[27] Angiography is of limited value, because findings may range from an avascular appearance to intense neovascularity within the tumor nodule.[40]

HISTOPATHOLOGY

Grossly, PXAs are well-demarcated, cystic tumors. The fluid within the cyst is invariably xanthochromic.[28] There may be leptomeningeal attachment, but the tumor is generally easily separated from normal brain.[2]

The histologic characteristics of PXA include pleomorphic tumor cells with large amounts of cytoplasm. Dark, multilobu-lated nuclei are common. Multinucleated giant cells with foamy, lipid-laden astrocytes are typical, and eosinophilic gran-ular bodies are common (Figure 86-2). Mitoses are occasion-ally seen, but necrosis is not usually a feature of PXAs.[16] Increased mitotic activity may suggest a predisposition to anaplastic transformation.[24] In addition, the presence of necro-sis in these tumors has been found to correlate with a more aggressive course.[1,17,18,28]

Tumors will invariably stain positive for glial fibrillary acidic protein (GFAP) and S-100 protein, confirming the astro-cytic lineage of PXAs. They are also strongly positive for class III β tubulin. Variants of PXAs include elements of neuronal differentiation, including gangliogliomas (the so-called PXA-GG). These tumors will stain positive for synaptophysin and neurofilament protein.[9]

A small percentage of PXAs undergo anaplastic transfor-mation that may ultimately lead to glioblastoma multiforme (GBM).[24] Although the exact percentage is not known, recur-ring PXAs exhibit high mitotic activity, hypercellularity, nuclear hyperchromatism, and endothelial proliferation.[24] PXAs that are necrotic but that do not exhibit these character-istics are an entity distinct from glioblastoma, although their prognosis is similarly unfavorable.[28]

THERAPY

The superficial nature of these lesions facilitates surgical resec-tion, which is the mainstay of treatment for PXA.[8,16,18] One study has shown that, in the absence of necrosis, gross-total resection provided a disease-free survival rate of 95% com-pared with a 68% survival rate for those who had a subtotal

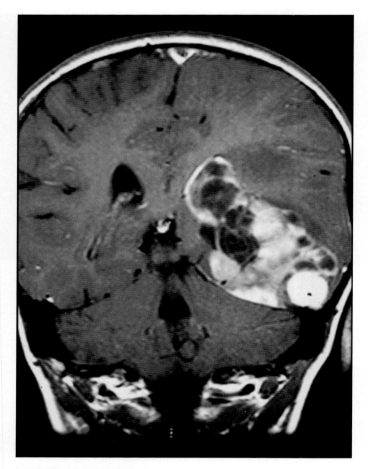

FIGURE 86-1 Coronal magnetic resonance imaging scan shows a pleomorphic xanthoastrocytoma in the temporal lobe, which extends into the trigone of the lateral ventricle. The solid component of the tumor and the walls of the multiple tumor cysts are enhanced with gadolinium.

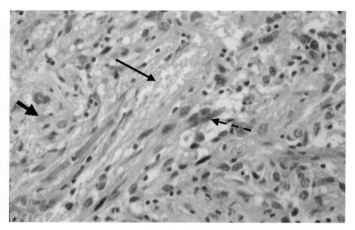

FIGURE 86-2 Histologic features of pleomorphic xanthoastrocytoma. *Small arrow,* Foamy cytoplasm in large astrocytes. *Large arrow,* Eosinophilic bodies. *Small broken arrow,* Multinucleated giant astrocytes.

PROGNOSIS AND RECURRENCE

After surgical resection, the prognosis for patients with PXA is generally favorable. The long-term survival rate for patients undergoing resection with or without radiation ranges from 50% to 77% at 15 years.[24,28] The presence of necrosis, however, significantly affects the survival profile. Necrosis has been shown to indicate a median survival rate of 1 year (compared with a median survival rate of 20 years without necrosis).[28] PXAs that harbor a necrotic component are classified differently from GBM, although PXAs can, in rare cases, transform to GBM. PXAs that have an aggressive histologic component, including increased mitotic activity (up to 4 mitoses per 10 high-power fields), trend toward anaplastic transformation that may lead to GBM.[24]

After initial resection, recurrence of PXA is unusual, unless the tumor is undergoing anaplastic transformation. Increased mitotic activity, hypercellularity, endothelial hyperplasia, and nuclear pseudopalisading are all features of more aggressive tumors.[7,11] Tumors that have these features upon initial resection should be monitored closely because these features are typically found in recurrent tumors and indicate an aggressive nature.[14,17,38,39]

CONCLUSION

PXA is a rare, astrocytic tumor that generally has a favorable prognosis. PXA usually occurs in adolescents and young adults who often have seizures. Surgical resection is the best treatment for good tumor control. There appears to be no benefit to adjunctive radiation therapy, and chemotherapy has not been adequately studied. PXAs that have a necrotic element are usually more aggressive and correlate with poorer survival. Although rare, PXA can progress to GBM, and the histologic characteristics of the tumor may indicate the potential for this progression.

resection.[28] When necrosis was included, gross-total resection provided a survival rate of 91% compared with 65% for subtotal resection, a difference that is not statistically significant. Other studies have shown that the completeness of resection does *not* correlate with recurrence or mortality rates in the first 10 years after the initial resection.[24]

Treatment of PXA with radiation therapy is controversial, and surgery followed by radiation has not been shown to provide an advantage over surgery alone.[24,36] Even in the face of recurrence, adjuvant radiation therapy has not been shown to be effective.[24,28] Indeed, for PXAs that are necrotic there may not be any advantage to surgery with or without radiation therapy.[28] Given the rarity of this tumor, chemotherapeutic regimens for PXA have not been studied, and in general, the standard therapies used for astrocytic tumors have been used against recurrent PXAs.

References

1. Allegranza A, Ferraresi S, Bruzzone M, et al: Cerebromeningeal pleomorphic xanthoastrocytoma. Report on four cases: clinical, radiologic and pathological features. (Including a case with malignant evolution). Neurosurg Rev 14:43–49, 1991.
2. Blom RJ: Pleomorphic xanthoastrocytoma: CT appearance. J Comput Assist Tomogr 12:351–352, 1988.
3. Bucciero A, De Caro M, De Stefano V, et al: Pleomorphic xanthoastrocytoma: clinical, imaging and pathological features of four cases. Clin Neurol Neurosurg 99:40–45, 1997.
4. Cervoni L, Salvati M, Santoro A, et al: Pleomorphic xanthoastrocytoma: some observations. Neurosurg Rev 19:13–16, 1996.
5. Davies KG, Maxwell RE, Seljeskog E, et al: Pleomorphic xanthoastrocytoma—report of four cases, with MRI scan appearances and literature review. Br J Neurosurg 8:681–689, 1994.
6. Evans AJ, Fayaz I, Cusimano MD, et al: Combined pleomorphic xanthoastrocytoma-ganglioglioma of the cerebellum. Arch Pathol Lab Med 124:1707–1709, 2000.
7. Gaskill SJ, Marlin AE, Saldivar V: Glioblastoma multiforme masquerading as a pleomorphic xanthoastrocytoma. Childs Nerv Syst 4:237–240, 1988.
8. Giannini C, Scheithauer BW, Burger PC, et al: Pleomorphic xanthoastrocytoma: what do we really know about it? Cancer 85:2033–2045, 1999.
9. Giannini C, Scheithauer BW, Lopes MB, et al: Immunophenotype of pleomorphic xanthoastrocytoma. Am J Surg Pathol 26:479–485, 2002.
10. Glasser RS, Rojiani AM, Mickle JP, et al: Delayed occurrence of cerebellar pleomorphic xanthoastrocytoma after supratentorial pleomorphic xanthoastrocytoma removal. Case report. J Neurosurg 82:116–118, 1995.
11. Grant JW, Gallagher PJ: Pleomorphic xanthoastrocytoma. Immunohistochemical methods for differentiation from fibrous histiocytomas with similar morphology. Am J Surg Pathol 10:336–341, 1986.
12. Herpers MJ, Freling G, Beuls EA: Pleomorphic xanthoastrocytoma in the spinal cord. Case report. J Neurosurg 80:564–569, 1994.
13. Heyerdahl Strom E, Skullerud K: Pleomorphic xanthoastrocytoma: report of 5 cases. Clin Neuropathol 2:188–191, 1983.
14. Iwaki T, Fukui M, Kondo A, et al: Epithelial properties of pleomorphic xanthoastrocytomas determined in ultrastructural and immunohistochemical studies. Acta Neuropathol 74:142–150, 1987.
15. Kawano N: Pleomorphic xanthoastrocytoma: some new observations. Clin Neuropathol 11:323–328, 1992.
16. Kepes JJ: Pleomorphic xanthoastrocytoma: the birth of a diagnosis and a concept. Brain Pathol 3:269–274, 1993.
17. Kepes JJ, Rubinstein LJ, Ansbacher L, et al: Histopathological features of recurrent pleomorphic xanthoastrocytomas: further corroboration of the glial nature of this neoplasm. A study of 3 cases. Acta Neuropathol 78:585–593, 1989.
18. Kepes JJ, Rubinstein LJ, Eng LF: Pleomorphic xanthoastrocytoma: a distinctive meningocerebral glioma of young subjects with relatively favorable prognosis. A study of 12 cases. Cancer 44:1839–1852, 1979.
19. Kleihues P, Burger PC, Scheithauer BW: The new WHO classification of brain tumours. Brain Pathol 3:255–268, 1993.
20. Kordek R, Biernat W, Sapieja W, et al: Pleomorphic xanthoastrocytoma with a gangliomatous component: an immunohistochemical and ultrastructural study. Acta Neuropathol 89:194–197, 1995.
21. Lim SC, Jang SJ, Kim YS: Cerebellar pleomorphic xanthoastrocytoma in an infant. Pathol Int 49:811–815, 1999.
22. Lindboe CF, Cappelen J, Kepes JJ: Pleomorphic xanthoastrocytoma as a component of a cerebellar ganglioglioma: case report. Neurosurgery 31:353–355, 1992.
23. Lipper MH, Eberhard DA, Phillips CD, et al: Pleomorphic xanthoastrocytoma, a distinctive astroglial tumor: neuroradiologic and pathologic features. AJNR Am J Neuroradiol 14:1397–1404, 1993.
24. Macaulay RJ, Jay V, Hoffman HJ, et al: Increased mitotic activity as a negative prognostic indicator in pleomorphic xanthoastrocytoma. Case report. J Neurosurg 79:761–768, 1993.
25. Mascalchi M, Muscas GC, Galli C, et al: MRI of pleomorphic xanthoastrocytoma: case report. Neuroradiology 36:446–447, 1994.
26. Nitta J, Tada T, Kyoshima K, et al: Atypical pleomorphic astrocytoma in the pineal gland: case report. Neurosurgery 49:1458–1461, 2001.
27. Osborn AG: Diagnostic neuroradiology. St. Louis, Mosby, 1994.
28. Pahapill PA, Ramsay DA, Del Maestro RF: Pleomorphic xanthoastrocytoma: case report and analysis of the literature concerning the efficacy of resection and the significance of necrosis. Neurosurgery 38:822–828; discussion 828–829, 1996.
29. Perry A, Giannini C, Scheithauer BW, et al: Composite pleomorphic xanthoastrocytoma and ganglioglioma: report of four cases and review of the literature. Am J Surg Pathol 21:763–771, 1997.
30. Perry A, Scheithauer BW, Szczesniak DM, et al: Combined oligodendroglioma/pleomorphic xanthoastrocytoma: a probable collision tumor—case report. Neurosurgery 48:1358–1361, 2001.
31. Rippe DJ, Boyko OB, Radi M, et al: MRI of temporal lobe pleomorphic xanthoastrocytoma. J Comput Assist Tomogr 16:856–859, 1992.
32. Rosemberg S, Rotta JM, Yassuda A, et al: Pleomorphic xanthoastrocytoma of the cerebellum. Clin Neuropathol 19:238–242, 2000.
33. Thomas C, Golden B: Pleomorphic xanthoastrocytoma: report of two cases and brief review of the literature. Clin Neuropathol 12:97–101, 1993.
34. Tien RD, Cardenas CA, Rajagopalan S: Pleomorphic xanthoastrocytoma of the brain: MR findings in six patients. AJR Am J Roentgenol 159:1287–1290, 1992.
35. Tonn JC, Paulus W, Warmuth-Metz M, et al: Pleomorphic xanthoastrocytoma: report of six cases with special consideration of diagnostic and therapeutic pitfalls. Surg Neurol 47:162–169, 1997.
36. van Roost D, Kristof R, Zentner J, et al: Clinical, radiological, and therapeutic features of pleomorphic xanthoastrocytoma: report of three patients and review of the literature. J Neurol Neurosurg Psychiatry 60:690–692, 1996.
37. Wasdahl DA, Scheithauer BW, Andrews BT, et al: Cerebellar pleomorphic xanthoastrocytoma: case report. Neurosurgery 35:947–950; discussion 950–941, 1994.
38. Weldon-Linne CM, Victor TA, Groothuis DR, et al: Pleomorphic xanthoastrocytoma. Ultrastructural and immunohistochemical study of a case with a rapidly fatal outcome following surgery. Cancer 52:2055–2063, 1983.
39. Whittle IR, Gordon A, Misra BK, et al: Pleomorphic xanthoastrocytoma. Report of four cases. J Neurosurg 70:463–468, 1989.
40. Yoshino MT, Lucio R: Pleomorphic xanthoastrocytoma. AJNR Am J Neuroradiol 13:1330–1332, 1992.
41. Zarate JO, Sampaolesi R: Pleomorphic xanthoastrocytoma of the retina. Am J Surg Pathol 23:79–81, 1999.

CHAPTER 87

HYPOTHALAMIC HAMARTOMAS

A. Leland Albright

DEFINITION AND LOCATION

Hamartomas are non-neoplastic congenital malformations that are composed of disordered neurons, glial cells, and myelinated tracts. They are not neoplasms. Hamartomas occurring in the region of the hypothalamus are designated as *hypothalamic hamartomas* (HHs), although their anatomic connection to the hypothalamus itself may be minimal. HHs range in size from 0.5 to 5 cm. They occur in two general locations, below the tuber cinereum and within the third ventricle. Those below the tuber cinereum are usually pedunculated; those within the third ventricle are sessile.

DIAGNOSIS

HHs present in one of two ways, either with precocious puberty (PP) or with seizures. There is a general correlation between the morphology of HHs and the clinical symptoms they induce: pedunculated lesions are more likely to be small (<2.0 cm), to lie below the tuber cinereum, and to cause PP but no other neurologic symptom. Sessile lesions are more often larger (2 to 5 cm) and associated with seizures, particularly gelastic seizures. Approximately two thirds of children with sessile HH have developmental delays, and half also have PP.

Precocious Puberty

PP is defined as the onset of pubertal changes earlier than normal, before 8 years of age in girls and 9.5 years in boys. PP usually occurs within the first 2 years of life. It may cause persistently dark areolae as a sign of estrogen excess. Infants with PP have secondary sexual characteristics, boys may have unusual muscularity, and both girls and boys may have personalities that are reminiscent of adolescent personalities, although normal young children may exhibit some of the same moodiness and irritability. Bone age and height are greater than normal. The diagnosis of PP can be confirmed by a peak serum luteinizing hormone level of more than 10 international units per liter after the administration of gonadotropin-hormone releasing hormone. Only sex hormones are likely to be affected by HHs; levels of growth hormone, thyroxine, cortisol, prolactin, and vasopressin are rarely abnormal.[5] HHs may induce PP either by secreting luteinizing hormone–releasing hormone or by producing transforming growth factor alpha.

PP induced by HH is almost never associated with mental retardation.

Seizures

The most common seizures associated with HHs are gelastic seizures, *laughing seizures*, characterized by facial expressions of laughing but without its emotional accompaniment. Such seizures typically begin early in life, often within the first 2 years. Children may have only gelastic seizures or have them associated with other seizure types, including generalized tonic-clonic seizures, partial complex seizures, or drop attacks. The frequency of seizures ranges from occasional to intractable and is typically the latter. Children with gelastic seizures often have associated cognitive deficits and affective or emotional abnormalities, including oppositional defiant disorders and attention-deficit or hyperactivity disorders.[6,14] As might be expected, cognitive scores correlate with the frequency of seizures.

Gelastic seizures appear to originate from the hamartoma itself. Depth electroencephalogram (EEG) recordings within HHs have demonstrated focal seizure origin from the hamartoma, and electrical stimulation has reproduced typical gelastic seizures.[7] Spectroscopy in patients with gelastic seizures and HH demonstrates no abnormalities of *N*-acetyl aspartate (NAA)-to-creatine ratios in the temporal lobes but decreased NAA/creatine levels within the hamartomas. In addition, although surface EEG recordings may indicate a temporal lobe focus, temporal lobectomies in such patients may improve seizures briefly, rarely providing long-term seizure control.

HHs are occasionally part of the Pallister-Hall syndrome, which consists of the constellation of HH, bifid epiglottis, and central or postaxial polydactyly. The syndrome may be familial (autosomal dominant) or sporadic. Children with Pallister-Hall syndrome may have growth hormone deficiency.

EPIDEMIOLOGY

The incidence and prevalence of HHs are not known. They are rare lesions and have been diagnosed far more commonly since the availability of computed tomography (CT) and magnetic resonance (MR) scans. Before 1980, approximately 37 cases of HH causing PP had been reported; since then, at least twice that number have been reported.

NEUROIMAGING

On CT scans, HHs are isodense, nonenhancing masses (Figure 87-1). Because of their similarity to normal brain tissue, not all HHs are detected on CT scans.

On MR scans (Figure 87-2), HHs are isointense to gray matter on T1-weighted (short TR) images. On T2-weighted (long TR) images, they are hyperintense. They are not enhanced after gadolinium administration. Sagittal and coronal MR images help clarify the relationship of the hamartoma to surrounding structures, including the hypothalamus and the basilar artery. Pedunculated hamartomas lie below the tuber cinereum (and could be regarded as hamartomas of that structure rather than of the hypothalamus.) Pedunculated HHs range from 5 to 20 mm in diameter. Sessile HHs range from 15 to 65 mm and may be located inferiorly below the tuber cinereum or centrally within the third ventricle, distorting it.[2] HHs within the third ventricle and hypothalamus are larger than those located below the tuber cinereum.

The MR appearance of HH is consistent and rarely changes during follow-up, although change in signal characteristics has been reported. Giant HHs are rarely cystic.

Single-photon emission computed tomography (SPECT) scans have demonstrated hyperperfusion in the region of HH.[12]

TUMOR HISTOLOGY

HHs that cause PP act as neurosecretory organs. Some neurons within HHs contain gonadotropin-releasing hormone (GnRH) granules, which cross axons and enter the hypophyseal-portal circulation.[10] Those neurons appear to be outside of normal neurophysiologic control and act as the pulsatile episodic secretory units necessary for the initiation and maintenance of puberty.

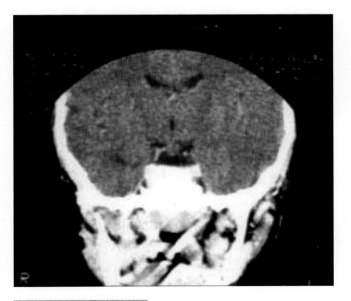

FIGURE 87-1 Coronal enhanced computed tomography scan demonstrating a hypothalamic hamartoma below the tuber cinereum.

THERAPY

PP needs to be treated, primarily because if it is not, the child's epiphyses fuse abnormally early, resulting in an unusually short adult height. In addition, the children are abnormally large during early childhood and may be ridiculed for either their size or sexual characteristics. Their parents are subjected to the emotional characteristics of adolescents until the PP is treated.

MEDICAL TREATMENT

Precocious Puberty

In the United States, HHs that cause PP are usually treated with long-acting GnRH analogues (e.g., Lupron). Because the initiation and continuation of puberty depends on the pulsatile release of GnRH, persistently high levels of exogenous GnRH analogues result in persistently high GnRH levels so that gonadotropin secretion is inhibited and puberty ceases. In most cases, such therapy stops the puberty, secondary sexual characteristics regress, and growth resumes at a normal rate.

Long-acting GnRH analogues are given in monthly injections until the time for normal puberty. After they are discontinued, puberty appears to occur normally. Long-term GnRH treatment is not known to cause adverse effects. Rarely, GnRH therapy is complicated by severe local reactions and failure of hormonal suppression. In such cases, surgical resection should be considered.

For children in countries where (expensive) GnRH is not available, resection of pedunculated HH is indicated.

Epilepsy

The seizures associated with HHs are notoriously difficult to control with medication. Few children become seizure free. The most commonly used medications have included dilantin, carbamazepine, valproate, vigabatrin, and lamotrigine. In children with PP and gelastic seizures, treatment of the PP with long-acting GnRH has occasionally been associated with cessation of the seizures. If satisfactory seizure control cannot be achieved with medical therapy, surgical intervention is appropriate to minimize or prevent the cognitive and behavioral sequelae associated with intractable gelastic seizures.

SURGERY

For Precocious Puberty

The surgical treatment of HH causing PP has improved in the past 12 years. In 1990, a review of 33 such cases treated by operations reported that 27 had subtotal resections, with clinical and hormonal success in only one case. Of the six who had total resections of HH, three were cured.[13] Since then, we and others have reported a high success rate in treating PP by complete resection of pedunculated HH.[1,3] The success of surgery for sessile HH would be expected to be less because of an impossibility of determining if all GnRH secreting neurons have been excised.

Pedunculated HH may be approached via a pterional or subtemporal approach.[1] It is important that whatever approach

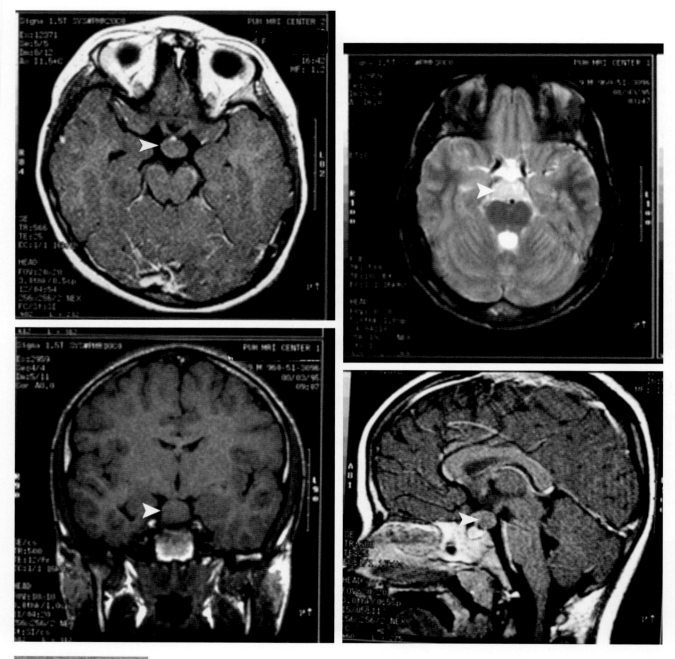

FIGURE 87-2   Magnetic resonance scans of hypothalamic hamartomas *(arrows)*. *Top left,* Axial T1 image. *Top right,* Axial T1 image. *Bottom left,* Coronal T1 image. *Bottom right,* Sagittal T2 image.

is used provide exposure of the oculomotor nerves on both sides of the hamartoma and of the posterior communicating and basilar arteries. Adhesions between the HH and basilar artery are not unusual.

For Epilepsy

The surgical treatment of epilepsy associated with HH has changed over the past 2 decades. Initial attempts to treat the epilepsy with either temporal lobectomies, corpus callosotomies, or corticectomies were relatively ineffective.[9] Cascino

et al performed video-EEG monitoring on seven patients with HH and gelastic seizures and identified cortical areas that were suspected of causing the seizures, but corticectomies of those sites did not alleviate the seizures.[4]

Sessile hamartomas within the third ventricle can be approached through a transcallosal-transforniceal route, with or without frameless stereotactic guidance.[12] HHs have a whitish, slightly gray appearance and bulge into the third ventricle from either wall of the hypothalamus or from its floor. Resection of the lesions is similar to resection of third ventricular astrocytomas: removal of the central core of the mass initially, then removal of tissue outward toward the periphery. As with many astrocytomas within the third ventricle, there is no evident plane between the hamartoma and the adjacent hypothalamus. Frameless stereotaxy wands are of some help in localization during this part of the procedure. Complete, or nearly complete, resections are needed to significantly reduce seizure frequency; several authors have correlated extent of resection with postoperative seizure control.

The largest surgical series of HH resections to treat seizures is that of Palmini, who treated 13 patients.[9] Postoperatively, two patients were completely seizure free, and the remaining 11 had a 90% or more reduction in their frequency of drop attacks and generalized tonic-clonic seizures, although minor seizures persisted in all 11. Palmini et al also observed dramatic improvements in behavior and cognition. Rosenfeld et al reported five patients treated by transcallosal resections; postoperatively all five had cessation of their preoperative seizures and none had postoperative neurologic deficits.[12]

RADIATION THERAPY

There is no published literature describing the use of radiation therapy to treat PP associated with HH.

Although there is no role for conventional fractionated irradiation in the treatment of HH-induced seizures, stereotactic radiosurgery (SR), particularly with the Gamma Knife®, appears to have some effectiveness. Regis et al treated 10 patients with HH and epilepsy with SR and found a clear correlation between dose and seizure control.[11] All patients with cured or improved seizures were treated with marginal doses of 17 Gy or higher. The use of radiosurgery in the pediatric population is constrained somewhat by the desire to avoid irradiation of children younger than 4 years in the Gamma Knife. Unfortunately, many children needing treatment fall into this age group.

EXPERIMENTAL THERAPY

Medically refractory seizures have been treated with stimulation of the left vagal nerve.[8] Murphy et al treated six patients with refractory seizures, four of whom had severe autistic behaviors. Three of the patients had marked improvements in seizure control, and the four with autistic behavior had marked behavioral improvement.

HHs have been also treated by radiofrequency thermocoagulation, although treatment of the entire HH is difficult with that technique.

RECURRENCE

If HHs are resected, they do not recur. Postoperative residual HHs do not increase in size, whether below the hypothalamus or intrahypothalamic, but may cause persistent symptoms of the type that were present preoperatively.

OUTCOME AND QUALITY OF LIFE ASSESSMENTS

Resection of pedunculated HHs results in cure of PP in most cases, perhaps 80%. Other hormones are not altered by the resection. All of the five children I have operated on to remove pedunculated HH causing PP have had cessation of their PP. They have been followed from 9.5 to 19.5 years, and all have subsequently gone through puberty at a normal age.

Until the mid-1980s, the surgical resection of HH to treat seizures was not only ineffective but was associated with considerable morbidity, including diabetes insipidus, hypopituitarism, cranial nerve palsies, and stroke. Since then, improved microsurgical techniques have been associated with significantly lower morbidity.[9,12]

References

1. Albright AL, Lee PA: Neurosurgical treatment of hypothalamic hamartomas causing precocious puberty. J Neurosurg 78:77–82, 1993.
2. Arita K, Ikawa F, Kurisu K, et al: The relationship between magnetic resonance imaging findings and clinical manifestations of hypothalamic hamartoma. J Neurosurg 91:212–220, 1999.
3. Boyko OB, Curnes JY, Oakes WJ, Burger PC: Hamartomas of the tuber cinereum: CT, MR, and pathologic findings. AJNR 12:309–314, 1991.
4. Cascino GD, Andermann, F, Berkovic SF, et al: Gelastic seizures and hypothalamic hamartomas: evaluation of patients undergoing chronic intracranial EEG monitoring and outcome of surgical treatment. Neurology 43:747–750, 1993.
5. Debeneix C, Bourgeois M, Trivin C, et al: Hypothalamic hamartomas: comparison of clinical presentation and magnetic resonance images. Horm Res 56:12–8, 2001.
6. Frattali CM, Liow K, Craig GH, et al: Cognitive deficits in children with gelastic seizures and hypothalamic hamartoma. Neurology 57:43–46, 2001.
7. Kusniecky R, Guthrie B, Mountz J, et al: Intrinsic epileptogenesis of hypothalamic hamartomas in gelastic epilepsy. Ann Neurol 43:273–275, 1998.
8. Murphy JV, Wheless JW, Schmoll CM: Left vagal nerve stimulation in six patients with hypothalamic hamartomas. Ped Neurol 23:167–168, 2000.
9. Palmini A, Chandler C, Andermann F, et al: Resection of the lesion in patients with hypothalamic hamartomas and catastrophic epilepsy. Neurology 58:1338–1347, 2002.
10. Price RA, Lee PA, Albright AL, et al: Treatment of sexual precocity by removal of a luteinizing hormone-releasing hormone secreting hamartoma. JAMA 251:2247–2249, 1984.
11. Regis J, Bartolomei F, deToffol B: Gamma knife surgery for epilepsy related to hypothalamic hamartomas. Neurosurgery 47:1343–1351, 2000.
12. Rosenfeld JV, Harvey AS, Wrennall J, et al: Transcallosal resection of hypothalamic hamartomas, with control of seizures, in children with gelastic epilepsy. Neurosurgery 48:108–118, 2001.
13. Starceski PJ, Lee PA, Albright AL, Migeon CJ: Hypothalamic hamartomas and sexual precocity. AJDC 144:225–228, 1990.
14. Weissenberger AA, Dell ML, Liow K, et al: Aggression and psychiatric comorbidity in children with hypothalamic hamartomas and their unaffected siblings. J Am Acad Child Adol Psych 40:696–703, 2001.

CHAPTER **88**

EPENDYMOMA

Thomas E. Merchant and Robert A. Sanford

Ependymoma is a rare tumor that primarily affects young children. Improvements in the treatment of ependymoma have been achieved through technical advances in surgery and radiation therapy and changes in clinical practice that define the current state of the art. Surgery and highly focused radiation therapy are likely to lead to further advances in the treatment of ependymoma, and these modalities will be further refined by risk classification based on tumor biology and advanced neuroimaging techniques. Advances in the treatment of ependymoma may be hampered by its rarity and the ability of patients to receive expert evaluation and treatment.

The standard of care for ependymoma is surgical resection and postoperative radiation therapy directed at the site of the primary tumor. Postoperative radiation therapy has not been accepted as a standard for children younger than age 3 because of the fear of side effects and despite evidence that delaying or avoiding irradiation with multiagent chemotherapy results in poor outcomes. Most practitioners now agree that at the present time chemotherapy has little role in the treatment of ependymoma.

Ependymoma accounts for approximately 10% of all childhood central nervous system (CNS) tumors, with fewer than 170 new cases diagnosed annually in the United States in children and adults younger than 25 years.[36] The mean age at the time of diagnosis ranges from 4 to 6 years,[8,13,32,46] and 25% to 40% of those diagnosed are younger than age 3.[5] The historical 5-year survival estimate is 50% to 64%, and the historical progression-free survival estimate is 23% to 45%.[8,13,34,37,38] Recurrences are typically local, and the median time to recurrence is 13 to 25 months.[8,13,27,32,34,37] Approximately 20% of failures involve distant recurrence, and late recurrences are possible. Fortunately, neuraxis dissemination at the time of diagnosis is rare and occurs in less than 5% of patients.[32]

Ependymoma develops from the neuroepithelial lining of the ventricles of the brain and the central canal of the spinal cord; 90% of tumors are located intracranially, with 30% occurring above the tentorium and 60% located in the infratentorial space.[36] Supratentorial ependymoma may arise from the lateral or third ventricle (60%) or from the cerebral hemisphere without ventricular connection (40%).[26,36] Infratentorial ependymoma arises from one of three specific sites within the fourth ventricle: the floor (60%), the lateral aspect (30%), or the roof (10%).[15,40] Tumors that arise from the floor of the fourth ventricle may extend through the foramen of Magendie and over the dorsal surface of the spinal cord. Those that arise from the lateral aspect of the fourth ventricle can extend out of the foramen of Luschka and into the cerebellopontine (CP) angle

and along the anterior aspect of the pons and medulla. Ependymoma may also arise primarily in the CP angle. Gross-total resection of posterior fossa ependymoma arising from the floor or lateral aspect of the fourth ventricle and CP angle can be difficult.

PROGNOSTIC FACTORS

Numerous studies have sought to identify prognostic factors for intracranial ependymoma; most have been single-institution, retrospective reports that span several decades and consequently include numerous changes in neuroimaging, neurosurgery, radiation oncology, chemotherapy, and supportive measures. Surgical resection appears to be the most important prognostic factor and will be exploited in the next series of protocols. Determining the significance of clinical and treatment factors requires prospective stratification and a sufficient number of patients and events to observe statistically meaningful differences.

The prognostic factors for ependymoma have been influenced by treatment era and include extent of disease at diagnosis, extent of resection, tumor location and grade, patient age, and the use of chemotherapy. There is no formally recognized staging system for ependymoma. Because of the risk of neuraxis dissemination, patients are classified as having localized or disseminated disease based on evaluations that include magnetic resonance imaging (MRI) of the brain and spine and lumbar cerebrospinal fluid (CSF) cytology. Long-term survival is rarely achieved for patients who have neuraxis dissemination, making knowledge of the extent of disease at diagnosis crucial to determining initial treatment options.

Extent of Resection

There is general agreement that extent of resection is the major determinant of outcome regardless of adjuvant therapy. Observation should not be considered an option for a patient with residual tumor after surgery, because patients who undergo subtotal resection have shorter event-free survival compared with those who undergo gross-total resection in all series despite adjuvant radiation therapy, chemotherapy, or the combination of the two.[8,12,13,26,27,32,34,37,38,46] The 5-year survival is 67% to 80% for patients with completely resected tumors, with a 5-year progression-free survival of 51% to 75%. Patients with incompletely resected tumors have a 5-year survival of 22% to 47% and a 5-year progression-free survival of 0% to 26%.

Extent of resection has been treated as a categoric variable (gross-total resection, near-total resection, subtotal resection) when it actually represents a continuous variable ranging from the most extensive resection with no residual disease present versus debulking procedures to establish a diagnosis and relieve symptoms. Gross-total resection for ependymoma has been defined as surgical removal of all grossly visible tumor at the time of surgery with or without evidence of microscopic residual tumor using the operating microscope. Gross-total resection must be confirmed by neuroimaging that shows no evidence of imaging abnormality that might be interpreted as tumor, within 72 hours postoperatively, before the development of postsurgical changes. Subtotal resection has been defined as gross residual tumor remaining after surgery that is visible to the neurosurgeon and by neuroimaging. Near-total resection has been defined[37] as a category with somewhat arbitrary values of 1.5 cm^2, similar to the medulloblastoma definitions, and 0.5 cm residual thickness of tumor bed enhancement.[22] Subtotal resection represented bulky residual tumor, and near-total resection was often characterized as a significant resection based on an estimate of the fraction of the resected tumor (i.e., 90% to 95%). Currently, subtotal resections resemble the near-total resections of the past, and patients undergoing near-total resection cannot be distinguished statistically from those who have undergone gross-total resection. This latter observation is important for the surgeon to understand, because patients with minimal residual tumor can be cured with irradiation. These facts should make the surgeon careful not to perform extensive resections that would lead to neurologic injury but not increase the probability of cure. It has been shown that for the degree of surgical resection, assessment by postoperative imaging is more important than the neurosurgeon's perspective on whether a gross-total or subtotal resection has been performed.[6,45]

Histologic Grade of the Tumor

Tumor grade is a controversial prognostic factor. Although numerous reports have suggested that patients with differentiated ependymoma achieve a better outcome than do those with anaplastic ependymoma,[18,20,24-26,31-33,43,47] some investigators believe that histologic grade has no prognostic significance.[37,38] One problem concerning tumor grade is the lack of agreement among individual pathologists. In a study from the Children's Cancer Group, 22 (69%) of 32 cases had a discrepancy in the diagnosis on central review.[37]

We recently reported histologic characterization of tumors and outcome in a contemporary series of 50 patients[24] where tumor grade was significantly related to progression-free survival after irradiation ($P < .001$). The 2-year event-free survival estimate ($\pm$ standard error) was 32% $\pm$ 14% for patients with anaplastic ependymoma and 84% $\pm$ 7% for patients with differentiated ependymoma. Statistical significance was maintained when the analysis was adjusted for age (<3 years), chemotherapy, and extent of resection. This study also demonstrated that anaplastic ependymoma was more likely to occur in the supratentorial brain ($P = .002$). The progression-free survival estimate after irradiation for patients with anaplastic ependymoma has been identified in a number of contemporary series.[23,47]

Histologic evaluation plays an important role in the design and interpretation of prospective trials and in determining the significance of prognostic factors in the current treatment era.

Cooperative multi-institutional protocols will enable us to determine the significance of the various factors that will be used to estimate prognosis and stratify individual treatments. The Children's Oncology Group Study (ACNS 0121) opened in 2003 used tumor grade to stratify treatment.

Age at Diagnosis

Age at the time of diagnosis has been described as an important prognostic factor. Children younger than 3 years old have a worse prognosis than older children, possibly because of more aggressive tumor biology, reluctance to give postoperative radiation therapy, or use of lower doses of radiation therapy.[13,34,39] For children younger than 3 years old at diagnosis, Pollack et al[34] reported a 5-year survival of 22% and a progression-free survival estimate of 12%. In older children, the 5-year survival estimate was 75%, and the progression-free survival was 60%. The first infant study by the Pediatric Oncology Group (POG) attempting to delay irradiation showed significant differences in outcome based on age.[4] This study also showed a 63% 5-year survival for young children (aged 24 to 35 months) in whom radiation therapy was delayed for 1 year, but a 26% 5-year survival for infants and very young children (aged 0 to 23 months) in whom radiation therapy was delayed for 2 years. The findings suggest that the poor survival estimates commonly reported for very young children are most likely related to the delay in the administration of radiation therapy, although infratentorial location and extent of resection were important cofactors. Increased survival was demonstrated in those who receive radiation therapy over those who did not.[25,44] One study suggested that the improvement in outcome may be radiation dose dependent (i.e., higher doses may improve outcome[23]), though no randomized trials have unequivocally demonstrated that improved outcome is caused solely by radiation therapy.

PATHOLOGY, BIOLOGY, AND MOLECULAR CHARACTERIZATION

Ependymoma is considered to be a tumor of glial progenitor cell origin, and according to most pathologists, confirming the diagnosis is not as difficult as it is for many of the other CNS tumors. However, the histologic grading of ependymoma is not entirely clear and has been difficult to reproduce. Evaluation in most centers consists of staining with hematoxylin and eosin for light microscopic evaluation with immunohistochemical staining and performance according to institutional preference. Electron microscopy is seldom used.

Differentiated ependymoma has been described as the classic lesion in which perivascular pseudorosettes are a requisite feature. Less cellular, more fibrillar regions are often present, and necrosis may be present. Unless very focal and unaccompanied by regions of high cellularity and mitotic activity, vascular endothelial proliferation should not be seen in a tumor classified as differentiated ependymoma. According to the World Health Organization (WHO) 2000 criteria,[16] the classification of grade II is made only when mitoses are rare or absent, occasional nonpalisading foci of necrosis are allowed, and nodules with greater cellularity and mitotic activity are permitted.

Anaplastic ependymoma includes tumors with clearly defined ependymal differentiation demonstrating perivascular pseudorosettes and increased cellularity, cytological atypia, and microvascular proliferation. The hypercellularity may be diffuse or focal and form well-circumscribed regions abutting those of lower cellularity. Cytologic atypia includes increased nuclear-to-cytoplasmic ratios and coarse chromatin. Vascular proliferation, usually of the glomeruloid variety, may be found within or adjacent to hypercellular regions. The cellular anaplastic regions are often more mitotically active, although no threshold for mitotic activity has been established. WHO 2000 criteria include increased cellularity, brisk mitotic activity associated with vascular proliferation, and pseudopalisading necrosis. The feature of necrosis is often required by some as an important feature of anaplasia and is largely based on WHO criteria and the grading of astrocytoma, which is why investigators use a combination of necrosis, endothelial proliferation, and mitotic index greater than 5 as negative predictive factors. Brisk mitotic activity and focal areas of atypia do not characterize a lesion as anaplastic.

Tumor grade occurs along a spectrum of cellular tissue with mitotically active areas more commonly seen in the highly cellular areas. Along the same lines, more subjective is the description of a tumor as focally anaplastic, which leads one to consider the effects of sampling and furthers the need for objective molecular characterization.

Histologic variants of ependymoma, including clear cell, myxoid, and papillary ependymoma to name a few, are most often seen in the supratentorial brain. The major concern with these subtypes is misclassification, because the treatment is otherwise the same among the possible variants.

Objective prognostic indicator systems have been described in the literature using the expression of proliferating cell nuclear antigens (PCNAs) and Ki-67 immunolabeling. One PCNA study on cell proliferation showed a significant statistical correlation between intensely positive nuclei and survival rates.[42] Ki-67 immunolabeling elucidates immunohistochemical cell proliferation characteristics, which often determine the degree of tumor aggression. The Ki-67 immunolabeling index was developed from a study of 74 pediatric ependymomas and has been shown to be a strong prognostic indicator.[1] Ki-67 appears to be more objective than the staining subjectivity that could occur in the PCNA method. Proliferation may also be confirmed with vimentin and CD31 in addition to Ki-67.

A number of studies have used molecular genetics and cytogenetics to examine ependymoma with the goal of characterizing these tumors for staging or therapeutic purposes. A number of karyotypic abnormalities have been documented, but definitive chromosomal defects have not been isolated.[2,17,21,28,35,49] Chromosomes 17 and 22 have been at the center of conflicting reports in the literature. A deletion in 17p was found in a significant number of specimens in one study, whereas losses in 22q were rare.[35] At approximately the same time, another study performed using fluorescence in situ hybridization (FISH) and polymerase chain reaction (PCR) disputed the role of 17p mutation as a primary event in ependymoma, suggesting that chromosome 22 loss may define instead a subset of adult ependymoma and that long-arm mutations may relate to the development or progression of pediatric ependymoma.[21]

A recent study showed that 75% of ependymoma cases coexpress ERB2 and ERBB4 receptors and that the co-expression of ERBB was associated with tumor proliferative activity—Ki-67 labeling index, extent of resection and poor outcome,[9] leading investigators to speculate that the ERBB receptor signaling is associated with aggressive tumor subtypes by promoting tumor cell proliferation.

Further studies evaluating specific assays for epidermal growth factor receptor (EGFR), ERBB, and global and focal assays for genomic abnormalities need to be conducted on large numbers of patients treated relatively homogeneously. Candidates include comparative genomic hybridization using PCR or array technology, loss of heterozygosity, DNA methylation, and other broad microarray technologies. Focal assays for Ki-67, ERBB, and other molecular assays should be given priority in treatment protocols.

NEUROIMAGING

MRI is central to the diagnosis and evaluation of ependymoma. MRI is critical to planning for surgery and radiation therapy and is the primary means for surveillance after treatment or monitoring the response to chemotherapy. Uncommonly, surgery is conducted with only a computed tomography (CT) study and without the benefit of MRI, especially when the tumor arises in the posterior fossa. Lack of preoperative MRI makes it difficult to accurately determine the extent of resection and to plan radiation therapy to the volume at risk.

In the evaluation of a patient with ependymoma, the standard of care is preoperative and postoperative MRI of the brain and the spine. Care should be taken to conduct the postsurgical examination within 72 hours of surgery, which minimizes postsurgical changes that can make it difficult to determine residual tumor and the extent of resection. The radiologist should be informed when hemostatic products have been placed in the tumor bed.

The determination of residual disease for ependymoma is based on abnormal anatomy. Ependymoma has a mixed pattern of enhancement and requires evaluation with all available imaging sequences, including enhanced and nonenhanced T1- and T2-weighted imaging, proton density, and fluid-attenuated inversion recovery (FLAIR) techniques capable of water suppression to define residual tumor.

The recommended frequency of imaging after treatment is based on knowledge that recurrence or progression most often occurs between 12 and 24 months after the initiation of radiation therapy and that early identification of recurrence may increase the likelihood of success in salvage maneuvers.

The identification of metastatic disease (neuraxis dissemination) can be problematic, because ependymoma and numerous conditions can mimic the appearance of metastatic disease, including bleeding, infection, and inflammatory changes caused by surgery and radiation therapy. Spinal imaging, if conducted postoperatively, should be deferred for approximately 7 to 10 days after the last invasive procedure, including resection, shunt placement, or revision and lumbar puncture. When the spine is examined, the MRI study should be performed of the entire spine, with contrast, and include at least two planes. If there is significant motion artifact or hemorrhage, the scan is not evaluable and must be repeated at a later time. Sedation or anesthesia is critical to the proper imaging evaluation of children with ependymoma.

In addition, tumor and operative-related changes in blood flow to meningeal vascularity can alter the appearance of vessels, mimicking disease in the sulci of the brain. Numerous case reports have been published identifying abnormalities on imaging mimicking the appearance of subarachnoid dissemination. Most cases of leptomeningeal disease have small nodular tumor or thick disease coating the subarachnoid space. Sugar coating in ependymoma rarely occurs, and the clinician should challenge this as a sign of metastatic disease, especially in a patient whose imaging study was preceded by an invasive procedure.

Complete responses of residual disease to radiation therapy and chemotherapy are uncommon, whereas partial responses are more common. After radiation therapy, tumor size may slowly diminish over a prolonged period of up to several years. Loss of contrast enhancement may occur as soon as 1 year after irradiation and is considered to be indicative of decreasing vascularity.

Recurrence during the first year after adequate radiation therapy is uncommon. Responses after chemotherapy also require time, generally on the order of 6 months as observed in the last baby POG study. Radiation is known to cause an increase in leukocyte-endothelial interactions, which may contribute to an increase in enhancement observed in some cases during the first few months after radiation therapy. Although this phenomenon is observed less commonly in ependymoma, it can be misinterpreted as progression and requires only careful observation.

Newer roles for neuroimaging in the evaluation of patients with ependymoma include the incorporation of MRI into radiation therapy treatment planning. At present, CT remains the basis for radiation dose calculations and must be used in the planning process to which MRI studies are registered using a variety of software tools to improve targeting and normal tissue structure definitions.

MR spectroscopy can be used as an adjunct to MRI in the evaluation of ependymoma, although limited data are available to demonstrate its usefulness.

Positron-emission tomography has yet to find a role in the evaluation of ependymoma.

SURGERY

Ependymoma is a relatively slow-growing tumor with a propensity for local invasion. Subarachnoid dissemination is rare and considered incurable. Because the predominant pattern of failure for ependymoma is local, aggressive measures of local control are essential. Several institutional retrospective reviews[8,13,26,27,32,34,38,46] and two prospective phase III trials[4,37] have shown that the extent of surgical resection is the most consistent prognostic factor for patients with ependymoma.

Sutton et al[46] retrospectively evaluated 45 patients with ependymoma and found that the 5-year survival estimate after total or near-total resection was 60%; the 5-year survival estimate after subtotal resection (defined as <90% tumor resection) was 21%. In a similar retrospective review of 40 patients, Pollack et al[34] found that 5-year survival after gross-total resection was 80%; after partial resection (i.e., less than gross-total resection), it was 22%.

Perilongo et al[32] retrospectively evaluated 92 children with ependymoma who participated in the Italian Pediatric Neuro-Oncology Group. For patients who had undergone gross-total resection, the 10-year survival estimate was 70%, and the progression-free survival estimate was 57%; for patients

who had undergone subtotal resection, the 10-year survival estimate was 32%, and the 10-year progression-free survival estimate was 11%. Finally, Robertson et al[37] prospectively treated 32 patients in the Children's Cancer Group (CCG) Protocol 921. They found that the 5-year progression-free survival was 66% for patients with residual tumor measuring 1.5 cm^2 and 11% for those with residual tumors measuring more than 1.5 cm^2, all of whom were treated with postoperative radiation.

Resection Alone

Successful treatment of newly diagnosed or recurrent intracranial ependymoma by resection alone has been reported by two independent groups.[14,30] Hukin et al[14] reported 10 pediatric cases in which gross-total resection was the only initial therapy for intracranial ependymoma (eight supratentorial tumors and two posterior fossa tumors). At a median follow-up of 48 months, seven patients were free of disease without further intervention, and three patients experienced tumor recurrence at 9, 10, and 20 months after resection. Two patients with recurrence were effectively treated with an additional surgical procedure and postoperative radiation therapy. Late failures have now occurred in two patients (personal communication).

Palma et al[30] reported on their success in treating supratentorial ependymoma with surgery alone. Of 12 surviving patients, 6 in their original series of 23 patients were treated with surgery alone, and only 1 experienced a recurrence after 10 years of follow-up. These findings indicate that some patients with intracranial ependymoma—probably those with low-grade supratentorial tumors—require resection only. Thus radiation therapy and its potential for late effects might be delayed until the time of recurrence for a very select group of patients such as those with low-grade supratentorial tumors, provided that no tumor is visible under the operating microscope or on postoperative MRI. This strategy will be permissible in the current COG ependymoma study, which included failure rate monitoring. It must be emphasized that this is currently not the standard of care.

Although complete resection is instrumental in the long-term, event-free, and overall survival of patients with childhood ependymoma, it is performed in only 42% to 62% of patients.[13,34,38,46] Complete resection is more easily accomplished for tumors in supratentorial locations and those originating from the roof of the fourth ventricle. Aggressive attempts to resect tumors in other locations, including those involving the lower cranial nerves, are associated with increased morbidity.

It is generally agreed that a complete resection—that is, one that results in a very low probability of leaving even microscopic residual tumor—is rarely achieved in ependymoma. Complete resection may be possible for patients with supratentorial tumors when a margin of normal tissue surrounding the tumor is also removed and test results of biopsy specimens of the operative cavity are negative. Biopsies of the operative cavity are seldom performed; however, such biopsies could be therapeutically beneficial and could contribute to the planning of radiation treatment.

Second Resection

Despite the high rate of incomplete initial resections, few studies have included a second surgical procedure for patients with residual disease.[7,41] The timing of a second resection is the subject of debate: some oncologists favor the use of chemotherapy between the initial and second resections.

The purpose of administering chemotherapy before a second resection is to make the tumor more amenable to resection and to prevent tumor progression during the interval between procedures. Foreman et al[7] reported second resections in five patients with residual tumors located in the fourth ventricle. One patient underwent an immediate second-look procedure, and the other four received short courses of chemotherapy before a second-look procedure. Gross-total resection was achieved with the second procedure in four of the five patients. No severe morbidity was reported after the second resection; three of the patients remained progression free at 23, 25, and 34 months after the second procedure and postoperative radiation therapy.

From April 1997 through April 2000, 40 pediatric patients were referred to St. Jude Children's Research Hospital for treatment of intracranial ependymoma[29]; 24 patients (60%) underwent complete resection, and 16 (40%) had residual tumor after their initial procedure and before referral. Of those 16, 12 were considered candidates for additional resection based on the location of the residual tumor and neurologic status at the time of evaluation.

A complete resection was performed in 10 patients and a near total resection in 2 patients with the second procedure. By combining the number of patients with a complete resection after their initial procedure with the number of those with complete resection after a second procedure, we increased the group's rate of complete resection to 85%.

The operative morbidity of these patients was also determined. Significant morbidity, defined as lower cranial neuropathy necessitating gastrostomy or tracheostomy, occurred in 4 of the 24 patients with initial complete resections and 4 of the 16 patients with initial incomplete resections. Significant morbidity occurred in only one patient who underwent a second resection. Of the 12 patients who underwent a second resection, 6 had tumors that progressed during the interval between surgical procedures, despite administration of chemotherapy. In a review of our overall series of personally operated-on cases, gross-total resection was accomplished in 77% and near-total in 11%.

Surgical Technique

The importance of gross-total surgical removal cannot be overstated. In our series, there is a threefold to fourfold survival advantage to gross-total versus a residual lump of tumor. In 45 of our cases we were able to achieve gross-total resection in 35 children (77%) and near-total (<1.5 mL) in 5 (11%). The largest residual in five cases was less than 2 mL.

To achieve these results, careful presurgical planning must be carried out. It is difficult to distinguish with any degree of certainty before the biopsy between ependymoma, medulloblastoma, and low-grade astrocytoma. However, increased density (hypercellularity) on CT and T1 images suggests a diagnosis of ependymoma. Interpretation of the extent of ependymoma is particularly treacherous on the MRI scan, because the tumor often has a portion that is enhanced by gadolinium and a portion that is not enhanced. Therefore it is important to compare closely the outline of the tumor on the T2 image with the T1 and then compare this with contrast

enhancement T1 images to determine the extent and the type of enhancement (patchy, diffuse, or dense). This information becomes critical in the postoperative period when evaluating the degree of surgical resection. The preoperative images need to be placed side by side with postoperative images. The postoperative images should be obtained within 24 to 48 hours to minimize the postsurgical artifact and give the best estimation of residual tumor. T2 images on the postoperative scans have now become quite inaccurate because of surgical artifact, as are the FLAIR sequences. When the preoperative images are compared side by side, residual tumor is usually apparent on the T1 images.

Ependymomas may be classified as supratentorial hemispheric, third ventricular, and posterior fossa. Surgical management of the supratentorial ependymoma is usually straightforward, because the tumor is always quite distinct from normal brain, making the margins clear. It is useful in supratentorial hemispheric tumor to attempt to determine the vascular supply. Occasionally an MR angiogram is useful. Arteriogram is never necessary. Frameless stereotaxy is useful to maximize the exposure and minimize the size of the craniotomy flap. The bone flap should be large enough that all the margins are visible at the time of surgery so that the surgeon does not work beneath a shelf of bone.

We use a fence-post technique with the frameless stereotaxic system for gliomas. It is not necessary for ependymomas, but often we do not know the diagnosis before the craniotomy. The fence posts must be inserted before mannitol and furosemide are given and before opening the dura. Using the frameless technique is simple; we use the stereotaxic system to plan our flap, the bone is removed, and before administering diuretic agents we make little linear incisions in the dura, divide the cortical surface, and under frameless guidance place multiple silastic catheters contouring the tumor margin. We do this with approximately four to six catheters, and following administration of osmotic diuretic agents we open the dura. In ependymoma, the fence-post technique is unnecessary because of its clear outline from the normal brain. It is a relief to get the diagnosis of ependymoma, because, compared with resecting a glioma from an eloquent area, all of these hemispheric lesions can be completely excised with minimal morbidity.

True intraventricular ependymomas are rare. Hemispheric ependymomas may compress or distort the ventricles but rarely are truly intraventricular.

Third ventricle ependymomas are rare as well. In this chapter we will not detail the various approaches to the third ventricle, but there are multiple approaches depending on whether the tumor is filling the anterior, middle, or posterior third ventricle.

Posterior fossa ependymoma may be subdivided by site of origin: cerebellar hemisphere, fourth ventricular (roof or floor), and CP angle.

In planning the surgical approach, again, the vascular supply is critical. Invariably, fourth ventricle ependymomas are supplied from the posterior-inferior cerebellar artery (PICA). Often, the feeding artery can be ascertained from the preoperative MRI scan. A MR angiogram may be useful in this respect.

The surgical procedure should be done with the patient prone with maximal tolerated flexion so that the floor of the fourth ventricle will be sloping away from the surgeon, enabling the surgeon to work parallel to the brainstem. If preoperative hydrocephalus exists, a tunnel ventriculostomy may be quite useful. We do not perform the ventriculostomy until all of the bone work is done and the posterior fossa dura is exposed. The nondominate lateral ventricle is cannulated and the catheter tunneled to be used in the postoperative period to monitor intracranial pressure and drain CSF as needed.

We favor a wide bony craniotomy with replacement of the bone at the end of the procedure. With large fourth ventricular tumors a C1 laminotomy should be done. The dura can then be opened at that level, being careful to allow very slow egress of fluid to stabilize the intracranial pressure if a ventricular drain has been placed; CSF is then alternatively released from the lateral ventricle and spine. Release of fluid too rapidly can result in blindness because of the hypoperfusion of the retina. The dura is opened in the standard fashion; cerebellar tonsils are separated, and the posterior and inferior cerebral arteries should be carefully traced until the feeding vessel is identified. The vascular supply invariably comes distally to the tonsillar loop. Once the branch to the tumor has been coagulated, this reduces the vascularity and thus intratumor bleeding to a great degree. This is especially important in small children and infants. Next, attention is turned to the superior portion of the tumor. I like to carefully maintain the margins circumferentially and debulk the superior portion of the tumor until the aqueduct is opened. At this point the posterior fossa will become quite decompressed. Attention is then turned to the inferior portion of the tumor, and it is debulked carefully. The floor of the fourth ventricle is slowly visualized. At this point, it is possible to tell whether the tumor is arising from the floor of the ventricle or the roof. If the tumor arises from the fourth ventricle, a portion of tumor is left on the floor. Hemostasis is obtained, and the entire tumor is painstakingly removed, alternating with debulking tumor and maintaining the plane between roof and the lateral cerebellar peduncle. Once the tumor has been completely removed except for the portion that is on the floor, I suggest attempting to carefully visualize the plane of the floor of the fourth ventricle. This can be done by viewing the floor of the fourth ventricle cephalad to the tumor and inferiorly. This allows mentally drawing a line below which the surgeon does not venture. We carefully bipolar the tumor within 1 to 2 mm of the floor. This can usually be done with minimal morbidity. It is treacherous, however, because if the small arterial feeders retract into the brainstem, obtaining hemostasis will often result in VI and VII cranial nerve palsies or involvement of the medial longitudinal fasciculus. If the procedure has been excessively long, significant blood loss has occurred, or the child has demonstrated repeated episodes of hypertension and bradycardia, once the fourth ventricle is debulked, it is sometimes better to return at a later date. Proceeding in an unstable child when the surgeon is fatigued is a recipe for a surgical disaster.

At the completion of tumor resection it is important that the cerebellar tonsils be completely dissected from the foramen magnum and adequate CSF is visualized in the spinal canal and around the brainstem. This gives the best chance of avoiding a permanent CSF diversionary procedure. It is also critical once the tumor is removed, to inspect the foramen of Luschka laterally, because a small tongue of tumor can be missed in this area, which necessitates a return to surgery.

Cerebellar hemisphere tumors are quite straightforward. They are well demarcated and should be easily gross totally excised. Also, it is important to not neglect the fact that the cerebellar tonsils must be completely decompressed at the end of the procedure. We use patch grafting of the dura in all cases

to maximize CSF circulation and check that the fourth ventricle is patent. Also, the bone is always replaced. I prefer titanium plates for holding bone securely away from the cerebellum, again, to maximize normal CSF flow. We have noted that if postoperative posterior fossa pressure monitoring is performed, the pressure is lower when the bone is supported with a generous space between the dura and the replaced bone.

CP angle ependymomas are one of the most challenging tumors faced in pediatric posterior fossa surgery. They take their origin from the lateral wall from the stem at the junction of the pons and the medulla, thus the name *CP angle*. Because they are so slow growing, they invariably envelop the cranial nerves V-X on the side of origin. When they grow, they rotate the brainstem so that the normal brainstem anatomy is distorted. They enter via the foramen of Lusaka, filling the fourth ventricle. In addition to having an arterial supply from the posterior inferior cerebellar artery, they may well have significant feeders from the anterior-inferior cerebellar artery. Because the tumors are large and principally infant, tumor blood loss at surgery becomes a significant consideration.

This is the one tumor whose diagnosis can be surmised from preoperative imaging. The surgeon should have adequate experience with this tumor before undertaking this surgical challenge.

The patient is placed prone, with the head rotated so that the lateral portion of the cerebellum is exposed. Rarely is a true skull-base approach necessary because an infant's skull is sufficiently horizontal that the tumor can be removed without removing much skull base. A curvilinear, rather than the traditional hockey stick, incision is used that extends to the midline, thereby minimizing the amount of paraspinous musculature to be displaced medially. The incision must take into account the fact that the tumor invariably goes down to the level of C1 or C2. Dissection of the muscle off the skull base must be done with care, because in this rotated position the vertebral artery is displaced upward and can be injured. Following removal of the bone, the bone is carefully removed over the descending sinus as close to the level of the jugular foramen as possible. The dura is opened; the intraspinal portion of the tumor can be removed with care taken to preserve the nerve roots. With removal of the spinal portion of the tumor, the vertebral and posterior-inferior cerebellar artery arteries are identified. At this point, if there is a large feeder to the tumor, it can be removed. A lateral debulking of the tumor proceeds until the ninth and tenth nerves are identified entering the jugular foramen. The seventh and eighth nerves are identified as they enter the foramen. Hearing is invariably lost even though the seventh and eighth nerves are anatomically preserved. Following identification of the nerves laterally, attention is given to the fourth ventricle; the entire tumor is removed from the fourth ventricle before attempting to remove any further portion of the tumor laterally. After the tumor has been removed from the fourth ventricle, the cerebellum can be elevated, the foramen of Lusaka can be identified, and the tumor removed here. Once the posterior fossa has been relaxed from this portion, the difficult part of the operation is gently teasing the tumor away from the ninth and tenth nerves. Once the nerves are followed medially to the level of brainstem, the tumor can be removed from the vertebral artery. Often the vertebral artery and basilar artery have been displaced away from the brainstem by up to 1 cm. Perforating vessels arise from the basilar artery and must be carefully preserved, or a brainstem infarct will result. This is a laborious and time-consuming procedure but can be accomplished with a high degree of success, greater than 90% in our series.

The major morbidity is cranial nerve dysfunction, which is transient 90% of the time. In the postoperative period the child remains intubated until adequately awake, and then the tube is removed and an otolaryngologist inspects the vocal cords. If vocal cords are completely paralyzed and the child is not handling secretions, a tracheostomy is necessary. If there is partial movement and the child is able to handle secretions, the child may be extubated. Within 48 hours of extubation swallowing tests are performed. Even though it is not unusual to avoid a tracheostomy, temporary gastrostomy is often required for feeding. Sixth, seventh, and eighth nerve palsies are also common; however, again, most of the time, the cranial nerves will recover within 3 to 6 months.

The most important consideration surgically is balancing the risk of permanent neurologic deficit with improved survival with gross or near-total resection. This is a tumor in which the surgeon should warn the family of the necessity of repeat surgery if tumor is present on the postoperative imaging.

RADIATION THERAPY

The avoidance of radiation therapy has been the hallmark of clinical trial designs for the treatment of ependymoma in young children. Strategies that delay or prevent irradiation have been justified on the basis of concerns about the effects of irradiation on neurologic, endocrine, and cognitive function. Although irradiation-induced deficits have not been well documented in cases of childhood ependymoma, this therapy has, in the past, paralleled that used for other more common childhood tumors such as medulloblastoma, for which the effects have been well documented. Since 1977, postoperative radiation therapy has been considered standard treatment for patients with ependymoma. Mork et al[25] were the first to demonstrate that postoperative radiation therapy improves outcome in ependymoma patients. These investigators reported a survival estimate of 17% for patients who underwent resection alone versus 40% survival estimate for those who underwent resection and postoperative irradiation. Radiation therapy has since been routinely administered to patients with ependymoma who are 3 years of age or older.

The role of radiation therapy has been evaluated in several studies in infants and children younger than age 3, including the POG 8633 study, which showed that young children with completely resected ependymoma in whom radiation therapy was delayed for 2 years experienced a significantly worse outcome (5-year survival estimate of 38%) than those in whom therapy was delayed for 1 year (5-year survival estimate of 88%).[4] These results support the use of radiation therapy, and from an oncologic point of view contradict the policy of delaying treatment for the time intervals specified in the study.

Optimal Radiation Dose, Volume, and Fractionation

Perhaps one of the more controversial topics in ependymoma until recently has been the volume of irradiation. With the advent of better imaging and surgical techniques, current evidence indicates that the predominant pattern of failure is local, regardless of tumor grade or location.[8,32,46] For infratentorial ependymomas, the entire posterior fossa does not need to be treated.[34] Vanuytsel[48] demonstrated that craniospinal is not better than focal radiation therapy. In addition, several retrospective studies have failed to demonstrate any benefits associated with the use of prophylactic craniospinal irradiation.[13,23,40,48]

Our current recommendation for nondisseminated ependymoma is local radiation therapy. Craniospinal radiation therapy is reserved for the less than 10% of children with neuraxis dissemination and has limited benefit owing to the lower total dose administered to tumor in the neuraxis.

Studies that have shown a dose-response level for ependymoma indicate a dose threshold of 45 to 50 Gy.[3,10] More recent studies suggest that dose escalation in subtotally resected tumors may be beneficial. The POG 9132 study used hyperfractionated radiation therapy to a total dose of 69.6 Gy (1.2 Gy twice daily) for the treatment of posterior fossa ependymoma. The investigators found that 19 patients who underwent subtotal resection had a better outcome (4-year event-free survival of 50%) than did a comparable group of patients who participated in the earlier POG 8532 study, which used a lower total dose of conventional radiation (4-year event-free survival of 24%).[19] Hyperfractionated radiation therapy did not improve survival estimates in patients with completely resected tumors.

The optimal dose of radiation remains unclear. The evaluation of a dose-response relationship for a given type of tumor requires prospective evaluation. Retrospectively, an increase in the dose of radiation administered to the primary site appears to improve local control.[23,44] In the United States, the initial results with hyperfractionated radiation therapy for those with residual tumor seemed promising, but this is not true with longer follow-up.

Conformal radiation therapy limits the highest doses to the primary site and decreases the dose received by normal tissues. Reducing the dose received by normal tissues is logical in children, but requires systematic definition of the treatment volume and prospective study to determine that irradiation using more limited volumes does not increase the risk of marginal treatment failures.

A phase II trial of conformal radiation therapy (CRT) was conducted at St. Jude from July 1997 through January 2003 to determine whether the targeted volume for radiation therapy could be reduced without affecting disease control or the pattern of failure. Patients with localized ependymoma were evaluated before and after CRT to determine neurologic, endocrine, and cognitive effects. A total of 88 children were enrolled with a median age of 2.8 years. Targeting included a 10-mm anatomically defined clinical target volume, and patients received radiation therapy to doses of 59.4 Gy ($n = 73$) or 54.0 Gy (age < 18 months and gross-total resection; $n = 15$). Gross-total resection was achieved in 74 patients before irradiation, near-total in 6, and subtotal in 8. With a median follow-up of 30.8 months at the time of its most recent report (June 2003), the 3-year actuarial event-free survival and local control estimates were 80.6% ± 6.8% and 89.5% ± 5.6%, respectively. These results are clearly the best results to date for ependymoma and indicate the importance of the extent of resection and improved targeting that can be achieved with conformal radiation techniques. Patients were evaluated before and after irradiation in an unprecedented manner that showed that IQ estimates (IQ + standard deviation [SD]) at baseline (93 + 18), 6 months (97 + 19), 12 months (97 + 19), 24 months (94 + 18), 36 months (98 + 19), and 48 months (97 + 19) were within the range of normal. Preirradiation growth hormone deficiency was observed in 29% of patients based on provocative testing. The results showed that the volume of irradiation may be safely reduced without affecting disease control rates in localized ependymoma.[22]

CHEMOTHERAPY

The role of chemotherapy continues to change. A number of agents have demonstrated activity against ependymoma with no clear impact on outcome, because even under optimal clinical circumstances that include gross-total resection and high-dose postoperative irradiation, the recurrence rate remains sufficiently high to warrant the investigation of agents with potential activity against ependymoma. The need is even greater for patients with metastatic disease in whom the prognosis is poor and the ability to give tumoricidal doses of radiation to the entire brain and spine is limited.

Recent reports of adjuvant combination chemotherapy in pediatric patients with newly diagnosed ependymoma have demonstrated encouraging responses without improving survival, suggesting a limited role. Several retrospective reviews have assessed the effectiveness of chemotherapy in the treatment of newly diagnosed ependymoma, and none have found that it improves overall survival.[3,8,13,23,32,34,46] The CCG 942 study is the only randomized trial that compared survival after irradiation alone with survival after irradiation and chemotherapy in pediatric patients (aged 2 to 16 years) with ependymoma. The investigators concluded that adjuvant chemotherapy with lomustine, vincristine, and prednisone did not improve outcome.[5] The CCG 921 study, a prospective randomized study of radiation therapy followed by either lomustine, vincristine, and prednisone or a combination of agents known as *8-in-1* (eight drugs in 1 day), used survival analyses to demonstrate that the outcome of patients who received chemotherapy was no better than that of historical controls.[37]

Standard versus Dose-Intensive Chemotherapy

The POG 9233 study compared standard chemotherapy (six 12-week cycles of cisplatin, cyclophosphamide, etoposide, and vincristine) and dose-intensive chemotherapy (eight 9-week cycles of the same agents with differences in relative intensity) in a group of infants with brain tumors, including ependymoma. Event-free survival estimates were significantly increased for patients with ependymoma treated with dose-intensive chemotherapy, yet there was no difference in overall survival estimates.

Grill et al[11] recently reported the results of a French Society of Pediatric Oncology trial in 73 children treated with multiagent chemotherapy for 16 to 18 months after maximal resection. Irradiation was not included in the treatment regimen. Progression-free survival estimates at 2 and 4 years were 33%

and 22%, respectively, with 50% of patients relapsing during the planned chemotherapy course.

Chemotherapy and Second Resection

Chemotherapy may make residual tumors more amenable to complete surgical resection. Foreman et al[7] used chemotherapy between the initial and second resections in four patients with ependymoma. After chemotherapy, all the patients had viable tumor; complete resections were performed in three of the four, all of whom remained progression-free at 23 to 34 months after second-look surgery. The subjective impression of the investigators was that the tumors were better defined and easier to dissect after chemotherapy.

Future Role of Chemotherapy

Chemotherapy may serve four important functions in the future: (1) to bridge the interval necessary while planning a second resection; (2) to make the tumor more amenable to resection and improve the rate of complete resection at the time of the second procedure; (3) to reduce the morbidity of the second resection; and (4) bridge the interval required to prepare a child who has suffered neurologic complications from tumor or surgery for daily radiation therapy and often anesthesia.

The selection of the best agents, the schedule of delivery, and the duration of chemotherapy necessary to achieve these goals are difficult to determine given the range of responses, the differences in toxicity profiles, and the lack of data from which to model such a study. Most investigators prefer to use combinations of drugs, including carboplatin or cisplatin, etoposide, cyclophosphamide, and vincristine. Concerns about the use of carboplatin, which has a better toxicity profile, persist among investigators, because this agent's equivalency to cisplatin has not been demonstrated.

CONCLUSION

Optimal local control has been repeatedly shown to be the single most important prognostic factor in the treatment of this disease, and achieving this goal begins with maximal surgical resection. Failure to perform a gross-total or near-total resection substantially decreases the likelihood of long-term disease control. A primary goal of the next Children's Oncology Group trial is to increase the number of patients whose tumors are gross totally or near totally resected. Second surgery is recommended for patients who undergo an initial subtotal resection. In an attempt to facilitate the second surgery, chemotherapy is administered between the first and second resections in the hopes of rendering the tumor more amenable to complete removal and, perhaps, reducing the likelihood of disease dissemination in the interim.

Following surgery, postoperative CRT is administered to all patients, with the exception of those with supratentorial, differentiated ependymomas whose tumors have been completely resected.

References

1. Bennetto L, Foreman N, Harding B, et al: Ki-67 immunolabelling index is a prognostic indicator in childhood posterior fossa ependymomas. Mol Chem Neuropathol 24:434–440, 1998.

2. Bhattacharjee MB, Armstrong DD, Vogel H, Cooley LD: Cytogenetic analysis of 120 primary pediatric brain tumors and literature review. Cancer Genet Cytogenet 97:39–53, 1997.

3. Chiu JK, Woo SY, Ater J, et al: Intracranial ependymoma in children: analysis of prognostic factors. J Neurooncol 13:283–290, 1992.

4. Duffner PK, Krischer JP, Sanford RA, et al: Prognostic factors in infants and very young children with intracranial ependymomas. Pediatr Neurosurg 28:215–222, 1998.

5. Evans AE, Anderson JR, Lefkowitz-Boudreaux IB, et al: Adjuvant chemotherapy of childhood posterior fossa ependymomas: craniospinal irradiation with or without adjuvant CCNU, vincristine, and presdnisone: a Children's Cancer Group study. Med Pediatr Oncol 27:8–14, 1996.

6. Fiez JA: Cerebellar contributions to cognition. Neuron 16:13–15, 1996.

7. Foreman NK, Love S, Gill SS, et al: Second-look surgery for incompletely resected fourth ventricle ependymomas: technical case report. Neurosurgery 40:856–860, 1997.

8. Foreman NK, Love S, Thorne R: Intracranial ependymomas: analysis of prognostic factors in a population-based series. Pediatr Neurosurg 24:119–125, 1996.

9. Gilbertson RJ, Bentley L, Hernan R, et al: ERBB receptor signaling promotes ependymoma cell proliferation and represents a potential novel therapeutic target for this disease. Clin Cancer Res 8:3054–3064, 2002.

10. Goldwein JW, Leahy JM, Packer RJ, et al: Intracranial ependymomas in children. Int J Radiat Oncol Biol Phys 19:1497–1502, 1990.

11. Grill J, Le Delay MC, Gambarelli D, et al: Postoperative chemotherapy without irradiation for ependymoma in children under 5 years of age: a multicenter trial of the French Society of Pediatric Oncology. J Clin Oncol 19:1288–1296, 2001.

12. Healey EA, Barnes PD, Kupsky WJ, et al: The prognostic significance of postoperative residual tumor in ependymoma. Neurosurgery 28:666–671, 1991.

13. Horn B, Heideman R, Geyer R, et al: A multi-institutional retrospective study of intracranial ependymoma in children: identification of risk factors. J Pediatr Hematol Oncol 21:203–211, 1999.

14. Hukin J, Epstein F, Lefton D, et al: Treatment of intracranial ependymoma by surgery alone. Pediatr Neurosurg 29:40–45, 1998.

15. Ikezaki K, Matsushima T, Inoue T, et al: Correlation of microanatomical localization with postoperative survival in posterior fossa ependymomas. Neurosurgery 32:38–44, 1993.

16. Kleihues P, Sobin LH: World Health Organization classification of tumors. Cancer 88:2887, 2000.

17. Kotylo PK, Robertson PB, Fineberg NS, et al: Flow cytometric DNA analysis of pediatric intracranial ependymomas. Arch Pathol Lab Med 121:1255–1258, 1997.

18. Kovalic JJ, Flaris N, Grigsby PW, et al: Intracranial ependymoma long-term outcome, patterns of failure. J Neurooncol 15:125–131, 1993.

19. Kovnar E, Curran W, Tomita, et al: Hyperfractionated irradiation for childhood ependymoma: improved local control in subtotally resected tumors (abstract). Childs Nerv Syst 14:489, 1998.

20. Kovnar E, Kun L, Burger P, et al: Patterns of dissemination and recurrence in childhood ependymoma: preliminary results of Pediatric Oncology Group Protocol #8532. Ann Neurol 30:457, 1991.

21. Kramer DL, Parmiter AH, Rorke LB, et al: Molecular cytogenetic studies of pediatric ependymomas. J Neurooncol 37:25–33, 1998.

22. Merchant TE: The Resurgence of Radiation Therapy for Very Young Children with Brain Tumors. American Society of Clinical Oncology 2003 Educational Book, 2003.

23. Merchant TE, Haida T, Wang MH, et al: Anaplastic ependymoma: treatment of pediatric patients with or without craniospinal radiation therapy. J Neurosurg 86:943–949, 1997.

24. Merchant TE, Jenkins JJ, Burger PC, et al: The influence of histology on the time to progression after irradiation for localized ependymoma in children. Int J Radiat Oncol Biol Phys 53:52–57, 2002.

25. Mork SJ, Loken AC: Ependymoma: a follow-up study of 101 cases. Cancer 40:907–915, 1977.

26. Nazar GB, Hoffman HJ, Becker LE, et al: Infratentorial ependymomas in childhood: prognostic factors and treatment. J Neurosurg 72:408–417, 1990.

27. Needle MN, Goldwein JW, Grass J, et al: Adjuvant chemotherapy for the treatment of intracranial ependymoma of childhood. Cancer 80:341–347, 1997.

28. Neumann E, Kalousek DK, Norman MG, et al: Cytogenetic analysis of 109 pediatric CNS tumors. Cancer Genet Cytogenet 71:40–49, 1993.

29. Osterdock RJ, Sanford RA, Merchant TE: Pediatric ependymoma (40 in 36 months). Paper presented at the annual meeting of American Association of Neurosurgeons (AANS)/Central Nervous System (CNS) Section on Pediatric Neurological Surgery; Coronado, Calif; December 6–9, 2000.

30. Palma L, Celli P, Mariottini A, et al: The importance of surgery in supratentorial ependymomas. Long-term survival in a series of 23 cases. Childs Nerv Syst 16:170–175, 2000.

31. Paulino AC, Wen BC, Hussey DH, et al: Intracranial ependymomas: an analysis of prognostic factors and patterns of failure (abstract). Cancer J Sci Am 6:104–105, 2000.

32. Perilongo G, Massimino M, Sotti G, et al: Analyses of prognostic factors in a retrospective review of 92 children with ependymoma: Italian Pediatric Neuro-oncology Group. Med Pediatr Oncol 29:79–85, 1997.

33. Pierre-Kahn A, Hirsch JF, Roux FX, et al: Intracranial ependymomas in childhood. Survival and functional results of 47 cases. Childs Brain 10:145–156, 1983.

34. Pollack IF, Gerszten PC, Martinez AJ, et al: Intracranial ependymomas of childhood: long-term outcome and prognostic factors. Neurosurgery 37:655–666, 1995.

35. Reardon DA, Entrekin RE, Sublet J, et al: Chromosome arm 6q loss is the most common recurrent autosomal alteration detected in primary pediatric ependymoma. Genes Chromosomes Cancer 24:230–237, 1999.

36. Ries LAG et al: Cancer Statistics Review, 1973–1997. Bethesda, Md, National Cancer Institute, 2000.

37. Robertson PL, Zeltzer PM, Boyett JM, et al: Survival and prognostic factors following radiation therapy and chemotherapy for ependymomas in children: a report of the Children's Cancer Group. J Neurosurg 88:695–703, 1998.

38. Rousseau P, Habrand J, Sarrazin D, et al: Treatment of intracranial ependymomas of children: review of a 15-year experience. Int J Radiat Biol Phys 28:381–386, 1994.

39. Sala F, Talacchi A, Mazza C, et al: Prognostic factors in childhood intracranial ependymomas. Pediatr Neurosurg 28:135–142, 1998.

40. Sanford RA, Gajjar A: Ependymomas. Clin Neurosurg 44:559–570, 1997.

41. Sanford RA, Kun LE, Heideman RL, et al: Cerebellar pontine angle ependymoma in infants. Pediatr Neurosurg 27:84–91, 1997.

42. Schiffer D, Chio A, Giordana MT, et al: Proliferating cell nuclear antigen expression in brain tumors, and its prognostic role

in ependymomas: an immunohistochemical study. Acta Neuropathol (Berl) 85:495–502, 1993.

43. Shaw EG, Evans RG, Scheithauer BW, et al: Postoperative radiotherapy of intracranial ependymoma in pediatric and adult patients. Int J Radiat Oncol Biol Phys 13:1457–1462, 1987.

44. Shuman RM, Alvord EC, Leech RW: The biology of childhood ependymomas. Arch Neurol 32:731–739, 1975.

45. Steen RG, Koury BSM, Granja CI, et al: Effect of ionizing radiation on the human brain: white matter and gray matter T1 in pediatric brain tumor patients treated with conformal radiation therapy. Int J Radiat Oncol Biol Phys 49:79–91, 2001.

46. Sutton LN, Goldwein J, Perilongo G, et al: Prognostic factors in childhood ependymomas. Pediatr Neurosurg 16:57–65, 1990–1991.

47. Timmermann B, Kortmann RD, Kuhl J, et al: Combined postoperative irradiation and chemotherapy for anaplastic ependymoma in childhood: results of the German Prospective Trials Hit '88/'89 and Hit '91 (abstract 122). Int J Radiat Oncol Biol Phys 42(suppl 1):185, 1998.

48. Vanuytsel LJ, Bessell EM, Ashley SE, et al: Intracranial ependymoma: long-term results of a policy of surgery and radiotherapy. Int J Radiat Oncol Biol Phys 23:313–319, 1992.

49. Von Haken MS, White EC, Daneshvar-Shyesther L, et al: Molecular genetic analysis of chromosome arm 17p and choromosome arm 22q DNA sequence in sporadic pediatric ependymomas. Genes Chromosomes Cancer 17:37–44, 1996.

CHAPTER **89**

MEDULLOBLASTOMA

Cormac O. Maher and Corey Raffel

Refinements in imaging, surgical technique, and adjuvant therapies have led to longer survival and an improving quality of life in patients with medulloblastoma. Although these gains are encouraging, medulloblastomas are still often lethal, with an overall long-term survival of approximately 60%. Surviving patients often suffer physical and cognitive impairment secondary to treatment. Advances in molecular biology should lead to more efficacious therapies in the future.

LOCATION

Medulloblastomas are primitive neuroectodermal tumors (PNETs) of the posterior fossa. By definition, therefore, medulloblastomas do not originate supratentorially. Most medulloblastomas arise in the cerebellar vermis and extend into the fourth ventricle. Medulloblastomas may also occur in the cerebellar hemispheres, although this is significantly less common than the midline location. Medulloblastomas in adults are more likely to arise in the cerebellar hemisphere.[32] There have been several case reports of medulloblastomas of the cerebellopontine angle.

Although medulloblastomas may extend from the vermis into one of the cerebellar hemispheres, isolated cerebellar hemispheric involvement is not common. The tumor usually fills the fourth ventricle, partially or entirely. In contrast to ependymomas, extension through the foramen of Luschka into the cerebellopontine angle or through the cerebral aqueduct into the third ventricle is unusual in medulloblastomas.

DIAGNOSIS

Patients with medulloblastoma may have symptoms of tumor mass effect on the cerebellum and nearby structures, symptoms of spinal "drop" metastases, or symptoms of hydrocephalus. Many patients have some combination of these symptoms. The clinical history of medulloblastoma is typically brief. Symptom onset is less than 6 weeks before patients seek treatment in approximately half of patients and less than 12 weeks in approximately 75% of patients.[54]

Regardless of histology, midline posterior fossa tumors in children characteristically cause symptoms of increased intracranial pressure (ICP) caused by hydrocephalus. At least 90% of patients with medulloblastomas have symptoms of hydrocephalus such as headache and recurrent vomiting. As a consequence, differentiation of those patients with medulloblastoma from those with other processes that may cause obstructive hydrocephalus is difficult by symptoms alone. Symptoms of hydrocephalus are typically worse in the morning and usually include headaches, nausea, and vomiting. Infants with hydrocephalus may be irritable, lethargic, and occasionally demonstrate progressive macrocephaly.[2,54] Older children usually complain of headaches and may consequently be referred for imaging sooner than infants. Older patients with a medulloblastoma arising in the cerebellar hemisphere may complain only of progressive loss of limb coordination.

Patients without hydrocephalus usually have truncal ataxia resulting from mass effect on the cerebellar vermis, especially when the diagnosis is delayed. Spinal drop metastases may cause back pain, urinary retention, or leg weakness.

In as many as 10% of cases, patients may have acute decompensation secondary to hemorrhage into the tumor, causing acute hydrocephalus or brainstem compression. Subarachnoid hemorrhage from hemorrhage into the fourth ventricle can also occur but is rare. Patients with medulloblastomas can occasionally have acute symptoms of brainstem compression necessitating immediate intervention.

On physical examination, papilledema is commonly noted in those patients presenting with hydrocephalus. Ataxia, nystagmus, and abnormalities of extraocular movements are also common findings. Diplopia generally represents impairment of cranial nerves IV or VI. The level of alertness is often affected and should be continuously assessed.

Imaging of the posterior fossa is indicated in any of these clinical settings. Although preoperative lumbar cerebrospinal fluid (CSF) sampling is often contraindicated in the presence of a posterior fossa tumor, intraoperative or postoperative CSF cytology is useful for staging these tumors.

EPIDEMIOLOGY

There are between 250 and 500 new cases of medulloblastoma diagnosed each year in the United States.[65] The median age at diagnosis is 5 to 7 years.[61] Although medulloblastomas may occur at any age, approximately 75% are diagnosed before the patient is 15 years of age,[54,61] and the approximate incidence in this age group is 0.5 per 100,000 children.[69] Medulloblastomas account for 15% to 30% of all brain tumors in children and 30% to 55% of posterior fossa tumors in children.[65] Furthermore, medulloblastoma is the most common primary brain tumor in children younger than 2 years.[24] Medulloblastomas have a predominance in males that varies from 1.3:1 to 2.7:1 in different series.[2,13,36,54]

Between 1% and 2% of all cases of medulloblastoma occur in association with a tumor syndrome.[20] Nevoid basal cell carcinoma syndrome (Gorlin syndrome) is a rare autosomal dominant syndrome that is associated with basal cell carcinomas, keratocysts of the jaw, spine and rib anomalies, calcification of the falx cerebri, and in approximately 4% of cases, medulloblastomas.[21,43] Most reported cases of medulloblastoma in the setting of Gorlin syndrome occur during the first 7 years of life, and annual screening with magnetic resonance imaging (MRI) has been advocated for patients with this syndrome.[43] Medulloblastoma accounts for approximately one quarter of all cerebral neoplasms in cases of Turcot syndrome.[53] Although medulloblastomas in patients with Turcot syndrome are usually diagnosed during the first 2 decades of life, they may occasionally occur in adulthood.[53]

IMAGING

On diagnostic imaging, medulloblastomas classically appear as well-defined, midline cerebellar mass lesions. Brainstem involvement is seen radiographically in a large minority of patients with medulloblastoma, and radiographic evidence of hydrocephalus is very common.[5,9]

Medulloblastomas typically appear hyperdense on noncontrast computed tomography (CT) scans because of their dense cellularity (Figure 89-1). This is an important means of differentiating medulloblastomas from cerebellar astrocytomas and ependymomas, which are generally hypodense and isodense, respectively, on noncontrast CT. Calcifications are noted in approximately 20% of medulloblastomas on CT scan and cystic

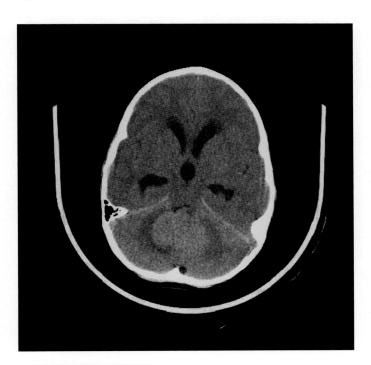

FIGURE 89-1   Computed tomography scan without contrast demonstrates a mildly hyperdense lesion in the posterior fossa with mass effect on the cerebellar hemispheres and the fourth ventricle, leading to obstructive hydrocephalus.

or necrotic regions in 20% to 50%.[64] A predominantly cystic cerebellar tumor, however, is more likely an astrocytoma in a child or a metastasis in an adult. Although intratumoral hemorrhage is a rare feature of medulloblastoma, it is more common in medulloblastomas than in cerebellar astrocytomas or ependymomas.

Most medulloblastomas have low to intermediate signal on T1-weighted MRI (Figure 89-2). T2 signal is characterized by heterogeneity secondary to intratumoral cysts, vessels, and calcifications. Medulloblastomas almost always enhance with gadolinium; the pattern of enhancement may be uniform or heterogeneous. Diffuse or patchy enhancement following contrast administration is seen in at least 90% of medulloblastomas (Figure 89-3).[5,9]

When time permits, preoperative imaging should evaluate the entire neuraxis for the presence of metastatic spread of the medulloblastoma to other sites in the central nervous system. Medulloblastoma spreads along CSF pathways. The most common intracranial sites of metastases, therefore, are the basilar and suprasellar cisterns, sylvian fissures, infundibular recess, lateral ventricles, and subfrontal region. Medulloblastoma metastases coating the cerebellum can often be seen on noncontrasted studies as blurring of the folia. Metastatic disease at other sites is best evaluated with contrasted images. Drop metastases in the spinal canal are common (20% at presentation), brightly enhanced, and are almost always extramedullary, although intramedullary metastases have been reported (Figure 89-4). Because of postoperative blood and protein artifacts, spinal imaging is best obtained preoperatively. If spinal imaging cannot be obtained preoperatively, imaging should be delayed for 2 weeks postoperatively to permit resolution of these artifacts.

For a medulloblastoma arising from the cerebellar vermis, the major differential diagnostic consideration on imaging is ependymoma. Unlike ependymoma, medulloblastomas typically do not extend through the foramina of Luschka. Calcification is also more common in ependymomas. Medulloblastomas are typically slightly hyperintense on CT, isointense or hypointense on T1-weighted MRI scans, and hyperintense on T2-weighted MRI scans. Medulloblastomas are usually strongly enhanced.

In the past, medulloblastomas were staged radiographically according to the Chang system, which assigns a stage based on tumor size (T stage) and metastatic spread (M stage).[12] The Chang system has been criticized for including tumor size despite studies demonstrating no clear correlation between preoperative tumor size and outcome. In addition, the Chang system does not include other factors such as age that are known to be predictive of outcome. Despite the failings of the Chang staging system, no other radiographic staging systems have been widely accepted.

Postoperative MRI is usually indicated within 2 days of surgery to assess the extent of tumor resection. Postoperative enhancement is a common finding on imaging performed between 1 day and 1 year following surgery and is most pronounced between postoperative days 3 and 21. Nodular enhancement is characteristic of residual tumor.

TUMOR HISTOLOGY

Bailey and Cushing first described medulloblastomas in 1925.[4] Based on histologic and embryologic investigations, Bailey and Cushing included medulloblastoma in a group of primitive

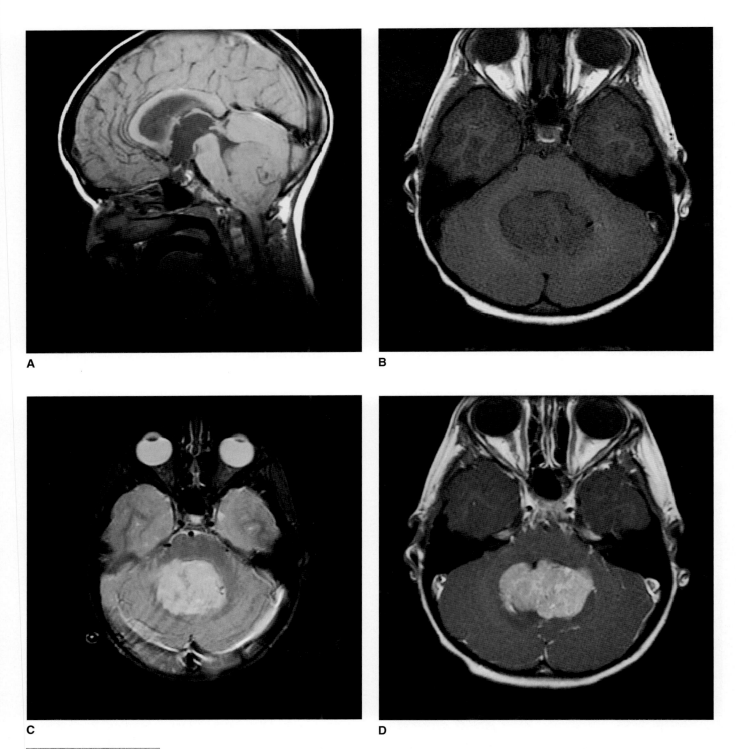

FIGURE 89-2 Typical appearance of medulloblastoma on magnetic resonance image. T1 sagittal section showing a lesion filling the fourth ventricle *(A)*. Medulloblastoma is usually hypointense to isointense on T1-weighted images *(B)*, hyperintense on T2-weighted images *(C)*, and strongly enhanced *(D)*.

brain tumors of childhood, thought to arise from the embryonal medulloblast. This classification scheme was later refined by Rubinstein and became widely accepted in the decades that followed.[63] Because medulloblastoma is histologically indistinguishable from retinoblastomas, neuroblastoma, and pineoblastomas, Rorke has suggested that the term *primitive neuroectodermal tumor* should be applied to each of these tumors instead of the formerly accepted nomenclature.[62] All medulloblastomas are grade IV tumors according to the current World Health Organization (WHO) classification.[27]

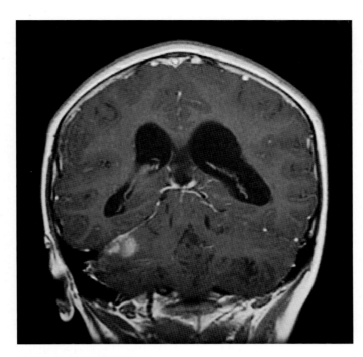

FIGURE 89-3 Postgadolinium T1-weighted coronal section magnetic resonance image demonstrating the typical appearance of a medulloblastoma of the cerebellar hemisphere. This location is more often found in adults than in children.

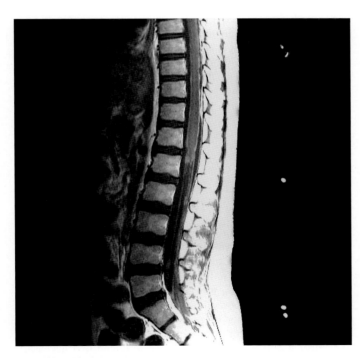

FIGURE 89-4 Gadolinium-enhanced sagittal magnetic resonance image demonstrating the typical appearance of a spinal "drop metastasis" at the level of the conus medullaris and the cauda equina.

Medulloblastoma has several histologic subtypes. The classic subtype is composed of small, densely packed undifferentiated cells with hyperchromatic nuclei and scant cytoplasm. These cells may cluster into Homer-Wright rosettes, but this is not a constant feature. The desmoplastic subtype is similar to the classic subtype but is further characterized by the presence of collagen bundles and scattered, less cellular areas, or "glomeruli." The desmoplastic subtype is found in approximately 6% of patients, is more common in adults, and may be associated with a more favorable prognosis.[32,68] The large cell medulloblastoma subtype is found in approximately 4% of cases and is characterized by large nuclei, prominent nucleoli, and abundant cytoplasm.[28] The large cell subtype is also associated with large areas of necrosis, a higher mitotic activity, and a more aggressive behavior as compared with the classic medulloblastoma. Although most medulloblastomas are grossly friable and soft, desmoplastic variants are firmer. All subtypes may calcify.

MOLECULAR BIOLOGY

Medulloblastoma has been extensively studied at the molecular level. Initial cytogenetic studies revealed loss of genetic material on the short arm of chromosome 17 in approximately one third of tumors.[7,41] The loss of heterozygosity (LOH) of 17p has been confirmed by restriction fragment length polymorphism (RFLP) analysis and shown to occur in up to one half of cases. Because the p53 gene is located on 17p, a number of investigators have examined the status of this gene in medulloblastoma.[7,59] Taken together, these studies clearly demonstrate that despite the deletion of one p53 allele in many of the tumors, the remaining p53 gene is rarely mutated in medulloblastoma. Interestingly, a small subset of tumors has only a small area of 17p loss that does not include the p53 gene.[7,14,59] This finding suggests the possibility that another tumor-suppressor gene is present on 17p. Indeed, fine mapping of the region has suggested that such a putative suppressor is located near the abr gene on 17p13.3.[49] This putative suppressor might be important in the oncogenesis of medulloblastoma.

Medulloblastomas are associated with two different inherited cancer syndromes: Gorlin syndrome and Turcot syndrome. Gorlin syndrome, also called *nevoid basal cell carcinoma syndrome,* is an autosomal dominant disorder.[30] Affected individuals develop multiple basal cell carcinomas, multiple odontogenic keratocysts of the jaws, palmar and plantar dyskeratoses, and skeletal anomalies, especially rib malformations. At least 40 cases of medulloblastoma have been reported in patients with this syndrome, suggesting an increased frequency of medulloblastoma in this population.[21] The gene for Gorlin syndrome has been mapped to chromosome 9q31.[23] In one study, however, only 5 of 36 cases of medulloblastoma examined had loss of 9q31, and only one of these had loss of the 9q marker most closely linked to the Gorlin gene.[66] Work has suggested that 9q deletions occur only in the desmoplastic subtype of medulloblastoma, raising the possibility of a Gorlin syndrome gene mutation being involved in the development of this subclass of tumor.[66] The gene for Gorlin syndrome has recently been identified as the PTCH gene, the human homologue of the *Drosophila* patched gene.[40] This *Drosophila* gene encodes a protein with 12 putative transmembrane domains; it may thus function as a membrane receptor or transporter.[35,51] The protein has an essential role in embryonic patterning in *Drosophila*—a similar role in humans may explain the congenital anomalies associated with Gorlin syndrome. PTCH mutations have been described in patients with Gorlin syndrome and in spontaneous basal cell carcinomas. In one study PTCH mutations were identified in 3 of 24 medulloblastomas.[60] These results suggest that PTCH mutations occur in approximately 10% of sporadic PNET, a finding in agreement with later reports.[71,74,75]

Turcot syndrome is a hereditary disorder in which affected individuals have multiple colonic polyps and a brain tumor. In one study, mutations in the APC gene were identified in a group of patients with Turcot syndrome in which the brain tumor was a medulloblastoma.[33] The relative risk for developing a medulloblastoma in the patients with Turcot and an APC gene mutation was 92 times that in the general population. Surprisingly, despite this association, APC gene mutations have not been identified often in spontaneously occurring medulloblastomas.[50,76]

Medulloblastomas have also been evaluated for oncogenic mutations in β-catenin, because these mutations result in the same phenotype as APC inactivation.[77] In one study 3 tumors out of 67 were found to have oncogenic mutations in β-catenin. These results suggest that alterations in the APC-β-catenin pathway may be important in the development of medulloblastoma.

Almost 20% of medulloblastomas contain double minute chromosomes, suggesting the possibility of gene amplification.[8] Gene amplification of 11 oncogenes has been investigated.[72] Of 20 primary medulloblastomas studied, only one tumor was found to have amplification of the c-erbB1 proto-oncogene, and no other tumor had amplification of any of the oncogenes examined. Interestingly, four established medulloblastoma cell lines were also tested, and three had proto-oncogene amplification. One had amplified c-myc, one N-myc, and one c-erbB1. These investigators suggest that in vitro culture may select for a small subpopulation of cells within the tumor that have preexisting amplification or that culture is more successful with tumors that have an amplified proto-oncogene.[8]

Members of the neurotrophin family (nerve growth factor, brain-derived neurotrophic factor, NT-3, and NT-4/5) and their family of high affinity receptors (trkA, trkB, and trkC) are important in the proliferation, differentiation, and survival of neuroepithelial cells. In addition to the trk receptors, a low affinity receptor for neurotrophins (p75[LNGFR]) has also been described in these cells. Because medulloblastoma is thought to arise from primitive neuroepithelial stem cells, neurotrophins and their receptors may be important in the development and growth of these tumors. Three studies have been performed examining the status of the low affinity nerve growth factor receptor in medulloblastoma.[42,44,56] Approximately one third of tumors studied had mRNA for this receptor. Expression of p75[LNGFR], however, may be restricted to the subset of PNETs demonstrating neuronal differentiation. Addition of nerve growth factor had no effect on the growth characteristics or morphology of a PNET cell line expressing the receptor. Interestingly, one study of a small number of tumors correlated good clinical outcome with high expression of full-length trkC mRNA.[67]

Two recent reports of gene expression in medulloblastoma have added insights to the basic biology of these tumors.[48,58] In the first of these, medulloblastoma samples were divided into two groups, depending on whether CSF dissemination of tumor was seen at the time the patient sought treatment.[48] Gene expression was analyzed on Affymetrix G110 cancer arrays, which are enriched for genes thought to be important in cancer biology. Fifty-nine genes were identified that had increased expression in the metastatic tumors compared with the non-metastatic tumors. An additional 29 genes were identified that had decreased expression in the metastatic tumors. Two of these genes, PDGFRA and SPARC, were shown by immunohistochemical staining to be expressed differentially between metastatic and nonmetastatic tumors. In addition, antibodies to PDGFRA blocked tumor cell migration in in vitro assays. These investigators were able to use the pattern of gene expression to predict which tumors caused CSF metastases in a blinded group of tumors. These results suggest that there may be genes important in the progression of medulloblastoma or that alterations in different pathways may be responsible for the differences in prognosis seen between tumors occurring without and with CSF dissemination.

The second study examined a group of "embryonal tumors" of the central nervous system, including medulloblastomas, extracerebellar PNETs, atypical teratoid-rhabdoid tumors, and malignant gliomas.[58] Gene expression was analyzed on Affymetrix HuGene FL arrays, containing 5920 known genes and 897 expressed sequence tags. The first finding from this data set was that each tumor type could be easily distinguished from the others based on gene expression pattern. Especially interesting was the ability to distinguish medulloblastomas from other CNS PNETs, suggesting that lumping these tumors together, as proposed by Rourke, may be inappropriate. The medulloblastomas often expressed genes normally expressed in the external granule cell layer (EGCL), lending credence to the hypothesis that EGCL precursors represent the cell of origin of medulloblastoma. Second, these investigators were able to distinguish "classic" medulloblastomas from desmoplastic medulloblastomas. The important genes with increased expression in the desmoplastic tumors were those involved in the sonic hedgehog-PTCH pathway. Lastly, using an eight-gene model, these investigators were able to accurately predict outcome in their patients with medulloblastoma. Genes associated with favorable clinical outcome included TRKC and other genes characteristic of cerebellar differentiation. In contrast, these genes were underexpressed in tumors with poor prognosis, and genes involved in cell proliferation were overexpressed.

SURGICAL TREATMENT

Hydrocephalus

Although hydrocephalus is noted preoperatively in most patients who have medulloblastoma, routine placement of a ventricular shunt or external ventricular drain (EVD) before resection is no longer indicated in most cases.[1,46] In addition to the risk of infection, upward transtentorial herniation is a rare but significant complication of preoperative ventricular drainage in the setting of posterior fossa mass lesions. Furthermore, earlier tumor detection and the use of corticosteroids to control ICP has made preoperative drainage less necessary than in the past. In cases where symptoms of hydrocephalus are significant and refractory to maximal medical therapy, an external ventricular drain should be placed promptly. To decrease the risk of upward herniation, CSF should be drained slowly and in a controlled manner.

Although most patients will have resolution of the hydrocephalus following tumor resection, approximately 40% of medulloblastomas will require placement of a ventricular shunt within 4 weeks of the tumor resection. When ventricular shunts are placed preoperatively, however, the overall rate of shunt dependency is substantially higher. Patients with postoperative lethargy, especially if progressively worsening, or patients with a large pseudomeningocele should be screened for hydrocephalus. Lee et al have identified three prognostic factors for permanent shunting: young age, dramatic preoperative ventricular dilation, and large tumors.[46] Importantly, patients with none of these characteristics rarely require permanent shunting. The theoretic risk of a ventriculoperitoneal shunt allowing seeding of the posterior fossa tumor into the peritoneum appears to be very small.[6]

Tumor Resection

Surgical resection of posterior fossa medulloblastomas is almost always indicated as an initial therapy.[54] Furthermore, the extent of surgical resection is prognostically significant for these tumors.[3,38] Any survival difference between a gross-total resection and near-total resection (>90% of tumor removed), however, has not been proved prospectively.[3] Aggressive resections, therefore, that violate the plane of the floor of the fourth ventricle in pursuit of a gross-total resection are not indicated.

Positioning of the patient for a posterior fossa tumor resection is dictated by patient age, tumor location, and the individual preferences of the surgeon. Most surgeons favor the lateral decubitus or modified prone (Concorde) position. A midline suboccipital craniotomy or craniectomy followed by a vertical approach through the vermis is the standard technique for exposing a midline lesion of the posterior fossa. The tumor is usually carefully dissected off of the floor of the fourth ventricle in a caudal-to-cranial direction. If extension of the tumor into the brainstem is anticipated preoperatively, intraoperative electromyogram (EMG) monitoring of the facial and abducens cranial nerves may be useful.[31] Medulloblastomas are usually soft and friable and are resected piecemeal. Typically, the rostral extent of medulloblastomas may be dissected by following a plane between the tumor and the superior medullary velum. Most of these tumors have a cap of CSF representing the superior fourth ventricle over the most rostral aspect of the tumor, serving as a useful surgical landmark.

Complications of posterior fossa tumor resection include infection, CSF leakage, cranial nerve palsy, and cerebellar mutism. The syndrome of cerebellar mutism following a vermian tumor resection was first described by Hirsch et al in 1979 and is now a well-known complication following the resection of any posterior fossa tumor, particularly medulloblastoma.[34] Cerebellar mutism is seen following approximately 8% of posterior fossa tumor removals.[16,57] This complication usually develops during the first postoperative week, often after a period of normal postoperative recovery, and may persist for several months (mean 6.8 weeks).[19] The mutism is followed in approximately 75% of cases with more slowly resolving dysarthric speech. Mutism may also be seen in association with a syndrome of pseudobulbar palsy.[57,73] Like isolated mutism, the syndrome of postoperative pseudobulbar palsy will usually abate after several weeks. Although various theories have been proposed, there is currently no consensus for either the etiology or the prevention of this syndrome. Minimizing midline cerebellar retraction or avoiding a midline vermian incision has been suggested to reduce the incidence.

RADIATION THERAPY

Medulloblastomas are radiosensitive tumors. Craniospinal radiation therapy in combination with surgery has improved survival and is indicated for most medulloblastomas. The incidence of spinal metastasis following spinal irradiation is 13%, as compared with a 75% incidence without postoperative irradiation.[36] Furthermore, the incidence of supratentorial metastasis increases when this region is not irradiated postoperatively.[10] The optimal radiation dose remains a subject of debate. Because of evidence that local control is improved with doses of at least 5000 cGy, this has become a standard regimen for the posterior fossa.[37] A typical plan also includes 4000 to 4500 cGy to the remainder of the intracranial compartment and 3000 to 3500 cGy to the spinal axis. Given the propensity of medulloblastoma to disseminate, radiosurgery is unlikely to supplant conventional craniospinal radiation therapy for patients with this tumor. However, initial reports suggest that radiosurgery can prevent local progression of small recurrent or residual medulloblastomas.[55]

The sequelae of radiation therapy in the developing nervous system can be profound, and have become increasingly important as the survival of patients with medulloblastoma has improved. Cognitive impairment, growth retardation, and leukoencephalopathy are all associated with the use of radiation therapy in children. The vast majority of children with medulloblastoma treated with adjuvant radiation therapy have a decrease in intelligence quotient (IQ).[39] Furthermore, the hypothalamic-pituitary axis is often depressed following posterior fossa irradiation, as evidenced by the high incidence of growth hormone deficiency in patients and an average height in the 25th percentile.[39]

CHEMOTHERAPY

Recent studies have suggested a role for chemotherapy as a postoperative adjuvant for medulloblastoma. Packer et al have reported an 85% overall 5-year survival in high-risk patients receiving chemotherapy in addition to surgery and radiation therapy.[52] The Pediatric Oncology Group demonstrated an improved 5-year survival with surgery, irradiation, and chemotherapy compared with surgery and irradiation alone.[45] Other prospective studies support the benefit of chemotherapy, particularly for patients with metastatic disease or locally unresectable tumors.[22] Chemotherapy may be useful in delaying radiation therapy in children younger than 3 years and in reducing the radiation dose.[17,26]

RECURRENCE

Although a recent study failed to demonstrate a survival benefit, most groups continue to advocate regular surveillance scanning following surgical resection.[47,70] A majority of medulloblastoma recurrences are asymptomatic and could potentially benefit from early treatment. Protocols for surveillance imaging vary. Mendel et al have suggested MRI of the head every 3 months for 2 years, then every 6 months for 2 years, then each year for 5 years.[47] Because late recurrences have been reported, the proper duration of surveillance scanning is not clear.

Most recurrences occur in the posterior fossa, usually in proximity to the site of the primary tumor, although spinal and supratentorial recurrences are also common. The mean time to recurrence is approximately 15 months.[15] The average life expectancy for children with recurrent medulloblastomas varies from 8 months to greater than 27 months.[47] However, long-term survivors have been reported.[15] Local posterior fossa recurrences of medulloblastoma may be treated surgically or with radiation.[18] Diffusely metastatic disease should be treated with chemotherapy.[11,25] Recurrent medulloblastoma will respond to "salvage" chemotherapy in approximately one half of cases, achieving a second remission in approximately one quarter.[11]

OUTCOME

Data from the Childhood Brain Tumor Consortium indicate that from 1930 to 1979 overall survival of patients with medulloblastoma did improve, although not significantly.[29] In recent years, however, with refinement of surgical and radiation therapy for these tumors and the introduction of chemotherapeutic measures, there is reason for greater optimism. Recent studies typically report 5-year survivals exceeding 70% and 5-year progression-free survival of better than 50%.[3,15,52] Predictors of shorter survival include age younger than 3 years at the time of diagnosis, the presence of drop metastases, and postoperative tumor volume.[3,22,38] Survival rates, however, do appear to be improving even for patients in these groups. Packer et al have reported an 85% progression-free survival in a group of patients with either subtotally resected tumors or metastatic spread.[52]

References

1. Albright AL: The value of precraniotomy shunts in children with posterior fossa tumors. Clin Neurosurg 30:278, 1983.
2. Albright AL: Posterior fossa tumors. Neurosurg Clin North Am 3:8818–891, 1992.
3. Albright AL, Wisoff JH, Zeltzler PM, et al: Effects of medulloblastoma resections on outcome in children: a report from the Children's Cancer Group. Neurosurgery 38:265–270, 1996.
4. Bailey P, Cushing H: Medulloblastoma cerebelli, a common type of midcerebellar glioma of childhood. Arch Neurol Psychiatry 14:192–224, 1925.
5. Barkovich AJ: Neuroimaging of pediatric brain tumors. Neurosurgery Clinics of North America 3:739–769, 1992.
6. Berger MS, Baumeister B, Geyer JR, et al: The risks of metastases from shunting in children with primary central nervous system tumors. J Neurosurg 74:872–877, 1991.
7. Biegel J, Burk CD, Barr FG, Emmanuel BS: Evidence for a 17p tumor-related locus distinct from p53 in pediatric primitive neuroectodermal tumors. Cancer Res 52:3391–3395, 1992.
8. Bigner S, Friedman H, Vogelstein B, et al: Amplification of the c-myc gene in human medulloblastoma cell lines and xenografts. Cancer Res 50:2347–2350, 1990.
9. Blaser S, Harwood-Nash DCF: Neuroradiology of pediatric posterior fossa medulloblastomas. J Neurooncology 29:23–34, 1996.
10. Bouffet E, Bernard JL, Frappaz D, et al: M4 protocol for cerebellar medulloblastoma: supratentorial radiotherapy may not be avoided. Int J Radiat Oncol Biol Phys 24:79–85, 1992.
11. Bouffet E, Doz F, Demaille MC, et al: Improving survival in recurrent medulloblastoma: earlier detection, better treatment or still an impasse? Br J Cancer 77:1321–1326, 1998.
12. Chang CH, Housepian EM, Herbert C: An operative staging system and a megavoltage radiotherapeutic technique for cerebellar medulloblastoma. Radiology 93:1351–1359, 1969.
13. Chatty E, Earler KM: Medulloblastoma: A report of 201 cases with emphasis on the relationship of histologic variants to survival. Cancer 28:977, 1971.
14. Cogen P, Daneshvar L, Metzger AK, et al: Involvement of multiple chromosome 17p loci in medulloblastoma tumorigenesis. Am J Hum Genet 50:584–589, 1992.
15. David K, Casey ATH, Hayward RD, et al: Medulloblastoma: is the 5-year survival rate improving? J Neurosurg 86:13–21, 1997.
16. Doxey D, Bruce D, Sklar F, et al: Posterior fossa syndrome: identifiable risk factors and irreversible complications. Pediatr Neurosurg 31:131–136, 1999.
17. Duffner P, Horowitz M, Krisher J, et al: Postoperative chemotherapy and delayed radiation in children less than three years of age with malignant brain tumors. N Engl J Med 24:1725–1731, 1993.
18. Elterman R, Bruce DA: The continued surveillance for recurrent medulloblastoma: primative neuroectodermal tumors. Pediatr Neurosurg 19:322, 1993.
19. Erashin Y, Mutluer S, Cagli S, Duman Y: Cerebellar mutism: report of seven cases and review of the literature. Neurosurgery 38:60–65, 1996.
20. Evans DG, Farndon PA, Burnell LD, et al: The incidence of Gorlin syndrome in 173 consecutive cases of medulloblastoma. Br J Cancer 64:959–961, 1991.
21. Evans DGR, Ladusaris EJ, Rimmer S, et al: Complications of the naevoid basal cell carcinoma syndrome: results of a population based study. J Med Genet 30:460–464, 1993.
22. Evans A, Jenkin RDT, Sposto R, et al: The treatment of medulloblastoma: results of a prospective randomized trial of radiation therapy with and without CCNU, vincristine, and prednisone. J Neurosurg 72:572–582, 1990.
23. Farndon P, Mastro RC, Evans D, Kilpatrick M: Location of gene for Gorlin syndrome. Lancet 339:581–582, 1992.
24. Farwell J, Dohrmann GJ, Flannery JT: Medulloblastoma in childhood: an epidemiological study. J Neurosurg 61:657–664, 1984.
25. Finlay J, Garvin J, Allen J: High-dose chemotherapy with autologous marrow rescue in patients with recurrent medulloblastoma/primitive neuroectodermal tumors. Prog Proc Am Soc Clin Oncol 13:176, 1994.
26. Gentet JC, Bouffet E, Doz F, et al: Preirradiation chemotherapy including "eight drugs in one day" regimen and high-dose methotrexate in childhood medulloblastoma: results of the M7 French Cooperative Study. J Neurosurg 82:608–614, 1995.
27. Giangaspero F, Bigner SH, Kleihues P, et al: Medulloblastoma. In Kleihues P, Cavenee WK (eds): Pathology and Genetics of Tumors of the Nervous System. Lyon, France, International Agency for Research on Cancer Press, 2000.
28. Giangaspero F, Rigobello L, Badiali M, et al: Large cell medulloblastomas. A distinctive variant with highly aggressive behavior. Am J Surg Pathol 16:687–693, 1992.

29. Gilles FH, Sobel EL, Leviton A, et al: Age-related changes in diagnoses, histological features, and survival in children with brain tumors: 1930–1979. Neurosurgery 37:1056–1067, 1995.

30. Gorlin R: Nevoid basal-cell carcinoma syndrome. Medicine 66:98–113, 1987.

31. Grabb PA, Albright AL, Sclabassi RJ, Pollack IF: Continuous intraoperative electromyography of cranial nerves during resection of 4th ventricular tumors in children. J Neurosurg 86:1–4, 1996.

32. Haie-Meder C, Song PY: Medulloblastoma: differences in adults and children. Int J Radiat Oncol Biol Phys 32:1255–1257, 1995.

33. Hamilton SR, Liu B, Parsons RE, et al: The molecular basis of Turcot's syndrome. N Engl J Med 332:839–847, 1995.

34. Hirsch JF, Renier D, Czernichow P, et al: Medulloblastoma in childhood. Survival and functional results. Acta Neurochir 48:1–15, 1979.

35. Hooper JE, Scott MP: The drosophila patched gene encodes a putative membrane protein required for segmental patterning. Cell 59:751–765, 1989.

36. Hubbard J, Scheithauer BW, Kispert DB, et al: Adult cerebellar medulloblastomas: the pathological, radiographic, and clinical disease spectrum. J Neurosurg 70:536–544, 1989.

37. Hughes E, Shillito J, Sallan SE, et al: Medulloblastoma at the Joint Center for Radiation Therapy between 1968 and 1984: the influence of radiation dose on the patterns of failure and survival. Cancer 61:1992–1998, 1988.

38. Jenkin D, Goddard K, Armstrong D, et al: Posterior fossa medulloblastoma in childhood: treatment results and a proposal for a new grading system. Int J Radiat Oncol Biol Phys 19:265–274, 1990.

39. Johnson D, McCabe MA, Nicholson HS, et al: Quality of long-term survival in young children with medulloblastoma. J Neurosurg 80:1004–1010, 1994.

40. Johnson R, Rothman A, Xie J, et al: Human homologue of Patched, a candidate gene for the basal cell nevus syndrome. Science 272:1668–1671, 1996.

41. Karnes P, Tran TN, Cuy MY, et al: Cytogenetic analysis of 39 pediatric central nervous system tumors. Cancer Genet Cytogenet 59:12–19, 1992.

42. Keles G, Berger M, Schofield D, Bothwell M: Nerve growth factor receptor expression in medulloblastomas and the potential role of nerve growth factor as a differentiating agent in medulloblastoma cell lines. Neurosurgery 32:274–280, 1993.

43. Kimonis VE, Goldstein AM, Pastakia B, et al: Clinical manifestations in 105 persons with nevoid basal cell carcinoma syndrome. Am J Med Genet 69:299–308, 1997.

44. Kokunai T, Sawa H, Tatsumi S, Tamaki N: Expression of nerve growth factor receptor by human primitive neuroectodermal tumors. Neurol Med Chir (Tokyo) 34:523–529, 1994.

45. Krischer JP, Ragab AH, Kun L, et al: Nitrogen mustard, vincristine, procarbazine, and prednisone as adjuvant chemotherapy in the treatment of medulloblastoma. J Neurosurg 74:905, 1991.

46. Lee M, Wisoff JH, Abbott R, et al: Management of hydrocephalus in children with medulloblastoma: prognostic factors for shunting. Pediatr Neurosurg 20:240–247, 1994.

47. Mendel E, Levy ML, Raffel C, et al: Surveillance imaging in children with primitive neuroectodermal tumors. Neurosurgery 38:692–694, 1996.

48. MacDonald TJ, Brown KM, LaFleur B, et al: Expression profiling of medulloblastoma: PDGFRA and the RAS/MAPK pathway as therapeutic targets for metastatic disease. Nat Genet 29:143–52, 2001.

49. McDonald J, Daneshvar L, Willert J, et al: Physical mapping of chromosome 1713.3 in the region of the putative tumor suppressor gene important in medulloblastoma. Genomics 23:229–232, 1994.

50. Mori T, Nagase H, Horii A, et al: Germ-line and somatic mutations of the APC gene in patients with Turcot's syndrome and analysis of APC mutations in brain tumors. Genes Chromosomes Cancer 9:168–172, 1994.

51. Nakano Y, Guerrero I, Hidalgo A, et al: A protein with several possible membrane-spanning domains encoded by the drosophila segment polarity gene patched. Nature 341:508–513, 1989.

52. Packer RJ, Sutton LN, Elterman R, et al: Outcome for children with medulloblastoma treated with radiation and cisplatin, CCNU, and vincristine chemotherapy. J Neurosurg 81:690–698, 1994.

53. Paraf F, Jothy S, van Meir EG: Brain-tumor-polyposis syndrome: two genetic diseases? J Clin Oncol 15:2744–2758, 1997.

54. Park T, Hoffman HJ, Hendrick EB, et al: Medulloblastoma: clinical presentation and management. J Neurosurg 58:543–552, 1983.

55. Patrice S, Tarbell NJ, Goumnerova LC, et al: Results of radiosurgery in the management of recurrent and residual medulloblastoma. Pediatr Neurosurg 22:197–203, 1995.

56. Pleasure S, Reddy R, Venkatakrishnan G, et al: Introduction of nerve growth factor (NGF) receptors into a medulloblasoma cell line results in expression of high-and low-affinity NGF receptors but not NGF-mediated differentiation. Proc Natl Acad Sci USA 87:8496–8500, 1990.

57. Pollack IF, Polinko P, Albright AL, et al: Mutism and pseudobulbar symptoms after resection of posterior fossa tumors in children: incidence and pathophysiology. Neurosurgery 37:885–893, 1995.

58. Pomeroy SL, Tamayo P, Gaasenbeek M, et al: Prediction of central nervous system embryonal tumour outcome based on gene expression. Nature 415:436–442, 2002.

59. Raffel C, Thomas GA, Tishler DM, et al: Absence of p53 mutations in childhood central nervous system primitive neuroectodermal tumors. Neurosurgery 33:301–306, 1993.

60. Raffel C, Jenkins RB, Fredrick L, et al: Sporadic medulloblastomas contain the PTCH mutations. Cancer Research 57:842–845, 1997.

61. Roberts RO, Lynch CF, Jones MP, Hart, MN: Medulloblastoma: a population-based study of 532 cases. J Neuropathol Exp Neurol 50:134–144, 1991.

62. Rorke LB: The cerebellar medulloblastoma and its relationship to primitive neuroectodermal tumors. J Neuropathol Exp Neurol 42:1–15, 1983.

63. Rubinstein L: Cytogenesis and differentiation of primitive central neuroepithelial tumors. J Neuropathol Exp Neurol 31:7–26, 1972.

64. Sandhu A, Kendall B: Computed tomography in management of medulloblastomas. Neuroradiology 29:444–452,1987.

65. Schoenberg BS, Shoenberg DG, Christine BW, Gomez MR: The epidemiology of primary intracranial neoplasms of childhood: a population study. Mayo Clin Proc 51:51, 1976.

66. Schofield DE: Diagnostic histopathology, cytogenetics, and molecular markers of pediatric brain tumors. Neurosurg Clin North Am 3:723–738, 1992.

67. Segal R, Goumnerova L, Kwon Y, et al: Expression of the neurotrophin receptor TrkC is linked to a favorable outcome in medulloblastoma. Proc Natl Acad Sci USA 91:12897–12871, 1994.

68. Shofield D, West W, Anthony D, et al: Correlation of heterozygosity at chromosome 9q with histological subtype in medulloblastomas. Am J Path 146:472–480, 1995.

69. Stevens MC, Cameron AH, Muir KR, et al: Descriptive epidemiology of primary central nervous system tumors in children: a population-based study. Clin Oncol (R Coll Radiol) 3:323–329, 1991.

70. Torres CF, Rebsamen S, Silber JH, et al: Surveillance scanning of children with medulloblastoma. N Engl J Med 330:892–895, 1994.

71. Vorechovsky I, Tingby O, Hartman M, et al: Somatic mutations in the human homologue of drosophila patched in primitive neuroectodermal tumors. Oncogene 15:361–366, 1997.

72. Wasson, JR, Zeltzer, P, Friedman, H, et al: Oncogene amplification in pediatric brain tumors. Cancer Res 50:2987–2990, 1990.

73. Wisoff JH, Epstein FJ: Pseudobulbar palsy after posterior fossa operation in children. Neurosurgery 15:707–709, 1984.

74. Wolter M, Reifenberger J, Sommer C, et al: Mutations in the human homologue of the drosophila segment polarity gene patched (PTCH) in sporadic basal cell carcinomas of the skin primitive neuroectodermal developmental abnormalities. Cancer Res 57:2581–2585, 1997.

75. Xie J, Johnson RL, Zhang X, et al: Mutations of the PATCHED gene in several types of sporadic extracutaneous tumors. Cancer Res 57:2369–2372, 1997.

76. Yong W, Raffel C, Deimling AV, Louis D: The APC gene in Turcot's syndrome. N Engl J Med 333:524, 1995.

77. Zurawel R, Chiappa SA, Allen C, Raffel C: Sporadic medulloblastomas contain oncogenic beta-catenin mutations. Cancer Res 58:896–899, 1998.

CHAPTER 90

SUPRATENTORIAL PRIMITIVE NEUROECTODERMAL TUMORS

Mandeep S. Tamber and Peter B. Dirks

Primitive neuroectodermal tumors (PNETs) are a group of highly malignant brain tumors that usually occur in the pediatric population. They comprise a spectrum of lesions that are histologically similar but arise in various locations of the central nervous system. A PNET in the infratentorial compartment is common and is more typically referred to as a medulloblastoma, but above the tentorium they are very uncommon and collectively referred to as *supratentorial PNETs (sPNETs)*. All PNETs are biologically aggressive tumors and tend to spread throughout CSF pathways. Despite their similar histology, there are important differences in prognosis based on PNET location, because medulloblastomas have a much better prognosis compared with their supratentorial counterparts. The scope of this chapter will be limited to discussion of those lesions found in the supratentorial compartment, sPNETs.

CONTROVERSIES IN TERMINOLOGY

Since the first description of PNET by Hart and Earle in 1973,[10] there has been an ongoing and unresolved controversy among neuropathologists with respect to their definition and cytogenesis. Whether they should be categorized according to their location and their pattern of differentiation (e.g., pineoblastoma) or whether they should be considered variants of a single lesion that can occur at any site in the neuraxis (e.g., PNET of the pineal region) has been widely debated. A number of hypotheses have been put forth, but as of yet, no single theory had been validated by clear cytogenetic or neuroembryologic data.

Rubinstein[21] proposed the traditional classification scheme for childhood primitive central neuroepithelial tumors. According to his initial classification, six intracranial tumors could be recognized based on their classic gross and histologic features—medulloepithelioma, cerebral neuroblastoma, polar spongioblastoma, ependymoblastoma, pineoblastoma, and the cerebellar neuroblastoma (classically known as the posterior fossa medulloblastoma). Apart from the medulloblastoma, each of these supratentorial PNETs have been given a putative cell of origin, often indicated by the name of the tumor. By inference, if malignant transformation occurred at one of the particular stages of the cytogenesis of the embryonic forebrain, it could theoretically give rise to PNETs with distinct differentiation potential, from the relatively undifferentiated and highly malignant medulloepithelioma (transformation of early progenitors) to the relatively more differentiated neuronal or glial lines (transformation of more committed progenitors).

Although Rubinstein's classification could account for up to 90% of the primitive embryonal tumors seen in childhood, Hart and Earle,[10] in their review of 23 primitive supratentorial tumors, emphasized that there also exists a group of largely undifferentiated neoplasms that do not fit into any of Rubinstein's categories. According to Hart and Earle, these largely undifferentiated brain tumors (>90% to 95% undifferentiated cells) share enough biologic and pathologic properties to justify classifying them as a single entity, the prototypic "primitive neuroectodermal tumor." This tumor would exist in addition to those tumors described by Rubinstein. The postulated cell of origin of this "PNET" was a primitive neuroepithelial cell capable of differentiating into neuronal, glial, and ependymal cell lines but whose location was not specified.[2,10]

Recently, Rorke[20] proposed that the term PNET be applied to a group of tumors, occurring most commonly in infancy and early childhood, that are primarily composed of undifferentiated neuroepithelial cells and that may contain subpopulations of cells clearly identifiable as astrocytes, ependymal cells, neurons, or other differentiated cells, regardless of the location of these tumors. Rorke suggested that these tumors are basically similar, regardless of their primary site of origin. Three major subclassifications of PNETs were detailed: PNET–not otherwise specified, composed of sheets of poorly differentiated cells; PNET with recognizable cells, along one or more lines of differentiation; and the medulloepithelioma with or without recognizable cells.

Presently, it is unclear whether there is a unique cell of origin in each location where these tumors occur, as per Rubinstein's hypothesis, or whether, as according to Rorke, these lesions arise from a primitive undifferentiated cell common to all parts of the central nervous system, such as those that exist in the subependymal germinal zone during embryologic development and early infancy. Until we have a reliable tumor marker that can identify a cell as, for example, a pineoblast or a neuroblast, the term PNET, as qualified by both location and differentiating features, may indeed be preferable.

What is clear from the previous discussion is that the PNET system is a hypothesis and not a defined morphologic system. Despite their histologic resemblance, so-called PNETs of the cerebral hemispheres and pineal region, collectively referred to as sPNETs, and other embryonal neuroepithelial tumors show clear differences in biologic and clinical behavior. Unfortunately, the underlying uncertainty over the pathologic definition of PNET undermines the validity of clinical studies of cases reported as PNET in the literature—any individual single institution retrospective series, without a clear statement of pathologic criteria, may not be comparable to other series.

EPIDEMIOLOGY

PNETs, if medulloblastomas are included, are the most common malignant intracranial neoplasm in the pediatric population. Medulloblastomas constitute approximately 20% of childhood brain tumors, whereas sPNETs account for only 2.5% to 6% of childhood tumors.[17] Based on Swedish data,[15] the annual incidence of sPNETs is approximately 2 cases per million population.

In various retrospective series, the mean age at first onset falls within the first decade of life.[7,26] In Albright et al's review of 27 sPNETs excluding pineoblastomas,[1] 33% of cases were between ages 1.5 and 3 years, 30% between 3 and 4 years, and 33% between 5 and 9 years. Similarly, in one of the few prospective studies in the literature, Cohen et al[6] report a similar age distribution for both pineal and nonpineal sPNETs—28% between ages 1.5 and less than 3 years, 30% between 3 and 4, and 30% of tumors occurring between ages 5 and 9. Unlike medulloblastoma, which has a clear male sex predilection, sPNETs do not exhibit a similar trend, hinting once again at potential biologic differences between supratentorial and infratentorial PNETs.

DIAGNOSIS

Because of their predilection for occurring in infants and very young children, the initial symptoms and signs of sPNETs are often nonspecific, nonlateralizing signs of elevated intracranial pressure. Therefore vomiting, lethargy, irritability, and anorexia are often patient complaints, with headaches in older children. Seizures may occur. Macrocephaly, full fontanelle, splitting of the cranial sutures, and sunsetting gaze may be seen on examination. A focal neurologic deficit may also occur.

Because these tumors have a propensity for rapid growth, the duration of symptoms is usually relatively short. In the series published by Horten and Rubinstein[11] regarding primary cerebral neuroblastoma, the mean duration of symptoms before diagnosis was 6 weeks. A retrospective review of 28 sPNETs from Korea[26] had children seeking neurosurgical attention within a mean of 4.9 months following symptom onset. Not only is the clinical history short, but when these lesions are brought to clinical attention, they are often large. PNETs of the pineal region (pineoblastomas) often have a more precipitous history than extrapineal or cerebral PNETs, related to earlier onset of obstructive hydrocephalus.

As alluded to earlier, these tumors have a well-established tendency to disseminate via cerebrospinal fluid (CSF) pathways. Therefore a thorough staging evaluation to document evidence of dissemination should be immediately undertaken. In many published series, a significant negative correlation between disseminated disease at diagnosis and outcome has

been documented. Every patient with a new diagnosis of PNET should be evaluated with gadolinium-enhanced magnetic resonance imaging (MRI) of the brain and spine. Usually assessment for CSF dissemination by cytology is reserved for postoperative management.

There is no generally accepted staging system for sPNETs. As is the case for medulloblastoma, the Chang classification[5] is often applied in the staging of sPNETs. M_0 stage, by definition, implies no gross subarachnoid or hematogenous metastases. If tumor cells are found in the CSF, then stage M_1 disease is declared. Gross nodular supratentorial or infratentorial nodular seeding (M_2 disease) or gross nodular seeding in the spinal subarachnoid space (M_3 disease) can be detected by gadolinium-enhanced MRI. Finally, extraneuraxial metastases define stage M_4 disease.

The exact incidence of dissemination throughout the CSF and subarachnoid space, whether at diagnosis or at the time of recurrence, has not been established, because complete staging evaluations have not been uniformly obtained in published reports. In the CCG study, metastatic spread at the time of diagnosis was seen in 4 of 26 patients with nonpineal sPNETs[6] and 4 of 24 patients with pineoblastomas.[13] Seven of 18 completely staged patients with nonpineal sPNETs in the series by Dirks et al[7] had either intracranial ($n = 4$) or spinal ($n = 3$) dissemination at the time of diagnosis. Horten and Rubinstein, in their review of primary cerebral neuroblastoma,[11] noticed asymptomatic tumoral dissemination through the CSF pathways in 38% of cases. Five out of twenty-two patients in a recently published series by Reddy et al[19] had evidence of disseminated disease at diagnosis, and all five of these patients died of progressive disease.

The incidence of metastatic disease in sPNETs appears to be lower than that seen in infratentorial PNETs (medulloblastomas). As shown by Zeltzer et al in the CCG-921 randomized phase III study comparing 8-in-1 chemotherapy both before and after radiation therapy with vincristine, CCNU, and prednisone after radiation therapy, 49% of the 168 patients aged 3 years and older with confirmed medulloblastoma and complete staging had evidence of metastases at diagnosis.[27] This discrepancy has been postulated to be due to the comparatively lower access of sPNETs to the CSF pathways.

IMAGING

Because sPNETs appear to be histologically similar irrespective of their primary site of origin in the neuraxis, so too can it be said of their radiographic appearance. In essence, there is no pathognomonic appearance that distinguishes the various sPNETs among themselves or from other malignant childhood brain tumors. Nevertheless, there are certain imaging characteristics that, when present, may lead the clinician to suspect a PNET in the differential diagnosis of an intracranial mass lesion (Figure 90-1).

Cranial computed tomography (CT) and MRI both show sharply circumscribed, expansile but not infiltrative, heterogeneous masses usually located in the deep frontoparietal white matter. They are often said to have a periventricular epicenter. The lesions are often very large. They tend to compress the surrounding brain parenchyma. A cystic component is common, representing either necrosis or old hemorrhage. Foci of calcification are also commonly observed, and there is a conspicuous

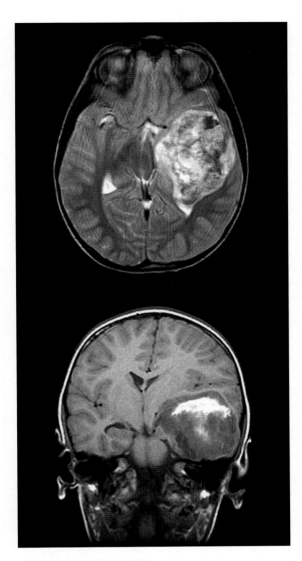

FIGURE 90-1 Four-year-old boy who had headache and signs of raised intracranial pressure. Magnetic resonance imaging reveals a large mass in the left temporal lobe, which proved to be a primitive neuroectodermal tumor.

lack of reactive vasogenic edema. These lesions show heterogeneous contrast enhancement on CT and MRI. On MRI scans, T1 signal characteristics are variable, depending on the presence and timing of intratumoral hemorrhage. They generally have high T2 signal, with the cystic components being slightly brighter than CSF, indicating a high protein content within the cyst. Pineoblastomas are difficult to distinguish from the more common pineal region germ cell tumors. Pineoblastomas also have a heterogeneous CT and MRI appearance. Because of their location, they often cause an obstructive hydrocephalus.

PATHOLOGY

Grossly, sPNETs may be described as well-circumscribed lesions with a sharp demarcation from adjacent normal brain parenchyma, typically showing foci of cystic degeneration, necrosis, calcification, and hemorrhage. The prototypic histologic appearance of sPNETs is that of a fairly uniform population of undifferentiated small blue cells, with scant cytoplasm, darkly staining nuclei, a high nuclear-to-cytoplasmic ratio, and frequent mitotic figures. There is often an underlying fine fibrillary stromal network. There may be foci of glial, neuronal, or ependymal differentiation apparent on either routine light microscopy or on electron microscopy (EM) or immunohistochemical studies. Blood vessels are abundant, often with evidence of endothelial proliferation; there may be areas of glial fibrillary acidic protein (GFAP) positively staining cells in the immediate vicinity of areas of endothelial proliferation. These tumors may invade the meninges and produce a malignant meningeal gliomatosis adjacent to the tumor. They often show evidence of microscopic invasion into the surrounding brain parenchyma.

According to Rorke's classification, the PNET–not otherwise specified is composed of sheets of uniform small primitive cells as described previously; typically, more than 90% of the cells in the preparation have to have this appearance to carry this designation. The medulloepithelioma, the most primitive of the sPNETs, thought to be derived from the neural tube epithelium itself, resembles the pattern of the medullary plate. The tissue may merge into sheets of primitive cells without differentiation, or show evidence of differentiation along one or multiple cellular lines—neuronal, astrocytic, oligodendroglial, or ependymal.

Rorke's PNET with neuronal differentiation (also called *cerebral neuroblastoma* by Rubinstein) may show a high frequency of Homer-Wright rosettes and focal differentiation into ganglion cells. Such cells may be neuron specific enolase (NSE)-positive in clusters but do not stain for GFAP. Horten and Rubinstein[11] proposed that cerebral neuroblastoma could be distinguished from other sPNETs histologically based on the absence of glial differentiation, less than 90% to 95% overall cellular nondifferentiation, and a lesser degree of cellular pleomorphism and endothelial hyperplasia in cerebral neuroblastomas when compared with PNETs differentiated along other cell lines. Furthermore, by their observations, they were able to categorize three distinct variants of cerebral neuroblastoma on the basis of the degree of connective tissue present. "Classic" neuroblastoma, which most closely resembles peripheral neuroblastoma, has a scant connective tissue stroma and a higher frequency of differentiated ganglion cells. Variants with a more prominent connective tissue stroma are named *desmoplastic*, and those with intermediate histology are called *transitional*.

PNET with astrocytic differentiation (Rubinstein's polar spongioblastoma) have cells aligned in rows of parallel palisades, with each row being separated by relatively acellular tissue. Foci of astrocytic differentiation are usually seen, hence the name. PNET with ependymal differentiation (ependymoblastoma according to Rubinstein) may show ependymal rosettes and tubules in addition to the background population of undifferentiated cells. PNETs may also differentiate along myoblastic and melanocytic cell lineages. Pineoblastomas have a microscopic signature similar to that of other PNETs. They tend to be densely populated tumors, composed of largely undifferentiated cells, and occasionally showing Homer-Wright rosettes. The general consensus in the literature is that the prognosis in sPNETs is not related to either the degree of differentiation within the tumor or the line along which differentiation is seen.[12]

Comparative genomic hybridization studies have provided further data to support the clinical observation that supratentorial PNETs are fundamentally different from infratentorial PNETs (medulloblastoma).[22] Three areas of the genome were found to be distinct by statistical analysis. Medulloblastomas showed a gain of isochromosome 17q in 37% of tumors analyzed; this copy number aberration was not seen in any sPNET analyzed. Similarly, 40% of sPNETs had loss of chromosome 14q, a finding absent in the medulloblastoma samples analyzed. Finally, loss of chromosome 19q was seen in 40% of sPNETs and only 2% of medulloblastomas analyzed. The common finding of loss of chromosomes 14q and 19q may implicate the involvement of a tumor-suppressor gene located on these chromosomes in the development of sPNETs.

By analyzing the pattern of gene expression in medulloblastoma and sPNETs, Pomeroy et al[18] were able to provide further data supporting the hypothesis that these two classes of embryonal tumors are molecularly distinct.

TREATMENT

Until recently, the prognosis for children with pineal and nonpineal sPNETs had been dismal, with most patients dying of their disease within 2 years of diagnosis.[10] Recent aggressive multimodality treatment regimens encompassing radiation therapy and chemotherapy, on a foundation of aggressive surgical resection, have produced slightly more encouraging results. Many of the treatment protocols applied in older series have been extrapolated from those used to treat medulloblastoma. Except for the recent CCG studies,[6,13] the contemporary literature is crowded with numerous retrospective case studies of a small number of patients treated in a heterogeneous fashion, which makes statistically meaningful analysis of the data extremely difficult. Nevertheless, despite the rarity of high quality prospective clinical series examining treatment issues in sPNETs, certain general therapeutic recommendations can be put forth.[12]

SURGERY

Aggressive surgical resection is felt to be the cornerstone of multimodality therapy in the contemporary management of sPNETs. Gross-total tumor resection has been advocated; however, the size, vascularity, multilobe, and deep location of these lesions often precludes such an approach. Gross-total resection should still be the goal, if this can be undertaken with an acceptable rate of perioperative morbidity and mortality, although the effect of this on prognosis is not well understood.

Several retrospective and prospective series have provided evidence to support the notion that the frequency of local (and possibly remote) recurrence may be related to the extent of initial surgical resection.[25] In Albright's report of 27 nonpineal sPNETs treated with aggressive surgery, radiation therapy, and chemotherapy,[1] progression-free survival with total resection appeared to be better than with less than total resection, although this finding was not found to be statistically significant, likely because of small numbers. Patients with less than 1.5 cm^2 of residual tumor on postoperative imaging fared slightly better than patients with more than 1.5 cm^2 of residual, with a 4-year survival of 40% ± 22% in the former group com-

pared with 13% ± 8% in the latter (P = .19). Similarly, a trend toward a better outcome with aggressive surgery was also borne out in the series of Reddy et al,[19] where the 5-year progression-free survival in those with complete or near complete resection versus partial resection or biopsy was 53% versus 25% (P = .22). In a recently published retrospective review of 28 sPNETs from Korea,[26] univariate analysis showed that the extent of resection was one of only two variables to correlate with survival. Dirks' review of the Hospital for Sick Children experience also showed a trend to better outcome with gross total excision.[7] Because of small numbers, it has been more difficult to prove the benefit of aggressive surgical resection in pineal region sPNETs. In the CCG study examining the multimodality treatment of pineoblastomas,[13] 2 of 6 patients with greater than 90% resection had delayed disease progression (2.7 and 5.9 years following diagnosis), whereas 4 of 11 patients with less than 90% resection who also had documented disease progression did so while undergoing adjuvant therapy postoperatively. However, the progression-free survival for patients with pineoblastoma treated with radiation therapy and chemotherapy was not statistically significant between those who had greater than or less than 90% resection (P > 0.3).

RADIATION THERAPY

Although radiation therapy has long been the cornerstone of treatment of malignant central nervous system neoplasms, concern over the late sequelae of neuraxis irradiation in children has led to the additional provision of chemotherapy to standard- and reduced-dose radiation therapy regimens, as well as to the evaluation of alternate modes of radiation delivery, including the use of hyperfractionation.

There have been few controlled studies examining the role of radiation therapy in the treatment of sPNETs. However, the utility of radiation therapy in managing these lesions can be inferred from various indirect observations. For instance, young age has consistently been demonstrated to be an adverse prognostic factor for pineal sPNETs.[7,13] Although infants may harbor tumors that are inherently biologically more aggressive, the difference in outcome between younger and older children may be due in part to the fact that infants and younger children tend to receive an attenuated dose of radiation, if they receive any at all, in an attempt to minimize the profound adverse neurocognitive sequelae of intense radiation therapy on the developing nervous system. In the recently published prospective trial examining the role of radiation therapy in the treatment of sPNETs,[24] the investigators made several important observations. Immediate postoperative radiation therapy followed by maintenance chemotherapy led to a superior outcome compared with children who received preirradiation chemotherapy, and progression of disease occurred predominantly in children who received preirradiation chemotherapy. The authors postulated that the poorer results seen in the preirradiation chemotherapy arm of the trial were due to the delay in initiating radiation therapy in those children who received preirradiation chemotherapy, rather than to any difference in the chemotherapeutic protocols themselves. Thus the authors recommended that radiation therapy should immediately follow surgery. Furthermore, it was noted that any modification of the established radiation therapy protocol (total neuraxis dose of 35.2 Gy with a boost to the primary tumor site of 20 Gy), either by reducing the total dose administered, omitting craniospinal irradiation altogether, or by restricting fields, was associated with a significantly diminished 3-year progression-free survival—49.3% in those children irradiated according to the protocol versus 6.7% in those with major violations.

The optimal dose of radiation to be used in the treatment of sPNETs has not yet been established, largely because of the disparity in the results of standard- versus low-dose regimens. Moreover, in some studies, radiation therapy has been used as the sole postoperative adjuvant treatment, whereas in others, radiation has been combined with a myriad of different chemotherapeutic regimens. The suggested tumor dose is 54 to 56 Gy, using conventional fractionation, initiated between 4 and 6 weeks postoperatively. Craniospinal irradiation with 23.4 to 36 Gy is also recommended, regardless of the patient's M stage at diagnosis, because of the known propensity of these tumors to disseminate in the subarachnoid space. Despite the relatively standard implementation of prophylactic craniospinal irradiation, it is difficult to definitively state how much this management philosophy has contributed to the recent gains in overall survival.

CHEMOTHERAPY

sPNETs are susceptible to chemotherapy because of their prominent vascularity, high growth fraction, and inherent biologic chemosensitivity. There has been insufficient historical evidence regarding chemotherapy and its correlation with improved survival, because there have not been any published series where patients have been treated in a standardized manner. Despite the recent prospective reports published by the CCG,[6,13] the role of adjuvant chemotherapy in the multimodality treatment of pineal and nonpineal sPNETs is still unclear, as all patients randomized in the CCG protocol received chemotherapy according to one regimen or another. In a retrospective review of older studies, there was no difference in survival between those treated with and without chemotherapy. However, long-term survival rates with adjuvant chemotherapy, whatever the regimen, have been higher in recent articles, suggesting that chemotherapy does have a definite role to play in the management of children with sPNETs.

In patients older than 3 years, both pineal and nonpineal sPNETs appear to be at least transiently responsive to neoadjuvant or adjuvant chemotherapy.[14] Pineal region sPNETs in infants and younger children may be less chemosensitive, according to data released in the CCG trial of 8-in-1 chemotherapy.[9] All eight infants with pineoblastomas treated with postoperative 8-in-1 chemotherapy alone developed progressive disease within 3 to 14 months from the start of treatment; the median time to death was 10 months.[6] Compared with the results seen for children with pineal-region sPNETs, infants with nonpineal sPNETs may have a better response rate to chemotherapy.[8]

The optimal chemotherapeutic regimen has yet to be elucidated. The results of the 1995 CCG randomized controlled trial revealed no difference in outcome for children treated with a regimen of craniospinal irradiation followed by eight cycles of CCNU, vincristine, and prednisone versus two cycles of 8-in-1 chemotherapy followed by craniospinal irradiation and then eight additional cycles of 8-in-1 chemotherapy. The 3-year progression-free survival was 57% ± 8% in the former treat-

ment arm, and 45% ± 8% in the latter. However, there was greater toxicity related to treatment in the 8-in-1 arm of the trial.

A recently published study investigating the role of high-dose cyclophosphamide, vincristine, and cisplatin with stem cell rescue following surgery and radiation therapy for medulloblastoma and sPNETs demonstrated that this protocol was both feasible and safe, with a low incidence of hematologic and infectious morbidity and without any toxic deaths.[23]

TREATMENT RECOMMENDATIONS

For infants with pineal region sPNETs, cumulative data suggest that chemotherapy alone is insufficient; however, given the severe and irreversible sequelae of cranial irradiation in infancy, there remains no reasonable alternative treatment with proven efficacy. Data on high-dose chemotherapy and stem cell rescue are forthcoming.

For older children with pineal region sPNETs, the survival data following postsurgical craniospinal irradiation and adjuvant chemotherapy is much more promising than that reported for infants, and is significantly better than previously thought. Thus this appears to be the optimal therapy, as long as the long-term sequelae of treatment are not prohibitive. Which chemotherapeutic agents should be used, at what dose, and whether neoadjuvant therapy offers any benefit compared with conventional adjuvant therapy remains to be elucidated.

A significant percentage of infants with nonpineal sPNETs may be effectively treated with surgery and chemotherapy alone.

Older children with nonpineal sPNETs should probably continue to be treated in a multimodality fashion with optimal surgical resection and craniospinal irradiation with a boost to the primary tumor site followed by adjuvant chemotherapy. As stated earlier, whether chemotherapy improves survival has yet to be determined.

RECURRENCE

Because of the propensity of sPNETs to disseminate widely along the entire neuraxis via CSF circulation pathways, recurrence in these lesions is not uncommon. Not surprisingly, disease recurrence may be at the primary tumor site, or at noncontiguous central nervous system sites. In general, early detection of asymptomatic recurrences carries a better prognosis than detection when symptoms or signs appear. At the time of relapse, a complete evaluation for the extent of recurrence is mandated; this includes complete gadolinium-enhanced MRI of the brain and spine.

The timing of recurrence is variable but often occurs early in the post-treatment phase. In Albright's series,[1] all but one of the recurrences occurred within the first 2 years post-treatment, and fully 50% were within the first year, while most patients were still undergoing treatment.

Biopsy or surgical resection may be necessary to confirm relapse; however, the need for surgical intervention must be individualized based on the initial tumor type, the location of relapse, the length of time between initial treatment and the reappearance of the lesion, and the overall clinical picture. Chemotherapy affords a low and transient response rate, even with high-dose regimens. Most patients die within 1 year of relapse. It is recommended that patients with sPNETs, including pineoblastomas, that recur after radiation alone be considered for treatment with known active chemotherapeutic agents, including vincristine, cyclophosphamide, cisplatin, carboplatin, and etoposide. Entry into studies of novel therapeutic approaches at the time of relapse after radiation therapy alone or radiation therapy and chemotherapy should be considered.

OUTCOME AND PROGNOSIS

In general, children with sPNETs have a poorer overall outcome when compared with medulloblastoma, a histologically identical tumor located within the posterior fossa. Even patients with poor risk medulloblastoma have been reported to have good outcomes, with 5-year disease-free survival reported to be 85% ± 6% in one recent report.[16] Patients in this study were treated with surgical resection followed by craniospinal irradiation with a local boost to the tumor bed and adjuvant chemotherapy that included vincristine, CCNU, and cisplatin. For children with sPNETs treated with an identical protocol, the 5-year progression-free survival was 37%, and the overall survival rate at 5 years was 53%.[19] Fundamental discrepancies in the biology of supratentorial and infratentorial primitive neuroectodermal tumors more than likely underlie the differences seen in their clinical behavior.

Furthermore, it should be emphasized that the prognosis following aggressive multimodality therapy is not uniform for all sPNETs. Within the supratentorial compartment, pineoblastomas appear to behave differently than nonpineal sPNETs.[7] It is possible to dissect out a subset of lesions, within the spectrum of sPNETs, that may have a more favorable prognosis.

In the first prospective randomized treatment trial for patients with sPNETs published by the CCG,[6,13] it was quite convincingly shown that the survival of older children with PNETs of the pineal region who were treated postoperatively with combined radiation therapy and chemotherapy was higher than previously thought. The estimated 3-year progression-free survival and overall survival rates in children older than 18 months of age at diagnosis were 61% ± 13% and 73% ± 12%, respectively. This was far superior to the 3-year progression-free survival of nonpineal (cortical) sPNETs in older children, which was found to be 33% ± 9%, a value far worse than that seen for pineoblastoma and medulloblastoma. Although pineal region of origin appears to be a favorable prognostic factor, it should be remembered that children younger than 18 months who were treated with chemotherapy without radiation therapy continue to have a dismal prognosis, with a 2-year progression-free survival of 9% ± 9%.

Some older literature suggests that among the nonpineal sPNETs, those that have a histology consistent with cerebral neuroblastoma may in fact have a natural history distinct from that of other cortical sPNETs.[3,4] In Berger's series[4] 7 of 11 patients with primary cerebral neuroblastoma were alive and stable without evidence of disease progression. Furthermore, patients with predominantly cystic tumors tended to fare better than those with solid tumors, with disease-free intervals ranging from 26 to 109 months after treatment for cystic lesions versus 52 months for solid lesions. In Rubinstein's cohort[3] a total of 42 patients were alive after a minimum follow-up of 3 years, with an overall 3-year survival rate of 60%.

With respect to ultimate clinical outcome, two variables appear to have a proportionately greater prognostic significance than any other: age and M stage at diagnosis.

Young age has consistently been shown to be an adverse prognostic factor in pineoblastoma.[13] The impact of age in nonpineal sPNETs is somewhat less clear. In the CCG study examining outcome in nonpineal sPNETs,[1] children aged 19 to 36 months, who received an attenuated dose of radiation had a significantly worse progression-free survival than older children who received full-dose irradiation. However, infants treated with 8-in-1 chemotherapy alone appeared to have a similar 3-year progression-free survival to that seen for older children treated with full-dose radiation.[9]

The most important prognostic factor for patients with nonpineal sPNETs in the CCG study[1] was M stage at diagnosis, with all patients who had M_1 stage disease or worse at diagnosis going on to develop progressive or recurrent disease. Three-year progression-free survival was 50% for M_0 disease versus 0% for M_1 or worse disease.[6] Although the number of patients with pineal region sPNETs and dissemination at diagnosis was small, a trend toward poorer prognosis with advanced M stage was also observed.[13]

References

1. Albright AL, Wiscoff JH, Zeltzer P, et al: Prognostic factors in children with supratentorial (nonpineal) primitive neuroectodermal tumors. Pediat Neurosurg 22:1–7, 1995.
2. Becker LE, Hinton D: Primitive neuroectodermal tumors of the central nervous system. Hum Pathol 14:538–550, 1983.
3. Bennett JP, Rubinstein LJ: The biological behavior of primary cerebral neuroblastoma: a reappraisal of the clinical course in a series of 70 cases. Ann Neurol 16:21–27, 1984.
4. Berger MS, Edwards MSB, Wara WM, et al: Primary cerebral neuroblastoma: long-term follow-up review and therapeutic guidelines. J Neurosurg 59:418–423, 1983.
5. Chang CH, Houseplan EM, Herbert C: An operative staging system for a megavoltage radiotherapeutic technique for cerebellar medulloblastomas. Radiology 93:1351–1359, 1969.
6. Cohen BH, Zeltzer PM, Boyett JM, et al: Prognostic factors and treatment results for supratentorial primitive neuroectodermal tumors in children using radiation and chemotherapy: a Children's Cancer Group randomized trial. J Clin Oncol 13:1687–1696, 1995.
7. Dirks PB, Harris L, Hoffman H, et al: Supratentorial primitive neuroectodermal tumors in children. J Neurooncol 29:75–84, 1996.
8. Duffner PK, Horowitz ME, Krischer JP, et al: Postoperative chemotherapy and delayed radiation in children less than three years of age with malignant brain tumors. N Engl J Med 328:1725–1731, 1993.
9. Geyer JR, Zeltzer PM, Boyett JM, et al: Survival of infants with primitive neuroectodermal tumors or malignant ependymomas of the CNS treated with eight drugs in 1 day: a report from the Children's Cancer Group. J Clin Oncol 12:1607–1615, 1994.
10. Hart MN, Earle KM: Primitive neuroectodermal tumors of the brain in children. Cancer 32:890–897, 1973.

11. Horten BC, Rubinstein LJ: Primary cerebral neuroblastomas. A clinicopathological study of 35 cases. Brain 99:735–756, 1976.
12. Jakacki RI: Pineal and nonpineal supratentorial primitive neuroectodermal tumors. Childs Nerv Syst 15:586–591, 1999.
13. Jakacki RI, Zeltzer PM, Boyett JM, et al: Survival and prognostic factors following radiation and/or chemotherapy for primitive neuroectodermal tumors of the pineal region in infants and children: a report of the children's cancer group. J Clin Oncol 13:1377–1383, 1995.
14. Kovnar EH, Kellie SJ, Horowitz ME, et al: Pre-irradiation cisplatin and etoposide in the treatment of high-risk medulloblastoma and other malignant embryonal tumors of the central nervous system: a phase II study. J Clin Oncol 8:330–336, 1990.
15. Lannering B, Marky I, Nordborg C: Brian tumors in childhood and adolescence in West Sweden 1970–1984. Epidemiology and Survival. Cancer 66:604–609, 1990.
16. Packer RJ, Sutton LN, Elterman R, et al: Outcome for children with medulloblastoma treated with radiation and cisplatin, CCNU, and vincristine chemotherapy. J Neurosurg 81:690–698, 1994.
17. Pollack IF: Brain tumors in children. N Engl J Med 331:1500–1507, 1994.
18. Pomeroy SL, Tamayo P, Gaasenbeek M, et al: Prediction of central nervous system embryonal tumor outcome based on gene expression. Nature 415:436–442, 2002.
19. Reddy AT, Janss AJ, Phillips PC, et al: Outcome for children with supratentorial primitive neuroectodermal tumors treated with surgery, radiation, and chemotherapy. Cancer 88:2189–2193, 2000.
20. Rorke LB: The cerebellar medulloblastoma and its relationship to primitive neuroectodermal tumors. J Neuropath and Experimental Neuro 42:1–15, 1983.
21. Rubinstein LJ: Embryonal central neuroepithelial tumors and their differentiating potential: a cytogenetic view of a complex neuro-oncological problem. J Neurosurg 62:795–805, 1985.
22. Russo C, Pellarin M, Tingby O, et al: Comparative genomic hybridization in patients with supratentorial and infratentorial primitive neuroectodermal tumors. Cancer 86:331–339, 1999.
23. Strother D, Ashley D, Kellie SJ, et al: Feasibility of four consecutive high-dose chemotherapy cycles with stem-cell rescue for patients with newly diagnosed medulloblastoma or supratentorial primitive neuroectodermal tumors after craniospinal radiotherapy: results of a collaborative study. J Clin Oncol 19:2696–2704, 2001.
24. Timmermann B, Kortmann RD, Kuhl J, et al: Role of radiotherapy in the treatment of supratentorial primitive neuroectodermal tumors in childhood: results of the Prospective German Brain Tumor Trials HIT 88/89 and 91. J Clin Oncol 20:842–849, 2002.
25. Tomita T, McLone DG, Yasue M: Cerebral primitive neuroectodermal tumors in childhood. J Neurooncol 6:233–243, 1988.
26. Yang HJ, Nam DH, Wang KC, et al: Supratentorial primitive neuroectodermal tumors in children: clinical features, treatment outcome and prognostic factors. Childs Nerv Syst 15:377–383, 1999.
27. Zeltzer PM, Boyett JM, Finlay JL, et al: Metastasis stage, adjuvant treatment, and residual tumor are prognostic factors for medulloblastoma in children: conclusions from the Children's Cancer Group 921 randomized phase III study. J Clin Oncol 17:832–845, 1999.

CHAPTER 91

DYSEMBRYOPLASTIC
NEUROEPITHELIAL TUMOR

Michael D. Taylor, Todd Mainprize, and Cynthia Hawkins

Dysembryoplastic neuroepithelial tumor (DNET) was first described in 1988 during a pathologic review of surgical specimens from patients undergoing epilepsy surgery. The authors identified a series of low-grade lesions that shared the common features of multinodular architecture, foci of dysplastic cortical disorganization, and the presence of a specific histopathologic element demonstrating a columnar structure perpendicular to the cortical surface. Subsequently, many other centers began to diagnose DNETs among their young patients with chronic pharmacoresistant epilepsy. DNET has been included in the recent World Health Organization (WHO) classification under the category of neuronal and mixed glial-neuronal tumors.

SIGNS AND SYMPTOMS

DNETs are usually diagnosed in children or young adults with long-standing, partial seizures that have an onset before the age of 20 years and who have no neurologic deficit or a stable congenital deficit, a normal intellect, and no stigmata of phacomatosis.[1] Although there is no known associated environmental exposure associated with DNET, it has very rarely been reported in children with neurofibromatosis type 1. There is a slight male predominance (23:16) in the original report.[2] The age of onset of symptoms (almost always seizures) was 1 to 19 years, with a mean of 9 years.[2] DNET does on occasion occur for the first time in adulthood. Many children have years of medical treatment for their seizure disorder before undergoing surgery, so that the age at operation ranged from 3 to 30 years (mean of 18 years).[2]

Almost all patients with a DNET have partial complex seizures, although approximately 15% of DNET patients with seizures can undergo secondary generalization.[2] The epilepsy syndromes in patients with DNET are disabling, with 75% of patients experiencing one or more seizures per day. Epilepsy in patients with DNET is classically pharmacoresistant. In the original description of DNET, 7.5% of patients undergoing epilepsy surgery harbored a DNET.[2] In other centers, the experience differs. In one report of 430 surgical specimens from patients with pharmacoresistant epilepsy, 92 patients had tumors on pathologic examination. Of those 92 tumors, the great majority (74 of 92) were DNETs, with gangliogliomas, low-grade astrocytomas, and oligodendrogliomas being seen infrequently.[6] The reason for this tremendous difference in rate is uncertain but may relate in part to increased recognition of DNETs in recent years. Some patients may have headaches (2 of 39 patients), and some may have elevated intracranial pressure and papilledema.[2] Other patients have been reported to have fixed, congenital neurologic deficits, including quadrantanopias and dysphasia.[13] Patients may also notice a skull prominence over the site of the lesion (see following discussion on imaging).[13] DNET can, rarely, cause acute intratumoral hemorrhage with a catastrophic clinical picture.[14] Indeed, evidence of small, asymptomatic, chronic hemorrhage can often be seen on pathologic examination (hemosiderin), and repeated small bleeds could lead to the incorrect impression of a cavernoma on magnetic resonance imaging (MRI). Most cases of DNET are diagnosed in the temporal lobe (62%) or frontal lobe (31%), with rare cases being reported elsewhere in the cerebral hemispheres, deep gray nuclei, and the posterior fossa. It is uncertain whether DNETs are in fact more common in the temporal and frontal lobes or whether lesions in these locations come more often to medical attention and surgery because of the known epileptogenicity of these regions.

IMAGING

Computed tomography (CT) imaging of DNET shows a well-demarcated, hypodense lesion, usually located in the temporal or frontal lobes.[1] Calcifications can be seen in up to 23% of cases, indicative of the chronicity of the lesion.[2] In patients with superficial tumors, there is commonly a deformity of the overlying bone (up to 60% of patients), and when the DNET is located in deep temporal structures, there may be enlargement of the middle cranial fossa.[9] It is important to note, however, that the CT scan can appear normal in up to 25% of patients later shown to have a DNET on MRI.[13]

The imaging modality of choice in patients with DNET is MRI with and without gadolinium enhancement. MRI shows a well-demarcated, hypointense signal on T1-weighted images, and a hyperintense signal on T2-weighted images (Figure 91-1).[8] Proton density images demonstrate a slightly higher signal intensity in the DNET than in cerebrospinal fluid and can be used to differentiate DNET from cystic lesions.[8] MRI shows much better than CT the cortical location of the tumor, which often resembles a "megagyrus."[1] Indeed, all cases of DNET are cortical or immediately subcortical. Gadolinium enhancement is present in some cases (around 18% of DNETs), and there may even be a ring enhancement in some cases.[1] Peritumoral

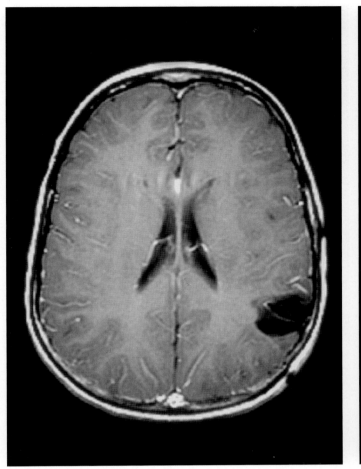

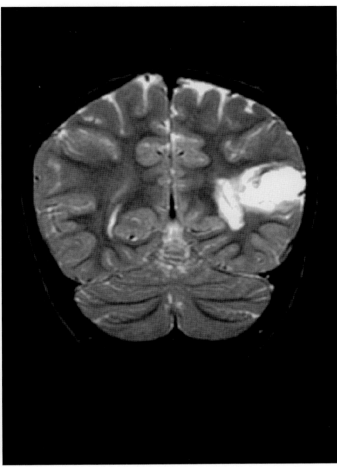

A

B

FIGURE 91-1 Magnetic resonance (MR) image of dysembryoplastic neuroepithelial tumor (DNET). Axial T1-weighted *(A)* and coronal T2-weighted *(B)* MR images with gadolinium contrast show a hypointense, nonenhanced, cortically based lesion typical of DNET.

edema is not seen and should suggest other entities such as low-grade glioma. Several authors have reported multifocal, noncontiguous DNET lesions and, as such, multiple lesions do not exclude a diagnosis of DNET.

PATHOLOGY

In the revised WHO classification of brain tumors, DNET has been included in the category of neuronal and mixed neuroglial tumors.[7] Grossly, at the time of surgery, the tumor appears as expanded cortex or a megagyrus and has a characteristic semi-liquid appearance, which may be associated with firmer nodules.[1] The tumor can be multifocal and, although it shows a marked predominance for temporal and frontal lobes, it can rarely be found elsewhere in the hemisphere, in the deep gray matter, and even in the posterior fossa.[10]

Microscopically, foci of cortical dysplasia are found adjacent to DNETs in 50% to 90% of cases, depending on the quality and extent of the specimen.[3,11] Among temporal lobe resections in patients with chronic epilepsy and DNET, the incidence of ipsilateral hippocampal sclerosis is uncertain, because

some authors did not ever find it, whereas others found it in up to 26% of cases.[6,13] On examination of the tumor itself, three histologic variants have been distinguished: the complex, simple, and nonspecific forms.[3] Although this subcategorization of DNETs has no clinical or therapeutic implications, it does reflect variable difficulties in terms of diagnosis.

In the simple form, the tumor consists of the so-called unique glioneuronal element (Figure 91-2). This element has a characteristic columnar appearance, oriented perpendicularly to the cortical surface. The columns are composed of bundles of axons lined by small oligodendrocyte-like cells (OLCs). The basic nature of these cells remains unresolved; they are S-100 positive and GFAP-negative, with subpopulations of cells staining for oligodendroglial or neuronal markers suggesting a mixed origin. Scattered GFAP-positive stellate astrocytes may also be seen. Between the columns, neurons appear to float in a pale, mucinous matrix.[1] Both within the tumor and in adjacent areas of cortical dysplasia, the neurons may show various degrees of cytologic atypia. However, DNETs do not contain atypical neurons that resemble ganglion cells or lymphocytes, features that are important in distinguishing them from gangliogliomas.

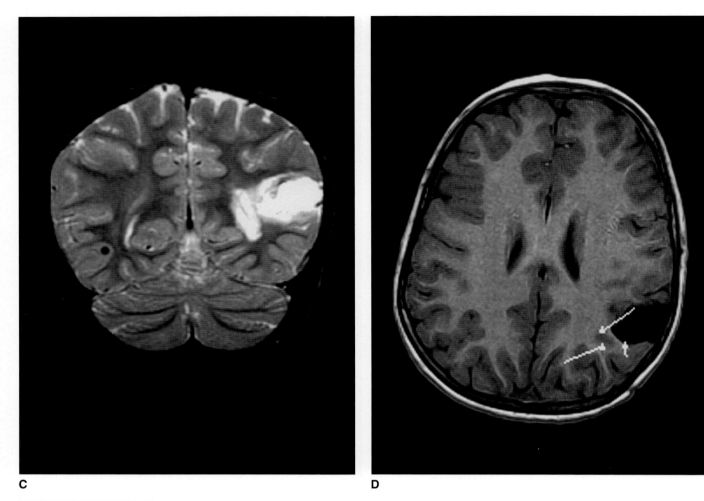

C   D

FIGURE 91-1 cont'd. *C,* The DNET is hyperintense on T2-weighted images. *D,* Because this patient had pharmacoresistent epilepsy, magnetoencephalography was done and shows interictal spikes arising from brain just posterior to the tumor.

In the complex form, glial nodules, which give the tumor a characteristic multinodular architecture, are seen in association with the glioneuronal element or foci of cortical dysplasia. The glial components have a highly variable appearance. They may be nodular or diffuse and usually resemble conventional categories of low-grade gliomas but may show nuclear atypia, mitoses, necrosis, or microvascular proliferation. In DNETs, however, the latter features do not seem to indicate a worse prognosis. Similarly the MIB-1 proliferative index has been reported to vary from 0% to 8% and does not seem to be of prognostic utility, nor is it helpful in distinguishing DNETs from ordinary gliomas.

The nonspecific form is the most controversial and is primarily championed by Daumas-Duport and colleagues. Others are skeptical of its existence, because it does not contain the glioneuronal element and cannot be objectively distinguished on morphologic criteria from ordinary gliomas. According to Daumas-Duport, a diagnosis of the nonspecific form of DNET should be considered when a histologically glial neoplasm is associated with all of the following: (1) partial seizures, with or without secondary generalization beginning before age 20; (2) no neurologic deficit or the presence of a stable and likely congenital neurologic deficit; (3) cortical topography of the lesion, best demonstrated on MRI; and (4) no mass effect on CT or MRI (except when related to a cyst).[3]

Abnormal hamartomatous vessels have been seen in cases of DNET that caused hemorrhage.[1,6] Angiography of patients with DNET has shown neovascularization of the tumor in a minority of cases.[2] Histologically, they are delicate, thin-walled, branching capillaries with an arcuate pattern that can be calcified, suggesting that they may have impaired vasoconstriction.[14] These delicate capillaries run freely through the mucoid matrix of the specific glioneuronal element where they can be vulnerable to the common microtrauma found in patients with recurrent seizures.[14]

The biology of DNET is poorly understood. There are conflicting opinions in the literature as to whether DNETs are true neoplasms or hamartomas. Several factors suggest that DNETs have a dysembryoplastic origin: the presence of foci of cortical dysplasia, young age at onset of symptoms, and the evidence of deformity of the overlying skull on neuroimaging.[1] It has been suggested that DNETs can arise from a transient embryologic structure known as the *fetal subpial granular layer* that involutes during the course of normal development.[1]

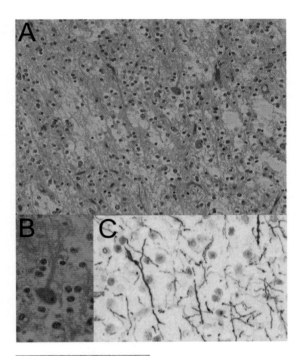

FIGURE 91-2 Pathology of dysembryoplastic neuro-epithelial tumor. *A,* The glioneuronal element is shown, with its characteristic columns of axon bundles lined by small, oligodendrocyte-like cells. Between the columns, neurons appear to float in a pale, mucinous matrix (hematoxylin and eosin [H&E] ×40). *B,* A magnified picture of a floating neuron is shown (H&E ×100). *C,* An immunohistochemical stain for neurofilament (NF) highlights the axon bundles (NF ×100).

However, serial growth of histologically verified DNETs on neuroimaging has been seen,[15] and there is a single report of malignant progression of a complex DNET,[4] suggesting that DNETs likely represent true neoplasms rather than hamartomatous lesions (see following discussion).

MANAGEMENT

The mainstay of treatment for patients with DNET is surgery. The initial report of DNETs detailed a very benign neoplasm.[2] Despite incomplete or subtotal removal of the tumor in 44% of cases, after a mean follow-up of 9 years, the authors did not observe any case in which there was evidence of clinical or radiologic progression.[2] Other authors have also reported excellent outcomes, including good outcomes in cases with multifocal disease where the distant foci were not removed.[9] This has not been the experience at some other centers, including our own, which has documented serial growth of histologically verified DNETs on neuroimaging.[15] Prayson and colleagues reported that 4 of 11 patients required at least one additional surgical procedure for tumor recurrence related to an incomplete initial excision 2.1 to 4.4 years earlier.[11] There is a single

report of malignant progression in which a complex DNET that exhibited the specific glioneuronal element recurred 11 years after a partial resection.[4] At the time of recurrence, this tumor was resected again, and the pathologic examination at that time revealed a glioblastoma multiforme.[4] These facts highly suggest that DNET is in fact a tumor and not a hamartoma as some authors have suggested. They further suggest that long-term follow-up of these patients is advisable, especially after incomplete resection. The question of what constitutes a complete resection of a DNET is also in doubt. Some cases that appear on postoperative MRI to have undergone a complete resection clearly show tumor at the margin of the resection on histopathologic examination, suggesting that a more diffuse abnormality remains.[5] Some patients with DNET have been treated with radiation in the past, and one patient died of radiation necrosis after whole-brain radiation therapy for DNET.[2] Radiation therapy is probably not indicated in the current management of typical DNETs.

The predominant complaint of patients with DNET is seizure disorder. The seizure disorder tends to be resistant to known antiepileptic medication. The original paper on DNETs reported a good seizure outcome, with 30 out of 39 patients seizure free, 3 having rare seizures, and 4 patients having significant reduction in seizure frequency despite a high incidence of incomplete resection in the whole cohort.[2] Other groups have not found excellent postsurgical seizure control. One group found that 6 out of 21 patients with DNET experienced no post surgical improvement in their seizure disorder.[12] These authors found that 3 out of 11 lesionectomy patients were seizure free, whereas 8 out of 10 patients were seizure free after lobectomy, suggesting that lobectomy may be more efficacious in the control of seizures in patients with DNET.[12] Another paper reports that 10 out of 77 patients operated on for DNET had persistent postoperative seizures occurring at least monthly.[5] Of these 10 patients, some had seizures arising in the ipsilateral hemisphere (and therefore perhaps amenable to surgical treatment), although others had evidence of a more diffuse disorder, with additional generalized seizures and cognitive and behavioral disturbances with multifocal and generalized electroencephalogram (EEG) abnormalities.[5] Repeat resection of a previously incompletely resected lesion resulted in freedom from seizures in at least one published case.[5] Among patients who do have a prolonged period of freedom from seizures postoperatively, the incidence of late relapse seems to be very low.[5]

CONCLUSION

DNET is a low-grade tumor, typically of the temporal or frontal lobe, which occurs in children and young adults with chronic, pharmacoresistant epilepsy. Current therapy consists of surgical resection. The long-term prognosis for these patients is excellent after complete surgical resection, although a minority of patients may have persistent symptoms or radiologic recurrence. The distinction of DNETs from conventional gliomas involves consolidation of clinical, radiologic, and pathologic information and is important to avoid unnecessary, aggressive radiation therapy or chemotherapy.

References

1. Daumas-Duport C: Dysembryoplastic neuroepithelial tumours. Brain Pathol 3:283–295, 1993.
2. Daumas-Duport C, Scheithauer BW, Chodkiewicz JP, et al: Dysembryoplastic neuroepithelial tumor: a surgically curable tumor of young patients with intractable partial seizures. Report of thirty-nine cases. Neurosurgery 23:545–556, 1988.
3. Daumas-Duport C, Varlet P, Bacha S, et al: Dysembryoplastic neuroepithelial tumors: nonspecific histological forms—a study of 40 cases. J Neurooncol 41:267–280, 1999.
4. Hammond RR, Duggal N, Woulfe JM, et al: Malignant transformation of a dysembryoplastic neuroepithelial tumor. Case report. J Neurosurg 92:722–725, 2000.
5. Hennessy MJ, Elwes RD, Binnie CD, et al: Failed surgery for epilepsy. A study of persistence and recurrence of seizures following temporal resection. Brain 123 Pt 12:2445–2466, 2000.
6. Honavar M, Janota I, Polkey CE: Histological heterogeneity of dysembryoplastic neuroepithelial tumour: identification and differential diagnosis in a series of 74 cases. Histopathology 34:342–356, 1999.
7. Kleihues P, Burger PC, Scheithauer BW: The new WHO classification of brain tumours. Brain Pathol 3:255–268, 1993.
8. Koeller KK, Dillon WP: Dysembryoplastic neuroepithelial tumors: MR appearance. AJNR Am J Neuroradiol 13:1319–1325, 1992.
9. Kuroiwa T, Bergey GK, Rothman MI, et al: Radiologic appearance of the dysembryoplastic neuroepithelial tumor. Radiology 197:233–238, 1995.
10. Leung SY, Gwi E, Ng HK, et al: Dysembryoplastic neuroepithelial tumor. A tumor with small neuronal cells resembling oligodendroglioma. Am J Surg Pathol 18:604–614, 1994.
11. Prayson RA, Morris HH, Estes ML, et al: Dysembryoplastic neuroepithelial tumor: a clinicopathologic and immunohistochemical study of 11 tumors including MIB1 immunoreactivity. Clin Neuropathol 15:47–53, 1996.
12. Raymond AA, Fish DR, Sisodiya SM, et al: Abnormalities of gyration, heterotopias, tuberous sclerosis, focal cortical dysplasia, microdysgenesis, dysembryoplastic neuroepithelial tumour and dysgenesis of the archicortex in epilepsy. Clinical, EEG and neuroimaging features in 100 adult patients. Brain 118:629–660, 1995.
13. Raymond AA, Halpin SF, Alsanjari N, et al: Dysembryoplastic neuroepithelial tumor. Features in 16 patients. Brain 117:461–475, 1994.
14. Thom M, Gomez-Anson B, Revesz T, et al: Spontaneous intralesional haemorrhage in dysembryoplastic neuroepithelial tumours: a series of five cases. J Neurol Neurosurg Psychiatry 67:97–101, 1999.
15. Yamaguchi N, Ohnishi H, Tachibana O, et al: [An enlarging dysembryoplastic neuroepithelial tumor during a 6-year period: a case report]. No Shinkei Geka 26:1097–1101, 1998.

CHAPTER **92**

PEDIATRIC MENINGIOMAS

Steve Casha, James M. Drake, and James T. Rutka

Meningiomas are the most common benign brain tumor encountered in the adult. They represent approximately 15% of adult brain tumors. They are thought to arise from arachnoid cap cells and occur in stereotypical locations, generally with a dural attachment.[3] Some exceptions include intraventricular and intraparenchymal meningiomas. When these slow-growing tumors become symptomatic or exhibit worrisome growth characteristics, surgical resection is the mainstay of therapy, with adjuvant radiation therapy and chemotherapy reserved for atypical or malignant variants or for tumors located in areas of high surgical morbidity and incompletely resected.

In the pediatric patient, meningiomas are far less common. Consequently, although several retrospective series have been published, they have generally had small numbers of patients and have taken place over long time spans within which significant technologic advances have occurred.[1,2,4–17,19,20,22–24,26,27] These studies have made several observations with regard to the differing behavior of pediatric meningiomas. Some of these observations have continued to be supported in subsequent series, whereas others have not remained substantiated. The published case series of pediatric meningiomas are summarized in Table 92-1. The upper range of age fluctuates; however, these articles examined characteristics of meningiomas occurring within the first 2 decades of life.

EPIDEMIOLOGY

Pediatric meningiomas represent a smaller proportion of brain tumors than do their adult counterparts. Literature series exhibit a range between 0.7% and 4.2% of pediatric brain tumors seen.[19,23] This range may be skewed by the referral pattern of the tertiary referral centers publishing these series; however, clearly these numbers are far below the adult proportion of approximately 13.4% to 27.3%.[15] Another perspective on this statistic is that pediatric meningiomas are reported to represent less than 2% of all meningiomas.[1,15] It must be recognized that it is not an uncommon occurrence to discover an asymptomatic meningioma on cranial imaging for another indication in the adult. Thus it is likely that our estimate of the true incidence of meningiomas in childhood is underestimated.

Meningiomas in the adult population are more common in women, accounting for 60% to 80% of these tumors.[15] This has prompted investigations into the effect of estrogen and progesterone on tumor growth. The weighted average male-to-female ratio in published pediatric series is 1.2 : 1, perhaps reflecting the minimal influence of sex hormones in this population (see

Table 92-1). A known external agent capable of inducing meningiomas in children is radiation therapy. Children who have received craniospinal irradiation for malignant tumors, such as medulloblastoma, will be at higher risk for developing meningiomas over time (Figure 92-1).

CLINICAL SIGNS AND SYMPTOMS

Clinical signs of pediatric meningiomas most commonly involve raised intracranial pressure with headache, nausea, vomiting, and papilledema. Other common signs of these rare tumors are seizures (up to 31%) and neurologic deficit (typically motor deficit or cranial nerve palsy).[1,12,15,17] Pediatric meningiomas are associated with the neurofibromatosis 2 (NF2) phenotype (Figure 92-2) in 7.1% to 42% of cases in the literature,[1,12,24,26] and one report found a 24.1% association with the NF1 phenotype[12] as well. These observations have led authors to recommend having a heightened suspicion for pediatric meningioma in NF patients as well as to recommend following pediatric patients with meningioma for the development of the NF phenotype. This latter point was illustrated in a report by Perry et al, where 27% of pediatric patients with meningioma were known to have NF at the time of tumor discovery, but an additional five patients developed NF on follow-up review, yielding a 42% association.[24]

Although these tumors occur in the same stereotypical locations as those seen in adults, their distribution among these sites differs. Pediatric meningiomas are more commonly seen in the posterior fossa compartment (14.5%), along the orbital nerve (5.5%), or in the ventricles (9.9%) and without dural attachment in the brain parenchyma or within the sylvian fissure (Table 92-2).[1,4–8,10–13,15–17,19,20,22,23,26,27] By comparison, in the adult, infratentorial and intraventricular meningiomas account for 10% and 5% of meningiomas, respectively.[25] A possible explanation for the distribution of childhood tumors is that these slow-growing tumors, when in the supratentorial compartment, are less likely to result in symptoms by mass effect and may not cause symptoms until later in life.

IMAGING CHARACTERISTICS

The diagnosis of meningioma is generally made through imaging. Historically, evidence of meningioma can be seen on plain film examinations of the skull with findings of bone erosion, abnormal calcification, and hyperostosis. Although

TABLE 92-1   Summary of Patient Demographics in Published Series of Pediatric Meningiomas

Author	Year	n	% of Pediatric Brain Tumors	Mean Age	Maximum Age	M:F
Crouse & Berg	1972	13	2.3	12.8	20	7:6
Cooper & Dohn	1974	7	—	11.0	14	2:5
Merten et al.	1974	48	—	10.9	19	27:21
Leibel et al.	1976	13	—	15.2	19	7:6
Herz et al.	1980	9	—	12.9	18	4:5
Sano et al.	1981	18	3.0	—	15	10:8
Deen et al.	1982	51	2.5	15	20	25:26
Chan & Thompson	1984	4	1.1	8.3	16	2:2
Drake et al.	1985	13	1.0	11.6	16	10:3
Nakamura & Becker	1985	7	0.7	11.6	16	4:3
Doty et al.	1987	13	3.2	8.8	16	7:6
Kolluri et al.	1987	18	4.2	—	15	9:9
Ferrante et al.	1989	19	2.8	9.1	16	13:6
Davidson & Hope	1989	22	—	—	16	13:9
Germano et al.	1994	23	2.9	13.3	21	14:9
Baumgartner & Sorenson	1996	—	—	—	—	—
Erdincler et al.	1998	29	2.4	10	15	18:11
Demirtas et al.	2000	13	2.7	—	16	—
Amirjamshidi et al.	2000	24	1.1	9.5	17	11:13
Perry et al.	2001	33	—	12	18	—
Sandberg et al.	2001	14	—	10.3	17	—
Im et al.	2001	11	1.9	9.9	14	5:6

M:F, Male-to-female ratio.

TABLE 92-2   Anatomic Location of Pediatric Meningiomas in Published Series

Author	Year	Supratentorial	Infratentorial	Intraventricular	Orbital
Crouse & Berg	1972	7	6	0	0
Cooper & Dohn	1974	6	0	1	0
Merten et al.	1974	24	9	8	6
Leibel et al.	1976	8	4	1	0
Herz et al.	1980	5	0	4	0
Sano et al.	1981	13	2	2	1
Deen et al.	1982	29	7	2	3
Chan & Thompson	1984	4	0	0	0
Drake et al.	1985	12	0	1	0
Nakamura & Becker	1985	7	0	0	0
Doty et al.	1987	11	0	2	0
Kolluri et al.	1987	14	2	1	1
Ferrante et al.	1989	17	2	0	0
Davidson & Hope	1989	13	5	1	3
Germano et al.	1994	16	3	3	1
Erdincler et al.	1998	22	6	3	0
Amirjamshidi et al.	2000	18	2	1	1
Sandberg et al.	2001	8	1	2	2
Im et al.	2001	7	1	2	1
Total		**241**	**50**	**34**	**19**
Proportion (%)		**70.1**	**14.5**	**9.9**	**5.5**

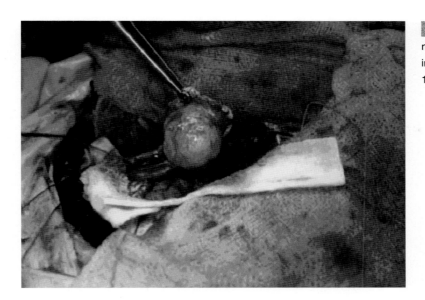

FIGURE 92-1 Intraoperative photograph of meningiomas being removed from temporal convexity dura in 16-year-old male who had received craniospinal irradiation 10 years previously for medulloblastoma.

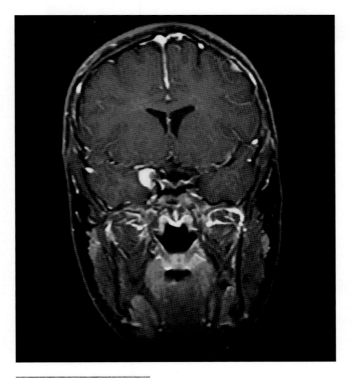

FIGURE 92-2 Fourteen-year-old male with neurofibromatosis 2 and right cavernous sinus meningiomas. This child also has numerous intraspinal dural-based lesions that are thought to be meningiomas. Such children are predisposed to developing meningiomas.

these findings are nonspecific and skull x-rays are always followed by further imaging, these investigations are still favored by some authors.[1,17] The computed tomography (CT) and magnetic resonance imaging (MRI) characteristics of pediatric meningioma are as generally experienced in the adult population and have been well described.[29] They are usually dural-based tumors that are slightly hyperintense to brain tissue on CT and T1 MRI, hypointense on T2 MRI (Figure 92-3). They

are usually enhanced and may exhibit a dural tail. In some series the pediatric tumor is less likely to exhibit a dural tail, more often demonstrates cysts, and is more likely to be seen in less common locations, particularly intraventricular, sylvian fissure without dural attachment, and intraparenchymal (as discussed previously).[17] Angiography is generally used in selected cases where preoperative detailed knowledge of the vascular anatomy is desirable or as a prelude to preoperative embolization of the tumor. This investigation may be of greater interest in the child, considering the issues of blood loss and the high operative mortality seen in early series.[16,20] Angiographically, these tumors classically exhibit a radial arterial blush pattern that empties slowly. Angiography may also be used in examining invasion of vascular structures, particularly venous sinuses, by tumor.

MANAGEMENT

The mainstay of treatment of meningiomas is surgical resection. A clear relationship has been established between the extent of surgical resection and recurrence and survival.[28] In the pediatric literature this principle is maintained. However, higher recurrence rates have been seen even after gross-total resection by some authors.[1,2,12,26] Most pediatric series report good clinical outcomes,[15] although the long follow-up required for these slow-growing tumors is often not reported. Adjuvant therapies are used in subtotally resected meningiomas, recurrent meningiomas, and histologically aggressive meningiomas. In the pediatric population some series have employed radiation therapy and stereotactic radiosurgery as an adjuvant in a small number of patients.[12,15,17,20] These data are not adequate to evaluate the role of this treatment in these tumors.

The outcome of meningioma treatment remains controversial. Although most authors indicate a good clinical outcome in their patients, some published series are remarkable for recurrence rates of 13.8% to 25%,[1,12,17] whereas others reported no recurrance.[15] Erdincler et al achieved an 86.2% gross-total resection rate; however, they still observed five deaths (17.2%) and eight patients (27.6%) who had moderate disability.

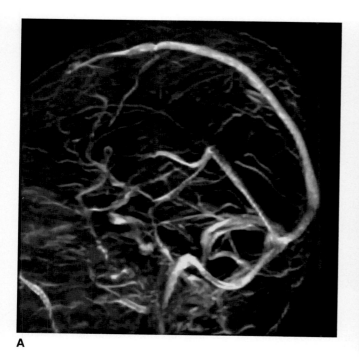

A

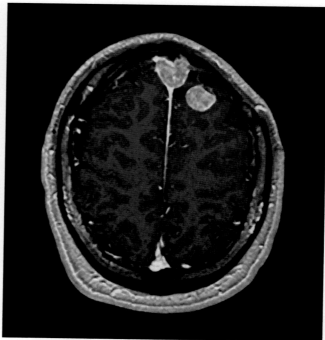

B

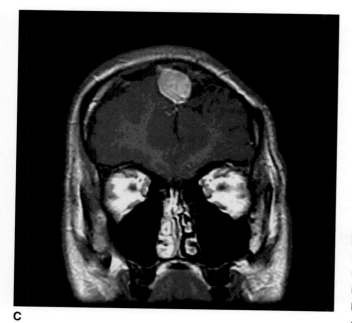

C

FIGURE 92-3 Sixteen-year-old male with atypical meningioma. *A,* Magnetic resonance (MR) venogram showing obstruction of the superior sagittal sinus anteriorly by tumor. *B,* Axial gadolinium-enhanced MR image showing tumor within the superior sagittal sinus and also a daughter lesion within the left frontal lobe. *C,* Coronal gadolinium-enhanced MR image showing meningiomas filling the superior sagittal sinus.

PATHOLOGY

Meningiomas have been pathologically classified in a variety of ways.[3] In most cases the light microscopic variations in tumor appearance have little to do with tumor behavior. However, some meningiomas are associated with a more aggressive course (e.g., clear cell, chordoid, and papillary meningioma). The World Health Organization (WHO) classification of meningiomas describes grades I to III based on the observation of loss of architecture, increased cellularity, nuclear pleomorphism, mitotic figures, focal necrosis, and brain infiltration.[21] Grade II is an atypical meningioma and grade III

an anaplastic meningioma. Perry et al found 40% grade I, 49% grade II, and 11% grade III meningiomas among their 33 pediatric patients and did not find any difference in NF1- or NF2-associated tumors.[24] Sandberg et al observed 36.4% grade II and 9.1% grade III among their 11 pediatric patients with meningioma.[26] Germano et al observed 71% grade I and 29% grade II, with no grade III lesions in 21 tumor specimens. These studies point to a high rate of aggressive morphology in pediatric meningiomas. By comparison, one large series of adult meningiomas found that in 657 tumors, 94.3% were benign, 4.7% were atypical, and 1% were anaplastic by the WHO criteria.[18] Previous pediatric studies have made similar conclusions using morphologic descriptions and recognizing the aggressive nature of some histologies. In particular Deen et al observed a 9.8% incidence of the papillary histology and a 2-year mean recurrence time in this group as compared with 9.4 years in other histologic types.[8] The literature regarding tumors in adults also reports increased recurrence rates and shorter mean recurrence times with more aggressive grade.[18]

Proliferative activity has become an increasingly used adjunct to traditional histopathology in the evaluation of meningiomas.[3] MIB-1 staining in pediatric meningiomas correlated with aggressive pathology and the tendency to recur in three studies.[17,24,26] Sandberg et al, in making this observation, concluded that a lack of difference in MIB-1 labeling in benign adult and pediatric meningiomas suggests that factors other than the rate of cellular proliferation may explain the more aggressive clinical features of childhood meningiomas.[26] One study observed a correlation of MIB-1 labeling with histologic grade but failed to find a significant correlation with prognosis or recurrence.[9] Perry et al examined genetic alterations in pediatric meningiomas as well as MIB-1 index. They found similar genetic alterations to adult tumors, particularly NF2 or merlin, DAL1 loss, and 1p and 14q deletions. They, however, demonstrated a greater occurrence of genotypically aggressive tumors (1p and 14q deletions).[24] These authors also found that progesterone receptor expression was inversely associated with histologic grade.

CONCLUSION

Meningiomas are not a common tumor in the pediatric population. They differ from their counterparts in adults in that they are more likely found in less common locations in the cranium, they lack the predilection for females seen in adults, and they are more likely to exhibit an aggressive histology and clinical behavior. Surgical resection is the mainstay of treatment of these tumors, although the recurrence rate even after gross-total removal may be higher in the pediatric population. The role of adjuvant radiation therapy and chemotherapy in this disease has not been rigorously evaluated.

References

1. Amirjamshidi A, Mehrazin M, Abbassioun K: Meningiomas of the central nervous system occurring below the age of 17: report of 24 cases not associated with neurofibromatosis and review of literature. Childs Nerv Syst 16:406–416, 2000.
2. Baumgartner JE, Sorenson JM: Meningioma in the pediatric population. J Neurooncol 29:223–228, 1996.
3. Black PM: Meningiomas. Neurosurgery 32:643–57, 1993.
4. Chan RC, Thompson GB: Intracranial meningiomas in childhood. Surg Neurol 21:319–322, 1984.
5. Cooper M, Dohn DF: Intracranial meningiomas in childhood. Cleve Clin Q 41:197–204, 1974.
6. Crouse SK, Berg BO: Intracranial meningiomas in childhood and adolescence. Neurology 22:135–141, 1972.
7. Davidson GS, Hope JK: Meningeal tumors of childhood. Cancer 63:1205–1210, 1989.
8. Deen HG, Jr, Scheithauer BW, Ebersold MJ: Clinical and pathological study of meningiomas of the first two decades of life. J Neurosurg 56:317–322, 1982.
9. Demirtas E, Ersahin Y, Yilmaz F, et al: Intracranial meningeal tumours in childhood: a clinicopathologic study including MIB-1 immunohistochemistry. Pathol Res Pract 196:151–158, 2000.
10. Doty JR, Schut L, Bruce DA, Sutton LN: Intracranial meningiomas of childhood and adolescence. Prog Exp Tumor Res 30:247–254, 1987.
11. Drake JM, Hendrick EB, Becker LE, et al: Intracranial meningiomas in children. Pediatr Neurosci 12:134–139, 1985.
12. Erdincler P, Lena G, Sarioglu AC, et al: Intracranial meningiomas in children: review of 29 cases. Surg Neurol 49:136–40; discussion 140–141, 1998.
13. Ferrante L, Acqui M, Artico M, et al: Cerebral meningiomas in children. Childs Nerv Syst 5:83–86, 1989.
14. Ferrante L, Acqui M, Artico M, et al: Paediatric intracranial meningiomas. Br J Neurosurg 3:189–196, 1989.
15. Germano IM, Edwards MS, Davis RL, Schiffer D: Intracranial meningiomas of the first two decades of life. J Neurosurg 80:447–453, 1994.
16. Herz DA, Shapiro K, Shulman K: Intracranial meningiomas of infancy, childhood and adolescence. Review of the literature and addition of 9 case reports. Childs Brain 7:43–56, 1980.
17. Im SH, Wang KC, Kim SK, et al: Childhood meningioma: unusual location, atypical radiological findings, and favorable treatment outcome. Childs Nerv Syst 17:656–662, 2001.
18. Jaaskelainen J, Haltia M, Servo A: Atypical and anaplastic meningiomas: radiology, surgery, radiotherapy, and outcome. Surg Neurol 25:233–242, 1986.
19. Kolluri VR, Reddy DR, Reddy PK, et al: Meningiomas in childhood. Childs Nerv Syst 3:271–273, 1987.
20. Leibel SA, Wara WM, Sheline GE, et al: The treatment of meningiomas in childhood. Cancer 37:2709–2712, 1976.
21. Louis D, Scheithauer B, Budka H, et al: Meningiomas. In Kleihues P, Cavenee W (eds): World Health Organization Classification of Tumours. Pathology and Genetics of Tumours of the Nervous System. Lyon, France, IRAC Press, 2000.
22. Merten DF, Gooding CA, Newton TH, Malamud N: Meningiomas of childhood and adolescence. J Pediatr 84:696–700, 1974.
23. Nakamura Y, Becker LE: Meningeal tumors of infancy and childhood. Pediatr Pathol 3:341–358, 1985.
24. Perry A, Giannini C, Raghavan R, et al: Aggressive phenotypic and genotypic features in pediatric and NF2-associated meningiomas: a clinicopathologic study of 53 cases. J Neuropathol Exp Neurol 60:994–1003, 2001.
25. Rohringer M, Sutherland GR, Louw DF, Sima AA: Incidence and clinicopathological features of meningioma. J Neurosurg 71:665–672, 1989.
26. Sandberg DI, Edgar MA, Resch L, et al: MIB-1 staining index of pediatric meningiomas. Neurosurgery 48:590–5; discussion 595–597, 2001.
27. Sano K, Wakai S, Ochiai C, Takakura K: Characteristics of intracranial meningiomas in childhood. Childs Brain 8:98–106, 1981.
28. Simpson D: The recurrence of intracranial meningiomas after surgical treatment. J Neurol Neurosurg Psychiatry 20:22–39, 1957.
29. Zimmerman RD, Fleming CA, Saint-Louis LA, et al: Magnetic resonance imaging of meningiomas. AJNR Am J Neuroradiol 6:149–157, 1985.

CHAPTER **93**

PINEAL REGION TUMORS IN CHILDREN

Tadanori Tomita

LOCATION

The pineal region comprises multiple structures in and around the pineal gland between the posterior third ventricle and the quadrigeminal cistern. The neural structures that surround the pineal gland are the quadrigeminal plate inferiorly, the cerebellar vermis posteriorly, and the splenium of the corpus callosum superiorly. Superolaterally to the pineal gland are the posterior thalami. Directly under the pineal gland is the posterior commissure and the superior colliculi, which form the roof of the aqueduct of Sylvius. Anteroinferiorly is the tegmentum of the midbrain, and the mammillary bodies more anteriorly. A hypothalamic sulcus traverses the lateral wall of the third ventricle from the foramen of Monro to the aqueduct of Sylvius, separating the thalamus above from the hypothalamus below. The roof of the third ventricle consists of the tela choroidea and fornix. The tela choroidea is a pial infolding and passes between the fornix and the roof of the third ventricle. This pial infolding of tela choroidea contains the internal cerebral veins and medial posterior choroidal arteries. The choroid plexus of the third ventricle attaches to the tela choroidea.

The great vein of Galen and its tributaries surround the pineal gland. The internal cerebral veins run parallel in the roof of the third ventricle and unite to form the great vein of Galen. The vein of Galen also receives the tributaries from the basal veins of Rosenthal, which run around the midbrain. The vein of Galen is located under the splenium and above the pineal gland and enters the straight sinus. At that point, it receives the precentral vein.

TUMOR HISTOLOGY AND HISTOGENESIS

Diverse types of tumor arise from the pineal gland and surrounding structures. They are classified into pineal (gland) origin and extrapineal tumors. Pineal and extrapineal origin tumors differ in histologic type. Those of pineal origin are germ cell tumors and pineal parenchymal cell tumors. Extrapineal tumors arise from the surrounding neural or mesenchymal structures and include astrocytomas, meningiomas, ependymomas, and choroid plexus papillomas. Therefore a wide variety of tumor histologic types can occur in the pineal region.

Germ Cell Tumors

Germ cell tumors derive from totipotential germ cells and span a wide range of differentiation and malignant characteristics. Histogenesis for the central nervous system (CNS) germ cell tumors remains controversial.[16,45] The primordial germ cells appear in the yolk sac wall in the third gestational week and migrate through the dorsal mesentery of the hindgut into the genital ridge in the sixth gestational week. These germ cells also migrate and disseminate widely throughout various tissues and organs in the early embryo. Outside of a gonadal location, they often remain in two midline locations: the mediastinum and around the third ventricle. The latter gives rise to extragonadal germ cell tumors in the pineal and hypothalamic regions. However, primordial germ cell elements were not found in the fetal pineal glands.[15] Sano postulated an origin for these CNS germ cell tumors to be a variety of displaced embryogenic tissues that become incorrectly enfolded into the brain at the time of neural tube formation.[45]

According to the WHO Classification of Tumors of the CNS of 1999, germ cell tumors are classified into germinomas, embryonal carcinomas, yolk sac tumors (endodermal sinus tumors), choriocarcinomas, teratomas (mature, immature, and teratoma with malignant transformation), and mixed germ cell tumors. Germinomas are composed of cells with suppressed differentiation potentials, whereas embryonal carcinomas are considered to be tumors of pluripotential cells. They further give rise to either embryonal tumors or extraembryonal tumors. Embryonal tumors consist of cells of all three germ layers. They are mature teratomas, immature teratomas, and teratoma with malignant transformation. Immature teratomas contain primitive elements derived from all or any of the three germ layers. They are composed of incompletely differentiating components resembling fetal tissue and behave in a malignant fashion. On rare occasions, mature teratomas harbor malignant components such as rhabdomyosarcoma and carcinoma, which are classified as teratoma with malignant transformation. In contrast, extraembryonal tumors include choriocarcinomas through trophoblastic differentiations or yolk sac tumors through yolk sac formation. Elements of various germ cell tumors may coexist in a single tumor, which is called a mixed germ cell tumor. Malignant germ cell tumors other than germinomas are classified into nongerminomatous germ cell tumor (NGGCT).

Pineal Parenchymal Tumors

Pineal parenchymal tumors are derived from pineal parenchymal cells within the pineal gland. They originate from pineocytes, which possess neurosecretory and photosensory functions. These tumors may differentiate into several cell lines, such as neuronal, astrocytic, retinoblastomatous, and mesenchymal components. Immunohistochemical or ultrastructural studies may disclose cellular differentiations and neurosecretory and photosensory functions. Pineal parenchymal tumors are classified into pineoblastoma and pineocytoma, depending on the cellular differentiations. Pineoblastomas are poorly differentiating malignant tumors and belong to the group of primitive neuroectodermal tumors (PNETs). Pineocytomas, in contrast, are differentiated to pineal parenchymal cells and are clinically benign. Some parenchymal tumors may have mixed components of pineoblastoma and pineocytoma.

Tumors of Glial and Miscellaneous Cell Origin

Glial tumors arise almost invariably from the glial tissue elements intimately surrounding the pineal gland. The most common pathologic type of glial tumors is astrocytoma, which often originates in the posterior thalamus or the midbrain. True astrocytomas of pineal gland origin are extremely rare, though glial cell tumors can occur in the pineal gland because astrocytes are normally present there.

Tumors of other histologic types also occur. They are glioblastomas, astroblastomas, ependymomas, oligodendrogliomas, choroid plexus papillomas, and medulloepitheliomas. Among tumors of mesenchymal origin, meningioma, hemangioma, or cavernoma may occur in the pineal region.

Non-Neoplastic Cysts

Pineal cysts, which result from focal degeneration of the pineal gland, contain gelatinous material within the cyst wall that consists of an outer fibrous layer, a middle layer of pineal parenchymal cells with variable calcification, and an inner layer of hypocellular glial tissue. Other developmental cysts include epidermoid and dermoid cysts. Arachnoid cysts consist of cerebrospinal fluid (CSF) cyst and cyst wall composed of arachnoid membrane.

SYMPTOMATOLOGY

Hydrocephalus resulting from obstruction of the aqueduct of Sylvius is the primary cause of symptoms. Common symptoms are headache, nausea, and emesis. Headaches usually occur intermittently initially but become more frequent and intense. Visual symptoms may be present. Double vision may be due to either abducens nerve palsy or tectal compression. Blurred vision is due to the tectal compression or visual obscuration secondary to papilledema. In the later stage of hydrocephalus, patients experience ataxic gait and altered mental status. Papilledema is a common sign of hydrocephalus secondary to pineal region tumors.

Common signs associated with pineal region tumor are due to direct compression on the quadrigeminal plate and pretectal region of the midbrain. Parinaud's sign is well known to be a pathognomonic sign for pineal region tumors. This syndrome is present in approximately 50% to 75% of patients with pineal region tumors and is characterized by upward gaze palsy, abnormal pupillary responses, spasms of convergence, or retraction nystagmus.

Synchronous germinomas in the pineal and suprasellar regions may cause diabetes insipidus and other hormonal dysfunctions and visual impairment.[53] Precocious puberty resulting from pineal region tumor occurs overwhelmingly in male patients with choriocarcinoma, because β-human chorionic gonadotropin (β-HCG) secreted by neoplastic syncytiotrophoblasts provokes androgen secretion by the testes.

DIAGNOSTIC STUDIES

Neuroimaging

Computed tomography (CT) and magnetic resonance imaging (MRI) are widely available and have revolutionized diagnosing pineal region tumors. Associated abnormalities, such as hemorrhage or calcifications, may be better appreciated with CT. MRI, however, is extremely useful for identification of tumor location and extension. The superior depiction of anatomic structures with MRI, on sagittal images in particular, demonstrates the relationship between the pineal gland, the quadrigeminal plate, and other structures. MRI often enables the determination of the pineal or extrapineal origin of the tumor, because the latter does not involve the pineal gland. The involvement of the midbrain, the thalamus, or other surrounding structures is often clearly determined. Tumor multiplicity or dissemination in the ventricular or subarachnoid spaces is also determined by these neuroimaging techniques.

Computed Tomography

Calcifications normally occur in the pineal gland. A normally calcified pineal gland is shown on CT scans of children as young as $6^1/_2$ years. The rate of occurrence of pineal calcifications visible on CT scans is 8% to 10% for children ages 8 to 14 years, 30% at age 15 years, and 40% at age 17 years.[60] Therefore the presence of calcification in children younger than 6 years is abnormal and needs to be investigated for a neoplastic process.

On CT scans, germinomas show soft tissue masses of hyperdensity relative to the surrounding brain tissue. Lobular soft tissue masses often surround the calcification. Cyst formation, however, is unusual. After intravenous infusion of contrast agent, germinomas tend to enhance homogeneously. NGGCTs tend to have similar homogeneous soft tissue density and are also similarly calcified as germinomas. Choriocarcinomas may have hemorrhagic foci. In contrast, the appearance of teratomas is often heterogeneous, with a variable degree of soft tissues, calcifications, and cyst formation. Pineoblastomas are relatively homogeneous and hyperdense on precontrast CT scans. After infusion of contrast material, enhancement ranges from dense to little or no enhancement. Calcifications are rare among pineoblastomas but, if present, are dispersed in the tumor.

Benign astrocytomas are often hypodense relative to the surrounding brain tissues on precontrast CT scans. Contrast enhancement is variable and often inhomogeneous. Dermoid and epidermoid tumors tend to be hypodense and are enhanced minimally after infusion of contrast material. Some epidermoid tumors may have density equal to that of CSF, and their appearance may mimic that of an arachnoid cyst or pineal cyst.

Magnetic Resonance Imaging

MRI has revolutionized the management of pineal region tumors. Because of the ability to obtain high-resolution images and multidimensional views with MRI, tumor location and extension are clearly shown. Although detection of calcification with MRI is poor, the nature of the soft tissue and cystic or hemorrhagic changes is well shown with the combination of T1-weighted, proton-density, and T2-weighted images.

MRI scans demonstrate associated anomalies. In cases of hydrocephalus, the site of obstruction of the CSF pathway is usually evident on magnetic resonance (MR) images. The secondary or disseminated diseases are detected on head and spine MR images. The suprasellar region should be carefully evaluated for concurrent germ cell tumors. From a surgical viewpoint, sagittal MR images provide surgeons with sufficient information about the floor of the third ventricle for third ventriculostomy and about the relationship between the tumor and deep venous structures for the selection of surgical approaches to the pineal region.

On MR images, teratomas are often heterogeneous with the presence of cyst formation and fat. Teratoma cysts are shown with high intensity on both T1- and T2-weighted images because of high proteinaceous content. Germinomas show low signal intensity to isointensity on T1-weighted images. They show high signal intensity or are isointense on T2-weighted images.[54] After infusion of contrast material, germinomas show intense enhancement. Malignant NGGCTs show variable signal intensity, partly because of the presence of hemorrhage.[55] Pineoblastomas are hypointense or isointense on T1-weighted images, and variable degrees of enhancement are noted. In general, MRI signal characteristics are usually nonspecific,[25,28,55] and correlation with the patient's age, sex, and other associated factors needs to be analyzed for diagnostic purposes. The concurrent presence of masses in both the anterior and posterior third ventricle strongly suggests germinomas. The frequency of this multiplicity has increased with the use of more sensitive neurodiagnostic methods.[53] Reported rates of occurrence of synchronous anterior and posterior third ventricle lesions among germ cell tumors are shown to be as high as 32% to 57%.[41,46,54] When pineal region tumor causes diabetes insipidus, the pituitary stalk and the tuber cinereum should be carefully investigated to disclose the multiplicity of the lesions. Among infants with either unilateral or bilateral retinoblastomas, 3% have pineal parenchymal tumor (trilateral retinoblastoma). Pineal region tumors are often associated with hydrocephalus. Conversely, pineal cysts, which are present in 2.4% of the normal population studied on MRI and in up to 40% on routine autopsy specimen, are rarely symptomatic and usually remain stable in size. They have a contrast-enhanced cyst wall that may be calcified and occasionally show radiographic evidence of tectal compression. However, the occurrence of hydrocephalus is very rare.

Laboratory Tests

Certain germ cell tumors secrete glycoproteins that are identified in the serum and the CSF. Their identification is important not only for diagnostic purposes but also for monitoring responses to treatment and relapses. It has become standard practice to perform serum and CSF assay for these tumor markers if CNS germ cell tumors are suspected. α-fetoprotein (AFP) is normally produced by the yolk sac endoderm, the fetal liver, and embryonic intestinal epithelium, but its production ceases by the time of birth. An AFP value less than 5 ng/mL in both serum and CSF is considered normal. In the CNS, yolk sac tumors show the greatest production of AFP. Embryonal carcinomas and immature teratomas produce AFP to a lesser extent. β-HCG is normally secreted by syncytiotrophoblastic giant cells. The normal value in the serum and CSF is less than 5 milli-international units per milliliter. Marked elevation of β-HCG is noted in choriocarcinomas, but mild elevations occur among germinomas and embryonal carcinomas. The biologic half-life is short, approximately 5 days for AFP and less than 24 hours for β-HCG; thus serial monitoring of these tumor markers is useful in determining the response to treatment. The values of β-HCG and AFP reflect the number of cells secreting these glycoproteins; this is useful when differentiating tumors with predominantly choriocarcinoma or yolk sac tumor but unable to confirm histologic diagnosis.[31]

Of CNS malignant germ cell tumors, 40% to 70% show positive tumor markers for either β-HCG or AFP or both.[31,54] The positive results for tumor markers are variable. Serum tumor titers tend to be higher than CSF titers, because the tumor should be in direct contact with the CSF to express positive CSF markers.

Placental alkaline phosphatase (PLAP) is a cell-surface glycoprotein produced by primordial germ cells. Germinomas often express PLAP. PLAP is distinguished from other common tissue alkaline phosphatases by its heat resistance and its inhibition by L-phenylalanine. Serum or CSF PLAP levels are measured with an enzyme-linked immunosorbent assay, but their sensitivity and specificity need further investigation. One report showed that five of nine patients with germinoma showed high levels of PLAP in the CSF.[38]

Cerebrospinal Fluid Cytology

The CSF, whenever available either by means of lumbar puncture or from the cerebral ventricle, should be analyzed with cytologic studies together with tumor markers for pineal region tumors. The reported frequency of CSF dissemination among malignant germ cell tumors varies from 10%[21] to 52%.[49] Pineoblastomas disseminate along the CSF pathway with a higher frequency of 17% to 50% at diagnosis and almost 100% at the terminal stage.[13,17,20,32]

Stereotactic or Ventriculoscopic Biopsy

Biopsy for pineal region tumors can be done by a stereotactic method. However, stereotactic procedures have a serious potential to result in hemorrhagic complications, because tumors originating from the pineal gland are surrounded by veins of the galenic system. Also, pineoblastomas and certain germ cell tumors may be extremely vascular. In my experience with 10 stereotactic biopsies of pineal region tumors, three patients (germinoma in two and pineoblastoma in one) had a serious hemorrhage into the tumor and ventricle, although other authors have reported no major complications.

Ventriculoscopic tumor biopsy from the third ventricle became popular because of recent advances in ventriculoscopic instrumentation. This procedure can be performed at the same time as third ventriculostomy, though the trajectory of the endoscope may need to be altered to access the pineal region.[36] The pineal region tumor is readily visualized in the posterior third ventricle through the endoscope, and hemostasis can be achieved with a bipolar cautery or laser. Controlling a major hemorrhage, however, is very difficult because of the limited field for ventriculoscopic instrumentation and poor visibility caused by hemorrhagic CSF.

Pathologic diagnosis can be determined for most tumors, although tumor samples obtained with either a stereotactic procedure or ventriculoscopy are small. For mixed malignant tumors, however, heterogeneous components may be overlooked; thus a small sample obtained with these methods may not indicate the true nature of these tumors.

EPIDEMIOLOGY

Pineal region tumors compose 3% to 8% of all intracranial tumors of children. Farwell and Flannery reported that the incidence of pinealoma and germinoma among children was 0.061 per 100,000 children per year.[14] The age-adjusted germ cell tumor incidence in Japan is reported to be 0.17 per 100,000 population per year.[26] Although the frequency of pineal region tumors is higher among the Japanese, a prospective study of actual population-based incidence done in Niigata Prefecture (Japan) and in Western Australia showed no significant difference in frequency between different races.[37] Among pineal region tumors, germ cell tumors are far more common in Asia, constituting 70% to 80%.[34] Germinomas are the most common variety among germ cell tumors and constitute 42%[31,45] according to some studies or 61% to 65% according to others.[15,21,34] The average United States incidence of CNS germinoma is considered to be 0.1 per 100,000 persons per year.[19] Germinomas and other germ cell tumors tend to occur in males, with a male-to-female ratio of 4 to 1 in the CNS.[31] Pineal germ cell tumors occur primarily in males, although the sexual distribution for hypothalamic germinomas is approximately equal between males and females, or females may be predominant.[15,21,31] Most germinomas occur in the first 3 decades, with a peak in the middle of the second decade corresponding to the onset of puberty. Approximately 65% occur between the ages of 10 and 21 years, and only 11% occur before the age of 9 years.

NGGCTs, including embryonal carcinomas, yolk sac carcinomas, and choriocarcinomas, are highly malignant but rare. Most cases of NGGCTs affect males in the first 2 decades of life. Choriocarcinomas tend to occur at a younger age (mean age 8 years) than do embryonal carcinomas and yolk sac tumors (mean age 14 and 17 years, respectively). Of choriocarcinomas, 35% occur before the age of 9 years, whereas only 10% to 12% of embryonal carcinomas and endodermal sinus tumors occur before the age of 9 years.

Teratomas in the pineal region often affect males. They are usually identified within the first 2 decades of life[42] but often occur in much younger children than do other germ cell tumors. Most teratomas occur in children younger than 9 years, but 20% occur between the ages of 16 and 18 years.

The documented rate of occurrence of mixed germ cell tumors has been increasing, partly because of a recent trend of aggressive tumor sampling and the availability of tumor marker studies. In a study by Matsutani et al, 49 (32%) of 153 intracra-

nial germ cell tumors were of mixed type.[31] The common components often present in mixed germ cell tumors are germinomas and teratoma, although germinoma and teratoma are the tumors that commonly occur as pure tumor types. The correct identification of mixed germ cell tumors and non–germ cell tumors requires adequate tumor sampling and proper preparation of the tissue for immunohistochemical and electron microscopic examination.[15]

Pineal parenchymal tumors occur at various ages. Pineoblastomas occur in infancy and early childhood, whereas pineocytomas occur in young adults.[32] Nomura reported that the highest incidence of pineoblastoma was noted in the 0- to 4-years age group.[34] Russel and Rubinstein reported that in 14 of 23 patients pineoblastomas occurred in the first 10 years of life.[42] In their series, pineoblastomas were more common in males, with a male-to-female ratio of 2 to 1.

The distribution of various pineal tumors by histology showed germ cell tumors had the highest frequency. There was regional difference in frequency between germ cell tumor and pineal parenchymal tumors. Their ratio was reported to be 5.8 to 1 in Asia and 2.5 to 1 in Western countries.[34]

TREATMENT AND OUTCOME

Hydrocephalus

Hydrocephalus may be controlled with either tumor mass reduction or a CSF diversion procedure. Surgical resection of a tumor in the pineal region would open the occluded aqueduct of Sylvius. Certain germ cell tumors can be considerably reduced in size in a short time following irradiation or chemotherapy, and hydrocephalus is resolved without surgery. However, these nonsurgical methods of tumor mass reduction require at least several weeks. Steroid therapy may be used for hydrocephalus while awaiting the efficacy of irradiation or chemotherapy. At present, the treatment of choice for hydrocephalus is the third ventriculostomy. The third ventriculostomy, if effective, will eliminate the necessity of a ventriculoperitoneal shunt, which poses the risk of peritoneal dissemination of tumor cells. At the same time, the posterior third ventricle can be inspected, and perhaps a tumor biopsy can be performed at the same time. Potential risks related to the third ventriculostomy include hemorrhage from the basilar artery and its branches and hypothalamic damage, particularly the development of diabetes insipidus if the tuber cinereum is damaged.

Craniotomy

Although initial experiences of direct surgical resection were quite discouraging due to high morbidity and mortality rates, the availability of the surgical microscope and more established surgical approaches have made it possible for neurosurgeons to resect these tumors effectively with minimal risks. In recent reports, surgical mortality is nearly zero. The purposes of craniotomy for pineal region tumors are histologic verification, maximum cytoreduction, and restoration of the CSF pathway. By means of direct visualization of the tumor, much larger tissue samples can be obtained for histologic verification. This is important for detailed histologic examination, because a small sample of tumor does not necessarily represent the entire picture of the tumor. Greater than 80% of childhood germ cell tumors are malignant. However, mature teratoma, pineocytoma, astrocytoma, and other benign tumors are often amenable to surgery. Patients do not need adjuvant therapy following resection of these benign tumors.

To access the pineal region, either a supratentorial or infratentorial route has been used. The supratentorial route includes an occipital transtentorial approach, posterior interhemispheric approach, posterior interhemispheric transcallosal approach, anterior interhemispheric transcallosal approach, and lateral transventricular approach. The infratentorial route is a supracerebellar approach.

Each approach has advantages and disadvantages and should be chosen on the basis of anatomic information provided from neurodiagnostic images, along with the surgeon's familiarity and confidence with the approach. Tumor location and extension and the deep venous system and surrounding neural structures need to be considered in planning the surgical approach. Also, other factors need to be taken into account, such as patient's age, presence or absence of hydrocephalus, and purpose of surgery (biopsy versus total resection). Childhood pineal region tumors tend to be large and extend in various directions, particularly to the lateral ventricle from the third ventricle. Also, the posterior fossa is small in children. Currently, most neurosurgeons choose the posterior interhemispheric transtentorial or supracerebellar approach.

Posterior Interhemispheric Transtentorial Approach

The prone position is used routinely, though some prefer a sitting position. I prefer to place patients in a prone position with the head turned slightly (approximately 15 degrees) away from the surgical side for patients who are old enough to receive head pins for a head holder. This position allows the occipital lobe to fall away from the falx by gravity without forcible brain retraction. If the patient is young, the head is rested on the well-padded, U-shaped head holder without turning the head. When hydrocephalus is present, the surgeon can control the brain retraction with intraoperative ventricular drainage. In the case of slit ventricles caused by an existing shunt, the retraction of the occipital and parietal lobes is more restricted. One should avoid forcible retraction of these lobes. The brain should be relaxed with administration of mannitol.

The posterior interhemispheric approach provides a wider surgical entry for access to the pineal region than an infratentorial approach. One can select from a wide range of entries through a craniotomy that extends from the inion to the entry site of the last cortical vein into the superior sagittal sinus, which is usually present 5 cm rostral to the lambda. At the entry of the interhemispheric fissure, there usually are no bridging veins posterior to the posterior parietal region. In my experience with 30 posterior interhemispheric approaches for pineal region tumor resection, only one patient had a significant draining vein from the occipital pole.

By sectioning the tentorial edge parallel to the straight sinus, one can achieve large exposure from the upper posterior fossa and the tectum of the brainstem to deep into the third ventricle by modifying the microscope trajectory. The veins of the galenic system overlie the tumor when approached from the occipital and posterior parietal regions. The microscope trajectory needs to be adjusted to a more horizontal angle to accommodate these anatomic structures and separate these veins from

the tumor surface. The only difficult area to expose is the contralateral side. As the veins of the galenic system are approached from the posterolateral angle, a portion of tumor located contralateral to the veins is difficult to expose.

When the third ventricle is totally occupied by a large tumor that further extends into the lateral ventricle either through the foramen of Monro or subchoroidally, an anterior interhemispheric transcallosal approach is preferable. This approach allows the surgeon to resect the tumor through the subchoroidal route. Because the tumor mass in the third ventricle has elevated the roof of the third ventricle, the subchoroidal space is widened in the medial wall of the lateral ventricle. The entire third ventricular space is readily accessed through the subchoroidal space. This approach is particularly useful for third ventricle tumors that extend bilaterally into the lateral ventricles.

Infratentorial Supracerebellar Approach

When a pineal region tumor is small and the primary reason for surgery is biopsy, the infratentorial supracerebellar approach is sufficient. The advantage of this approach is the midline trajectory, approaching the center of the tumor between the cerebellum and tentorial opening. The superior vermian veins need to be sectioned along with the precentral vein to access the pineal location. The deep venous system is above and to the side of the tumor; thus it does not interfere with tumor resection. If the tumor is present above the galenic system, however, it is very difficult to remove through this approach. If a sitting position is used, gravity works in the surgeon's favor as the tumor falls away from the galenic system above, and cerebellar retraction needs minimum force. A serious concern when using a sitting position is the development of air embolism and hypotension. Moreover, obtaining a sitting position in a young child, who cannot tolerate the head pins for three-point head fixation, is difficult. When a sitting position is used, associated hydrocephalus needs to be decompressed before craniotomy. Otherwise, gravity would force the CSF to gush from the open third ventricle, which could result in acute collapse of the ventricular system and subdural hematoma or pneumocephalus. Some surgeons prefer the Concorde (modified prone) position over a sitting position.

In infants or young children, the posterior fossa is small. Thus the surgical field through a posterior fossa craniotomy is often restricted. Depression of the cerebellum to expand the surgical opening results in postoperative cerebellar swelling. In particular, exposing the portion of the tumor situated in the anterior medullary velum between the superior vermis and the inferior colliculi requires undesirable forcible depression of the vermis. The width of the surgical field at its depth is limited by the tentorial opening. Therefore it is difficult to remove tumors located above the deep venous system or located laterally beyond the tentorial opening or extending into the lateral ventricle.

Surgical Complications

With a posterior interhemispheric approach, retraction of the occipital lobe can cause hemianopia, though this is almost always transient. In the presence of hydrocephalus, brain relaxation is attained by CSF drainage through ventriculostomy. With an infratentorial supracerebellar approach, retraction of the cerebellum together with sectioning of the superior vermian veins may result in a postoperative cerebellar swelling. Manipulation of the quadrigeminal plate at tumor resection may result in persistent or worsened Parinaud's syndrome. This is due not only to mechanical manipulation but also to vascular insults of the quadrigeminal plate. The consequences to the surgical occlusion of the galenic system are not known, but venous infarcts of the thalamus and basal ganglia may occur.

ADJUVANT THERAPIES

Germ Cell Tumors

Irradiation

Germinomas are extremely radiosensitive. Only a 1600 cGy radiation dose can totally eradicate the tumor.[5] After treatment with fractionated radiation therapy (RT) alone for biopsy-proved pineal germinomas, the disease-free survival rate for 5 to 15 years' survival is 100% to 80%, respectively.[8,12,18,31,48] In the past, patients with pineal region tumor were treated by means of diagnostic irradiation with a dose of 2000 cGy when germinoma was suspected. Responders to this "diagnostic RT" subsequently received up to 5000 to 5500 cGy total dose. These patients had a 5-year survival rate of 73% to 83% after the completion of RT.[12,33,43]

The dose and field of irradiation for CNS germinomas have been controversial. The irradiation doses for germinomas generally range from 5000 to 5500 cGy in the literature. Some authors contend that the dose should be lowered for this radiosensitive tumor because comparative disease-free survival rates were achieved with a dose to the primary tumor site of less than 4800 cGy.[22,50] However, a lack of long-term control was noted among patients who were treated with a lesser radiation dose ranging from 3000 to 4600 cGy.[3]

The field of irradiation also remains controversial regarding whether it should be limited to the primary tumor site and its margin or include the whole brain or craniospinal axis. Some recommend stereotactic irradiation or brachytherapy. Experience of CNS germinomas treated with Gamma Knife® radiosurgery have shown a 90% response rate, but complete response was noted in only 10% of patients.[24] It is recommended to irradiate the craniospinal axis when there is evidence of CSF dissemination.[49]

Although germinomas are radiosensitive, one should be aware of a late toxicity of ionizing irradiation to the developing CNS. The younger the patient and the greater the dose and field of the irradiation, the greater the sequelae. Even a dose of 2000 cGy to the child's brain is quite substantial. Intellectual retardation and endocrine dysfunction are relatively common sequelae, occurring in approximately 25% after irradiation for pineal germinomas in childhood.[44]

Germinomas recur in approximately 10% of patients despite their well-established radiosensitivity. Recurrences may be due to an inadequate initial radiation field. The risk of recurrence of germinomas in the leptomeninges without prior irradiation to the spine is in the range of 6% to 20%.[31,58] However, Shibamoto et al showed that the survival rate was not substantially different between cytology-positive and cytology-negative patient groups after RT with a variable radiation field and dose.[49] Other factors for radiation failure are presence of radioresistant tumor components, such as teratoma or NGGCT. Germinomas with an elevated β-HCG may be less radiosensi-

tive than pure germinomas.[31,56] Following RT to germinomas, recurrent tumors may be of the more differentiating type. When a ventriculoperitoneal shunt is placed, peritoneal dissemination can occur despite a disease-free CNS.

In contrast to pineal germinomas, malignant NGGCTs are resistant to RT. The 5-year survival rate after RT ranges from 10%[31] to 45.5%.[18] The Japanese Intracranial Germ Cell Tumors Study Group reported a median survival of 18 months and a rate of dissemination through the CSF or hematogenous dissemination of 45% among patients with NGGCTs who had been treated with postoperative RT.[31]

To reduce radiation dose and field for patients with germinomas and to achieve improved tumor control for patients with NGGCTs, chemotherapy has been incorporated into protocols for CNS germ cell tumors.

Chemotherapy

Patients with malignant germ cell tumors of systemic organs have shown an excellent response to multiagent chemotherapy. There is substantial evidence of chemosensitivity among primary and recurrent germ cell tumors in the pineal location. This is partly due to the lack of the blood-brain barrier in the pineal gland, which allows penetration of chemotherapeutic agents. The use of chemotherapy for pineal germ cell tumors has been widely accepted for pineal germ cell tumors.

Allen et al reported their experience with cyclophosphamide-based neoadjuvant chemotherapy for newly diagnosed germ cell tumors in 1987.[2] Ten of eleven patients with germinomas had a complete response to neoadjuvant chemotherapy. These patients subsequently received a reduced dose of RT that included the craniospinal axis. Subsequently, multiple reports indicated high response rates of malignant germ cell tumors to neoadjuvant chemotherapy.[9,47,59] Allen also reported a 100% response rate of germinomas to single-agent chemotherapy with carboplatin in 10 patients.[1]

A prospective international cooperative study of multiagent chemotherapy without RT for newly diagnosed CNS germ cell tumors showed extremely encouraging data.[6] In this study, 71 patients (45 with germinoma and 26 with NGGCT) received four cycles of carboplatin, etoposide, and bleomycin. Those (*n* = 39) with a complete response received two further cycles, and the others received two cycles of chemotherapy intensified by the addition of cyclophosphamide. Fifty-five patients (78%) showed a complete response with six cycles of chemotherapy without RT. The rate of complete response showed no difference between the germinoma group (84%) and the NGGCT group (78%).

Matsutani et al reported the results of the Japanese Pediatric Brain Tumor Study Group.[30] They used a postsurgical combination chemotherapy followed by RT. The chemotherapy consisted of etoposide with carboplatin or cisplatin for germinoma and the intermediate-prognosis group and a combination of ifosfamide, cisplatin, and etoposide for the poor-prognosis group. A complete response was noted in 83.6% of the patients with germinoma and 77.8% of those with germinoma with syncytiotrophoblastic giant cells. In this study, of eight malignant teratomas or mixed tumors of intermediate prognosis, none showed complete response but six had partial response, although among six mixed tumors with poor prognosis, two had a complete response and four had progressive disease.

Despite initial excellent responses to chemotherapy, both international and Japanese studies showed high recurrence rates following chemotherapy without RT. The Japanese Pediatric Brain Tumor Study Group reported that despite initial complete response, 50% of patients with germinoma had recurrence within 1.5 years when RT was not given.[30] Similarly, in the international cooperative study, subsequent follow-up without RT showed recurrences in 28 (51%) of the 55 patients with a complete response to neoadjuvant chemotherapy, which occurred between 8 and 49 months (median 18 months).[6] Most recurrences were treated with a combination of RT and chemotherapy. In this study, patient's age, tumor location, CSF dissemination, extent of tumor resection, and positive tumor markers did not influence the outcome of the patients. However, a statistically significant difference was noted between the pathologic types: the 5-year survival rates were 84% for the germinoma group and 62% for the nongerminoma group.

Chemotherapy is effective for not only primary tumor but also disseminated germinomas. In patients who received a CSF diversion shunt for malignant germ cell tumor, chemotherapy reduces the risk of peritoneal spread of tumor cells.[18]

Although patients with NGGCT show an excellent short-term response to chemotherapy, there is no statistically significant difference in the recurrence rate between the group treated with postoperative RT and the group treated with postoperative RT and chemotherapy.[31]

Nevertheless, the use of neoadjuvant chemotherapy is quite useful from a surgical viewpoint. Certain malignant NGGCTs are extremely vascular. These tumors can be treated initially with chemotherapy, which not only reduces the size of the mass but also reduces the vascularity in the tumor. Second-look surgery for residual tumor after neoadjuvant chemotherapy is strongly recommended before further treatment.[6] The residual tumor can be resected at the second-look surgery. The tissues obtained after chemotherapy are often necrotic without viable tumor cells or chemoresistant components such as teratoma. The dose and field of irradiation are reduced by the use of chemotherapy.[10,31] At present, we have adopted an institutional protocol with "diagnostic" chemotherapy for suspected germinomas. By this method, limited-field RT is used for the patient whose tumor is totally resolved following chemotherapy. If there is persistent disease, however, it will be resected surgically to identify tumor type.

Although chemotherapy is well tolerated by children, side effects need to be watched for. The most common ones are infectious complications and bone marrow suppression. The international cooperative study showed that 10% died of chemotoxicity.[6] The Japanese Pediatric Brain Tumor Study Group showed no mortality, although 42 of 143 had severe leucopenia.[30]

Pineal Parenchymal Tumors

Pineoblastomas commonly affect infants and young children. They tend to recur and disseminate. Pineocytomas, however, are considered benign, and surgical excision can lead to cure. Histologically, pineoblastomas may have multiple cellular differentiations. Among these, neuronal differentiation in pineoblastomas is considered an indicator of benign prognosis,[35] although others did not observe a correlation between the prognosis and the degree of differentiation.[32] Nevertheless, the prognosis of children with pineoblastoma remains extremely poor. In the literature, 76% of 76 children with pineoblastoma reported were dead by the time of publication.[13]

Patients with pineoblastoma have been treated with postoperative adjuvant therapy, including RT and chemotherapy. For very young children, postoperative adjuvant chemotherapy was used in both the Pediatric Oncology Group and Children's Cancer Group. All 11 patients younger than 3 years treated by the Pediatric Oncology Group with combination chemotherapy of cyclophosphamide, vincristine, cisplatin, and etoposide failed between 2 and 11 months.[13] All children younger than 18 months treated with chemotherapy of eight drugs in one day by the Children's Cancer Group had progressive disease with a median time of 4 months from the treatment.[20] In contrast, the group of patients who were older than 18 months and received craniospinal RT and chemotherapy had a better survival rate. These patients had a 3-year progression-free survival rate of 61%. The sites of relapse were commonly in the primary location and in the CSF. According to Ashley et al, children with pineoblastoma responded in some degree to postoperative high-dose cyclophosphamide therapy, attaining a prolonged remission lasting from 63 to 131 weeks after up-front cyclophosphamide treatment followed by RT that included craniospinal axis irradiation and autologous marrow rescue chemotherapy.[4] However, cyclophosphamide therapy for recurrent pineoblastomas was not effective.

The influence of the extent of surgical resection of pineoblastoma on patient's survival is not well known, although a gross-total resection of other PNETs, medulloblastomas in particular, provides a better outcome. Gutierrez et al found that the maximum tumor resection did not show advantageous effects on patient's outcome.[17] Jakacki et al also concluded that the extent of resection of pineoblastoma did not correlate with outcome among patients who were treated with postoperative RT and chemotherapy.[20] The lack of correlation between the extent of tumor resection and the outcome may be related to a high propensity of CSF dissemination of these tumors. Pineocytomas with a pineoblastic component are regarded as malignant and treated accordingly. Pineocytomas are in general considered benign and rarely disseminate, although some authors consider them to be malignant and recommend RT. D'Andrea et al reported that pineocytomas in children are aggressive with a high propensity for leptomeningeal dissemination, needing both RT and chemotherapy.[11] Others, however, contend that these reported cases are probably inadequately sampled or misclassified.[29] When total resection is achieved, no adjuvant therapy is recommended.[27,57]

Astrocytomas

Astrocytomas of the quadrigeminal plate usually have indolent progression. They are often observed among patients with late-onset aqueductal stenosis, often managed with CSF diversion alone. The literature indicates that progression of disease can occur in 25% of patients during follow-up.[40,52] When they show progression, treatment is needed. Some recommend treating these tumors with limited-field RT or stereotactic radiosurgery.[23] However, these tumors are not necessarily radiosensitive. Potential malignant transformation secondary to the irradiation needs to be considered. It is possible to resect these tumors surgically, particularly those with exophytic extension with minimal morbidity.[7,39] But if the tumor is of an intrinsic nature, the incision to the quadrigeminal plate should be started from the rostral dome at the midline. One should avoid traumatizing the inferior colliculi to avoid auditory dysfunctions.

References

1. Allen JC, Da Rosso RC, Donahue B, et al: A phase II trial of preirradiation carboplatin in newly diagnosed germinoma of the central nervous system. Cancer 74:940–944, 1994.
2. Allen JC, Kim JH, Packer RJ: Neoadjuvant chemotherapy for newly diagnosed germ-cell tumors of the central nervous system. J Neurosurg 67:65–70, 1987.
3. Amendola BE, McClatchey K, Amendola MA: Pineal region tumors: analysis of treatment results. Int J Radiat Oncol Biol Phys 10:992–997, 1984.
4. Ashley DM, Longee D, Tien R, et al: Treatment of patients with pineoblastoma with high dose cyclophosphamide. Med Pediatr Oncol 26:387–392, 1996.
5. Aydin F, Ghatak NR, Radie-Keabe K, et al: The short-term effect of low-dose radiation on intracranial germinoma: a pathological study. Cancer 69:2322–2326,1992.
6. Balmaceda C, Heller G, Rosenblum M, et al: Chemotherapy without irradiation: a novel approach for newly diagnosed CNS germ cell tumors—results of an international cooperative trial. J Clin Oncol 15:2908–2915, 1996.
7. Bognar L, Fischer C, Turjman F, et al: Tectal plate gliomas. III. Apparent lack of auditory consequences of unilateral inferior collicular lesion due to localized glioma surgery. Acta Neurochir (Wien) 127:161–165, 1994.
8. Calaminus G, Bamberg M, Baranzelli MC, et al: Intracranial germ cell tumors: a comprehensive update of the European data. Neuropediatrics 25:26–32, 1994.
9. Cataneda VL, Parmley RT, Geiser CF, et al: Postoperative chemotherapy for primary intracranial germ cell tumor. Med Pediatr Oncol 18:299–303, 1990.
10. Chang TK, Wong TT, Hwang B: Combination chemotherapy with vinblastine, bleomycin, cisplatin, and etoposide (VBPE) in children with primary intracranial germ cell tumors. Med Pediatr Oncol 24:368–372, 1995.
11. D'Andrea AD, Packer RJ, Rorke LB, et al: Pineocytomas of childhood. A reappraisal of natural history and response to therapy. Cancer 59:1353–1357, 1987.
12. Dearnaley DP, A'Hern RP, Wittaker S, et al: Pineal CNS germ cell tumors: Royal Marsden Hospital Experience 1962–1987. Int J Radiat Oncol Biol Phys 18:773–781, 1990.
13. Duffner PK, Cohen ME, Sanford RA, et al: Lack of efficacy of postoperative chemotherapy and delayed radiation in very young children with pineoblastoma. Med Pediatr Oncol 25:38–44, 1995.
14. Farwell JR, Flannery JT: Pinealomas and germinomas in children. J Neurooncology 7:13–19, 1989.
15. Felix I, Becker LE: Intracranial germ cell tumors in children: an immunohistochemical and electron microscopic study. Pediatr Neurosurg 16:156–162, 1990–1991.
16. Glenn OA, Barkovich AJ: Intracranial germ cell tumors: a comprehensive review of proposed embryologic derivation. Pediatr Neurosurg 24:242–251, 1996.
17. Gutierrez FA, Tomita T, Leestma J, et al: Pineoblastomas in children. Concepts Pediatr Neurosurg 10:118–128, 1990.
18. Hoffman HJ, Otsubo H, Hendrick EB, et al: Intracranial germ cell tumors in children. J Neurosurgery 74:545–551, 1991.
19. Horowitz MB, Hall WA: Central nervous system germinomas. Arch Neurol 48:652–657, 1991.
20. Jakacki RI, Zeltzer PM, Boyett JM, et al: Survival and prognosis factors following radiation and/or chemotherapy for primitive neuroectodermal tumors of the pineal region in infants and children: a report of the Childrens Cancer Group. J Clin Oncol 13:1377–1383, 1995.
21. Jennings MT, Gelman R, Hochberg F: Intracranial germ-cell tumors: natural history and pathogenesis. J Neurosurg 63:155–167, 1985.
22. Jereb B, Zupancic N, Petric J: Intracranial germinoma: report of seven cases. Pedatr Hematol Oncol 7:183–188, 1990.
23. Kihlstrom L, Lindquist C, Lindquist M, et al: Stereotactic radiosurgery for tectal low-grade gliomas. Acta Neurochir 62(suppl):55–57, 1994.
24. Kobayashi T, Kida Y, Mori Y: Stereotactic Gamma knife radiosurgery for pineal and related tumors. J Neuroncology 54:301–309, 2001.
25. Korogi Y, Takahashi M, Ushio Y: MRI of pineal region tumors. J Neurooncol 54:251–261, 2001.
26. Kuratsu J, Ushio Y: Epidemiological study of primary intracranial tumors: a regional study in Kumamoto Prefecture in Southern part of Japan. J Neurosurg 84:946–950, 1996.
27. Lapras C: Surgical therapy of pineal region tumors. In Neuwelt EA (ed): Diagnosis and Treatment of Pineal Region Tumors. Baltimore, Williams & Wilkins, 1984.
28. Levrier O, Farnarier P, Peragut JC, et al: Value of MRI in the morphological evaluation of tumors of the third ventricle. J Neuroradiol 19:23–37, 1992.
29. Mana H, Nakazato Y, Jouvet A, et al: Pineocytoma. In Kleihues P, Cavenee WK (eds): Pathology and Genetics of Tumours of the Central Nervous System. Lyon, France, IARC Press, 2000.
30. Matsutani M: The Japanese Pediatric Brain Tumor Study Group: combined chemotherapy and radiation therapy for CNS germ cell tumors—Japanese experience. J Neurooncol 54:311–316, 2001.
31. Matsutani M, Sano K, Takakura K, et al: Primary intracranial germ cell tumors: a clinical analysis of 153 histologically verified cases. J Neurosurg 446–455, 1997.
32. Mena H, Rushing EJ, Ribas JL, et al: Tumors of pineal parenchymal cells: a correlation of histological features, including nucleolar organizer regions, with survival in 35 cases. Hum Pathol 26:20–30, 1995.
33. Nakagawa K, Aoki Y, Akanuma A, et al: Radiation therapy of intracranial germ cell tumors with radiosensitivity assessment. Radiat Med 10:55–61, 1992.
34. Nomura K: Epidemiology of germ cell tumors in Asia of pineal region tumor. J Neurooncol 54:211–217, 2001.
35. Numoto RT: Pineal parenchymal tumors: cell differentiation and prognosis. J Cancer Res Clin Oncol 120:683–690, 1994.
36. Oi S, Shibata M, Tominaga J, et al: Efficacy of neuroendoscopic procedures in minimally preferential management of pineal region tumors: a prospective study. J Neurosurgery 93:245–253, 2000.
37. Ojeda VJ, Ohama E, English DR: Pineal neoplasms and third ventricular teratomas in Niigata (Japan) and Western Australia: a comparative study of their incidence and clinicopathological features. Med J Aust (Sydney) 146:357–359, 1987.
38. Ono N, Naganuma H, Inoue HK, et al: Cerebrospinal fluid placental alkaline phosphatase in the intracranial germinomas: results of enzyme antigen immunoassay. Neurol Med Chir (Tokyo) 31:563–567, 1991.
39. Pendl G, Vorkapic P, Koniyama M: Microsurgery of midbrain lesions. Neurosurgery 26:641–648, 1990.
40. Pollaack IF, Pang D, Albright AL: The long-term outcome in children with late-onset aqueductal stenosis resulting from benign intrinsic tectal tumors. J Neurosurg 80:681–688, 1994.
41. Rich TA, Cassady JR, Strand RD, et al: Radiation therapy for pineal and suprasellar germ cell tumors. Cancer 55:932–940, 1985.
42. Russel DS, Rubinstein LJ: Pathology of tumours of the nervous system. Baltimore, Williams & Wilkins, 1977.
43. Saitoh M, Tamaki N, Kokunai T, et al: Clinicobiological behavior of germ-cell tumors. Childs Nerv Syst 7:246–250, 1991.
44. Sakai N, Yamada H, Andoh T, et al: Primary intracranial germ-cell tumors: a retrospective analysis with special reference to

long-term results of treatment and behavior of rare types of tumors. Acta Oncol 27:43–50, 1988.

45. Sano K: Pathogenesis of intracranial germ cell tumors reconsidered. J Neurosurg 90:258–264, 1999.

46. Satoh H, Uozumi T, Kiya K, et al: MRI of pineal region tumours: relationship between tumours and adjacent structures. Neuroradiology 37:624–630, 1995.

47. Sebag-Montefiore D, Douek E. Kingston J, et al: Intracranial germ cell tumours. I. Experience with platinum based chemotherapy and implications for curative chemoradiotherapy. Clin Oncol 4:345–350, 1992.

48. Shibamoto Y, Mitsuyuki A, Yamashita J, et al: Treatment results of intracranial germinomas as a function of the irradiated volume. Int J Radiat Oncol Biol Phys 15:285–290, 1988.

49. Shibamoto Y, Oda Y, Yamashita J, et al: The role of cerebrospinal fluid cytology in radiotherapy planning for intracranial germinoma. Int J Radiat Oncol Biol Phys 29:1089–1094, 1994.

50. Shibamoto Y, Takahashi M, Abe M: Reduction of the radiation dose for intracranial germinomas: a prospective study. Br J Cancer 70:984–989, 1994.

51. Shinoda J, Yamada H, Sakai N, et al: Placental alkaline phosphatase as a tumor marker for primary intracranial germinoma. J Neurosurg 68:710–720, 1988.

52. Squires LA, Allen JC, Abbott R, et al: Focal tectal tumors: management and prognosis. Neurology 44:953–956, 1994.

53. Sugiyama K, Uozumi T, Kiya K, et al: Intracranial germ-cell tumor with synchronous lesions in the pineal and suprasellar regions: report of six cases and review of the literature. Surg Neurol 38:114–120, 1992.

54. Sumida M, Uozumi T, Kiya K, et al: MRI of intracranial germ cell tumours. Neuroradiology 37:32–37, 1995.

55. Tien RD, Barkovich AJ, Edwards MSB: MR imaging of pineal tumors. Am J Neuroradiol 11:557–565, 1990.

56. Uematsu Y, Tsuura Y, Miyamoto K, et al: The recurrence of primary intracranial germinoma with STGC (syncytiotrophoblastic giant cell). J Neurooncol 13:247–256, 1992.

57. Vaquero J, Ramiro J, Martinez R, et al: Clinicopathological experience with pineocytomas: report of five surgically treated cases. Neurosurgery 27:612–618, 1990.

58. Wara W, Jenkin D, Evans A, et al: Tumors of the pineal and suprasellar region: Children's Cancer Study Group treatment results 1960–1975. Cancer 43:698–701, 1979.

59. Yoshida J, Sugita K, Kobayashi T, et al: Prognosis of intracranial germ cell tumours: effectiveness of chemotherapy with cisplatin and etoposide (CDDP and VP-16). Acta Neurochirur 120:111–117, 1993.

60. Zimmerman RA, Bilaniuk LT: Age-related incidence of pineal calcification detected by computed tomography. Radiology 142:659–662, 1982.

CHAPTER 94

PITUITARY TUMORS
IN CHILDREN

Ratan D. Bhardwaj and James T. Rutka

The pituitary, sellar, and parasellar regions play host to a diverse spectrum of lesions in the pediatric population. There is virtually no histologic restraint to the kinds of pathologic processes that can be encountered in this part of the neuraxis. Many of these lesions are neoplastic in nature, whereas others are malformative lesions, and still others represent inflammatory processes. Despite the diversity of pathologic processes represented, all are unified by a somewhat stereotypic and double-edged clinical presentation that features endocrinologic concerns on the one hand complicated by mass-related neurologic issues on the other. Accordingly, when dealing with suspected pathology in the sellar region, all diagnostic and therapeutic interventions must comprehensively address the duality of the clinical problem. This is especially true in the case of pituitary adenomas, where the need for intervention and timing and mode of therapy (surgical, pharmacologic, radiotherapeutic) will vary, depending on the endocrinologic and neurologic status of the patient.

In this chapter, the diagnosis and management of pediatric pituitary adenomas are comprehensively reviewed. Whereas pediatric pituitary adenomas are numerically far less significant than other neoplasms occurring in this region, they do represent an important and potentially curable class of disease. Other neoplastic, cystic, and non-neoplastic processes that occur in the region are also discussed briefly, particularly because they may masquerade as primary pituitary adenomas and often emerge as diagnostic contenders in the differential diagnosis of a sellar mass.

ANATOMY OF THE SELLAR REGION

An understanding of the anatomy in the vicinity of the pituitary gland is important in appreciating the manner in which many pathologic entities in this area ultimately occur. The pituitary gland is located within the sella turcica and attaches to the hypothalamus via the pituitary stalk. The roof of the sella turcica is formed by the diaphragma sellae (a shelf of dura mater stretched between the clinoid processes), through which the pituitary stalk, or infundibulum, passes.[11] The anterior lobe of the pituitary gland is the adenohypophysis, which is glandular tissue comprising three parts: the pars distalis, pars intermedia, and pars tuberalis. The pars distalis is responsible for the meticulous homeostatic regulation and synthesis of hormones and is also the site for the majority of intrasellar neoplasia. The

normal anterior pituitary comprises five histologically and functionally distinct cell types. These are lactotrophs, somatotrophs, corticotrophs, thyrotrophs, and gonadotrophs, which are distinguished functionally by their secretion of prolactin (PRL), growth hormone (GH), adrenocorticotropic hormone (ACTH), thyroid-stimulating hormone (TSH), and the gonadotropins (luteinizing hormone [LH] and follicle-stimulating hormone [FSH]), respectively. Although susceptibilities vary, each of these cell types is subject to neoplastic transformation, giving rise to tumors that retain the morphologic characteristics, secretory capacity, and nomenclature of the cell of origin. From an endocrine standpoint, the vascular supply to the adenohypophysis is via a confluence of capillary networks forming the portal system, which is crucial for the transfer of trophic hypothalamic hormones to the adenohypophysis.

An understanding of the normal developmental patterns of the pituitary gland is necessary to delineate pathologic change from normal growth and development. During fetal development, the cells in the adenohypophysis are well differentiated and produce all of the trophic hormones. The pituitary gland is a bulbous structure with a superior convex surface in the neonatal period. After the first few months of life, the gland lengthens, and the superior border flattens or becomes slightly concave, which is the normal shape observed during adolescence and adult years. During puberty, gonadotroph hypertrophy causes an increase in the size of the pituitary gland, which is more prominent in girls than in boys. After puberty, the mean height of the pituitary gland decreases in both sexes.

The neurohypophysis, which includes the median eminence, pituitary stalk, and posterior lobe of the pituitary, is of neural origin and is responsible for the release of the hypothalamic hormones vasopressin and oxytocin. The former is essential for water homeostasis and the latter during labor and lactation. The posterior pituitary is seldom the site of clinically significant primary disease, although neurohypophyseal dysfunction is common in the setting of hypothalamic mass lesions.

The optic chiasm is a major landmark that, in its typical position, is situated immediately above the central portion of the diaphragma sellae and pituitary gland. Lesions growing from the pituitary gland will often begin compressing the optic chiasm from below, producing a variety of characteristic visual deficits.

The sella is bounded laterally by the cavernous sinus on each side, through which the carotid artery, oculomotor nerve, trochlear nerve, ophthalmic and maxillary divisions of the trigeminal nerve, and the abducens nerve transit. Compression or infiltration of the cavernous sinuses produces characteristic cranial nerve palsies that can precisely localize the pathology to the region.

EPIDEMIOLOGY

Despite their frequency in adults, pituitary tumors are relatively rare in the pediatric population. Only 2% to 3% of all pediatric brain tumors are in fact pituitary adenomas.[10] Hoffman, in his review of the experience of the Hospital for Sick Children in Toronto during a 25-year period, found that only 1.2% of their supratentorial tumors were pituitary adenomas.[5]

Among pituitary tumors, there are differences in the frequency of different adenoma types. From an endocrine standpoint, pituitary tumors can be broadly classified as being either hormone secreting or hormonally inactive. In the pediatric population, some 95% of pituitary tumors will be hormone secreting. Lactotroph adenomas, which produce PRL, tend to be the most common, followed in frequency by corticotroph adenomas and somatotroph adenomas. Thyrotroph adenomas are distinctly rare. Clinically nonfunctioning adenomas are uncommon, accounting for only 5% of all pituitary tumors. Most of these are of gonadotropic origin and, although some may secrete small amounts of LH or FSH, do not activate a clinically recognizable endocrinopathy and are therefore considered clinically nonfunctional. The various subpopulations of pediatric pituitary adenomas were recently reported and analyzed by three large institutions (Centre Foch, Mayo Clinic, and UCSF). These results are summarized in Table 94-1.[2,4,9,10]

With respect to age- and sex-related incidence, some generalizations can be made from the experience of large pediatric hospitals. Seldom will pituitary adenomas occur before the age of 5 years. Among prepubertal children (ages 5 to 11) corticotroph adenomas tend to be most common, whereas pubertal and postpubertal children are more apt to harbor prolactinomas.[9] Somatotroph adenomas, including those that cause gigantism, tend to occur at or after puberty. Across all age groups, females tend to be affected more often than males, although this tends to be far more conspicuous with prolactinomas than is the case with corticotroph and somatotroph adenomas.

The overwhelming majority of pituitary tumors are sporadic lesions. Less than 3% of these lesions are familial in origin, occurring in the context of the MEN-1 syndrome. The condition is a variably penetrant autosomal dominant condition.

DIAGNOSIS

In view of the aforementioned anatomic relationships of the sella, pituitary tumors will occur with a predictable constellation of signs and symptoms referable to either mass effects or pituitary dysfunction. Accordingly, a two-step diagnostic approach is mandatory in all patients harboring sellar disease. First, the clinician must arrive at an anatomic or neurologic diagnosis, and second, one must also establish an endocrinologic diagnosis, both of which must be fully congruent with the clinical setting at hand.

Neurologic Manifestations

Neurologic manifestations can include generalized features of increased intracranial pressure (ICP) or more discrete features of focal mass effects. Clinical manifestations of raised ICP may occur as a direct result of the sheer size of the lesion, or secondarily from hydrocephalus caused by third ventricular compression. Children are often quite resilient, and symptoms of elevated ICP may be quite subtle, including headache, behavioral change, or declining school performance. Depending on the duration of the process, other generalized symptoms such as vomiting, irritability, seizures, listlessness, failure to thrive, and decreased level of consciousness may eventually intercede.

Of the focal manifestations of pituitary tumors, the visual system is often hardest hit and a consultation from a neuro-ophthalmologist is often appropriate. Visual-field deficits, with bitemporal hemianopsia being the classic hallmark, are often presenting signs. Other visual-field defects, including superior temporal quadrant defects, anterior chiasmatic syndromes, junctional scotomas, and monocular hemianopsia, can also occur depending on the precise growth trajectory of the tumor. Impairments in visual acuity, though typically later in occurrence, are still encountered. These tend to be asymmetric and can sometimes take the form of a relative afferent pituitary defect. Fundoscopic abnormalities, including various patterns of optic atrophy and papilledema, should be carefully sought

TABLE 94-1	Pediatric Pituitary Adenomas According to Hormonal Type in Three Institutional Series*					
Tumor Type	Centre Foch		Mayo Clinic		UCSF	
	Number	%	Number	%	Number	%
Prolactinoma	18	27.3	15	41.7	60	50.4
Cushing's Disease	36	54.5	16	44.4	45	37.8
Gigantism/Acromegaly	8	12.1	3	8.3	10	8.4
Nonfunctioning	4	6.1	2	5.6	4	3.4
Total	66	100	36	100	119	100

*The Centre Foch series included patients younger than 16 years; the Mayo Clinic series included patients younger than 18 years; and the UCSF series included patients who were younger than 20 years (*n* = 136). For purposes of comparison with the other two series, the UCSF data presented in this table are from only patients younger than 18 years (*n* = 119).
UCSF, University of California, San Francisco.

during the examination. Abnormalities of ocular motility are also common, and generally reflect cavernous sinus compression or invasion. Diplopia can be due to either third or sixth cranial nerve palsies, the former also manifesting with varying degrees of papillary enlargement and ptosis. See-saw nystagmus, a binocular synchronous alternating depression and extorsion of one eye with elevation and intorsion of the other eye, is another ocular motility manifestation of pituitary tumors, particularly those with diencephalic compression. Finally, numbness or paresthesias in the ophthalmic and maxillary divisions of the trigeminal nerve can occur as a result of cavernous sinus involvement.

Occasionally, pituitary tumors can assume massive proportions, extending into the anterior, middle, and occasionally posterior cranial fossas. Such lesions can generate the full spectrum of focal neurologic deficits.

Endocrinologic Manifestations

Endocrinologic manifestations can take the form of hormone excess or hormone deficiency. The latter is essentially a mass-related feature resulting from compression of the nontumorous pituitary gland or stalk. Because approximately 95% of pediatric pituitary adenomas are hormone secreting, a hypersecretory state is often the most conspicuous aspect of the presentation. Specific adenoma subtypes will be addressed in the following discussion, along with their endocrinologic manifestations and diagnostic tests.

Hyperprolactinemia: Prolactinomas

Patients with prolactin-secreting adenomas mostly have growth arrest, in the form of short stature, and pubertal arrest.[6,9] Specifically, females are at risk for menstrual dysfunction and galactorrea, whereas males have hypogonadism. All patients harboring prolactinomas in a Mayo Clinic study had a raised level of serum prolactin.[6] Hyperprolactinemia may also occur as a result of the stalk section effect. If the pituitary stalk is compressed, so that the delivery of the prolactin inhibitor (dopamine) to the adenohypophysis is interfered with, then hyperprolactinemia may occur. Thus hyperprolactinemia occurring as a result of a prolactinoma versus the stalk section effect must be distinguished. The most common hormone deficiency associated with prolactinomas is GH.[15]

In children, prolactinomas are quite rare, but when present can grow to large size (Figure 94-1). In many instances, chil-

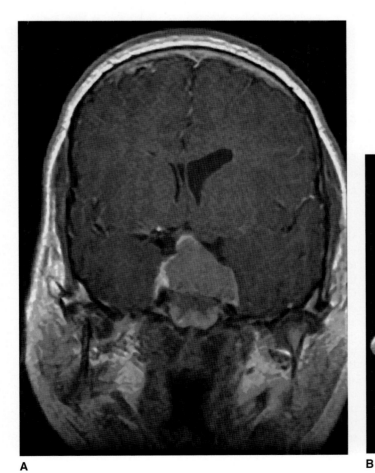

A

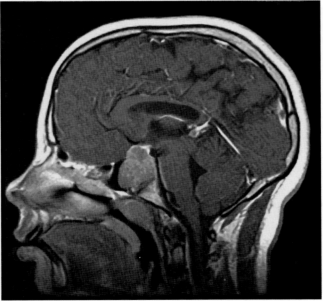

B

FIGURE 94-1 Coronal (A) and sagittal (B) magnetic resonance images after gadolinium administration to an 11-year-old girl with large macroadenoma of the pituitary. The patient experienced precocious puberty and galactorrhea. The serum prolactin level was markedly elevated. Unfortunately, this lesion was resistant to bromocriptine, cabergoline, and pergolide, and the patient required transsphenoidal resection of her tumor.

dren will have visual impairment as a result of compression of the optic apparatus. The diagnosis may not be entertained, especially in young children when other conditions such as optic gliomas and craniopharyngiomas occur more commonly in this age group. A plea is therefore made for clinicians to perform a prolactin level test in all children with large pituitary lesions so that the diagnosis of a prolactinoma is not missed.

Hypercortisolemia: Corticotroph Adenomas and Cushing's Disease

The first step in diagnosing a patient with hypercortisolemia (Cushing's syndrome) is to find the etiology. In the subset of causes of Cushing's syndrome in the pediatric population, 85% of cases resulted from Cushing's disease.[8] Patients diagnosed with Cushing's disease, thus having ACTH-releasing corticotroph adenomas, exhibit cushingoid features. Most often, these features in children are short stature, rapid weight gain, menstrual irregularities, skin striae, and mental status changes.[9] To demonstrate that hypersecretion of cortisol is present, tests such as the 24-hour urinary free cortisol, 17-hydroxycorticosteroid, and creatinine excretion tests are performed.[8] The normal diurnal variation in secretion of cortisol is also lost in Cushing's disease. The high- and low-dose dexamethasone suppression tests are also administered, with the dose of dexamethasone given according to body weight, and these tests have important diagnostic implications. These dynamic tests measure cortisol secretion following a test bolus of dexamethasone to help localize the site of pathology to a central site (e.g., the hypothalamus), to the pituitary gland (e.g., microadenoma) (Figure 94-2), or to a distant target organ (e.g., the cortex of the adrenal gland). In Cushing's disease, there is suppression of cortisol secretion with high-dose dexamethasone testing but no suppression with low-dose dexamethasone testing, suggesting a higher feedback threshold but nonetheless a retained negative feedback responsiveness. In contrast, patients harboring an adrenal neoplasm and having hypercortisolemia on that basis will tend to have suppressed ACTH levels and not to show cortisol suppression, regardless of the dexamethasone dose. Corticotropin-releasing hormone (CRH) may also be given to stimulate the pituitary axis, with subsequent plasma cortisol and corticotropin levels being measured at numerous intervals. A potentially important test is inferior petrosal sinus sampling, which aids the diagnosis in cases of ambiguous laboratory or imaging results. Specifically, this technique is valuable in aiding with the lateralization of ACTH-secreting microadenomas.

Hypersomatotropism: Somatotroph Adenomas and Gigantism or Acromegaly

Some of the most dramatic clinical presentations occur as a result of GH hypersecretion. The oversecretion of GH before the epiphyseal plates have closed results in the clinical manifestation of gigantism, or excessive linear growth. The status of the epiphyseal growth plate is important, because hypersecretion of GH may allow for accelerated growth velocity provided that fusion of the growth plate has not already occurred. Once the growth plate has fused after puberty, the changes are similar to the acromegaly seen in adults. Because GH has such an immense spectrum of physiologic activity, its sustained hypersecretion affects a myriad different organs, such as the

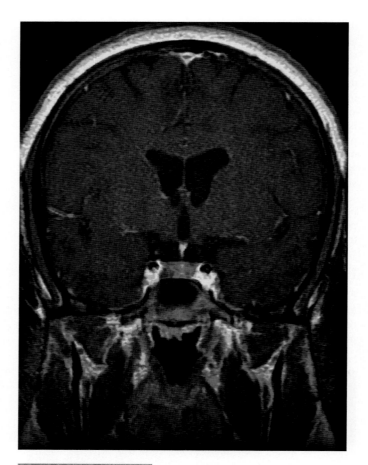

FIGURE 94-2   Coronal magnetic resonance scan in a 14-year-old boy with Cushing's disease. As is often the case with basophil adenomas of the pituitary, these lesions are small and can be difficult to detect on imaging studies. In this case, the adenoma is appreciated in the right inferior aspect of the gland.

skin and connective tissues, and the musculoskeletal, cardiovascular, and respiratory systems. Some of the classic characteristics of acromegaly are coarse facial features, soft-tissue thickening, and enlargement of hands and feet. Thus the excess GH production that occurs with somatotroph adenomas in children is manifested by rapid linear growth, acromegalic features, and menstrual irregularities.[9] With respect to the laboratory diagnosis of GH excess, the basal levels of GH should be measured and are often high in patients with somatotroph adenomas. Because growth hormone is secreted in a pulsatile fashion, a single elevated random GH level is insufficient to either secure or exclude a diagnosis of hypersomatotropism. Instead, one needs to demonstrate failure of GH suppressibility during an oral glucose tolerance test, as well as an elevated age- and sex-appropriate insulin-like growth factor 1 (IGF-1) level (somatomedin-C).

Secondary Hyperthyroidism: Thyrotroph Adenomas

The thyrotroph is the rarest of all secretory adenomas. It warrants attention, because its presence has been increasingly recognized as a cause for hyperthyroidism. Its greater recognition along with the ultrasensitive TSH assays should allow these tumors to be better diagnosed and managed in the future. Most thyrotroph adenomas will have the clinical signs of classic hyperthyroidism and often in the setting of goiter. The hallmark laboratory test is the TSH value, which is in this case high or abnormally "normal."

Hypopituitarism

With the presence of some sellar neoplasms, the compression or infiltration of the hypothalamus or pituitary stalk can lead to the clinical manifestation of hypopituitarism. This may result in the deficient secretion of some or all of the pituitary hormones. In the pediatric setting, pubertal arrest and short stature may occur. Various clinical manifestations relating to the specific loss of some or all of GH, ACTH, TSH, LH, FSH, and PRL can occur and thus cause secondary GH deficiency, adrenal insufficiency, hypothyroidism, and hypogonadism.

IMAGING

Crucial information in the early management of a child with a pituitary lesion is gained from neuroimaging. At the present time, magnetic resonance imaging (MRI) has eclipsed computed tomography (CT) as the preferred modality in the initial investigation of a cooperative patient with a suspected pituitary lesion. High-resolution T1- and T2-weighted spin echo MR images with and without gadolinium enhancement are routinely used in the evaluation of sellar masses (Figure 94-3). It should also be noted that the pituitary gland is not static in growth. It is known that the pituitary is in fact a very dynamic gland, which undergoes dramatic changes in size and shape throughout life, as has been previously outlined, and this must be taken into consideration when searching for abnormalities in the vicinity. For example, the pituitary gland can appear quite enlarged at the time of puberty, especially in adolescent females.

It should also be noted that CT imaging is still useful in many situations. This modality can resolve calcium well, which may be important in delineating a craniopharyngioma, which often contains calcified deposits, from other sellar pathologies. The superior imaging of bone is also of great assistance in gaining appreciation of the anatomy of bone in the parasellar region, particularly when dealing with pituitary tumors in the setting of reoperation, when anatomic landmarks may be distorted. In particular, this is important in visualizing the transsphenoidal corridor when contemplating this route of exposure. The extent of hydrocephalus is also easily visualized with CT, and the fast imaging times may be beneficial if the patient is uncooperative.

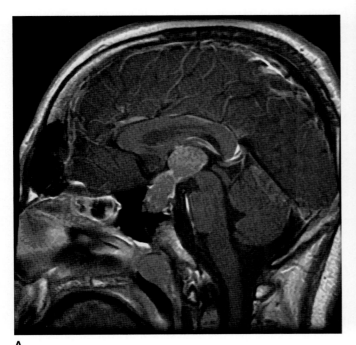

A

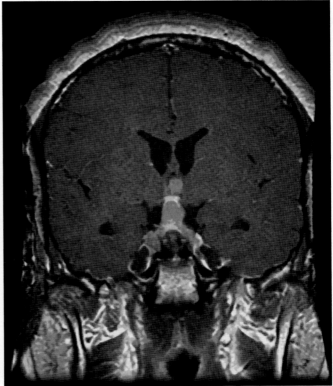

B

FIGURE 94-3 Sagittal *(A)* and coronal *(B)* magnetic resonance images of a 16-year-old boy with gigantism caused by a growth hormone–secreting adenoma. Note the large size of the tumor, which extends through the diaphragma sellae and invaginates into the third ventricle.

TUMOR HISTOLOGY

Adenomas of the pituitary gland are common epithelial neoplasms that originate from adenohypophyseal cells. In most cases, they are slow-growing benign lesions, but great variability in growth rate, size, and morphology can always occur. On the basis of size, microadenomas are tumors smaller than 10 mm and macroadenomas are greater than 10 mm in diameter. This tremendous variability in the growth characteristics of these tumors has been reflected in the current radiologic classification of pituitary tumors. Based on the work of Hardy and Veniza, this is a five-tier classification that grades tumors on the basis of size and growth characteristics. Microadenomas are grade 0 or grade I tumors, whereas macroadenomas are grade II to IV, depending on the degree of invasion or destruction of the skull base. Systems based on immunocytologic and electron microscopy additionally provide further detailed and sophisticated classifications of pituitary adenomas.[12] Kovacs and colleagues have proposed the current World Health Organization (WHO) classification of pituitary tumors,[7] which is a comprehensive classification that incorporates functionality, tumor pathology, radiologic features, and estimates of tumor aggressiveness based on proliferation markers. This classification system specifically applies five descriptive levels to each adenoma subtype: (1) clinical presentation and secretory activity, (2) size and invasiveness, (3) histologic features, (4) immunohistochemical profile, and (5) ultrastructural subtype. This scheme attempts to integrate all complimentary classification systems to provide a synopsis of all relevant pathologic and clinical aspects of the given adenoma.[12]

DIFFERENTIAL DIAGNOSIS

Craniopharyngiomas are benign tumors of squamous epithelium origin. They are thought to arise from squamous cell rests of the pars tuberalis. They tend to be cystic tumors with solid elements and necrotic debris. Calcification is often present, and the cyst commonly contains cholesterol-laden fluid. Histopathologic examinations have shown that the posterior extent of the tumor may blend imperceptibly into important structures such as the hypothalamus.[11] These lesions typically make themselves known on the basis of signs of increased ICP, visual dysfunction, endocrine disturbance, or hypothalamic dysfunction.

Germ cell tumors possess elements of pluripotential or totipotential capabilities and thus are able to display a wide span of differentiation and propensity for malignancy. On a histopathologic basis, germ cell tumors can be divided into germinomas and nongerminomas. Germinomas represent two thirds of intracranial germ cell tumors, whereas nongerminomas include teratoma, embryonal carcinoma, and choriocarcinoma.[11] All germ cell tumors are malignant and capable of metastasis, except for benign teratoma.[11] Measurements of serum tumor markers such as β-human chorionic gonadotropin, α-fetoprotein, and placental alkaline phosphatase may be important in aiding the diagnosis of malignant germ cell tumors. Clinical signs may include hypopituitarism, diabetes insipidus, and precocious puberty.

Optic chiasmatic and hypothalamic gliomas are low-grade astrocytomas histologically, but they seem to be more aggressive and invasive than optic nerve gliomas.[11] Lesions affecting the hypothalamus can cause refractory obesity. A history of profound thirst and increased urination may be present when diabetes insipidus occurs.

Rathke's cleft cysts (Figure 94-4), believed to be embryologic remnants of Rathke's pouch, are benign epithelium-lined intrasellar cysts.[11] Most patients with Rathke's cleft cysts have local compressive symptoms and signs, such as headache, hypopituitarism, hyperprolactinemia, visual disturbance, and diabetes insipidus. Arachnoid cysts are benign cysts of developmental origin that occur variably throughout the neuroaxis. Hydrocephalus, secondary to third ventricular compression, may often be the initial sign. Visual and endocrine dysfunction may also be present.

Inflammatory conditions, namely sarcoidosis and histocytosis X, may also occur in the region of the sella.

THERAPY: GENERAL CONSIDERATIONS

Notwithstanding the fact that each of the different pituitary tumor types will be accompanied by a different set of therapeutic imperatives, the general goals of pituitary tumor management include the following:

1. Normalization of hormone hypersecretion
2. Amelioration of mass effects
3. Treatment of hormone deficiency
4. Prevention of or forestalling recurrence

Fortunately, in the current era of microsurgical, pharmacologic, and radiotherapeutic management, absolute realization of these goals is becoming an increasingly feasible expectation. It is important to recognize, however, that no one mode of management will be appropriate for all pituitary tumors, and that some pituitary tumors will require multimodality therapy to achieve control. An overview of the modalities of treatment is presented here, followed by recommendations for management of individual tumor types.

Medical Management: Receptor-Mediated Pharmacotherapy

Numerous pharmacologic agents are available for the treatment of pituitary tumors. In some instances, such as dopamine agonist therapy for prolactinomas, these agents have usurped surgery as the treatment of choice. In other instances, pharmacologic agents can be used adjuvantly following an incomplete surgical response.

Dopamine Agonist Therapy

Dopamine is the physiologic inhibitor of PRL secretion. Accordingly, dopaminergic therapy has emerged as a powerful therapy for prolactinomas. Bromocriptine is the prototypic dopamine agonist and has been shown to effectively suppress PRL secretion, restore gonadal function, and shrink prolactinomas. Its side effects, however, include nausea, dizziness, and headache, which may be debilitating enough to withdraw treatment. Cabergoline is a new, longer-lasting dopamine agonist

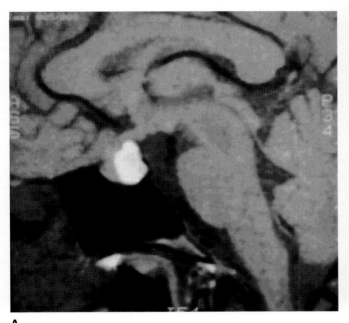

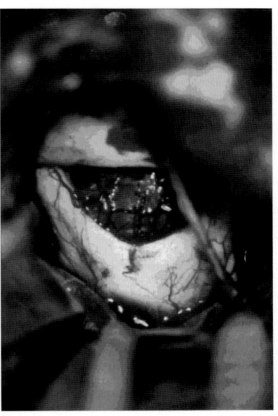

A B

FIGURE 94-4 Rathke's cleft cyst in a 3-year-old girl with endocrine dysfunction. *A,* Sagittal magnetic resonance image showing relationship of lesion to pituitary gland. *B,* Intraoperative view showing lesion in prechiasmatic space. Note olfactory nerve coursing over optic nerve and tract.

that appears to be more effective than bromocriptine in both normalizing serum prolactin and in restoring gonadal function. It also appears to be better tolerated than bromocriptine. Quinagolide and pergolide, which are both dopamine agonists, are other choices available in the medical treatment of hyperprolactinemia.[16]

Somatostatin Analog Therapy

The hypothalamic hormone somatostatin is the physiologic inhibitor of pituitary somatotrophs and thyrotrophs. Pharmacologically more stable analogs of somatostatin have proved effective for somatotroph adenomas and thyrotroph adenomas. Unlike the dramatic shrinkage that occurs in prolactinomas treated with dopamine agonists, the same rarely occurs with somatostatin analogs. Still, these agents are important postoperative adjuvants for somatotroph and thyrotroph adenomas. Octreotide is the best-studied somatostatin analog, and it has been proved effective in reducing GH secretion by somatotroph adenomas.[13] Headaches and arthralgias disappear quickly, and rapid improvements from acromegalic symptoms have also been shown to occur. Side effects associated with octreotide therapy are gallstone formation, nausea, abdominal pain, and diarrhea.

Growth Hormone Antagonists

A new avenue toward treating GH hypersecretion from somatotroph adenomas may lie with pegvisomant, a genetically engineered growth hormone-receptor antagonist. It functions as an analogue of human growth hormone and prevents the correct dimerization of the receptor. A 12-week, double-blind, placebo-controlled clinical trial recently demonstrated the amelioration of the biochemical and clinical manifestations of acromegaly with pegvisomant therapy.[14] The onset of efficacy was rapid, with maximal reduction of GH occurring within the first 2 weeks. Pegvisomant was also well tolerated.

Pharmacologic Agents for Hypercortisolemia

Some medical therapies are available for the treatment of Cushing's disease. Ketoconazole is able to suppress cortisol secretion in the adrenal gland. Metyrapone and valproate can be used as well.

Surgery

Aside from prolactinomas, where dopaminergic therapy is the treatment of choice, surgery will be the initial therapy of choice for the remaining pituitary tumors in children. Surgical approaches to pituitary tumors include transsphenoidal and transcranial approaches. The transsphenoidal approach, being the most direct and least invasive corridor of access, is the preferred route in the overwhelming majority of cases. Of the many virtues of the transsphenoidal approach, its safety and low complication rate are among the most important. With its lack of visible scars, lower mortality and morbidity than conventional transcranial approaches, and patient's better tolerance, transsphenoidal surgery is appealing to both patient and physician. It is certainly among the safest and most effective procedures in contemporary neurosurgical practice. As determined by several retrospective cumulative series, mortality and major morbidity rates are 0.5% and 2.2%, respectively.[17] When performing transsphenoidal surgery in the child, the neurosurgeon must be aware of the relatively smaller nasal passages and sphenoid sinus, which may pose problems with the approach.

Less than 5% of pituitary tumors will require a transcranial approach (i.e., pterional, subfrontal, anterior interhemispheric). Transcranial routes are required either primarily or as a staged second procedure after a transsphenoidal approach when there is significant lateral intracranial extension that extends beyond the midline accessibility of the available corridor in the transsphenoidal approach.

A new advance in the combined realm of imaging and surgery—intraoperative imaging—is also changing the treatment of pituitary lesions. The ability to perform and obtain MRI within minutes of completion of a surgical resection in the surgical operating room is now available. The notion is that this capability would allow the surgeon to have a second look within the same surgical procedure in the event that an incomplete tumor resection has occurred, based on MRI. Therefore the rate of surgical success, via complete versus partial tumor resection, may be improved by obtaining MRI scans inside the operating theater.[3]

Radiation Therapy and Stereotactic Radiosurgery

Radiation therapy has been shown to be effective in treating pituitary adenomas, but this modality is considered to pose too great a threat of radiation damage on the developing brain as a first-line therapy modality.[9] Thus it has an extremely limited role in the management of pediatric pituitary tumors, because most can be managed by surgical and medical means.

RECOMMENDED THERAPY, OUTCOME, AND RECURRENCE FOR SPECIFIC TUMOR TYPES

Prolactinomas

The initial therapy with prolactinomas is medical treatment. Medical management for prolactin-secreting macroadenomas

in the form of bromocriptine, a dopamine agonist, has been shown to be effective in shrinking tumor size (all patients demonstrated a 33% or greater decrease in tumor size) and improving vision.[15] Other medical options have also been described previously. If the tumor fails to shrink with medical therapy alone or if the tumor is so large at diagnosis that its mass is compressing vital neural structures, then surgery is indicated. In some refractory cases, radiation therapy may also be used. A trial looking at the management of macroprolactinomas in the child and adolescent age group reported that the operative cure rate was 50% over the long term and that the rate of recurrence was 38%.[6]

Somatotroph Adenomas

Surgery is the initial therapy of choice, with adjuvant medical therapy being used if necessary. The goal of treatment is to achieve suppression of GH to less than 1 ng/mL during the oral glucose tolerance test and to normalize the IGF-1 values. In one study following adolescents and children with GH-secreting adenomas, the rate of endocrinologic remission following surgery in long-term follow-up was 46.7%.[1] The recurrence rate was found to be 13.3% in this study.

Corticotroph Adenomas

For ACTH-secreting microadenomas (Cushing's disease), surgical therapy should be instituted rapidly to avoid severe impairment of growth, which invariably follows the disease. If surgery is unsuccessful, radiosurgery or bilateral adrenalectomy could be considered. One large study that specifically looked at Cushing's syndrome in children and adolescents found that 98% of patients who underwent transsphenoidal surgery entered remission, and only 5% had a recurrence.[8]

Thyrotroph Adenomas

Surgery is the treatment of choice within this subgroup. Again, radiation therapy may be needed as an adjuvant therapy. Medical treatment, in the form of octreotide, can be helpful in normalizing thyroid hormone levels.

Clinically Nonfunctioning Tumors

Surgery is the main form of therapy in the management of clinically nonfunctioning tumors.

Rehabilitation

Following transsphenoidal resection of pituitary adenomas, the majority of patients will not require hormone-replacement therapy, provided that hypopituitarism was not present preoperatively. Still, ongoing surveillance for and replacement of any hormone deficits is an essential task.

References

1. Abe T, Tara LA, Ludecke DK: Growth hormone-secreting pituitary adenomas in childhood and adolescence: features and results of transnasal surgery. Neurosurgery 45:1–10, 1999.

2. Dyer EH, Civit T, Visot A, et al: Transsphenoidal surgery for pituitary adenomas in children. Neurosurgery 34:207–212, 1994.

3. Fahlbusch R, Ganslandt O, Buchfelder M, et al: Intraoperative magnetic resonance imaging during transsphenoidal surgery. J Neurosurg 95:381–390, 2001.

4. Gupta N, Rutka JT: Pituitary tumors in children. In Thapar K, Kovacs K, Scheithauer BW, et al (eds): Diagnosis and Management of Pituitary Tumors. Totowa, Humana Press, 2001.

5. Hoffman HJ: Pituitary adenomas. In American Association of Neurological Surgeons (ed): Pediatric Neurosurgery: Surgery of the Developing Nervous System. New York, Grune & Straton, 1982.

6. Kane LA, Leinung MC, Scheithauer BW: Pituitary adenomas in childhood and adolescence. J Clin Endocrinol Metab 79:1135–1140, 1994.

7. Kovacs K, Scheithauer BW, Horvath E, et al: The World Health Organization classification of adenohypophyseal neoplasms. A proposed five-tier scheme. Cancer 78:502–510, 1996.

8. Magiakou MA, Mastorakos G, Oldfield EH, et al: Cushing's syndrome in children and adolescents. NEJM 331:629–636, 1994.

9. Mindermann T, Wilson CB: Pediatric pituitary adenomas. Neurosurg 36:259–269, 1995.

10. Partington MD, Davis HG, Laws ER, et al: Pituitary adenomas in childhood and adolescence. J Neurosurg 80:209–216, 1994.

11. Rutka JT, Hoffman HJ, Drake JM, et al: Suprasellar and sellar tumors in childhood and adolescence. Neurosurg Clin North Am 3:803–820, 1992.

12. Thapar K, Kovacs K: Neoplasms of the sellar region. In Bigner DD, McLendon RE, Bruner JM (eds): Russell & Rubenstein's Pathology of Tumors of the Nervous System. London, Arnold, 1998.

13. Thapar K, Kovacs K, Stefaneanu L, et al: Antiproliferative effect of the somatostatin analogue octreotide on growth hormone-producing pituitary tumors: results of a Multicenter Randomized Trial. Mayo Clin Proc 72:893–901, 1997.

14. Trainer PJ, Drake WM, Katznelson L, et al: Treatment of acromegaly with the growth hormone-receptor antagonist pegvisomant. N Engl J Med 342:1171–1177, 200015.

15. Tyson D, Reggiardo D, Sklar C, et al: Prolactin-secreting macroadenomas in adolescents. AJDC 147:1057–1061, 1993.

16. Webster J, Piscitelli G, Polli A, et al: A comparison of cabergoline and bromocriptine in the treatment of hyperprolactinemic amenorrhea. N Engl J Med 331:904–909, 1994.

17. Zervas NT: Surgical results for pituitary adenomas: results of an international survey. In Black PM, Zervas NT, Ridgeway EC, et al (eds): Secretory Tumors of the Pituitary Gland. New York, Raven Press, 1984.

CHAPTER **95**

CRANIOPHARYNGIOMA

Rose Du, Michael W. McDermott, and Nalin Gupta

LOCATION

Craniopharyngiomas are neuroepithelial tumors that occur in the parasellar region and commonly involve the optic apparatus, hypothalamus, and pituitary stalk, leading to neurologic deficits attributable to these structures. Although craniopharyngiomas are histologically benign, they are locally invasive, and their involvement of neural structures in the suprasellar region greatly complicates their management. Treatment options include surgical resection, radiation therapy, radiosurgery, intracavitary radiation, or chemotherapy. Any of these treatment modalities, however, can exacerbate neurologic and endocrine deficits, a factor that has led to considerable controversy regarding the optimal management plan for craniopharyngioma. The rate of recurrence with any form of treatment ranges from 25% at 5 years to up to 50% at 10 years. If recurrence cannot be controlled, local invasion and growth can result in death.

Craniopharyngiomas are classified anatomically according to their relationship to the optic chiasm: prechiasmatic, retrochiasmatic, subchiasmatic, or laterally expansile.[28] Thirty percent of craniopharyngiomas extend anteriorly, 25% extend laterally into the middle fossa, and 20% are retroclival. Most craniopharyngiomas are intrasellar and extrasellar (75%), but some are purely suprasellar (20%) or purely intrasellar (5%). Intraventricular craniopharyngiomas that arise within the third ventricle and extend downward through the sphenoid bone into the nasopharynx are very uncommon.[24]

DIAGNOSIS

General

The relationship of the tumor to the optic chiasm influences the clinical picture. Retrochiasmatic tumors, in particular, push the chiasm anteriorly against the tuberculum sellae leading to early visual changes. In addition, these tumors tend to fill the third ventricle and cause hydrocephalus, which typically causes headache, nausea, and vomiting. Large tumors can compress the pituitary stalk or adenohypophysis, leading to endocrine abnormalities such as diabetes insipidus, hyperprolactinemia, or panhypopituitarism. Subtle endocrinopathies often escape clinical detection for long periods and are apparent only in hindsight.

Signs and Symptoms

The most common symptoms at presentation are visual and endocrine abnormalities. In a retrospective study of patients (adults and children) treated at the University of Erlangen from 1983 to 1997, 47% had visual symptoms, 24% had symptoms referable to anterior pituitary dysfunction, and 5% had diabetes insipidus.[29] Other symptoms included headache without hydrocephalus (8%), headache secondary to hydrocephalus (8%), and undefined neurologic symptoms (5%). Visual symptoms underestimated the effect upon visual function, because 75% of patients demonstrated documented abnormalities on formal ophthalmologic examination. Mental status changes are unusual in children but occur in 25% of adults. Frontal lobe involvement can lead to dementia, apathy, and abulia. Temporal lobe involvement can lead to seizures and amnesia.[48]

Visual Loss

The classic visual field deficit described for an expanding sellar mass is a superior temporal quadrantanopia. Eccentric growth of craniopharyngiomas can lead to this and other patterns of visual loss. Patients often note decreased clarity of vision, diplopia, blurred vision, subjective visual field deficits, and even reported cases of unilateral or bilateral blindness. Yasargil et al noted that 68% of their patients had preoperative visual deficits.[76] The most common abnormality was a bitemporal hemianopsia (28% of the total), followed by homonymous hemianopsia (13%), homonymous quadrantanopia (13%), blindness (6%), and a variety of other deficits.

Fewer children appear to have visual loss at diagnosis.[19,48,76] The explanation for this discrepancy is unclear; it may be due to the lack of awareness among children of a progressive narrowing of the peripheral fields. Toddlers, in particular, can become virtually blind before the extent of visual loss becomes apparent. All patients with craniopharyngiomas should have assessment of visual acuity and a complete visual-field examination before any treatment and then at intervals after treatment at follow-up evaluations.

Endocrine Abnormalities

Craniopharyngiomas usually affect hormonal secretion by direct compression or destruction of the hypothalamus or pituitary stalk. Direct mass effect on the pituitary gland itself can also occur, but pure intrasellar craniopharyngiomas are rare. Hormonal abnormalities occur in 43% to 90% of patients at diagnosis.[48] All of the adenohypophyseal hormones can be affected, including growth hormone; luteinizing hormone (LH) or follicle-stimulating hormone (FSH); adrenocorticotropic hormone (ACTH); and thyroid stimulating hormone. Deficiencies in LH and FSH lead to delayed or arrested puberty in adolescents, loss of libido, or secondary amenorrhea in adults. Low growth-hormone levels will result in growth retardation and delayed bone age. Hypothyroidism leads to poor growth, weight gain, cold intolerance, and fatigability. Forty percent of children demonstrate decreased height velocity or short stature at diagnosis, either from growth-hormone deficiency, central hypothyroidism, delayed puberty, or a combination of these three. Impingement on the pituitary stalk leads to decreased amounts of prolactin inhibitory factors such as dopamine. This "stalk effect" results in hyperprolactinemia. In Fahlbusch's reported data, preoperative endocrine dysfunction was more common than the symptoms suggested: hypogonadism, 77%; hyperprolactinemia, 41%; adrenal failure, 32%; hypothyroidism, 25%; and diabetes insipidus, 16%.[17] In the subset of pediatric patients ($n = 30$), the preoperative endocrine abnormalities were similar, except hypogonadism, which was more common (91%), and hyperprolactinemia (17%) and diabetes insipidus (10%), which were less common. Lastly, some children have "hypothalamic obesity" caused by damage of the ventromedial hypothalamus (VMH), with resultant dysregulation of energy balance.[28,40,41]

Any hormonal deficiency should be evaluated and treated before definitive treatment. A complete endocrinologic assessment is necessary before surgery and is invaluable when varying degrees of endocrine dysfunction may develop (Table 95-1). All patients should receive stress-dose steroids before surgery on the assumption that normal ACTH regulation is blunted. Hypothyroidism can take several days to correct and therapy should be begun preoperatively. However, adrenocorticoid insufficiency can be precipitated if thyroid replacement is begun before steroid is given. Any electrolyte abnormalities should also be identified and corrected before surgery.

EPIDEMIOLOGY

The incidence of craniopharyngioma is 1.3 per 1,000,000 person years. It constitutes 5% to 10% of pediatric brain tumors and 1% to 4% of adult brain tumors.[6] It is the most common neuroepithelial intracranial tumor in children and comprises 56% of pediatric sellar and suprasellar tumors.[46] It is seen more commonly in adults, however, because the overall incidence of brain tumors is higher in adults than in children. The distribution of craniopharyngiomas is bimodal with respect to age. There is a peak during childhood (5 to 14 years) and later in adulthood (65 to 74 years in the Central Brain Tumor Registry of the United States (CBTRUS)—50 to 74 years in the Los Angeles County Cancer Surveillance Program).[6,17]

IMAGING

Plain radiographs are no longer used for diagnosis but if performed will demonstrate sellar changes and associated calcifications. Computed tomography (CT) and magnetic resonance imaging (MRI) are the current modalities of choice. Sixty-six

TABLE 95-1

Endocrinologic Evaluation for Sellar Masses

Pituitary Function	Tests
Adrenal axis	Morning cortisol level
	24-hour urine free cortisol level
	Cosyntropin stimulation test in questionable cases
Thyroid axis	Free T4 level
	Thyroid-stimulating hormone level
	Thyrotropin-releasing hormone stimulation test in questionable cases
Gonadal axis	Follicle-stimulating hormone level
	Luteinizing hormone level
	Sex steroids: estradiol in women, testosterone in men
Growth hormone	Somatomedin-C (IGF-I) level
	Growth hormone level is pulsatile, so a single random level is not reliable
Prolactin	Prolactin level
Antidiuretic hormone	Serum sodium
	Urine specific gravity
	Urine output

IGF, Insulin-like growth factor.

percent of adults and 90% of children have abnormalities such as tumor-associated calcification, sellar enlargement, or erosion of the clinoid processes or dorsum sellae on plain radiographs. Tumor-associated calcification is seen in 40% of adults and 80% of children. Sellar enlargement is seen in 65% of patients, whereas sellar erosion is seen in 44%.[14] The presence of abundant suprasellar calcification, best demonstrated by CT, is important information for the surgeon, because this feature makes removal more difficult. The calcification can be obvious with large confluent areas or small punctuate or curvilinear areas. Sellar enlargement and erosion are also well seen on CT (Figure 95-1). The tumor often appears as a lobulated, heterogeneous, and cystic suprasellar mass. The cyst fluid is isodense or hypodense. The solid portion and cyst capsule are enhanced with contrast.

Calcification is more difficult to detect on MRI, but MRI provides far more detail regarding the relationship of the tumor to adjacent anatomic and vascular structures, which are useful in determining the mode of treatment and extent of surgery. High-resolution sequences of the sellar region, with and without contrast enhancement, should be obtained in all cases. The signal characteristics of craniopharyngiomas on MRI are typically heterogeneous and depend upon the amount of cystic and solid components, as well as the amount of cholesterol, keratin, hemorrhage, and calcification (Figure 95-2). On T1-weighted images, the cystic component is hypointense, whereas the cyst rim is enhanced following contrast administration (Figure 95-3). The solid component is isointense but enhances after contrast agent is administered. The tumor is almost always hyperintense on T2-weighted images.[14,48]

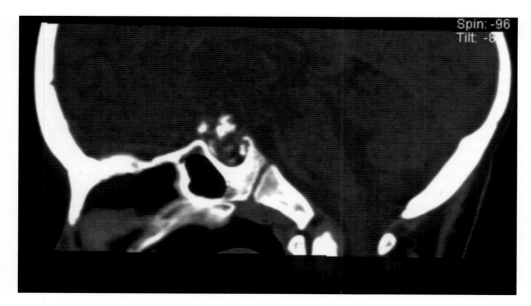

FIGURE 95-1   Computed tomography image (reformatted in the sagittal plane, "bone window" density) demonstrating calcification within the sella and in the suprasellar area. A larger cystic portion of the tumor is not visible above the calcified portion.

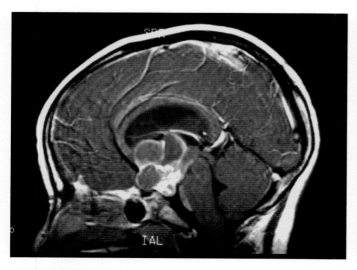

FIGURE 95-2   Sagittal T1-weighted magnetic resonance image of a multicystic craniopharyngioma. The solid component of the tumor is inferior with several cysts extending superiorly into the region of the third ventricle. The pituitary sella is directly below the tumor, and the brainstem is directly behind the cystic area.

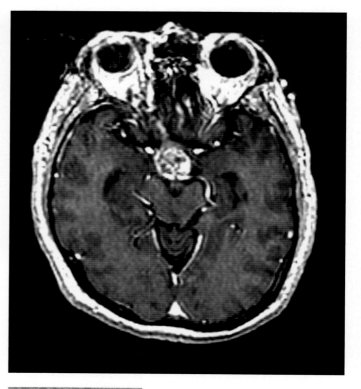

FIGURE 95-3   Axial T1-weighted magnetic resonance image with contrast showing a small, mainly solid craniopharyngioma in the suprasellar area immediately anterior to the brainstem. The central component is heterogeneous in nature.

The differential radiographic diagnosis of cystic suprasellar masses include Rathke's cleft cyst (absence of a solid component, not lobulated, nonenhanced, more homogeneous), pituitary adenomas (sella enlarged, more homogeneous, and less cystic), meningiomas (rarely cystic), optic pathway gliomas (usually not calcified), and aneurysms (laminated thrombus).[18]

PATHOLOGY

Etiology

The anterior pituitary is derived from epithelial tissue (Rathke's pouch), which originates from the primitive oropharynx, or sto-modeum.[46,49,61] This outpouching of epithelial tissue eventually terminates at the cranial base adjacent to the posterior pituitary, which is itself an extension of the floor of the third ventricle and therefore a central nervous system structure. Craniopharyngiomas are believed to develop from squamous cell rests found along the path of the adenohypophysis. Some have proposed a metaplastic origin from the adenohypophysis for the papillary subtype of craniopharyngioma.[46]

Histopathology

Craniopharyngiomas are classified into three histologic types: adamantinomatous, papillary, and mixed.[64] The most common type, adamantinomatous tumors, are cystic and filled with dark brown fluid resembling machine oil. The epithelium resembles tumors of long bones or adamantinomas, hence the name. Microscopically, the epithelium consists of a basal layer of small basophilic cells. The intermediate layer is of variable thickness and is composed of a loose collection of stellate cells whose processes traverse the intercellular spaces. The top layer consists of keratinized squamous cells that desquamate into the cyst cavity, resulting in a cyst fluid that is rich in membrane lipids such as cholesterol and keratin from the cytoskeleton. The cyst contents can cause chronic inflammation within the cyst walls. The desquamated cells often calcify and, rarely, progress to metaplastic bone formation. Squamous papillary craniopharyngiomas are composed of stratified squamous epithelium, which has papillary projections of epithelial cords into the surrounding tissues. The cell layers are solid and compact with no stellate regions. These tumors rarely calcify or desquamate. They occur mostly in adults. Mixed craniopharyngiomas, the third type, have features of both the adamantinomatous and papillary types.

Although the adamantinomatous type is common in all age groups, the squamous papillary type is rare in children. In pediatric patients, 92% to 96% had adamantinomatous tumors, 0% squamous papillary, 0% to 4% mixed, and 4% tumors that were not classified.[46,74] In adults, 63% to 66% had adamantinomatous tumors, 27% to 28% squamous papillary, 6% to 7% mixed, and 3% tumors that were not classified. Malignant change is extremely rare with only a handful of cases reported in the literature.[36] Other cases reported in the literature were presumably from transplantation of tumor fragments during surgery or from meningeal seeding.[3,20,30,31,37,43,56]

Tumor Biology

Thapar et al reported that the estrogen receptor gene was expressed in the proliferative epithelial component of 19 adamantinomatous and 4 papillary craniopharyngiomas, suggesting hormonal involvement in the genesis or progression of craniopharyngiomas.[67] However, there was no correlation between the mRNA hybridization signal for the estrogen receptor and clinical outcome. Raghavan et al measured the proliferative activity of craniopharyngiomas based on their MIB-1 immunostaining for the Ki-67 nuclear antigen but found no correlation with morphologic features or clinical outcomes.[55] Barbosa et al studied acetylcholinesterase and butyrylcholinesterase histochemical activities in several brain tumors and found a high level of acetylcholinesterase activity and a low level of butyrylcholinesterase activity in all three craniopharyngiomas studied.[2] Low levels of butyrylcholinesterase were correlated with slow growth in the tumors studied, but the correlation between the butyrylcholinesterase level and clinical outcome was not studied. Finally, Vidal et al found strong cytoplasmic immunoreactivity for vascular endothelial growth factor (VEGF) in epithelial cells of both adamantinomatous and papillary craniopharyngiomas. Microvessel density, a measure of angiogenesis, was correlated with an increased risk of recurrence.[71] However, not every recurrent tumor had a high microvessel density, indicating that other factors are involved in the prognosis of these tumors.

Little is known about the genetic basis for the development of craniopharyngiomas. Matsuo et al demonstrated the expression of prostaglandin H synthetase-2 (PHS-2) in a variety of brain tumors, including two out of four craniopharyngiomas, suggesting that PHS-2 may play a role in tumorigenesis, but the significance of this isolated finding remains unclear.[44] Sarubi et al, studied 22 adamantinomatous craniopharyngiomas for mutations in three genes associated with odontogenic tumors, $Gs\alpha$, $Gi2\alpha$, and patched (PTCH), but found no mutation in any of the three genes.[63] Nozaki et al studied the occurrence of p53 mutations in a variety of tumors including four craniopharyngiomas but found no p53 mutation in craniopharyngiomas.[52] The genetic and molecular basis for craniopharyngiomas remains poorly understood and will require further research if targeted therapeutics can be developed for clinical use.

THERAPY

General

The optimal treatment choice that results in cure with minimal morbidity remains a controversial topic and is the subject of ongoing debate.[45,60,69] The individual modalities of treatment include surgical resection, cyst aspiration, radiation therapy, stereotactic radiosurgery, intracavitary irradiation, and new approaches such as chemotherapy and the use of interferon-alpha (IFN-α). There are two main views regarding the optimal treatment modality. Some believe that radical resection offers the best chance for long-term survival by avoiding the additional morbidity of additional surgery and external-beam radiation therapy. Others believe that radical resection leads to unacceptable morbidity and recommend an approach focused on subtotal resection and adjunctive therapy. The two approaches have not been compared directly in a clinical trial.

Surgery

The three goals in the surgical treatment of craniopharyngiomas are diagnosis, decompression, and prevention of recurrence if cure is not possible. Hydrocephalus and endocrine abnormalities are associated with high perioperative morbidity and must be treated first. Hydrocephalus can be treated acutely with either an external ventricular drain or more permanently with a ventriculoperitoneal shunt before definitive surgery. Patients with craniopharyngiomas who have acute visual deterioration or symptoms of elevated intracranial pressure from tumor-associated mass effect also require urgent surgical decompression. Because endocrine abnormalities such as hypothyroidism may take several days to correct, a patient who is stable should have elective surgery after all endocrine abnormalities are managed. Those patients with large tumors and cerebral edema will benefit from dexamethasone.

In general, for smaller tumors where complete resection is possible without injury to critical structures, surgery remains the treatment of choice. The surgical approach is determined by the anatomic location and the consistency of the tumor (cystic versus solid, extent of calcification). The most common approaches are bifrontal or extended frontal, unilateral subfrontal, pterional, transsphenoidal, transcallosal or transventricular, and subtemporal. Each of these approaches has its advantages and disadvantages, although some are better suited for tumors in specific locations.

The bifrontal and subfrontal approaches are used for primarily suprasellar tumors such as prechiasmatic and large retrochiasmatic lesions that extend anteriorly and fill the third ventricle. The extended bifrontal frontal approach is the preferred approach at our institution. A bifrontal craniotomy is followed by a supraorbital osteotomy and removal of the superior orbital rim. Although time consuming, this added step has the advantage of minimizing frontal lobe retraction and improving visualization of the tumor. The pterional approach allows a more lateral view than the subfrontal approach and is used for large retrochiasmatic tumors with both anterior and posterior extensions.[48,61] This approach can be combined with the unilateral subfrontal approach. Retrochiasmatic tumors have the lowest rates of gross-total resection; a finding related to their involvement of the hypothalamus and intimate relationship with the optic apparatus. For purely intraventricular tumors, an interhemispheric transcallosal approach is used.[48,61] A staged surgical approach can also be used to combine the intraventricular approach with the subfrontal or pterional approach at a later date to resect portions of the tumor within the sella.

The transsphenoidal approach is used for cystic infradiaphragmatic lesions, as well as symmetric and well-defined suprasellar and retrosellar lesions with an enlarged sella and tumors without calcification that are not adherent to parasellar structures.[10,48,51] The transsphenoidal approach results in lower surgical morbidity and postoperative visual loss than the various intracranial routes.[58] In two recent studies involving 45 patients, no patient had a deterioration in vision after transsphenoidal surgery.[17,58] The disadvantages include the limited lateral exposure and the possibility of a cerebrospinal fluid leak. If suprasellar calcifications are found, complete tumor removal is unlikely via the transsphenoidal approach, and a subfrontal approach is necessary.[61]

For tumors that are mainly cystic, stereotactic aspiration of cyst can be followed by tumor resection or radiation therapy with instillation of radioisotopes into the cyst cavity.[25,50,61] Cyst aspiration can also serve to relieve hydrocephalus.[25] Regardless of surgical approach, any open procedure should be followed by a postoperative MRI scan to document the degree of resection. This study should be done within 48 hours of surgery, before postoperative enhancement appears and confuses the interpretation of the study.

Complications of Surgery

The surgical resection of craniopharyngiomas is associated with significant risks to endocrine function and vision. The most common postoperative complication is diabetes insipidus, which occurs in 59% to 93% following surgery.[17,27,28,58,62,68,76] All patients undergoing open resection should be warned of the very high likelihood of requiring lifelong therapy to treat partial or complete diabetes insipidus. Fahlbusch et al noted that normal preoperative anterior pituitary function was maintained in approximately 50% of patients after surgery, and the incidence of hypogonadism increased only from 77% to 80%.[17] However, other series note that panhypopituitarism occurs in

75% to 100% of patients who undergo surgical resection.[11,12,33] Visual deterioration occurred in 2% to 45% of patients who underwent surgical resection.[17,53]

Hypothalamic injury leads to debilitating consequences such as obesity, disorders of temperature regulation, somnolence, cardiorespiratory instability, and diabetes insipidus. Following surgery, up to 40% of patients experience debilitating weight gain of 12 to 20 kg/year, which persist without plateau. Suppression of insulin secretion has been shown to be effective in preventing or reversing this complication.[42] Minor surgical trauma to the hypothalamus can also cause sleep disorders, memory problems, apathy, and appetite changes.[7,61]

Neuropsychologic and behavioral disturbances were found in 36% to 60% of children who underwent radical resection.[1,33,59,72] A decrease in school performance and learning disability occurs in up to a third of children.[59,72,78] Merchant et al found a drop in IQ scores of 9.8 points in 15 pediatric patients.[45] Whereas neuropsychologic outcome is most often studied in children, adults can have neuropsychologic sequelae as well. Donnet et al found in a study of 22 adults that 9% had severe memory and intellectual deficits and 14% had moderate learning deficits.[13] Van Effenterre et al, in contrast, found in a study of 122 patients that the rate of normal neuropsychologic function was 91% as assessed by patients and their families.[69]

Conventional and Stereotactic Fractionated Radiation Therapy

Radiation therapy is often used as an adjuvant to partial resection of the tumor or in cases of tumor recurrence. Conventional fractionated external-beam irradiation consists of the delivery of multiple daily doses of radiation to the target to achieve a high cumulative total dose of radiation. Total doses typically range from 50 to 65 Gy divided into fractionated doses of 180 to 200 cGy per day. Doses less than 54 Gy are reported to have a higher recurrence rate in children (50%) and adults (33%), whereas doses greater than 54 Gy have a lower recurrence rate in children (15%) and adults (17%).[57] Recently, Varlotto et al recommended that craniopharyngioma should be treated with a total dose of 60 Gy based on data suggesting reduced rates of progression-free survival in those patients receiving less than 57 Gy.[70]

Fractionated stereotactic radiation therapy is similar to conventional external fractionated irradiation but also uses stereotactic guidance. It has the advantage of treating tumors larger than 3 cm and those that are close to important structures.[48,66] It spares the frontal and temporal lobes of a child, thereby reducing the risk of mental retardation and behavioral problems in children as well as the risk of radiation-induced neoplasms. Experience with this modality is limited.

Radiosurgery

Stereotactic radiosurgery has mainly been used as an adjunct therapy to surgery, cyst aspiration, and conventional radiation therapy, especially in cases of recurrent craniopharyngiomas. Radiosurgery employs a single treatment session and uses multiple intersecting beams to increase the total radiation dose at the target and reduce the dose to the adjacent structures such as the hypothalamus and optic nerves. The radiation source is either a linear accelerator (LINAC) or multiple cobalt-60 sources (Gamma Knife®, Elekta AB). Two features that limit radiosurgery are large tumor volume and inability to distinguish a boundary between the tumor and a critical structure such as the optic nerve. Other treatment modalities such as cyst aspiration for cystic tumors are thus sometimes used to reduce tumor size before radiosurgery.[9]

Historically, the total radiation dose used is determined by balancing the dose required to control the tumor while avoiding damage to the optic apparatus. The radiation doses used for the tumor margins have varied from 9.5 to 16.5 Gy as reported in a number of recent series.[8,9,35,47,57] The optic apparatus in these reports received 13 Gy or less, but in more recent studies this has been further reduced to 8 Gy or less.[8,9,35,47] With radiosurgery, tumor control rates range from 70% to 92%, although mean follow-up periods of 6 months to 28 months are too short to state long-term effect with confidence.[8,9,35,47,77] Chung et al reported three patients who developed enlargement of the cystic portion of the tumor 5 to 17 months after Gamma Knife radiosurgery and required cyst aspiration.[9] The mechanism of the cyst enlargement remains unclear. Smaller tumors were found to be more likely to respond.[47]

Stereotactic radiosurgery is associated with relatively low morbidity. Diabetes insipidus, panhypopituitarism, and visual loss occurred in 0% to 4%, 0% to 2%, and 0% to 4% of patients who had undergone radiosurgery, respectively.[9,47,77] Chung et al reported good to excellent outcomes (independent living) in all patients with mainly solid or cystic tumors and in 50% of those with mixed solid and cystic tumors.[9] Visual deterioration occurred in 10% to 66% of patients.[16,35] Given its effects on vision, stereotactic radiosurgery should be applied only to small tumors less than 2 cm and more than 4 to 5 mm away from the optic apparatus.[39]

Complications of Radiation Therapy

Radiation therapy results in endocrine dysfunction and visual defects similar to those observed following surgery, but the severity of these complications, particularly with respect to diabetes insipidus, appears to be reduced. In a retrospective study of 72 patients at UCSF from 1972 to 1999 treated for initial disease, 32% had visual deficits after subtotal resection followed by irradiation, although 81% of these had visual deficits before treatment, and 72% retained the same functional status. For 36 patients treated for recurrent disease, only 53% retained the same functional status with no difference associated with extent of surgical resection, whereas 78% had permanent deficits. A majority of patients had impaired endocrine function. Sixty-four percent required thyroid hormone replacement, 56% required cortisol, 44% required sex hormones, 17% had diabetes insipidus, and 1% had elevated prolactin levels. The endocrinologic sequelae of radiation therapy are comparable with other series that report 6% to 38% with diabetes insipidus after radiation therapy, much lower than for patients who have undergone total resection.[16] The incidence of endocrinologic sequelae is correlated with both age and maximum dose of radiation, being 80% in children and 26% in adults for doses greater than 6.1 Gy and 36% in children and 13% in adults for doses less than 6.1 Gy.[57]

Partial or whole-brain irradiation significantly affects intellectual function in children with much greater effects noted in younger children.[75] In children younger than 3 years treated with either partial or whole-brain irradiation for various brain tumors not including craniopharyngiomas, 60% were mentally retarded with IQ less than 69. The incidence of mental retardation or dementia and vascular complications of radiation therapy for craniopharyngioma is highly correlated with the maximum dose: 40% in children and 45% in adults for doses greater than 61 Gy and 0% for doses less than 61 Gy.[57] In children who had received radiation therapy, 32% to 33% had poor school performance or required special schooling because of moderate to severe learning disability after treatment.[22,78] Merchant et al found a drop in IQ scores of 1.25 points in 15 children treated with limited surgery and irradiation compared with 9.8 points in the surgery-only group.[45] Although the results of the damaging effects of radiation on the intellectual function of young children younger than 3 years has not been studied specifically in craniopharyngiomas, we do not employ radiation therapy in children younger than 3 years of age who have undergone a subtotal resection unless they become symptomatic.

Other complications of radiation therapy include radiation-induced neoplasms (glioblastoma, sarcoma, meningioma), radiation necrosis, vascular occlusion, radiation vasculitis, optic neuritis, dementia, calcification of basal ganglia, hypothalamic-pituitary dysfunction, and hypothalamic obesity.[16,41,48]

Intracavitary Therapy

Intracavitary therapy refers to the instillation of an agent through a surgically placed catheter directly into the cyst cavity. Intracavitary therapy of cystic craniopharyngiomas was first reported by Leksell and Liden in 1952[38] and has been used both as primary and adjuvant therapy for recurrent cases. Radioisotopes such as [90]yttrium, [32]phosphorus, or [186]rhenium can be instilled into the cavity so that a high dose of radiation can be delivered to the surrounding secretory epithelial layer. From a review of the literature by Blackburn et al, 121 of 149 cysts treated in 127 patients shrank or were obliterated in the follow-up period of 0.2 to 13 years. However, the distinction between recurrence of a cyst versus recollection of the initial lesion varied among the different studies.[4] In a study of 30 patients treated with [32]phosphorus where cyst regression was defined as more than 50% reduction in volume, 88% were found to have cyst regression with response occurring within 3 months of surgery and continued decrease in cyst size up to 2 years after surgery.[54] Overall survival rate was 55% at 5 years and 45% at 10 years with a mean survival of 9 years.[73] Because of varying reports of effects upon endocrine and visual function, and the difficulties handling radioactive compounds, this technique has not been widely adopted.

Chemotherapy

The use of chemotherapeutic agents in the treatment of craniopharyngiomas is still under investigation. The best described technique is intracavitary instillation with bleomycin, an antibiotic with antineoplastic actions based on the inhibition of DNA, RNA, and protein synthesis. Takahashi et al first reported the administration of bleomycin in seven children with craniopharyngiomas.[65] Of these, four underwent partial excision and three underwent biopsy of the tumor. Bleomycin was administered 2 weeks postoperatively at a dose of 1 to 5 mg every other day. Injection of bleomycin was discontinued when the cystic fluid changed from a machine oil–like fluid to an almost colorless fluid. All patients with cystic tumors survived at 2 to 7 years' follow-up. Those with mixed or solid tumors did poorly and died within 2 years of treatment. Hoffman et al reported 21 cases of pediatric cystic craniopharyngiomas that were treated with the administration of intracavitary bleomycin.[28] Daily doses from 2 to 10 mg were given. Fifty-seven percent had reduction in cyst size. One complication occurred from the action of bleomycin on the hypothalamus, leading to seizures. Similar results were recently reported by Hader et al, who found greater than 50% reduction in cyst size at a mean follow-up period of 3 years in 57% of children treated with bleomycin.[23]

Intracavitary bleomycin has the advantage of avoiding direct injury to the hypothalamus and pituitary gland, which can occur with radiation therapy and surgery. Other advantages include prevention of cyst reaccumulation and thickening of the cyst wall, which may aid subsequent tumor resection. The main disadvantage is that it mainly works only for tumors that are entirely cystic, in which case radical surgery is less likely to result in hypothalamic or pituitary injury.[25] Other complications include headaches, hypopituitarism, and peritumoral edema.[23]

IFN-α has been shown to have significant effect on squamous cell carcinoma. Because squamous cell carcinoma shares the same epithelial origin as craniopharyngioma, IFN-α is also being investigated for craniopharyngiomas. A phase II trial of IFN-α for progressive, recurrent, or unresectable craniopharyngiomas in children younger than 21 years has been reported by Jakacki et al.[32] Treatment consisted of an induction phase consisting of 8,000,000 units/m² daily for 16 weeks. Patients without progressive disease at 16 weeks then continued with maintenance therapy at the same dose three times a week for 32 weeks. Time to progression after discontinuation of IFN-α was 6 to 23 months. IFN-α toxicity occurred in 60% in the first 8 weeks of treatment but resolved with discontinuation or dose reduction. Toxicities included hypoadrenal crisis with fever, neutropenia, transaminitis, fatigue, rash, insomnia, and seizures.[32] A definitive study examining the efficacy of IFN-α has not been done.

RECURRENCE AND OUTCOME

On the basis of postoperative imaging, gross-total resection (GTR) varies widely in various series, ranging from 29% to 77% of cases.[15–17,62,69,72] Recurrence has been reported to occur in 8% to 100% of patients after initial GTR, reflecting the heterogeneity of patient groups. The mean duration of follow-up in these studies ranges from 5 to 10 years.[15,17,26,33,72] Recurrence following GTR probably occurs because of undetected residual tumor. Small rests of epithelium may not be detected intraoperatively or with postoperative high-quality imaging and can eventually develop into recurrent tumors. Although postoperative MRI is viewed as the gold standard to decide whether a GTR has been achieved, Van Effenterre et al argue that the intraoperative impression of the surgeon is more sensitive for small fragments of tumor than is postoperative imaging.[69] Although most groups would not offer radiation following a GTR, adjuvant therapy following GTR has not been explored in detail.

In many cases, only a portion of the tumor can be removed because of calcifications or adhesions to vessels and vital structures such as the optic nerve and chiasm.[17,61] In patients undergoing subtotal resection without radiation therapy, the recurrence rate is 43% to 75%, with mean follow-up of 5 to 7 years.[17,34,72] For partial resection followed by radiation therapy, the recurrence rate was 43% to 54% during a mean follow-up period of 65 to 84 months, which is comparable with the rate for GTR.[17,72] The management of recurrent tumors is often fraught with difficulties. If a focal recurrence is present on imaging studies, repeat surgical exploration may be warranted. Not surprisingly, recurrent tumors are more difficult to resect and have a GTR rate of 13% to 50% via the transcranial approach[15,17,72] and 53% through the transsphenoidal route.[17] The latter group represents a closed area that limits the extension of the tumor and is more amenable for repeat surgery. Overall, 81% of patients who underwent surgery (intracranial or transsphenoidal) were independent on follow-up review at 65 months.[17] Duff et al, using rigorous criteria, noted good outcomes in 60% of patients, with a mean follow-up of 10 years.[15] These data suggest that although significant morbidity is possible, the majority of patients are able to function at near normal levels. Van Effenterre et al, however, do report tumor-related mortality of 11% in a large group of patients followed for a mean of 7.5 years.[69]

Survival of patients with craniopharyngiomas treated with radiation therapy for initial or recurrent disease is comparable to that for patients treated with different modalities (Tables 95-2 and 95-3). Overall survival rates for two recent series of patients treated in a variety of ways at 5, 10, and 15 years was 100%, 68% to 86%, and 59% to 86%, respectively.[5,33] At UCSF, the overall survival rates for patients treated for initial disease with surgery followed by radiation therapy at 5, 10, and 15 years were 88%, 80%, and 77%, respectively, whereas disease-specific survival probabilities at 5, 10, and 15 years were 97%, 92%, and 92%, respectively (unpublished data). Overall survival rates for patients with recurrent tumors treated with radiation therapy at 5 and 10 years were similar at 87% and 82%, respectively, and disease-specific survival rates at 5 and 10 years were 97% and 91%, respectively. Recently, the group at St. Jude Children's Hospital reported their results.[45] They argue that relying on surgery to avoid endocrine and cognitive deficits is illusory, because many patients have endocrine abnormalities. Furthermore, long-term control and improved functional capacity following irradiation is an achievable goal. These results lead some to argue that radical resection should not be the primary goal for all tumors.

Radiation therapy has been shown to be an effective adjuvant treatment to subtotal surgical resection for initial disease as well as for recurrent disease, as compared with treatment with surgery alone. In patients treated with primary surgery, recurrence occurred in a median time of 19 months.[15] In those treated with radiation combined with surgery at UCSF, recurrences occurred from 3 to 125 months, with a median of 41 months. The recurrence rate did not differ between those treated with radiation therapy for initial and recurrent disease. Overall freedom-from-progression rates in patients treated with initial disease at 5, 10, and 15 years were 89%, 83%, and 79%, respectively. Relapse-free survival rates at 5, 10, and 15 years were 91% to 100%, 82% to 83%, and 83%, respectively, in recurrent tumors treated with surgery and radiation therapy, and 67%, 0%, and 0%, respectively, for recurrent tumors treated with surgery alone. For recurrent tumors, surgery combined with radiation therapy can achieve a much better result than surgery alone. However, Bulow et al found that when patients

TABLE 95-2	Outcomes of Primary Surgery with Gross-Total Resection for Craniopharyngiomas			
Series	Year	Number of Patients	Recurrence-Free Survival	Percent Survival
Van Effenterre[69]	2002	122	95% at 5 years 75% at 10 years	90% at 10 years 95% at 5 years
Duff[15]	2000	121	77% at 5 years	88% at 10 years 74% at 15 years
Kalapurakal[33]	2000	14	92% at 5 years 60% at 10 years 60% at 10 years	100% at 5 years 86% at 10 years 86% at 10 years
Fahlbusch[17]	1999	73	87% at 5 years 81% at 10 years	93% at 10 years
Villani[72]	1997	17	82% at 7 years	94% at 7 years
Hetelekidis[26]	1993	5	0% at 10 years	100% at 10 years

TABLE 95-3	Outcomes for Subtotal Resection Combined with Radiation Therapy for Patients Treated for Primary and Recurrent Disease				
Series	Year	Primary Disease vs. Recurrence	Number of Patients	Recurrence-free Survival	Percent Survival
UCSF	2002	Primary	72	89% at 5 years 83% at 10 years 79% at 15 years	88% at 5 years 80% at 10 years 77% at 15 years
		Recurrence	36	91% at 5 years 82% at 10 years	87% at 5 years 82% at 10 years
Habrand[22]	1999	Primary and Recurrence	37	78% at 5 years 57% at 10 years	91% at 5 years 65% at 10 years
Gurkaynak[21]	1994	Primary	23	74% at 5 years 62% at 10 years	NA
Hetelekidis[26]	1993	Primary	37	86% at 10 years	86% at 10 years

UCSF, University of California, San Francisco.

who died within 6 months of therapy are excluded, the advantage of radiation therapy no longer becomes statistically significant. There was also no difference in rate of recurrence with respect to age or extent of surgery.[5]

CONCLUSION

Despite recent advances in treatment options, craniopharyngiomas remain a challenging disease. In choosing the optimal mode of treatment, one must take into consideration not only the efficacy of the treatment but also the acceptability of the long-term sequelae. This is particularly true in the pediatric population. No definitive recommendation can be made at this time regarding the optimal treatment strategy. In general, GTR should be attempted for tumors where the chance of hypothalamic injury can be minimized. If the hypothalamus is involved, subtotal resection combined with external-beam irradiation should be done to achieve tumor control. Other therapies such as intracavitary therapy, chemotherapy, and radiosurgery are still either under investigation or are limited to tumor subtypes (e.g., cystic tumors). Finally, more data are needed for each mode of therapy to understand long-term psychologic and social consequences in the pediatric population.

References

1. Anderson CA, Wilkening GN, Filley CM, et al: Neurobehavioral outcome in pediatric craniopharyngioma. Pediatr Neurosurg 26:255–260, 1997.
2. Barbosa M, Rios O, Velasquez M, et al: Acetycholinesterase and butyrylcholinesterase histochemical activities and tumor cell growth in several brain tumors. Surg Neurol 55:106–112, 2001.
3. Barloon TJ, Yuh WT, Sato Y, Sickels WJ: Frontal lobe implantation of craniopharyngioma by repeated needle aspirations. AJNR Am J Neuroradiol 9:406–407, 1988.
4. Blackburn TP, Doughty D, Plowman PN: Stereotactic intracavitary therapy of recurrent cystic craniopharyngioma by instillation of 90yttrium. Br J Neurosurg 13:359–365, 1999.
5. Bulow B, Attewell R, Hagmar L, et al: Postoperative prognosis in craniopharyngioma with respect to cardiovascular mortality, survival, and tumor recurrence. J Clin Endocrinol Metab 83:3897–3904, 1998.
6. Bunin GR, Surawicz TS, Witman PA, et al: The descriptive epidemiology of craniopharyngioma. J Neurosurg 89:547–551, 1998.
7. Carpentieri SC, Waber DP, Scott RM, et al: Memory deficits among children with craniopharyngiomas. Neurosurgery 49:1053–1057, 2001.
8. Chiou SM, Lunsford LD, Niranjan A, et al: Stereotactic radiosurgery of residual or recurrent craniopharyngioma, after surgery, with or without radiation therapy. Neuro-oncol 3:159–166, 2001.
9. Chung WY, Pan DH, Shiau CY, et al: Gamma knife radiosurgery for craniopharyngiomas. J Neurosurg 93 Suppl 3:47–56, 2000.
10. de Divitiis E, Cappabianca P, Gangemi M, et al: The role of the endoscopic transsphenoidal approach in pediatric neurosurgery. Childs Nerv Syst 16:692–696, 2000.
11. De Vile CJ, Grant DB, Hayward R, et al: Growth and endocrine sequelae of craniopharyngioma. Arch Dis Child 75:108–114, 1996.
12. De Vile CJ, Grant DB, Kendall BE, et al: Management of childhood craniopharyngioma: can the morbidity of radical surgery be predicted? J Neurosurg 85:73–81, 1996.
13. Donnet A, Schmitt A, Dufour H, et al: Neuropsychological follow-up of twenty two adult patients after surgery for craniopharyngioma. Acta Neurochir (Wien) 141:1049–1054, 1999.
14. Donovan JL, Nesbit GM: Distinction of masses involving the sella and suprasellar space: specificity of imaging features. AJR Am J Roentgenol 167:597–603, 1996.
15. Duff JM, Meyer FB, Ilstrup DM, et al: Long-term outcomes for surgically resected craniopharyngiomas. Neurosurgery 46:291–305, 2000.
16. Einhaus SL, Sanford RA: Craniopharyngiomas. In Albright L, Pollack I, Adelson D (eds): Principles and Practice of Pediatric Neurosurgery. New York, Thieme, 1999.
17. Fahlbusch R, Honneger J, Paulus W, et al: Surgical treatment of craniopharyngiomas: experience with 168 patients. J Neurosurg 90:237–250, 1999.
18. Fischbein NJ, Dillon WP, Barkovich AJ: Teaching Atlas of Brain Imaging. New York, Thieme, 2000.
19. Fisher PG, Jenab J, Gopldthwaite PT, et al: Outcomes and failure patterns in childhood craniopharyngiomas. Childs Nerv Syst 14:558–563, 1998.
20. Gupta K, Kuhn MJ, Shevlin DW, Wacaser LE: Metastatic craniopharyngioma. AJNR Am J Neuroradiol 20:1059–1060, 1999.
21. Gurkaynak M, Ozyar E, Zorlu F, Akyol FH, Atahan IL: Results of radiotherapy in craniopharyngiomas analysed by the linear quadratic model. Acta Oncol 33:941–943, 1994.
22. Habrand JL, Ganry O, Couanet D, et al: The role of radiation therapy in the management of craniopharyngioma: a 25-year experience and review of the literature. Int J Radiat Oncol Biol Phys 44:255–263, 1999.
23. Hader WJ, Steinbok P, Hukin J, et al: Intratumoral therapy with bleomycin for cystic craniopharyngiomas in children. Pediatr Neurosurg 33:211–218, 2000.
24. Harwood-Nash DC: Neuroimaging of childhood craniopharyngioma. Pediatr Neurosurg 21 Suppl 1:2–10, 1994.
25. Hayward R: The present and future management of childhood craniopharyngioma. Childs Nerv Syst 15:764–769, 1999.
26. Hetelekidis S, Barnes PD, Tao ML, et al: 20-year experience in childhood craniopharyngioma. Int J Radiat Oncol Biol Phys 27:189–195, 1993.
27. Hoffman HJ, De Silva M, Humphreys RP, et al: Aggressive surgical management of craniopharyngiomas in children. J Neurosurg 76:47–52, 1992.
28. Hoffman HJ, Drake JM, Stapleton SR: Craniopharyngiomas and pituitary tumors. In Choux M, Di Rocco C, Hockley AD, et al (eds): Pediatric Neurosurgery. New York, Churchill Livingstone, 1999.
29. Honegger J, Buchfelder M, Fahlbusch R: Surgical treatment of craniopharyngiomas: endocrinological results. J Neurosurg 90:251–257, 1999.
30. Israel ZH, Pomeranz S: Intracranial craniopharyngioma seeding following radical resection. Pediatr Neurosurg 22:210–213, 1995.
31. Ito M, Jamshidi J, Yamanaka K: Does craniopharyngioma metastasize? Case report and review of the literature. Neurosurgery 48:933–935; discussion 935–936, 2001.
32. Jakacki RI, Cohen BH, Jamison C, et al: Phase II evaluation of interferon-alpha-2a for progressive or recurrent craniopharyngiomas. J Neurosurg 92:255–260, 2000.
33. Kalapurakal JA, Goldman S, Hsieh YC, et al: Clinical outcome in children with recurrent craniopharyngioma after primary surgery. Cancer J 6:388–393, 2000.
34. Khoo LT, Flagel J, Liker M, et al: Craniopharyngiomas: surgical management. In Petrovich P, Brady LW, Apuzzo ML, et al (eds): Combined Modality Therapy of Central Nervous System Tumors. Berlin, Springer, 2001.
35. Kobayashi T, Tanaka T, Kida Y: Stereotactic gamma radiosurgery of craniopharyngiomas. Pediatr Neurosurg 21 Suppl 1:69–74, 1994.
36. Kristopaitis T, Thomas C, Petruzzelli GJ, Lee JM: Malignant craniopharyngioma. Arch Pathol Lab Med 124:1356–1360, 2000.
37. Lee JH, Kim CY, Kim DG, Jung HW: Postoperative ectopic seeding of craniopharyngioma. Case illustration. J Neurosurg 90:796, 1999.
38. Leksell L, Liden K: A therapeutic trial with radioactive isotope in cystic brain tumor: radioisotope techniques I. Med Physiol Appl 1:1–4, 1952.
39. Lunsford LD, Pollock BE, Kondziolka DS, et al: Stereotactic options in the management of craniopharyngioma. Pediatr Neurosurg 21 Suppl 1:90–97, 1994.
40. Lustig RH: Hypothalamic obesity: the sixth cranial endocrinopathy. Endocrinologist 12:210–217, 2002.
41. Lustig RH, Post SR, Srivannaboon K, et al: Risk factors for obesity in children surviving brain tumors. J Clin Endocrinol Metab 88:611–616, 2003.
42. Lustig RH, Rose SR, Burghen GA, et al: Hypothalamic obesity caused by cranial insult in children: altered glucose and insulin dynamics and reversal by a somatostatin agonist. J Pediatr 135:162–168, 1999.
43. Malik JM, Cosgrove GR, VandenBerg SR: Remote recurrence of craniopharyngioma in the epidural space. Case report. J Neurosurg 77:804–807, 1992.
44. Matsuo M, Yonemitsu N, Zaitsu M, et al: Expression of prostaglandin H synthetase-2 in human brain tumors. Acta Neuropathol 102:181–187, 2001.

45. Merchant TE, Kiehna EN, Sanford RA, et al: Craniopharyngioma: the St. Jude Children's Research Hospital experience 1984–2001. Int J Radiat Oncol Biol Phys 53:533–542, 2002.

46. Miller DC: Pathology of craniopharyngiomas: clinical import of pathological findings. Pediatr Neurosurg 21 Suppl 1:11–17, 1994.

47. Mokry M: Craniopharyngiomas: a six year experience with Gamma Knife radiosurgery. Stereotact Funct Neurosurg 72 Suppl 1:140–149, 1999.

48. Moore K, Couldwell WT: Craniopharyngioma. In Bernstein M, Berger MS (eds): Neuro-oncology: The Essentials. New York, Thieme, 2000.

49. Moore K, Persaud TVN: The Developing Human: Clinically Oriented Embryology. Philadelphia, WB Saunders, 1993.

50. Nakamizo A, Inamura T, Nishio S, et al: Neuroendoscopic treatment of cystic craniopharyngioma in the third ventricle. Minim Invasive Neurosurg 44:85–87, 2001.

51. Norris JS, Pavaresh M, Afshar F: Primary transsphenoidal microsurgery in the treatment of craniopharyngiomas. Br J Neurosurg 12:305–312, 1998.

52. Nozaki M, Tada M, Matsumoto R, et al: Rare occurrence of inactivating p53 gene mutations in primary non-astrocytic tumors of the central nervous system: reappraisal by yeast functional assay. Acta Neuropathol 95:291–296, 1998.

53. Pierre-Kahn A, Sainte-Rose C, Renier D: Surgical approach to children with craniopharyngiomas and severely impaired vision: special considerations. Pediatr Neurosurg 21 (Suppl 1):50–56, 1994.

54. Pollock BE, Lunsford LD, Kondziolka D, et al: Phosphorus-32 intracavitary irradiation of cystic craniopharyngiomas: current technique and long-term results. Int J Radiat Oncol Biol Phys 33:437–446, 1995.

55. Raghavan R, Dickey WT, Jr, Margraf LR, et al: Proliferative activity in craniopharyngiomas: clinicopathological correlations in adults and children. Surg Neurol 54:241–247, 2000.

56. Ragoowansi AT, Piepgras DG: Postoperative ectopic craniopharyngioma. Case report. J Neurosurg 74:653–655, 1991.

57. Regine WF, Mohiuddin M, Kramer S: Long-term results of pediatric and adult craniopharyngiomas treated with combined surgery and radiation. Radiother Oncol 27:13–21, 1993.

58. Rilliet B, de Paul Djientcheu V, Vernet O, et al: Craniopharyngiomas, results in children and adolescents operated through a transsphenoidal approach compared with an intracranial approach. Front Radiat Ther Oncol 33:114–122, 1999.

59. Riva D, Pantaleoni C, Devoti M, et al: Late neuropsychological and behavioural outcome of children surgically treated for craniopharyngioma. Childs Nerv Syst 14:179–184, 1998.

60. Rutka JT: Craniopharyngioma. J Neurosurg 97:1–2, 2002.

61. Samii M, Tatagiba M: Surgical management of craniopharyngiomas: a review. Neurol Med Chir (Tokyo) 37:141–149, 1997.

62. Sanford RA: Craniopharyngioma: results of survey of the American Society of Pediatric Neurosurgery. Pediatr Neurosurg 21 (Suppl 1):39–43, 1994.

63. Sarubi JC, Bei H, Adams EF, et al: Clonal composition of human adamantinomatous craniopharyngiomas and somatic mutation analyses of the patched (PTCH), Gsalpha and Gi2alpha genes. Neurosci Lett 310:5–8, 2001.

64. Sidawy MK, Jannotta FS: Intraoperative cytologic diagnosis of lesions of the central nerous system. Am J Clin Pathol 108(Suppl 1):S56–66, 1997.

65. Takahashi H, Nakazawa S, Shimura T: Evaluation of postoperative intratumoral injection of bleomycin for craniopharyngioma in children. J Neurosurg 62:120–127, 1985.

66. Tarbell NJ, Barnes P, Scott RM, et al: Advances in radiation therapy for craniopharyngiomas. Pediatr Neurosurg 21 (Suppl 1):101–107, 1994.

67. Thapar K, Stefaneanu L, Kovacs K, et al: Estrogen receptor gene expression in craniopharyngiomas: an in situ hybridization study. Neurosurgery 35:1012–1017, 1994.

68. Tomita T, McLone DG: Radical resections of childhood craniopharyngiomas. Pediatr Neurosurg 19:6–14, 1993.

69. Van Effenterre R, Boch AL: Craniopharyngioma in adults and children: a study of 22 surgical cases. J Neurosurg 97:3–11, 2002.

70. Varlotto JM, Flickinger JC, Kondziolka D, et al: External beam irradiation of craniopharyngiomas: long-term analysis of tumor control and morbidity. Int J Radiat Oncol Biol Phys 54:492–499, 2002.

71. Vidal S, Kovacs K, Lloyd RV, et al: Angiogenesis in patients with craniopharyngiomas: correlation with treatment and outcome. Cancer 94:738–745, 2002.

72. Villani RM, Tomei G, Bello L, et al: Long-term results of treatment for craniopharyngioma in children. Childs Nerv Syst 13:397–405, 1997.

73. Voges J, Sturm V, Lehrke R, et al: Cystic craniopharyngioma: long-term results after intracavitary irradiation with stereotactically applied colloidal beta-emitting radioactive sources. Neurosurgery 40:263–269; discussion 269–270, 1997.

74. Weiner HL, Wisoff JH, Rosenberg ME, et al: Craniopharyngiomas: a clinicopathological analysis of factors predictive of recurrence and functional outcome. Neurosurgery 35:1001–1010, 1994.

75. Weiss M, Sutton L, Marcial V, et al: The role of radiation therapy in the management of childhood craniopharyngioma. Int J Radiat Oncol Biol Phys 17:1313–1321, 1989.

76. Yasargil MG, Curcic M, Kis M, et al: Total removal of craniopharyngiomas. Approaches and long-term results in 144 patients. J Neurosurg 73:3–11, 1990.

77. Yu X, Liu Z, Li S: Combined treatment with stereotactic intracavitary irradiation and gamma knife surgery for craniopharyngiomas. Stereotact Funct Neurosurg 75:117–122, 2000.

78. Zuccaro G, Jaimovich R, Mantese B, et al: Complications in paediatric craniopharyngioma treatment. Childs Nerv Syst 12:385–390, 1996.

CHAPTER 96

GERM CELL TUMORS IN CHILDREN

Toshihiko Wakabayashi and Jun Yoshida

The histopathologic entity of primary intracranial germ cell tumors includes a number of subtypes such as germinoma, germinoma with syncytiotrophoblastic giant cells (STGCs), mature teratoma, immature teratoma, yolk sac tumor, choriocarcinoma, and mixed germ cell tumors that include several types of components of germ cell tumors.[11] Even though the symptoms and radiologic appearances are similar, the prognoses and outcome of primary intracranial germ cell tumors are extremely different and depend on tumor type.[2,6,22]

In this chapter, the characteristic findings of germ cell tumors in children are described. In addition, the prognostic factors for survival and quality of life are presented. Finally, we summarize the most recent data from the literature on primary intracranial germ cell tumors treated with surgery, radiation therapy, and chemotherapy.

EPIDEMIOLOGY

Intracranial germ cell tumors consist of rare and varied histologic types of brain tumors. A higher incidence of germ cell tumors in Asian countries compared with Western countries has been reported. The incidence of pineal region tumors in Asia is higher (3.0%) than in Europe and the United States (0.4 to 1.0%). Of the germ cell tumors limited to the pineal region in Japanese and Korean studies, pure germinoma was found in 70.3% and 80.2%, respectively. In European and U.S. studies, pure germinomas constitute 53.6% and 58.3% of pineal region germ cell tumors, respectively. Age and sex distributions of pineal region germ cell tumors show a high incidence in males and in children. The sex ratio of the occurrence of germ cell tumor in the pineal region shows a marked male predominance, with a male to female ratio of 51:5.5. Males predominate for all the different subtypes of germ cell tumors. As for age distribution, germinoma, embryonal carcinoma, and malignant teratoma have a peak age incidence at 10 to 14 years, whereas choriocarcinoma and teratoma are widely distributed through ages 10 to 20 years.

As for the germ cell tumors in the suprasellar region, the sex ratio between males and females is almost equal. Compared with the pineal region, there is a tendency for suprasellar germ cell tumors to be nongerminomatous germ cell tumors, especially immature teratoma.

LOCATION

As with other extragonadal germ cell tumors, intracranial germ cell tumors tend to arise in the midline. More than 80% of intracranial germ cell tumors arise in the region of the pineal gland, followed by tumors in the suprasellar region. Other sites of origin of intracranial germ cell tumors include intraventricular, basal ganglia, thalamic, cerebral hemispheric, bulbar, intramedullary, and intrasellar. Multifocal germ cell tumors usually involve the pineal region and suprasellar compartment simultaneously (synchronously) or sequentially (metachronously).

DIAGNOSIS

Clinical Features

The clinical manifestations of germ cell tumors and their duration vary with histologic type and location. Tumors of the pineal region often compress and obstruct the cerebral aqueduct, resulting in progressive hydrocephalus with intracranial hypertension. Also, pineal region tumors may compress and invade the tectal plate, producing a characteristic paralysis of upward gaze and convergence known as Parinaud's syndrome. Suprasellar tumor typically compresses the optic chiasm, causing visual field deficits, and often disrupts the hypothalamus as suggested by the occurrence of diabetes insipidus and manifestations of pituitary failure, which include growth retardation and delayed sexual maturation. Germ cell tumors may also cause precocious puberty by pineal or hypothalamic destruction or by the elaboration of human chorionic gonadotropin (HCG), a stimulant of testosterone production that is secreted by neoplastic syncytiotrophoblasts located in the tumor.

Tumor Markers

Tumor marker levels in the serum or cerebrospinal fluid (CSF) provide quite reliable data for the diagnosis of the germ cell tumor type, even for primary intracranial mass lesions. HCG-β is mostly elevated with the diagnosis of germinoma with STGCs. In cases of choriocarcinoma, the levels of HCG-β sometimes exceed 10,000 ng/mL in the serum, and they correlate well with a poor prognosis. α-Fetoprotein (AFP) is another reliable marker for the diagnosis of yolk sac tumor, and levels greater than 4000 milli-international units per milliliter are indicative of a poor prognosis. Sometimes the serum levels of carcinoembryonic antigen (CEA) are elevated in cases of embryonal carcinoma. Finally, placental alkaline phosphatase (PLAP) is positive at times in immunohistochemical studies of germinoma.

Imaging

The diagnosis of germinoma may be suggested on plain computed tomography (CT) when nodular clusters of calcification in the pineal region are present. Usually, hydrocephalus can be seen because of obstruction of the aqueduct by the mass. Germ cell tumors usually appear as solid masses that are isodense or slightly hyperdense relative to gray matter. Following contrast administration, the germ cell tumors typically show prominent enhancement on CT or magnetic resonance imaging (MRI). Suprasellar germ cell tumors may initially cause only enhancement of the pituitary stalk until a later stage, when the tumor may infiltrate the optic chiasm. In cases of teratoma, cystic regions may also be identified as part of the mass. An intratumoral hemorrhage seen on imaging studies strongly suggests the diagnosis of choriocarcinoma.

Histology

Whereas germinoma and teratoma typically occur as pure tumor subtypes, choriocarcinoma, yolk sac tumor, and embryonal carcinoma occur as mixed germ cell tumor types. Of all the pineal region germ cell tumors in Japan, the most common tumor subtype is germinoma, accounting for 70.3% of tumors, followed by immature teratoma at 14.7%.

TREATMENT

Most malignant germ cell tumors other than germinoma are associated with a poor prognosis; however, recent progress in surgical techniques and effective chemoradiation therapy has improved the prognosis.

Surgery

The surgical procedures that are used for germ cell tumors include a shunt operation or third ventriculostomy for hydrocephalus, tumor biopsy, or aggressive tumor resection. It remains somewhat controversial as to whether surgery of germ cell tumors should be the first line of therapy. For example, in Western countries there is a tendency to select surgery, but in Asian countries radiation therapy or chemotherapy is selected as the first treatment, because radiochemosensitive germinoma is predominantly found for tumors in the pineal region. Certainly the role of radical surgery for germinoma has never been proved. However, for nongerminomatous germ cell tumors, total resection of the mass lesion may improve the prognosis.

Radiation Therapy

Radiation therapy has long been known to be effective for germinoma. After the diagnosis is made, germinomas are treated by radiation therapy that comprises treatment of the whole ventricle or focal boost cranial irradiation. Whole-brain irradiation was used in the past, but this practice has largely disappeared. If spinal seeding has been demonstrated, the spine is incorporated into the radiation fields. Because of some of the deleterious effects of radiation therapy on the central nervous system (CNS), current approaches have explored the possibility of reducing or even eliminating radiation therapy.[15] Recently, it has been recommended that the radiation dose and volume for germinomas be reduced to 24 to 30 Gy in a localized field (including the entire ventricular systems).[3,21] The 5-year cumulative survival rate in patients who received reduced radiation therapy with chemotherapy has been almost equal to that of those who were treated with full-dose irradiation alone. Finally, in cases of other malignant germ cell tumors, the prognosis is still unsatisfactory, even after full-dose irradiation with chemotherapy.

Chemotherapy

In efforts to reduce radiation dose and to improve prognosis, combination chemotherapy with radiation therapy has been generally accepted.[1] Of the chemotherapeutic agents used to treat germ cell tumors, cisplatin, carboplatin, vinblastine, etoposide, bleomycin, or CCNU are generally effective. Several drug combinations such as PVB (cisplatin, vinblastine, bleomycin), PE (cisplatin, etoposide), and ICE (ifosfamide, carboplatin, etoposide) have been shown to have particular promise. Today, PE therapy may be the chemotherapy treatment of choice for germ cell tumors. Interestingly, chemotherapy alone without radiation therapy is currently not recommended, because recurrences have been reported in many patients.[13]

OUTCOME—SURVIVAL

Outcome for germ cell tumors varies widely among differing histologies. Of the cumulative survival rates for various types of germ cell tumors, germinoma shows the highest survival rate at 89.2%. In the case of germinoma, it is known that diffuse dissemination of disease at diagnosis is not a risk factor for a poor prognosis. Embryonal carcinoma, yolk sac tumor, and choriocarcinoma have worse survival rates than the other types of germ cell tumors (Table 96-1).[12]

FUNCTIONAL OUTCOME

Functional outcome after treatment for germ cell tumors can be assessed by examining performance status, neurologic deficits, hormonal dysfunction, and brain injury after radiation therapy.

Performance Status

Yoshida et al analyzed performance status after radiochemotherapy for germ cell tumors. They showed a performance status score of 75% for pure germinoma, 75% for germinoma with STGCs, and 57% for nongerminomatous germ cell tumors. In this report, the response rate for all germ cell tumors was 67%.[25] In long-term survivors, if patients had received radiation therapy with a total dose of more than 30 Gy, cognitive dysfunction was found in some cases. In general, intellectual decline correlates directly with total radiation dose.

Follow-up MRI studies in patients who have received cranial irradiation will typically show cerebral atrophy. In one study that examined patients treated for germ cell tumors with a mean follow-up of 99 months, only 13% of patients maintained a performance status of 100%.[20]

Though not included as an assessment item for performance status, sterility caused by cisplatin therapy, which is an indispensable chemotherapeutic agent for germ cell tumors, should be seen as a major problem for long-term survivors. In addition, etoposide, which is one of the major drugs used in the treatment for germ cell tumors, is known to induce secondary neoplasms, albeit at a low rate.

Neurologic Deficits

After neurosurgical treatment for tumor excision or insertion of a CSF shunt, hydrocephalus is usually well controlled. For tumors originating around the optic pathway, there may be a high frequency of visual impairments affecting acuity and fields. Some patients will demonstrate limitations in upward gaze palsy as a result of involvement of tumor with the quadrigeminal plate. High-tone hearing loss has been observed after cisplatin therapy, which can also cause peripheral neuropathy.

Hormonal Disorder

For patients with suprasellar lesions, hormone replacement therapy is a common requirement after treatment, affecting almost 80% of patients. Diabetes insipidus or anterior pituitary dysfunction is common. Treatment of the former with DDAVP (1-deamino-8-D-arginine vasopressin [desmopressin]) is usually long term. Saki et al emphasized that pituitary dysfunction present before treatment persisted or even worsened after patients went into remission, except for patients with small and localized masses on admission.[17]

Cerebral Injury after Radiation Therapy

Cerebral injury from radiation therapy is usually seen following whole-brain irradiation of 30 Gy or more. On MRI, generalized brain atrophy, multiple cerebral lacunae infarction, and high signal intensity areas in the white matter representing demyelination are generally observed. Associated with cerebral atrophy are mental and physical deterioration, hypothalamic or endocrinologic dysfunction, and impaired quality of life. A feared complication of radiation therapy is a radiation-induced secondary neoplasm. Sawamura et al also described 4 patients from a total of 84 intracranial germ cell tumor patients (4.7%) who developed radiation-induced neoplasms, including two glioblastomas and two meningiomas.[20] Moreover, there is another report describing a 12% occurrence of secondary neoplasms over a 20-year period.[13]

As an illustrative case, we describe a 14-year-old boy with a solid mass in the suprasellar area who underwent biopsy and proved to have an immature teratoma. Chemoradiation therapy was given, and a total radiation dose of 60 Gy was administered. After these treatments, MRI showed complete remission of tumor. The patient did well in school until 6 years after the initial treatment when he complained of headache and depression. A follow-up MRI study revealed a low-intensity lesion in the right basal ganglia with mild brain atrophy. After 6 months, a repeat MRI scan showed progressive brain atrophy (Figure 96-1). This case is typical for delayed brain injury induced by radiation therapy.

SUBCLASSIFICATION OF INTRACRANIAL GERM CELL TUMORS

According to the World Health Organization (WHO) classification of intracranial germ cell tumors, germinoma, embryonal carcinoma, yolk sac tumor (endodermal sinus tumor), choriocarcinoma, mature teratoma, immature teratoma, teratoma with malignant transformation, and mixed germ cell tumors are the main types.[11]

Germinomas

Pure Germinoma

Pure germinoma may be cured with a better than 90% 5-year survival rate using radiation therapy alone. In the report of Japan's Brain Tumor Registry in 2000, a remarkable improvement in cumulative survival for germinoma by radiation therapy was shown.[4] Several issues concerning quality of life, however, are known to be induced by radiation therapy. Therefore combined chemoradiation therapy has been used to reduce the total radiation dose to the brain. Nowadays, it is generally accepted that patients with germinoma can be cured by preirradiation chemotherapy followed by reduced doses of irradiation.

According to the analyses by the Brain Tumor Registry in 2000, relative survival rates for germinoma at 1-year, 2-year, and 5-year intervals were 96.6%, 94.3%, and 91.2%, respectively.[4] Brandes et al showed a 5-year survival rate of 96%.[3] Recently, Sano also showed 5- and 10-year survival rates of 96% and 93%, respectively.[19]

Germinoma with Syncytiotrophoblastic Giant Cells

Approximately 13% of germinomas contain syncytiotrophoblastic giant cells (STGC) positive for HCG-β.[21,22] This type of tumor has been shown to have a different response to chemoradiation therapy. Although the response rate is high, the

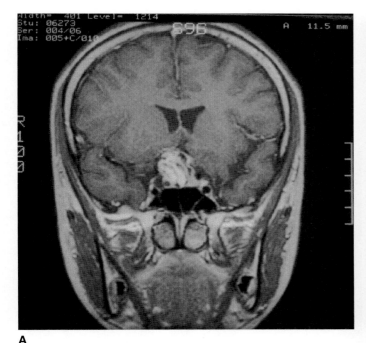

A

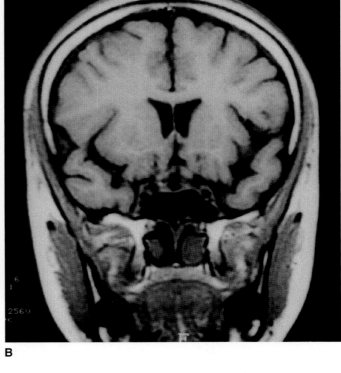

B

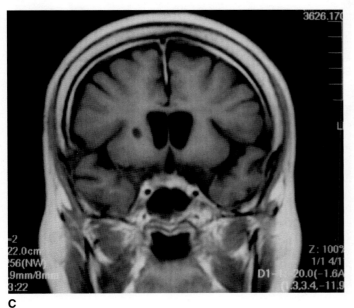

C

FIGURE 96-1   *A,* A 14-year-old boy complained of visual disturbance. Magnetic resonance imaging (MRI) with gadolinium enhancement revealed an enhanced solid mass in the suprasellar (neurohypophysis) region. Histologic examination revealed an immature teratoma. Extensive chemoradiation therapy was performed, and total radiation dose was 60 Gy (whole-brain 40 Gy + boost 20 Gy). *B,* After treatment, MRI revealed complete remission of tumor. The patient's condition was excellent and, after graduating from high school, he worked in computer programming. *C,* Six years after initial treatment, the patient complained of headache and slight depression. Follow-up MRI revealed a low-intensity lesion in the right basal ganglia with mild brain atrophy. After 6 months, his mental status gradually became worse. He is suspected to have brain damage induced by radiation therapy.

tumor mass tends to regress much more slowly, and a complete response rate is generally lower than for pure germinoma. Also, germinomas with elevated HCG-β levels in serum or CSF are considered to have a higher risk of recurrence.[9] One report of patients with germinoma with elevated CSF HCG-β levels showed a 40% recurrence rate even after complete conventional radiation therapy.

To illustrate this point, a 15-year-old male who complained of headache received an MRI scan with gadolinium that showed an enhanced solid mass in the pineal lesion. CSF and serum HCG-β levels were elevated. After treatment with chemotherapy and focal radiation therapy, the MRI revealed complete remission. Four years after treatment, this patient had

cerebellar ataxia. Repeat MRI showed complete remission of the original pineal lesion but diffuse dissemination of disease in the brain and spinal cord (Figure 96-2).

Teratoma

Mature Teratoma

It is generally accepted that mature teratoma should be treated by surgical resection without additional therapy. The completeness of tumor resection has been established as the most powerful prognostic parameter for this disease.[7] According to the analyses of the Brain Tumor Registry of Japan in 2000, it was reported that the relative survival rate of teratoma at 5 years was 81.2%.[4] Brandes et al showed a 5-year survival rate of 100%.[3]

Immature Teratoma

In this tumor, one finds mature teratoma along with primitive, malignant elements. Even after total gross-total resection, most cases show recurrence, and adjuvant therapy is essential to prolong survival. If serum HCG or AFP levels are elevated, prognosis is generally less favorable. However, Yoshida et al have described immature teratomas in which HCG and AFP tumor makers are negative, and the tumors are resistant to PE combination chemotherapy.[25] Matsutani et al analyzed the long-term outcome of patients with immature teratoma and showed a 10-year survival rate of 70.7%.[12] Brandes et al reported a 5-year survival rate of 67%.[3]

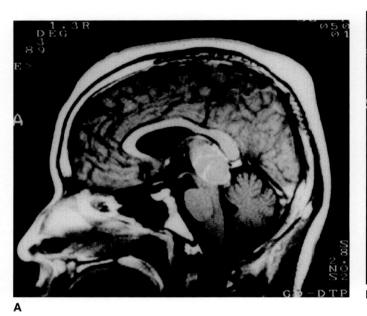

A

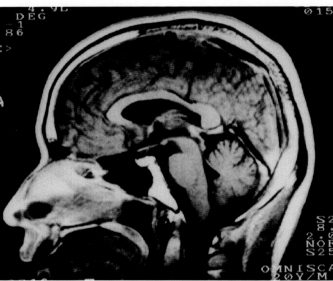

B

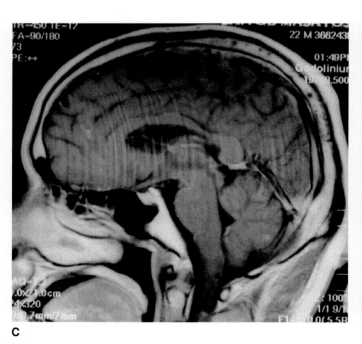

C

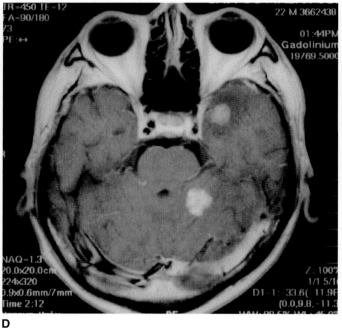

D

FIGURE 96-2   *A,* A 15-year-old patient complained of headache. Magnetic resonance imaging (MRI) with gadolinium showed an enhanced solid mass in the pineal region. The level of β-human chorionic gonadotropin was elevated in both cerebrospinal fluid and serum. *B,* After treatment with chemoradiation, MRI revealed complete remission. *C,* Four years after treatment, the patient complained of a floating sensation and showed cerebellar ataxia. Repeated MRI still showed complete remission in the original pineal lesion. Multiple intramedullary dissemination is not only in the brain *(D)* but also in the spinal cord *(E).*   *Continued*

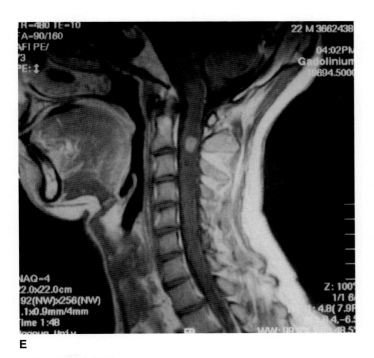

FIGURE 96-2 cont'd.

As a case illustration, a 3-year-old boy sought treatment for vomiting. MRI with gadolinium showed an enhanced solid and cystic mass in the right occipital region. At surgery, a gross-total excision was performed, and histologic examination revealed an immature teratoma. Extensive chemoradiation therapy was performed. One year after treatment, follow-up MRI revealed a local recurrence with dissemination in the contralateral ventricle. After several months, regrowth of the original tumor with diffuse CSF dissemination was seen (Figure 96-3).

Teratoma with Malignant Transformation

Teratoma with malignant transformation includes the mature teratoma with a malignant component such as carcinoma or sarcoma inside the tumor mass. This tumor subtype is associated with a poor prognosis and a less than 50% chance of 5-year survival. The elements that may demonstrate malignant transformation include adenocarcinoma, squamous cell carcinoma, sarcoma, or mesenchymal carcinoma. That is why aggressive chemoradiation therapy has been performed. Despite heavy treatment strategies, Dearnaley et al reported a 5-year survival rate of only 18.2%.[5]

Other Malignant Germ Cell Tumors

Other malignant germ cell tumors include yolk sac tumors, choriocarcinomas, and embryonal carcinomas. Despite extensive surgical resection and aggressive postoperative treatment, these tumors show a poor response rate, early tumor recurrence, and frequent CSF dissemination into the spine. The prognosis for these patients remains poor at a 20% to 40% chance of a 5-year survival.[12]

For these highly malignant germ cell tumors, extensive resection may be associated with improved survival, and neoadjuvant chemotherapy and high-dose craniospinal radiation therapy must be given.[8,23,24]

Yolk Sac Tumors (Endodermal Sinus Tumor)

Yolk sac tumors are rare, constituting less than 0.1% of all intracranial tumors. This tumor usually shows a remarkable elevation of AFP levels in serum or CSF. This tumor has a tendency to disseminate within the CSF pathways. According to the analyses of the Brain Tumor Registry in Japan in 2000, it was reported that the 1-year, 2-year, and 5-year survival rates for patients with yolk sac tumors were 50.0%, 39.7%, and 27.2%, respectively.[4] One report suggests that extensive tumor resection followed by repeated intensive chemotherapy (PVB + PE) may improve prognosis.[16]

Choriocarcinoma

The rare tumor choriocarcinoma is mainly located in the pineal region and has a predominance in males. Choriocarcinoma usually exists as a part of a mixed germ cell tumor.

Clinically, intratumoral bleeding may occur as the initial symptom. The serum HCG levels correlate well with tumor progression, and it is a reliable tumor marker. According to the analyses of the Brain Tumor Registry in Japan in 2000, the 1-year, 2-year, and 5-year survival rates of choriocarcinomas are 55.9%, 44.8%, and 44.9%, respectively.[4] Jennings et al showed that none of 10 choriocarcinoma patients survived longer than 1 year.[10] To attain longer survival rates, radical surgery followed by intensive radiation therapy (total dose 52.2 Gy) and chemotherapy using ifosfamide, carboplatin, and etoposide (ICE therapy), has been proposed.[18]

Embryonal Carcinoma

Intracranial embryonal carcinoma usually exists as a part of mixed gem cell tumor with immature teratoma or choriocarcinoma. HCG-β or AFP may be positive in serum or CSF. This tumor is located mainly in the pineal region but sometimes within the suprasellar region. CSF dissemination is common. The 1-year, 2-year, and 5-year survival rates for embryonal carcinomas are 80.4%, 56.4%, and 50.6%, respectively.[4] Sawamura et al treated nine patients with embryonal carcinoma before 1990.[21] No patients survived longer than 2 years after diagnosis. Packer et al treated six patients with embryonal carcinoma using radiation therapy, either alone or with adjuvant chemotherapy. All patients initially responded to therapy, but only one survived longer than 1 year.[14]

Mixed Germ Cell Tumors

Mixed germ cell tumors are composed of various combinations of two or more types of germ cell tumor elements. More than half of the described mixed germ cell tumors show combinations of germinoma and teratoma with or without immature components. The prognosis of mixed germ cell tumors relates to the most malignant element present. According to a report by Sano, germinoma components are found in 79%, teratoma components in 63%, yolk sac tumor components in

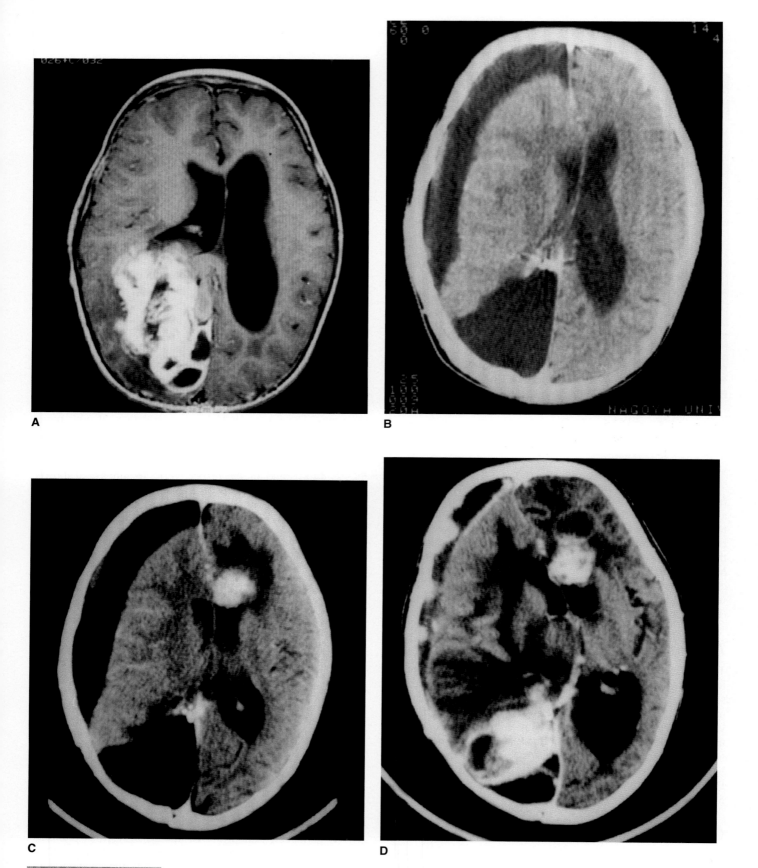

FIGURE 96-3 *A,* A 3-year-old boy experienced frequent vomiting. Magnetic resonance imaging (MRI) with gadolinium showed an enhanced solid and partly cystic mass in the right occipital lesion. *B,* After gross-total removal of the tumor, histologic examination revealed an immature teratoma. Extensive chemoradiation therapy was performed. *C,* One year after treatment, the 4-year-old patient had no symptoms, but follow-up MRI revealed local recurrence with dissemination at the contralateral lateral ventricle. *D,* After several months, MRI showed local recurrence of tumor with diffuse dissemination to cerebrospinal fluid.

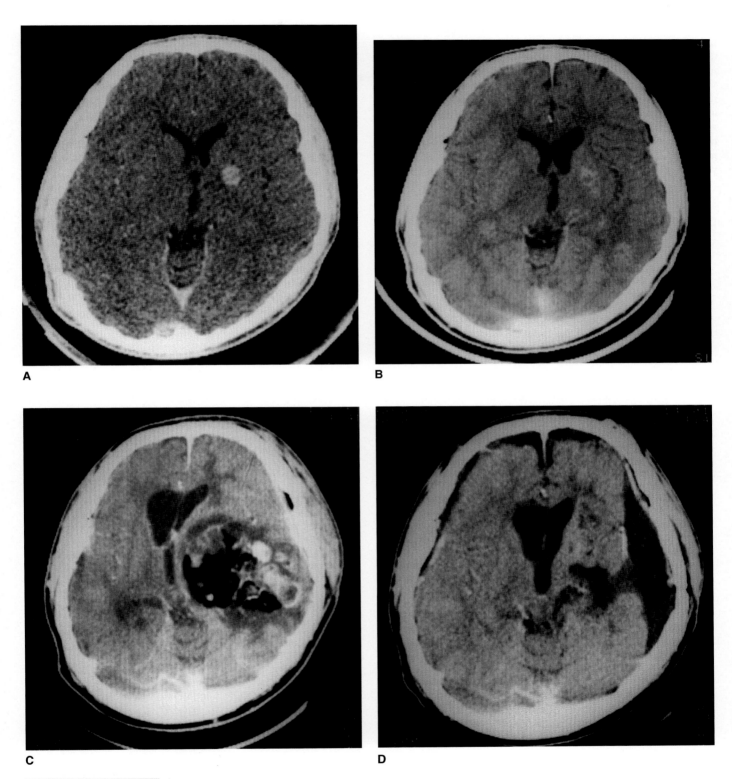

FIGURE 96-4   *A,* An 8-year-old boy showed mild right hemiparesis. Computed tomography (CT) revealed an enhanced solid mass in the left basal ganglia. A specimen was obtained by stereotactic biopsy, and histologic examination revealed a choriocarcinoma. Extensive chemoradiation therapy was performed and the patient's condition was quite good. *B,* After treatment, CT scan revealed reduced mass effect and a less enhanced tumor. *C,* Six years after initial treatment, the patient had a headache with progressive left hemiparesis, and follow-up magnetic resonance imaging revealed local recurrence, with an irregularly enhanced huge mass. *D,* After gross-total removal of tumor, subsequent CT showed no tumor, but histologic examination revealed a teratoma. The patient received no additional treatment and at 4-year follow-up review showed no recurrence.

33.3%, and embryonal carcinoma components in 15.8% of mixed germ cell tumors.[19] Matsutani et al analyzed the long-term outcome of patients with mixed tumors whose predominant characteristics were germinoma and teratoma combined with minor elements of pure malignant tumor. The analysis revealed a 3-year survival rate of 70%.[12] Brandes et al reported a 5-year survival rate of 69% for immature teratoma mixed with germinomas.[3] At least one report of a mixed germ cell tumor treated by extensive tumor resection followed by repeated intensive chemotherapy led to a survival of 4.5 years.[16]

The following is a case of a patient with a choriocarcinoma and teratoma located in the left basal ganglia who had right hemiparesis. The patient received extensive chemoradiation therapy and after treatment saw a marked reduction in tumor size. Six years after initial treatment, this patient complained of headache with progressive left hemiparesis, and follow-up MRI revealed local recurrence with an irregularly enhanced huge mass in the same area. After repeat gross-total excision of tumor (Figure 96-4), the histologic examination revealed a mature teratoma. This patient has now been followed for more than 4 years and shows no recurrence.

References

1. Aoyama H, Shirato H, Ikeda J, et al: Induction chemotherapy followed by low-dose involved-field radiotherapy for intracranial germ cell tumors. J Clin Oncol 20:857–865, 2002.
2. Balmaceda C, Modak S, Finlay J: Central nervous system germ cell tumors. Semin Oncol 25:243–250, 1998.
3. Brandes AA, Pasetto LM, Monfardini S: The treatment of cranial germ cell tumours. Cancer Treat Rev 26:233–242, 2000.
4. Committee of Brain Tumor Registry of Japan, 10th ed: Neurol Med Chir 40 (Supplement), 2000.
5. Dearnaley DP, A'Hern RP, Whittaker S, Bloom HJ: Pineal and CNS germ cell tumors: Royal Marsden Hospital experience 1962–1987. Int J Radiat Oncol Biol Phys 18:773–781, 1990.
6. Diez B, Balmaceda C, Matsutani M, Weiner HL: Germ cell tumors of the CNS in children: recent advances in therapy. Childs Nerv Syst 15:578–585, 1999.
7. Gobel U, Schneider DT, Calaminus G, et al: Germ-cell tumors in childhood and adolescence. GPOH MAKEI and the MAHO study groups. Ann Oncol 11:263–271, 2000
8. Hoffman HJ, Otsubo H, Hendrick EB, et al: Intracranial germ-cell tumors in children. J Neurosurg 74:545–551, 1991.
9. Inaguma T, Nishio S, Ikezaki K, Fukui M: Human chorionic gonadotrophin in CSF, not serum, predicts outcome in germinoma. J Neurol Neurosurg Psychiatry 66:654–657, 1999.
10. Jennings MT, Gelman R, Hochberg F: Intracranial germ-cell tumors: natural history and pathogenesis. J Neurosurg. 63: 155–167, 1985.
11. Kleihues P, Cavenee WK (eds): Pathology and genetics of tumours of the nervous system. In: Germ Cell Tumours. Lyon, France, International Agency for Research on Cancer, 2000.
12. Matsutani M, Sano K, Takakura K, et al: Primary intracranial germ cell tumors: a clinical analysis of 153 histologically verified cases. J Neurosurg 86:446–455, 1997.
13. Nakajima T, Kumabe T, Jokura H, Yoshimoto T: Recurrent germinoma in the optic nerve: report of two cases. Neurosurgery 48:214–218, 2001.
14. Packer RJ, Sutton LN, Rorke LB, et al: Intracranial embryonal cell carcinoma. Cancer 54:520–524, 1984.
15. Paulino AC, Wen BC, Mohideen MN: Controversies in the management of intracranial germinomas. Oncology 13:513–521, 1999.
16. Sakai N, Yamada H, Andoh T, et al: Long-term survival in malignant intracranial germ-cell tumors: a report of two cases and a review of the literature. Childs Nerv Syst 9:431–436, 1993.
17. Saki N, Tamaki K, Kurai H, et al: Long-term outcome of endocrine function in patients with neurohypophyseal germinomas. Endocr J 47:83–89, 2000.
18. Sakurada K, Kayama T, Kawakami K, et al: A successfully operated case of choriocarcinoma with recurrent intratumoral hemorrhage. No Shinkei Geka 2881:67–72, 2000.
19. Sano K: Pathogenesis of intracranial germ cell tumors reconsidered. J Neurosurg 90:258–264, 1999
20. Sawamura Y, Ikeda J, Shirato H, et al: Germ cell tumours of the central nervous system: treatment consideration based on 111 cases and their long-term clinical outcomes. Eur J Cancer 34:104–110, 1998.
21. Sawamura Y, Shirato H, de Tribolet N (eds): Intracranial germ cell tumors. In Sawamura Y: Prognosis of CNS GCTs. New York, Springer-Verlag (Wien), 1998.
22. Sawamura Y, Shirato H, Ikeda J, et al: Induction chemotherapy followed by reduced-volume irradiation for newly diagnosed central nervous system germinoma. J Neurosurg 88:66–72, 1998.
23. Schild SE, Haddock MG, Scheithauer BW, et al: Nongerminomatous germ cell tumors on the brain. Int J Radiat Oncol Biol Phys 36:557–563, 1996.
24. Wolden SL, Wara WM, Larson DA, et al: Radiation therapy for primary intracranial germ-cell tumors. Int J Radiat Oncol Biol Phys 32:943–949, 1995.
25. Yoshida J, Sugita K, Kobayashi T, et al: Prognosis of intracranial germ cell tumours: effectiveness of chemotherapy with cisplatin and etoposide (CDDP and VP-16). Acta Neurochir (Wien) 120:111–117, 1993.

CHAPTER 97

CHOROID PLEXUS TUMORS

Nabeel Al-Shafai, Raafat Yahya, and James T. Rutka

Choroid plexus tumors (CPTs) are defined as papillary neoplasms originating from the epithelium of the choroid plexus within the ventricles. They are classified into mainly two types: benign choroid plexus papillomas (CPPs) (World Health Organization [WHO] grade I) and choroid plexus carcinomas (CPCs) (WHO grade III).[1,3,23] An intermediate group lies between the two groups and is referred to as *atypical CPTs*. However, it is very rare for benign papillomas to convert to carcinomas.[8,31]

In 1883 Guerard was the first to describe CPTs in the literature. In 1906 Bielschowsky and Unger reported the first surgical resection of a CPT. Later, Cushing and Dandy described these tumors in much more detail.[11,12]

Anatomically, the choroid plexus is the junction between the brain pia and the ventricular ependymal layer in all four ventricles. Embryologically, it is derived from the specialization of ventricular neuroepithelium along certain neural tube segments. Interestingly, there is a common ontogeny between choroid epithelium and cells of glial origin. On occasion this may create a source of diagnostic confusion.[5,32] Physiologically, the choroid plexus is specialized in cerebrospinal fluid (CSF) production.

EPIDEMIOLOGY

CPTs are seen in all age groups, with an overall incidence of 0.5% to 0.6% of all brain tumors (10% to 20% in infants). However, they are primarily tumors of childhood with higher incidence rates ranging from 1.8% to 2.9% in the pediatric population.[10,14,21] Haddad et al and Galassi et al have reported that CPTs constitute 12.8% to 14% of all tumors in infants.[16,19] Laurence reported that 45% of CPTs occur in the first year of life and 74% in the first decade of life.[24] He also concluded that 50% were in the lateral ventricles, 37% in fourth ventricle, 9% in the third ventricle, and the remainder in other locations. There has been no sex predilection shown in many of these studies. They are always solitary tumors. However, rare case reports have been published documenting multiple CPPs.[43] Overall, CPCs constitute 29% to 39% of all choroid neoplasms.[14,22,42] CPPs are more commonly found in the fourth ventricle in adults.

CLINICAL FEATURES

Intracranial hypertension is the most common feature.[14,21,24,28] This is because ventriculomegaly is secondary to obstructive hydrocephalus or CSF overproduction. Hydrocephalus was present in 78% of cases at the Hospital for Sick Children[21] and 95% of cases at the Brigham and Children's Hospital in Boston.[14]

Patients with CPTs have nausea, vomiting, irritability, headache, visual difficulty, and seizures. Frequently occurring neurologic signs include craniomegaly, papilledema, and decreased level of consciousness in a subset of approximately 25% of these patients in some series. Ellenbogen reported two groups of patients based on the duration of symptoms. The first group was younger than age 2, who presented with a brief history of symptoms less than 2 months in duration, versus a second group that comprised older children who had prolonged symptom histories before diagnosis.

Although CPPs are considered slow-growing tumors, rapid neurologic deterioration can occur secondary to hydrocephalus or from intratumoral hemorrhage.[30,35] Lateralizing signs are found in a minority of patients secondary to asymmetric ventricular dilation.

RADIOLOGY

Imaging studies reveal the diagnosis of a ventricular tumor in most cases. In the past, skull films may have shown split sutures and punctate tumoral calcifications. Cerebral angiography demonstrates the hypervascularity of these lesions. In CPCs, arteriography can demonstrate arteriovenous shunting and neovascularization. Enlargement of the posterior choroidal artery is a common feature of CPTs in general. Third ventricular lesions are supplied by the medial posterior choroidal artery, and fourth ventricular lesions receive their supply from medullary or vermian branches of the posterior-inferior cerebellar artery (PICA).

Computed tomography (CT) and magnetic resonance imaging (MRI) are the diagnostic imaging procedures of choice.[40,46] Cerebral angiography may be useful if preoperative embolization is a consideration.[13,46] Otherwise, magnetic resonance (MR) angiography and venography have supplanted conventional angiography. By CT, CPTs appear as hyperdense lesions on unenhanced scans (Figures 97-1 and 97-2). They are enhanced homogeneously in the case of CPPs, and heterogeneously in CPCs. By MRI, CPTs are isointense to hypointense lesions on T1-weighted images and isointense, decreased, or hyperintense on T2-weighted images. Imaging features suggestive of CPCs include dense heterogeneous enhancement, ventricular entrapment, subarachnoid seeding, necrosis, cyst formation, subependymal tracking of tumor, and parenchymal

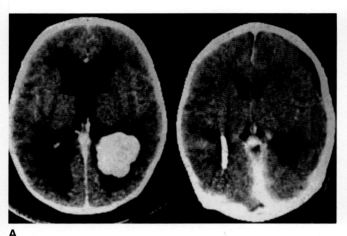

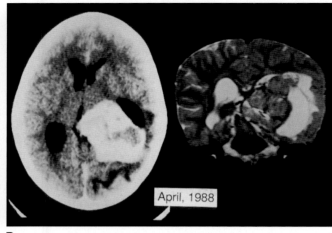

A   **B**

FIGURE 97-1 Computed tomography (CT) appearance of choroid plexus tumors. *A*, Axial contrast-enhanced CT showing choroid plexus papillomas with homogeneous enhancement *(left)*. Note dilated ventricles. Following surgery and cerebrospinal fluid shunting, the tumor has been completely removed, and the child is well *(right)*. *B*, Axial *(left)* contrast CT and T2-weighted magnetic resonance image *(right)* of choroid plexus carcinoma showing a large, irregular mass in trigone of left lateral ventricle with brain invasion and surrounding edema.

edema suggesting brain invasion. Imaging features found in CPPs and CPCs are engulfment of choroids plexus by the mass rather than displacement, punctate calcification, subarachnoid hemorrhage, vascular voids, and frondlike contour of the lesion. When CPCs are suspected, MRI of the spine may be a valuable preoperative diagnostic study to rule out drop metastases.

PATHOLOGY

CPPs are cauliflower-like masses in appearance. They are described as exaggerated soft fronds of normal choroid plexus. They have a rough globular shape with an irregular surface and intervening encapsulated areas. Old hemorrhagic areas are sometimes seen. CPPs tend to expand the ventricles rather than invade the ependyma.

CPPs are similar to normal choroid plexus histopathologically (Figure 97-3).[37,38] However, CPPs show numerous papillae covered with a simple columnar or cuboidal epithelium. They have a fibrovascular stroma containing connective tissue and small blood vessels. The stromal features are essential to distinguish CPPs from the papillary form of ependymomas.[32]

CPCs are essentially similar to CPPs, with some notable differences.[17,37] They tend to be softer and more friable than CPPs grossly. CPCs are characterized by brain invasion and cytologic atypia. Brain invasion is recognized by transgression of the ependymal lining by tumor cells and the extension of tumor into the periventricular parenchyma. The cytologic criteria of malignancy are nuclear atypia, increased nuclear to cytoplasmic ratio, prominent and numerous mitotic figures, and a loss of the normal papillary architecture (Figure 97-4).[20]

The epithelial nature of some CPCs could produce a diagnostic challenge with conditions such as metastatic adenocarcinoma (which is extremely rare) and medulloepithelioma, which could look very similar. Electron microscopy plays an essential role in these situations, demonstrating the ultrastruc-

tural details such as cilia and blepharoplasts, which are not characteristics of CPTs.

By immunohistochemistry, S-100 is positive in most CPTs.[9,20,29,33] However, S-100 protein and glial fibrillary acidic protein (GFAP) are not very helpful to distinguish these tumors from normal glial and choroid plexus tissue. Other markers such as vimentin, GFAP, and the cytokeratins lack specificity as well. Prealbumin or transthyretin (TTR) is immunohistochemically localized to the choroid plexus. In some reports 20% of CPTs were TTR negative. Paulus and Janisch reported that certain immunohistochemical features can be used to determine patient prognosis and outcome.[33] For instance, a poor prognosis is expected in patients whose tumor cells are negative for TTR. In addition, patients whose tumors had less than 50% of the cells staining heavily for S-100 are expected to have a poor prognosis.

PATHOGENESIS

The pathogenesis of CPTs is unknown. There is no satisfying explanation for their frequency in the pediatric age group. There is one report of two cases in one family.[48] Certain syndromes like Aicardi syndrome have an association with CPTs, but causal relationships have not been determined.[34,43,44] Cytogenetic analyses have not shown a predictive relationship between karyotypes, pathologic diagnosis, or outcome.

Some studies have shown the presence of CPTs in transgenic animals. Large T antigen, the major regulator of late viral gene products of the simian virus 40 (SV-40), when expressed in mice, induces the formation of choroid plexus neoplasms.[2] The large T antigen is expressed only in the choroid plexus and appears to interact with the product of the p53 gene.[27] More recently, the expression of transgenes of the viral oncoproteins E6 and E7 from human papilloma virus have also been shown to produce tumors in 71% of offspring, of which 26% of the tumors were CPTs.[2]

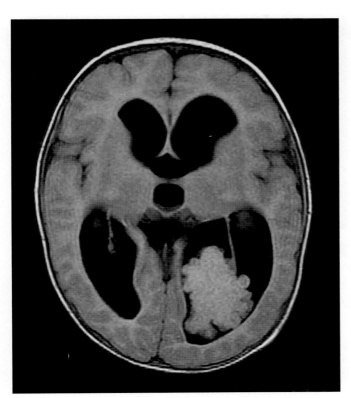

A

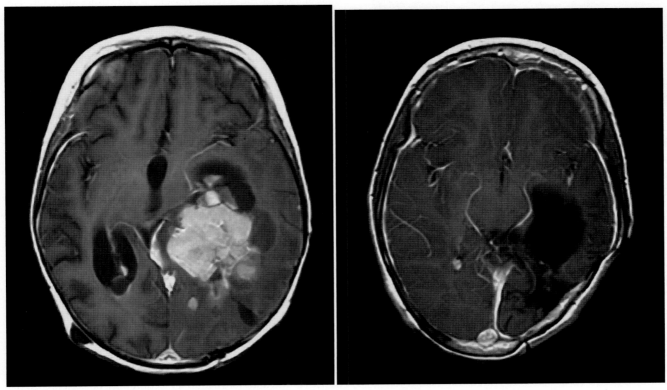

B

FIGURE 97-2 Magnetic resonance imaging (MRI) appearance of choroid plexus tumors. *A,* Axial T1-weighted MRI showing variegated, frondlike mass in left lateral ventricle supplied by vascular pedicle. The lesion proved to be a choroid plexus papilloma. *B,* Axial contrast-enhanced MRI of choroid plexus carcinoma *(left)* showing irregular tumor infiltrating brain parenchyma. After surgery, chemotherapy, and repeat surgery, a gross-total resection has been achieved.

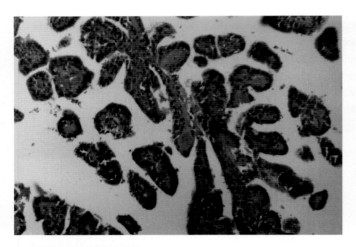

FIGURE 97-3 Histopathology of choroid plexus carcinoma showing multiple papillary structures that simulate the normal pattern of architecture of the choroid plexus (hematoxylin and eosin stain).

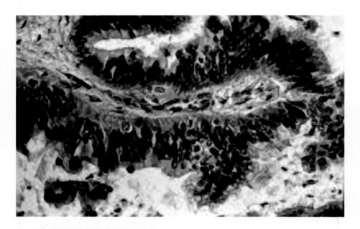

FIGURE 97-4 Histopathology of choroid plexus carcinoma showing irregular papillary structures with marked cytoplasmic and nuclear pleomorphism. MIB stain showing marked up-regulation in cell proliferation index.

The hydrocephalus associated with CPTs can be due to increased CSF production or obstruction of the CSF pathways.[6,47] However, despite total removal of the tumor abolishing both mechanisms, up to 78% of these patients may still be shunt dependent.[21,25] Arachnoidal scarring, blood in the ventricles, and postoperative meningitis can all contribute to the impaired absorption of CSF, resulting in communicating-type hydrocephalus, which is treated by insertion of a ventriculoperitoneal shunt.[26]

TREATMENT

The management of patients with CPTs is aimed initially at relieving the most common clinical feature, namely, intracranial hypertension. CSF shunting or drainage for hydrocephalus

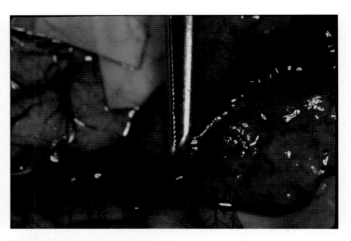

FIGURE 97-5 En bloc resection of choroid plexus papillomas (CPPs) is facilitated by early identification of the vascular pedicle leading to the tumor mass. Upon coagulation of the pedicle, the CPP typically shrinks and can be removed as a single mass lesion.

becomes urgent if the patient is acutely deteriorating. The need for permanent CSF diversion depends on several factors mentioned previously and depends on the patient's condition.

CPTs are potentially difficult tumors to remove because of their extreme vascularity and the small blood volume of the infant or child. The tumor vessels arborize rapidly so that facile coagulation of the arterial vessels is sometimes difficult. The strategy in surgical approaches to CPPs is to identify and expose the vascular pedicle early leading to an en bloc excision of the tumor (Figure 97-5).[36,39]

For CPTs of the lateral ventricles, a temporal-parietal flap is the approach of choice, providing access to the temporal pole and angular gyros posteriorly. The steps include draining CSF initially to decompress the brain and drain any trapped compartment of the lateral ventricle. Corticectomy followed by cerebrotomy posterior to the angular gyrus should give access to the entire trigone and allow identification of the tumor pedicle, which needs to be coagulated. However, wider exposures might be necessary if the tumor extends anteriorly and reaches the foramen of Monro. In this circumstance, the ventricle is approached anteriolaterally, and an incision is made in the frontal convolutions. This might be more challenging, because the vascular pedicle comes posterioinferiorly in this location and would be hidden from the surgeon's view. Therefore an alternative approach could be transsuperior or middle temporal gyrus cerebrotomy.[21]

For CPTs of the fourth ventricle, a standard midline posterior fossa approach exposing the vermis and both tonsils is used. Triventricular obstructive hydrocephalus is almost always present. Dealing with the hydrocephalus and then the tumor in a two-stage operation is a common approach. Factors to remember relating to anatomic landmarks are that (1) these tumors arise from the caudal part of the roof of the fourth ventricle, (2) the anterior medullary velum may be adherent to the tumor, (3) the tumor can extend to the lateral recess or the foramen of Magendie, and (4) the blood supply from branches of the PICA is visualized from a medial angle.[18]

Once the laterally derived blood supply of the tumor is interrupted, bleeding is considerably reduced, and the tumor delivers itself as the surgeon develops a plane between the tumor and the cerebellum bilaterally. The final stage is to remove the tumor from its attachment at the floor of the fourth ventricle.

For third ventricular tumors, a midline interhemispheric transcallosal craniotomy is the approach of choice. This is a rare location for CPTs. The anterior aspect of the ventricle is entered through an opening in the corpus callosum extending from the rostrum to the supraoptic recess. This facilitates the separation of the tumor from the tela choroidea, where it is usually attached, and the accompanying bridging vessels are identified and divided. This particular approach could be associated with hydrocephalus or shunt-related large subdural collection. This has been postulated by Boyd and Steinbok to be related to a persistent ventriculosubdural fistula. They suggest preventing this condition by the use of pial stay sutures to close the cortical incision reinforced with Tisseal glue.[4]

The treatment of CPCs in terms of surgical approaches parallels that of CPPs. However, they are distinguished by the following features: (1) tumor vascularity is exuberant, (2) tumor and brain lack a well-developed plane between them, and (3) there is excessive friability of the tissue, all of which render them more challenging surgically.

Chemotherapy before CPC excision (after biopsy) has proved to be extremely helpful in reducing tumor volume and vascularity, leading to a safer and more complete surgical removal of the tumor during the second stage operation.[42] Souweidane et al published a case report of a patient with CPC who had a volumetric response to chemotherapy, with 29.5% reduction in the tumor volume.[41] Recently, Fitzpatrick et al[15] reviewed all patients with CPC reported since 1985. The single most important predictor of outcome in these patients was the extent of tumor resection. Although having limited statistical significance, the study showed that 4 of the 37 patients who had gross-total resection were not treated with chemotherapy and survived between 18 and 114 months, thus validating the question of the value of chemotherapy in this particular group of patients. Chemotherapy is useful in cases of subtotal resection, because it delays the use of radiation therapy in the young child and may allow a subsequent gross-total resection.

OUTCOME

The literature supports a morbidity rate that averages between 8% and 9.5% as the operative mortality for CPTs.[21,26] In essence, patients with CPPs should be cured following complete surgical excision.

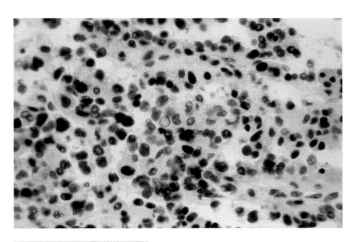

FIGURE 97-6 MIB index of choroid plexus carcinoma showing the majority of cells stained positively for the marker of cell proliferation.

Unfortunately, the outcome of patients with CPCs is not so good.[14,42] The 5-year survival rate for patients with CPCs is on the order of 30% to 50%. Although the numbers are not very encouraging except in isolated case reports, the use of adjuvant therapy as well as the timing of multimodal therapy may prove to be important to the patient's survival.

The CPT's proliferative potential, as determined by MIB-1, can prove to be a useful diagnostic criterion, as well as a prognostic indicator in CPTs (Figure 97-6).[23,45]

Clinicopathologic correlative studies have shown that CPCs in children are characterized by a higher MIB-1 labeling index and greater cell cycle dysregulation than are CPPs. Carlotti et al reported that chemotherapy may work in part on CPCs to decrease their proliferative potential and expression of cell cycle regulatory proteins.[7]

CONCLUSION

The optimum treatment of patients with CPTs requires logical decision making and surgical skills of the neurosurgeon who plays a pivotal role in caring for these patients. Recent developments in neurosurgical technology have reduced the morbidity and mortality of patients undergoing CPT surgery. Unfortunately, the survival for patients with CPCs is far from acceptable. However, presurgical chemotherapy has provided an important strategy for caring for these patients.

References

1. Ang LC, Taylor AR, Bergin D, Kaufmann JC: An immunohistochemical study of papillary tumors in the central nervous system. Cancer 65:2712–2719, 1990.
2. Arbeit JM, Munger K, Howley PM, et al: Neuroepithelial carcinomas in mice transgenic with human papillomavirus type 16 E6/E7 ORFs. Am J Pathol 142:1187, 1993.
3. Berger C, Thiesse P, Lellouch-Tubiana A, et al: Choroid plexus carcinomas in childhood: clinical features and prognostic factors. Neurosurgery 42:470–475, 1998.
4. Boyd MC, Steinbok P: Choroid plexus tumors: problems in diagnosis and management. J Neurosurg 66:800–805, 1987.
5. Buchino JJ, Mason KG: Choroid plexus papilloma. Report of a case with cytologic differential diagnosis. Acta Cytol 36:95–97, 1992.
6. Buxton N, Punt J: Choroid plexus papilloma producing symptoms by secretion of cerebrospinal fluid. Pediatr Neurosurg 27:108–111, 1997.
7. Carlotti CG, Jr, Salhia B, Weitzman S, et al: Evaluation of proliferative index and cell cycle protein expression in choroid

plexus tumors in children. Acta Neuropathol (Berl) 103:1–10, 2002.

8. Chow E, Jenkins JJ, Burger PC, et al: Malignant evolution of choroid plexus papilloma. Pediatr Neurosurg 31:127–130, 1999.

9. Cruz-Sanchez FF, Rossi ML, et al: Choroid plexus papillomas: an immunohistological study of 16 cases. Histopathology 15:61–69, 1989.

10. Cushing H: Intracranial Tumors, Springfield, Charles C. Thomas, 1932.

11. Dandy W: Diagnosis, localization and removal of tumours of the third ventricle. Bull Johns Hopkins Hosp 33:188, 1922.

12. Davis LE, Cushing H: Papillomas of the choroid plexus with a report of six cases. Archs Neurol Psychiat (Chicago) 13:681, 1925.

13. Do HM, Marx WF, Khanam H, Jensen ME : Choroid plexus papilloma of the third ventricle: angiography, preoperative embolization, and histology. Neuroradiology 43:503–506, 2001.

14. Ellenbogen RG, Winston KR, Kupsky WJ: Tumors of the choroid plexus in children. Neurosurgery 25:327, 1989.

15. Fitzpatrick LK, Aronson LJ, Cohen KJ : Is there a requirement for adjuvant therapy for choroid plexus carcinoma that has been completely resected? J Neurooncol 57:123–126, 2002.

16. Galassi E, Godano U, Cavallo M, et al: Intracranial tumors during the 1st year of life. Childs Nerv Syst 5:288, 1989.

17. Gaudio RM, Tacconi L, Rossi ML: Pathology of choroid plexus papillomas: a review. Clin Neurol Neurosurg 100:165–186, 1998.

18. Gupta N, Humphreys RP, Jay V, Rutka JT: Choroid Plexus Papillomas and Carcinomas. In Youmans (ed): Neurological Surgery, 4th ed. Toronto, WB Saunders, 1996.

19. Haddad SF, Menezes AH, Bell WF, et al: Brain tumors occurring before 1 year of age: a retrospective review of 22 cases in an 11-year period (1977–1987). Neurosurgery 29:8, 1991.

20. Ho DM, Wong TT, Liu HC: Choroid plexus tumors in childhood. Histopathologic study and clinico-pathological correlation. Childs Nerv Syst 7:437–441, 1991.

21. Humphreys RP, Nemoto S, Hendrick EB, et al: Childhood choroid plexus tumors. Concepts Pediat Neurosurg 7:1, 1987.

22. Johnson DL: Management of choroid plexus tumors in children. Pediatr Neurosci 15:195, 1989.

23. Kato T, Fujita M, Sawamura Y, et al: Clinicopathological study of choroid plexus tumors: immunohistochemical features and evaluation of proliferative potential by PCNA and Ki-67 immunostaining. Noshuyo Byori 13:99–105, 1996.

24. Laurence KM: The biology of choroid plexus papilloma and carcinoma of the lateral ventricle. In Vinken PJ, Bruyn GW (eds): Handbook of Clinical Neurology. New York, Elsevier, 1974.

25. Lena G, Genitori L, Molina J, et al: Choroid plexus tumors in children. Review of 24 cases. Acta Neurochir(Wien) 106:68, 1990.

26. MacDonald JV: Persistent hydrocephalus following the removal of papillomas of the choroid plexus of the lateral ventricles. J Neurosurg 30:736, 1969.

27. Marks JR, Lin J, Hinds P, et al: Cellular gene expression in papillomas of the choroid plexus from transgenic mice that express the simian virus 40 large T antigen. J Virol 63:790, 1989.

28. Matson DD, Crofton FD: Papilloma of choroid plexus in childhood. J Neurosurg 17:1002, 1960.

29. McComb RD, Burger PC: Choroid plexus carcinoma. Report of a case with immunohistochemical and ultrastructural observations. Cancer 51:470, 1983.

30. Murphy M, Grieve JP, Stapleton SR: Presentation of a choroid plexus papilloma mimicking an extradural haematoma after a head injury. Childs Nerv Syst 18:457–459, 2002.

31. Niikawa S, Ito T, Murakawa T, et al: Recurrence of choroid plexus papilloma with malignant transformation—case report and lectin histochemistry study. Neurol Med Chir (Tokyo) 33:32–35, 1993.

32. Park SH, Park HR, Chi JG: Papillary ependymoma: its differential diagnosis from choroid plexus papilloma. J Korean Med Sci 11:415–421, 1996.

33. Paulus W, Janisch W: Clinicopathologic correlations in epithelial choroid plexus neoplasms: a study of 52 cases. Acta Neuropathol (Berl) 80:635–641, 1990.

34. Pianetti Filho G, Fonseca LF, Silva MC: Choroid plexus papilloma and Aicardi syndrome: case report. Arq Neuropsiquiatr 60:1008–1010, 2002.

35. Piguet V, de Tribolet N: Choroid plexus papilloma of the cerebellopontine angle presenting as a subarachnoid hemorrhage: case report. Neurosurgery 15:114–116, 1984.

36. Raimondi AJ, Gutierrez FA: Diagnosis and surgical treatment of choroid plexus papilloma. Childs Brain 1:81, 1975.

37. Russell DS, Rubenstein LJ: Pathology of Tumors of the Nervous System, 5th ed. London, Williams & Wilkins, 1989.

38. Sarkar C, Sharma MC, Gaikwad S, et al: Choroid plexus papilloma: a clinicopathological study of 23 cases. Surg Neurol 52:37–39, 1999.

39. Schijman E, Monges J, Raimondi AJ, Tomita T: Choroid plexus papillomas of the III ventricle in childhood. Their diagnosis and surgical management. Childs Nerv Syst 6:331–334, 1990.

40. Shin JH, Lee HK, Jeong AK, et al: Choroid plexus papilloma in the posterior cranial fossa: MR, CT, and angiographic findings. Clin Imaging 25:154–162, 2001.

41. Souweidane MM, Johnson JH Jr, Lis E: Volumetric reduction of a choroid plexus carcinoma using preoperative chemotherapy. J Neurooncol 43:167–171, 1999.

42. St. Clair SK, Humphreys RP, Pillay PK, et al: Current management of choroid plexus carcinoma in children. Pediatr Neurosurg 17:225, 1991–1992.

43. Taggard DA, Menezes AH: Three choroid plexus papillomas in a patient with Aicardi syndrome. A case report. Pediatr Neurosurg 33:219–223, 2000.

44. Uchiyama CM, Carey CM, Cherny WB, et al: Choroid plexus papilloma and cysts in the Aicardi syndrome: case reports. Pediatr Neurosurg 27:100–104, 1997.

45. Vajtai I, Varga Z, Aguzzi A: MIB-1 immunoreactivity reveals different labelling in low-grade and in malignant epithelial neoplasms of the choroid plexus. Histopathology 29:147–151, 1996.

46. Wagle V, Melanson D, Ethier R, et al: Choroid plexus papilloma: magnetic resonance, computed tomography, and angiographic observations. Surg Neurol 27:466–468, 1987.

47. Wilkins RH, Rutledge BJ: Papillomas of the choroid plexus. J Neurosurg 18:14, 1961.

48. Zwetsloot CP, Kros JM, Paz y Greuze HD: Familial occurrence of tumors of the choroid plexus. J Med Genet 28:492, 1991.

CHAPTER 98

COLLOID CYSTS IN CHILDREN

R. Loch Macdonald

Colloid cysts are benign, surgically curable lesions. They have attracted in some ways a disproportionate level of interest as a result of their propensity to cause sudden, unexpected death. The first description of a colloid cyst is attributed to Wallmann.[48] They were later called *paraphysial* or *neuroepithelial cysts* based on theories of origin of the cyst from the paraphysis or primitive neuroepithelium. The original term, colloid cyst, remains most appropriate.

EPIDEMIOLOGY

Incidence, Prevalence, and Geography

Colloid cysts constitute 0.3% to 2% of all brain tumors.[4,16] Review of 1000 magnetic resonance imaging (MRI) studies of asymptomatic, normal individuals disclosed one confirmed low-grade oligodendroglioma, one pilocytic astrocytoma, and no colloid cysts.[17] Among the 870,000 inhabitants of eastern Finland, 40 patients with colloid cysts were discovered among 2000 with brain tumors (2% of tumors) over 15 years, leading to an estimated incidence of three per one million person years.[16] In the Netherlands 78 cases were identified among the 15.5 million inhabitants in 5 years.[49] The incidence was estimated at one per one million population per year. Prevalence was estimated at 1 per 8500 persons based on autopsy and routine neuroimaging studies. There is no known racial predilection or geographic variation in incidence, although in view of their rarity and the variation in medical care throughout the world, whether such variations exist cannot be stated.

Age and Sex Distribution

Yenermen et al reviewed 54 of their own cases and 200 from the literature, to which can be added additional cases.[29,50] Of 271 in whom age at diagnosis was given, 39 (14%) were younger than age 20, 73 (27%) were in the third decade of life, 70 (26%) in the fourth, 58 (21%) in the fifth, 23 (9%) in the sixth, and 6 (2%) in the seventh or eighth decade. The mean age was 36 years in three series totaling 106 cases.[1,29,36] There were 179 males and 156 females.[16,29,49,50] Patients younger than age 18 represented 0% to 17% of patients in nine series (mean 53 of 556 patients [10%]).[1,4,9,10,16,18,29,36,50] The youngest reported patient was 2 months old, and the oldest 78.[15,29] I found 61 patients reported in the literature who were younger than age 18,[1,3,6,8,25,28–30,41,43,50,51] and in addition to general information from various reports on colloid cysts, the pediatric cases are

repeatedly referred to throughout this chapter. The mean age was 12 years old, and the distribution by sex was reported as 32 females and 26 males.

PATHOLOGY AND PATHOGENESIS

Location

The vast majority of colloid cysts occur in the anterior third ventricle. They are attached to the anterior superior portion of the third ventricle immediately above the foramen of Monro. Virtually all pediatric cases have been at this site. Other reported sites of occurrence are the posterior third ventricle,[19,44] septum pellucidum, and fourth and lateral ventricles.[24,37]

Gross Pathology and Size

The gross pathology is characterized by a smooth, green or whitish, well-defined, spherical or ellipsoid cyst with varying degrees of adherence to the anterior roof of the third ventricle and adjacent structures. The surface may be covered in small vessels, but most are relatively avascular. The foramen of Monro is varied in size; normally it is approximately 1 cm in diameter. The choroid plexus travels from the lateral ventricle forward and through the posterior edge of the foramen of Monro into the roof of the third ventricle and may be adherent to the cyst. Size ranges from a few millimeters to 9 cm,[15] although the latter size is exceptional, and the majority of symptomatic lesions are 1 to 2.5 cm in diameter. The mean size of 49 cysts in one general series was 2 cm[50] and 1.4 cm in another series of 37 cases.[29] Among 36 children in whom size was reported, maximum diameter was 1.8 cm. The cyst wall is thin, and the contents are white or green material that varies in consistency from mucouslike liquid to gelatinous material and even soft cheeselike material.

Microscopy

Microscopy demonstrates two layers to the cyst wall (Figure 98-1). There is an outer, fibrous layer containing collagen and an inner layer of epithelium. The epithelium usually is simple cuboidal or columnar but occasionally has areas of pseudostratification. Some of the cells are ciliated, and electron microscopy has demonstrated that approximately 30% have cilia. There may be goblet cells and cells staining with periodic acid-Schiff stain.[22] Pathologists have generally not assessed the

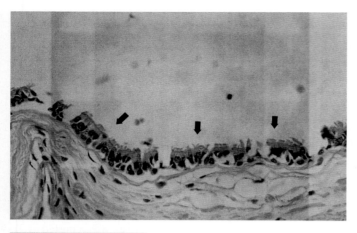

FIGURE 98-1 Photomicrograph of the wall of a colloid cyst. The epithelium is a simple, cuboidal and columnar, ciliated layer *(arrows)* on an outer layer of fibrous tissue (hematoxylin and eosin stain, ×350).

proliferative rate of the cyst epithelium by immunoreactivity to Ki-67 (MIB-1). It generally is assumed that these are benign, non-neoplastic cells and that the cysts that enlarge do so by desquamation of cells and material into the cyst. There are no reports of malignant transformation or of spread of colloid cysts through cerebrospinal fluid pathways or outside the nervous system. Recurrences are reported after surgical resection, but these are most likely the result of inadequate resection of the cyst wall. The immunohistochemical features of colloid cysts include immunoreactivity to cytokeratins, epithelial membrane antigen, and vimentin and no reactivity to glial fibrillary acidic protein, neuron-specific enolase, and neurofilament.[19,22,23,32]

Pathogenesis of Colloid Cysts

The etiology of colloid cysts is unknown. There are several theories of the pathogenesis of colloid cysts. Sjoval proposed an origin from the paraphysis.[27] The paraphysis is a structure in the roof of the third ventricle of lower vertebrates that is derived from neuroectoderm (neuroepithelium) and that is present only transiently in human embryos. It is unlike a colloid cyst in that it is extraventricular and has a nonciliated, low columnar epithelium. Other inconsistencies with the theory of origin from the paraphysis are the reports of cysts lined by epithelium identical to those in colloid cysts but located in other areas such as the fourth and lateral ventricles and the different immunohistochemical profiles of colloid cysts and other structures derived from neuroectoderm.[5,44]

Shuangshoti and Netsky noted that tissues in the region that could give rise to colloid cysts are all derived from the embryonic neuroepithelium and include choroid plexus, ependyma, and the paraphysis.[44] Only ependyma normally contains ciliated cells. It was suggested, therefore, that colloid cysts might arise from abnormal partitioning of ependymal cell collections from the developing ventricular system, which would explain other paraventricular locations. Some features, however, were suggested to be inconsistent with this origin. Mucin-secreting cells are characteristic of colloid cysts,[19] and the tissue of origin might therefore be expected also to contain

such cells. Whether choroid plexus contains such cells has been debated.[19,44] Ependyma probably does.[44] Other differences between colloid cyst and choroid plexus epithelium are that the contents of colloid cysts stain with periodic acid-Schiff reagent, whereas normal choroid plexus does not.[19,22]

Finally, the immunoreactivity of colloid cysts differs from choroid plexus and ependyma and has led to the conclusion that colloid cysts are derived from the primitive neuroectoderm that forms the tela choroidea of the roof of the third ventricle.[19] Other immunohistochemical and ultrastructural studies, however, noted similarities between colloid cysts and enteric and Rathke's cleft cysts, suggesting they could be derived from endodermal tissue from the primitive foregut or stomodeum that gives rise to the adenohypophysis.[22,23] This is supported by the similar histologic appearance of these cysts with some endodermally derived epithelia.

CLINICAL FEATURES

Symptoms and Signs

The classic symptom onset is with intermittent attacks of headache associated with vomiting and visual blurring.[18,27,50] Kelly characterized three clinical courses as (1) headache with or without symptoms or signs of increased intracranial pressure, (2) progressive dementia with or without headache, and (3) intermittent or paroxysmal attacks of headache with asymptomatic intervals of varying duration.[18] Eleven of his twenty-nine patients (38%) had headaches, vomiting, and papilledema. Other series noted this symptom complex in 42% of 123 cases (range from 20 of 54 [37%] to 17 of 36 [47%]).[1,36,50] The headache in these cases is a manifestation of the increase in intracranial pressure that can be intermittent, perhaps because of fluctuations in the degree of hydrocephalus or adjacent brain swelling from episodes of venous engorgement with sleep, postural changes, Valsalva maneuvers, and such. Review of the literature notes headache as an initial symptom in 187 of 231 (81%) patients and at some time during the history in 96%.[36,50] Another review of 1300 patients from the literature, with 939 having adequate clinical history, showed three fourths experienced headache, one third nausea and vomiting, and one fifth each visual or mental disturbances or decreased level of consciousness.[16]

Symptoms and signs in the absence of headache included nausea, vomiting, episodes of drowsiness, alteration in consciousness including transient coma, and lower-extremity weakness with falling to the ground (drop attacks). These symptoms usually were accompanied by papilledema. No headache was recorded in 3 of 36 cases in one series (8%).[36] Among 61 pediatric cases from the literature, 41 (67%) patients had headaches and various other symptoms; 3 were asymptomatic; 9 had inadequate information; 5 infants had increasing head circumference, splayed sutures, and a tense anterior fontanelle; and 2 patients had no history of headache.

Headaches may occur in paroxysms with asymptomatic intervals of days to years. This was remarked upon in 14 of 61 (23%) pediatric cases and in one third of 36 patients in another series.[36] Often, much is made of precipitation of such attacks by positional change, but this particular feature is not common. It occurred in 9 of 187 cases (5%) in three series and a similar percentage of pediatric cases.[10,18,49] A less common but characteristic symptom complex is episodes of sudden weakness of the lower limbs causing the patient to fall, usually without losing consciousness (drop attacks), a feature noted in 13% of 141 patients in three series (range from 1 in 38 to 11 in 74).[18,27,49]

Normal-pressure hydrocephalus is characterized by memory loss, gait ataxia, and urinary incontinence. Occurrence of colloid cysts with this syndrome generally is confined to adults in whom age-related atrophy or chronicity of hydrocephalus has resulted in ventriculomegaly without increased pressure. I was unable to find any cases with this symptom in the pediatric population.

A review of the literature found that the duration of symptoms was 1 day or less in 20 cases of 258 (8%).[29,50] Six of these patients died suddenly. Symptoms lasted 1 to 30 days in 40 patients (15%), 1 to 12 months in 81 (32%), and longer in 109 (44%). The duration of symptoms is variable, but there are cases of sudden deterioration and death within hours of symptom onset.[45,50] Among 37 cases seen in a major Swedish neurosurgical center, the mean duration of symptoms was 14 months.[29] The mean duration of symptoms was 9 months in 50 pediatric cases.

In summary, the vast majority of colloid cysts in children cause headaches and additional symptoms. The pediatrician or general practitioner may have difficulty deciding which of the many patients with headaches requires investigation. A history and neurologic examination should be performed to determine if there are other symptoms or signs of increased intracranial pressure. Whether there is papilledema is important, but its absence unfortunately does not exclude serious intracranial pathology. The temporal course of the headaches and the presence of other symptoms and signs of increased intracranial pressure, such as vomiting; papilledema; visual blurring; sixth nerve palsy; confusion or decreased level of consciousness; or in infants, increasing head circumference, bulging fontanelle, and split sutures, probably warrant investigation. The situation is rendered extremely problematic by reports of children who have died within days of onset of headache.[28,40,43]

Sudden Death and Acute Deterioration

Sudden death is a well-recognized complication of a colloid cyst.[7,49] Symptom onset with sudden deterioration and death at some time during the course of symptoms occurred in 5% of 78 cases in a population-based study[49] and in 10% of another series of 31 patients.[27] More patients deteriorate rapidly and are saved by emergency medical care. Children with colloid cysts are at particular risk. Among pediatric cases, there were 23 patients of 61 (38%) who deteriorated acutely at some time during their illness. This was the first indication of the colloid cyst in 7 of the 23. Seven died without receiving medical attention, eleven died despite medical intervention, and five were saved. Twenty-five of seventy-four (34%) collected from the entire population of the Netherlands over 5 years acutely deteriorated at some stage in their illness.[49] Four died immediately, and five remained severely disabled despite ventricular drainage. In the comprehensive literature review of Hernesniemi and Leivo, 21% of 939 patients had depressed consciousness, and 37% of their 35 patients deteriorated acutely. Five died.[16]

Büttner et al reviewed 98 cases of sudden death from colloid cysts and added two of their own.[7] Patients ranged in age from 6 to 79 years, with a mean of 30, and there were 15

children. There were 41 females and 42 males. Cyst size ranged from 0.8 to 8 cm in diameter (mean 2.1 cm). Of note, two cysts were less than 1 cm and three were 1 cm in diameter. In 56 cases in which it was recorded, onset of symptoms before death ranged from a few hours to 17 years. Medical management is certainly complicated by the fact that symptoms were recorded for less than 24 hours in 15 patients and less than 7 days in 31, and that, although well-documented cases of deterioration with or without death in the absence of preceding headache are rare, they probably do occur. It is apparent that in the patient with a colloid cyst, acute onset of severe headache, particularly if accompanied by vomiting, can lead to death within hours. Another review of sudden deaths noted that not all patients who died had enlarged ventricles and that sudden death was not predicted by cyst size, degree of ventricular dilation on computed tomography (CT) or MRI, or duration of symptoms.[42] Mechanisms of sudden death include acute hydrocephalus with increased intracranial pressure. It also has been postulated that in some cases without ventricular enlargement there may be cardiovascular abnormalities induced by compression of centers around the third ventricle that mediate cardiovascular reflexes.

The frequency of colloid cyst as a cause of sudden death could be estimated from a series of 10,995 consecutive deaths in which 19 were found to be due to intracranial neoplasms and only 1 was a colloid cyst.[13] Because colloid cysts make up less than 5% of intracranial tumors, it could be suggested that colloid cysts are relatively more likely to cause sudden death than other types of intracranial tumors.

Asymptomatic Colloid Cysts

Colloid cysts are being discovered incidentally with increasing frequency. Often CT or MRI is performed because of chronic headache in the absence of other symptoms or signs, and in some cases the headaches are not attributed to the cyst or the patient does not have headache. Whether the cyst should be treated is based on various factors, including the size of the cyst, age of the patient, and whether there is associated hydrocephalus on the CT or MRI scan. In most cases, consultation with a neurosurgeon would be warranted. Among a series of 68 patients thought to be asymptomatic, the mean age was 57. The main indications for imaging were headaches in 19 and cerebral infarction in 8. Forty-nine (85%) were hyperdense on CT scan as compared with 181 of 259 (70%) in a literature review. Furthermore, 22 (32%) were 0.1 to 0.5 cm, 37 (54%) 0.5 to 1.0 cm, and 9 (13%) greater than 1.0 cm in diameter. The ventricles were of normal proportions in 69%.[38] Cysts judged to be asymptomatic were smaller, found in older patients, and were more often hyperdense on CT scan. It is generally accepted that cysts larger than 1 cm in diameter should be treated regardless of symptoms. Small cysts have been found incidentally at autopsy. Larger cysts also have been found incidentally at autopsy, however, and these have been postulated to be due to slow enlargement of the cyst allowing for compensatory mechanisms.[10,39,51] Tiny lesions might be followed with serial imaging studies. The smallest symptomatic cysts recorded are 0.7 and 0.8 cm in diameter.[29,50] The previous information as well as natural history data reviewed in the following text suggest that, in the absence of extenuating circumstances, all but the smallest asymptomatic colloid cysts should be treated in the pediatric population.

Associated Conditions

The vast majority of colloid cysts are sporadic. Mathiesen et al reported a mother and son who both had colloid cysts and noted two reports in the literature of twins and nontwin brothers with colloid cysts.[29] Tada and Nakamura described a patient with basal encephalomeningocele, anophthalmia, agenesis of the corpus callosum, and colloid cyst.[46] They found 13 cases in the literature with encephalomeningocele and 7 with agenesis of the corpus callosum and ocular abnormalities but none with colloid cysts. One 15-year-old female with Asperger's syndrome (a variant of autism) and ligamentous laxity had a lesion consistent with a colloid cyst on a routine CT scan.[47] A 14-year-old female with nevoid basal cell carcinoma had a symptomatic colloid cyst removed transcallosally.[35] This syndrome includes multiple nevoid basal cell epitheliomas, jaw cysts, bifid ribs, cerebellar medulloblastoma and calcification of the dura, meningiomas, hydrocephalus, and partial agenesis of the corpus callosum.

DIAGNOSTIC TESTS

Computed Tomography

The diagnosis of colloid cyst can be made confidently in most cases on CT or MRI (Figures 98-2 and 98-3). Some other lesions that enter into the radiologic differential diagnosis are listed in Table 98-1. Most colloid cysts are hyperdense, spherical or ellipsoid masses located at the anterior end of the third ventricle at the level of the foramen of Monro. Most are homogeneous, although central hypodensity has been noted. Laidlaw and Kaye reviewed CT characteristics of 144 cases reported in the literature and found that 100 (69%) were hyperdense on CT scan, 34 were isodense (24%), and 10 (7%) were hypodense.[24] Administration of contrast resulted in enhancement of the cyst wall, which gives a ringlike pattern of enhancement, in 10 of

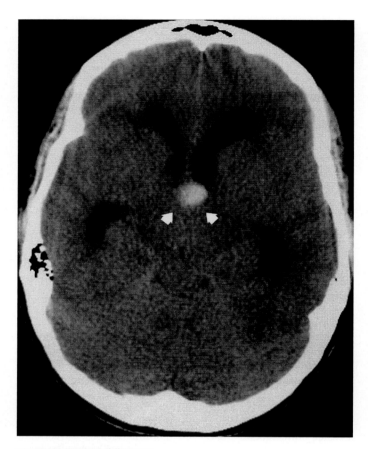

FIGURE 98-2   Unenhanced computed tomography scan of the brain of a typical hyperdense colloid cyst *(arrows)* that is associated with acute obstructive hydrocephalus.

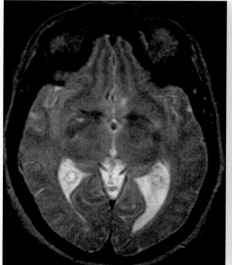
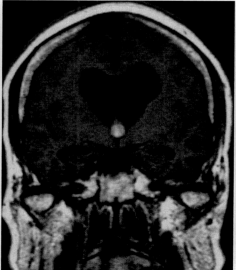
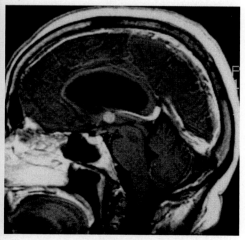

FIGURE 98-3   Magnetic resonance images of a colloid cyst. The cyst is hypointense on the axial T2 image *(left)*, is hyperintense on the coronal T1 image *(center)*, and demonstrates some enhancement of the cyst wall on a sagittal T1 image *(right)*.

TABLE 98-1

Radiologic Differential Diagnosis of Lesions of the Anterior Third Ventricle and Other Cystic Lesions

Neoplasms
Colloid cyst
Central neurocytoma
Neuroepithelial tumors
    Ependymoma
    Subependymoma
    Oligodendroglioma
    Hypothalamic astrocytoma
    Subependymal giant cell astrocytoma (in tuberous
       sclerosis)
Choroid plexus papilloma, carcinoma
Craniopharyngioma
Suprasellar extension of pituitary adenoma
Intraventricular meningioma
Lymphoma (primary central nervous system or metastatic)
Metastasis
Histiocytosis X
Dermoid, epidermoid
Germ cell tumors (germinoma, teratoma, endodermal sinus
tumor, choriocarcinoma, embryonal carcinoma)

Vascular Lesion
Basilar bifurcation aneurysm
Cavernous malformation
Arteriovenous malformation

Infectious Lesion
Cysticercosis cyst

Inflammatory Lesion

Other Lesions Reported
Xanthogranuloma of choroid plexus
Bullet
Arachnoid cyst
Sarcoidosis

---

31 cases (32%) from two series.[24] Hypodense cysts may be difficult to visualize on plain CT scans, but their presence may be suspected if there is enlargement of the lateral ventricles out of proportion to the third and fourth ventricles. Alternatively, they may be easily detected on MRI. There usually is no calcification visible on the CT images. Sixteen pediatric cases did not differ greatly from those observed overall: Eleven were hyperdense on plain CT scan, three were isodense, and two were hypodense.

Magnetic Resonance Imaging

MRI demonstrates colloid cysts optimally and has the advantages of ability to easily obtain multiplanar images, to assess for the degree and acuity of hydrocephalus, and to differentiate from other lesions such as basilar bifurcation aneurysms or

other tumors (see Figure 98-3). Among 26 asymptomatic lesions, 17 (65%) were hyperintense on T1-weighted images, 8 (31%) were isointense, and 1 (4%) was hypointense.[38] On T2-weighted images, 2 (8%) were hyperintense, 7 (27%) were isointense, and 17 (65%) were hypointense. Symptomatic lesions were similar on T1 but were hypointense on T-weighted images in 12 of 27 cases (44%).[39] Very few reports detail imaging characteristics in children.

Other Radiology

Skull radiography is not necessary for the diagnosis of colloid cysts. Cerebral angiography seldom is required. It might be indicated to exclude a vascular lesion such as a high basilar artery bifurcation aneurysm, although MRI usually will suffice in excluding this possibility.

Laboratory Investigations

Laboratory tests are of no specific value in diagnosis of colloid cysts. Similarly, cerebrospinal fluid yields no useful information and usually is clear, colorless, and without abnormalities.[18] Furthermore, lumbar puncture, the usual route by which cerebrospinal fluid is obtained, has been temporally related and is probably the proximate cause of sudden death in numerous patients with colloid cysts. Lumbar puncture is absolutely contraindicated in the patient with a colloid cyst.[10,16,29] No patient with headaches and signs of increased intracranial pressure, especially papilledema or altered consciousness, should have a lumbar puncture before cranial CT or MRI has been done to exclude an intracranial space–occupying lesion. A probable exception to this is the infant with open sutures and fontanelles in which intradural infection is much more likely and the risk of deterioration much less.

NATURAL HISTORY

Information on the natural history of colloid cysts can be obtained from the previous discussion regarding sudden deterioration and death. The mortality without intervention may be astonishingly high if one considers that one third of pediatric patients identified in the literature deteriorated and would have died without intervention. Even with medical care, albeit not optimally administered in retrospect, one sixth died. The overall duration of symptoms in all pediatric cases was 9 months. Hernesniemi and Leivo's large literature review found that one in five patients deteriorated hours to years into their illness and one in three of their own patients also did.[16] Death would be common in these cases without emergency ventricular drainage.

Pediatric patients have seldom been diagnosed with colloid cysts and followed with serial imaging studies. Mathiesen et al followed seven adult and pediatric patients for 6 to 37 months.[29] Five cysts enlarged and two remained unchanged in size. Of the cysts that enlarged, one was in an elderly patient who developed symptoms of normal-pressure hydrocephalus. One patient followed was a 9-year-old child with a hyperdense cyst that increased from 3 to 7 mm over 2 years and then underwent uneventful transcallosal resection.

Pollock et al followed 68 patients with radiologically diagnosed colloid cysts.[38] The mean age was 57 years (range from

7 to 88 years), and cyst size ranged from 0.4 to 1.8 cm with a mean of 0.8 cm in diameter. Forty-nine of 58 (84%) were hyperdense on CT. Mean follow-up was 6.6 years, which included 40 patients for 2, 28 for 5, and 14 for 10 years. Symptomatic progression occurred in 8% at 10 years. There were no sudden deaths. One cyst (3% of 34) grew 0.2 cm over 7 years but remained asymptomatic. A second patient developed hydrocephalus on imaging 8 years after diagnosis. This 57-year-old woman refused surgery and developed acute obstructive hydrocephalus 5 months later. She deteriorated and died 4 years later in a nursing home. These patients are different from the population with colloid cysts as a whole, and in particular the pediatric population, in that they are older, they are more likely to have hyperdense cysts on CT, and the cysts are smaller than average. Multivariate analysis of these patients with a concurrent cohort of 87 symptomatic lesions showed that symptomatic cysts were associated with younger age (44 vs. 57 years), larger size (1.3 vs. 0.8 cm), presence of ventricular dilation (83% versus 31%), and increased signal intensity on T2-weighted MRI.[39] The results were interpreted as suggesting that patients with colloid cysts develop symptoms when the cyst enlarges rapidly, obstructing the ventricular system and producing hydrocephalus and increased intracranial pressure. Slow enlargement allows accommodation to occur, and the patient may remain asymptomatic. The authors could categorize patients into groups that tend to reflect current management. Patients who are younger, who have cysts more than 1 cm in diameter with ventriculomegaly, and whose cysts exhibit increased signal on T2 generally are symptomatic and require surgery. Older patients with cysts smaller than 1 cm, and more confidently smaller than 0.8 cm, who have no hydrocephalus, and whose cysts are less likely hyperintense on T2 are often asymptomatic and might be followed. CT hyperdensity is more common in the latter group as well (77% versus 90%).

MANAGEMENT

General Treatment

Patients with altered consciousness and acute hydrocephalus require emergency neurosurgical consultation. Ventricular drainage by placement of catheters into one or both lateral ventricles is indicated as an emergency procedure, often done at the bedside in an intensive care unit, in most cases. The goal is to drain cerebrospinal fluid to relieve acute hydrocephalus, reduce intracranial pressure, and restore neurologic function. The risks are insignificant in this situation and include intracerebral or intraventricular hemorrhage, aggravation of brain shift and neurologic injury from draining one lateral ventricle, and not the contralateral one, and inadvertent puncture of the cyst and spillage of inflammatory contents into the ventricles, causing aseptic meningitis and scarring of the ventricular system and permanent hydrocephalus and infection. External ventricular drainage is a temporizing measure to stabilize the patient until a definitive procedure can be carried out. Cranial CT imaging usually is adequate initially to establish the diagnosis, although MRI usually is necessary for surgical planning. Lumbar puncture is absolutely contraindicated and has been followed closely by death in numerous cases. Once hydrocephalus has been addressed, a definitive surgical attack on the cyst itself can be planned at leisure. Medical decision making is difficult in the symptomatic patient who is alert. I have a low threshold for admission to hospital and preoperative ventricular drainage. Additional management issues arise in determining whether symptoms such as headache are caused by small cysts that are not associated with hydrocephalus and in the management of the asymptomatic patient. In general, I recommend surgical treatment for all lesions in pediatric patients with the exception of those with the smallest cysts.[29,39] If observation is recommended, the patient and caregivers must be aware that at present there is no accurate method of predicting which cysts will lead to neurologic deterioration. Deterioration may occur when any cyst reaches a maximum diameter, probably of 0.7 to 0.8 mm, and headache will usually but not always precede any catastrophe. No evidence at present indicates that serial CT or MRI can prevent deterioration. The patient or caregivers should report worrisome symptoms immediately.

Surgical Options, Cerebrospinal Fluid Diversion

Treatment of colloid cysts is surgical. The indications for external ventricular drainage have been discussed previously, and although drainage may be life-saving, it should not be instituted indiscriminately, because some surgical procedures become more difficult when the ventricles have collapsed. Options for treatment include permanent cerebrospinal fluid diversion with a shunt or direct procedures to aspirate or remove the cyst. Direct procedures include stereotactic aspiration, endoscopic procedures, or craniotomy and resection by a transcortical, transventricular, or interhemispheric, transcallosal approach.

Shunting as the primary treatment is seldom indicated in children or young adults. Shunting may be indicated for the very elderly or medically infirm in whom the risks of open surgery are felt to outweigh the benefits of cyst removal. In addition, hydrocephalus does not always resolve following cyst removal, and shunting may be necessary in patients with persistent, symptomatic hydrocephalus who have undergone cyst removal. Shunting was required in 9% of 115 patients (range from 1 in 20 to 3 in 18) undergoing surgical removal of colloid cysts in four series.[8,11,16,21] If a shunt is placed, ventricular catheters must be inserted in both lateral ventricles, because the cyst generally obstructs the outlets of both lateral ventricles (the foramina of Monro). An attractive option, however, is to place a ventricular catheter in one lateral ventricle and perforate the septum pellucidum either with the catheter or endoscopically at the time of shunt placement so that the lateral ventricles communicate. When an open surgical procedure is performed it is advisable to fenestrate the septum pellucidum so that if shunting becomes necessary subsequently, the ventricles will communicate and unilateral shunting will be adequate. Disadvantages of shunting are that patients who have not had the cyst removed may be at risk of sudden neurologic deterioration if the shunt malfunctions and acute hydrocephalus develops. Ryder et al suggested that these patients might also be at risk of acute deterioration because of pressure on or effects of venous obstruction from the cyst itself on the adjacent hypothalamic structures, even in the presence of a functioning shunt.[42] I am not aware of any such cases, and this possibility probably does not need to be among the factors entering into the decision to place a shunt. Among eight shunted patients in one series, there were two shunt infections, two malfunctions requiring revisions, and one patient who underwent craniotomy to remove the cyst.[8]

Craniotomy, Transcallosal Approach

The main advantage of craniotomy approaches are that these are at present the only methods that allow complete removal of a colloid cyst. Endoscopic techniques and instrumentation are improving, however, and may permit cyst removal in the future. The advantage of complete removal is that recurrence generally does not occur. Disadvantages compared with less invasive procedures such as stereotactic aspiration and endoscopic procedures are debated in the neurosurgical literature and include risks inherent in any major operation (infection, postoperative hematomas), seizures, and neurologic deficits. I prefer transcallosal resection, but transcortical surgery is an acceptable alternative, and endoscopy is improving. The risk of recurrence with stereotactic aspiration makes this procedure much less desirable in the child. All are reported in the pediatric population.[12,29]

The transcallosal approach is done through a small, right frontal craniotomy. It does not require ventricular enlargement. Under the surgical microscope the plane between the falx cerebri and the medial aspect of the frontal lobe is developed. A small opening is made in the corpus callosum and the lateral ventricle entered. The cyst usually can be seen projecting through the foramen of Monro. The cyst is opened, its contents suctioned out, and the capsule is removed using microsurgical dissection techniques. A small remnant of capsule adherent to critical structures has been left in many cases without apparent long-term consequence or recurrence.[21,26,29] The main risks include hemiparesis, usually worse in the lower extremity, because of injury to the anterior cerebral artery or venous infarction from injury to the bridging veins, but other focal neurologic deficits may occur. The most commonly cited risk and thus main disadvantage of the transcallosal approach when compared with the transcortical, transventricular procedure is adversely affecting cognition. This must be weighed against the risk of epilepsy that may be higher with the transcortical approach, although a valid comparison of the two approaches has not been made, and both continue to be used with good results.[24]

Disconnection syndrome can develop after corpus callosum section, but this usually has been observed in cases where extensive sectioning was done for epilepsy. For removal of colloid cysts, however, only a small incision generally is made. Sophisticated testing of interhemispheric information transfer in 11 patients operated on transcallosally did not reveal any significant deficits.[2] In contrast, Jeeves et al tested three adults who had transcallosal procedures and noted that all had asymptomatic defects in interhemispheric transfer of tactile but not visual data. These defects might be important in, for example, musicians. Memory loss, usually specific for short-term and transient, is more common. Three series of patients (n = 63) undergoing transcallosal colloid cyst resection reported transient hemiparesis in 2 (3%), transient memory difficulty in 11 (17%), permanent memory deficit in 1 (2%), and postoperative infection in 6%.[16,26,29] Seizures were not reported. Overall outcome was excellent or good in 61 (97%), poor in 1, and resulted in death in 1.

The transcortical, transventricular approach is easier when the lateral ventricles are enlarged, but it can be performed, usually with stereotactic guidance, when there is no hydrocephalus. The most commonly cited risk, and hence the main disadvantage as compared with the transcallosal approach, is epilepsy. Among four series of patients (n = 99) operated on with this approach, 6 patients (6%) developed seizures.[8,10,14,21] Transient hemiparesis occurred in 1 (1%)[21] and transient new memory loss in 6 (6%). Overall outcome seemed excellent or good in 95 patients.

Endoscopy

Endoscopic aspiration with removal of some portion of the wall of the cyst usually is done under general anesthesia with the endoscope inserted through a burr hole anterior to the coronal suture and several centimeters off the midline. A transcortical, transventricular trajectory is taken, similar to that used for open surgery. Advantages compared with stereotactic aspiration are that vessels can be visualized, thereby reducing the risk of bleeding, and that part of the cyst wall can be removed such that the recurrence rate might be lower. Disadvantages are that removal of the cyst wall cannot be complete enough with current techniques to reassure the surgeon that no recurrence will occur. Three series reported on 34 patients undergoing endoscopic cyst removal, including one 12-year-old female.[12,26,41] Successful evacuation was obtained in 30 patients. Complications included transient hemiparesis and short-term memory loss in two patients and noninfectious meningitis in one. Postoperative shunting was performed in one patient. The follow-up period was a mean of approximately 30 months in 24 patients and was marked by one recurrence 18 months after endoscopy. Whether the advantages of endoscopy, which are reportedly shorter recovery and hospital stays and such general advantages of less invasive procedures, will outweigh the risks of recurrence is uncertain at present.

Stereotactic Aspiration

Stereotactic aspiration can be performed under local or general anesthesia. A stereotactic frame is applied to the head, and a CT or MRI scan obtained. An instrument is then advanced through a burr hole into the cyst under stereotactic guidance and its contents aspirated. No attempt can be made to remove the cyst wall. The disadvantage is that recurrence rates may be high and complications are not unheard of. Three series included 45 patients.[20,33,34] Complete aspiration was achieved in 26 (58%). Complications included permanent memory deficit in one and permanent hemiparesis in one. Small cysts and those that are hyperdense on CT scan (the majority) are difficult to aspirate.[20] Mathiesen et al took a relatively less favorable view of stereotactic aspiration.[30] They reported 16 such patients, including one 18-year-old. Repeat procedures were required in 13 (81%), including repeated aspirations in 5, shunt placement in 3, and open surgical resection in 5. Three patients became comatose after aspiration because of hydrocephalus and cyst recurrence 1, 64, and 180 months, respectively, after stereotactic aspiration. Complications of 26 aspiration procedures included three patients with headache, temporary memory deficit, and mild personality change; one patient with coma 1 day after surgery caused by inadequate aspiration; and one patient with a disabling pain syndrome. Time to need for another procedure was within 1 month for 5 patients and 1 to 180 months for 8 patients, including 7 of 16 who had recurrence more than 8 years postaspiration, a finding of particular concern for the pediatric population.

Medical Management, Adjuvant Therapy

Medical therapy is limited to anticonvulsants in the relatively few patients who develop epilepsy after cyst treatment and is restricted to acute measures to reduce intracranial pressure before insertion of a ventricular drain; these include intubation, hyperventilation, and administration of mannitol and furosemide intravenously. There are no indications for radiation therapy or chemotherapy at present.

Recurrence and Long-Term Follow-Up

There were no recurrences among 31 transcallosal resections in patients followed for a mean of 4 years.[16] Follow-up information is not reported optimally in many series. Review of the literature, however, suggests that recurrence is rare after craniotomy and resection. Cases are cited by Rodziewicz et al[41] and McKissock.[31] The recurrence rate after stereotactic aspiration has been discussed earlier in this chapter and most likely exceeds that of surgery. Endoscopy remains uncertain in this regard.

In Hernesiemi and Leivo's review of the world literature, patients treated in the microsurgical era by transcortical microsurgery had an excellent or good outcome in 128 of 139 cases (92%), and 2 patients (1%) died.[16] For transcallosal microsurgery, 95 of 106 (90%) had an excellent or good outcome, and 4 (4%) died. Stereotactic aspiration or endoscopy resulted in 139 of 153 excellent or good outcomes (91%) with no mortality. Management outcome, which includes those patients dying before intervention—although most likely still an underestimate because they may not get to hospital—is worse.[16] Among 856 operated cases, 584 were reported to have an excellent or good (68%) outcome, and 81 died (11%). In the Netherlands over 5 years, 74 patients were diagnosed.[49] There was an overall 12% mortality. The outcome among 60 pediatric cases was 20 dead, 25 alive, and 15 with outcome unknown.

References

1. Antunes JL, Louis KM, Ganti SR: Colloid cysts of the third ventricle. Neurosurgery 7:450–455, 1980.
2. Apuzzo MLJ, Chikovani OK, Gott PS, et al: Transcallosal, interfornicial approaches for lesions affecting the third ventricle: surgical considerations and consequences. Neurosurgery 10:547–554, 1982.
3. Aronica PA, Ahdab-Barmada M, Rozin L, et al: Sudden death in an adolescent boy due to a colloid cyst of the third ventricle. Am J Forensic Med Pathol 19:119–122, 1998.
4. Batnitzky S, Sarwar M, Leeds NE, et al: Colloid cysts of the third ventricle. Radiology 112:327–341, 1974.
5. Bertalanffy H, Kretzschmar H, Gilsbach JM, et al: Large colloid cyst in lateral ventricle simulating brain tumor. Case report. Acta Neurochir (Wien) 104:151–155, 1990.
6. Brun A, Egund N: The pathogenesis of cerebral symptoms in colloid cysts of the third ventricle: a clinical and pathoanatomical study. Acta Neurol Scand 49:525–535, 1973.
7. Buttner A, Winkler PA, Eisenmenger W, et al: Colloid cysts of the third ventricle with fatal outcome: a report of two cases and review of the literature. Int J Legal Med 110:260–266, 1997.
8. Cabbell KL, Ross DA: Stereotactic microsurgical craniotomy for the treatment of third ventricular colloid cysts. Neurosurgery 38:301–307, 1996.
9. Cairns H, Mosberg WH, Jr: Colloid cyst of the third ventricle. Surg Gynecol Obstet 92:545–570, 1951.
10. Camacho A, Abernathey CD, Kelly PJ, et al: Colloid cysts: experience with the management of 84 cases since the introduction of computed tomography. Neurosurgery 24:693–700, 1989.
11. Carmel PW: Tumours of the third ventricle. Acta Neurochir (Wien) 75:136–146, 1985.
12. Decq P, Le Guerinel C, Brugieres P, et al: Endoscopic management of colloid cysts. Neurosurgery 42:1288–1294, 1998.
13. DiMaio SM, DiMaio VJ, Kirkpatrick JB: Sudden, unexpected deaths due to primary intracranial neoplasms. Am J Forensic Med Pathol 1:29–45, 1980.
14. Fritsch H: Colloid cysts—a review including 19 own cases. Neurosurg Rev 11:159–166, 1988.
15. Gemperlein J: Paraphyseal cysts of the third ventricle. Report of two cases in infants. J Neuropathol Exp Neurol 19:133–134, 1960.
16. Hernesniemi J, Leivo S: Management outcome in third ventricular colloid cysts in a defined population: a series of 40 patients treated mainly by transcallosal microsurgery. Surg Neurol 45:2–14, 1996.
17. Katzman GL, Dagher AP, Patronas NJ: Incidental findings on brain magnetic resonance imaging from 1000 asymptomatic volunteers. JAMA 282:36–39, 1999.
18. Kelly R: Colloid cysts of the third ventricle. Analysis of twenty-nine cases. Brain 74:23–65, 1951.
19. Kondziolka D, Bilbao JM: An immunohistochemical study of neuroepithelial (colloid) cysts. J Neurosurg 71:91–97, 1989.
20. Kondziolka D, Lunsford LD: Stereotactic management of colloid cysts: factors predicting success. J Neurosurg 75:45–51, 1991.
21. Kondziolka D, Lunsford LD: Microsurgical resection of colloid cysts using a stereotactic transventricular approach. Surg Neurol 46:485–490, 1996.
22. Kuchelmeister K, Bergmann M: Colloid cysts of the third ventricle: an immunohistochemical study. Histopathology 21:35–42, 1992.
23. Lach B, Scheithauer BW, Gregor A, et al: Colloid cyst of the third ventricle. A comparative immunohistochemical study of neuraxis cysts and choroid plexus epithelium. J Neurosurg 78:101–111, 1993.
24. Laidlaw J, Kaye AH: Colloid cysts. In Kaye AH, Laws ER, Jr. (eds): Brain Tumors: An Encyclopedic Approach, 1st ed. New York, Churchill Livingstone, 1995.
25. Lane CD, Lignelli GJ: Colloid cyst of the third ventricle. Penn Med 88:40–44, 1985.
26. Lewis AI, Crone KR, Taha J, et al: Surgical resection of third ventricle colloid cysts. Preliminary results comparing transcallosal microsurgery with endoscopy. J Neurosurg 81:174–178, 1994.
27. Little JR, MacCarty CS: Colloid cysts of the third ventricle. J Neurosurg 39:230–235, 1974.
28. Macdonald RL, Humphreys RP, Rutka JT, et al: Colloid cysts in children. Pediatr Neurosurg 20:169–177, 1994.
29. Mathiesen T, Grane P, Lindgren L, et al: Third ventricle colloid cysts: a consecutive 12-year series. J Neurosurg 86:5–12, 1997.
30. Mathiesen T, Grane P, Lindquist C, et al: High recurrence rate following aspiration of colloid cysts in the third ventricle. J Neurosurg 78:748–752, 1993.
31. McKissock W: The surgical treatment of colloid cyst of the third ventricle. A report based upon twenty-one personal cases. Brain 74:1–9, 1951.

32. Miettinen M, Clark R, Virtanen I: Intermediate filament proteins in choroid plexus and ependyma and their tumors. Am J Pathol 123:231–240, 1986.

33. Mohadjer M, Teshmar E, Mundinger F: CT-stereotaxic drainage of colloid cysts in the foramen of Monro and the third ventricle. J Neurosurg 67:220–223, 1987.

34. Musolino A, Fosse S, Munari C, et al: Diagnosis and treatment of colloid cysts of the third ventricle by stereotactic drainage. Report on eleven cases. Surg Neurol 32:294–299, 1989.

35. Nishino H, Gomez MR, Kelly PJ: Is colloid cyst of the third ventricle a manifestation of nevoid basal cell carcinoma syndrome? Brain Dev 13:368–370, 1991.

36. Nitta M, Symon L: Colloid cysts of the third ventricle. A review of 36 cases. Acta Neurochir (Wien) 76:99–104, 1985.

37. Parkinson D, Childe AE: Colloid cyst of the fourth ventricle. Report of a case of two colloid cysts of the fourth ventricle. J Neurosurg 9:404–409, 1952.

38. Pollock BE, Huston J, III: Natural history of asymptomatic colloid cysts of the third ventricle. J Neurosurg 91:364–369, 1999.

39. Pollock BE, Schreiner SA, Huston J, III: A theory on the natural history of colloid cysts of the third ventricle. Neurosurgery 46:1077–1081, 2000.

40. Read EJ, Jr: Colloid cyst of the third ventricle. Ann Emerg Med 19:1060–1062, 1990.

41. Rodziewicz GS, Smith MV, Hodge CJ, Jr: Endoscopic colloid cyst surgery. Neurosurgery 46:655–660, 2000.

42. Ryder JW, Kleinschmidt-DeMasters BK, Keller TS: Sudden deterioration and death in patients with benign tumors of the third ventricle area. J Neurosurg 64:216–223, 1986.

43. Saulsbury FT, Sullivan JS, Schmitt EJ: Sudden death due to colloid cyst of the third ventricle. Clin Pediatr (Phila) 20:218–219, 1981.

44. Shuangshoti S, Netsky MG: Neuroepithelial (colloid) cysts of the nervous system. Further observations on pathogenesis, location, incidence, and histochemistry. Neurology 16:887–903, 1966.

45. Shulman K, Shapiro K: Colloid cysts of the third ventricle in infancy and childhood. In American Association of Neurological Surgeons (ed): Pediatric Neurosurgery: Surgery of the Developing Nervous System, 1st ed. New York, Grune & Stratton, 1982.

46. Tada M, Nakamura N: Sphenoethmoidal encephalomeningocele and midline anomalies of face and brain. Hokkaido Igaku Zasshi 60:48–56, 1985.

47. Tantam D, Evered C, Hersov L: Asperger's syndrome and ligamentous laxity. J Am Acad Child Adolesc Psychiatry 29:892–896, 1990.

48. Wallmann H: Eine Colloidcyste im dritten hirnventrikel und ein lipom im plexus chorioides. Virchows Archiv 13:385–388, 1858.

49. Witt Hamer PC, Verstegen MJ, de Haan RJ, et al: High risk of acute deterioration in patients harboring symptomatic colloid cysts of the third ventricle. J Neurosurg 96:1041–1045, 2002.

50. Yenermen MH, Bowerman CI, Haymaker W: Colloid cyst of the third ventricle. A clinical study of 54 cases in the light of previous publications. Acta Neuroveg 17:211–277, 1958.

51. Zilkha A: Computed tomography of colloid cysts of the third ventricle. Clin Radiol 32:397–401, 1981.

CHAPTER **99**

ATYPICAL TERATOID/ RHABDOID TUMORS

Michael D. Taylor and Lucy B. Rorke

In 1978 Beckwith and Palmer described a histologic variant of Wilms tumor that occurred primarily in infants and was associated with an especially poor prognosis.[2] It was subsequently called *malignant rhabdoid tumor*—rhabdoid because the tumor looked like a rhabdomyosarcoma, but the cells did not demonstrate typical morphologic or immunohistochemical features of muscle.[8] A central nervous system (CNS) tumor composed of rhabdoid cells was first reported in 1985,[6] but the unique clinical and pathologic features were not well-defined until 1995 or 1996.[14,15] Because approximately 70% of these tumors contain fields indistinguishable from medulloblastoma or primitive neuroectodermal tumor, pathologists generally gave one or the other diagnosis. However, careful study of these tumors with routine hematoxylin and eosin (H&E) stains disclosed fields of rhabdoid cells with or without areas of primitive neuroepithelial cells, and in a quarter to a third of tumors, mesenchymal or epithelial elements were seen as well. Thus although such a combination of disparate tissue types suggested that these tumors were teratomas, they lacked the standard features required for such a diagnosis. The diagnostic term that seemed most appropriate was *atypical teratoid/rhabdoid tumor* (AT/RT), and so they were christened.

EPIDEMIOLOGY

AT/RT of the CNS most commonly arises in infants, the majority of patients being 3 years of age or younger at the time of diagnosis,[15] although rarely it occurs in adults as well.[15] The mean age at diagnosis ranges from 17 to 29 months.[7,15] These tumors are slightly more common in boys (3 : 2 male-to-female ratio). Approximately 1% to 2% of all brain tumors in children are of this type,[12,15] although some investigators report that 6.7% of CNS tumors in infants 0 to 2 years were AT/RTs.[12]

CLINICAL PRESENTATION OF CENTRAL NERVOUS SYSTEM AT/RT

Because rhabdoid tumors were originally found in the kidney, such tumors have been described in many different organs and soft tissues, as well as in the CNS. AT/RTs in the CNS are most commonly infratentorial (63%), 27% are supratentorial, and 8% are multifocal.[15] Although the cerebellum and cerebral hemispheres are the most common locations, these tumors have

a predilection for the cerebellopontine angle. They may also arise in the spinal cord, pineal gland, and suprasellar region.[7,15] A posterior fossa location is more common in children younger than 3 years old (70%), as opposed to older children (33%); the few examples in adults are almost exclusively in the cerebrum.[10,15] A small group of children have both renal and CNS rhabdoid tumors, which most likely represent metachronous tumors and are probably due to a germline mutation in the *hSNF5* gene (see the following discussion of AT/RT's molecular pathology).

Infants whose cranial sutures have not yet fused tend to have nonspecific symptoms such as lethargy, vomiting, or failure to thrive.[15] Older children have head tilts (fourth-nerve palsy), diplopia (sixth-nerve palsy), facial weakness (seventh-nerve palsy), headaches, or hemiplegia.[15] Many children with posterior fossa AT/RT have hydrocephalus at symptom onset because of obstruction of the fourth ventricle. The constellation of clinical signs and symptoms in children with AT/RT is similar to those in children with primitive neuroectodermal tumor–medulloblastoma (PNET-MB). One third of children with AT/RT have leptomeningeal spread of tumor at diagnosis, a rate similar to that seen in children with PNET-MB.[15] There is no difference in age between those children who have disseminated disease and those who do not.[15] Examination of the cerebrospinal fluid (CSF) at the time of diagnosis revealed malignant cells in 9 of 29 patients in one study, and CSF may be positive when craniospinal imaging is negative.[7]

IMAGING

The imaging procedure of choice in children with AT/RT is craniospinal magnetic resonance imaging (MRI) with or without gadolinium. The tumor shows low signal intensity on T1-weighted images and isointense or decreased signal on T2-weighted images (Figure 99-1).[15] Cysts and hemorrhages are commonly seen. Noncommunicating hydrocephalus and transependymal edema may be seen, especially with tumors located in the posterior fossa that block the fourth ventricle or its outlet foramina. The main tumor is inhomogeneously mass enhanced after administration of gadolinium. Leptomeningeal spread appears as diffuse enhancement of the meninges or enhanced clumps along the spinal cord and cauda equina. All of these features are similar to those seen in PNET-MB, and in fact, no imaging features differentiate AT/RT from the

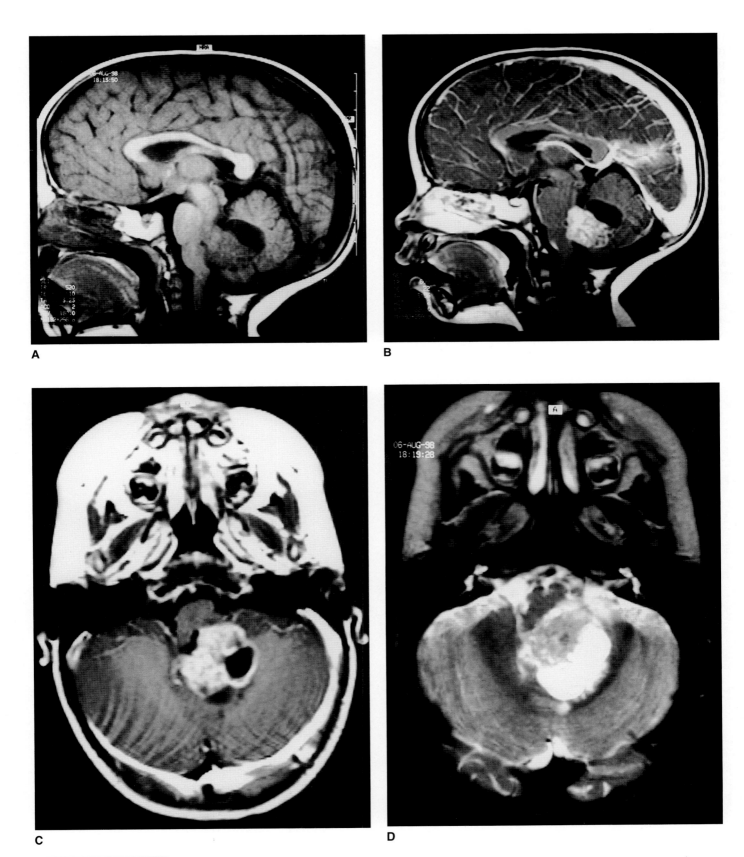

FIGURE 99-1 *A* and *B,* Sagittal T1-weighted magnetic resonance images of a patient with a posterior fossa atypical teratoid-rhabdoid tumor. Images without *(A)* and with *(B)* gadolinium enhancement show an isointense to hypointense lesion in the fourth ventricle that is diffusely enhanced with the administration of gadolinium. *C,* Axial image shows the partially cystic, diffusely enhanced tumor filling the fourth ventricle. *D,* The tumor is hyperintense on T2-weighted images.

PNET-MB. Some children may undergo computed tomography (CT) scanning as part of their diagnostic evaluation. As with PNET-MB, the AT/RT appears as a hyperdense lesion on an unenhanced CT scan, presumably because of the high cellularity of the tumor.[15]

GROSS AND MICROSCOPIC PATHOLOGY

Macroscopic features of these tumors differ in no way from those of PNET-MB. They are soft, pinkish red, necrotic, or hemorrhagic. Those with a prominent mesenchymal component may be firm and contain tan-white foci. Tumors primarily in the cerebellopontine angle may incorporate cranial nerve roots in the vicinity. Leptomeningeal deposits display no specific distinguishing features and are basically similar to PNET-MB. On section, these tumors tend to be infiltrative and have poorly demarcated margins.

Microscopic characteristics of AT/RT are variable, although it is evident that they must contain rhabdoid cells (Figure 99-2). Some tumors consist of only this cell type, whereas more commonly there is a mixture of rhabdoid fields and areas indistinguishable from classic PNET-MB (Figure 99-3). Although this portion may rarely contain Flexner-Wintersteiner or Homer-Wright rosettes, neither desmoplastic nor the nodular-neuroblastic histologic types have been observed. Basically, the PNET-MB portions simply consist of small primitive-appearing neuroepithelial cells.

The typical rhabdoid cell is of medium to large size and consists of an eccentric nucleus adjacent to which is eosinophilic cytoplasm equal to or larger than the nucleus. This tends to be round or slightly bulbous and may have a faint pink rim accentuating a denser pink core. Many nuclei contain a prominent nucleolus (see Figure 99-2B). Mitotic figures are common. The rhabdoid cells may range from small to giant size, the latter sometimes containing two nuclei.

Rhabdoid and PNET fields tend to remain separate, as do the epithelial and mesenchymal components, although there are no sharply delineated margins. A recognizable epithelial component, which may be adenomatous or squamous, occurs in approximately a quarter of the tumors, although a much higher number of tumor cells express epithelial antigens (Figure 99-4). A small group of these tumors may mimic choroid plexus carcinoma, and this possibility should be kept in mind. In addition, approximately one third of tumors contain neoplastic mesenchymal elements that, in the extreme, mimic sarcomas (Figure 99-5).

These tumors often exhibit large areas of necrosis and hemorrhage, but intrinsic vasculature generally manifests no distinguishing features.

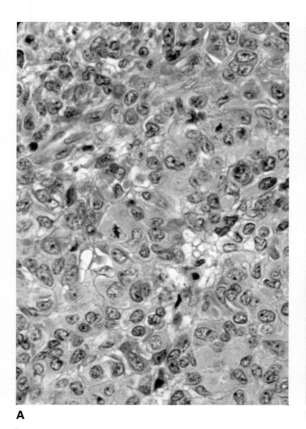
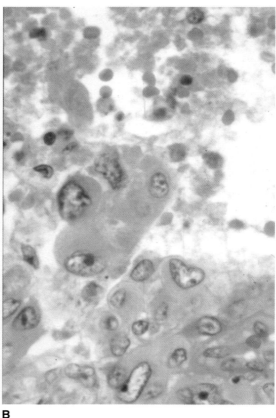

A   **B**

FIGURE 99-2   *A,* Field of rhabdoid cells demonstrating characteristic features, specifically, eccentrically placed nucleus with prominent nucleolus, distinct cell borders, homogeneous cytoplasm, and prominent mitotic activity (hematoxylin and eosin [H&E]). *B,* Higher magnification of rhabdoid cells showing a medium to large cell body and round nucleus with prominent nucleolus (H&E).

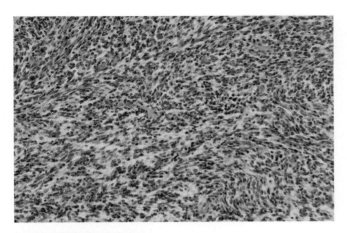

FIGURE 99-3 Field composed of primitive neuroecto-dermal cells in atypical teratoid-rhabdoid tumor in a cerebellar tumor (hematoxylin and eosin).

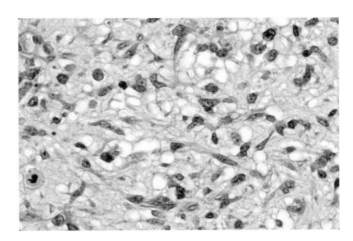

FIGURE 99-5 Field of multiprocessed mesenchymal cells in cerebellar atypical teratoid-rhabdoid tumor from the same tumor shown in Figure 99-4 (hematoxylin and eosin).

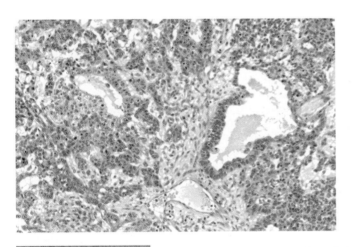

FIGURE 99-4 Glandular pattern in an area of cerebellar atypical teratoid-rhabdoid tumor (hematoxylin and eosin).

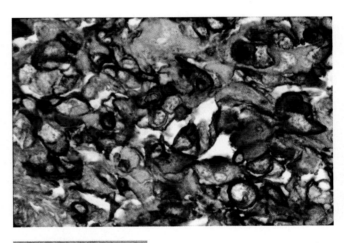

FIGURE 99-6 Immunoperoxidase preparation of atypical teratoid-rhabdoid tumor demonstrating expression of epithelial membrane antigen (EMA).

Confidence in making a specific histologic diagnosis of AT/RT may be enhanced by studying the tumor with a panel of monoclonal antibodies. Most helpful are the following: epithelial membrane antigen (EMA), vimentin, smooth muscle actin (SMA), keratin (K), glial fibrillary acidic protein (GFAP), and neurofilament protein (NFP) (Figures 99-6 and 99-7). Desmin is expressed rarely by the neuroepithelial cells but not by rhabdoid cells. Markers for germ cells are consistently negative.

The pattern of expression of these antigens is complex; hence attention must be paid to which cellular component is expressing the antigen. The rhabdoid cells typically express vimentin and EMA but express SMA less often. They may also express K, GFAP, or NFP.

The neuroepithelial cells express only GFAP or NFP, whereas the epithelial component expresses K plus or minus EMA; vimentin and SMA are typically expressed by the mesenchymal cells.

Ultrastructural findings vary, depending upon sampling. The classic, but not pathognomonic, finding in the rhabdoid cell consists of large bundles of intermediate filaments in the cytoplasm (Figure 99-8).

MOLECULAR PATHOLOGY

More than 10 years ago it was established that CNS AT/RTs often show loss or deletion of the long arm of chromosome 22q[4] (Figure 99-9). This was often the only karyotypic change seen in this tumor, and it was thought that a tumor-suppressor gene was localized to that region. Moreover, it was suggested that loss of one copy of chromosome 22q could distinguish an AT/RT from a PNET-MB, which is often associated with loss of 17p or isochromosome 17q. Subsequently, Versteege et al identified deletions and truncating mutations of the hSNF5 gene on chromosome 22q11 in a series of cell lines derived from renal rhabdoid tumors.[18] The hSNF5 protein is highly conserved and is not greatly changed between flies, mice, and humans. The hSNF5 protein is the smallest member of a family of proteins

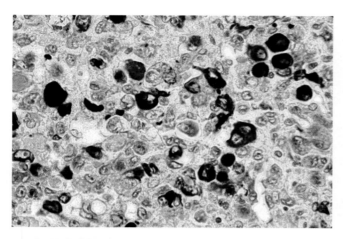

FIGURE 99-7   Immunoperoxidase preparation of atypical teratoid-rhabdoid tumor demonstrating expression of neurofilament protein (NFP) in rhabdoid cells.

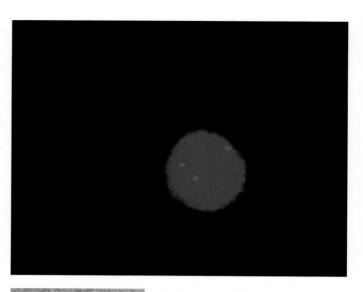

FIGURE 99-9   Interphase nuclei from an atypical teratoid-rhabdoid tumor demonstrating loss of one copy of the rhabdoid tumor gene (hSNF5 or INI1) in red, as compared with two copies of the 22q12 control probe in green.

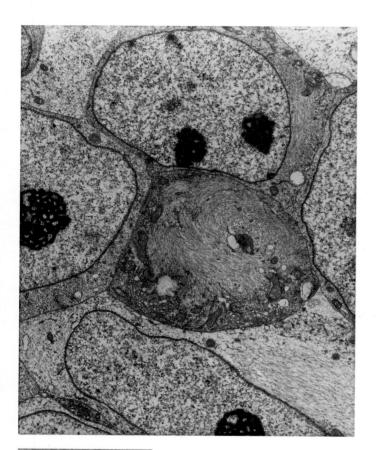

FIGURE 99-8   Electron micrograph of rhabdoid cell showing large bundle of intermediate filaments in perikaryon. (Magnification ×4500.)

that form a complex, which regulates the DNA through changes in the nucleosome (a fundamental unit of DNA). By "winding" and "unwinding" DNA, this complex changes the configuration of genomic DNA, thus allowing or denying transcription factors access to the DNA and changing gene expression patterns.

Biegel et al subsequently identified somatic mutations of hSNF5 in a series of CNS AT/RTs.[5] Some children with AT/RT are born with heterozygous germline mutations of the hSNF5 gene, suggesting that these children were predisposed to develop AT/RT.[5] In most cases, these germline mutations are *de novo* (a new mutation, not inherited from the parents), but in some instances they may be inherited from phenotypically normal parents.[5,17] Individuals and families with germline mutations of hSNF5 are also at increased risk to develop carcinoma of the choroid plexus.[17] However, it remains to be determined whether these are true choroid plexus tumors or AT/RTs, which may sometimes be misdiagnosed as a choroid plexus carcinoma.

Heterozygous mSNF5 plus or minus "knockout" mice develop tumors resembling AT/RTs, supporting the role of hSNF5 as a tumor-suppressor gene.[13] Although most AT/RTs show evidence of some genetic derangement at the hSNF5 locus, mutational analysis of the hSNF5 gene in a series of PNETs-MBs revealed mutations in only 4 of 52 tumors.[3] Of those four, two were reclassified as AT/RT on reexamination of the pathology, but there was insufficient clinical material to establish an accurate diagnosis in the other two cases. This suggests that tumors diagnosed as PNET-MB with hSNF5 are most likely AT/RT. Such confusion is not surprising, given the large number of AT/RTs that contain fields indistinguishable from PNET-MB. Although mutation or deletion of hSNF5 is not currently sufficient for a diagnosis of AT/RT, it appears to be related to the clinical outcome, and hence searching for it is becoming part of the diagnostic evaluation.

TREATMENT

Surgery

The initial treatment for most children with AT/RT is surgery. Children *in extremis* with severe hydrocephalus require a CSF diversionary procedure, either a ventriculostomy, a ventriculo-peritoneal shunt, or more recently, an endoscopic third ven-triculostomy.[16] Most children undergo a craniotomy, with maximal safe resection of tumor. The interface of the AT/RT and cerebellum may be abrupt or infiltrative and ill defined.[7] Total, or near-total, resection of the tumor is feasible in approx-imately 50% of patients.[15] Although surgery is excellent for dealing with acute mass effect, children who receive surgery alone with no adjuvant therapy typically die within 1 month of surgery.[15] There are no high-quality, prospective data on the value of surgical resection in the management of AT/RT, but in patients with PNET-MB, progression-free survival in children without disseminated disease at diagnosis is 20% better if the amount of postoperative residual tumor is less than 1.5 cm^3 in diameter, as compared with children in whom the amount of residual tumor is greater than 1.5 cm^3.[1]

Chemotherapy

Most children with AT/RT receive chemotherapy at some point during their clinical course, especially those younger than age 2 years, for whom radiation therapy is not an option. Several different chemotherapeutic regimens have been tried, including baby Pediatric Oncology Group (POG) protocols, eight drugs in 1 day, single-agent cyclophosphamide, and single-agent ifos-famide.[15] Most of these regimens were chosen based on their efficacy in treating PNET-MB. However, patients with AT/RT respond poorly to chemotherapy, and only 6 of 33 children who received only chemotherapy after surgery or chemotherapy before radiation therapy had a response, as defined by greater than 50% reduction in tumor mass.[15] In addition, most responses were short-lived, the longest being 10 months.[15] Some AT/RTs have been documented to enlarge during the course of chemotherapy.[7] Two children treated with high-dose chemotherapy followed by autologous bone marrow transplant had a good response, with one child surviving 19 months and another alive and well at 46 months of follow-up.[9] There is one report where chemotherapy previously described for use in patients with parameningeal rhabdomyosarcoma was adminis-tered to three patients with AT/RT. Therapy included surgery, radiation therapy, chemotherapy, and triple intrathecal chemo-therapy. All three patients were reported to be alive and well,

with no evidence of disease at 5 years, 2 years, and 9 months, respectively.[11] This exciting result awaits confirmation in larger, prospective trials.

Radiation Therapy

Most children with AT/RT are younger than 2 years; thus, because of toxicity of radiation to young brains, radiation therapy is initially withheld. Currently, the goal is to temporize with chemotherapy until the child is at least 2 or 3 years of age, at which time radiation effects are less severe. Because chil-dren with AT/RT commonly have leptomeningeal dissemina-tion or else develop it at the time of relapse, it is desirable to administer craniospinal radiation therapy, in addition to treat-ment of the primary tumor. Some authors have advocated a boost of radiation to the primary tumor by conventional means or by stereotactic radiation surgery at the time craniospinal therapy is administered. However, radiation therapy does not seem to alter the progression of disease in children with AT/RT; indeed, an objective response to radiation therapy was obtained in only 2 of 10 patients.[7,15] Despite these dismal statistics, chil-dren who are between 2 and 3 years of age and older will receive radiation therapy at some point in the course of their disease.

OUTCOME

The prognosis for children with AT/RT is dismal. The median time to progression is 4.5 months and the median reported sur-vival times range from 6 to 11 months.[7,15] Currently, the patient reported surviving longest was a 3-year-old girl who survived 5.5 years after developing a thalamic tumor that was treated with craniospinal irradiation. At relapse, the disease may be local (31%), in the leptomeninges (11%), or both (58%).[15] At postmortem examination, 10 of 11 children with AT/RT had widespread leptomeningeal disease. Obviously, current treat-ments for this tumor in the form of surgery, chemotherapy, or irradiation are not sufficient. Identification and characterization of the rhabdoid tumor predisposition gene on chromosome 22q may allow development of more focused, effective therapeutic agents that may increase survival time.

References

1. Albright AL, Wisoff JH, Zeltzer PM, et al: Effects of medul-loblastoma resections on outcome in children: a report from the Children's Cancer Group. Neurosurgery 38:265–271, 1996.
2. Beckwith JB, Palmer NF: Histopathology and prognosis of Wilms tumors: results from the First National Wilms' Tumor Study. Cancer 41:1937–1948, 1978.
3. Biegel JA, Fogelgren B, Zhou JY, et al: Mutations of the INI1 rhabdoid tumor suppressor gene in medulloblastomas and primi-tive neuroectodermal tumors of the central nervous system. Clin Cancer Res 6:2759–2763, 2000.
4. Biegel JA, Rorke LB, Packer RJ, et al: Monosomy 22 in rhabdoid or atypical tumors of the brain. J Neurosurg 73:710–714, 1990.
5. Biegel JA, Zhou JY, Rorke LB, et al: Germ-line and acquired mutations of INI1 in atypical teratoid and rhabdoid tumors. Cancer Res 59:74–79, 1999.

6. Briner J, Bannwart F, Kleihues P, et al: Malignant small cell tumor of the brain with intermediate filaments—a case of primary cere-bral rhabdoid tumor. Pediatr Pathol 3:117–118, 1985.
7. Burger PC, Yu IT, Tihan T, et al: Atypical teratoid/rhabdoid tumor of the central nervous system. A highly malignant tumor of infancy and childhood frequently mistaken for medulloblastoma: a Pediatric Oncology Group study. Am J Surg Pathol 22:1083–1092, 1998.
8. Haas JE, Palmer NF, Weinberg AG, et al: Ultrastructure of malig-nant rhabdoid tumor of the kidney. A distinctive renal tumor of children. Hum Pathol 12:646–657, 1981.
9. Hilden JM, Watterson J, Longee DC, et al: Central nervous system atypical teratoid tumor/rhabdoid tumor: response to intensive therapy and review of the literature. J Neurooncol 40:265–275, 1998.

10. Lutterbach J, Liegibel J, Koch D, et al: Atypical teratoid/rhabdoid tumors in adult patients: case report and review of the literature. J Neurooncol 52:49–56, 2001.

11. Olson TA, Bayar E, Kosnik E, et al: Successful treatment of disseminated central nervous system malignant rhabdoid tumor. J Pediatr Hematol Oncol 17:71–75, 1995.

12. Rickert CH, Paulus W: Epidemiology of central nervous system tumors in childhood and adolescence based on the new WHO classification. Childs Nerv Syst 17:503–511, 2001.

13. Roberts CW, Galusha SA, McMenamin ME, et al: Haploinsufficiency of Snf5 (integrase interactor 1) predisposes to malignant rhabdoid tumors in mice. Proc Natl Acad Sci USA 97:13796–13800, 2000.

14. Rorke LB, Packer R, Biegel J: Central nervous system atypical teratoid/rhabdoid tumors of infancy and childhood. J Neurooncol 24:21–28, 1995.

15. Rorke LB, Packer RJ, Biegel JA: Central nervous system atypical teratoid/rhabdoid tumors of infancy and childhood: definition of an entity. J Neurosurg 85:56–65, 1996.

16. Sainte-Rose C, Cinalli G, Roux FE, et al: Management of hydrocephalus in pediatric patients with posterior fossa tumors: the role of endoscopic third ventriculostomy. J Neurosurg 95:791–797, 2001.

17. Taylor MD, Gokgoz N, Andrulis IL, et al: Familial posterior fossa brain tumors of infancy secondary to germline mutation of the hSNF5 gene. Am J Hum Genet 66:1403–1406, 2000.

18. Versteege I, Sevenet N, Lange J, et al: Truncating mutations of hSNF5/INI1 in aggressive paediatric cancer. Nature 394:203–206, 1998.

CHAPTER 100

LANGERHANS CELL HISTIOCYTOSIS

Abhaya V. Kulkarni and Cynthia Hawkins

Langerhans cell histiocytosis (LCH) is a dendritic cell-related disorder of varied biologic behavior. It has a spectrum of clinical presentations and a clinical course that ranges from very benign (in most cases) to highly aggressive (in a few). LCH continues to be surrounded by some confusion. Numerous terms and conditions are associated with LCH, including eosinophilic granuloma (EG), histiocytosis X, Hand-Schüller-Christian (HSC) disease, and Letterer-Siwe (LS) disease. Further, the very nature and etiology of this condition is uncertain: is it a neoplastic or a reactive phenomenon?[21] Although some progress has been made in clarifying the terminology, the issue of etiology remains unresolved.

TERMINOLOGY

The term *EG* describes a defined pathologic entity in which the predominant histologic features are the presence of Langerhans cells and eosinophils.[23] It is usually used to refer to a single LCH lesion. *HSC disease* has been used in varying contexts over the past century, originally describing a clinical triad of exophthalmos, diabetes insipidus, and calvarial bone lesions. However, many cases with such a triad represent pathologically heterogeneous entities, only some of which have the typical features of LCH.[24] In current usage, the term *HSC* is more commonly used to describe multifocal LCH. *LS disease* has been used to describe another clinical syndrome consisting mainly of (1) hepatosplenomegaly, (2) hemorrhagic diatheses, (3) lymphadenopathy, (4) localized bone lesions, (5) secondary anemia, and (6) hyperplasia of nonlipoid-storing macrophages in various organs, especially the spleen, liver, lymph nodes, bones, lungs, skin, thymus, and lymph follicles of the intestines.[1] This is seen mainly in infants and generally has a poor prognosis. As with HSC, LS is not specific for a given pathologic entity but rather describes a clinical picture. The term *histiocytosis X* was originally attributed to Lichenstein, who used it to group the conditions that had previously been termed *EG, HSC,* and *LS*.[23] The problem, however, with this terminology, as argued by Lieberman et al, is that HSC and LS are clinical syndromes and do not describe specific pathologic conditions.[24]

For the purposes of this chapter, the terminology used to describe LCH will be limited to unifocal LCH, multifocal-unisystem LCH, and multifocal-multisystem LCH (which will include some cases of what might be referred to as HSC and LS). A detailed discussion of the historical context of the use of these various terms can be found in a comprehensive article by Lieberman et al.[24]

EPIDEMIOLOGY

LCH is more common in children than in adults, with most cases being diagnosed before the age of 15 years.[24] The incidence is estimated at between 0.2 and 1 per 100,000 children under 15 years of age.[43] Large series of these lesions also tend to demonstrate a preponderance in males, sometimes as high as 60% to 70% of cases.[24] It is also more common in whites of Northern European descent.

SITES OF INVOLVEMENT

Most cases (approximately 65%) of LCH are unifocal, and bone is, by far, the most common site of involvement, accounting for more than 90% of all such lesions.[24] The most common bones involved include skull, femur, pelvis, ribs, and vertebrae (each accounting for roughly 10% to 15%). Among the cases of vertebral involvement, the thoracic spine is most commonly involved, followed by the lumbar and cervical spine.[3] In the rare unifocal case without bone involvement, the most common sites are lung, lymph node, or skin.

In multifocal LCH, the pattern of tissue involvement is similar to unifocal LCH, with exclusive bone lesions accounting for roughly 60% of cases.[24] More than 50% of such cases will have skull lesions. A substantial minority (25%) of multifocal LCH involves both bone and soft tissue (i.e., multisystem, which WHO classifies as multifocal, multisystem), whereas exclusive soft-tissue involvement is less common (approximately 15%).[24]

When soft tissue is involved in multifocal LCH, the most common sites are, again, lung, lymph node, and skin.

Rare sites of involvement with LCH that are relevant to neuro-oncology include the hypothalamus (usually as part of a multifocal presentation, but also reported as a unifocal lesion),[7] the orbit,[9,40] the cerebral hemispheres,[16,18,27] the choroid plexus,[19] the cerebellum,[15] and the skull base.[4] The remainder of this chapter will concentrate on cranial and vertebral involvement of LCH.

SIGNS AND SYMPTOMS

The presenting clinical picture varies according to the site of involvement. Skull lesions tend to occur as new cranial lumps, usually with some pain or tenderness.[35] Spinal lesions almost always cause local pain, sometimes with associated back stiffness, torticollis, or kyphoscoliosis.[3,26,38] Rarely, spinal LCH can cause neurologic deficits secondary to spinal cord or nerve root compression.[2,25] Hypothalamic pituitary involvement is seen in approximately 10% of LCH patients and usually with a clinical picture of diabetes insipidus, most commonly in the setting of multifocal disease. There may also be other endocrinologic deficits, including panhypopituitarism.[7] Other, less common central nervous system (CNS) manifestations include extraparenchymal space-occupying lesions from the meninges or choroid plexus and more global neurologic and neuropsychologic sequelae. The latter occurs in approximately 1% of the overall LCH population but in up to 10% of patients with diabetes insipidus. Symptoms range from tremor to severe ataxia, dysarthria, and dysphagia to intellectual impairment or behavioral changes. Patients with multifocal, multisystem disease are usually infants who have fever, hepatosplenomegaly, lymphadenopathy, pancytopenia, and skin and bone lesions.

PATHOLOGY

The gross appearance of bone LCH is that of an expanding, circumscribed lesion that usually extends through the adjacent cortical bone. There may be associated pathologic fractures or subperiosteal new bone formation. The lesion itself varies from tan to hemorrhagic red, with solid or cystic components.[24]

Microscopically, the key feature is the presence of Langerhans cells. These are recognized histologically by their slightly eccentric, convoluted nuclei with linear grooves and inconspicuous nucleoli and their moderately abundant eosinophilic cytoplasm. The Langerhans cells are found in a background of variable numbers of eosinophils, histiocytes, neutrophils, lymphocytes, and plasma cells (Figure 100-1). Multinucleated giant cells or areas of necrosis are sometimes also seen, but mitoses are a rare finding. Older lesions may show areas of fibrosis. The Langerhans cells show positive immunohistochemical staining for CD1a and S-100. However, the characteristic feature and diagnostic gold standard for Langerhans cells is the ultrastructural identification of Birbeck granules (Figure 100-2), which are 34 nm wide tubular or tennis-racket-shaped intracytoplasmic pentalaminar structures with a zipper-like central core.[24] Langerhans cell sarcoma is also recognized, although it is extremely rare. It is characterized by multiorgan involvement and is diagnosed pathologically when the Langerhans cells display overtly malignant cytologic features. Further, there are abundant mitotic figures, and the polymorphic infiltrate found in LCH is typically absent. Rare reports of the pathologic findings in the ill-defined cerebellar lesions associated with the neurodegenerative syndrome describe variable perivascular rarefaction, perivascular histiocytes, and gliosis, but no LCH cells.

ETIOLOGY

Many etiologies have been proposed for LCH including immunologic, viral, and neoplastic causes; however, its origin remains unknown. Further, studies of the pathogenesis of LCH have been hampered by the difficulty in culturing the cells and by the lack of a good animal model of the disease. LCH is included in the classification of histiocytic disorders, where it falls into the category of disorders of varied biologic behavior, rather than the frankly malignant disorders, and into the subcategory of dendritic cell–related, as opposed to macrophage-related. LCH has been shown to be a monoclonal proliferation of CD1+ histiocytes in all forms of the disease, from the solitary lytic lesions of bone to the disseminated multisystem disease of infancy.[44,46,47] Although monoclonal proliferations of hematopoietic cells are usually neoplastic, this is not always the case, and the significance of clonality in LCH is unclear.

The role of viruses in the pathogenesis of LCH is also debated. It has been postulated that proliferation of Langerhans cells might be a reaction to some form of viral infection,[29] though no viral genome has been consistently found in LCH tissues.[28,30] There is some consensus in the belief that altered immune responses and immune dysfunction may play a role in the pathophysiology of the disease; however, there is no evidence that these patients have a primary defect in their immune systems.

NEUROIMAGING

Skull Lesions

On plain x-ray films, skull lesions tend to be well-demarcated, rounded, osteolytic lesions of the calvarium without a sclerotic rim.[35] Computed tomography (CT) demonstrates that the outer table is usually more destroyed than the inner table by a hypodense lesion that is strongly enhanced (Figures 100-3 and 100-4). Within the center of the osteolytic lesion, residual bone can sometimes be seen. With magnetic resonance imaging (MRI), skull LCH is characteristically isointense to gray matter on T1-weighted and hyperintense on T2-weighted images. Aside from lesional enhancement, it is also common to see enhancement of the adjacent dura and galea.

Technetium bone scintigraphy demonstrates increased uptake, especially in the periphery of the lesion with a central defect. However, in some cases multiple lesions can be missed by nuclear scanning, requiring the use of plain x-ray skeletal surveys to assess for the presence of other bone lesions, especially of the long bones.[3,12,43]

Spinal Lesions

The radiographic and MRI characteristics of LCH of the spine are similar to those previously mentioned for skull lesions. More than 80% of cases involve the vertebral body, with only a minority involving either the pedicles or lamina.[3] Involvement is usually limited to a single vertebral level, but it is not uncommon for the involved vertebrae to be partially or completely collapsed (vertebra plana).[3] Although it is a classic imaging feature of LCH, vertebra plana is not a specific sign and is also seen in Ewing's sarcoma and spinal infection.[3]

Intracranial Lesions

Imaging of hypothalamic LCH usually reveals a suprasellar mass in the floor of the third ventricle that is slightly hyper-

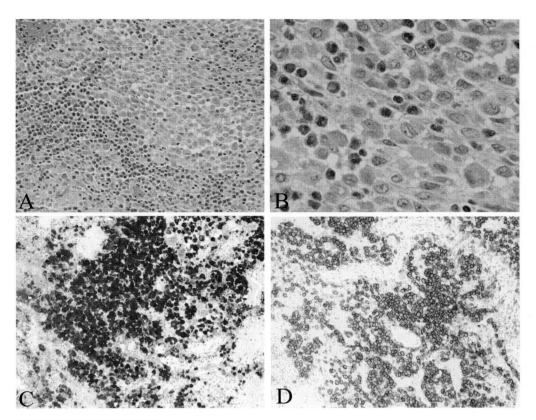

FIGURE 100-1 Langerhans cell histiocytosis. *A,* Mixed infiltrate composed of histiocytes, eosinophils, lymphocytes, and neutrophils (hematoxylin and eosin [H&E] stain ×100). *B,* High power view showing the typical nuclear grooving (H&E ×600). *C,* Immunohistochemical labeling with S-100 protein. *D,* Immunohistochemical labeling with CD1a.

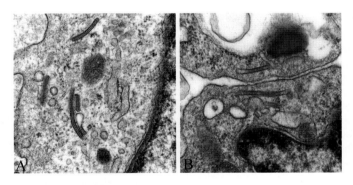

FIGURE 100-2 Electron microscopy of Langerhans cell histiocytosis showing multiple Birbeck granules with typical penta-laminar structure *(A)* and rod or tennis racket shapes *(B).*

dense on CT imaging with bright and homogeneous enhancement.[7] On MRI, the lesions tend to be hypointense on T1-weighted and hyperintense on T2-weighted images with bright gadolinium enhancement. In the extremely rare case of intracerebral LCH, the imaging characteristics appear to be similar to that of hypothalamic LCH, with the added feature of edema surrounding the lesion.[18] The appearance is very nonspecific.

TREATMENT

Unifocal Langerhans Cell Histiocytosis of the Skull

The initial management of the patient with suspected LCH involves confirming the diagnosis. In a patient with a skull lesion, this usually includes ruling out multifocal involvement and then performing an open removal of the lesion. In most cases this will not only provide the diagnosis but can also be curative. If total removal of the lesion can be performed (and this is usually the case), then no further therapy is warranted, and the patient can simply be observed. There are also reports of spontaneous regression, with complete healing of the bone, of skull lesions that appeared to be radiologically consistent with LCH.[36] Lesions that are painful may respond to intralesional steroid injection. Indomethacin has also been suggested as a steroid alternative. Regardless of the initial therapy, these patients require clinical and imaging follow-up, because they can develop recurrent or multifocal lesions over time (usually within weeks to months). This can occur despite successful removal of an initial unifocal lesion.[17,42]

Unifocal Langerhans Cell Histiocytosis of the Spine

Confirming the diagnosis of a spinal lesion as LCH requires a biopsy specimen. This can usually be accomplished through a

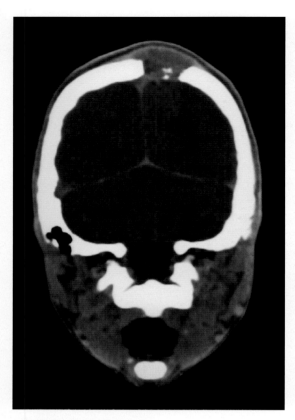

FIGURE 100-3 Coronal computed tomography scan of Langerhans cell histiocytosis demonstrating an osteolytic lesion near the vertex. Note the small amount of residual bone within the lesion.

percutaneous CT-guided needle biopsy.[41] In the absence of multifocal involvement, treatment of spinal LCH is determined by various factors. First, in the rare case of neurologic deficit from spinal cord compression, decompressive surgery may be warranted.[25] Second, in the presence of a potentially unstable lesion, some form of spinal immobilization is required (e.g., cervical collar, halo vest, or thoraco-lumbar bracing). There have been reports of simply observing spinal LCH lesions after immobilization with good results.[26] Also, it has been reported that in long-term follow-up review many of these lesions tend to heal very well. In fact, even in the presence of vertebral collapse, restoration in vertebral body height has been reported, sometimes to near normal levels.[26,38]

Further treatment options for spinal LCH include local radiation therapy or chemotherapy. For unifocal LCH of the spine, relatively low dose radiation therapy (8 to 12 Gy) has been used with efficacy.[38] Although the doses involved are generally not thought to lead to impaired spinal growth in children, caution must still be exercised in recommending radiation therapy for the very young. An alternative to radiation therapy is chemotherapy (e.g., vinblastine). This has been reported in the treatment of young children with good results.[17,22] Although the use of steroids has also been reported, its efficacy in the treatment of LCH is unclear.[22]

Unifocal Langerhans Cell Histiocytosis—Intracranial

Occurrence of LCH as a unifocal intracranial lesion is very rare. When reported, the regions involved included the hypothalamus (although this more commonly occurs with multifocal involvement), cerebellum,[15] or cerebral hemispheres.[7,18] In the absence of multifocal lesions, the diagnosis is virtually impossible to predict based on the nonspecific imaging findings alone. Therefore these lesions are usually subject to the treatment algorithm applied to suspected brain tumors, which would involve either an attempt at open resection or biopsy. This can be a particularly difficult task for hypothalamic lesions, which usually need to be accessed by either an open craniotomy or, if feasible, an endoscopic transventricular route. However, once the diagnosis of LCH is confirmed, the treatment options can be better defined. Following a gross-total resection of an intracranial LCH lesion, most patients should be observed without any further therapy.[7,8,18] In the setting of a biopsy or incomplete resection, the options include radiation therapy and chemotherapy. The relative efficacy of each is not entirely clear, given the relatively small series appearing in the literature. In younger children, where the avoidance of radiation therapy (particularly in the suprasellar region) is very desirable, chemotherapy may be the preferred option. Patients with hypothalamic involvement also require a thorough endocrinologic evaluation and appropriate hormone replacement therapy.

Multifocal Langerhans Cell Histiocytosis

When making the diagnosis of multifocal LCH, it is important to fully assess the extent of body involvement. The prognosis is thought to be substantially worse in the presence of soft-tissue involvement (e.g., lymph nodes, liver, spleen, skin) than if only multifocal bone lesions are present.[12] A typical screening for extent of systemic involvement would include a detailed history and physical examination, complete blood count, coagulation and liver profiles, nuclear scintigraphy, and skeletal survey. Further, the Histiocyte Society recommends that all LCH patients at initial diagnosis undergo the following evaluations: height, weight, pubertal status, water deprivation test for diabetes insipidus, baseline hormone studies (T4, thyroid-stimulating hormone, cortisol, follicle-stimulating hormone, luteinizing hormone, and prolactin), baseline age-appropriate tests of intellectual and motor development, and behavioral tests, as well as brain MRI with a contrast agent.

With only multifocal bone involvement, chemotherapy is generally given.[43] There is some evidence to suggest that chemotherapy for multifocal bone involvement reduces the incidence of recurrence.[43] However, some have recommended that a subset of such patients can simply be observed, reserving chemotherapy for only those with involvement of critical bone structures (e.g., the spine).[12]

In the presence of multisystem disease, chemotherapy is the treatment of choice.[12,17,33,43] The most often reported chemotherapeutic regimen for multifocal LCH has been vinblastine, usually with concomitant prednisone. Other agents that have been used include methotrexate, etoposide, 6-mercaptopurine, cyclosporine, and cyclophosphamide.[11,12,31,45] A recent randomized trial (LCH-I) found no significant difference in outcome between vinblastine and etoposide.[10] However, during this study it was noted that children whose disease fails

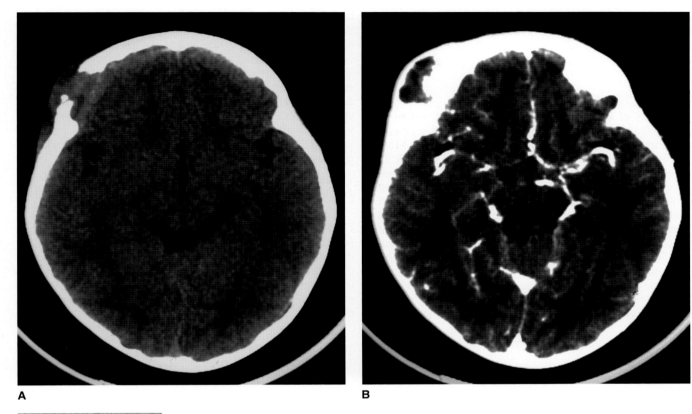

A B

FIGURE 100-4 Axial computed tomography of Langerhans cell histiocytosis, without *(A)* and with *(B)* contrast enhancement. An osteolytic lesion with strong contrast enhancement is present in the right frontotemporal region.

to enter remission after an initial 6-week treatment period are at significantly increased risk of ultimate treatment failure. Identification of this new prognostic factor may lead to the development of improved treatments for higher-risk patients while sparing lower-risk patients unnecessary toxicity. Long-term follow-up review of patients enrolled on LCH-I will also provide important information about the impact of successful treatment on reducing the long-term side effects of LCH such as diabetes insipidus.

Following the successful completion of LCH-I, a follow-up study was developed that built upon the results of LCH-I. LCH-II was a randomized phase III trial for patients with multisystem LCH considered to be at higher risk of disease progression or recurrence. LCH-II sought to more clearly define the additive role of etoposide in the treatment of high-risk LCH, using a different approach than was taken in LCH-I. The LCH-II clinical trial compared, in a randomized fashion, the effectiveness of the combination of vinblastine, oral prednisone, and mercaptopurine to the same combination with the addition of etoposide. Also in LCH-II, patients were stratified into lower or higher risk groups based on their extent of disease at the time of diagnosis. Almost 700 patients were registered onto LCH-II. The results of LCH-II are expected to be published soon.

There are currently two open treatment protocols for LCH, established by the Histiocyte Society. LCH-III, an international, multicenter, prospective clinical study, opened on April 1, 2001. It comprises a randomized clinical trial for multisystem "high-risk" patients, a randomized clinical trial for multisystem

"low-risk" patients, and a pilot study for patients with single-system multifocal bone disease and localized "special sites." LCH-S-98, available since autumn of 1998, is a nonrandomized phase II study that seeks to confirm the activity of 2-chlorodeoxyadenosine treatment in children with refractory or progressive LCH whose disease progressed after combination therapy with prednisolone, vinblastine, and etoposide. Other investigational agents include indium-labeled anti-CD1a antibody and cytokine inhibitors.

Depending on the severity of disease, a chemotherapeutic regimen may be required for a prolonged period of time (sometimes several years). Complications from this type of medical management include hematologic disorders (e.g., neutropenia, secondary leukemia), Cushing's syndrome (with steroid use), infection, and local skin complications from intravenous drug administration.[12,14] In the most severe cases of multifocal LCH, the use of myeloablative therapy and bone marrow transplant has been reported.[34] Although radiation therapy, high-dose steroids, and various chemotherapeutic agents have been tried in patients with LCH-associated progressive CNS deterioration, none of these agents resulted in significant clinical improvement.

In addition to systemic chemotherapy, local treatment might also be required for certain lesions in multifocal disease. For example, local involvement of the spine might warrant immobilization, local radiation therapy, or surgery (see previous discussion). Local radiation therapy might also be considered for particularly painful bone lesions elsewhere that do not respond to chemotherapy.[12] An alternative local therapy that can also be considered is intralesional injection of steroids.[5,12,43]

OUTCOME

The prognosis of LCH is highly dependent on the extent of body involvement and, in particular, whether soft tissue is involved. In unifocal LCH, the prognosis is excellent. More than 95% of cases are self-limiting with minimal or even no local therapy.[39,43] In the spine there is also evidence that conservatively treated lesions can heal very well with at least partial restoration of vertebral body height.[38] Multifocal LCH with only bone involvement appears to carry a similarly good prognosis.[43] However, as previously mentioned, recurrent lesions (either local or elsewhere) have been reported in both unifocal and multifocal bone LCH and occur with an incidence of approximately 15% to 20%.[43] A recent report suggests that the incidence of recurrence might be somewhat higher in skeletally mature patients as compared with younger ones.[37] Most such recurrences tend to occur within 2 years,[24,37] although rare

reports of recurrence several years after remission have been noted.[13] Therefore long-term follow-up is necessary. It has also been reported that, on rare occasions, recurrent LCH might occur with hypothalamic involvement and diabetes insipidus.[43]

The prognosis is much worse for patients with multisystem LCH with soft-tissue involvement (especially of critical organs), those diagnosed at a young age, and those with a poor early response to chemotherapy.[32] Despite aggressive treatment with chemotherapy and radiation therapy, there is a mortality incidence of close to 20%.[12,32] In infants with organ dysfunction, the mortality rate is close to 100%.[20]

CONCLUSION

LCH is a highly varied clinical condition that most commonly presents with bone lesions. In the absence of multisystem involvement, the prognosis is very good, and the treatment is generally kept as conservative as possible. With multisystem involvement, particularly in infants, the disease tends to a much more malignant course and warrants appropriately aggressive therapy.

References

1. Abt AF, Denenholz EJ: Letterer-Siwe's disease: splenohepatomegaly associated with widespread hyperplasia of nonlipoid-storing macrophages-discussion of the so-called reticuloendothelioses. Am J Dis Child 51:499–522, 1936.
2. Acciarri N, Paganini M, Fonda C, et al: Langerhans cell histiocytosis of the spine causing cord compression: case report. Neurosurgery 31:965–968, 1992.
3. Bertram C, Madert J, Eggers C: Eosinophilic granuloma of the cervical spine. Spine 27:1408–1413, 2002.
4. Brisman JL, Feldstein NA, Tarbell NJ, et al: Eosinophilic granuloma of the clivus: case report, follow-up of two previously reported cases, and review of the literature on cranial base eosinophilic granuloma. Neurosurgery 41:273–278; discussion 278–279, 1997.
5. Capanna R, Springfield DS, Ruggieri P, et al: Direct cortisone injection in eosinophilic granuloma of bone: a preliminary report on 11 patients. J Pediatr Orthop 5:339–342, 1985.
6. Chu T, Jaffe R: The normal Langerhans cell and the LCH cell. Br J Cancer Suppl 23:S4–S10, 1994.
7. d'Avella D, Giusa M, Blandino A, et al: Microsurgical excision of a primary isolated hypothalamic eosinophilic granuloma. Case report. J Neurosurg 87:768–772, 1997.
8. Forrest E, Gallacher SJ, Hadley D, et al: Central nervous system histiocytosis X—imaging and responses to chemotherapy. Scott Med J 38:148–149, 1993.
9. Furuta S, Sakaki S, Hatakeyama T, et al: Pediatric orbital eosinophilic granuloma with intra- and extracranial extension—case report. Neurol Med Chir (Tokyo) 31:590–592, 1991.
10. Gadner H, Grois N, Arico M, et al: A randomized trial of treatment for multisystem Langerhans' cell histiocytosis. J Pediatr 138:728–734, 2001.
11. Gadner H, Heitger A, Grois N, et al: Treatment strategy for disseminated Langerhans cell histiocytosis. DAL HX-83 Study Group. Med Pediatr Oncol 23:72–80, 1994.
12. Ghanem I, Tolo VT, D'Ambra P, Malogalowkin MH: Langerhans cell histiocytosis of bone in children and adolescents. J Pediatr Orthop 23:124–130, 2003.

13. Grimm RA, Muss HB, Patterson RB, et al: Reactivation of Hand-Schuller-Christian disease six and thirteen years after discontinuation of systemic therapy. Med Pediatr Oncol 9:17–21, 1981.
14. Haupt R, Fears TR, Rosso P, et al: Increased risk of secondary leukemia after single-agent treatment with etoposide for Langerhans' cell histiocytosis. Pediatr Hematol Oncol 11:499–507, 1994.
15. Iraci G, Chieco-Bianchi L, Giordano R, Gerosa M: Histiocytosis "X" of the central nervous system. Clinical and pathological report of a case with predominant cerebellar involvement. Childs Brain 5:116–130, 1979.
16. Itoh H, Waga S, Kojima T, et al: Solitary eosinophilic granuloma in the frontal lobe: case report. Neurosurgery 30:295–298, 1992.
17. Karagoz Guzey F, Bas NS, Emel E, et al: Polyostotic monosystemic calvarial and spinal langerhans' cell histiocytosis treated by surgery and chemotherapy. Pediatr Neurosurg 38:206–211, 2003.
18. Katati MJ, Martin JM, Pastor J, Arjona V: Isolated primary Langerhans' cell histiocytosis of central nervous system. Neurocirugia (Astur) 13:477–478, 2002.
19. Kim EY, Choi JU, Kim TS, et al: Huge Langerhans cell histiocytosis granuloma of choroid plexus in a child with Hand-Schuller-Christian disease. Case report. J Neurosurg 83:1080–1084, 1995.
20. Kusuma Kumary P, Priyakumari T, Chellam VG, et al: Langerhans cell histiocytosis in children less than 2 years of age. Indian Pediatr 36:29–36, 1999.
21. Ladisch S: Langerhans cell histiocytosis. Curr Opin Hematol 5:54–58, 1998.
22. Levy EI, Scarrow A, Hamilton RC, et al: Medical management of eosinophilic granuloma of the cervical spine. Pediatr Neurosurg 31:159–162, 1999.
23. Lichtenstein L: Histiocytosis X: integration of eosinophilic granuloma of bone, "Letterer-Siwe disease," and "Schüller-Christian disease," as related manifestations of a single nosologic entity. AMA Arch Pathol 56:84–102, 1953.
24. Lieberman PH, Jones CR, Steinman RM, et al: Langerhans cell (eosinophilic) granulomatosis. A clinicopathologic study encompassing 50 years. Am J Surg Pathol 20:519–552, 1996.

25. Maggi G, de Sanctis N, Aliberti F, Nunziata Rega A: Eosinophilic granuloma of C4 causing spinal cord compression. Childs Nerv Syst 12:630–632, 1996.

26. Mammano S, Candiotto S, Balsano M: Cast and brace treatment of eosinophilic granuloma of the spine: long-term follow-up. J Pediatr Orthop 17:821–827, 1997.

27. Marafioti T, Cardia E: Solitary eosinophilic granuloma of cerebral lobes. Value of immunohistochemistry for a diagnostic interpretation. Zentralbl Pathol 140:391–396, 1994.

28. McClain K, Jin H, Gresik V, Favara B: Langerhans cell histiocytosis: lack of a viral etiology. Am J Hematol 47:16–20, 1994.

29. McClain K, Weiss RA: Viruses and Langerhans cell histiocytosis: is there a link? Br J Cancer Suppl 23:S34–S36, 1994.

30. Mierau GW, Wills EJ, Steele PO: Ultrastructural studies in Langerhans cell histiocytosis: a search for evidence of viral etiology. Pediatr Pathol 14:895–904, 1994.

31. Minkov M, Grois N, Broadbent V, et al: Cyclosporine: a therapy for multisystem langerhans cell histiocytosis. Med Pediatr Oncol 33:482–485, 1999.

32. Minkov M, Grois N, Heitger A, et al: Response to initial treatment of multisystem Langerhans cell histiocytosis: an important prognostic indicator. Med Pediatr Oncol 39:581–585, 2002.

33. Moore JB, Kulkarni R, Crutcher DC, Bhimani S: MRI in multifocal eosinophilic granuloma: staging disease and monitoring response to therapy. Am J Pediatr Hematol Oncol 11:174–177, 1989.

34. Morgan G: Myeloablative therapy and bone marrow transplantation for Langerhans' cell histiocytosis. Br J Cancer Suppl 23:S52–S53, 1994.

35. Okamoto K, Ito J, Furusawa T, et al: Imaging of calvarial eosinophil granuloma. Neuroradiology 41:723–728, 1999.

36. Oliveira M, Steinbok P, Wu J, et al: Spontaneous resolution of calvarial eosinophilic granuloma in children. Pediatr Neurosurg 38:247–252, 2003.

37. Plasschaert F, Craig C, Bell R, et al: Eosinophilic granuloma. A different behaviour in children than in adults. J Bone Joint Surg Br 84:870–872, 2002.

38. Raab P, Hohmann F, Kuhl J, Krauspe R: Vertebral remodeling in eosinophilic granuloma of the spine. A long-term follow-up. Spine 23:1351–1354, 1998.

39. Sartoris DJ, Parker BR: Histiocytosis X: rate and pattern of resolution of osseous lesions. Radiology 152:679–684, 1984.

40. Schick U, Hassler W: Pediatric tumors of the orbit and optic pathway. Pediatr Neurosurg 38:113–121, 2003.

41. Shabb N, Fanning CV, Carrasco CH, et al: Diagnosis of eosinophilic granuloma of bone by fine-needle aspiration with concurrent institution of therapy: a cytologic, histologic, clinical, and radiologic study of 27 cases. Diagn Cytopathol 9:3–12, 1993.

42. Song A, Johnson TE, Dubovy SR, Toledano S: Treatment of recurrent eosinophilic granuloma with systemic therapy. Ophthal Plast Reconstr Surg 19:140–144, 2003.

43. Titgemeyer C, Grois N, Minkov M, et al: Pattern and course of single-system disease in Langerhans cell histiocytosis data from the DAL-HX 83- and 90-study. Med Pediatr Oncol 37:108–114, 2001.

44. Willman CL: Detection of clonal histiocytes in Langerhans cell histiocytosis: biology and clinical significance. Br J Cancer Suppl 23:S29–S33, 1994.

45. Yu LC, Shenoy S, Ward K, Warrier RP: Successful treatment of multisystem Langerhans cell histiocytosis (histiocytosis X) with etoposide. Am J Pediatr Hematol Oncol 16:275–277, 1994.

46. Willman CL, Busque L, Griffith BB, et al: Langerhans'-cell histiocytosis (histiocytosis X)—a clonal proliferative disease. N Engl J Med 331:154–160, 1994.

47. Yu RC, Chu C, Buluwela L, Chu AC: Clonal proliferation of Langerhans cells in Langerhans cell histiocytosis. Lancet 343:767–768, 1994.

CHAPTER 101

PEDIATRIC SKULL BASE TUMORS

Henry E. Aryan, Hal S. Meltzer, Derek A. Bruce, and Michael L. Levy

This chapter focuses on tumors that occur in the base of the skull or its immediate proximity; it does not include primary central nervous system (CNS) tumors that occur in the basal area of the intracranial intradural space. The tumors to be discussed are rare in neurosurgical practice for two reasons. Many of the lesions are not treated by extensive surgery and thus seen by the neurosurgeon, and the incidence of most of the tumors seen in this area is low.

Unlike tumors in adults, the majority of tumors excised in children are not malignant, although they may be locally invasive and tend to recur if not completely excised. The surgical challenges are to obtain adequate exposure to prevent damage to functional structures and to growth centers of the face and teeth. Because of the rarity and variable pathology of skull base tumors in children, the ideal therapies are only now being defined. As with so many disease processes in children, the best strategy for therapy includes a multispecialty approach that includes pediatric neurosurgery, craniofacial or otorhinolaryngology surgery, neuroradiology, pediatric anesthesia, neuropathology, hematology or oncology, radiation therapy, speech therapy, neuropsychologists, and social workers. It is a mistake for a neurosurgeon to undertake the treatment of children with these lesions in isolation. After therapy, the long-term survival rate is good if the selection of primary therapy is appropriate. Most of these tumors need combined therapy including surgery, radiation therapy, or chemotherapy.

LOCATION AND TUMOR HISTOLOGY

To understand the symptoms and signs of and the therapy for skull base lesions requires knowledge of the formation and anatomy of the structures at the base of the skull. The tissues, cartilage, bone, muscle, nerves, blood vessels, sinus mucosa, notochord, lymphoid tissue, and orbital structures may all be the origin of tumors (Table 101-1). The anterior neuropore of the embryo closes in a long slit running from the foramen caecum to the base of the pituitary gland. Neural tissue or pluripotential tissue can be isolated from the CNS in this area and give rise to teratomas, nasal or tongue gliomas, and dermoids or epidermoids of the nose or orbits. Teratomas in the tongue or pharyngeal area are presumably the result of neuronal or pluripotential tissue having been pinched off as neural tube or skin closure occurred or as mesoderm development occurred. Primary tumors of the upper nasal mucosa include olfactory neuroblastomas and neuroendocrine carcinoma. These tumors occur in the ethmoid and maxillary sinuses and nasal septum. Olfactory neuroblastomas arise from primary olfactory neurons and neuroendocrine carcinoma from the epithelium of the exocrine glands found in the normal nasal mucosa.

The point of origin of olfactory neuroblastoma appears to be the upper portion of the nasal septum. This tumor commonly has an intracranial component, whereas neuroendocrine carcinoma rarely penetrates the cranium. Neuroblastomas occur at the skull base, usually as metastatic lesions to the orbit in infants, but occasionally occur as a primary tumor at any age of childhood. These tumors arise from autonomic neurons or neuronal precursors. Neurofibromas and schwannomas usually arise from the branches of the fifth nerve. They may also be plexiform, involving the orbit, face, or deep tissues of the skull base. These can occur in patients with neurofibromatosis or as isolated tumors. Gliomas of the optic nerve within the orbit occur as sporadic tumors but are often associated with neurofibromatosis type 1. Primary melanoma can occur from mucosal and sinus tissues, and metastatic lesions from the eye can seed to the skull base. Primitive neuroectodermal tumors (PNETs), whose cell of origin is uncertain, can occur in the skull base as either primary or metastatic lesions. Meningiomas that occur in this area are usually from the optic foramen or arise in the olfactory groove or planum sphenoidale. Occasionally, meningiomas unattached to the dura are reported. Large pituitary tumors, usually prolactin-secreting, can invade the skull base and destroy the upper clivus and medial aspect of the middle fossa. Very rarely, ectopically located pituitary tumors or craniopharyngiomas may occur in the sphenoid sinus or pharynx.

The midline portion of the skull base is formed from cartilage, which can give rise to chondromas and chondrosarcomas. The latter may be intradural or extradural in origin, with the pathology of the intracranial lesions usually showing mesenchymal chondrosarcoma. The common tumors that arise from bone are fibrous dysplasia, osteoma, osteoblastoma, osteosarcoma (often secondary to previous radiation therapy), giant cell tumors, and aneurysmal bone cysts. Primary Ewing's sarcoma can occur, but more commonly the disease is metastatic. The facial bones and skull are sites for both local and generalized histiocytosis X. Primary rhabdomyosarcoma can arise from any of the muscles attached to the skull base or orbit or in the middle ear. The most common location for skull base rhabdomyosarcoma in children is in the orbit.

TABLE 101-1

Skull Base Tumors in Children

Type of Lesion	Tumor
Developmental	Teratoma
	Choriostoma
	Epidermoid
	Dermoid
	Nasal Glioma
	Lipoma
Neoplastic	
Neural	Optic glioma
	Neuroblastoma
	Olfactory neuroblastoma
	Schwannoma
Mesenchymal	Meningioma
	Neurofibroma
	Fibromatosis
	Angiofibroma
	Myxoma
	Rhabdomyosarcoma
	Ewing's sarcoma
	Nonrhabdoid sarcoma
Osteocartilaginous	Osteoma
	Ossifying fibroma
	Osteoblastoma
	Osteosarcoma
	Fibrous dysplasia
	Giant cell tumor
	Aneurysmal bone cyst
	Chondroma
	Chondrosarcoma
Notochordal	Chordoma
Vascular	Glomus tumors
	Hemangioma
	Hemangiopericytoma
Epithelial	Carcinoma

There are a variety of other mesenchymal tissues within the sinuses and skull base that give rise to tumors. All of these tumors are rare, but the more common are myxomas, angiofibromas, myofibromatosis, fibromatosis, malignant fibrous histiocytomas (which may occur after irradiation), nonrhabdoid sarcomas, and very rarely, childhood carcinomas. Besides Ewing's sarcoma, rhabdomyosarcoma, and osteosarcoma, a variety of sarcomatous lesions are reported in children and teenagers; these include myofibrosarcoma, myxosarcoma, fibromyxoid sarcoma, synovial sarcoma, and epithelioid sarcoma. The notochord precedes the development of the clivus. Thus tumors that arise from notochordal remnants, chordomas, can arise in the clivus centrally and off the midline in the petrous apex, temporal bone, and cavernous sinus region. These lateral tumors are believed to result from branching of the notochord. Chordomas also occur in the upper cervical spine and foramen magnum region. Although rare, paragangliomas arising from the sympathetic and parasympathetic neurons or vascular glomus tissue occur. The vagus nerve is more often the site of origin in children. Some of these tumors may produce vasoactive compounds and cause systemic hypertension. Other vascular tumors include hemangioma and hemangiopericytoma. Lymphomas and leukemias are occasionally seen as primary lesions of the skull base occurring in the orbit, the sphenoid bone, or the clivus. Plasmocytomas and pseudotumor are rarely reported in children. Other mass lesions that enter the differential diagnosis are encephaloceles, mucoceles, and cholesterol cysts, the latter occurring in the petrous apex.

Age has a strong association with the likely pathologic diagnosis. In the infant, teratomas and hamartomas are the most common lesions, followed by nasal gliomas and dermoid cysts and tract. Neurofibromas are occasionally seen in infants; the most common sarcoma is rhabdomyosarcoma. The metastatic lesion that is most common is orbital neuroblastoma, which is often bilateral. The primary melanomas of the retina can metastasize to the skull base. Also, in the first year of life, Langerhans histiocytosis can affect the skull base, rather than the vault, and is usually misdiagnosed on imaging studies as rhabdomyosarcoma. The major differential of a mass at this age is encephalocele. In the toddler and young child, chordomas arise and can be seen through the rest of childhood. Sinus tumors such as the rare myxoma can occur at this age, as can neurofibromas. Metastatic tumors are most commonly Ewing's sarcoma or neuroblastoma. Some of the rare sarcomas begin to occur in the child older than 10 years of age; angiofibromas, chordomas, giant cell tumors of bone, aneurysmal bone cysts, and fibrous dysplasia are the most common tumors. Angiofibromas occur almost exclusively in males. Secondary tumors are usually seen after primary radiation treatment in infancy for a malignant tumor. Osteogenic sarcoma is reported after treatment of retinoblastoma and malignant fibrous histiocytoma after radiation therapy for rhabdomyosarcoma.

DIAGNOSIS

The most common symptom onset of skull base tumors in children is an abnormality of the visual system such as diplopia, visual loss, or proptosis. The reason is that the majority of true skull base lesions in children occur centrally in the anterior skull base and clivus. The structures at most risk are the globe of the eye producing proptosis; the optic nerves producing visual loss; and the cranial nerves that exit from the clivus close to the midline and run through the cavernous sinus (III, IV, VI), producing diplopia or amblyopia. Headaches do occur but are not the most common complaint. Swallowing difficulties and focal neurologic deficits, such as extremity weakness or ataxia, can occur as a result of mass effect and distortion of the medulla or brainstem. Other common symptoms are stuffy nose, nosebleeds, repeated ear infections, and loss of hearing as a result of eustachian tube obstruction. Visible mass lesions on the face, forehead, or nose are apparent in a number of the tumors. In others, the mass is visible only on inspection of the nasal passages or the oropharynx. Primary pituitary dysfunction is rare. Once again, the age of the child and the type of the lesion dictate the signs and symptoms.

In the newborn child with a large teratoma or hamartoma, respiratory difficulties predominate, because these lesions typically involve the paramidline structures of the tongue, retropharynx, and neck. Emergency tracheostomy is often performed in the first or second day of life to alleviate airway obstruction. The teratomas or hamartomas that occur in this region have an unusual propensity to grow very rapidly in the first few days of life and thus are often misdiagnosed as malignant lesions. They are visible as mass lesions in the posterior pharynx or neck. Although usually benign, atypical and malignant teratomas do occur. Bilateral orbital swelling is usually due to neuroblastoma, with vision becoming affected from mass effect in the orbit. Nasal gliomas can cause nasal obstruction and respiratory distress. They may be totally intranasal or can appear as a mass at the base of the nose. Dermoids and epidermoids may be difficult to distinguish from nasal gliomas. In those with a sinus tract, the skin opening is usually distal to the inferior margin of the nasal bone and drains desquamated epithelium.

In toddlers and children younger than age 10, the most common sign is an extraocular nerve palsy that results from compression of cranial nerves III, IV, or VI at the superior orbital fissure, in the cavernous sinus, or more posteriorly at the petrous apex. Headache, visual loss, and ear infections are common, followed by swallowing problems or long-tract signs from compression of the midbrain, pons, or medulla by tumor mass. In older children and teenagers, visual disturbance, headache, stuffy nose, and epistaxis predominate. Systemic symptoms can occur from tumors that secrete biologically active compounds such as chemodectomas or pituitary lesions. The former may result in systemic hypertension, and in the latter the symptoms are usually of excess prolactin secretion. Occasionally Cushing's syndrome results from ectopic pituitary tissue in the sphenoid sinus. Easy fatigability, anemia, clotting problems, bruising, or repeated infections occur with leukemia or lymphoma.

INCIDENCE AND PREVALENCE

The frequency of skull base lesions in childhood is low. Tumors of the cranial base account for 8% of all pediatric brain tumors. The rarity of these diseases, even in a busy pediatric neurosurgical practice, means that no one group will gain a large experience. Therefore it is important that the experiences be shared to minimize complications and that data be pooled regarding best therapy. The age of symptom onset of skull base disease in children ranges across the whole of childhood (Table 101-2). The pathology of the lesions is different at each age.

Among infants (1 to 2 years of age), the most common primary malignant tumor is rhabdomyosarcoma. Metastatic neuroblastoma is relatively common and usually occurs with bilateral orbital swelling. Langerhans histiocytosis is also seen in the first year of life. Most of these lesions occur in the cranial vault, but they can occur in the middle fossa and invade the bone and pterygoid fossa. Langerhans histiocytosis also affects the facial bones at this age. Occasionally, a true malignant or immature teratoma is encountered. The origin of these lesions is unclear, because those that occur in the tongue do not have any intracranial component. Biopsy specimen, because it demonstrates cerebral tissue, is often read as encephalocele. The lesions do not exit from any of the usual areas where encephaloceles are found, and the rapid rate of growth does not fit with that diagnosis. Although extending intracranially, they

TABLE 101-2

Skull Base Tumors by Age of Presentation

Age Group	Tumor
Infants (less than 1 year old)	Teratoma
	Hamartoma
	Rhabdomyosarcoma
	Neuroblastoma
Children (1–9 years old)	Chordoma
	Rhabdomyosarcoma
	Nonrhabdoid sarcoma
Older Children (10 years old and older)	Angiofibroma
	Fibromatosis
	Giant cell tumor of bone
	Chordoma
	Nonrhabdoid sarcoma

rarely extend intradurally. If the lesion is recognized, complete one-step resection is possible, even in the infant. Excision of larger lesions that grow into the neck and around the carotid artery may be postponed until the end of the first year of life. Large solitary neurofibromas of the fifth cranial nerve can also be present at birth. They occur as a mass in the upper part of the anterior triangle of the neck. Diagnosis is usually made by biopsy. As with the teratomatous lesions, if the tumor is large, it is safer to do a tracheotomy and delay surgery for a few months until the baby has grown. Lymphoma and leukemia can also occur as skull base lesions in infants.

Among children (2 to 9 years of age), the common malignant tumors are rhabdomyosarcoma; nonrhabdoid sarcomas; esthesioneuroblastoma; chondrosarcoma; Ewing's sarcoma, usually metastatic but also primary; and neuroblastoma, usually metastatic. Aggressive fibromatosis and chordoma are the most common benign lesions. The nonrhabdoid sarcomas, chondrosarcoma, fibromatosis, and chordoma are best treated by primary resection if possible. The outcome is best with total surgical resection. This is also true for esthesioneuroblastoma and Ewing's sarcoma, but these lesions usually require chemotherapy and radiation therapy. Esthesioneuroblastoma may be shrunk using chemotherapy before radical resection. Rhabdomyosarcomas should also be completely resected if possible, but because of the good response to radiation therapy and chemotherapy, the first surgery is usually gross debulking. If there is residual mass after irradiation and chemotherapy, a second surgery to resect residual tumor is done. Secondary tumors following radiation therapy for retinoblastoma can occur at this age. The most common pathology is osteogenic sarcoma.

Among children ages 10 to 16 years, the most common malignant lesion is still rhabdomyosarcoma, but at this age a variety of nonrhabdoid sarcomas are seen, with pathology ranging from myxosarcoma to fibrosarcoma and malignant fibrous histiocytoma. These lesions arise in the maxillary ethmoid or sphenoid sinuses and invade the skull base. Metastases from these lesions are rare, and the problem is usually one of local recurrence. Ewing's sarcoma and esthesioneuroblastoma occur and are treated by surgery plus irradiation and chemotherapy. Nasal carcinoma, adenocystic carcinoma, and mucoepithelial carcinoma are also seen.

NEURO-ONCOLOGY IMAGING

The primary diagnostic study is either computed tomography (CT) or magnetic resonance imaging (MRI). Although many of these lesions can be identified by plain skull x-rays, these do not supply sufficient information to guide surgical intervention. In many of the skull base tumors, both CT and MRI performed without and with contrast are necessary to delineate bone and soft tissue involvement by the tumor. For most tumors, MRI best delineates the extent of tumor infiltration into areas such as the carotid canal of the petrous bones and the extradural space around the upper cervical cord. However, the extent of bone destruction of the clivus or facial region cannot be assessed by MRI, because bone structures are poorly seen with MRI. A CT scan is required to allow the surgeon to envisage the true state of the bones of the face, the clivus, the occipital condyles, and the upper cervical vertebrae.

Knowing the anatomy of the residual facial bones is necessary during tumor resection and in preparing for reconstruction. Maintaining accurate, three-dimensional orientation while drilling the clivus, arch of C1, and the dens can be very difficult and lead to inadequate exposure if the surgeon expects either absent or very involved bone but finds apparently solid bone in the operative field; having both CT and MRI scans minimizes this problem. The upper cervical spine needs to be imaged in children with chordomas, chondrosarcomas, or other lesions that involve the foramen magnum. The whole spine may need to be imaged in those cases in which a malignant lesion is in immediate proximity to the cerebrospinal fluid (CSF) spaces. The finding of diffuse intradural disease will have an impact on the appropriateness of extensive surgery. Magnetic resonance (MR) angiography and MR venography studies can be helpful to define the involvement of the carotid arteries, the vertebral and basilar arteries, the cavernous sinus, and jugular bulbs and veins. Some idea of the vascularity of the tumor can be obtained from MRI, especially if large flow voids are seen within the tumor.

Angiography, either conventional or CT angiography, may be used to identify the anatomy of the vascular supply and the vascularity of the tumor. Angiography is usually necessary in patients with angiofibromas, giant cell tumors of bone, and certain metastatic lesions. The location and distortion or compression of the carotid arteries can be seen on MR angiography. If flow is low, MR angiography may be inadequate to define whether the carotid artery is patent. In these cases, angiography is needed to ascertain the status of the vessel.

Because of the nature of skull base lesions in children, it is unusual to require balloon occlusion testing of the cerebral circulation unless there is a potential need to sacrifice one carotid. Because most of the lesions are extradural in origin and rarely invasive, the carotid artery is not at risk for invasion by the tumor. Even in those tumors that enter the region of the cavernous sinus, the tumor is usually extradural and not intradural and can be removed without damage to the arteries.

The carotid vessels are in proximity to the surgical field, but in cases other than malignant tumors they are rarely directly involved by the tumor, despite marked distortion of the vessels by the tumor mass. If the tumor is highly vascular, preoperative embolization may be of value in limiting blood loss. This has been used for large angiofibromas, giant cell tumors of bone, chemodectomas, and metastatic melanoma. Embolization depends on the distribution of the feeding vessels. If these are from the external carotid artery, extensive and safe embolization is possible and helpful. It is the most superior portion of the tumor that is likely to be fed by the internal carotid and the least able to be embolized.

Ultrasonography can supply diagnostic information for lesions within the orbit. It is rarely the only imaging study required for lesions that have expanded to involve the skull base, because it supplies inadequate information about the surrounding structures. Other imaging studies are rarely useful. Myelography and cisternography can be helpful in the postoperative planning of the radiation portals around residual tumor but is rarely of value preoperatively. Cerebral blood flow studies are rarely indicated unless there is a plan to resect one carotid artery. The use of venous catheterization to sample blood from the tumor to aid in the diagnosis can be helpful in the rare secreting chemodectomas and in locating ectopic pituitary lesions. Infusion of chemotherapy directly to the tumor in an effort to shrink the lesion has not been reported in skull base tumors. As the choice of drugs is increased, this may become a viable option to produce a preliminary decrease in tumor bulk before resection in the chemotherapy-responsive tumors, as is currently done with rhabdomyosarcoma and esthesioneuroblastoma.

THERAPY

Most malignant tumors in children are not treated by skull base resections, because such lesions are often sensitive to chemotherapy, radiation therapy, or both. Indeed, the most frequently encountered lesions are rarely treated by the pediatric neurosurgeon. These are retinoblastoma, which is usually limited to the retina, neuroblastoma, rhabdomyosarcoma, and Ewing's sarcoma. Diagnosis of tumor type is necessary and can often be performed with blood and urine samples, as in the case of neuroblastoma. The other tumors require diagnostic biopsy, which may be transnasal or by percutaneous image-guided needle biopsy.

In the case of rhabdomyosarcoma, resection is performed at the time of biopsy. The extent of the resection depends on the involvement of surrounding structures. If there is local residual tumor after combined therapy, a more extensive second resection may be indicated. Isolated recurrent rhabdomyosarcoma is a candidate for repeat surgical resection. Parameningeal rhabdomyosarcomas have a high incidence of intracranial subarachnoid seeding, and thus imaging of the whole craniospinal axis and sampling of the CSF for cytology are necessary before there is any consideration of an extensive operative resection. The results of treatment of these lesions with combined therapy, surgery, irradiation, and chemotherapy has markedly improved the outcome in these tumors. The complications of these combined therapies can be severe, but the incidence of untreatable complications is less than 5%.

Primary Ewing's sarcoma is treated by resection, followed by chemotherapy, irradiation, or both, regardless of the completeness of resection. Surgery alone is the primary therapy for benign lesions and some of the low-grade malignant lesions. There are many possible surgical approaches to the skull base region. Before selecting an approach, a complete diagnostic evaluation of the tumor and its relationship to surrounding structures is required. Consideration of the age of the child is important when formulating a differential diagnosis. The majority of skull base lesions in children arise from the extradural space and usually do not penetrate the dura. The dura in children is elastic and growing; thus epidural tumors can expand the dura so that portions of tumor that may look intradural on the imaging studies are still epidural.

The first surgical approach should almost always be extradural, even when portions of the tumor appear to be intradural and even intraparenchymal. If there is indeed intradural tumor that cannot be removed at the initial surgery, a second surgical approach can be planned, but at least an extradural tumor has not been inadvertently made intradural by the surgeon. This mistake could result in the conversion of a curable tumor to an incurable one. Malignant lesions, both primary and metastatic, are not usually treated by radical surgery but by chemotherapy plus radiation therapy. Neuroblastoma, rhabdomyosarcoma, and Ewing's sarcoma are the most common lesions, and 5-year disease-free survival rates are as high as 80%, depending on the stage of the tumor at initial diagnosis. Patients with skull base extension or distant metastases do worse than those with localized disease. Surgery has a role in the treatment of recurrent tumors in this area.

Secondary malignant tumors that arise after therapy for retinoblastoma and rhabdomyosarcoma, usually osteogenic sarcoma and malignant fibrous histiocytoma, respectively, are treated by surgical resection to remove the entire tumor, if possible. Chemotherapy as an adjunct is used for both types of lesions, but in the absence of total surgical removal, the value of adjuvant therapy is unclear. For adjuvant therapy of malignant fibrous histiocytoma or other radiation-induced tumors, local irradiation by brachytherapy has a role dependent on the location and geometry of the lesion. Gamma Knife® therapy can provide palliation to nonresectable or repeatedly recurrent areas of tumor, and despite being the result of previous radiation therapy, radiation-induced tumors do respond to further radiation therapy. Although distant metastases may occur as late sequelae, the predominant problem is one of local control. Optic gliomas that do not involve the optic chiasm are treated by surgical resection if vision is very poor or absent. If vision is useful, chemotherapy or local radiation therapy may shrink the tumor, prevent further growth, and preserve vision.

Fibrous dysplasia is not treatable by chemotherapy or radiation therapy and thus surgical control is usually the only option. It is rare that the clival involvement causes any symptoms or signs, and surgery is usually indicated to prevent or to reverse optic nerve compression, proptosis, or craniofacial deformity. Resection of the total mass of fibrous dysplastic tissue is rarely possible and rarely necessary. Malignant change is rare, and involvement of cranial nerves other than II, III, IV, and VI is unusual. In very vascular areas of unresectable fibrous dysplasia, transarterial embolization to decrease flow in an effort to decrease pain may benefit some patients. Angiofibromas are treated by surgical resection, as are myxomas, myofibromatosis, fibromatosis, aneurysmal bone cysts, giant cell tumors of bone, and osteoblastomas. Preoperative embolization may be helpful to decrease intraoperative hemorrhage in angiofibromas, giant cell tumors, and aneurysmal bone cysts. Giant cell tumors may recur, presumably because complete

resection was not achieved. Skull base irradiation is then given, by means of proton beam therapy if possible or, if unavailable, by routine stereotactic irradiation. Esthesioneuroblastomas, if large, are pretreated with chemotherapy to reduce tumor bulk before resection. Resection is usually followed by radiation therapy and more chemotherapy.

Mesenchymal chondrosarcomas require postresection radiation and usually chemotherapy as well. Radiation therapy may have to include the whole spinal axis if the tumor is intradural. Melanoma, if local, is treated with radiation therapy after resection. There is also a role for chemotherapy and immunotherapy, although the best timing is not known. This additional therapy is usually reserved for recurrence or the appearance of distal metastases. Meningiomas, if they recur or cannot be totally resected, are treated either with Gamma Knife or routine radiation therapy. There is little long-term follow-up data on Gamma Knife therapy in children, and whether this form of radiation minimizes side effects and the appearance of secondary tumors has not been established.

Hemangiomas and hemangiopericytomas are treated with radiation therapy if complete resection cannot be achieved or if they recur. Chordomas and chondrosarcomas are rarely curable with surgery alone unless identified when small and localized. The best results of ancillary therapy are with proton beam therapy. The results seem to depend on delivery of high doses of radiation, with the best results occurring with doses of more than 7500 Gy. Because adjuvant therapy is needed for most children with these tumors, the case should be discussed preoperatively with the radiation therapist so that an appropriate plan for resection can be made. This team approach is important, because often the easiest part of the tumor to remove surgically is not the area that the radiation therapist needs resected to ensure that the maximal dose of radiation can be delivered. The need to obtain the best geometry of any residual tumor and a clear CSF space around the area to be irradiated are the minimal requirements that need to be accomplished by the surgeon. It is this cooperation between the radiation therapist and the surgical team that will probably determine the outcome for the child in many cases of chordoma. These tumors should not be operated upon without this type of consideration and planning.

Gamma Knife therapy has been and is being used for chordoma and chondrosarcoma, but the results are not as good as those for proton beam therapy. In addition, because of the geometry of the residual disease and the size of the area to be treated, Gamma Knife irradiation is not always applicable. Whether routine stereotactic irradiation will prove equally beneficial to proton beam therapy remains to be seen, but because of the Bragg peak effect with the proton beam, it is likely that this will remain the only way to give very high doses to tumor proximal to neural tissue without excessive dosage to the CNS tissue. Chemotherapy has not been shown to be of value for the treatment of chordoma or chondrosarcoma. Malignant chordomas have been reported, but even in this setting, chemotherapy seems to be of little value. Chordomas metastasize in 8% to 48% of cases, and neither CNS nor distant metastases are very responsive to chemotherapy. Chemodectomas are best treated by complete resection. However, the results of partial resection followed by irradiation are similar to that of radical surgery, with a 90% 10-year survival rate. Preoperative embolization can be a useful adjunct to decrease intraoperative blood loss. Neurofibromas are treated primarily by resection, but for extensive plexiform lesions and in patients with neurofibromatosis, chemotherapy may be of some value.

REHABILITATION

Outcome

Outcome depends on size, location, and pathologic type of the tumor. Because most of the lesions treated surgically are either of low-grade malignancy or are benign, the recurrence rates are low (26%). Surgical mortality and morbidity are also low in the hands of an appropriate team. Because long-term survival is common, the choice of surgical approach and the avoidance of new deficits is very important. This end is attained by having a clear plan of treatment before the initiation of any therapy.

Carcinomas are not common in children; the only one that is relatively commonly encountered is nasopharyngeal carcinoma. This is a rare occurrence in the United States, but in the Middle East and Southeast Asia, where nasopharyngeal carcinoma is more common, 8% to 15% of these tumors occur in children. The 5- and 10-year survival rates with irradiation alone or with irradiation and chemotherapy are 50%. The role of radical surgery in these children has not been explored. The other carcinoma seen in children in this area is the neuroendocrine carcinoma; this tumor is rarely reported in children younger than age 16 years. Treatment for olfactory neuroblastoma (esthesioneuroblastoma) depends on the stage of the tumor and the ability to attain a complete resection.

Radiation therapy may be given before surgery, after surgery, or not at all if complete resection is achieved. The 5-year survival rate is 50%, with better results in smaller lesions. The results of therapy of skull base sarcomatous lesions in children is good, with 5-year progression-free survival rates of 70% to 80% in patients with rhabdomyosarcoma, Ewing's sarcoma, and low-grade fibrosarcoma. The extensive rhabdomyosarcomas, those categorized in group III or IV, have a high recurrence rate and median survival of only 3.5 and 2 years, respectively. There may be a role for skull base resection in these lesions. Primary Ewing's sarcoma is rare but does occur and is best treated by surgical excision followed by radiation therapy. Low-grade sarcomas such as fibrosarcoma, myxosarcoma, myofibrosarcoma, and chondrosarcoma are usually treated by maximal local excision with or without radiation therapy, depending on whether surgical resection is complete and the age of the child and the actual lesion pathology. Many low-grade sarcomas seem to respond to proton beam therapy better than routinely delivered x-ray therapy, which is conceivably purely a dose-related phenomenon. With stereotactic delivery of radiation therapy, the results may improve to equal those of the proton beam therapy (20% to 30% of cases recur after proton beam therapy).

A high cure rate is expected for retinoblastoma and metastatic lesions such as neuroblastoma after enucleation in the former and chemotherapy, irradiation, or both in the latter. Thus radical surgery plays little role in the primary therapy of these tumors. The major problems that result from radiation therapy are poor facial growth and secondary tumors such as osteosarcoma and malignant fibrous histiocytoma. Lymphomas, plasmocytomas, and leukemias are treated by chemotherapy plus radiation therapy with 70% to 80% cure rates; the role of surgery is usually only to establish a tissue diagnosis. This is also true of pseudotumor of the sphenoid sinus. Large angiofibromas (stage IIIA and IIIB) have been operated on by a number of approaches, and in many units still are operated on by otorhinolaryngologists on their own using a degloving facial exposure. The recurrence rates in these large lesions are reported at 20% to 30% at 6 years. Although the numbers are small, we have had no recurrences in stage IIIB tumors, and an extended transcranial, subfrontal operation is more likely than a subcranial approach to achieve complete resection of that portion of the tumor that is intradural and in the posterior portion of the sphenoid sinus and cavernous sinus. With repeat surgery, most recurrent angiofibromas can be cured. By the time chordomas are diagnosed in children they are usually large, making total surgical resection impossible in many cases.

Surgical cure rates are hard to define because of the small numbers of reported cases. Progression-free 3-year survival rates of less than 10% are reported. Local radiation therapy or focused beam irradiation have been used, resulting in a 5-year survival rate of less than 50%. In contrast, recent results with proton beam irradiation in children show a disease-free survival rate of 68% at 5 years. Of the remaining living patients from our series treated with proton beam therapy, one has had a recurrence, which may be related to inadequate surgical decompression of the nervous tissue and thus limitation of radiation dosage. To improve the results, close cooperation is necessary between the radiation therapist and the surgical team. Complications include pituitary dysfunction, sinusitis, hearing loss, radiation necrosis, and possibly, second tumors.

Given that the outcome for chondrosarcoma, chordoma, and possibly giant cell tumors is better after proton beam therapy than after standard irradiation, it is conceivable that the use of proton beam therapy might also result in better survival rates for other low-grade sarcomas of the skull base. However, if confirmed, it would produce a dilemma, because few proton beam therapy machines are available worldwide and many patients simply do not have the resources to travel for such expensive therapy, even within the United States or Europe. For Third World countries with limited resources and health care budgets, it is important to establish how efficacious other, more available therapies are, such as standard x-ray therapy, when combined with modern surgical techniques. This is also an important issue in the United States, because health care costs are being strictly controlled. If surgical results are better in one location versus another, all of these rare tumors should be referred to these few centers. In light of the serious side effects of radiation in children, if a benefit cannot be shown, the answer is that these additional therapies should not be used. If proton beam therapy is superior, all children with responsive lesions should be directed to proton beam units for therapy. At present, even for patients in the United States, this is impossible given the few available centers. The only way to obtain useful data regarding the best therapy is to develop a registry and to require reporting of these rare tumors, their treatment, and the complications involved so that all outcomes can be available for critical study. Unfortunately, it seems unlikely that funding could be obtained for such a project.

Chemotherapy has rarely been reported for chordomas, but there is one report of limited local control with etoposide, ifosfamide, carboplatin, and mesna. Metastases from chordomas do occur in children but within the spinal subarachnoid space, at the surgical site and distally, with an incidence of 3% to 48%.

Although no long-term benefit has been reported, transient local control has been reported using chemotherapy. Chemotherapy has not yet established a firm base in the treatment of skull base lesions that are treated with primary surgery. Currently, chemotherapy is used for many nonrhabdosarcomas, primitive neuroepithelial tumors, Ewing's sarcomas, and olfactory neuroblastomas. Neurofibromas, other than the plexiform ones, rarely grow after near-total or total excision; this is also true for osteomas, aneurysmal bone cysts, and optic gliomas. Infants with hamartoma, teratoma, and immature teratoma have all been cured with surgical resection. Future growth can be normal if the tumor is resected before major deformity occurs. Once significant deformation of bone occurs, reconstructive surgery is often required.

CHAPTER 102

TUMORS OF THE SKULL

Tien T. Nguyen and J. Gordon McComb

The types of skull tumors most commonly encountered—epidermoid and dermoid cysts, eosinophilic granulomas, and fibrous dysplasia—are not neoplastic. True neoplastic tumors constitute only a small fraction of lesions that affect the skull. Benign neoplasms, such as osteomas and osteoblastomas, are usually seen in adults and account for merely 1% of all bone tumors. Primary malignant tumors occur even more rarely, with osteosarcoma being the most common, followed by chondrosarcoma, and then fibrosarcoma.

SIGNS AND SYMPTOMS

Patients commonly have a visible or palpable scalp mass, but some lesions are discovered on imaging studies obtained for another reason. Generally, asymptomatic tumors tend to be benign and nongrowing or slow growing. Pain or tenderness to palpation may be a symptom of benign but locally aggressive lesions (e.g., eosinophilic granuloma, osteoid osteoma, and aneurysmal bone cyst) or malignant tumors as a response to significant local tissue reaction. If the mass is located at the skull base and involves one or more foraminae, cranial nerve deficits can occur.

DIAGNOSTIC STUDIES

Evaluation of a patient with a skull mass starts with a physical examination followed by imaging studies. Plain skull x-ray studies are still useful, because they allow the assessment of the general radiologic features, size, and location of the tumor, and the presence of additional lesions. However, computed tomography (CT) is the method of choice for studying the cortical bone detail, pattern of destruction, and matrix mineralization and is better in delineating lesions located in complicated areas such as the orbit and skull base. Magnetic resonance imaging (MRI) is complementary to CT and valuable for defining extracortical growth and the relationship of the tumor to neurovascular structures. Scintigraphy of the skeleton is useful for assessing polyostotic involvement, as can be seen with malignant tumors, fibrous dysplasia, and eosinophilic granuloma. This technique is relatively nonspecific but may help in the diagnosis of osteoid osteoma if the "double density" sign is present.

Images of the mass can show evidence of osteoblastic, osteolytic, or mixed activity. The features of the bone margins and the involved diploe of a lytic lesion are important to note.

Sclerotic reactive bone at the margins is usually present in tumors that are slow growing. Rapidly growing lesions do not allow time for the surrounding bone to reform and thus have minimal or no sclerosis at the margins. Tumors that expand the diploe or erode the inner and outer tables of the skull disproportionately are often benign. The pattern of mineralization within the lesion matrix is also helpful in differentiating between benign bone- and cartilage-producing tumors. Malignancy is suspected if the lesions are multiple, have irregular margins, and equally destroy both tables of the skull.

TREATMENT

Treatment is usually excisional biopsy. Reconstruction of the skull is often necessary following a large resection. Surgery is also indicated for neural decompression and correction of cosmetic deformities. Certain locally aggressive tumors and malignant lesions are treated adjuvantly with irradiation or chemotherapy.

NON-NEOPLASTIC SKULL TUMORS

Epidermoid and Dermoid

Epidermoid and dermoid cysts are the most common tumors, accounting for up to 60% of the calvarial masses in the pediatric population.[52,72] The lesions result when cutaneous ectodermal rests are included in the developing cranium. They grow within the diploe and expand and erode the outer and inner tables of the skull. Both epidermoid and dermoid cysts are lined by stratified squamous epithelium and contain keratin from desquamation. Because a dermoid also has skin appendages, its cyst may contain hair and sebum as well. Because the primitive ectoderm has the capacity to form all the epidermal and dermal elements, these cysts embryologically can all be dermoids. Some reports, especially in the older literature, do not differentiate between epidermoid and dermoid cysts. Also, the tissue sent for histopathologic examination may not reflect the lesion in its entirety, or the dermal elements may have been destroyed by inflammation.

Intradiploic epidermoids and dermoids are similar clinically and radiologically. They both typically occur as a painless mass. A plain radiograph shows a rounded osteolytic lesion with well-defined, sclerotic margins (Figure 102-1A). The hypodense mass can be seen on CT scans eroding the inner

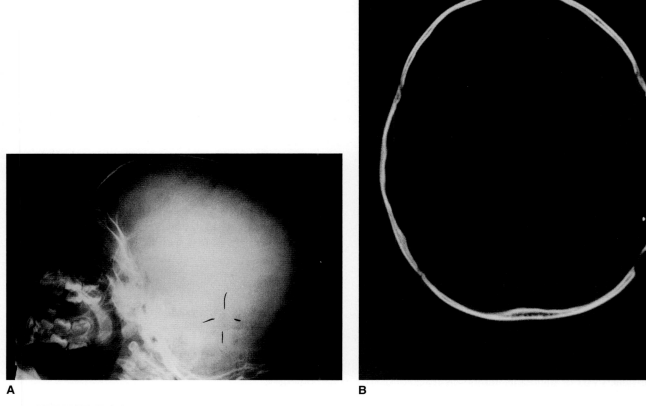

A   **B**

FIGURE 102-1 Dermoid cyst. This 17-month-old girl presented with a left parietal, enlarging, nontender mass. *A,* The lateral skull x-ray film shows a round osteolytic lesion with a sclerotic margin. *B,* The computed tomography scan reveals more erosion of the outer table of the skull than the inner table, resulting in a beveled margin.

skull table more than the outer table and sometimes expanding both (Figure 102-1*B*).[4] Capsular calcification or enhancement occurs in rare instances.

The majority of dermoid cysts are located off the midline in the supraorbital region and along cranial sutures, but some cysts may arise in the midline, commonly at the anterior fontanel and occipital region (Figure 102-2).[52,64] Dermoid cysts of the skull can also be seen in association with congenital dermal sinus (CDS).[15] The CDS is a tract lined by stratified squamous epithelium. The tract is found in the midline in the region of the nasion or in the occipital area, with none entering the skull in the region occupied by the superior sagittal sinus.[17,72] The tract may end just below the skin surface or extend intracranially through the foramen cecum to the crista galli from the nasion. The CDS can be associated with one or more inclusion cysts that vary in size from barely more than the diameter of the tract to a large tumor and can occur at any point along the tract; it has a preference, however, for the terminus. Because the abnormal connection between the dermal-ectoderm and neural-ectoderm that forms the CDS is small during early embryologic development, the disturbance in the

mesoderm condensing around the tract is minimal. As a result, the distortion of the adjacent skull is insignificant, and detection of a bone defect with imaging studies can often be difficult. Also, the opening of the CDS on the skin surface may be so small as to escape detection, except with close inspection. Surrounding angiomatous changes may sometimes be present with these lesions, particularly in the occipital location. Hair may be seen to protrude from the orifice. Debris or purulent material may drain from the site. The depth to which the CDS penetrates and whether it is associated with one or more dermoid cysts will determine the clinical manifestation. A CDS often goes unnoticed until the patient has infection, most commonly subcutaneous; however, one can also see extradural or intradural abscesses and meningitis. Often, it is helpful to get both CT and MRI scans for evaluation of a CDS. The diagnosis of a CDS, however, is clinical, and imaging studies are only augmentative. A negative imaging study does not exclude the need to explore the tract to its end; however, such studies can be helpful in ascertaining if the CDS is associated with one or more dermoid cysts. Complete surgical excision of the mass with the capsule results in cure.

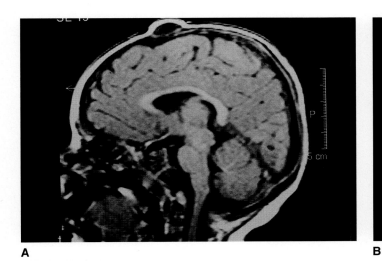

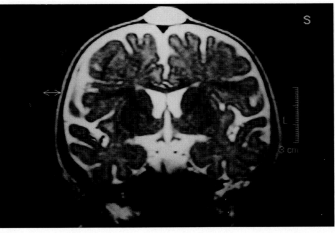

A B

FIGURE 102-2 Dermoid cyst. *A*, T1-weighted and *B*, T2-weighted magnetic resonance images of an 8-month-old girl with an anterior fontanel mass progressively increasing in size. Magnetic resonance imaging findings vary depending on the content of the cyst.

Eosinophilic Granuloma

Histiocytosis X can affect any organ of the body, but especially the calvarium.[79] Even though the etiology is unknown, the presence of non-neoplastic Langerhans histiocytes, eosinophils, and large multinucleated giant cells within the granulomas may reflect defective immunoregulation. Histiocytosis X is categorized in three forms, depending on the extent of systemic disease. Eosinophilic granuloma is the mildest and most common form (60% to 80%) and is usually a benign solitary lesion, although multiple skull lesions can occur. Patients with Hand-Schüller-Christian disease have a triad of granulomatous lesion of the skull, exophthalmos, and diabetes insipidus, but these are rarely observed all together in the same patient. Letterer-Siwe disease is a fulminant, malignant process during infancy with widespread lytic bone and visceral involvement and a high mortality rate. Isolated eosinophilic granuloma and Hand-Schüller-Christian disease often affect older children, usually 5 to 10 years of age, and have an excellent prognosis with treatment.[79]

Eosinophilic granulomas of the calvarium affect more males than females and are often located in the parietal and frontal regions.[52,63,79] Patients often have a painful skull mass with a history of recent growth. The classic finding on plain radiographs is a sharply demarcated, punched-out lesion without sclerotic margination (Figure 102-3*A*). The lesion may have a beveled edge, because destruction of the outer table is usually more extensive than of the inner table. A calcified sequestration is rarely present in the center of the lesion, resulting in a "target" appearance, which was once considered diagnostic but may be seen in other conditions.[30] A nuclear bone scan may show a focus of increased tracer uptake, but false-negatives are known to occur in a third of cases.[3,80]

Diagnosis is often obtained at the time of excisional biopsy (Figure 102-3*B*). Once the diagnosis is confirmed, further evaluation is necessary because of possible multiple bone and organ involvement and entails examination of the skin, a chest x-ray, skeletal survey, complete blood count, and liver function studies.[41] Single lesions are treated by excision and curettage, but in up to a third of cases new lesions can develop within

several years.[69] Younger patients have a higher risk of recurrence than adults; accordingly, continued follow-up is necessary. Multiple lesions can be treated with low-dose radiation therapy (300 to 1000 rads) or chemotherapy.[56] A course of repeated intralesion injection of steroid has resulted in long-term control of tumors that irradiation and chemotherapy have failed to control.[39]

Fibrous Dysplasia

Fibrous dysplasia represents 2% to 5% of all bone tumors and often affects the skull and facial bones, with a predilection for the sphenoid, frontal, and maxilla bones.[47] It is a benign disease that is characterized by progressive replacement of normal bone by fibrous connective tissue. On histologic examination, the tissue is composed of loose fibrous connective tissue intermixed with trabeculae of woven bone. The onset of fibrous dysplasia is often during childhood. It becomes most active during the period of the child's rapid bone growth, and its progression customarily ceases after puberty. Continued growth into adulthood does occur and is more often observed in females than males.[20] The monostotic form of fibrous dysplasia is clinically relatively silent and is usually detected incidentally in early adulthood. Polyostotic fibrous dysplasia, compared with the monostotic type, is diagnosed at a younger age, most likely because of the more widespread bone disease and its rapid progression. The polyostotic form is susceptible to spontaneous malignant transformation into sarcomas, which occurs in fewer than 1% of all cases.[21,73] The association of the polyostotic form with café-au-lait spots and endocrine dysfunction is known as McCune-Albright syndrome. Most patients with this syndrome are female and experience precocious puberty.

Painless localized enlargement of the skull on one side is the most common difference noted initially by patients with fibrous dysplasia. Involvement of the skull base can cause symptoms of neurovascular compression. The appearance of the mass on CT scan is variable and has been classified as sclerotic (homogeneously dense), cystic (radiolucent surrounded

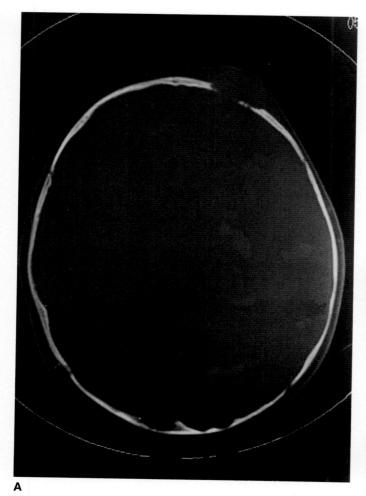

A

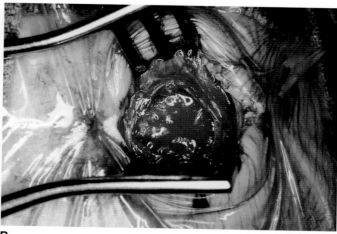

B

FIGURE 102-3 Eosinophilic granuloma. *A,* Computed tomography scans of a 6-month-old girl with multiple enlarging skull lesions tender to palpation. Destruction of the outer skull table is greater than that of the inner table. *B,* The appearance of an eosinophilic granuloma in a 4-month-old boy during surgery. The tumor was excised and the bone edges curettaged.

by a dense rim), or pagetoid (radiodense and radiolucent areas, with typical ground-glass appearance) (Figure 102-4).

Complete resection of the growth followed by craniofacial reconstruction is the treatment of choice (Figure 102-5). The goals of surgical treatment are to correct the deformation, stop further impairment of function, and prevent malignant degeneration. Prophylactic decompression of the optic nerve is unnecessary for optic canal stenosis without visual compromise.[43] Most instances of visual loss result from pressure by cysts or mucoceles associated with fibrous dysplasia and not from the isolated narrowing of the optic canal.[59,65] Because the procedure itself carries a high risk of causing blindness, it should be undertaken only when there is documented evidence of progressive visual loss. In general, lesions not amenable to complete resection should be observed. Radiation therapy is found to cause an increase in the rate of malignancy and is contraindicated.[50]

Ossifying Fibroma

Ossifying fibromas are benign, slow-growing tumors of the skull discovered often incidentally on radiographs but occasionally because of symptoms caused by their rapid enlargement. They may be a rare form of fibrous dysplasia having a similar distribution. The differences between the two can be seen histologically by the presence of calcified psammomatoid bodies and a prominent rim of osteoblasts outlining the lamellar trabeculae of woven bone in an ossifying fibroma, features that are absent in fibrous dysplasia.[78,87] An ossifying fibroma appears as a homogeneous, dense mass on x-ray studies, analogous to fibrous dysplasia, but its borders are more discrete (Figure 102-6).[25] Treatment is by total excision of the area of abnormality.

Aneurysmal Bone Cyst

Aneurysmal bone cysts are non-neoplastic expansile tumors of the diploic space affecting mostly long bones, but they arise in the skull in 2% to 6% of cases.[55,76] Two thirds of these cysts originate in the maxilla or mandible, and those involving the calvarial vault often occur in the occipital and temporal bones.[76] Most of the lesions occur by the end of the second decade of life as a rapidly enlarging mass.[2,76] Symptoms of intracranial hypertension and cranial nerve deficit are not unusual, and pain

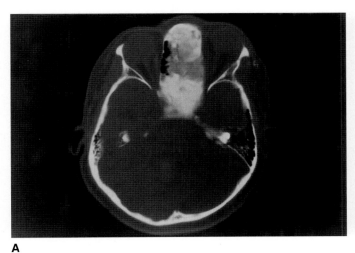

A

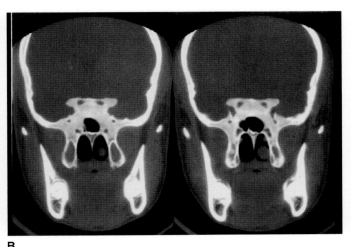

B

FIGURE 102-4 Fibrous dysplasia. *A,* Axial and *B,* coronal computed tomography scans of a 15-year-old boy obtained after an episode of difficulty with mental concentration. The appearance of this lesion is atypical of fibrous dysplasia because it is symmetric. The sphenoid bone is thickened with a ground-glass appearance. Even though the optic canals are narrow, ophthalmologic examination showed no abnormalities. The child was followed regularly without change in his examination results to date.

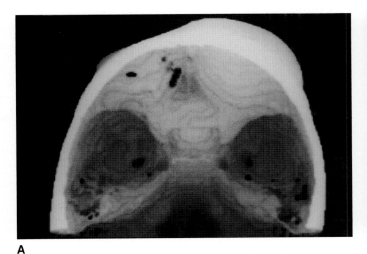

A

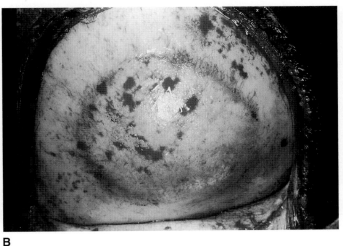

B

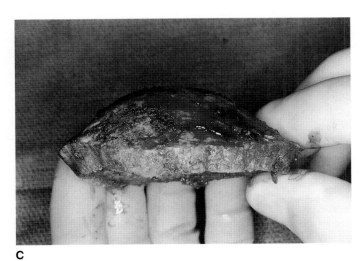

C

FIGURE 102-5 Fibrous dysplasia. *A,* Three-dimensional computed tomography reconstruction of a child with a disfiguring left frontal mass. *B,* The appearance of the lesion upon reflecting the scalp. *C,* The thickened calvarium was excised and the skull was reconstructed using hydroxyapatite and titanium bars and mesh.

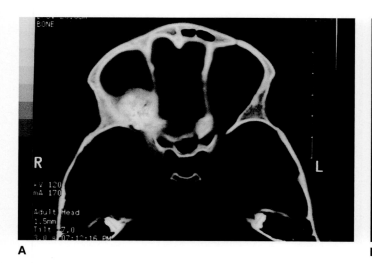
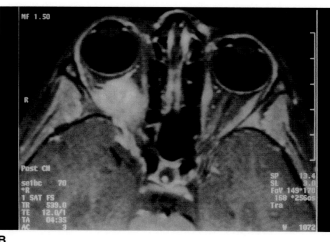

FIGURE 102-6 Ossifying fibroma. *A,* An axial computed tomography scan of a 9-year-old girl with painless proptosis shows a dense lesion involving the walls of the orbit. *B,* A postcontrast T1-weighted magnetic resonance image shows the mass is localized with relatively sharp margins.

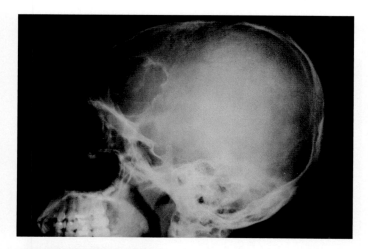

FIGURE 102-7 Aneurysmal bone cyst. A lateral skull x-ray study of a left-frontal, enlarging, and tender mass in a 12-year-old girl shows an expansile lesion with loculation and sclerotic margins. At the time of surgery, old blood was found within the cysts.

may be a factor. The blood-filled cysts have walls composed of trabecular bone lined by connective tissue and giant cells. A skull x-ray study and CT scan will show the multiloculated expansile bone lesions with characteristic fluid levels (Figure 102-7).

Treatment is surgical, with the goal of complete resection. Aneurysmal bone cysts are highly vascular, and preoperative angiography for possible embolization is recommended. Residual abnormal bone and recurrence is best treated with repeat excision. Radiation therapy is usually reserved for lesions not amenable to surgical removal.[49] Endovascular injection of sclerosing agents has shown promise as a primary treatment.[14,38] Approximately 30% of cranial aneurysmal bone cysts are associated with another primary osseous disease, such as giant cell tumors, chondroblastomas, and osteoblastomas.[51]

BENIGN NEOPLASMS

Osteoma

Osteomas are benign bone tumors with a predilection for membranous bones and are the most common primary bone neoplasms of the calvarium.[81] They arise from mesenchymal matrix within mature cortical bone and with growth protrude outward, forming a hemispheric mass of compact bone. The new bone is macroscopically indistinguishable from the adjacent outer skull table (Figure 102-8). However, under the microscope, proliferating osteoblasts are seen around the periphery where the lesion is "immature."

Patients with osteomas are typically 25 to 50 years of age, rarely children.[32] They typically have a slow-growing, firm, and nontender mass arising from the skull. Painful sinusitis can occur when osteomas obstruct drainage from the paranasal sinuses. A plain radiograph will reveal localized, protuberant, dense cortical bone with smooth contours. The lesion is almost always homogeneously hyperdense on CT, but on rare occasions is lytic.[58] During the tumor's active growth phase, it will have an intense focal increased uptake of isotope on scintigraphy. A patient with multiple cranial osteomas may have Gardner's syndrome and require evaluation for colonic polyposis and other soft tissue tumors (see Figure 102-8).[86]

Some surgeons advocate complete resection of symptomatic osteomas. However, because of the low risk of recurrence, simply reducing the mass with a high-speed drill to achieve a normal contour may be adequate treatment. Asymptomatic lesions should just be observed.[33]

Hemangioma

Hemangiomas are benign, slow-growing neoplasms of vascular origin, arising mostly in the vertebral bodies. Calvarial hemangiomas are relatively rare, accounting for a fraction of 1% of all bone neoplasms and 10% of benign primary neoplasms of the skull.[10,66] They occur more often in females than males and usually in older children and adults. Patients can be

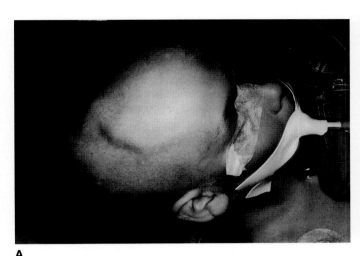

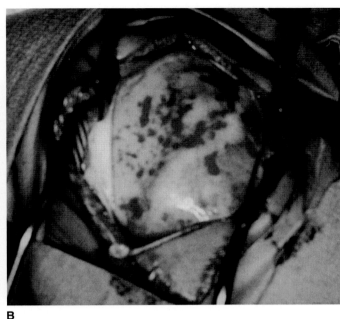

A   B

FIGURE 102-8 Osteoma. *A*, This child with Gardner's syndrome had firm and nontender frontal skull masses. *B*, Appearance of the protuberant tumors at the time of surgery. The masses were rendered flat with a high-speed drill.

asymptomatic or have a hard scalp mass that, in certain cases, is painful. The lesions are commonly located in the frontoparietal region and are unifocal in the majority of cases.

Calvarial hemangiomas are intradiploic lesions with scalloping and even expansion of the inner and outer skull tables. Lesions of the skull are usually cavernous, as opposed to capillary, and are composed of numerous large sinusoidal vessels interspersed among bone trabecula.[35] The radiating spicules of bone produce, on plain x-ray studies, a honeycomb or sunburst pattern within a round or ovoid area of lucency.[8] The radiographic features are nearly pathognomonic. A CT or MRI scan may reveal an intracranial extension exerting mass effect or as the cause of an epidural hematoma.[82] A hemangioma may appear hypervascular on an angiogram; however, a study revealing no abnormalities does not exclude its diagnosis.[46]

The majority of incidentally found hemangiomas have no significant sequelae and do not require any intervention. However, biopsy may be necessary if the clinical and radiographic diagnosis is uncertain. Surgical resection is reserved for symptomatic lesions and for cosmetic reasons. Excision or curettage is considered curative. Radiation therapy has been used for surgically inaccessible lesions with success.

Giant Cell Tumor

Giant cell tumors account for 4% to 5% of primary bone tumors, with a higher incidence in females and patients with Paget's disease.[48] Patients usually seek treatment between 20 and 40 years of age because of pain and swelling at the involved site. The mass is typically large by the time of its discovery. The tumor often affects the long bones and affects the skull in less than 1% of cases.[19] In the skull, the sphenoid and temporal bones are preferentially involved, possibly because they derive from endochondral ossification akin to long bones.[5,9,89]

The tumor appears grossly as a soft, brown mass with areas of hemorrhage. Under the microscope, characteristic osteoclast-like giant cells are seen dispersed among mononuclear stromal cells. Giant cell tumors are histologically benign but can behave aggressively, with a tendency for recurrence and metastasis, especially to the lungs.[9] Malignancy occurs in 5% to 10% of patients and can arise *de novo* or may be the result of radiation-induced transformation.[12,24,54] Radiographic features are analogous to those of an aggressive tumor, showing cortical expansion, osteolysis, and nonsclerotic margins. The local recurrence rate is 30% to 40%, even with wide surgical excision.[26] Use of adjuvant radiation therapy is controversial, because its efficacy has not been proved and it potentially increases the risk of malignant transformation.[19] Because the tumor is highly vascular, preoperative embolization to reduce bleeding during surgery should be considered.

Chordoma

Chordomas are tumors of the axial skeleton, arising from primitive notochord remnants, and constitute 2% to 4% of all primary bone tumors. Chordoma is a slow-growing tumor, with the onset of symptoms usually not until the third to sixth decades of life and rarely during childhood. The tumor typically originates in either the sacrum or clivus and is seldom found in the vertebrae between the two ends of the spinal axis. Whereas chordomas preferentially originate in the sacrum of adults, they occur most often in the clivus of young children.[29] Children thus have cranial nerve palsies and long-tract signs. Because of its deep location, infiltrative nature, and propensity for recurrence and metastasis, the management of clival chordomas is formidable.

Radiographic studies reveal a well-demarcated osteolytic mass with sclerotic bone reaction. The lesion can be seen infiltrating adjacent structures on MRI. The soft tissue component is hyperintense on T2-weighted images and hypointense on T1-weighted images and, when contrast is administered, has a lobulated, honeycomb appearance.[23] Microscopically, the tumor cells are physaliferous because they contain vacuoles of varying sizes in the cytoplasm. The prognosis depends on the extent of resection and age of the child at diagnosis. Chordomas in patients younger than 5 years tend to progress aggressively, have atypical histology, and metastasize.[11] The combined treatment with surgery and irradiation for skull base tumors results in 50% long-term survival for children and nearly 70% for adults.[18,88] Systemic chemotherapy with ifosfamide and doxorubicin and intrathecal or intraventricular injection of hydrocortisone, ARA-C, and methotrexate may benefit patients with a metastases.[75] Patients with a relapse have poor survival rates despite salvage operations.[27]

Osteoid Osteoma

Osteoid osteomas are benign osteoblastic neoplasms that can occur in people of any age. More males than females are affected by a 3:1 ratio. The tumor may occur in any bone but rarely occurs in the skull. It has a central nidus, composed of vascular osteoid tissue, surrounded by sclerotic bone. The nidus is usually no larger than 2 cm in diameter. This is seen on plain radiographs as a spot of radiolucency located in the center of an area of uniform sclerosis.[36] Radiotracer uptake is intense at the nidus and less by the sclerotic bone, producing a "double-density" sign on scintigraphy that is considered diagnostic.

Pain, present in the majority of cases, is characteristically dull, aching, more severe at night, and increases in intensity and duration with time. Nonsteroidal anti-inflammatory drugs (NSAIDs) relieve the pain attributed to the elevated levels of prostaglandin E_2 in the nidus.[31] Surgical extirpation of the nidus treats the neoplasia and the pain.

Osteoblastoma

Benign osteoblastomas are rare and account for only 1% of all bone tumors. A wide age range is affected but they occur relatively frequently in children and have a male predominance. Ten to twenty percent of all osteoblastomas occur in the skull.[57] The lesion consists of a vascularized stroma with immature osteoid tissue and proliferating osteoblasts and, in some instances, can be histologically indistinguishable from an osteoid osteoma. However, the clinical and radiologic differences between osteoblastoma and osteoid osteoma are definite. Osteoblastomas are usually nontender, but if pain is present it is not responsive to NSAIDs. Plain radiographs and CT scans of both lesions show an osteolytic lesion, but osteoblastomas typically measure greater than 2 cm. Also unlike osteoid osteomas, the radiolucent lesions of osteoblastomas have minimal reactive sclerosis and a variable-size central calcification, reflecting new bone formation.[16,53] A bone scan would demonstrate an intense focus of activity but without a double-density sign. Complete resection of the tumor is recommended because of possible recurrence and malignant transformation.[13,28]

Intraosseous Meningioma

Meningiomas of osseous origin are rare and are thought to arise from arachnoid cell rests.[77,84] Histologic examination shows islands of meningocytes surrounded by fibrosis. The tumor usually manifests symptoms during the fourth decade of life, rarely during childhood. Some cases of intraosseous meningioma may be linked to neurofibromatosis. The orbit is affected most often, resulting in proptosis.[60] Within the cranial vault, common locations are the middle ear, near suture lines, and a possibly previous fractures.[77] As for fibrous dysplasia, a CT scan shows an expansile growth of bone with hyperostosis and a ground-glass appearance. However, whereas the inner table of skull is smooth in fibrous dysplasia, the inner table of an intraosseous meningioma is irregular, especially at the site of origin.[34] Treatment is with complete resection.

Melanotic Neuroectodermal Tumor of Infancy

Melanotic neuroectodermal tumors are pigmented osteolytic neoplasms that primarily arise from the maxilla and mandible of infants within the first year of life. The skull can also be affected, with a predilection for the anterior fontanel.[85] Histologically, these tumors consist of large melanin-containing cells admixed with neuroblast-like cells.[37,40] The lesion is thought to derive from neural crest cells and can be associated with elevated levels of serum and urinary catecholamines.[6,37,85] The tumor is benign but is known to grow rapidly, and rare examples of malignant degeneration, brain invasion, and metastases have been reported.[67,68] It appears as an irregular, but well-circumscribed radiolucency on radiography. The recurrence rate can be as high as 60% after what appears to be complete surgical resection.[40,67]

Chondroma, Chondroblastoma, and Chondromyxoid Fibroma

Chondroma, chondroblastoma, and chondromyxoid fibroma are benign cartilaginous neoplasms occurring most commonly during young adulthood. Chondromas (or enchondromas) and chondromyxoid fibromas are thought to arise from ectopic hyaline cartilaginous rests, whereas chondroblastomas, even though they are histologically composed of neoplastic chondroblasts and chondroid matrix, are considered by some authors to be bone-forming neoplasms.[1,61] Because the three tumors typically affect bones of endochondral origin, the calvarial vault, formed by intramembranous ossification, is seldom affected. But the skull base, particularly the temporal bone, which contains areas of synchondrosis, is the site most commonly involved.[45] On CT scan, these tumors appear as well-circumscribed lytic lesions with surrounding sclerosis and variable amounts of mineralization in "rings and arcs."[70] Chondroblastomas and chondromyxoid fibromas are typically tender to palpation. Chondromas are usually asymptomatic, but pain, if present, may indicate malignant degeneration.[62] Multiple chondromas, whether or not associated with Ollier's disease or Maffucci's syndrome, have a high rate of malignant transformation.[7,83]

MALIGNANT TUMORS

Sarcoma

Sarcomas involving the skull include osteosarcoma (or osteogenic sarcoma), chondrosarcoma, fibrosarcoma, and

Ewing's sarcoma. These tumors usually arise from the long bones of the body and affect the skull rarely. Sarcomas in the skull are more commonly metastatic than of primary origin. Except for osteosarcoma, patients typically have pain at the site of the lesion. On plain radiographs and CT scans, sarcomas generally appear as osteolytic lesions with irregular, poorly marginated borders and no reactive sclerosis. MRI is necessary for evaluating intracranial extension, often present at the time of diagnosis. Conventional angiography may aid in the planning of surgery and allows for possible arterial embolization of hypervascular lesions. The treatment is total resection, including resection of tumor-infiltrated dura mater, followed by chemotherapy or radiation therapy. Yet, despite gross-total resection and adjuvant therapy, the recurrence rate remains high. Long-term survival and functional outcome depend on the size and location of the tumor, the histologic grade, and the presence of metastasis.

Osteosarcoma, the most common malignant primary skull tumor, occurs in young adults and, less commonly, in children. This sarcoma represents approximately 1% to 2% of all skull tumors, with the incidence increasing in patients with fibrous dysplasia or Paget's disease and previous irradiation.[22] Calcification of the tumor matrix within a destructive bone mass suggests the diagnosis (Figure 102-9).[42,44]

Ewing's sarcoma, derived from the red bone marrow, is the most lethal of these bone tumors. Unlike osteosarcoma, it is a disease of children and adolescents. A plain skull x-ray study may show laminated periosteal reaction with a typical onion-skin pattern.

Chondrosarcoma is a malignant tumor of cartilaginous origin and is composed of chondroid and immature cartilage. It may arise *de novo* or secondarily within a chondroma. Because the x-ray studies and CT scans of chondrosarcoma may be indistinguishable from those of a chondroma, malignant transformation cannot be determined from imaging studies. However, the presence of pain should alert the physician to possible malignancy. A relatively good prognosis can be obtained with surgery and radiation therapy.[71]

Fibrosarcoma can also be a primary or secondary bone tumor, arising from preexisting lesions or after local radiation therapy. It is composed of malignant fibroblasts embedded in a collagen matrix.

Metastases

In both children and adults, metastases or direct invasion by extracranial tumors are the most common malignancies of the skull. In adults, cancers of the prostate, breast, and lung are found to metastasize to the skull most often. Neuroblastoma is the most likely source of metastasis to the skull in children, because it is the most common extracranial solid tumor in this age group. Leukemias, lymphomas, and multiple myeloma involve the cranium when the bone marrow is invaded by circulating malignant cells. Plain x-ray studies and CT scans of

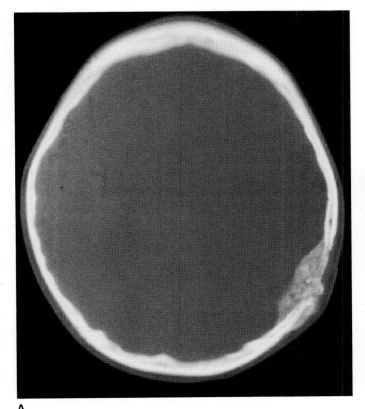

A

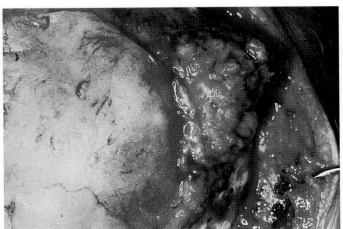

B

FIGURE 102-9 Osteosarcoma. *A,* Computed tomography scan shows equal destruction of the inner and outer skull tables and intracranial extension of the tumor. *B,* Appearance of the osteosarcoma during surgery. The tumor eroded through the skull and infiltrated the overlying scalp and underlying dura mater.

metastases generally show multiple small lesions that can be osteoblastic or osteoclastic. Metastatic lesions from prostate and breast cancer induce sclerosis and thickening of the skull, whereas neuroblastomas, lung tumors, and melanomas appear as lucent lesions on radiographs. Surgical intervention is indicated only for neural decompression or for biopsy when the primary source is unknown. Otherwise, they are treated with radiation or systemic chemotherapy.

DIFFERENTIAL DIAGNOSES

Skull masses that affect young children can result from trauma. A calcified cephalohematoma develops when a subperiosteal hematoma, usually caused by trauma at birth, mineralizes. Most occur in early infancy, are located in the parietal region, and do not cross sutural lines. The protuberance diminishes as the skull grows and remodels; only rarely is surgical intervention indicated. A calcified cephalohematoma can be prevented by aspirating the subperiosteal blood. Growing skull fractures (or leptomeningeal cysts) usually occur in children younger than 3 years who have suffered a skull fracture that is diastatic to the extent that the underlying dura mater is lacerated.[74] Congenital skull lesions seen in neonates and young children include pacchionian granulations, parietal foramina, sinus pericranii, cutis aplasia congenita, and rudimentary encephaloceles. In adults, hyperparathyroidism, osteomyelitis, and Paget's disease should also be included in the differential diagnoses of skull lesions.

References

1. Aigner T, Loos S, Inwards C, et al: Chondroblastoma is an osteoid-forming, but not cartilage-forming neoplasm. J Pathol 189:463–469, 1999.
2. Ameli NO, Abbassioun K, Azod A, Saleh H: Aneurysmal bone cyst of the skull. Can J Neurol Sci 11:466–471, 1984.
3. Antonmattei S, Tetalman MR, Lloyd TV: The multiscan appearance of eosinophilic granuloma. Clin Nucl Med 4:53–55, 1979.
4. Arana E, Latorre FF, Revert A, et al: Intradiploic epidermoid cysts. Neuroradiology 38:306–311, 1996.
5. Arseni C, Horvath L, Maretsis M, Carp N: Giant cell tumors of the calvaria. J Neurosurg 42:535–540, 1975.
6. Atkinson GO, Jr, Davis PC, Patrick LE, Winn KJ, et al: Melanotic neuroectodermal tumor of infancy. MR findings and a review of the literature. Pediatr Radiol 20:20–22, 1989.
7. Banna M, Parwani GS: Multiple sarcomas in Maffucci's syndrome. Br J Radiol 42:304–307, 1969.
8. Bastug D, Ortiz O, Schochet SS: Hemangiomas in the calvaria: imaging findings. AJR Am J Roentgenol 164:683–687, 1995.
9. Bertoni F, Unni KK, Beabout JW, Ebersold MJ: Giant cell tumor of the skull. Cancer 70:1124–1132, 1992.
10. Bizzozero L, Solaining Talamonti C, Villa F, et al: Cavernous hemangioma of the skull. Case report and review of the literature. J Neurosurg Sci 41:419–421, 1997.
11. Borba LA, Al-Mefty O, Mrak RE, Suen J: Cranial chordomas in children and adolescents. J Neurosurg 84:584–591, 1996.
12. Boutou-Bredaki S, Agapios P, Papachristou G: Prognosis of giant cell tumor of bone. Histopathological analysis of 15 cases and review of the literature. Adv Clin Path 5:71–78, 2001.
13. Cabezudo JM: Recurrent benign osteoblastoma of the parietal bone. Neurosurgery 25:1012–1013, 1989.
14. Chartrand-Lefebvre C, Dubois J, Roy D, et al: Direct intraoperative sclerotherapy of an aneurysmal bone cyst of the sphenoid. AJNR Am J Neuroradiol 17:870–872, 1996.
15. Cheek WR, Laurent, JP: Dermal sinus tracts. Concepts Pediatr Neurosurg 6:63–75, 1985.
16. Choudhury AR, al Amin MS, Chaudhri KA, al Moutaery KR: Benign osteoblastoma of the parietal bone. Childs Nerv Syst 11:115–117, 1995.
17. Crawford R: Dermoid cyst of the scalp: intracranial extension. J Pediatr Surg 25:294–295, 1990.
18. Crockard HA, Steel T, Plowman N, et al: A multidisciplinary team approach to skull base chordomas. J Neurosurg 95:175–183, 2001.
19. Dahlin DC: Caldwell Lecture. Giant cell tumor of bone: highlights of 407 cases. AJR Am J Roentgenol 144:955–960, 1985.
20. Davies ML, Macpherson P: Fibrous dysplasia of the skull: disease activity in relation to age. Br J Radiol 64:576–579, 1991.
21. Di Rocco C, Marchese E, Velardi F: Fibrous dysplasia of the skull in children. Pediatr Neurosurg 18:117–126, 1992.
22. Dodick DW, Mokri B, Shaw EG, et al: Sarcomas of calvarial bones: rare remote effect of radiation therapy for brain tumors. Neurology 44:908–912, 1994.
23. Doucet V, Peretti-Viton P, Figarella-Branger D, et al: MRI of intracranial chordomas. Extent of tumour and contrast enhancement: criteria for differential diagnosis. Neuroradiology 39: 571–576, 1997.
24. Emley WE: Giant cell tumor of the sphenoid bone. A case report and review of the literature. Arch Otolaryngol 94:369–374, 1971.
25. Engelbrecht V, Preis S, Hassler W, et al: CT and MRI of congenital sinonasal ossifying fibroma. Neuroradiology 41:526–529, 1999.
26. Epstein N, Whelan M, Reed D, Aleksic S: Giant cell tumor of the skull: a report of two cases. Neurosurgery 11:263–267, 1982.
27. Fagundes MA, Hug EB, Liebsch NJ, et al: Radiation therapy for chordomas of the base of skull and cervical spine: patterns of failure and outcome after relapse. Int J Radiat Oncol Biol Phys 33:579–584, 1995.
28. Figarella-Branger D, Perez-Castillo M, Garbe L, et al: Malignant transformation of an osteoblastoma of the skull: an exceptional occurrence. Case report. J Neurosurg 75:138–142, 1991.
29. Fink FM, Ausserer B, Schrocksnadel W, et al: Clivus chordoma in a 9-year-old child: case report and review of the literature. Pediatr Hematol Oncol 4:91–100, 1987.
30. Fisher AJ, Reinus WR, Friedland JA, Wilson AJ: Quantitative analysis of the plain radiographic appearance of eosinophilic granuloma. Invest Radiol 30:466–473, 1995.
31. Greco F, Tamburrelli F, Ciabattoni G: Prostaglandins in osteoid osteoma. Int Orthop 15:35–37, 1991.
32. Greenspan A: Benign bone-forming lesions: osteoma, osteoid osteoma, and osteoblastoma. Clinical, imaging, pathologic, and differential considerations. Skeletal Radiol 22:485–500, 1993.
33. Haddad FS, Haddad GF, Zaatari G: Cranial osteomas: their classification and management. Report on a giant osteoma and review of the literature. Surg Neurol 48:143–147, 1997.
34. Hansen-Knarhoi M, Poole MD: Preoperative difficulties in differentiating intraosseous meningiomas and fibrous dysplasia around the orbital apex. J Craniomaxillofac Surg 22:226–230, 1994.
35. Heckl S, Aschoff A, Kunze S: Cavernomas of the skull: review of the literature 1975–2000. Neurosurg Rev 25:56–62; discussion 66–57, 2002.

36. Helms CA, Hattner RS, Vogler JB, 3rd: Osteoid osteoma: radionuclide diagnosis. Radiology 151:779–784, 1984.

37. Hoshino S, Takahashi H, Shimura T, et al: Melanotic neuroectodermal tumor of infancy in the skull associated with high serum levels of catecholamine. Case report. J Neurosurg 80:919–924, 1994.

38. Ikeda H, Niizuma H, Yoshimoto T: Aneurysmal bone cyst of the skull. Surg Neurol 25:145–148, 1986.

39. Jones RO, Pillsbury HC: Histiocytosis X of the head and neck. Laryngoscope 94:1031–1035, 1984.

40. Kapadia SB, Frisman DM, Hitchcock CL, et al: Melanotic neuroectodermal tumor of infancy. Clinicopathological, immunohistochemical, and flow cytometric study. Am J Surg Pathol 17:566–573, 1993.

41. Kilpatrick SE, Wenger DE, Gilchrist GS, et al: Langerhans' cell histiocytosis (histiocytosis X) of bone. A clinicopathologic analysis of 263 pediatric and adult cases. Cancer 76:2471–2484, 1995.

42. Kornreich L, Grunebaum M, Ziv N, Cohen Y: Osteogenic sarcoma of the calvarium in children: CT manifestations. Neuroradiology 30:439–441, 1988.

43. Lee JS, FitzGibbon E, Butman JA, et al: Normal vision despite narrowing of the optic canal in fibrous dysplasia. N Engl J Med 347:1670–1676, 2002.

44. Lee YY, Van Tassel P, Nauert C, et al: Craniofacial osteosarcomas: plain film, CT, and MR findings in 46 cases. AJR Am J Roentgenol 150:1397–1402, 1988.

45. LeMay DR, Sun JK, Mendel E, et al: Chondromyxoid fibroma of the temporal bone. Surg Neurol 48:148–152, 1997.

46. Lobato RD, Lamas E, Amor T, Rivas JJ: Primary calvarial hemangioma: angiographic study. Surg Neurol 10:389–394, 1978.

47. Lustig LR, Holliday MJ, McCarthy EF, et al: Fibrous dysplasia involving the skull base and temporal bone. Arch Otolaryngol Head Neck Surg 127:1239–1247, 2001.

48. Magitsky S, Lipton JF, Reidy J, et al: Ultrastructural features of giant cell tumors in Paget's disease. Clin Orthop 213–219, 2002.

49. Marcove RC, Sheth DS, Takemoto S, et al: The treatment of aneurysmal bone cyst. Clin Orthop 157–163, 1995.

50. Mark RJ, Poen J, Tran LM, et al: Postirradiation sarcomas. A single-institution study and review of the literature. Cancer 73:2653–2662, 1994.

51. Martinez V, Sissons HA: Aneurysmal bone cyst. A review of 123 cases including primary lesions and those secondary to other bone pathology. Cancer 61:2291–2304, 1988.

52. Martinez-Lage JF, Capel A, Costa TR, et al: The child with a mass on its head: diagnostic and surgical strategies. Childs Nerv Syst 8:247–252, 1992.

53. Martinez-Lage JF, Garcia S, Torroba A, et al: Unusual osteolytic midline lesion of the skull: benign osteoblastoma of the parietal bone. Childs Nerv Syst 12:343–345, 1996.

54. Marui T, Yamamoto T, Yoshihara H, et al: De novo malignant transformation of giant cell tumor of bone. Skeletal Radiol 30:104–108, 2001.

55. Matt BH: Aneurysmal bone cyst of the maxilla: case report and review of the literature. Int J Pediatr Otorhinolaryngol 25:217–226, 1993.

56. Matus-Ridley M, Raney RB, Jr, Thawerani H, Meadows AT: Histiocytosis X in children: patterns of disease and results of treatment. Med Pediatr Oncol 11:99–105, 1983.

57. McLeod RA, Dahlin DC, Beabout JW: The spectrum of osteoblastoma. Am J Roentgenol 126:321–325, 1976.

58. Mehta JS, Sharr MM, Penney CC: Unusual radiological appearance of a skull osteoma. Br J Neurosurg 13:332–334, 1999.

59. Michael CB, Lee AG, Patrinely JR, et al: Visual loss associated with fibrous dysplasia of the anterior skull base. Case report and review of the literature. J Neurosurg 92:350–354, 2000.

60. Michel RG, Woodard BH: Extracranial meningioma. Ann Otol Rhinol Laryngol 88:407–412, 1979.

61. Mii Y, Miyauchi Y, Morishita T, et al: Ultrastructural cytochemical demonstration of proteoglycans and calcium in the extracellular matrix of chondroblastomas. Hum Pathol 25:1290–1294, 1994.

62. Murphey MD, Flemming DJ, Boyea SR, et al: Enchondroma versus chondrosarcoma in the appendicular skeleton: differentiating features. Radiographics 18:1213–1237; quiz 1244–1215, 1998.

63. Ochsner SF: Eosinophilic granuloma of bone; experience with 20 cases. Am J Roentgenol Radium Ther Nucl Med 97:719–726, 1966.

64. Pannell BW, Hendrick EB, Hoffman HJ, et al: Dermoid cysts of the anterior fontanelle. Neurosurgery 10:317–323, 1982.

65. Papadopoulos MC, Casey AT, Powell M: Craniofacial fibrous dysplasia complicated by acute, reversible visual loss: report of two cases. Br J Neurosurg 12:159–161, 1998.

66. Peterson DL, Murk SE, Story JL: Multifocal cavernous hemangioma of the skull: report of a case and review of the literature. Neurosurgery 30:778–781; discussion 782, 1992.

67. Pettinato G, Manivel JC, d'Amore ES, et al: Melanotic neuroectodermal tumor of infancy. A reexamination of a histogenetic problem based on immunohistochemical, flow cytometric, and ultrastructural study of 10 cases. Am J Surg Pathol 15:233–245, 1991.

68. Pierre-Kahn A, Cinalli G, Lellouch-Tubiana A, et al: Melanotic neuroectodermal tumor of the skull and meninges in infancy. Pediatr Neurosurg 18:6–15, 1992.

69. Rawlings CE, III, Wilkins RH: Solitary eosinophilic granuloma of the skull. Neurosurgery 15:155–161, 1984.

70. Robbin MR, Murphey MD: Benign chondroid neoplasms of bone. Semin Musculoskelet Radiol 4:45–58, 2000.

71. Rosenberg AE, Nielsen GP, Keel SB, et al: Chondrosarcoma of the base of the skull: a clinicopathologic study of 200 cases with emphasis on its distinction from chordoma. Am J Surg Pathol 23:1370–1378, 1999.

72. Ruge JR, Tomita T, Naidich TP, et al: Scalp and calvarial masses of infants and children. Neurosurgery 22:1037–1042, 1988.

73. Ruggieri P, Sim FH, Bond JR, Unni KK: Malignancies in fibrous dysplasia. Cancer 73:1411–1424, 1994.

74. Scarfo GB, Mariottini A, Tomaccini D, Palma L: Growing skull fractures: progressive evolution of brain damage and effectiveness of surgical treatment. Childs Nerv Syst 5:163–167, 1989.

75. Scimeca PG, James-Herry AG, Black KS, et al: Chemotherapeutic treatment of malignant chordoma in children. J Pediatr Hematol Oncol 18:237–240, 1996.

76. Sheikh BY: Cranial aneurysmal bone cyst "with special emphasis on endovascular management." Acta Neurochir (Wien) 141:601–610; discussion 610–601, 1999.

77. Shuangshoti S: Primary meningiomas outside the central nervous system. In Al-Mefty O (ed): Meningiomas. New York, Raven Press, 1991.

78. Slootweg PJ: Maxillofacial fibro-osseous lesions: classification and differential diagnosis. Semin Diagn Pathol 13:104–112, 1996.

79. Stull MA, Kransdorf MJ, Devaney KO: Langerhans cell histiocytosis of bone. Radiographics 12:801–823, 1992.

80. Taillefer R, Levasseur A, Robillard R: Ga-67 imaging in eosinophilic granuloma. Clin Nucl Med 6:270–271, 1981.

81. Tucker WS, Nasser-Sharif FJ: Benign skull lesions. Can J Surg 40:449–455, 1997.

82. Uemura K, Takahashi S, Sonobe M, et al: Intradiploic haemangioma associated with epidural haematoma. Neuroradiology 38:456–457, 1996.

83. Unni KK, Dahlin DC: Premalignant tumors and conditions of bone. Am J Surg Pathol 3:47–60, 1979.

84. Van Tassel P, Lee YY, Ayala A, et al: Case report 680. Intraosseous meningioma of the sphenoid bone. Skeletal Radiol 20:383–386, 1991.

85. Walsh JW, Strand RD: Melanotic neuroectodermal tumor of the neurocranium in infancy. Childs Brain 9:329–346, 1982.

86. Watne AL, Lai HY, Carrier J, Coppula W: The diagnosis and surgical treatment of patients with Gardner's syndrome. Surgery 82:327–333, 1977.

87. Wenig BM, Vinh TN, Smirniotopoulos JG, et al: Aggressive psammomatoid ossifying fibromas of the sinonasal region: a clinicopathologic study of a distinct group of fibro-osseous lesions. Cancer 76:1155–1165, 1995.

88. Wold LE, Laws ER, Jr: Cranial chordomas in children and young adults. J Neurosurg 59:1043–1047, 1983.

89. Wolfe JT, III, Scheithauer BW, Dahlin DC: Giant-cell tumor of the sphenoid bone. Review of 10 cases. J Neurosurg 59:322–327, 1983.

CHAPTER 103

EPIDURAL SPINAL TUMORS

Paul Steinbok, Stephen John Hentschel, Robert D. Labrom, Michael Sargent, Caron Stralendorf, Karen Goddard, and Glenda Hendson

Spinal tumors may be classified by location within the spinal canal as follows: intramedullary tumors, which involve the substance of the spinal cord; intradural extramedullary tumors, which involve intradural structures apart from the spinal cord itself; and extradural tumors, which involve the structures outside the dura.

This chapter considers tumors of the extradural compartment, which includes the bony structures of the spinal canal and the tissues of the epidural space, mainly fat and blood vessels. Tumors that commonly cause spinal cord compression are discussed in detail, whereas tumors of bone origin are discussed in another chapter. The special characteristics of extradural tumors in the child, as opposed to the adult, are highlighted. A logical and clinically relevant algorithm for managing a child who has the final diagnosis of an epidural spinal cord tumor is presented.

EPIDEMIOLOGY

Tumors of the spinal cord and spinal elements constitute 5% to 10% of all pediatric central nervous system neoplasms, with an incidence of approximately 1 per 1,000,000 overall population per year. There is a near equal distribution of extradural, intradural extramedullary, and intramedullary tumors. If congenital lesions are excluded, there is an even distribution over the first 15 years of life. The location of these tumors generally follows the relative sizes of the cervical, thoracic, lumbar, and sacral segments, with the most common level being thoracic. There is no definite relationship between race and environmental factors and the occurrence of such tumors.

Table 103-1 lists the approximate frequency of pediatric neoplasms involving the extradural compartment. The vast majority are malignant neoplasms, but rarely a benign lipoma occurs in the extradural space. Tumors such as schwannomas and, in particular, plexiform neurofibromas may also grow into the spinal canal from extradural locations. In addition, there are primary bone tumors that secondarily involve the extradural space, but these are not discussed here because they do not typically occur as epidural masses. They include osteoid osteoma, osteoblastoma, aneurysmal bone cyst, giant cell tumor, eosinophilic granuloma, osteochondroma, and enchondroma. Extradural neoplasms are the leading cause of nontraumatic pediatric paraparesis in North America. Overall, up to 20% of patients with Ewing's sarcoma, 10% with neuroblastoma, and 8% with osteogenic sarcoma will develop spinal cord compression during the course of their illness.[6] Approximately 3% to 5% of children with a systemic malignancy will develop spinal cord compression, and in nearly 50% it will occur as an initial sign. A report from St. Jude Children's Research Hospital found that the incidence of spinal cord compression in children with cancer was 2.7%.[2] Table 103-2 lists the frequency of various tumors to occur as spinal cord compression in that study.

CLINICAL FEATURES

The onset of symptomatology may be quite insidious in some cases or precipitous in others. The most common features are pain and weakness. Pain may be localized to the back or may be radicular, involving a limb or the chest. Radicular pain is common with extradural tumors in children, because these tumors in the child typically involve the neural foramina, and such pain may be present before the onset of spinal cord compression. Local back pain develops from expansion or invasion of bone or from spinal deformity. Worrisome features of back pain include a progressive and unrelenting nature, pain that is worse at night, and pain associated with a rigid back in a young child. In infants and nonverbal children, pain may manifest as irritability or refusal to walk or use one or more limbs. Weakness is usually related to spinal cord compression and is part of an upper motor neuron syndrome, with associated spasticity, increased deep tendon reflexes, and Babinski responses. Lower motor neuron weakness occurs if the conus medullaris, cauda equina, or nerve root is involved. The child is rarely the one to notice the weakness, and often parents do not recognize the fact that the child is weak until the weakness is severe. In the very young child, weakness may manifest as regression in walking or other developmental skills.

Bladder dysfunction may be present and typically occurs earlier than bowel dysfunction. In infants and younger children who are not toilet trained, it is difficult to know what is normal bladder and bowel function. Urinary dysfunction may manifest as recurrent urinary tract infections. A child with back pain requires taking a careful history, directed toward eliciting evidence of bladder or bowel dysfunction. Such dysfunction has been reported in up to 60% of patients with spinal cord compression secondary to extradural tumors.

A sensory level may be identified on examination, but this is rarely noticed by the patient. Scoliosis occurs in approximately 5% of children with extradural tumors. Features of

TABLE 103-1

Tumor Type for Tumors Causing Spinal Cord Compression

Tumor	Frequency
Neuroblastoma	26%
Ewing's sarcoma	21%
Rhabdomyosarcoma	13%
Osteogenic sarcoma	12%
Lymphoma	8%
Other sarcoma	5%
Germ cell	5%
Leukemia	3%
Wilms	2%
Other	5%

From Raffel C: Spinal cord compression by epidural tumors in childhood. Neurosurg Clin N Am 3:925–930, 1992.

TABLE 103-2

Frequency of Various Tumor Types to Occur as Metastatic Spinal Cord Compression in Children with Cancer

Tumor	% of Total Tumor Type
Ewing's sarcoma	16%
Osteosarcoma	8%
Neuroblastoma	7%
Rhabdomyosarcoma	5%
Non-Hodgkin's lymphoma	4%
Germ cell	4%
Hodgkin's lymphoma	2%
Leukemia	1%
Wilms	1%

From Ch'ien LT, Kalwinsky DK, Paterson G, et al: Metastatic epidural tumors in children. Med Pediatr Oncol 10:455–462, 1982; Klein SL, Sanford RA, Muhlbauer MS: Pediatric spinal epidural metastases. J Neurosurg 74:70–75, 1991.

scoliosis that point to a neurologic etiology include a convex curve to the left, rapid progression, and a curve of greater than 50 degrees. Kyphotic deformities may also be present but tend to occur late in the disease and usually indicate a pathologic fracture. Occasionally, a local swelling or fullness can be identified deep to the skin adjacent to one or more spinous processes, and this may occur when the tumor has grown posteriorly from the spinal canal into the paravertebral muscles.

Spinal cord compression tends to occur early in the course of the disease in Ewing's sarcoma, neuroblastoma, Hodgkin's disease, and lymphoma, whereas in osteosarcoma and rhabdomyosarcoma it tends to present later in the course of disease. In lymphoma this is in contrast to the adult experience, where spinal cord compression occurs late in the disease process.

INITIAL INVESTIGATIONS

In the child with back or radicular pain and no identifiable neurologic abnormalities, anteroposterior and lateral radiographs directed to the area of the pain are the initial investigations. Almost 10% of children with back pain and scoliosis will be found to have an underlying pathologic cause, but an intraspinal tumor is only rarely the problem. The majority of these patients with an underlying pathologic cause will have abnormal plain radiographs, most commonly spondylolysis or spondylolisthesis.

If plain films are abnormal, or if there is evidence of spinal cord or cauda equina dysfunction on examination, further investigations are required. If the plain radiographs are normal and there is no previous history of malignancy, a radionuclide bone scan is the next investigation of choice, followed by computed tomography (CT) if there is a focus of increased activity on the bone scan. This approach will demonstrate the large majority of causes of back pain in children, including mechanical lesions such as spondylolysis and Scheuermann's disease, as well as benign tumors such as osteoblastoma. Epidural and paravertebral lesions including tumor and abscess may also be identified.

Abnormalities on plain radiographs of the spine may be noted in around 50% of children with intraspinal tumors, including those with known primary malignancy. Findings include abnormal curvature; vertebral body destruction, which is usually lytic but may be sclerotic; widened spinal canal; eroded pedicle; enlarged intervertebral foramen; paraspinal soft tissue mass; and dystrophic calcification (Figure 103-1). Increased separation and thinning of the ribs is common with posterior mediastinal neurogenic tumors.

Magnetic resonance (MR) scanning is the investigation of choice for identifying spinal extradural tumors. MR scanning can image the spinal canal longitudinally and has the ability to produce images in multiple planes, which is valuable for defining the precise location of the lesion within and outside the spinal canal. The MR scan will demonstrate very well the epidural spinal lesion in both T1- and T2-weighted images. Fat suppression or other special techniques such as short tau inversion recovery (STIR) may be necessary for full characterization of vertebral and intraspinal lesions. MR-compatible surface markers may be placed to assist surgical localization. Depending on the age and cooperation of the child, deep sedation or general anesthetic may be required for completion of the MR scan. Whereas MR imaging (MRI) is the modality of choice for identifying the intraspinal extradural tumor, CT scans of the lesion demonstrate better the adjacent bone anatomy.

The typical MR findings of an epidural tumor are an intraspinal soft tissue mass elevating the dura and compressing the subarachnoid space, with obtuse margins between the mass and the underlying cerebrospinal fluid (CSF) (Figure 103-2). In series including predominantly adult patients, epidural masses posterior to the spinal cord tend to be associated with hemopoietic malignancy, whereas anterior epidural metastases are associated with vertebral metastases. Most epidural tumors have intermediate signal, higher than CSF on T1-weighted images but lower than CSF on T2-weighted images. The cord may be displaced or compressed. Edema, characterized by increased T2 signal, may be shown in the spinal cord. Where epidural tumors involve bone, there will usually be abnormal

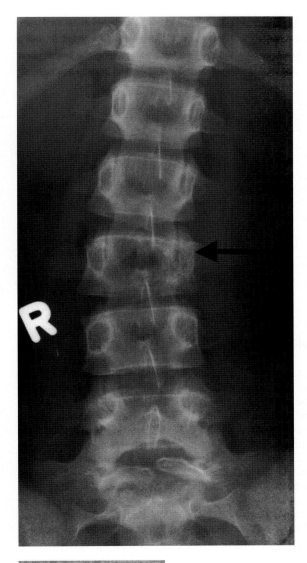

FIGURE 103-1 Anteroposterior radiograph of the lumbar spine in an 11-year-old girl shows scoliosis resulting from destruction of the left L3 vertebral body and pedicle *(arrow)* by a paraspinal rhabdomyosarcoma. Computed tomography and magnetic resonance imaging confirmed epidural extension.

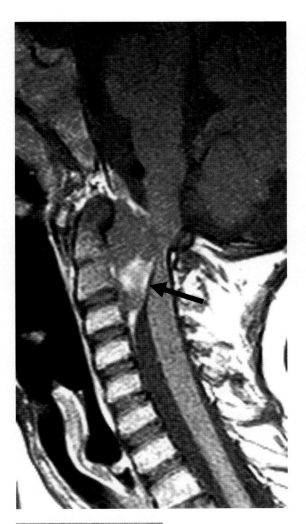

FIGURE 103-2 Sagittal T1-weighted magnetic resonance imaging scan in a 2-year-old boy with torticollis shows a tumor displacing and compressing the cervicomedullary junction of the cord. The obtuse interface between this epithelioid sarcoma and the cerebrospinal fluid in the underlying subarachnoid space indicates its epidural location. Areas of bright signal in the mass *(black arrow)* are due to intravenous contrast enhancement.

vertebral signal or enhancement. Intravenous contrast enhancement using gadolinium chelates causes T1 shortening with increased signal on T1-weighted images in many tumors. This enhancement is useful in younger children but in older children and in adults with fatty marrow, it may mask metastases.

Spinal ultrasound can be used to assess the contents of the spinal canal in infants younger than 3 months where the posterior elements are still cartilaginous, but it provides little additional information about the tumor. Spinal ultrasound may be useful during surgery for the tumor.

Before the advent of MRI, myelography with CT scanning was the procedure of choice for investigating patients with suspected intraspinal tumors. Assuming that MR scanning is available, CT myelography is rarely necessary, given the requirement for lumbar puncture and the associated risk of neu-

rologic deterioration resulting from release of CSF. However, if there has been spinal fixation surgery, as often is the case with a tumor recurrence, CT myelography may be preferred to MRI because of metal-related artifact and signal loss.

Further imaging investigations are directed according to the expected pattern of spread of the known or presumed tumor type. Where primary or secondary malignancy is suspected, coordination of imaging with the local pediatric oncology and radiology services helps to ensure that appropriate testing is performed and to minimize unnecessary procedures.

Imaging may be required to evaluate local, regional, or distant disease. Ultrasonography provides noninvasive screening of the abdomen, including the liver, kidneys, and adrenals, but delineation of retroperitoneal and paraspinal disease is limited and requires cross-sectional imaging using CT or MRI

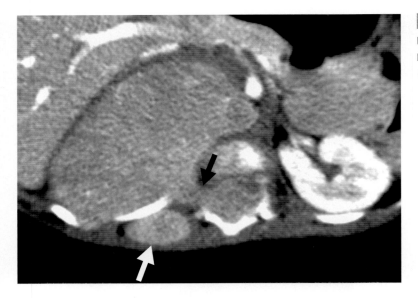

FIGURE 103-3   Axial contrast-enhanced computed tomography scan of a 1-year-old girl's chest shows a posterior mediastinal neuroblastoma invading the spinal canal *(black arrow)* and displacing the dura and cord to the right.

(Figure 103-3). Chest radiography is usually performed, but CT of the chest is the technique of choice to look for metastatic lesions in the lungs of children with sarcomas and for mediastinal lymph nodes with lymphoma or neuroblastoma. Routine imaging of the brain is rarely indicated.

Scintigraphy using various radionuclides is valuable in the evaluation of both primary and metastatic tumors of childhood. Single-photon emission computed tomography (SPECT) is essential. The initial perfusion and blood pool images of a three-phase technetium-99m labeled diphosphonate (MDP) bone scan may highlight soft-tissue and bone tumors because of their increased vascularity. Increased activity on delayed images indicates sites of increased bone turnover, which may be normal, lytic, or sclerotic on plain radiograph or CT scan. Photopenic lesions are less common. Because the main value of the bone scan is to identify bone lesions remote from the primary spinal epidural tumor, delayed images should always include the whole body. Increased activity is nonspecific and may be caused by other lesions such as infection or trauma. Hence plain radiographs may be needed to help characterize remote lesions found on scintigraphy.

The primary soft-tissue tumor of neuroblastoma accumulates bone-seeking radiopharmaceuticals in approximately 70% of cases. Radiolabeled ^{123}I or ^{131}I meta-iodolbenzylguanidine (MIBG) is taken up by 85% of neuroblastomas. MIBG is a guanethidine derivative of norepinephrine and epinephrine, which is taken up by catecholaminergic cells. MIBG and MDP scans are complementary techniques for the evaluation of disease metastatic to bone marrow and cortex.

Neuroblastoma will demonstrate accumulation of ^{18}F-fluorodeoxyglucose (FDG) on positron-emission tomography (PET) scanning, but its role remains to be defined. Thallium-201 scanning is used in the evaluation of musculoskeletal tumors.

Angiography is rarely required in the assessment of epidural masses in children. It may be warranted for diagnosis, if the differential includes hemorrhage from a vascular malformation. Angiography may also be performed for preoperative planning with or without embolization.

TUMOR HISTOLOGY

The most common nonosseous, malignant tumors in the extradural space are neuroblastomas, Ewing's sarcoma, rhabdomyosarcomas, lymphomas, and leukemias. These are small-blue-round-cell tumors (Figure 103-4). The diagnosis of the small-blue-round-cell tumors is based on a combination of light microscopic, immunohistochemical, and electron microscopic features and genetic studies, which may be either cytogenetic, molecular, or both (Tables 103-3 and 103-4). With routine preparations they may be difficult to differentiate from each other and often require detailed ancillary investigations. The genetic studies are not just diagnostic but may be of prognostic significance and are required in the management of patients with extradural lesions.

MANAGEMENT

The goals of management of a child with a spinal epidural mass include diagnosis of the tumor type, pain relief, preservation of spinal cord function and spinal stability, and eradication of the lesion. Combinations of surgery, chemotherapy, or radiation therapy may be required (Figure 103-5).

After diagnosis of an extradural spinal tumor, the initial strategies vary depending on whether the child has a history of a known malignant process and whether there is evidence of spinal cord or cauda equina compression. In the presence of a prior diagnosis of malignancy, the spinal tumor is usually presumed to be a metastasis from the original malignancy, and the initial investigations are directed toward identifying other metastatic lesions. When there is no such history, the diagnosis of the tumor type becomes an important goal. Elevation of serum and urine catecholamine levels, vanillylmandelic acid, and homovanillic acid and a positive MIBG scan indicate neuroblastoma. Elevations of beta human chorionic gonadotropin (BHCG) or alpha fetoprotein indicate a malignant germ cell tumor. A complete blood count (CBC) or marrow biopsy may

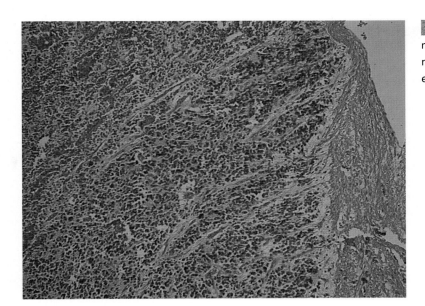

FIGURE 103-4 Neuroblastoma showing a markedly cellular tumor composed of neuroblasts and neuropil—so-called small-blue-round-cell tumor. (Hematoxylin and eosin stain ×100.)

indicate evidence of leukemia. Chest radiograph, abdominal ultrasound, or CT scan may identify lymphoma or an intrathoracic or suprarenal neuroblastoma. If these simple tests are negative, a biopsy for tissue diagnosis is required. This may be achieved as part of a resection of the tumor, if such a resection is indicated, as discussed later. In the absence of indications for resective surgery, needle biopsy may be undertaken to establish the diagnosis and will provide a diagnosis in most cases.[11] This should be performed in such a way that potential surgical margins are not disrupted. Furthermore, it is important to obtain enough biopsy material to allow molecular genetic analysis of the tumor, because the results of such analysis will determine the definitive management. Once a pathologic diagnosis is established, definitive management of the tumor may be initiated.

Approximately 2% to 3% of pediatric patients with sarcomas or neuroblastoma, 2% with lymphoma (non-Hodgkin's), and fewer than 0.5% with leukemia will clinically present initially with spinal cord or cauda equina compression.[2] In such cases, high doses of steroids, for example, dexamethasone 1 to 2 mg/kg per dose every 6 hours for 96 hours, are started in an attempt to reduce the neurologic deficits. There is one potential negative consequence of early steroid treatment and that relates to patients with undiagnosed lymphoma. In such cases, prolonged steroid use before obtaining tissue for diagnosis may render biopsies difficult to interpret because of a partially treated state.

The major factors that must be considered in deciding initial medical therapy (chemotherapy or radiation therapy) versus surgical resection are the type of neoplasm and the extent of spinal cord or cauda equina compression. In patients with neuroblastoma, germ cell tumors, and lymphoma, surgery for epidural masses is not indicated unless patients have severe spinal cord or cauda equina compression.[6] For these tumors, in the absence of severe spinal cord or cauda equina compression, there is no difference in the outcome between medical and surgical therapy. This is not the case for sarcomas, with the possible exception of Ewing's sarcoma. The extent of spinal cord compression has to be considered in the decision-making

process. Historically, patients with a 50% or more block on myelogram were shown to have a better neurologic recovery with surgery than with medical therapy. However, with modern chemotherapy, good neurologic outcomes have been reported after medical therapy, even in children with complete paraplegia. Current absolute indications for surgical resection of pediatric spinal extradural tumors include non-Ewing's sarcoma with signs of spinal cord compression, primary spinal instability resulting from destruction of osseous elements by tumor, and progression of neurologic deficit during medical therapy. A relative indication for surgical resection is severe spinal cord or cauda equina compression, indicated by complete loss of neurologic function or rapid progression to a nonambulatory state over a 12-hour period regardless of tumor type (Table 103-5).

There is a distinctive difference between pediatric and adult forms of spinal cord or cauda equina compression that influences surgical management. In the pediatric population, the tumors tend to enter the spinal canal through the intervertebral foramen and thus occur posterolaterally, whereas in adults the tumors tend to involve the vertebral body and occur anteriorly. This allows access to the lesion via a posterior approach in the pediatric patient, whether it be by laminectomy or laminotomy. Immediate spinal stability is generally not a concern with the posterior approaches, although this may be an issue in the longer term.

Another distinctive difference between adult and pediatric patients with spinal cord compression is that adults with complete neurologic deficits have a very poor chance of significant neurologic recovery. This is not the case with children, in whom the situation is far from hopeless, with 50% of patients improving to an ambulatory status regardless of the method of therapy.[6]

The long-term sequelae of multilevel laminectomies in the pediatric population are well known to consist of scoliosis, kyphosis, and spondylolisthesis. Risk factors include the level of the surgery (the more cephalad the more risk), asymmetric radiation fields, higher doses of radiation therapy, facet disruption, vertebral body destruction, and young age (<2 years old).[9]

TABLE 103-3   Pathology of Common Extradural Tumors

Tumor	Histology	Special Stains and Immunohisto-chemistry	Electron Microscopy	Genetic Marker and Significance
Neuroblastoma	Undifferentiated small round cells in nests, surrounded by neuropil and separated by delicate septa. Homer-Wright rosettes may be present characterized by central neuropil surrounded by 1 or 2 layers of neuroblasts. The tumor cells are small and round, have a high nuclear-cytoplasmic ratio, speckled chromatin, nucleoli, and a thin rim of cytoplasm. Mitotic activity is usually brisk. Neuroblastomas showing maturation contain ganglion cells and Schwann cells.	*Neuronal markers*: Neuron specific enolase Synaptophysin Neurofilament Protein gene product 9.5 Ganglioside GD2 Chromogranin A *Schwann cells*: S-100 protein	Varies with the degree of differentiation. Immature neuroblasts have irregular, lobulated, or indented nuclei, a high nuclear-cytoplasmic ratio, and a thin rim of cytoplasm. Within the cytoplasm are ribosomes, mitochondria, and heterogeneous osmiophilic granules. The more differentiated cells have more abundant cytoplasm and a variable number of dense core neurosecretory granules (50–200 nm in diameter) in the cell processes and on the periphery of the cytoplasm. Microtubules and neurofilaments may be present.	*Flow cytometry*: Hyperdiploid (+) Diploid (–) *Chromosome 1p Abnormality*: Absent (+) Present (–) *Double minutes, homogeneous staining regions*: Absent (+) Present (–) *N-myc amplification*: Not amplified (+) Amplified (–) *TrkA expression*: Present (+) Absent (–) *trisomy 17q*: Present (–) Absent (+)
Ewing's sarcoma/ peripheral PNET	Sheets or lobules of monotonous round to oval, light and dark cells. Pseudorosettes may be present. The tumor nuclei have smooth contours, inconspicuous nucleoli, and finely dispersed chromatin. The cytoplasm is faintly vacuolated or clear.	Periodic acid Schiff (PAS) Vimentin Neuron-specific enolase Synaptophysin MIC2 (CD99)	Light and dark cells with a high nuclear-cytoplasmic ratio. Nuclei are uniform. Abundant glycogen in the cytoplasm. There is relative paucity of organelles.	*Cytogenetics or RT-PCR*: t(11,22)(q24;q12) t(21,22)(q22;q12)
Rhabdomyosarcoma	*Embryonal subtype*: Diffuse infiltrate of round to elongated cells with eccentric, hyperchromatic nuclei and abundant eosinophilic cytoplasm. Occasional cells have cross-striations. *Alveolar subtype*: Small round cells in sheets or nests separated by fibrovascular septa. Cells adjacent to the septa are cohesive. The central spaces contain larger, more non-cohesive, and multinucleate cells.	Myoglobin Desmin Myoglobin Muscle-specific actin Myogenin MyoD Muscle-specific actin	In less differentiated cells the myosin-ribosome complex (rudimentary sarcomere) is identified. These are short parallel bundles of rigid 15 nm myosin filaments with attached ribosomes in single file. In more differentiated tumors there are myosin (thick) and actin (thin) filaments that form hexagonal arrays on cross section. Z, M, and I bands may be present.	*Cytogenetics or RT-PCR for alveolar rhabdomyosarcoma*: t(2,13)(q35;q14) t(1,13)(p36;q14)

PNET, Primitive neuroectodermal tumor; RT-PCR, reverse transcription polymerase chain reaction; TrkA, tyrosine kinase receptor A; (+) favorable prognosis; (–) unfavorable prognosis.

TABLE 103-4   **Pathology of Common Hematologic Extradural Tumors**

Tumor	Histology	Special Stains and Immunohistochemistry	Genetic Marker and Significance
Acute lymphoblastic leukemia (ALL) and lymphoblastic lymphoma	Infiltrate of monotonous, noncohesive blasts. The tumor cells have nuclei that are smaller than those of the macrophages but larger than small lymphocytes. The nuclear membranes are convoluted, the chromatin is finely dispersed, the nucleoli are inconspicuous, and the cytoplasm is scant. Mitotic figures are frequent.	PAS Nonspecific esterase Terminal deoxynucleotidyl transferase (TDT)	*For precursor B-ALL:* t(9;22)(q34;q11.2) (−) t(4;11)(q21;q23) (−) t(1;19)(q23;p13.3) (−) t(12;21)(p13;q22) (+) Hyperdiploid >50 (+) Hypodiploidy (−) *Flow cytometry:* B-cell markers or T-cell markers, depending on precursor cell: B cell: CD19, cytoplasmic CD79a, cytoplasmic 22, CD 10, cyt-mu. T cell: CD1a, CD2, CD3, CD4, CD5, CD7, CD8.
Burkitt's lymphoma (small noncleaved cell lymphoma)	Infiltrate of cells with round to oval nuclei with distinct membranes, clumped chromatin, and 2–5 prominent, centrally placed nucleoli. The cytoplasm is basophilic and contains lipid. Mitotic figures and apoptotic cells are abundant. Numerous benign macrophages give a "starry sky" appearance.	B-cell markers: CD19 CD20	t(8;14)(q24;q32) t(2;8)(q11;q24) t(8;22)(q24;q11)
Diffuse large B-cell lymphoma	Moderate to large cells with oval to round vesicular nuclei, fine chromatin and 2–4 nucleoli. The cytoplasm is scanty, amphophilic to basophilic. Cells can be multilobated. The immunoblastic cells have large nuclei, centrally located nucleoli, and an appreciable amount of basophilic cytoplasm.	B-cell markers: CD19 CD20 CD22 CD79a	t(14;18)(q32;q21)
Anaplastic large cell lymphoma	Diffuse infiltrate of large cells with abundant cytoplasm and pleomorphic, often horseshoe- or kidney-shaped nuclei. The nuclear chromatin is clumped and the nucleoli are basophilic. The cytoplasm is clear, basophilic, or eosinophilic.	Acid phosphatase Nonspecific esterase ALK1 CD30 EMA T-cell markers: CD3, CD2, CD4, CD45Ro	t(2;5)(p23;35) t(1;2)(q23;p22) t(2;3)(p23;q35) inv(2)(p23q35)
Hodgkin's lymphoma	Reed-Sternberg (RS) cells in a background of non-neoplastic lymphocytes, eosinophils, neutrophils, histiocytes, plasma cells, fibroblasts, and collagen fibers. Classic RS cells are large, have abundant, slightly basophilic cytoplasm and at least 2 nuclear lobes or nuclei. The nuclei are large, with a prominent nuclear membrane and usually 1 prominent eosinophilic nucleolus.	RS cells: Leu M1 CD30	

PAS, Periodic acid Schiff; (+) favorable prognosis; (−) unfavorable prognosis.

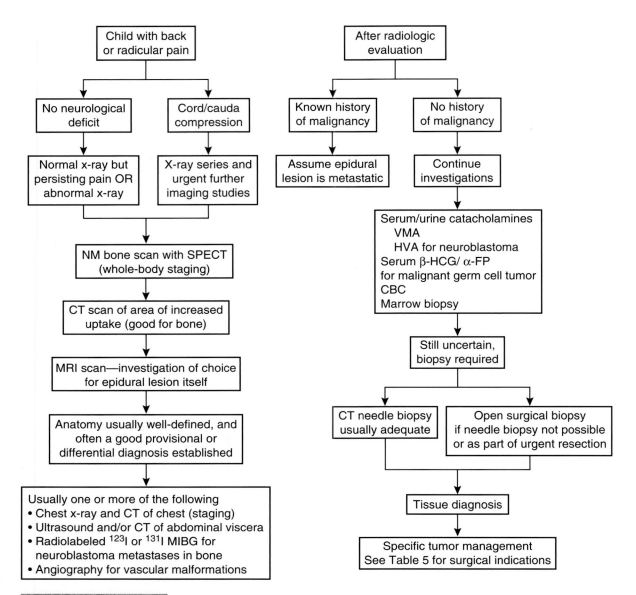

FIGURE 103-5 Algorithm for management of a child with the final diagnosis of an epidural spinal cord tumor. CBC, Complete blood count; CT, computed tomography; β-HCG, human chorionic gonadotropin; HVA, homovanillic acid; MIBG, metaiodobenzylguanidine; MRI, magnetic resonance imaging; NM, nuclear medicine; SPECT, single photon emission computed tomography; VMA, vanillymandelic acid.

TABLE 103-5

Surgical Indications in Spinal Cord Compression

Absolute Indications
Non-Ewing's sarcoma
Progression of neurologic deficit on medical therapy
Spinal instability

Relative Indications
Complete neurologic deficit of <72 hours' duration
Progress to nonambulatory state over <12 hours

One study found a 46% incidence of spinal column deformity if laminectomies were performed before 15 years of age, compared with a 6% incidence between 15 and 24 years of age, and a 0% incidence if performed after 25 years of age. Correlation with sex, neurologic status, length of time since surgery, or even the number of laminae removed has been inconsistent.[9] In an attempt to avoid these problems, laminoplastic procedures, where the posterior elements are replaced, are often performed instead of laminectomies. The ability to perform these procedures with minimal complications such as spondylosis, stenosis, or significant bone resorption has been well documented. Some studies have also shown a lower incidence of spinal deformity with laminoplasty compared with laminectomy in the short term, but it has not been demonstrated that the long-term outcome in terms of spinal deformity is any better.

Neuroblastoma

Neuroblastoma is the most common extracranial solid malignant neoplasm in the pediatric population. This tumor is responsible for 30% of pediatric spinal neoplasms and 50% of malignant neoplasms in the neonatal age group. These tumors arise from neural crest tissue, either from the sympathetic nervous system or from tissue embryologically destined for the sympathetic nervous system. Forty percent arise from the adrenal gland, with the remainder from the abdominal, thoracic, cervical, and pelvic sympathetic chains, in descending order of frequency. Of the tumors that occur as intraspinal lesions, the majority involve the thoracic spine, most likely because the thoracic vertebral segments surround a large percentage of the spinal cord rather than because of a particular predilection for this part of the spine.[5] Of the patients who have involvement of the spinal canal on initial imaging, half will have symptomatic spinal cord compression.[5] These tumors usually enter the intervertebral foramen and occur as a dumbbell tumor from a paravertebral location or, less commonly, they may be metastatic to the epidural space via hematogenous or lymphatic spread.

In general, the initial treatment of epidural neuroblastoma is chemotherapy, even when there is neurologic deficit. Induction chemotherapy usually consists of a combination of carboplatin, etoposide, cyclophosphamide, and doxorubicin. With chemotherapy alone, 58% of patients have reduction in the epidural mass, and 92% show neurologic improvement. Laminectomy for spinal cord or cauda equina decompression can be prevented in at least 60% of patients.[12] If there is no response or evidence of progression in neurologic signs on chemotherapy, immediate surgical decompression is recommended. Numerous reports indicate that the results of chemotherapy are at least as good as those for laminectomy,[12] and some studies have shown that the neurologic recovery with chemotherapy is greater.[3]

Radiation therapy in the emergency setting is not recommended unless progressive or persistent neurologic signs continue despite chemotherapy and surgery. Although neuroblastoma is a radiosensitive tumor, the role of radiation continues to evolve and depends on the risk group of the patient. Radiation therapy is a major contributor to significant late sequelae, and this limits its use in many of the modern protocols. Radiation therapy is limited to those patients with progressive clinical deterioration despite other modalities, persistent viable disease and unfavorable biology after completion of chemotherapy, or persistent disease following surgery for local recurrence. It may also be appropriate to irradiate sites of metastatic disease, depending on the extent of disease.

Interestingly, the survival rate tends to be higher among those patients with spinal involvement, and disseminated disease is unusual if the patient has spinal cord compression. It is also known that some tumors may mature to a more benign form, ganglioneuroma, or regress over time spontaneously.

Ewing's Sarcoma

Ewing's sarcoma is the most common bone neoplasm in the population younger than 10 years. Eighty percent of patients with Ewing's sarcoma seek treatment when younger than age 20. These neoplasms probably arise from neural crest cells and not from endothelial or hematopoietic cells as was originally believed. Genetic analysis demonstrates a relationship with peripheral primitive neuroectodermal tumor (PNET), with both tumors sharing the same reciprocal translocation (11;22) (q24;q12). They are associated with and may arise from postganglionic parasympathetic neural tissue and are able to synthesize choline acetyl transferase. These are primitive tumors that may involve the spinal canal via primary spinal or metastatic disease. Approximately 5% of all cases of Ewing's sarcoma are of the primary spinal variety, but if sacral lesions are excluded, this drops to less than 1%.[15] Rarely, Ewing's sarcoma occurs as an extraosseous extradural tumor, and such variants tend to occur in an adult population.

The mainstay of treatment of epidural Ewing's sarcoma is chemotherapy. Randomized clinical trials during the past 15 years led to the general acceptance of the combination of vincristine, doxorubicin, and cyclophosphamide as standard therapy for Ewing's sarcoma. More recently, a Children's Cancer Group (CCG)–Pediatric Oncology Group (POG) randomized trial in 1993 showed superior results with the addition of ifosfamide and etoposide, and this five-drug regimen has become the standard chemotherapeutic approach. Dose intensification and interval compression of therapy are presently being evaluated to improve the outcome of children with Ewing's sarcoma. Although some studies have shown up to a 60% initial tumor response to chemotherapy (with one third of these being complete resolution of the mass),[7] others have not shown as dramatic responses using chemotherapy for the initial management of spinal cord compression. Many centers use chemotherapy in a neurologically stable patient, followed by resection of residual tumor, but they consider surgical resection initially if the patient is losing neurologic function. A significant prognostic factor in Ewing's sarcoma has been shown to be the degree of response of the tumor to initial combination chemotherapy.[4,14] It has been stated that the advantages of preoperative chemotherapy include rendering unresectable neoplasms resectable and that, administered early, it may help eradicate circulating cells and micrometastases.

Patients with spinal, vertebral, and paraspinal Ewing's sarcoma require radiation therapy for local control. The dose of radiation therapy used in the treatment of Ewing's sarcoma in this site generally should be in the region of at least 4500 cGy. The dose can possibly be reduced in patients with small tumors (smaller than 8 cm) and those who have an excellent response to chemotherapy. However, this is still controversial. It is difficult to treat these tumors adequately with standard techniques and also respect the normal tissue tolerance of the spinal cord. Therefore special techniques to focus the radiation very precisely are often indicated to treat these tumors. New techniques such as intensity-modulated radiation therapy (IMRT) and proton therapy may be the means of delivering an adequate dose of radiation to ensure local control and at the same time reduce morbidity.

Local control rates of 100% and 5-year disease-free survival rates of 86% have been reported for nonsacral tumors, whereas for sacral lesions the respective numbers are 63% and 25%. The sacral tumors generally appear later and tend be much larger and less amenable to complete resection. Other studies have not found such a discrepancy between sacral and nonsacral neoplasms.

Surgical indications include those mentioned for all tumors as well as residual disease after chemotherapy and possibly a sacral location. One study found that patients with spinal cord compression caused by Ewing's sarcoma treated by laminectomy survived an average of 3 years longer and had better post-treatment neurologic status than did those treated with chemotherapy or radiation therapy, although the results were not statistically significantly different.[6] Of the surgical patients who were not ambulating independently preoperatively, 85% were able to do so postoperatively.

Sarcomas

Approximately 1% of patients with osteosarcoma have a primary spinal site. In a recent report from the Cooperative Osteosarcoma Study Group, 11 of 22 patients were younger than 18 years of age. Median survival for the whole group was 23 months. Wide resection followed by chemotherapy with or without radiation therapy was associated with a statistically significant increase in survival versus those patients who received a debulking surgical procedure followed by adjuvant therapy.[8] Patients with osteogenic sarcoma develop spinal metastases in approximately 10% of cases and tend to seek treatment late in the course of the disease with spinal cord compression and multiple metastases.[6] The prognosis for these patients is extremely poor. At St. Jude Children's Research Hospital, 11 of 16 patients with metastatic osteosarcoma were not candidates for therapy, because they all had advanced disease and multiple metastases.[6] However, two of the five patients undergoing treatment had laminectomies and both made a significant improvement in neurologic function. The other three were treated with radiation therapy or chemotherapy, and none improved.

Rhabdomyosarcoma accounts for 8% of malignant solid neoplasms in children and arises from immature mesenchymal cells that ultimately are destined to become skeletal muscle. The goals of therapy should be gross-total resection, because prognosis has been shown to be improved with complete resection followed by chemotherapy.[1] Complete surgical margins are difficult to achieve, and radiation therapy is essential in these cases, paying careful attention to the dose and the volume of radiation. Chemotherapy usually includes the classic VAC (vincristine, actinomycin D, and cyclophosphamide) in combination with ifosfamide, etoposide, topotecan, or sometimes, a new experimental agent.

Hematologic Malignancies

Lymphomas may invade the epidural space by way of paraspinal lymphatics, vertebral body involvement, or through the intervertebral foramen. Primary spinal lymphoma is rare, tends to be more common in males, usually originates from the thoracic spine, and has a better prognosis than metastatic lymphoma. Lymphomas are exquisitely chemosensitive and respond dramatically to steroids alone; therefore it is essential that the diagnosis be made and biopsies obtained before the commencement of therapy. Chemotherapy regimens are usually cyclophosphamide based. A common combination includes CHOP (cyclophosphamide, adriamycin, vincristine, prednisone) or BACOP (bleomycin, adriamycin, cyclophosphamide, vincristine, prednisone).[10] Radiation therapy is generally reserved for progressive disease. These tumors are very sensitive to radiation therapy, and treatment generally consists of doses in the range of 3000 to 3600 cGy in fractions of 180 cGy. Surgical intervention is rarely required. The indications for surgery include diagnostic biopsies, recurrent cord compression after maximal radiation therapy and chemotherapy (an unusual event), spinal instability, and vertebral body collapse.

Leukemia can cause epidural masses by invading the epidural fat and connective tissues. In one review, 10 of 44 cases of granulocytic sarcoma (chloroma) of the spine were in patients younger than age 18, most cases being males with acute myelogenous leukemia. Chemotherapy is the treatment of choice, and surgery or radiation therapy are rarely necessary.

CONCLUSION

A multidisciplinary approach is essential in the diagnosis and treatment of children with epidural spinal tumors. Immunohistochemistry and newer molecular genetic techniques are aiding in prompt and accurate diagnoses and allowing the rapid commencement of appropriate surgical intervention or chemotherapy. For many of these tumor groups, newer therapies and options are being explored, including targeting with monoclonal antibodies, adoptive immunotherapy, and different maturational agents. However, spinal involvement remains an oncologic emergency, and prompt therapy, often multimodal, is required to preserve the neurologic function and prevent long-term sequelae.

References

1. Beer S, Menezes A: Primary tumors of the spine in children: natural history, management, and long-term follow-up. Spine 22:649–658, 1997.
2. Ch'ien L, Kalwinsky D, Paterson G, et al: Metastatic epidural tumors in children. Med Pediatr Oncol 10:455–462, 1982.
3. De Bernardi B, Pianca C, Pistamiglio P, et al: Neuroblastoma with symptomatic spinal cord compression at diagnosis: treatment and results with 76 cases. J Clin Oncol 19:183–190, 2001.
4. Jurgens H, Exner U, Gadner H, et al: Multidisciplinary treatment of primary Ewing's sarcoma of bone. A 6-year experience of a European Cooperative Trial. Cancer 61:23–32, 1988.
5. Katzenstein H, Kent P, London W, et al: Treatment and outcome of 83 children with intraspinal neuroblastoma. J Clin Oncol 19:1047–1055, 2001.
6. Klein S, Sanford R, Muhlbauer M: Pediatric spinal epidural metastases. J Neurosurg 74:70–75, 1991.
7. Oberlin O, Patte C, Demeocq F, et al: The response to initial chemotherapy as a prognostic factor in localized Ewing's sarcoma. Eur J Cancer Clin Oncol 21:436–467, 1985.
8. Ozaki T, Flege S, Liljenqvist U, et al: Osteosarcoma of the spine. Cancer 94:1069–1077, 2002.
9. Papagelopoulos P, Peterson H, Ebersold M, et al: Spinal column deformity and instability after lumbar or thoracolumbar laminectomy for intraspinal tumors in children and young adults. Spine 22:442–451, 1997.
10. Perry J, Deodhare S, Bilbao J, et al: The significance of spinal cord compression as the initial manifestation of lymphoma. Neurosurgery 32:157–162, 1993.

11. Pierot L, Boulin A: Percutaneous biopsy of the thoracic and lumbar spine: transpedicular approach under fluoroscopic guidance. AJNR. Am J Neuroradiol 20:23–25, 1999.

12. Plantaz D, Rubie H, Michon J, et al: The treatment of neuroblastoma with intraspinal extension with chemotherapy followed by surgical removal of residual disease. A prospective study of 42 patients: results of the NBL 90 Study of the French Society of Pediatric Oncology. Cancer 78:311–319, 1996.

13. Raffel C: Spinal cord compression by epidural tumors in childhood. Neurosurg Clin North Am 3:925–930, 1992.

14. Rosen G, Marcove R, Caparros B, et al: Primary osteogenic sarcoma: the rationale for preoperative chemotherapy and delayed surgery. Cancer 43:2163–2177, 1979.

15. Sharafuddin MJ, Haddad FS, Hitchon PW, et al: Treatment options in primary Ewing's sarcoma of the spine: report of seven cases and review of the literature. Neurosurgery 30:610–618; discussion 618–619, 1992.

CHAPTER 104

SPINAL COLUMN TUMORS IN PEDIATRIC PATIENTS

Douglas L. Brockmeyer and Wayne M. Gluf

Primary tumors of the spinal column in children are relatively uncommon, constituting less than 1% of all childhood tumors. They demonstrate a wide spectrum of pathologic types and can occur anywhere in the spinal axis. There are three general categories of primary pediatric spinal column tumors: (1) benign primary bone tumors, (2) benign tumors of nonosseous elements, and (3) malignant tumors involving the spine. The initial symptoms of spinal tumors in children depend on a variety of factors, including the patient's age and the tumor type. Patients may be evaluated by either plain radiographs or by several different, but complementary, radiographic modalities.

Defining the appropriate treatment for a specific spinal column tumor in the pediatric population can be difficult and may present unique challenges to the clinician. In general, the goals of treatment are threefold: complete excision of the lesion (when possible), preservation of neurologic function, and consideration of stability in a growing spine. These issues, along with those discussed previously, are the focus of this chapter.

CLINICAL PRESENTATION

The most common symptom for a child with a primary tumor of the spinal column is back pain.[2] It must be understood that back pain is abnormal in children, and continued complaints about it should lead to a radiographic investigation. However, the decision as to what exactly constitutes back pain in children is often difficult to arrive at. Nonverbal infants and toddlers who are unable to convey their symptoms accurately can have the nonspecific symptoms of fussiness, irritability, sleep interruption, and inconsolable crying. These symptoms often lead to delays in diagnosis. Therefore spinal column tumor should be suspected in young children who are just "not well," and a low threshold for radiographic screening should be maintained.

Older children with back pain can communicate their discomfort, and their pain may be interpreted more accurately. But common pitfalls in symptom interpretation still exist. Continued localized back pain not responsive to analgesics or rest should be investigated radiographically. One must first rule out the existence of paraspinous trigger points or myofascial pain syndromes before ordering radiographic studies. Myofascial pain syndromes are fairly common among preadolescents and adolescents. Another caveat is that the pain associated with osteoid osteoma will typically improve dramatically with salicylates.

Children harboring a primary spinal column tumor may also have scoliosis or kyphosis. These children should undergo radiographic investigation. A spinal column tumor should be highly suspected if painful scoliosis is present. Another significant finding is the rapid increase in a kyphoscoliotic curve. Typically, the scoliosis caused by spinal tumors is different from the juvenile idiopathic type, and any deviations should be investigated radiographically.

The last occurring symptom of a spinal column tumor in children is neurologic deficit. Deficits may include sensorimotor, bowel, or bladder changes. The sensorimotor changes can occur in either a myelopathic or radiculopathic pattern depending on the location and size of the tumor.[2] Syrinxes associated with a spinal column tumor may give a suspended sensory or motor level, and paresthesias are not uncommon. The earlier comments regarding preverbal children apply here as well, because sensory changes may lead to bizarre or confusing behavior patterns. In general, any unexplained neurologic deficit in a child should be investigated with an appropriate radiographic study.

RADIOGRAPHIC IMAGING

Plain radiographs of the appropriate area are typically the first imaging study obtained in patients with spinal pain. The radiographic abnormalities seen in spinal tumors can be subtle, and an experienced radiologist is usually called for. These changes may include an increased interpedicular distance or morphologic changes in the pedicle. Plain spine radiographs also allow for the quantification and assessment of kyphoscoliosis. Flexion and extension views of the cervical or lumbar spine (depending on the location of pain) can be obtained to look for spinal instability if that is a concern. Many times, flexion and extension radiographs are critical in making decisions about spinal stability either before or after surgery. In the overall population of spinal tumor patients, plain radiographs are often normal and thus further imaging is required.

If an abnormality is found on the plain spine radiographs, the next study that is typically obtained is a computed tomography (CT) scan through the abnormal area. CT provides excellent information regarding the bone anatomy of the lesion and its surroundings. The lesions may be lytic, blastic, or noninvasive to the surrounding bone. Some information regarding soft tissue anatomy and its involvement by tumor may be gained also. Many times the preoperative CT information is critical in determining the potential stability or instability of a patient's spine after surgery. Similarly, postoperative CT documentation of the extent of bone removal is also important.

Radionucleotide bone scanning can be a useful adjunct in either localizing a lesion in a patient with bone pain or determining if multiple lesions are present. Abnormalities found on bone scan should be followed up with either CT or magnetic resonance imaging (MRI).

The last major imaging modality for children with primary spinal tumors is MRI. When investigating patients who are suspected of having tumor in or around the spine, gadolinium should be administered. Detailed information about the size, nature, and location of the lesion; its enhancement characteristics; and the involvement of surrounding structures can be obtained. Depending on the type of lesion involved, MRI of the entire spinal or neural axis may be recommended to evaluate for other lesions. Postoperative or postadjuvant therapy MRI is also important in documenting the extent of lesion removal or change. Surveillance MRI is the gold standard in following patients with malignant disease.

TUMOR TYPES

Benign Primary Bone Tumors

Osteoid Osteoma and Osteoblastoma

Both benign osteoplastic processes of the spine, osteoid osteoma and osteoblastoma, are distinguished from one another by their size. By definition, osteoid osteomas are less than 1.5 cm in diameter, and osteoblastomas are greater than 1.5 cm in diameter.[3,11,13] They both tend to occur in the cervical or lumbar cancellous posterior elements, particularly the pedicle and lamina. Taken together, these two lesions account for approximately 1% of all primary bone tumors. Osteoid osteomas tend to occur in the second decade of life and osteoblastomas in the third decade. As mentioned previously, the pain they cause is commonly, but not invariably, relieved by salicylates.[2] The pain may ebb and flow and is often worse at night. Painful scoliosis may also occur, especially with osteoblastoma.

The radiographic characteristics of these lesions are similar. On plain radiographs, they demonstrate a lytic bone lesion with a dense, sclerotic border. However, until the sclerotic border forms, the lesions are radiographically not apparent, which may lead to a delay in diagnosis. To assist in making the diagnosis, a bone scan is helpful, because focal uptake of radionucleotide leads to further imaging. CT and MRI typically demonstrate a lesion with a discrete nidus of loose, soft, or granular tumor tissue with a dense, sclerotic border.

Although spontaneous cures have been known to occur, both of these lesions almost always require surgical excision. Complete surgical excision leads to both a cure and resolution of pain for the patient.[2] Excision of an osteoid osteoma is usually a simple matter and rarely requires fusion of the involved level. However, excision of a large osteoblastoma may lead to spinal instability, and management decisions must be made with this in mind.

Osteochondroma

Osteochondroma, the most common benign tumor of bone, arises in any cartilaginously formed part of the skeleton. It especially tends to occur in the diaphyseal ends of long bones. Anywhere between 3% and 7% of osteochondromas occur in the vertebral column.[19] They typically occur in the posterior elements of the thoracic or lumbar spine and rarely occur in the cervical spine. The disease tends to occur in the second decade of life, when growth is most rapid; at that point, the tumor also undergoes rapid growth.

The patient may have local pain, but most often the lesion is silent. Osteochondromas are commonly discovered incidentally and occasionally may be found during palpation of a bony mass on the spinous process. On rare occasions, they produce myelopathic or radicular symptoms by arising from the inner surface of the lamina, pedicle, or vertebral body and causing compression of the neural elements.

Osteochondromas may be very difficult to detect on plain films and appear as a lesion of radiolucency. CT shows a sessile lesion of decreased density surrounded by a cartilaginous cap, which may contain calcifications. Bone scan may demonstrate increased activity, especially during periods of skeletal growth in childhood.

Typically, surgical excision of these lesions is curative. Patients with multiple osteochondromas have an increased incidence (10%) of malignant transformation to osteosarcoma or chondrosarcoma, for which the prognosis is significantly worse.[12]

Aneurysmal Bone Cyst

Aneurysmal bone cysts are benign bone tumors that occur primarily in the second decade of life. Their origins are unclear. They contain a small amount of osteoid tissue with multiple hemosiderin-laden macrophages, multinucleated giant cells, and fibrous tissue. They may occur as solitary lesions or in the presence of another benign or malignant process of bone, such as fibrous dysplasia or giant cell tumor. It has been suggested that these lesions may even be reactive or degenerative in nature.[8] More than half of aneurysmal bone cysts are located in the spine, with an even distribution between the vertebral bodies and the posterior elements. They grow rapidly and, in the process, may strip the periosteum away from bone.

Patients typically complain of local pain and swelling with posteriorly placed lesions and myelopathic or radiculopathic symptoms resulting from cord or root compression with anteriorly placed lesions.

The radiographic appearance of these lesions can be very distinctive, with an eccentrically placed cystic (sometimes multicystic) expansile mass lesion. Plain radiographs will show radiolucent areas with preservation of a thin rim of bone. CT and MRI show a cystic, expansile lesion, perhaps with fluid levels indicative of previous hemorrhage. Arteriography typically demonstrates a very vascular tumor, sometimes involving the soft tissue.

Treatment consists of surgical removal. Preoperative embolization with transarterial or direct delivery of embolic material can be extremely helpful in reducing intraoperative blood loss. Complete excision of these lesions may be very challenging because of intraoperative hemorrhage or difficult-to-access tumor. Incomplete excision is associated with a rather high recurrence rate; therefore every effort must be made for a gross-total removal (Figure 104-1). Because of the risk of malignant transformation, radiation therapy should be reserved only for residual lesions that are in a surgically inaccessible location.

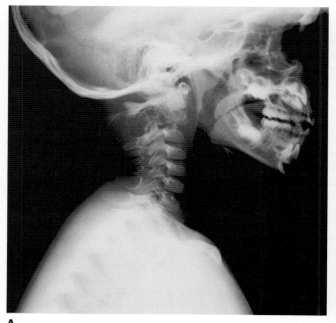

A

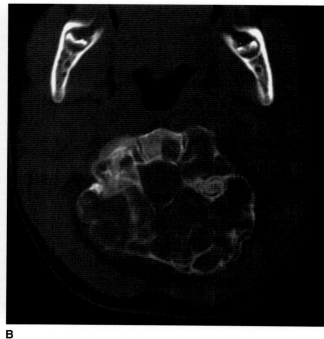

B

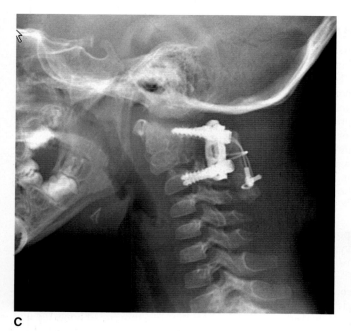

C

FIGURE 104-1 A 4-year-old girl with a large aneurysmal bone cyst involving C2. *A,* Plain lateral cervical spine film demonstrating a large cystic lesion involving C2. *B,* Axial computed tomography slice through C2 depicting the multicystic nature of the lesion. *C,* Postoperative plain lateral cervical spine film showing the extent of lesion resection and instrumentation and fusion used to stabilize the upper cervical spine.

Hemangioma

Hemangiomas of the vertebral body are relatively common, benign lesions in adults and are very rare in children. They consist of normal blood vessels of various sizes, causing a characteristic radiographic appearance of pronounced vertical trabeculae. These tumors may extend into the posterior elements of the spinal column.[2] Hemangiomas have been known to enlarge rapidly during pregnancy or the immediate postpartum period, sometimes associated with a large soft-tissue component.

Painful symptoms occur with the expansion of bone or collapse of a severely involved vertebral level. Surgical intervention is usually not indicated, except in cases of neurologic compromise. Preoperative embolization may be a useful surgical adjunct.

Giant Cell Tumor

Giant cell tumors, otherwise known as *osteoclastomas,* are aggressive, rapidly growing tumors of bone that are rarely found in children. Most giant cell tumors occur in extraspinal locations. In North America they constitute less than 2% of all vertebral tumors, yet in Asian countries they make up almost 20% of primary spinal growths. After discovery in the spine, these benign lesions have been known to spread to remote locations. They typically occur in the vertebral body as an expanding radiolucent mass with clear margins. CT and MRI typically show a large soft-tissue lesion in the vertebral body with a thin periosteal bone margin. Because of their high growth rate, symptoms (pain and neurologic compromise) may progress rapidly.

Surgical removal of these lesions can be very challenging because of their large size. Issues regarding postoperative spinal instability are common and need to be considered in the overall management strategy of the tumor. Radiation may slow the growth of unresectable or residual lesions. Recurrence is possible even with gross-total excision.

Benign Tumors of Nonosseous Elements

Eosinophilic Granuloma

Eosinophilic granulomas arise from the reticuloendothelial system. They are part of the Hand-Schüller-Christian and Letterer-Siwe disease complexes. They are not common and occur in children and adolescents. Minor local pain is usually the initial symptom, but spinal cord or nerve root compression may cause neurologic symptomatology. A lytic lesion in the anterior vertebral body is the most common pathology, with the lesion sometimes leading to complete vertebral body collapse, leaving only the endochondral ossification centers. The radiographic finding associated with this phenomenon is known as *vertebra plana* and represents the end stage of eosinophilic granuloma. However, over time, the collapsed vertebral body may reconstitute itself, depending on the age of the patient and the potential for cancellous bone formation. Older children and adolescents have less of this potential. These lesions may also extend over several vertebral levels and have been known to extend to the posterior spinal elements and ribs.

Radiographs typically demonstrate a lytic bone lesion in the anterior vertebral body that is "cold" on bone scans. CT and MRI show a lytic, soft tissue tumor that may extend into the spinal canal or neural foramen.

Because these lesions invariably heal on their own, surgical excision is reserved for patients who have significant neurologic compromise. Low-dose radiation therapy may be used as well, leading to rapid tumor disappearance.[4,18] In the case of very large lesions that take over the entire vertebral body, radiation therapy may lead to unwanted vertebral collapse and spinal instability. In those cases, prophylactic surgical excision of the lesion and spinal reconstruction may be indicated.

Malignant Tumors Involving the Spine

Ewing's Sarcoma

Ewing's sarcoma is the most common nonprimary malignant tumor involving the spine in children, accounting for approximately 10% of all such lesions. Although originally thought to derive from the reticuloendothelial system, it is now known to derive from neuroectodermal tissue.[15] The cells in question are thought to be from postganglionic parasympathetic tissue, because they can synthesize choline acetyl transferase and have no sympathetic precursors. Grossly, Ewing's sarcomas appear gray, firm, and friable. On histologic inspection, they typically demonstrate primitive cells with hyperchromatic nuclei, little

cytoplasm, and few mitoses. Often there is hemorrhage and necrosis. Occasionally, there are Homer-Wright rosettes and a background of fibrous stroma. Poorly differentiated Ewing's sarcoma demonstrates larger nuclei, more cellular pleomorphism, and a greater number of mitoses when compared with the differentiated variety.

Ewing's sarcoma commonly affects the sacral region, with thoracolumbar lesions seen less often.[5] Cervical lesions are rare but can occur (Figure 104-2). The tumors grow rapidly, producing unremitting nighttime pain and neurologic deficit as the initial symptoms. Because of tumor bulk and the soft tissue involvement, systemic symptoms such as weight loss and fever may also occur. Radiographic studies demonstrate a lytic spine mass with nonsclerotic, poorly defined borders. CT and MRI are used to determine the extent of the lesion and to plan possible surgical therapy.

Surgery, chemotherapy, and if indicated, radiation therapy all play a significant role in the control of Ewing's sarcoma. Although the extent of surgical resection of Ewing's sarcoma has never been proved to improve prognosis, surgery is important in establishing a histologic diagnosis, attempting neural element decompression, and possibly assisting with pain control. Two studies have looked at tumor location, specifically the sacrococcygeal area, as an independent indicator of 5-year survival and have had conflicting results.[5,14] It is well known that it is sometimes difficult, if not impossible, to obtain gross-total resection of a Ewing's sarcoma at the initial surgery. For that reason, a generous biopsy specimen or subtotal debulking is preferable, with a mind toward second-look surgery after chemotherapy and irradiation. If a decompressive multilevel

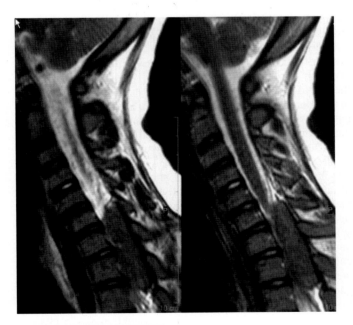

FIGURE 104-2 An 11-year-old boy with an extradural Ewing's sarcoma involving the mid to lower cervical spine. These T2-weighted magnetic resonance images show the extent of intracanal involvement and cord compression. The patient was treated with resection of the tumor therapy and fusion of the involved levels, along with postoperative radiation therapy and chemotherapy.

laminectomy is indicated to achieve neural decompression, it should be performed with the potential risks of spinal instability and kyphosis in mind. Chemotherapy commonly consists of vincristine, dactinomycin, cyclophosphamide, and doxorubicin.[7,20] With aggressive multimodality treatment, a 5-year progression-free survival rate of more than 50% can be anticipated.

Osteosarcoma

Although rare, osteosarcoma, otherwise known as *osteogenic sarcoma*, is still the most common primary malignant tumor of bone. Most cases occur in adults and are related to Paget's disease or prior radiation therapy. Approximately 2% of cases occur in the spine. These tumors are highly malignant and in most cases occur with distant metastases. Vertebral bodies of the lumbosacral spine are typically involved, with significant neurologic deficits present at the time of diagnosis. Total surgical excision of osteosarcoma is usually not possible. The recurrence rate after chemotherapy and radiation therapy is high, and the prognosis is poor.[2]

Lymphoma

Hodgkin's and non-Hodgkin's lymphoma account for approximately 10% of childhood malignancies. When childhood lymphoma involves the spine, it may occur in the vertebral column, intradural-extramedullary space, extradural space, or leptomeningeal compartment. The vertebral body is preferentially involved when spinal column disease is present. Patients experience back pain, neurologic deficit, or signs of systemic illness. A spinal cord compression syndrome is uncommon as a primary sign of disease but occurs commonly in patients with more advanced lymphoma. The estimated overall incidence of spinal cord compression in children with lymphoma is between 1.2% and 7%.[6] Spinal cord symptomatology may occur from growth of extradural, transforaminal, or vertebral body tumor. "Primary" spinal lymphoma, that is, lymphoma localized to the spinal column, has been reported. It typically affects boys in the thoracic spine.[16] It should be noted that the prognosis for patients with primary spinal lymphoma is better than that for patients with metastatic lymphoma with spread to the cord.[17]

Children with spinal column lymphoma typically have a prodrome of back pain before developing neurologic symptomatology. During the prodromal phase, plain radiographs are usually not helpful, because the disease is typically confined to the soft tissues or epidural space. One study found plain radiographs unhelpful in more than two thirds of patients with spinal disease.[9] MRI is the study of choice to determine the nature and extent of involvement of spinal lymphoma. Spinal column lymphoma typically appears hyperdense on T1-weighted images and exhibits variable enhancement with gadolinium. CT can help determine the exact extent of bone involvement in these patients.

The treatment of spinal column lymphoma is controversial. Many reports suggest that surgical decompression of the spinal cord via laminectomy and debulking or complete resection of the tumor is beneficial; other reports state that irradiation and chemotherapy should be the mainstays of treatment for this radiosensitive disease. In general, indications for surgical treatment consist of spinal cord compression with neurologic deficit, especially if it is progressive. Patients with complete paraplegia lasting longer than 24 hours probably have no chance for neurologic recovery following surgical decompression, although the 24-hour guideline is not absolute. Successful chemotherapeutic agents include methotrexate, doxorubicin, and vincristine.

Neuroblastoma

Neuroblastoma is the most common extracranial malignancy in children, accounting for approximately 30% of pediatric spinal tumors and as many as 50% of malignant tumors in neonates.[10] Vertebral column metastases and spinal cord compression from extradural tumor often occur with new-onset disease. These tumors arise in locations near the sympathetic nervous system but are more commonly found in the abdomen; approximately 40% of these tumors arise from the adrenal gland. Radiographic evidence of spinal cord compression is present in more than 10% of patients who have neuroblastoma. Several studies have shown that neuroblastoma in children may spontaneously regress or at least transform into a less malignant histologic type.[1] Neuroblastoma may arise within the spinal canal or result from the spread of tumor from intra-abdominal or paravertebral masses. It can also spread hematogenously or through the lymphatic system. Paraspinous or sympathetically derived tumors tend to involve the vertebral body or grow intraforaminally in a dumbbell shape and commonly result in spinal cord compression. Adrenally derived tumor also tends to involve the vertebral body, but spinal cord involvement is not common.

Patients typically have pain from epidural nerve root involvement. More significant compression of the spinal cord leads to myelopathy and paraparesis or paraplegia. Plain spinal radiographs are positive in approximately 60% of patients at diagnosis. Findings include an increased interpeduncular distance, with destruction of the pedicles, marked enlargement of the intravertebral foramen or foramina, scalloping of the vertebral body, and possibly calcification in the paraspinous region involving the tumor. MRI shows an intermediate-intensity lesion on T1-weighted images, with avid enhancement of gadolinium. MRI is the imaging study of choice in patients with neuroblastoma. CT may be helpful in determining the extent of bone involvement.

The diagnosis of neuroblastoma encompasses several laboratory tests. Urinalysis shows increased levels of at least two catecholamine derivatives, including homovanillic acid, vanillylmandelic acid, dopamine, or norepinephrine. The histologic appearance of the tumor is remarkable for eosinophilia, paranuclear halos, and cellular pleomorphism. The tumor's gross appearance is a well-encapsulated fleshy mass.

The treatment of neuroblastoma involves surgical decompression of the spinal cord in cases where there is significant pain or neurologic deficit, along with multiagent chemotherapy. Results with radiation have been inconsistent. More extensive, or even staged, procedures are required for patients with large tumor masses. Often, the latter of the staged procedures are performed after at least one round of chemotherapy. The prognosis for patients diagnosed with neuroblastoma depends on the tumor stage, the site of the tumor, and age at diagnosis. Patients older than 1 year with advanced disease or with adrenally derived tumors have a much worse prognosis than children younger than 1 year or with nonadrenally derived tumors. Several serum or genetic markers, such as C-myc amplification, may also be prognostic.

Chordoma

Chordomas are rare lesions in children resulting from malignant transformation of embryonic notochordal elements. They arise either in the sacrococcygeal or clival area and can cause significant neurologic deficits. Radiologic imaging reveals a lesion that destroys and replaces bone. Foamy, physaliphorous cells predominate on histology and are pathognomonic of the lesion. Complete surgical resection of these lesions is often extremely difficult to achieve, and postoperative radiation therapies consisting of proton beam or other heavy ion treatments are commonly employed. Local control can be achieved in some cases, but in most cases the clinical course is rapidly progressive and fatal.

References

1. Balakrishan V, Rice MS, Simpson DA: Spinal neuroblastomas. J Neurosurg 40:631–638, 1974.
2. Beer SJ, Menezes AH: Primary tumors of the spine in children: natural history, management, and long-term follow-up. Spine 22:649–659, 1997.
3. Brockmeyer D et al: Nine-year-old female with neck pain. Pediatr Neurosurg 28:320–325, 1998.
4. Green NE, Robertson WW, Kilroy AW: Eosinophilic granuloma of the spine with associated neural deficit. J Bone Joint Surg Am 62:1198–1202, 1980.
5. Grubb MR et al: Primary Ewing's sarcoma of the spine. Spine 19:309–313, 1994.
6. Herman TS: Involvement of the central nervous system by non-Hodgkins lymphoma. Cancer 43:390–397, 1979.
7. Kissane JM et al: Ewing's sarcoma of bone. Hum Pathol 14:773–779, 1983.
8. Lichtenstein L: Aneurysmal bone cyst. In Lichtenstein L (ed): Bone Tumors. St. Louis, Mosby, 1977.
9. MacVicar D, Williams MP: CT scanning in epidural lymphoma. Clin Radiol 43:95–102, 1991.
10. Mayfield JK, Riseborough EJ, Jaffe H, et al: Spinal deformity in children treated for neuroblastoma. J Bone Joint Surg Am 63:183–193, 1981.
11. McLeod RA, Dahlin DC, Beabout JW: The spectrum of osteoblastoma. AJR Am Roentgenol 126:321–335, 1976.
12. Palmer FJ, Blum PW: Osteochondroma with spinal cord compression. J Neurosurg 52:845, 1980.
13. Pettine KA, Klassen RA: Osteoid-osteoma and osteoblastoma of the spine. J Bone Joint Surg Am 68:354–361, 1986.
14. Pilepich MV et al: Ewing's sarcoma of the vertebral column. Int J Radiat Oncol Biol Phys 7:27–31, 1981.
15. Pizzo PA, Poplack DG: Principles and Practice of Pediatric Oncology. Philadelphia, Lippincott-Raven, 1997.
16. Raco A, Cervoni L, Salvat M, et al: Primary spinal epidural non-Hodgkin's lymphomas in childhood: a review of 6 cases. Acta Neurochir 139:526–528, 1997.
17. Rao TV, Narayanaswamy KS, Shankar SK, et al: "Primary" spinal epidural lymphomas. Acta Neurochir 62:307–317, 1982.
18. Seimon LP: Eosinophil granuloma of the spine. J Pediatr Orthop 1:371–376, 1981.
19. Storrs BB: Spinal column tumors. In Albright L, Pollack I, Adelson D (ed): Principles and Practice of Pediatric Neurosurgery. New York, Thieme, 1999.
20. Zucker JM et al: Intensive systemic chemotherapy in localized Ewing's sarcoma in childhood. Cancer 52:415–423, 1983.

CHAPTER 105

PEDIATRIC INTRADURAL AND EXTRAMEDULLARY SPINAL CORD TUMORS

John C. Wellons III and W. Jerry Oakes

In 1888 Sir William Macewen, a Scottish neurosurgeon and well-known pioneer in the field of craniospinal surgery, reported the removal of five extradural spinal tumors via laminectomy in a lecture to the Glasgow Medical Society. The first patient, a 9-year-old boy, underwent surgical resection in 1882. All but one patient (who died) made a significant degree of functional recovery.[25] In 1887 Sir Victor Horsley, another pioneer in the field, successfully removed the first intradural, extramedullary spinal cord tumor, which had been initially diagnosed by Sir William Gowers.[8] Today's neurosurgeon, aided in diagnosis by magnetic resonance imaging (MRI) and in resection by modern microneurosurgical techniques, continues to redefine and improve the body of knowledge regarding pediatric spinal cord tumors. The pre-MRI literature reports the incidence of spinal cord tumors at up to 2.5 per 100,000 people and from 3 to 12 times less common than brain tumors in the general population.[1] With the advantage of MRI, spinal cord tumors are now thought to make up 15% of primary central nervous system (CNS) tumors.[18] In the general population, intradural extramedullary tumors tend to occur more commonly with radiculopathy or motor weakness.[1,12] Children tend to have less specific symptoms than adults (e.g., irritability, weight loss) as well as scoliosis, gait problems (either decompensation or inability to achieve milestones), and bowel or bladder disturbances.[1,2] Children more commonly have multiple-level involvement than adults, and an increased frequency of multiple levels is seen in patients with neurofibromatosis.[1] Extramedullary lesions tend to be a slightly different group in children than in adults, with lesions such as dermoids and epidermoids being relatively more common in children.[2] The following tumors are examples that are found in the intradural, extramedullary space in children. Primary treatment in all cases is judicious surgical extirpation.

MYXOPAPILLARY EPENDYMOMA

Myxopapillary ependymomas occur in the cauda equina and directly involve the filum terminale. Extension may occur into the conus medullaris, along the nerve roots, or through the subarachnoid space. The most common initial symptom in children with myxopapillary ependymoma is an exacerbation of low-back pain, but other symptoms include lower extremity weakness, numbness or pain, difficulty with ambulation, and bowel or bladder incontinence.[34] Symptoms of 13 months, and up to 18 months, have been reported before diagnosis, most commonly the result of the difficulty young children have in describing and localizing the pain or problem.[5,13]

Patients with myxopapillary ependymomas tend to seek treatment in their third or fourth decade.[34] Up to 50% of all spinal ependymomas in adults are myxopapillary ependymomas, but this number is reduced in children to 8% to 14%.[13,34] Chan et al report that 7 of 14 spinal ependymomas treated during a 62-year period at The Hospital for Sick Children in Toronto were histologically proved myxopapillary ependymomas.[5] Again, of the eight spinal ependymomas that St. Jude's hospital in Memphis treated between 1974 and 1999, four were myxopapillary ependymomas.[30] Twenty-eight percent of all spinal ependymomas, both in adults and children, treated by Gagliardi et al were localized to the filum terminale, and 12% of these were in children.[13]

The imaging technique of choice is MRI with and without contrast. The most common imaging characteristic is that of a sausage-shape lesion within the cauda equina, isointense on T1- and hyperintense on T2-weighted MRI. Enhancement with intravenous gadolinium does occur[35] (Figure 105-1). If the child is unable to lie still for the procedure, sedation is warranted. If contraindications to MRI exist, computed tomography (CT) myelography is the next choice.

Histologically, myxopapillary ependymoma appears as a "sheet-like arrangement of epithelial cells" that is interrupted by pools of mucin-containing blood vessels. The tumor cells can "extend elongated cellular processes to the margins of these bloated fibrovascular cores," which may give the tumor a "ragged appearance" on microscopic examination.[29] Immunohistochemistry tends to mirror other central nervous system ependymomas that weakly stain positive for glial fibrillary acidic protein (GFAP). Cytokeratin, S-100, and epithelial membrane antigen (EMA) have also been reported in ependymomas in general but are not common.[29]

The literature would support that outcome from these tumors for children tends to be excellent under the circumstances of either (1) a gross-total resection (GTR), or (2) a subtotal resection followed by local radiation therapy. Myxopapillary ependymomas are amenable to resection when they are separate from the conus medullaris and surrounding nerve

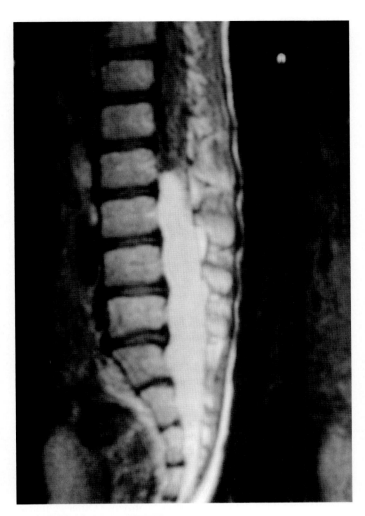

FIGURE 105-1 Sagittal T1-weighted lumbar magnetic resonance image with gadolinium enhancement revealing a myxopapillary ependymoma below the conus medullaris.

roots. On occasion, the filum may be sectioned above and below the tumor and the lesion lifted out *en bloc* with minimal subarachnoid dissection. Not uncommonly, there are dense adhesions between the lesion and surrounding nerve roots, making determination of origin and safe resection difficult. If the lesion is integrated within the conus medullaris, judgment should be exercised. Gross-total excision may cure the patient but may be inadvisable to undertake given the substantial risk of bowel or bladder problems postoperatively.

Because of the control achieved with radiation therapy (XRT), tumor may be left in an effort to preserve neurologic function.[30] In this setting, local irradiation is warranted.[14] If a GTR is thought to have occurred, serial imaging only and no adjuvant therapy would be called for. Yoshii et al report that no benefit is incurred with XRT after a GTR in the adult population.[47] Few publications are found in the literature speaking directly to this topic. Chan et al, who treated seven children, found that the two patients who underwent a GTR of the lesion followed by radiation therapy each continued to be "alive and well" at 1- and 17-year follow-up, respectively. The five other

children underwent "gross total resection" followed by no postoperative radiation therapy. Of these, two had recurrence in the spine and received reoperation. One received postoperative irradiation. Another in this group recurred intracranially (suprasellar region) and received radiation therapy only. All remain "alive and well" at the time of article publication, with follow-up ranging from 2 months to 17 years.[5]

Gagliardi et al report four children who underwent tumor resection, two of whom underwent GTR and had no recurrence. Of the other two with subtotal resections, one then underwent postoperative radiation therapy and the other did not. That patient underwent a secondary operation for tumor recurrence 3 years after the first operation. All four children were alive at the time of publication (mean 6.5 years).[13] Nagib and O'Fallon report that all three of their patients underwent a GTR, but that one tumor recurred away from the initial tumor bed and received a "piecemeal" resection. This child received a GTR at second surgery followed by radiation therapy. All three patients at follow-up remain tumor-free (30, 32, and 36 months, respectively).[34] Merchant et al reviewed four children with myxopapillary ependymomas and reported that all four received a subtotal resection followed by postoperative radiation therapy. Craniospinal irradiation is mentioned as being given to three of the patients, all of whom had subarachnoid dissemination. Chemotherapy (4-hydroxycyclophosphamide, carboplatin, and topotecan) was given to two of these children, both of whom also had radiation therapy. One died 7 months after diagnosis, and the others remained tumor free.[30] Finally, Scott also reports the successful treatment of a 17-year-old male with a myxopapillary ependymoma with a subtotal resection followed by radiation to the area.[40]

Myxopapillary ependymomas do occur in children, albeit rarely, and tend to have longer symptomatology, which tends to focus more on an exacerbation of long-standing lower back pain. Treatment consists of a reasonably aggressive surgical excision with radiation therapy reserved for local treatment in the event of a subtotal resection. Further surgical resection for recurrences has been successful, as has radiation therapy for later related intracranial masses. At this time chemotherapy or further experimental therapy play a questionable role in management.

MENINGIOMA

Large pediatric spinal meningioma series do not exist in the literature. Spinal cord meningiomas tend to occur more commonly in the adult population, reaching up to 46% of spinal neoplasms.[16] In adults, these lesions tend to appear in the dorsal or lateral thoracic intradural extramedullary space and are amenable to surgical resection.[16] In children, these rare lesions tend to occur in the cervical or thoracic region and have a less typical pattern.[20,33,46] Meningioma occurrence in the lumbosacral area is the least common but not unheard of.[23] Spinal meningiomas may occur not only in the intradural, extramedullary space (83%) but also in the extradural space (14%) and intradural, intramedullary space (3%).[16] A clear association exists between neurofibromatosis type 2 and spinal meningiomas.[26,38]

Because spinal cord meningiomas occur more commonly in the cervical or thoracic spine, myelopathy, spasticity, and paraplegia or quadriplegia are the most common symptoms in addition to pain. Once again, the pain in children is often difficult for them to characterize, contributing to diagnostic delay. Often, prolonged courses of delayed gait development, gait regression, or gradual weakness developing over 3 to 6 months are reported.[20,23,46] In adults, meningiomas tend to more commonly cause localized radicular pain in addition to weakness.[16] Otherwise, sensory disturbances or bowel and bladder dysfunction may be identified as well.

Spinal meningiomas, like intracranial meningiomas, are rare in children. Sheikh et al report that the incidence of the latter is approximately 2% of all pediatric brain tumors.[42] In a large series of intraspinal tumors in children, DeSousa et al found only 3 of 81 were meningiomas.[9] In 1964, before the advent of MRI, Slooff et al reported that of the 337 total spinal meningiomas his group encountered in patients age 0 to 80 years and older, only 0.6% (2 patients) fell in the age group 0 to 9 years and 1.5% (5 patients) occurred in the age group 10 to 19 years.[43] Constantini and Epstein report 2.4% in a combined review of the New York University pediatric experience and previous published studies.[7] Interestingly, Grant and Austin report that an unusual 17% of pediatric spinal tumors encountered in their 1956 study were meningiomas.[17]

MRI provides the most useful radiologic examination. Typically, these tumors appear isointense on T1- and T2-weighted sequencing and commonly are enhanced with gadolinium administration. The presence of a dural tail or enhanced dura adjacent to the lesion makes spinal meningioma a suspect but does not confirm it.[35]

In adults, spinal meningiomas tend to be either psammomatous, meningothelial, or fibroblastic, with the former being the most common.[1,16,29] The few reports of pediatric spinal meningiomas that do mention histology indicate psammomatous and meningotheliomatous patterns as well as malignant meningioma.[20,23,33] The hallmark of psammomatous meningiomas is the presence of a cellular whorl growth pattern with central psammoma bodies.[29] Meningothelial meningiomas, also known as syncytial meningiomas, are characterized by large nucleoli surrounded by polygonal cytoplasmic borders. Intranuclear cytoplasmic inclusions or whorl formations may appear as well.[29] Increased cellularity and the presence of mitotic figures push the diagnosis to one of malignancy.[23] Immunohistochemically, the majority of meningiomas stain positive for EMA and vimentin. S-100, cytokeratins, and carcinoembryonic antigen (CEA) may also be identified.[29]

Surgical resection is the mainstay of therapy for these lesions. The typical approach is through a multilevel posterior laminectomy or laminoplasty using microsurgical techniques (Figure 105-2). Intraoperative ultrasound may assist with limiting the number of bone levels removed. Critical surgical concepts include early separation of the meningioma from its dural-based blood supply and, in the setting of ventral or lateral-based lesions, minimizing iatrogenic spinal cord damage through aggressive debulking of the exposed tumor in lieu of cord retraction. This then allows the tumor to come into the exposed field rather than risking paraplegia or other neurologic compromise.

Radiation appears to have been used in the cases of recurrence and following a secondary debulking if possible. Gezen et al surgically resected 36 spinal cord meningiomas in adults. Two recurred at 5 and 8 years postoperatively and underwent re-resection followed by radiation therapy. Neither had re-

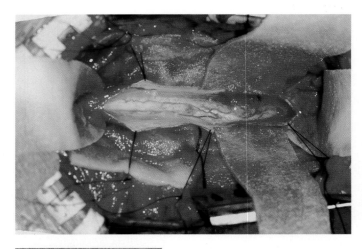

FIGURE 105-2 Intraoperative photograph of a meningioma arising from a dorsal thoracic rootlet and impinging on the spinal cord.

recurred at the time of publication.[16] Tumor recurrence also appears to be related to subtotal resection. In a 1996 study, Klekamp and Samii reported that all adult patients with partially removed spinal meningiomas had recurrence within 5 years of initial surgical resection and that only 84% of tumors believed to be totally resected recurred in that time frame. Of the 88 patients, 10 were noted to have clinical recurrence. No mention was made of any other therapy other than secondary resection at the time of recurrence.[22] In DeSousa et al, 3 of 81 spinal tumors were meningiomas, and 2 recurred (1 cervical and 1 filum terminale meningioma). Both patients were given "palliative radiation therapy" and apparently showed no improvement. One died 6 years after treatment.[9] Other pediatric case reports have inadequate follow-up periods to judge recurrence and make no mention of adjuvant therapy.[20,33,46] Of note, Liu et al do report a malignant spinal meningioma filling the subarachnoid space from the thoracic to sacral area in a 3-year-old male. He underwent biopsy followed by craniospinal irradiation. Only 3 months of follow-up were reported.[23] Few long-term studies examining recurrence exist in either the adult or pediatric literature. Recurrences range from 1.3% to 32%.[16] For cranial and spinal meningiomas, 15-year recurrence rates for adult and pediatric patients with subtotal resections approach 90%.[31] The vast majority of symptomatic patients show progressive improvement after surgical removal. After an adequate recovery period, serial imaging should be performed. Recurrence of symptoms or other localizing signs to the spinal cord should prompt repeat MRI and further treatment.

Pediatric spinal cord meningiomas are rare, but the treatment may be extrapolated from the adult literature. They do tend to be less typical in their location but are still responsive to surgical therapy. If the tumors do not easily dissect from the surrounding spinal cord or nerve root (excluding the thoracic region), consideration should be given to the preservation of neurologic function and the performance of a subtotal resection. This caution should be tempered, however, with the knowledge of the high likelihood of recurrence in this setting. Subtotal resections are more likely to recur and are treatable by secondary resection. There are insufficient data to recommend radiation therapy for anything other than symptomatic unresectable recurrent lesions or meningiomas of malignant histology.

NEUROFIBROMA AND SCHWANNOMA

Intradural extramedullary neurofibromas and schwannomas are considered together here; differences are emphasized when appropriate. Although sporadically occurring spinal schwannomas exist, most of these lesions in children are associated with the autosomal dominant hereditary disorder neurofibromatosis.[19,21] The reader is referred to Chapter 108, Neurocutaneous Syndromes, for further details on the diagnostic criteria and associated central nervous system lesions found in neurofibromatosis type 1 (NF1) and neurofibromatosis type 2 (NF2). Neurofibromas and schwannomas make up nearly 4% to 11% of spinal cord tumors in published pediatric series.[7,9] Both neurofibromas and schwannomas appear in the cervical, thoracic, and lumbosacral spine; occur for the most part on dorsal sensory roots; and may be found at multiple levels in the same patient.[19,21,29,45]

Neurofibromas found in the syndrome of NF1 may be peripheral or paraspinous in origin and fusiform or plexiform in nerve or root involvement.[10,38] NF1 affects 1 in 3000 to 4000 people and is inherited in an autosomal dominant pattern, with nearly 50% of the cases caused by spontaneous mutation.[38] Intradural extramedullary neurofibromas occur in nearly 20% of patients with NF1.[11,35] Most paraspinous neurofibromas are fusiform.[38] Multiple nerve roots may be involved, and often, surgical exposure for single lesions reveals multiroot neurofibromas not seen on imaging (Figure 105-3).

NF2, once primarily known as central neurofibromatosis, occurs in 1 in 50,000 people.[18,19] Extracranial involvement is common, and this includes the presence of nerve root schwannomas. These tend to arise from a single nerve root, be well circumscribed, and be amenable to resection.[10,38] A propensity toward the lumbar region may exist, but all levels of spinal involvement have been noted.[29]

Both of these slow-growing lesions may enlarge to surprising dimensions, causing a great degree of spinal cord displacement before becoming symptomatic. Symptoms tend to be similar to other intradural, extramedullary lesions; however, radicular pain may occur more often because of nerve root involvement.

A classic radiographic finding of neurofibromas and schwannomas on plain lateral spine roentgenograms is the trumpeting, or widening, of the involved neural foramen. The lesions take on a dumbbell shape because of the intradural extramedullary component of the tumor, the foraminal portion more limited in its growth, and an extradural paraspinal portion. On T1-weighted MRI, neurofibromas and schwannomas tend to be isointense and are brightly enhanced with contrast.[35]

Whereas schwannomas tend to be separate lesions from the nerve, stretching most of the originating nerve over its encapsulated mass, neurofibromas tend to involve the entire nerve with a "hyperplasia of the schwannian and fibroblastic supporting elements of the nerve."[37] The schwannoma consistency and organizational pattern may be either spindle-shaped with compact, parallel alignment (Antoni A tissue) or loose, edematous cells in an irregular pattern separated by microcystic and mucinous regions (Antoni B tissue).[29] Schwannomas will stain positive for the immunohistochemical marker S-100.[29]

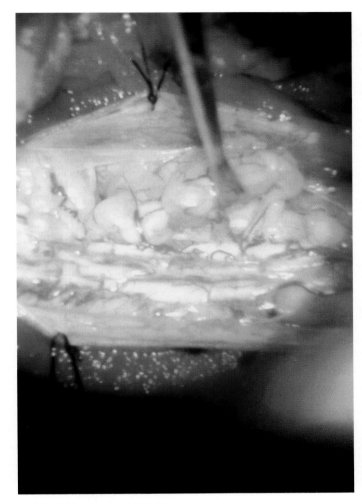

FIGURE 105-3 Intraoperative photograph of multiple spinal intradural, extramedullary neurofibromas through a midline laminectomy.

Symptomatic lesions or large asymptomatic lesions with significant spinal encroachment may be removed generally through a midline laminectomy. Smaller intradural lesions without significant cord compression or solely extradural, paraspinous lesions (with rare exception) are left alone and observed.[38] Despite dermatomal overlap, resection of even small lesions is associated with some sensory loss at that level. The involved sensory root or rootlet will need to be manipulated frequently during an operation, potentially resulting in either direct injury to the involved nerve or indirect injury from damage to the microvasculature and resulting infarction. For the large paraspinous components of the dumbbell lesions, tumor may be followed into the foramen and resected, or a more complex extraspinal approach may be incorporated.[15,28,39]

Any benefit of the addition of traditional radiation therapy to the surgical treatment of these lesions, either initially or with recurrences, is unknown but unlikely. Malignant schwannomas have been known to form in regions of previous radiation therapy.[44] Chemotherapy for neurofibromas is reserved for progressive unresectable symptomatic plexiform neurofibromas with inconsistent benefit. Past alternative treatments in early clinical trials include antihistamines, maturation agents, or antiangiogenic drugs (ketotifen fumarate, cis-retinoic acid, interferon-alpha, thalidomide, or oral farnesyl protein transferase inhibitor) and have unproven results. Of these, tumor growth may have stopped or slowed, but no study has demonstrated a decrease in tumor size of greater than 50% on imaging.[36] New directions offer treatment on a cellular and molecular level that involve genetic-targeted therapy or cytokines thought crucial in tumor growth.[36] Clinical trials are ongoing. Malignant schwannomas have also been treated solely with chemotherapy with poor results. In combination with surgery, however, chemotherapy may increase survival for patients with these aggressive lesions.[6,44]

The recurrence of symptoms should be a concern for either regrowth of the resected lesion, which is more likely in the setting of a partially resected tumor (remaining paraspinous component), or enlargement of an adjacent lesion. These children may already be undergoing an imaging regimen and certainly should be followed with serial imaging postoperatively. The role of adjuvant therapy for these children in this setting is not known.

The vast majority of neurofibromas and schwannomas are associated with NF1 and NF2. The intradural extramedullary space is the most common spinal region for these to occur. In the absence of symptoms or significant radiologic cord compression, these lesions are usually observed. Symptoms are those of spinal cord compression in addition to radicular pain, and treatment consists of surgical resection through a laminectomy with or without a more aggressive approach to any extradural, paraspinous involvement. Radiation or chemotherapy as primary or adjuvant therapy has been performed, but its contribution is not clear. Future therapies targeted at the molecular, cellular, and even genetic abnormalities may prove to be efficacious.

DERMOID AND EPIDERMOID

Dermoids and epidermoids (also referred to as *dermoid* and *epidermoid cysts*) make up a small subsection of pediatric spinal cord tumors. Constantini and Epstein report an incidence of a little more than 6% in an analysis of their own series and the current literature.[7] DeSousa et al found that 8 of 81 (9.8%) children with spinal cord tumors had either a dermoid or epidermoid.[9] Predictably, as age demographics increase, the relative incidence of these two lesions decreases as the number of other intradural, extramedullary lesions seen in adulthood increases (e.g., meningioma and schwannoma).[1]

Intraspinal dermoids and epidermoids tend to remain extramedullary and gradually displace the neural elements as they enlarge. Rare lesions may directly invade the spinal cord. These lesions tend to occur in the lumbosacral area[3,24,29] and are also associated with dermal sinus tracts that are noticed either on physical inspection after birth or with recurring bouts of meningitis.[32,41] These lesions have also occurred many years after a lumbar puncture with a hollow needle and no stylet during which a small plug of epidermis is deposited within the spinal canal.[4,9] Dermoids and epidermoids are also well-known lesions in the spina bifida population and occur years after closure of the myelomeningocele if small dermal elements are included within the repair.[24,27,41]

In the non–spina bifida population, these lesions cause motor or sensory problems as well as bowel or bladder distur-

bances. Pain along the spine, especially at night, is worrisome, as well as long-standing irritability, decreased ability to walk, or development of scoliosis.[3,32] In the spina bifida population, loss of baseline sensation, motor ability (declining ambulation or upper extremity weakness), or bowel or bladder function (including multiple urinary tract infections) in the face of a functioning shunt is worrisome for development of a tethered cord. The presence of a dermoid or epidermoid in this setting must be ruled out with imaging.[3,27]

Dermoids are hyperintense on T1-weighted MRI and usually hypointense on T2-weighted imaging, depending on the intracystic contents. No enhancement is seen. Epidermoids tend to be hypointense on T1- and hyperintense on T2-weighted imaging, similar to cerebrospinal fluid (CSF).[35] In the differentiation of arachnoid cysts versus epidermoids, diffusion-weighted MRI or fluid-attenuated inversion recovery (FLAIR) sequencing may be performed. With diffusion-weighted imaging, epidermoids will have more restrictive flow than arachnoid cysts because of the intracystic contents. In FLAIR sequencing, CSF collections will have similar density to the CSF in the ventricular system, whereas epidermoids will not.

Microscopically, intraspinal dermoid cysts are lined by simple squamous epithelium and include dermis that may contain hair follicles, hair, sebaceous glands, oil, and other skin appendages indicative of dermal inclusion. Epidermoids are lined by compound squamous epithelium and grow via the accumulation of keratin.[29]

If a dermal sinus tract is present, this lesion must be circumferentially excised and the tract followed through the muscle fascia and into the thecal sac. The lesion may then end in the intradural, extramedullary space or extend into the spinal cord itself. Removal of the cyst must be done in a way to minimize spillage of cyst contents into the subarachnoid space. This material may be caustic and may cause symptomatic chemical meningitis.[24] The periphery, or wall, of the lesion should be carefully peeled from the surrounding structures. However, if the wall is not easily freed from the adjacent neural tissue, conventional wisdom suggests a subtotal resection rather than risk neurologic compromise. For spina bifida patients who have been identified for surgical exploration and resection of a presumed dermoid or epidermoid, the approach should be similar to that for a tethered cord, with recognition of the abnormal anatomy and limited resection capability. In the setting of recurrence in either population, a secondary resection may be undertaken with the knowledge of increased risk of neurologic compromise with overaggressive resection. Neither radiation therapy nor chemotherapy plays a role in the treatment of these lesions.

Bailey reports only one patient with recurrence in 10 dermoids operated on who has worsened neurologically, and Lunardi et al report that 10 of 16 adult patients returned to a normal working life.[3,24] In the spina bifida population, the long-term outcome is less certain, and Scott et al report a more significant rate of symptom fluctuation and hospitalization.[41]

Dermoid and epidermoid tumors tend to be cystic and occur in the lumbosacral area near the conus medullaris and cauda equina. Along with their incidence in the general pediatric population, they are a well-defined entity in children with spina bifida who may fare less well in long-term outcome. Judicious surgical resection continues to be the only known manner of treatment. Patients should undergo reimaging if symptoms recur.

CONCLUSION

Surgical resection remains the treatment of choice for both primary and recurrent intradural, extramedullary spinal cord tumors. Because of the benign tendency of these lesions, postoperative local irradiation plays a role in situations of either residual myxopapillary ependymomas after a subtotal resection or after a re-resection of a recurred spinal meningioma. Successful adjuvant therapy for schwannomas or neurofibromas may lie in a genetic or molecular-based attack on the underpinnings of NF1 or NF2. It is reasonable to attempt salvage chemotherapy or radiation therapy in malignant or unresectable lesions. Dermoid or epidermoid cysts should be resected in a manner to not harm the underlying neural tissue. A high degree of suspicion of tumor should be held for a child with spina bifida who has worsening neurologic function in the face of a functioning ventricular shunt. Initially, serial postoperative imaging may play a role in all of these lesions and certainly in the setting of symptomatic recurrence. In general, chances remain excellent for a good long-term functional outcome.

References

1. Alter M: Statistical aspects of spinal cord tumors. In Vinken PJ, Bruyn GH (eds): Handbook of Clinical Neurology. Amsterdam, North-Holland, 1975.
2. Anderson FM, Carson MJ: Spinal cord tumors in children. A review of the subject and presentation of twenty-one cases. J Pediatr 43:190–207, 1953.
3. Bailey IC: Dermoid tumors of the spinal cord. J Neurosurg 33:676–681, 1970.
4. Batnitzky S, Keucher TR, Mealey J, et al: Iatrogenic intraspinal epidermoid tumors. JAMA 237:148–150, 1977.
5. Chan HSL, Becker LE, Hoffman HJ, et al: Myxopapillary ependymoma of the filum terminale and cauda equina in childhood: report of seven cases and review of the literature. Neurosurgery 14:204–210, 1984.
6. Chandler CL, Uttley D, Wilkins PR, et al: Primary spinal malignant schwannoma. Br J Neurosurg 8:341–345, 1994.
7. Constantini S, Epstein FJ: Intraspinal tumors in infants and children. In Youmans JR (ed): Neurological Surgery, 4th ed. Vol 4. Philadelphia, WB Saunders, 1996.
8. Critchley, M: Sir William Gowers, 1845–1915: A biographical appreciation. London, Heinemann, 1949.
9. DeSousa AL, Kalsbeck JE, Mealy J, et al: Intraspinal tumors in children: a review of 81 cases. J Neurosurg 51:437–445, 1979.
10. Donner TR, Voorhies RM, Kline DG: Neural sheath tumors of major nerves. J Neurosurg 81:362–373, 1994.
11. Egelhoff JC, Bates DJ, Ross JS, et al: Spinal MR findings in neurofibromatosis types 1 and 2. AJNR 13:1071–1077, 1990.
12. El-Mahdy W, Kane PJ, Powell MP, et al: Spinal intradural tumours: part I—extramedullary. Br J Neurosurg 13:550–557, 1999.
13. Gagliardi M, Cervoni L, Domenicucci M, et al: Ependymomas of the filum terminale in childhood: report of four cases and review of the literature. Childs Nerv Syst 9:3–6, 1993.
14. Garcia DM: Primary spinal cord tumors treated with surgery and postoperative irradiation. Int J Radiat Oncol Biol Phys 11:1933–1939, 1985.
15. George B, Lot G: Neurinomas of the first two cervical nerve roots: a series of 42 cases. J Neurosurg 82:917–923, 1995.
16. Gezen F, Kahraman S, Canakci Z, et al: Review of 36 cases of spinal cord meningioma. Spine 25:727–731, 2000.
17. Grant FC, Austin GM: The diagnosis, treatment, and prognosis of tumors affecting the spinal cord in children. J Neurosurg 13:535–545, 1956.
18. Greenberg MS: Handbook of Neurosurgery. Lakeland, Fla, Greenberg Graphics, 1994.
19. Halliday AL, Sobel RA, Martuza RL: Benign spinal nerve sheath tumors: their occurrence sporadically and in neurofibromatosis types 1 and 2. J Neurosurg 74:248–253, 1991.
20. Kaya U, Ozden B, Turantan MI, et al: Spinal epidural meningioma in childhood: a case report. Neurosurgery 10:746–747, 1982.
21. Kim P, Ebersold MJ, Onofrio BM, et al: Surgery of spinal nerve schwannoma. J Neurosurg 71:810–814, 1989.
22. Klekamp J, Samii M: Surgical results of spinal meningiomas. Acta Neurochir 65:77–81, 1996.
23. Liu HC, De Armond SJ, Edwards MSB: An unusual spinal meningioma in a child: case report. Neurosurgery 17:313–316, 1985.
24. Lunardi P, Missori P, Gagliardi FM, et al: Long-term results of the surgical treatment of spinal dermoid and epidermoid tumors. Neurosurgery 25:860–864, 1989.
25. Macewen W: An address on the surgery of the brain and spinal cord. Br Med J 2:302–309, 1888.
26. Mautner VF, Lindenau M, Baser ME, et al: The neuroimaging and clinical spectrum of neurofibromatosis 2. Neurosurgery 38:880–886, 1996.
27. Mazzola CA, Albright AL, Sutton LN, et al: Dermoid inclusion cysts and early spinal cord tethering after fetal surgery for myelomeningocele. N Engl J Med 347:256–259, 2002.
28. McCormick PC: Surgical management of dumbbell and paraspinal tumors or the thoracic and lumber spine. Neurosurgery 38:67–75, 1996.
29. McLendon RE, Bigner DD, Bigner SH, Provenzale JM: Pathology of Tumors of the Central Nervous System, A Guide to Histologic Diagnosis. New York, Arnold, 2000.
30. Merchant TE, Kiehna EN, Thompson SJ, et al: Pediatric low-grade and ependymal spinal cord tumors. Pediatr Neurosurg 32:30–36, 2000.
31. Mirimanoff RO, Dosretz DE, Lingood RM, et al: Meningioma: analysis of recurrence and progression following neurosurgical resection. J Neurosurg 62:18–24, 1985.
32. Myles ST, Hamilton MG: Congenital cysts: neurenteric, arachnoid, dermoid. In Albright L, Pollack I, Adelson D (eds): Principles and Practice of Pediatric Neurosurgery. New York, Thieme, 1999.
33. Naderi S, Yilmaz M, Canda T, et al: Ossified thoracic spinal meningioma in childhood: a case report and review of the literature. Clin Neurol Neurosurg 103:247–249, 2001.
34. Nagib MG, O'Fallon MT: Myxopapillary ependymoma of the conus medullaris and filum terminale in the pediatric age group. Pediatr Neurosurg 26:2–7, 1997.
35. Osborn AG: Diagnostic Neuroradiology. St. Louis, Mosby, 1994.
36. Packer RJ, Gutmann DH, Rubenstein A, et al: Plexiform neurofibromas in NF1: toward biologic-based therapy. Neurology 58:1461–1470, 2002.
37. Poirier J, Gray F, Escourolle R: Manual of Basic Neuropathology, 3rd ed. Philadelphia, WB Saunders, 1990.
38. Pollack IF, Mulvihill JJ: Neurofibromatosis. In Albright L, Pollack I, Adelson D (eds): Principles and Practice of Pediatric Neurosurgery. New York, Thieme, 1999.
39. Sen CN, Sekhar LN: An extreme lateral approach to intradural lesions of the cervical spine and foramen magnum. Neurosurgery 27:197–204, 1990.

40. Scott M: Infiltrating ependymomas of the cauda equina: treatment by conservative surgery plus radiotherapy. J Neurosurg 41:446–448, 1974.

41. Scott RM, Wolpert SM, Bartoshesky LE, et al: Dermoid tumors occurring at the site of previous myelomeningocele repair. J Neurosurg 65:779–783, 1986.

42. Sheikh BY, Siqueira E, Dayel F: Meningioma in children: a report of nine cases and review of the literature. Surg Neurol 45: 328–335, 1996.

43. Slooff JL, Kernohan JW, MacCarty CS: Primary intramedullary tumors of the spinal cord and filum terminale. Philadelphia-London, WB Saunders, 1964.

44. Sordillo PP, Helson L, Hajdu SI, et al: Malignant schwannoma: clinical characteristics, survival, and response to therapy. Cancer 47:2503–2509, 1981.

45. Thakkar SD, Feigen U, Mautner VF: Spinal tumours in neurofibromatosis type 1: an MRI study of frequency, multiplicity and variety. Neuroradiology 41:625–629, 1999.

46. Wantanabe M, Chiba K, Morio M, et al: Infantile spinal cord meningioma: case illustration. J Neurosurg (Spine 2) 94:334, 2001.

48. Yoshii S, Shimizu K, Ido K, et al: Ependymoma of the spina cord and the cauda equina region. J Spinal Dis 12:157–161, 1999.

CHAPTER 106

INTRAMEDULLARY SPINAL TUMORS

Joseph H Piatt, Jr.

Intramedullary spinal neoplasia represents a particularly cruel clinical problem, especially in childhood, because it causes pain, deformity, and progressive disability without blunting the patient's awareness of self and circumstances until, in malignant instances, the very last stages of the illness. In the past the obscurity of the symptoms often delayed the diagnosis, and the initial surgical management often contributed to the morbidity of the disease. Fortunately, universal access to magnetic resonance imaging (MRI) has simplified and has probably shortened the diagnostic process. Improvements in surgical instrumentation and electrophysiologic monitoring methods have bolstered the surgeon's confidence in approaching intramedullary tumors and have probably enhanced outcomes as well. These recent advances in patient care may season this chapter with satisfaction and hope.

EPIDEMIOLOGY

Intramedullary spinal cord tumors are rare in childhood, as they are in adulthood, and valid epidemiologic data are scarce. An estimate of the incidence of intramedullary tumors in childhood can be derived from the population-based data of Farwell and Dohrmann.[38] Between 1935 and 1973 there were 488 central nervous system tumors among children recorded in a Connecticut state registry. There were 21 intramedullary tumors in this registry, for a brain-to-spinal cord ratio of 22:1. This ratio is quite close to the commonly cited ratio of 20:1 for the relative masses of these two organs. Based on an annual incidence of pediatric brain tumors of 2 to 5 per 100,000 population,[126] the incidence of pediatric intramedullary tumors may be estimated at 1 to 2 per 1,000,000 population.

Virtually every type of tumor that has been described in the brain has been described in the spinal cord as well, but the predominant histologic categories are astrocytoma and ependymoma. In adulthood ependymoma is the most common histologic diagnosis, but in childhood astrocytoma predominates. In the population-based data of Farwell et al, the ratio of astrocytoma to ependymoma was 2:1.[37] Other reports are tarnished by referral bias, but ratios have ranged from as low as 15:11 to as high as 17:2.[2,28,49,58,81,96,102,103] In the very large personal series of Epstein, the ratio was 3:1.[36] In a major multicenter study of childhood intramedullary astrocytoma in France, 35% of astrocytic tumors were malignant.[13] Between 5% and 10% of spinal cord astrocytic tumors are frank glioblastoma multiforme.[13,37,81]

Malignant spinal cord ependymomas, in contrast, are very rare.[9] Low-grade intramedullary astrocytomas can be either pilocytic or fibrillary. Contradictory observations have been reported regarding the relative proportions of these histologic subtypes.[13,89,91,119] Because pilocytic tumors typically displace adjacent neural tissue, whereas fibrillary tumors typically infiltrate it, the distinction could in theory have clinical significance, and clinicopathologic correlates have been reported both in children[13] and in adults.[91]

LOCATION

Intramedullary gliomas are distributed uniformly over the length of the spinal cord in rough proportion to segmental cross-sectional area. Tumors involving the entire length of the spinal cord, so-called *holocord tumors*, are also well described. Most such tumors are low-grade astrocytomas,[17,34,35,101] but gangliogliomas[106] and oligodendrogliomas[104] have been described as well. Tumors arising at the cervicomedullary junction are discussed elsewhere in this volume. Also outside the scope of this chapter are intradural extramedullary myxopapillary ependymomas arising from the filum terminale and the rare extracanalicular ependymal tumors arising in the subcutaneous tissues in the intergluteal cleft at the former site of the caudal medullary vestige.[5,21,94,136,143]

DIAGNOSIS

The clinical manifestations of intramedullary tumors can be musculoskeletal, neurologic, or pain related. Diagnosis can be confounded by the rarity of these lesions and, in the pediatric age group, by difficulty in obtaining description of symptoms and cooperation with examination. Before the proliferation of MRI facilities in the past decade, many incorrect diagnoses were often entertained for many months before the true nature of the condition became apparent.[2] Intramedullary spinal cord tumors have been mistaken for spinal muscular atrophy, transverse myelitis, poliomyelitis, congenital lordosis, congenital scoliosis, congenital pes plana, congenital hip dysplasia, ruptured intervertebral disk, Guillain-Barré syndrome, epidural abscess, Pott's disease, muscular dystrophy, celiac syndrome, irritable bowel syndrome, subarachnoid hemorrhage, "growing pains," developmental regression, and conversion reaction.[3,24,45,117] The diagnosis of "progressive cerebral palsy" is a contradiction in terms and always deserves further investigation.[50] Another pitfall in diagnosis has been to approach acquired torticollis and back pain in childhood with the same light regard that they may merit in adulthood. These symptoms always require diagnostic investigation in the pediatric age group.

The neurologic manifestations of intramedullary tumors are what might be expected from basic principles of neuroanatomy and neurophysiology. The most common neurologic symptoms are gait disturbance, loss of fine motor skills in a hand, or in young children loss of previously acquired motor milestones.[24,28,114] There can be segmental signs related to the site of the tumor itself, namely, weakness and atrophy in muscles innervated by the involved segments, impairment of pain and temperature sensation (the sensory modalities sustained by fibers that cross at a segmental level), and obliteration of muscle stretch reflexes. Horner's syndrome may announce the presence of a cervicothoracic spinal cord tumor, and although it is not exclusively predictive of an intramedullary process, in the pediatric age group it is at least predictive of a neoplastic process. There can also be so-called *long-tract signs* related to compression of ascending and descending axon bundles with weakness and spasticity in muscles innervated by caudal segments and impairment of various sensory modalities to varying degrees below the level of the lesion. Impairment of one sensory modality in a certain body region with preservation of other modalities is often described as a "dissociated" sensory loss and is typical of intramedullary disease processes. Long-tract compression tends to exaggerate the segmental muscle stretch reflexes, suppress the superficial abdominal reflexes and the cremasteric reflexes, and cause emergence of the Babinski sign. Bladder, bowel, and sexual function can be impaired either on the basis of long-tract compression or on the basis of disruption of critical segmental reflex circuits.

The musculoskeletal manifestations of intramedullary tumors are at once more obvious and more confusing, and they typify the symptoms of the slowly progressive, histologically benign lesions. Spinal deformity is a common but very nonspecific symptom.[7,22,24,81,121,128] It is attributable to disruption of the neural control of the muscular mechanisms that sustain spinal posture, so in this sense it might be considered a neurologic sign. In distinction from the much more common idiopathic scoliosis of adolescence, the scoliosis associated with spinal cord tumors is often accompanied in its later stages by pain and rigidity resulting from nerve root compression and traction at the level of the mass.[22,115] In the cervical region this phenomenon occurs as acquired torticollis.[16,24,66,139] Myelopathic gait disturbances can masquerade as developmental phenomena like in-toeing and as congenital hip dysplasia. In the young child neurologic impairment can, over months and years, lead to deformities ranging from foot size and leg-length discrepancies to joint contractures to frank dysplasias of bones and joints.

Pain is the most common initial complaint among children with intramedullary tumors,[24,28,114,117,118,128,133] but there is no particular quality of the pain that is pathognomonic. It can be axial and either focal or diffuse, depending on the number of spinal segments involved by the tumor. It can be radiating, although it is seldom constrained to the distribution of a single nerve root. It can be dull and constant, or it can be paroxysmal and

severe.[117] Radiating pain in the thoracic and upper lumbar segments can be very confusing from a semiological standpoint and can lead to frustrating diagnostic investigations of thoracic and abdominal viscera.[31,117] Explosive onset of axial pain typifies spinal subarachnoid hemorrhage, a rare symptom of intramedullary tumors reported in association with astrocytoma, ependymoma, and hemangioblastoma.[10,33,60] The phenomenology of pain among children with spinal tumors has been examined by Sun Hahn and McLone.[133]

The propensity of some intramedullary tumors to disseminate throughout the leptomeninges can lead to hydrocephalus—commonly a grim complication of the later stages of the illness but occasionally a confusing initial symptom. In one large personal series, hydrocephalus developed in 25 of 171 patients (15%) at some time in the course of their disease.[116] Twenty-three of these twenty-five patients were children, perhaps in this series an artifact of referral. Only 6 patients (4%) actually initially had hydrocephalus, but among the 20 patients with malignant tumors in this series, 4 (20%) had hydrocephalus at diagnosis. Thirteen of the twenty patients with malignancies (65%) developed hydrocephalus at some time, whereas only 12 of 151 patients (7%) with histologically benign tumors did so. In the benign cases the hydrocephalus was not associated with leptomeningeal disease but with the presence of rostral spinal cord cysts at the cervicomedullary junction.[116] Although oligodendroglioma is a rare spinal cord primary tumor, it seems to have a propensity for leptomeningeal dissemination and hydrocephalus—31% of cases in a 1980 literature review.[40]

IMAGING

To exaggerate the importance of MRI in the diagnosis and management of intramedullary spinal cord tumors is scarcely possible. Ready access to this technology in almost all regions of the United States ensures that patients usually appear in the office of the specialist with an MRI study ordered by the primary physician already in hand. Nevertheless, radiographic findings deserve mention for the light that they shed on the disease process. Skeletal radiographic changes are not uncommonly seen. In older series accumulated before computer-assisted imaging was available, roughly half of all patients had abnormal radiographs.[9,81] A chronic expansile process within the spinal canal can cause remodeling of the surrounding osseous elements. In an anteroposterior view of the spinal column, the medial aspects of the pedicles may be flattened, and the interpedicular width of the spinal canal may be enlarged. In normal anatomy, beginning high in the thoracic spine, the interpedicular distance increases steadily at each succeeding lower segment all the way to S1. An interpedicular measurement at one segment that is greater than the measurement at a lower segment is abnormal, although this observation is not specific for intramedullary processes such as tumor and syrinx. It can be seen in the setting of diastematomyelia, in which case dysplastic changes in the posterior elements will invariably be present as well. It can also be seen in conjunction with the dural ectasia associated with neurofibromatosis. Expansile changes can be seen less commonly on lateral views of the spine. As discussed previously, scoliosis is a common presentation of intramedullary tumors and is, of course, manifested radiographically.

For many decades the mainstay of diagnosis of intramedullary tumors was myelography, supplemented beginning in the 1980s by computed tomography (CT). This imaging modality is obsolete and will not be discussed further. Likewise, ultrasonography has seen limited use outside the operating room as a follow-up imaging modality for laminectomized patients.[14] Without a doubt the superior anatomic detail and superior clinical utility of modern MRI has consigned these other technologies to the dust bin.

The MRI characteristics of the most common intramedullary tumors of childhood, the astrocytic tumors, are heterogeneous, as are the growth patterns and biologic behavior of this class of neoplasms. Some astrocytic tumors, namely the pilocytic astrocytomas, push adjacent neural tissue aside as they grow. Other astrocytic tumors, the fibrillary astrocytomas and the malignant astrocytomas, infiltrate adjacent tissue. These growth patterns are reflected more or less faithfully in the MRI: pilocytic astrocytomas have distinct borders, and the infiltrative astrocytomas have indistinct borders. Spinal cord edema, manifest as high signal changes on T2-weighted images, may be present adjacent to any astrocytic tumor regardless of its growth patterns, but for infiltrative tumors to distinguish peritumoral edema from the leading edge of infiltration is impossible. Syringes at the rostral or caudal pole or within the tumor itself are not uncommonly seen, and peritumoral edema probably represents a presyrinx state in some instances. Contrast enhancement patterns are variable and correlate in only a limited fashion with histology. Bright, homogeneous contrast enhancement generally signifies a benign tumor of the pilocytic type. Nonenhanced lesions may be benign or malignant, and faint, inhomogeneous enhancement is worrisome, although not diagnostic, for malignancy (Figure 106-1). Enhancement of the surface of the spinal cord remote from the lesion signifies leptomeningeal dissemination, which is usually but not exclusively a feature of malignancy.

Closely related to the purely astrocytic tumors in biology and management are gangliogliomas.[106] These tumors typically involve many segments or even the entire cord, and remodeling of the osseous confines of the spinal canal is seen. Associated syrinx cavities are common, but adjacent spinal cord edema is seldom present. On T1-weighted images without contrast, the lesions are isointense or of mixed signal intensity, and they enhance inhomogeneously. Interestingly, enhancement of the adjacent spinal cord surface is common.

Ependymoma is less prevalent among childhood intramedullary tumors than astrocytoma and ganglioglioma,[89] but it is sufficiently common, and the MRI appearance is sufficiently distinctive, that preoperative diagnosis may sometimes be possible.[39] These tumors generally have crisp borders. They consistently display high intensity on T2-weighted images, and they exhibit consistent contrast enhancement, uniform or inhomogeneous in roughly equal proportions. A diagnostic feature present in a minority of cases is a rim of hemosiderin manifest as a thin layer of very low signal intensity on T2-weighted images.

Within the pediatric age range, intramedullary hemangioblastoma is seen predominantly among adolescents, and despite its low prevalence outside the context of von Hippel-Lindau disease, its imaging features can occasionally suggest the diagnosis before surgery.[118] Like the ependymoma, the hemangioblastoma has a clearly demarcated border with adjacent spinal cord tissue. There is bright contrast enhancement on T1-weighted images. The lesion exhibits high signal on T2-weighted images, and adjacent edema and syringes are virtually always present. Unlike ependymoma, and contrary to intuition, hemangioblastoma never exhibits the surrounding

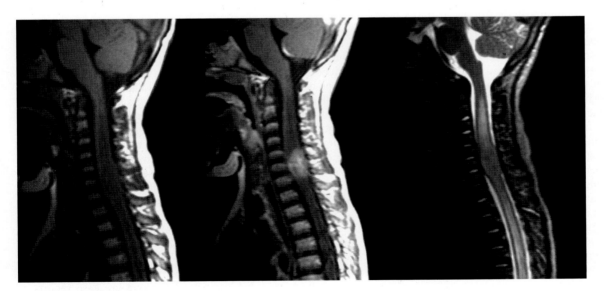

FIGURE 106-1 This 4-year-old boy had a 10-day history of headache, neck pain and immobility, right upper-extremity weakness, and a right Horner's syndrome. T1-weighted sagittal magnetic resonance imaging of the cervical spine showed a low-intensity expansile intramedullary lesion in the lower cervical region with indistinct borders *(left)*. There was faint contrast enhancement *(center)*. On a T2-weighted sagittal image there were high-intensity changes within the spinal cord rostral and caudal to the lesion *(right)*. Hemilaminectomy revealed that the tumor had breached the pia and was enveloping the dorsal rootlets on the right side. The diagnosis was anaplastic astrocytoma. Despite radiation therapy, chemotherapy, and treatment of complicating hydrocephalus, this child died 7 months later.

rim of low signal intensity on T2-weighted images indicative of hemosiderin. Virtually pathognomonic of hemangioblastoma is the presence of vascular flow voids on the surface of the adjacent spinal cord and the surrounding subarachnoid spaces. Vascular structures were seen on MRI in 8 of 19 cases in a recent series.[118] This dilation of spinal cord vessels and the associated intense tumor stain make hemangioblastoma recognizable on spinal cord angiography, and even since the introduction of MRI, angiography has been useful for the planning of the surgical attack.[118,140]

Intramedullary spinal cord tumors have an imaging differential diagnosis. In one large institutional series, 9 of 212 patients undergoing surgery did not actually have neoplastic disease.[76] The list of lesions that have masqueraded as intramedullary tumors includes demyelinating disease, sarcoid, tuberculoma, Leigh disease, amyloid angiopathy, inflammatory pseudotumor, and spinal cord infarction.[48,64,76,146] If the clinical circumstances do not provide sufficient guidance, an imaging clue is that non-neoplastic processes often fail to expand the cord in proportion to the volume of the associated MRI signal abnormality.[76]

TUMOR HISTOLOGY

The histopathologic characteristics of intramedullary spinal cord tumors are not so distinct from those of their intracranial counterparts that description of the microscopic appearances of each type needs repetition in this chapter. The reader may look into the chapters on each corresponding intracranial tumor type elsewhere in this text. Table 106-1 is a list of the various histologies that have been described for intramedullary tumors in childhood with selected citations.

A recent trend in histopathologic diagnosis deserves mention. Ependymoma and astrocytoma have long been reported to be the most common intramedullary tumors both among adults and among children, whereas ganglioglioma of the spinal cord has been considered a curiosity. In recent years, however, study of the pathologic material from the very large referral practice of Epstein et al has raised the standing of ganglioglioma in relation to other intramedullary tumor types in childhood. In 2000 Miller reviewed 294 surgical specimens from the clinical practice at New York University, among which were 117 specimens from pediatric patients.[89] As expected, ependymomas predominated among the adult cases, but in the pediatric material ganglioglioma was as common as astrocytoma, and both of these diagnoses were more prevalent than ependymoma. That ganglioglioma was not recognized more frequently in the adult material suggests that the surprising prevalence of this diagnosis in the pediatric material was not simply a matter of local diagnostic sensibilities. Miller attributed the unique New York University perspective to systematic identification of neoplastic ganglion cells by immunohistochemical staining for synaptophysin and by examination of more complete tissue specimens than have been available in other series.[89,90] Because the biologic behavior of the glial component is generally what determines the prognosis for ganglioglioma, distinction of this lesion from low-grade astrocytoma has little impact on patient care, at least in a surgical practice guided by the intention to achieve radical resection in every case.

Intramedullary hemangioblastoma is largely a tumor of adulthood, except in the setting of Von Hippel-Lindau disease.

TABLE 106-1

Histologies of Childhood Intramedullary Tumors

Astrocytoma
   Malignant astrocytoma and glioblastoma
Ganglioglioma
Ependymoma
Oligodendroglioma
Hemangioblastoma
Schwannoma[11,12,42,129]
Gliofibroma[57,85,142]
Subependymoma[99]
Primitive neuroectodermal tumor
   Primary intramedullary[73]
   Intramedullary metastasis without leptomeningeal
     seeding[8,147]
Primary atypical teratoid/rhabdoid tumor[134]
Myolipoma[67]
Angiolipoma[82]
Myxoma[105]
Epidermoid cyst[18,62,120,138]
Dermoid cyst[137]
Lipoma[77]
Enterogenous cyst[93,131]
Teratoma[20,44,46,130]
Germ cell tumor[55]
Endodermal sinus tumor[72]
Paraganglioma/secretory gangliocytoma[4]
Ganglioneuroma[100]
Lymphoma[84]
Chloroma/granulocytic sarcoma[69]

Only 15% of intramedullary hemangioblastomas come to attention before the patient is 18 years of age.[15,118] Roughly one third to one half of all spinal hemangioblastomas are associated with Von Hippel-Lindau disease,[15,33] and patients with Von Hippel-Lindau disease seek treatment for their hemangioblastomas roughly a decade earlier, on the average, than nonsyndromic patients.[118] So the pediatric patient, in most instances an adolescent, with an intramedullary hemangioblastoma is very likely to have Von Hippel-Lindau disease, and the associated stigmata should be sought by ophthalmologic consultation, MRI of the entire central nervous system, and CT of the abdomen.

Neurofibromatosis types 1 and 2 (NF1 and NF2) are the other neurocutaneous syndromes occasionally associated with intramedullary tumors. The histology of intramedullary neoplasia in these conditions seems to be different. In NF1 astrocytic tumors predominate.[78,144] There are case reports of intramedullary schwannoma and subependymoma in NF1 in childhood as well.[11,99] NF2 has been associated with ependymoma and, in one case report, with ganglioglioma.[32,68,78,87,125,135]

The border between dysplastic developmental lesions and true intramedullary tumors becomes indistinct in some cases, particularly in the setting of dysraphism. Dermoid and epidermoid cysts and lipomas, typical lesions associated with spinal dysraphism, have been described many times as isolated intramedullary tumors without any associated osseous dysplasia or cutaneous stigmata.[18,62,71,77,120,137,138] Intramedullary teratomas have been seen both in isolation and in relation to dysraphism, specifically to diastematomyelia.[20,27,44,46,75,130] And on the far end of the spectrum, immature teratomas and primary intramedullary germ cell tumors have been described.* The relationship between developmental disturbance and frank neoplasia in the spine has been reviewed.[43,97]

TREATMENT

The treatment of intramedullary tumors crossed a technologic threshold in the early 1980s. The impact of MRI has been mentioned, but ultrasonic tissue aspirators, surgical lasers, intraoperative ultrasound, and electrophysiologic monitoring all came on the neurosurgical scene about the same time.[14,34,54,70,83,95,107,108] Although there has been some dissent on electrophysiologic monitoring,[1] the employment of these technical adjuncts has become nearly universal and has come to define modern treatment.

There may be a *de facto* standard of care in diagnostic and surgical technologies, but many critical questions in patient care must still be addressed without a satisfying evidentiary basis. Nadkarni and Rekate recently attempted a structured literature review of the management of intramedullary tumors,[98] but in the total absence of published class I evidence, their review was nothing more than a reflection of contemporary neurosurgical manners. To a degree unusual in any field of medicine, the maker of manners in the care of intramedullary tumors of childhood has been one individual, Fred J. Epstein, first at New York University and later at the Institute for Neurology and Neurosurgery at the Beth Israel Medical Center in New York City. Most of the recent, major publications on the topic of intramedullary neoplasia in childhood have been descriptions of various aspects of his referral practice.† The latest report of his pediatric experience[25] includes more cases than all other English-language, institutional reports from the modern technologic era combined, and more than twice as many cases as the multicenter investigation presented by Bouffet et al.[13] Such a concentration of clinical material at one center has had, no doubt, great benefit for the patients fortunate enough to be treated there, and it has also facilitated the advancement of adjuvant surgical technologies.[36,70,95,111] But it has not yielded generalizable data on treatment outcomes useful to workers in other environments.

The theme of Epstein's work has been radical surgical excision. That intramedullary ependymomas have discrete borders amenable to radical excision has long been recognized. Epstein extended this approach to the astrocytomas (and gangliogliomas) prevalent in childhood. He asserted that, with the aid of modern technologies and a skilled eye, even intramedullary astrocytomas can be resected from inside outward to their borders with normal spinal cord tissue while preserving function. In practice, however, in 23% of his pediatric series he stopped short of a complete resection.[25] Thus the foundation of his work in this field was a claim not only to technical virtuosity but also to surgical judgment. That his clinical

results were truly superior to the results of his predecessors seems likely but is impossible to establish objectively from the published evidence. The applicability of his results to other contemporary surgical practices is likewise impossible to establish.

Even though the most prominent authority in the field abominated the use of radiation,[24,25,41] and even though other authors agree,[58,81,110] contemporary reports still mention the use of adjuvant radiation therapy for incompletely resected benign lesions.[19,56,58,65,96,103,113,119,123] The evidentiary support for adjuvant irradiation is even weaker for benign intramedullary tumors than for benign brain tumors, a vexatious matter discussed elsewhere in this text. About the morbidities there is less uncertainty. Radiation stunts the growth of the musculoskeletal elements of the spine in younger patients.[109] It makes reoperation more difficult and compromises the healing of reopened wounds. There are also concerns about the induction by radiation of malignancy in benign astrocytomas, a phenomenon described as occurring with tumors in the head but not yet, apparently, in the spine among pediatric patients.[29]

The management of malignant intramedullary tumors is a matter of great frustration but of fairly general consensus. The prevailing approach is biopsy or limited resection followed by radiation therapy. The role of adjuvant chemotherapy has been discussed but not so far investigated extensively.[6,30,51,80,141] Because survival is often so short, decompression by wide laminectomy and dural grafting may have a palliative effect, preserving neurologic function until later stages of tumor growth. Whereas admitting that radical resection does not seem to provide improved function or prolonged survival, Epstein et al nevertheless recommended aggressive surgery for malignant astrocytomas to improve diagnostic tissue sampling and to facilitate pain control.[23]

Intramedullary tumors commonly cause spinal deformity, but deformity often appears or grows worse after treatment.[28,81,114] In Epstein's series of children and young adults, 31% of patients needed spinal fusion after treatment.[25] Many factors contribute, but a potential factor within the control of the surgeon is the technique used for opening the spinal canal. Conventional laminectomy removes intervertebral ligaments that play some role in spinal stability. Wide laminectomy may disrupt the zygapophyseal joints as well. Prolonged periods of postoperative bracing have been recommended without evidence of efficacy.[81,96] Yasargil has described resection of intramedullary tumors through a hemilaminectomy exposure that preserves the interspinous and supraspinous ligaments, the contralateral yellow ligaments, and all the contralateral muscle attachments.[145] Another popular approach has been osteoplastic laminotomy,[53,112] apparently first described by Raimondi.[112] This technique requires exposure of both sides of the posterior elements of the spine with sparing of the supraspinous ligament. Cuts are made in the lamina on both sides, medial to the zygapophyseal joints, over the length of the exposure using a power drill with a footplate to prevent injury to the contents of the spinal canal. An intervertebral level is selected for division of the supraspinous, interspinous, and yellow ligaments, and the lamina segments above and below are reflected superiorly and inferiorly as pedicle flaps based on the supraspinous ligaments at the ends of the exposure. At the conclusion of the tumor resection, the lamina flaps can be replaced and secured by various techniques. There is no question that osseous healing of osteoplastic laminotomies occurs regularly. Whether this technique actually mitigates subsequent spinal deformity has

---

*See references 47, 52, 55, 61, 72, 86, 92, 124, 127, 132.
†See references 24, 25, 36, 39, 41, 63, 70, 74, 76–79, 89, 95, 106, 116, 118.

not been established conclusively, but encouraging anecdotal data have been presented.[26]

RECURRENCE

The management issues raised by recurrence of an intramedullary tumor are identical to the issues associated with a recurrent intracranial tumor of similar histology. Local recurrence of a benign lesion can sometimes be controlled by reoperation without radiation therapy or chemotherapy.[25] Because of the adverse effects of radiation on the growth and development of the spinal column, reoperation alone may be wise particularly in younger patients, a recommendation articulated enthusiastically by Epstein et al.[24] Use of chemotherapy as a tactic for avoiding or deferring radiation therapy may be successful for recurrence in the spine, as it has been in the head.[30,51] A prospective, multicenter trial in France yielded favorable results with a regimen of carboplatin, procarbazine, vincristine, cyclophosphamide, etoposide, and cisplatin.[30] Of eight children with progressive low-grade intramedullary lesions, seven exhibited clinical and radiographic responses, and the other child stabilized. At a median follow-up of 3 years, five of eight children were free of progression without radiation therapy.[30]

OUTCOME AND QUALITY OF LIFE

The methodologic obstacles to assessment of the outcomes of the treatment of intramedullary tumors in childhood are daunting, if not finally insurmountable. With very few notable exceptions,[13,30] the entire literature consists of retrospective reviews of institutional series that are compromised by many forms of bias. Because intramedullary tumors are so uncommon, these series often span several decades, during which time attitudes and technologies may have evolved. Again, because there are so few cases to discuss, many reports fail to analyze outcomes by age or by histologic type. Because surgery of intramedullary tumors places such heavy demands on technique and judgment, reports that describe the outcomes of a single surgeon are of doubtful relevance to the practices of other surgeons. Reports that describe the outcomes from one particular department of radiation therapy are likewise compromised by unanswerable questions about referral and selection for treatment. Indigestible though they may be, data describing overall survival and progression-free survival are presented in Table 106-2.

A report from the French Society for Neurosurgery deserves special mention because it appears to be the only published attempt at a population-based study of treatment results for childhood intramedullary tumors.[13] Bouffet et al present a retrospective review of 73 consecutive pediatric patients treated at 13 neurosurgical centers between 1971 and 1994 for intramedullary astrocytoma. Histopathologic diagnoses were reviewed centrally. Overall, 5- and 10-year survival rates for the entire series were 66% and 60%, respectively. Survival rates at last follow-up review for patients with pilocytic astrocytoma ($n = 28$), fibrillary astrocytoma ($n = 21$), anaplastic astrocytoma ($n = 21$), and glioblastoma ($n = 3$) were 82%, 69%, 40%, and 0%, respectively. Independent predictors of survival in a multivariate analysis using the Cox proportional hazards model were histology and duration of symptoms before diagnosis. Extent of resection and administration of postoperative radiation therapy had no detectable effect on survival.

The suggestion that aggressive resection of intramedullary tumors may improve outcome has been a stimulus to surgical virtuosity, but evidence that aggressive resection has a favor-

TABLE 106-2   Pediatric Intramedullary Tumors—Survival

Author	Year	Cases	Histology	Ages	1 y	Overall 5 y	Overall 10 y	Event-free 5 y	Event-free 10y	Comment
Reimer[114]	1985	27	Astrocytoma	≤20 y		0.81	0.55			
Reimer[114]	1985	5	Malignant astrocytoma	≤20 y	0					
Hardison[49]	1987	26	Mixed	Pediatric		0.39		0.14		
Cohen[23]	1989	19	Malignant astrocytoma	Mostly pediatric	0.3					
Rossitch[119]	1990	12	Astrocytoma	Pediatric	1		0.75	0.73	0.73	
Sandler[123]	1992	21	Astrocytoma	Median = 21 y			0.68			
Lang[74]	1993	30	Ganglioglioma	Mostly pediatric		0.84		0.36		
Huddart[56]	1993	27	Mixed astrocytic	All		0.59	0.52	0.38	0.26	Radiation therapy department
O'Sullivan[103]	1994	28	Mixed	≤17 y			0.8		0.73	Radiation therapy department
Constantini[24]	1996	27	Mixed	≤3 y				0.76		
Jyothirmayi[65]	1997	23	Mixed astrocytic	All		0.55	0.39	0.75	0.55	Median follow-up period 11 y
Przybylski[110]	1997	18	Mixed astrocytic	Pediatric			0.82			
Bouffet[13]	1998	73	Mixed astrocytic	Pediatric		0.66	0.6			
Lonjon[79]	1998	20	Ependymoma	Pediatric		0.9	0.9	0.93	0.7	
Constantini[25]	2000	164	Mixed	≤21 y				0.78 (lg) 0.3 (hg)		

hg, High grade; lg, low grade.

able effect on survival or objective measures of function has been elusive. Numerous retrospective reviews at other institutions have failed to demonstrate a relationship between extent of resection and survival.[13,56,58,59,103,119,123] In addition to the methodologic weaknesses mentioned previously, many of these reports have relied on surgeons' perceptions of extent of resection without the benefit of postoperative MRI. In Epstein's most recent report, patients who underwent only partial (<80%) resections experienced early progression, although few of these patients had received adjuvant radiation therapy despite the presence of significant residual disease. There was no difference in progression-free survival rates between gross-total (>95%) and subtotal (>80%) resections.[25] This observation should soften the surgeon's resolve to excise every remaining scrap of tumor whatever the risk to the patient. Knowing when to quit in the resection of intramedullary tumors clearly remains a critical matter of surgical judgment.

As a measure of outcome, *survival* is an indisputable endpoint, and with attention to definitions, *"progression-free"* survival can acquire a satisfying degree of objectivity. But measurement of functional outcomes after the treatment of intramedullary spinal cord tumors remains at a very rudimentary level. In 1985 Cooper and Epstein presented 6- and 5-point scales for assessing lower and upper limb function, respectively, in adults who had undergone resection of intramedullary tumors. McCormick et al used a 4-point functional scale based on neurologic symptoms and signs, gait, and activities of daily living to describe outcomes of adults undergoing treatment for intramedullary ependymoma.[88] Goh et al and Constantini et al used a 5-point modified McCormick scale to analyze outcomes of pediatric intramedullary tumors.[25,41] These scales all had the advantage of a small number of grades, but each grade generally carried a complex and not very precise definition. None of these scales was validated by analysis of interobserver variability or by comparison with other standard measures of functional outcome. Innocenzi et al circumvented these criticisms by using a 3-point scale condensed from the Karnofsky Performance Scale.[58] In none of the reports cited were assessments administered by investigators not directly associated with the surgical team. The strongest statement about functional outcome that the current literature can support is that patients who are minimally affected before surgery generally retain a high level of function after surgery, whereas patients who are profoundly disabled before surgery seldom make startling recoveries.[25,26,58,122]

FUTURE DIRECTIONS

The relentless advance of technology in imaging, surgical instrumentation, and radiation therapy will continue to improve the outlook for children with intramedullary tumors. Harnessing these technologic advances, however, will require prospective, multicenter clinical trials incorporating standardized diagnostic and treatment methods and employing standardized measures of outcome with validated instruments.

References

1. Albright AL: Intraoperative spinal cord monitoring for intramedullary surgery: an essential adjunct? Pediatr Neurosurg 29:112, 1998.
2. Auberge C, Ponsot G, Lemerle J, et al: [Intramedullary tumors in children. Apropos of 30 cases]. Arch Fr Pediatr 36:1024–1039, 1979.
3. Aysun S, Cinbis M, Ozcan OE: Intramedullary astrocytoma presenting as spinal muscular atrophy. J Child Neurol 8:354–356, 1993.
4. Azzarelli B, Luerssen TG, Wolfe TM: Intramedullary secretory gangliocytoma. Acta Neuropathol 82:402–407, 1991.
5. Bale PM: Ependymal rests and subcutaneous sacrococcygeal ependymoma. Pathology 12:237–243, 1980.
6. Balmaceda C: Chemotherapy for intramedullary spinal cord tumors. J Neurooncol 47:293–307, 2000.
7. Banna M, Pearce GW, Uldall R: Scoliosis: a rare manifestation of intrinsic tumours of the spinal cord in children. J Neurol Neurosurg Psychiatry 34:637–641, 1971.
8. Barnwell SL, Edwards MS: Spinal intramedullary spread of medulloblastoma. Case report. J Neurosurg 65:253–255, 1986.
9. Barone BM, Elvidge AR: Ependymomas. A clinical survey. J Neurosurg 33:428–438, 1970.
10. Bhandari YS: Subarachnoid hemorrhage due to cervical cord tumor in a child. Case report. J Neurosurg 30:749–751, 1969.
11. Bhayani R, Goel A: Multiple intramedullary schwannomas—case report. Neurol Med Chir (Tokyo) 36:466–468, 1996.
12. Binatli O, Ersahin Y, Korkmaz O, et al: Intramedullary schwannoma of the spinal cord. A case report and review of the literature. J Neurosurg Sci 43:163–167, 1999.
13. Bouffet E, Pierre-Kahn A, Marchal JC, et al: Prognostic factors in pediatric spinal cord astrocytoma. Cancer 83:2391–2399, 1998.
14. Braun IF, Raghavendra BN, Kricheff II: Spinal cord imaging using real-time high-resolution ultrasound. Radiology 147:459–465, 1983.
15. Browne TR, Adams RD, Roberson GH: Hemangioblastoma of the spinal cord. Review and report of five cases. Arch Neurol 33:435–441, 1976.
16. Bussieres A, Cassidy JD, Dzus A: Spinal cord astrocytoma presenting as torticollis and scoliosis. J Manipulative Physiol Ther 17:113–118, 1994.
17. Chacko AG, Chandy MJ: Favorable outcome after radical excision of a "Holocord" astrocytoma. Clin Neurol Neurosurg 102:240–242, 2000.
18. Chandra PS, Manjari T, Devi BI, et al: Intramedullary spinal epidermoid cyst. Neurol India 48:75–77, 2000.
19. Chandy MJ, Babu S: Management of intramedullary spinal cord tumours: review of 68 patients. Neurol India 47:224–228, 1999.
20. Chidambaram Balasubramaniam B, Balasubramaniam V, Shankar SK, et al: Giant intramedullary teratoma in an infant. Pediatr Neurosurg 33:21–25, 2000.
21. Ciraldo AV, Platt MS, Agamanolis DP, et al: Sacrococcygeal myxopapillary ependymomas and ependymal rests in infants and children. J Pediatr Surg 21:49–52, 1986.
22. Citron N, Edgar MA, Sheehy J, et al: Intramedullary spinal cord tumours presenting as scoliosis. J Bone Joint Surg Br 66:513–517, 1984.
23. Cohen AR, Wisoff JH, Allen JC, et al: Malignant astrocytomas of the spinal cord. J Neurosurg 70:50–54, 1989.

24. Constantini S, Houten J, Miller DC, et al: Intramedullary spinal cord tumors in children under the age of 3 years. J Neurosurg 85:1036–1043, 1996.

25. Constantini S, Miller DC, Allen JC, et al: Radical excision of intramedullary spinal cord tumors: surgical morbidity and long-term follow-up evaluation in 164 children and young adults. J Neurosurg 93:183–193, 2000.

26. Cristante L, Herrmann HD: Surgical management of intramedullary spinal cord tumors: functional outcome and sources of morbidity. Neurosurgery 35:69–74, 1994.

27. Cybulski GR, Von Roenn KA, Bailey OT: Intramedullary cystic teratoid tumor of the cervical spinal cord in association with a teratoma of the ovary. Surg Neurol 22:267–272, 1984.

28. DeSousa AL, Kalsbeck JE, Mealey J, Jr, et al: Intraspinal tumors in children. A review of 81 cases. J Neurosurg 51:437–445, 1979.

29. Dirks PB, Jay V, Becker LE, et al: Development of anaplastic changes in low-grade astrocytomas of childhood. Neurosurgery 34:68–78, 1994.

30. Doireau V, Grill J, Zerah M, et al: Chemotherapy for unresectable and recurrent intramedullary glial tumours in children. Brain Tumours Subcommittee of the French Society of Paediatric Oncology (SFOP). Br J Cancer 81:835–840, 1999.

31. Eden KC: Dissemination of a glioma of the spinal cord in the leptomeninges. Brain 61:298–310, 1938.

32. Egelhoff JC, Bates DJ, Ross JS, et al: Spinal MR findings in neurofibromatosis types 1 and 2. AJNR Am J Neuroradiol 13:1071–1077, 1992.

33. Emery E, Hurth M, Lacroix-Jousselin C, et al: [Intraspinal hemangioblastoma. Apropos of a recent series of 20 cases]. Neurochirurgie 40:165–173, 1994.

34. Epstein F: Spinal cord astrocytomas of childhood. Adv Tech Stand Neurosurg 13:135–169, 1986.

35. Epstein F, Epstein N: Surgical management of holocord intramedullary spinal cord astrocytomas in children. J Neurosurg 54:829–832, 1981.

36. Epstein FJ, Farmer JP, Schneider SJ: Intraoperative ultrasonography: an important surgical adjunct for intramedullary tumors. J Neurosurg 74:729–733, 1991.

37. Farwell JR, Dohrmann GJ: Intraspinal neoplasms in children. Paraplegia 15:262–273, 1977.

38. Farwell JR, Dohrmann GJ, Flannery JT: Central nervous system tumors in children. Cancer 40:3123–3132, 1977.

39. Fine MJ, Kricheff, II, Freed D, et al: Spinal cord ependymomas: MR imaging features. Radiology 197:655–658, 1995.

40. Fortuna A, Celli P, Palma L: Oligodendrogliomas of the spinal cord. Acta Neurochir 52:305–329, 1980.

41. Goh KY, Velasquez L, Epstein FJ: Pediatric intramedullary spinal cord tumors: is surgery alone enough? Pediatr Neurosurg 27:34–39, 1997.

42. Gorman PH, Rigamonti D, Joslyn JN: Intramedullary and extramedullary schwannoma of the cervical spinal cord—case report. Surg Neurol 32:459–462, 1989.

43. Grawe A, Nisch G, Siedschlag WD: [Dysontogenetic tumors of the spinal canal. Clinical aspects and long- term follow-up]. Zentralbl Neurochir 51:82–84, 1990.

44. Hader WJ, Steinbok P, Poskitt K, et al: Intramedullary spinal teratoma and diastematomyelia. Case report and review of the literature. Pediatr Neurosurg 30:140–145, 1999.

45. Haft H, Ransohoff J, Carter S: Spinal cord tumors in children. Pediatrics 23:1152–1159, 1959.

46. Hamada H, Kurimoto M, Hayashi N, et al: Intramedullary spinal teratoma with spina bifida. Childs Nerv Syst 17:109–111, 2001.

47. Hanafusa K, Shibuya H, Abe M, et al: Intramedullary spinal cord germinoma. Case report and review of the literature. Rofo Fortschr Geb Rontgenstr Neuen Bildgeb Verfahr 159:203–204, 1993.

48. Hanci M, Sarioglu AC, Uzan M, et al: Intramedullary tuberculous abscess: a case report. Spine 21:766–769, 1996.

49. Hardison HH, Packer RJ, Rorke LB, et al: Outcome of children with primary intramedullary spinal cord tumors. Childs Nerv Syst 3:89–92, 1987.

50. Haslam RH: "Progressive cerebral palsy" or spinal cord tumor? Two cases of mistaken identity. Dev Med Child Neurol 17:232–237, 1975.

51. Hassall TE, Mitchell AE, Ashley DM: Carboplatin chemotherapy for progressive intramedullary spinal cord low-grade gliomas in children: three case studies and a review of the literature. Neuro-oncology 3:251–257, 2001.

52. Hata M, Ogino I, Sakata K, et al: Intramedullary spinal cord germinoma: case report and review of the literature. Radiology 223:379–383, 2002.

53. Hejazi N, Hassler W: Microsurgical treatment of intramedullary spinal cord tumors. Neurol Med Chir (Tokyo) 38:266–271, 1998.

54. Herrmann HD, Neuss M, Winkler D: Intramedullary spinal cord tumors resected with CO2 laser microsurgical technique: recent experience in fifteen patients. Neurosurgery 22:518–522, 1988.

55. Hisa S, Morinaga S, Kobayashi Y, et al: Intramedullary spinal cord germinoma producing HCG and precocious puberty in a boy. Cancer 55:2845–2849, 1985.

56. Huddart R, Traish D, Ashley S, et al: Management of spinal astrocytoma with conservative surgery and radiotherapy. Br J Neurosurg 7:473–481, 1993.

57. Iglesias JR, Richardson EP, Jr, Collia F, et al: Prenatal intramedullary gliofibroma. A light and electron microscope study. Acta Neuropathol 62:230–234, 1984.

58. Innocenzi G, Raco A, Cantore G, et al: Intramedullary astrocytomas and ependymomas in the pediatric age group: a retrospective study. Childs Nerv Syst 12:776–780, 1996.

59. Innocenzi G, Salvati M, Cervoni L, et al: Prognostic factors in intramedullary astrocytomas. Clin Neurol Neurosurg 99:1–5, 1997.

60. Iob I, Andrioli GC, Rigobello L, et al: An unusual onset of a spinal cord tumour: subarachnoid bleeding and papilloedema. Case report. Neurochirurgia (Stuttg) 23:112–116, 1980.

61. Itoh Y, Mineura K, Sasajima H, et al: Intramedullary spinal cord germinoma: case report and review of the literature. Neurosurgery 38:187–190, 1996.

62. Jadhav RN, Khan GM, Palande DA: Intramedullary epidermoid cyst in cervicodorsal spinal cord. J Neurosurg 90:161, 1999.

63. Jallo GI, Danish S, Velasquez L, et al: Intramedullary low-grade astrocytomas: long-term outcome following radical surgery. J Neurooncol 53:61–66, 2001.

64. Johnson DL, Erickson RE: Leigh's disease presenting as an intramedullary mass lesion. Neurosurgery 30:774–776, 1992.

65. Jyothirmayi R, Madhavan J, Nair MK, et al: Conservative surgery and radiotherapy in the treatment of spinal cord astrocytoma. J Neurooncol 33:205–211, 1997.

66. Kiwak KJ, Deray MJ, Shields WD: Torticollis in three children with syringomyelia and spinal cord tumor. Neurology 33:946–948, 1983.

67. Knierim DS, Wacker M, Peckham N, et al: Lumbosacral intramedullary myolipoma. Case report. J Neurosurg 66:457–459, 1987.

68. Kobata H, Kuroiwa T, Isono N, et al: Tanycytic ependymoma in association with neurofibromatosis type 2. Clin Neuropathol 20:93–100, 2001.

69. Kook H, Hwang TJ, Kang HK, et al: Spinal intramedullary granulocytic sarcoma: magnetic resonance imaging. Magn Reson Imaging 11:135–137, 1993.

70. Kothbauer K, Deletis V, Epstein FJ: Intraoperative spinal cord monitoring for intramedullary surgery: an essential adjunct. Pediatr Neurosurg 26:247–254, 1997.

71. Kumar S, Gupta S, Puri V, et al: Intramedullary dermoids in children. Indian Pediatr 27:626–629, 1990.

72. Kurisaka M, Moriki A, Mori K, et al: Primary yolk sac tumor in the spinal cord. Childs Nerv Syst 14:653–657, 1998.

73. Kwon OK, Wang KC, Kim CJ, et al: Primary intramedullary spinal cord primitive neuroectodermal tumor with intracranial seeding in an infant. Childs Nerv Syst 12:633–636, 1996.

74. Lang FF, Epstein FJ, Ransohoff J, et al: Central nervous system gangliogliomas. Part 2: Clinical outcome. J Neurosurg 79:867–873, 1993.

75. Larbrisseau A, Renevey F, Brochu P, et al: Recurrent chemical meningitis due to an intraspinal cystic teratoma: case report. J Neurosurg 52:715–717, 1980.

76. Lee M, Epstein FJ, Rezai AR, et al: Nonneoplastic intramedullary spinal cord lesions mimicking tumors. Neurosurgery 43:788–794, 1998.

77. Lee M, Rezai AR, Abbott R, et al: Intramedullary spinal cord lipomas. J Neurosurg 82:394–400, 1995.

78. Lee M, Rezai AR, Freed D, et al: Intramedullary spinal cord tumors in neurofibromatosis. Neurosurgery 38:32–37, 1996.

79. Lonjon M, Goh KY, Epstein FJ: Intramedullary spinal cord ependymomas in children: treatment, results and follow-up. Pediatr Neurosurg 29:178–183, 1998.

80. Lowis SP, Pizer BL, Coakham H, et al: Chemotherapy for spinal cord astrocytoma: can natural history be modified? Childs Nerv Syst 14:317–321, 1998.

81. Lunardi P, Licastro G, Missori P, et al: Management of intramedullary tumours in children. Acta Neurochir 120:59–65, 1993.

82. Maggi G, Aliberti F, Colucci MR, et al: Spinal intramedullary angiolipoma. Childs Nerv Syst 12:346–349, 1996.

83. Maiuri F, Iaconetta G, Gallicchio B, et al: Intraoperative sonography for spinal tumors. Correlations with MR findings and surgery. J Neurosurg Sci 44:115–122, 2000.

84. Mathur S, Law AJ, Hung N: Late intramedullary spinal cord metastasis in a patient with lymphoblastic lymphoma: case report. J Clin Neurosci 7:264–268, 2000.

85. Matsumura A, Takano S, Nagata M, et al: Cervical intramedullary gliofibroma in a child. A case report and review of the literature. Pediatr Neurosurg 36:105–110, 2002.

86. Matsuyama Y, Nagasaka T, Mimatsu K, et al: Intramedullary spinal cord ganglioneuroma. Spine 20:2338–2340, 1995.

87. Mautner VF, Tatagiba M, Lindenau M, et al: Spinal tumors in patients with neurofibromatosis type 2: MR imaging study of frequency, multiplicity, and variety. AJR Am J Roentgenol 165:951–955, 1995.

88. McCormick PC, Torres R, Post KD, et al: Intramedullary ependymoma of the spinal cord. J Neurosurg 72:523–532, 1990.

89. Miller DC: Surgical pathology of intramedullary spinal cord neoplasms. J Neurooncol 47:189–194, 2000.

90. Miller DC, Lang FF, Epstein FJ: Central nervous system gangliogliomas. Part 1: Pathology. J Neurosurg 79:859–866, 1993.

91. Minehan KJ, Shaw EG, Scheithauer BW, et al: Spinal cord astrocytoma: pathological and treatment considerations. J Neurosurg 83: 590–595, 1995.

92. Miyauchi A, Matsumoto K, Kohmura E, et al: Primary intramedullary spinal cord germinoma. Case report. J Neurosurg 84:1060–1061, 1996.

93. Mizuno J, Fiandaca MS, Nishio S, et al: Recurrent intramedullary enterogenous cyst of the cervical spinal cord. Childs Nerv Syst 4:47–49, 1988.

94. Morantz RA, Kepes JJ, Batnitzky S, et al: Extraspinal ependymomas. Report of three cases. J Neurosurg 51:383–391, 1979.

95. Morota N, Deletis V, Constantini S, et al: The role of motor evoked potentials during surgery for intramedullary spinal cord tumors. Neurosurgery 41:1327–1336, 1997.

96. Mottl H, Koutecky J: Treatment of spinal cord tumors in children. Med Pediatr Oncol 29:293–295, 1997.

97. Muraszko K, Youkilis A: Intramedullary spinal tumors of disordered embryogenesis. J Neurooncol 47:271–281, 2000.

98. Nadkarni TD, Rekate HL: Pediatric intramedullary spinal cord tumors. Critical review of the literature. Childs Nerv Syst 15:17–28, 1999.

99. Nakasu S, Nakasu Y, Saito A, et al: Intramedullary subependymoma with neurofibromatosis—report of two cases. Neurol Med Chir (Tokyo) 32:275–280, 1992.

100. Ng TH, Fung CF, Goh W, et al: Ganglioneuroma of the spinal cord. Surg Neurol 35:147–151, 1991.

101. Nunes ML, Coutinho LM, Janisch C, et al: Congenital intramedullary tumor with neonatal manifestations. J Child Neurol 14:467–469, 1999.

102. Oi S, Raimondi AJ: Hydrocephalus associated with intraspinal neoplasms in childhood. Am J Dis Child 135:1122–1124, 1981.

103. O'Sullivan C, Jenkin RD, Doherty MA, et al: Spinal cord tumors in children: long-term results of combined surgical and radiation treatment. J Neurosurg 81:507–512, 1994.

104. Pagni CA, Canavero S, Gaidolfi E: Intramedullary "holocord" oligodendroglioma: case report. Acta Neurochir 113:96–99, 1991.

105. Pasaoglu A, Patiroglu TE, Orhon C, et al: Cervical spinal intramedullary myxoma in childhood. Case report. J Neurosurg 69:772–774, 1988.

106. Patel U, Pinto RS, Miller DC, et al: MR of spinal cord ganglioglioma. AJNR Am J Neuroradiol 19:879–887, 1998.

107. Platt JF, Rubin JM, Chandler WF, et al: Intraoperative spinal sonography in the evaluation of intramedullary tumors. J Ultrasound Med 7:317–325, 1988.

108. Prestor B, Golob P: Intra-operative spinal cord neuromonitoring in patients operated on for intramedullary tumors and syringomyelia. Neurol Res 21:125–129, 1999.

109. Probert JC, Parker BR, Kaplan HS: Growth retardation in children after megavoltage irradiation of the spine. Cancer 32:634–639, 1973.

110. Przybylski GJ, Albright AL, Martinez AJ: Spinal cord astrocytomas: long-term results comparing treatments in children. Childs Nerv Syst 13:375–382, 1997.

111. Raghavendra BN, Epstein FJ, McCleary L: Intramedullary spinal cord tumors in children: localization by intraoperative sonography. AJNR Am J Neuroradiol 5:395–397, 1984.

112. Raimondi AJ, Gutierrez FA, Di Rocco C: Laminotomy and total reconstruction of the posterior spinal arch for spinal canal surgery in childhood. J Neurosurg 45:555–560, 1976.

113. Rauhut F, Reinhardt V, Budach V, et al: Intramedullary pilocytic astrocytomas—a clinical and morphological study after combined surgical and photon or neutron therapy. Neurosurg Rev 12:309–313, 1989.

114. Reimer R, Onofrio BM: Astrocytomas of the spinal cord in children and adolescents. J Neurosurg 63:669–675, 1985.

115. Richardson FC: A report of 16 tumors of the spinal cord in children: the importance of spinal rigidity as an early sign of disease. J Pediatr 57:42–54, 1960.

116. Rifkinson-Mann S, Wisoff JH, Epstein F: The association of hydrocephalus with intramedullary spinal cord tumors: a series of 25 patients. Neurosurgery 27:749–754, 1990.

117. Robertson PL: Atypical presentations of spinal cord tumors in children. J Child Neurol 7:360–363, 1992.

118. Roonprapunt C, Silvera VM, Setton A, et al: Surgical management of isolated hemangioblastomas of the spinal cord. Neurosurgery 49:321–327, 2001.

119. Rossitch E, Jr, Zeidman SM, Burger PC, et al: Clinical and pathological analysis of spinal cord astrocytomas in children. Neurosurgery 27:193–196, 1990.

120. Roux A, Mercier C, Larbrisseau A, et al: Intramedullary epidermoid cysts of the spinal cord. Case report. J Neurosurg 76:528–533, 1992.

121. Russo CP, Katz DS, Corona RJ, Jr, et al: Gangliocytoma of the cervicothoracic spinal cord. AJNR Am J Neuroradiol 16:889–891, 1995.

122. Samii M, Klekamp J: Surgical results of 100 intramedullary tumors in relation to accompanying syringomyelia. Neurosurgery 35:865–873, 1994.

123. Sandler HM, Papadopoulos SM, Thornton AF, Jr, et al: Spinal cord astrocytomas: results of therapy. Neurosurgery 30:490–493, 1992.

124. Sasaki T, Amano T, Takao M, et al: A case of intramedullary spinal cord tumor producing human chorionic gonadotropin. J Neurooncol 56:247–250, 2002.

125. Sawin PD, Theodore N, Rekate HL: Spinal cord ganglioglioma in a child with neurofibromatosis type 2. Case report and literature review. J Neurosurg 90:231–233, 1999.

126. Schoenberg BS, Schoenberg DG, Christine BW, et al: The epidemiology of primary intracranial neoplasms of childhood. A population study. Mayo Clin Proc 51:51–56, 1976.

127. Seol HJ, Wang KC, Kim SK, et al: Intramedullary immature teratoma in a young infant involving a long segment of the spinal cord. Childs Nerv Syst 17:758–761, 2001.

128. Shariff SY, Brennan P, Allcutt D: Intraspinal tumours in children—clinical presentation. Ir Med J 90:264–265, 1997.

129. Sharma SC, Ray RC, Banerjee AK: Intramedullary spinal schwannoma. Indian Pediatr 26:290–292, 1989.

130. Shimauchi M, Yamakawa Y, Maruoka N, et al: Intramedullary teratoma of the thoracic spinal cord associated with anomalies of the vertebrae and ribs—case report. Neurol Med Chir (Tokyo) 28:1005–1009, 1988.

131. Silvernail WI, Jr, Brown RB: Intramedullary enterogenous cyst. Case report. J Neurosurg 36:235–238, 1972.

132. Slagel DD, Goeken JA, Platz CA, et al: Primary germinoma of the spinal cord: a case report with 28-year follow-up and review of the literature. Acta Neuropathol 90:657–659, 1995.

133. Sun Hahn Y, McLone DG: Pain in children with spinal cord tumors. Childs Brain 11:36–46, 1984.

134. Tamiya T, Nakashima H, Ono Y, et al: Spinal atypical teratoid/rhabdoid tumor in an infant. Pediatr Neurosurg 32:145–149, 2000.

135. Ueki K, Sasaki T, Ishida T, et al: Spinal tanycytic ependymoma associated with neurofibromatosis type 2—case report. Neurol Med Chir (Tokyo) 41:513–516, 2001.

136. Vagaiwala MR, Robinson JS, Galicich JH, et al: Metastasizing extradural ependymoma of the sacrococcygeal region: case report and review of literature. Cancer 44:326–333, 1979.

137. Verdu A, de la Cruz M, Pascual-Castroviejo I, et al: Intramedullary dermoid of the cervical spinal cord in a child. J Neurol Neurosurg Psychiatry 49:462–463, 1986.

138. Viale ES: Intramedullary epidermoid tumours. Remarks on the radical removal. Neurochirurgia (Stuttg) 20:116–118, 1977.

139. Visudhiphan P, Chiemchanya S, Somburanasin R, et al: Torticollis as the presenting sign in cervical spine infection and tumor. Clin Pediatr (Phila) 21:71–76, 1982.

140. Wang C, Zhang J, Liu A, et al: Surgical management of medullary hemangioblastoma. Report of 47 cases. Surg Neurol 56:218–226, 2001.

141. Weiss E, Klingebiel T, Kortmann RD, et al: Intraspinal high-grade astrocytoma in a child—rationale for chemotherapy and more intensive radiotherapy? Childs Nerv Syst 13:108–112, 1997.

142. Windisch TR, Naul LG, Bauserman SC: Intramedullary gliofibroma: MR, ultrasound, and pathologic correlation. J Comput Assist Tomogr 19:646–648, 1995.

143. Wolff M, Santiago H, Duby MM: Delayed distant metastasis from a subcutaneous sacrococcygeal ependymoma. Case report, with tissue culture, ultrastructural observations, and review of the literature. Cancer 30:1046–1067, 1972.

144. Yagi T, Ohata K, Haque M, et al: Intramedullary spinal cord tumour associated with neurofibromatosis type 1. Acta Neurochir 139:1055–1060, 1997.

145. Yasargil MG, Tranmer BI, Adamson TE, et al: Unilateral partial hemi-laminectomy for the removal of extra- and intramedullary tumours and AVMs. Adv Tech Stand Neurosurg 18:113–132, 1991.

146. Yuh WT, Marsh EE, III, Wang AK, et al: MR imaging of spinal cord and vertebral body infarction. AJNR Am J Neuroradiol 13:145–154, 1992.

147. Zumpano BJ: Spinal intramedullary metastatic medulloblastoma. Case report. J Neurosurg 48:632–635, 1978.

CHAPTER 107

PERIPHERAL NERVE TUMORS IN CHILDREN

W. Bradley Jacobs, Rajiv Midha, and Mubarak Al-Gahtany

Peripheral nerve tumors (PNTs) are not common lesions. Although it is widely recognized that these lesions do occur in the pediatric population, PNTs occur with less frequency there than in the adult population. The differential diagnosis of a suspected PNT in a child follows the same general framework as for adult patients (Table 107-1), but there are several key differences between PNTs in the pediatric population and their adult counterparts. For instance, as will be discussed in detail later, lesions with a neural histogenesis, such as neuroblastoma, occur in a much larger proportion of pediatric patients with PNTs than in adults, whereas nerve sheath tumors are relatively less common. This chapter highlights the specific nuances of PNTs that are unique to the pediatric population.

CLASSIFICATION

PNTs can arise from components of the nerve sheath (Schwann cells, perineurial fibroblasts) or from neuroectodermal cells. In addition, a number of rare tumors with a non-nerve sheath or non-neural histogenesis may also infiltrate the peripheral nerves of children. The spectrum of PNTs presented in Table 107-1 is a modification of Reed and Harkin's classic taxonomy of PNTs.[19] Each of these lesions has the potential to arise in children, but the relative distribution of lesions is quite different from that in adults. For instance, although schwannomas and neurofibromas represent the vast majority of peripheral nerve neoplasms in the adult population, they account for less than 50% of childhood peripheral nerve neoplasms.[6] In the same manner, because of their embryonal nature, neuroblastic PNTs compose a relatively larger portion of childhood PNTs, with 99.5% of all peripheral neuroblastic tumors occurring in the first 2 decades of life[3] and accounting for approximately one third of childhood PNTs.[6]

CLINICAL PRESENTATION AND DIFFERENTIAL DIAGNOSIS

Pediatric PNTs commonly occur as a painless soft-tissue mass in the abdomen or within an extremity or as an incidental mass lesion on routine chest x-ray films. The general differential diagnosis of a soft-tissue mass is extensive and includes infectious or inflammatory lesions, vascular malformations, soft-tissue neoplasia, and in the case of abdominal or thoracic lesions, organ-specific neoplasia. When considering this differential diagnosis in pediatric patients, it should be noted that soft-tissue neoplasms comprise a heterogeneous spectrum of mesenchymal tumors that are of particular importance in pediatric oncology. This is highlighted by the fact that 6% to 8% of all childhood malignancies are of soft-tissue origin, versus fewer than 1% in adults.[11]

Often, specific features of the clinical history, findings on physical examination, or diagnostic investigations can help to identify the soft-tissue lesion associated with a peripheral nerve and hence a potential peripheral nerve neoplasm. Whereas exact numbers are difficult to determine, estimates suggest that 14% of all pediatric soft-tissue tumors arise from the peripheral nervous system.[6] For instance, a family history or clinical stigmata of neurofibromatosis 1 (NF1) or neurofibromatosis 2 (NF2) raises suspicion of neurofibromas or schwannomas, respectively. NF1 and NF2 are autosomal dominant phakomatoses that arise because of germline mutations of chromosomes 17q and 22q, respectively, and are associated with the development of numerous tumors, including PNTs. Further detailed discussion of the diagnostic criteria, phenotype, and specific molecular genetic aberrations of NF1 and NF2 are found elsewhere in this text.

Unfortunately, there are no pathognomonic features that permit absolute differentiation among PNTs on clinical grounds alone. Most pediatric PNTs are painless, with a slow and insidious growth pattern. New-onset pain, greatly increased pain, rapid increase in tumor size, or sudden progressive loss of function along the involved nerve should raise suspicion of malignant degeneration of a previously benign neurofibroma or *de novo* formation of a malignant lesion, such as a malignant peripheral nerve sheath tumor (MPNST). Furthermore, because of the risk of malignant degeneration in children with NF1,[24] all PNTs in NF1 patients should be viewed with suspicion. Children may also complain of some degree of mild subjective sensory loss or paresthesias as an initial sign of a PNT, although objective loss of function in the distribution of the affected nerve is relatively rare. The extremely slow rate of growth, with subsequent gentle stretch and elongation of the involved fascicles, accounts for the relatively well-preserved neural function that is observed, even in the context of rather large pediatric PNTs.

Peripheral neuroblastic lesions arise from the sympathetic nervous system and, accordingly, have a clinical presentation different from other peripheral nerve neoplasms. In addition to their presentation as abdominal, mediastinal, or thoracic mass lesions, this group of neoplasms may cause Horner's syndrome, owing to the involvement of cervical sympathetic nerves, or diarrhea related to release of vasoactive intestinal polypeptide. Spinal cord compression with consequent myelopathy is also possible by infiltration of dumbbell-shaped neuroblastic tumors through the neural foramina into the vertebral canal (Figure 107-1).

ELECTRODIAGNOSTIC AND IMAGING INVESTIGATIONS

Although the specific imaging characteristics of pediatric PNTs are similar to their counterparts in adults, the diagnostic

TABLE 107-1

Classification of Peripheral Nerve Tumors

Nerve Sheath Origin
Benign
    Schwannoma
    Neurofibroma
    Perineurioma
Malignant
    Malignant peripheral nerve sheath tumor (MPNST)

Neural Origin
Neuroblastoma
Ganglioneuroma
Ganglioneuroblastoma

Non-Neural Origin
Lipofibromatous hamartoma
Intraneural lesions (lipoma, ganglion cyst, hemangioma)

Metastases to Peripheral Nerve

imaging investigation of PNTs can be a challenging proposition in the pediatric population because of the patient's size and noncompliance.[2] Magnetic resonance imaging (MRI) is the imaging modality of choice because it is noninvasive, demonstrates proximal and distal lesions with equal efficacy, provides unparalleled image resolution, and can often definitively identify the nerve of origin.

Nerve conduction studies (NCSs) and electromyography (EMG) may also be performed in the diagnostic evaluation of a pediatric PNT. However, these studies are technically difficult in infants and young children and do not often contribute salient information to the specific diagnostic decision-making process because there are no neurophysiologic characteristics that differentiate among PNTs; in fact, often NCSs and EMG show no abnormality. Therefore the role of NCSs and EMG in the evaluation of pediatric PNTs is limited. NCSs and EMG can, however, provide objective electrophysiologic measures of baseline nerve function and thus may be of use for documentation of baseline nerve function in cases where neurologic function is to be monitored over time for deterioration and for evaluation of treatment.

TUMORS OF NERVE SHEATH ORIGIN

Benign Nerve Sheath Tumors

The classification of peripheral nerve sheath tumors has traditionally been an area of great dispute, and a detailed nosologic discussion of schwannomas, neurofibromas, and perineuriomas is beyond the scope of this chapter. It should suffice to say that the nerve sheath itself consists of three interconnected and tubular compartments—the epineurium, perineurium, and endoneurium—with perineurial fibroblasts and Schwann cells within the sheath. Schwann cells are derived from neural crest cells, and perineurial fibroblasts are of mesenchymal origin. Although it is known that schwannomas arise from Schwann cells (which produce the peripheral nerve's myelin coating) and perineuriomas from perineurial fibroblast (which gives rise to the epineurium, perineurium, and endoneurium), the histogenesis of the neurofibroma remains obscure and may be derived

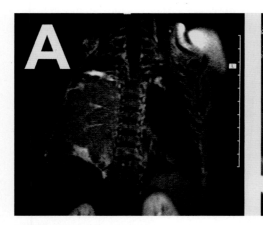
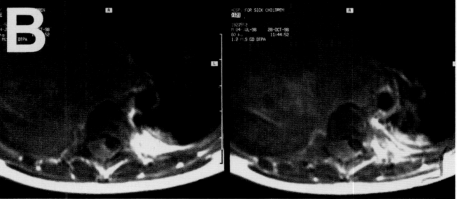

FIGURE 107-1 Coronal T1-weighted (A) and axial T1-weighted (B) magnetic resonance images of a thoracic dumbbell neuroblastoma. The axial images reveal extension of the tumor through the neural foramina and severe compression of the thoracic spinal cord. (Courtesy of Dr. James Drake.)

from an intermediate cell or a combination of both the Schwann cell and perineurial fibroblast.

Tumors of nerve sheath origin are less common in the pediatric population, but as a group they continue to account for a significant portion of childhood PNTs (approximately 50%).[6] The specific nuances of individual childhood peripheral nerve sheath tumors are discussed later.

Schwannoma

Although schwannomas are one of the most common PNTs in adults, they are not common in the pediatric population. In one large series, only 3% of schwannomas occurred in patients in their first 2 decades of life,[29] whereas another case series showed that 5% of all pediatric peripheral nerve neoplasms were schwannomas.[6] Indeed, because of their relative rarity, pediatric patients who have one or more confirmed schwannomas should be evaluated for a possible NF2 mutation.[16]

Classically, schwannomas are palpable, painless masses, although a small percentage of children may experience spontaneous pain related to a schwannoma. Referred dysesthesia when tapping or percussing over the mass (Tinel's sign) is also a very common clinical finding. Although mild subjective sensory loss or paresthesias is an initial symptom of schwannomas, objective loss of function in the distribution of the affected nerve is relatively rare because of the slow rate of growth of these lesions.

The pathology of pediatric schwannomas is identical to that of schwannomas in the adult population. Briefly, on macroscopic examination schwannomas are often oval and well circumscribed with a prominent tumor capsule. Involvement of a single nerve fascicle in the mass of the tumor, with the remaining fascicles tethered over the tumor capsule, is readily apparent. Sectioning of the gross specimen reveals a yellow, fleshy appearance. Light microscopy reveals two distinct cellular organizational structures referred to as Antoni A and Antoni B tissue. Antoni A regions are cellular and composed of spindle-shaped cells in a palisading fashion. An area of densely packed palisading Antoni A cells is known as a *Verocay body*. Antoni B tissue is composed of spindle-shaped cells in loosely meshed, areolar areas with a clear mucinous matrix.

Pediatric schwannomas should be managed in a fashion identical to their counterparts in adults. Surgical extirpation is the mainstay of therapy and is described in detail elsewhere in this text. Because schwannomas are slow-growing benign lesions, complete resection provides a cure in practically all cases. Although there are no outcome data that focus solely on pediatric schwannomas, in the largest adult series to date 90% of patients improved or remained clinically stable after surgical resection.[7] Given that the biologic and clinical behavior of pediatric schwannomas appears identical to that in cases in adults, a similar success rate should be achieved in pediatric cases.

Neurofibroma

The incidence of neurofibromas in the pediatric population, unlike schwannomas, more closely approximates that of the adult population. In a large series by Coffin et al,[6] neurofibromas accounted for 43% of all pediatric peripheral neurogenic tumors and, because of the low incidence of schwannomas in

children, 90% of all benign pediatric peripheral nerve sheath tumors. By way of comparison, in large adult surgical series, neurofibromas account for 40% to 67% of benign peripheral nerve sheath tumors.[1,7] The proportion of NF1-associated neurofibromas is approximately the same in pediatric and adult surgical series (approximately 30%),[6,7] suggesting that an association with this phakomatosis does not account for the increased proportion of pediatric neurofibromas relative to schwannomas.

As with adult neurofibromas, two different morphologic types of neurofibromas are found in the pediatric population. The first is the fusiform neurofibroma, which usually arises from a single nerve fascicle as an isolated proliferation of neoplastic cells within the sheath of an associated nerve. Fusiform neurofibromas develop as a nodular swelling on a nerve. These are often solitary lesions, but may be multiple and occur as part of NF1. Plexiform neurofibromas constitute the second type of neurofibroma. These tumors form a network-like growth, arise from multiple nerve fascicles, often involve multiple branches of a large nerve, and lead to a diffuse mass of thickened nerves. Plexiform neurofibromas do not necessarily involve a nerve plexus such as the brachial or lumbosacral plexi. Plexiform neurofibromas are almost exclusively associated with NF1.

The pathology of pediatric fusiform and plexiform neurofibromas are identical to that of the lesions in adults and are discussed in detail elsewhere in this book. Briefly, on macroscopic examination fusiform neurofibromas usually have a capsule, are well circumscribed, firm, and demonstrate a glistening tan surface on sectioning. Plexiform neurofibromas are elongated, multinodular tumors that involve many fascicles of a single nerve, or many branches of a nerve plexus. Microscopic examination reveals cells with spindle-shaped nuclei separated by a more myxomatous stroma than is typical of schwannomas. The cytoarchitecture is most akin to the Antoni B regions of schwannomas. An extensive collagen network is also often present and has been said to be similar in appearance to "shredded carrots." Mitoses and nuclear atypia are rare. As neurofibromas enlarge, they typically encase multiple nerve fascicles, and thus, nerve fibers can be histologically observed within the tumor mass. This feature differentiates neurofibromas from schwannomas, which displace rather than encase nerve fascicles. Although fusiform neurofibromas arise from single fascicles, plexiform neurofibromas arise from multiple fascicles of a single nerve, each of which is expanded by neoplastic cells.

Sporadic (Non-Neurofibroma 1) Neurofibromas

Pediatric neurofibromas that occur outside of NF1 are almost exclusively solitary, fusiform lesions and found in association with nerves ranging from small unidentifiable cutaneous nerves, to larger peripheral nerves, spinal nerve roots, and the brachial and lumbosacral plexi. As with schwannomas, a painless, palpable mass is the most common occurrence. However, neurofibromas are more likely to be associated with radicular pain than are other nerve sheath tumors.[7] Children with neurofibromas may also complain of sensory loss, paresthesias, or weakness in the distribution of the involved nerve. Although demonstrable objective loss of function still occurs in only a minority of patients, it does occur more commonly with neurofibromas than with schwannomas.[7]

Neurofibroma 1–Associated Neurofibromas

Neurofibromas are the most consistent feature of NF1, and both fusiform and plexiform varieties occur in association with NF1. A large portion of NF1 patients develop cutaneous (dermal) neurofibromas by the time they reach adulthood. These lesions are fusiform neurofibromas of tiny cutaneous nerves. They are soft, discrete, often violaceous nodules that lie within the dermis and epidermis. They can occur on any cutaneous surface, are rarely painful, and exhibit a nonlinear growth pattern, with years of slow growth followed by periods of rapid expansion. These lesions rarely undergo malignant degeneration, but unfortunately, because of their usual occurrence in large numbers, they can be severely disfiguring.

NF1-associated deep, fusiform neurofibromas very seldom occur in the first decade but begin to appear thereafter, with a peak incidence late in the third decade.[7] No male or female predilection exists for NF1-associated neurofibromas. Like other neurofibromas, these lesions may be palpable, painless masses. However, loss of function (motor or sensory) in the distribution of the involved nerve appears to be more common among NF1-associated neurofibromas, with only approximately 20% of cases exhibiting normal preoperative function.[7]

The treatment of choice for pediatric fusiform neurofibromas (non-NF1 and NF1-associated) is complete surgical resection and follows the same surgical principles as outlined for neurofibromas in adults.

Plexiform neurofibromas are the most common peripheral neoplasm in children with NF1.[17] The prevalence of these lesions continues to increase as patients reach adulthood, as illustrated by the fact that computed tomography screening documented plexiform neurofibromas in the thorax of 4% of children with NF1,[22] whereas a separate study noted that 20% of adults with NF1 had similar lesions.[27] Most patients were asymptomatic. Plexiform neurofibromas are large, soft subcutaneous swellings with poorly defined margins starting in early childhood. Often the overlying skin is hyperpigmented or hypertrophied, with occasional hypertrichosis. Although severe intractable pain may be associated with plexiform neurofibromas, this is the exception rather than the norm.[15] Motor and sensory abnormalities along the affected nerve are very common.[7,15]

Plexiform neurofibromas are recognized as a significant cause of morbidity and mortality in patients with NF1. Surgery is still the only viable option for patients in whom a tumor is causing intractable pain or disability, although results are often less than satisfactory. A recent large series of patients with surgically treated pediatric plexiform neurofibromas noted that, although severe neurologic complications occurred in only 4.6% of patients, overall freedom from progression was only 54% at a median follow-up time of 6.8 years.[17] Prognostic factors for tumor recurrence were age younger than 10 years at the time of initial surgery; presence of residual tumor after surgery; and location of the tumor on the head, neck, or face.

The risk of sarcomatous degeneration is high among nondermal NF1-associated neurofibromas and is a particularly worrisome feature of plexiform neurofibromas. In general, patients with NF1 have a 3% to 5% risk of conversion of a plexiform neurofibroma to an MPNST, whereas non-NF1 plexiform neurofibromas undergo malignant degeneration in less than 1% of cases.[25] A recent report suggests that the relative risk of an NF1 patient developing an MPNST is 133 times greater in relation to the general population.[13] Therefore, considering the potentially long life span of pediatric patients with NF1, these children need careful long-term follow-up evaluation. Any hint of symptomatology that suggests malignant progression (increased deficit, increased pain, rapid increased size) should trigger aggressive investigation and surgical therapy.

Perineurioma

The perineurioma is a benign tumor composed of neoplastic perineurial cells. It exhibits proliferating perineurial cells throughout the endoneurium, resulting in the formation of characteristic "pseudo-onion bulbs." The clinical presentation is most commonly due to progressive muscle weakness, with or without atrophy. Perineuriomas typically occur during childhood and adolescence[14]; however, this lesion is exceedingly rare in both the pediatric and adult populations, representing much less than 1% of all peripheral nerve neoplasms. Macroscopically, perineuriomas produce a segmental, tubular enlargement of the affected peripheral nerve, whereas the microscopic appearance is one of proliferating perineurial cells throughout the endoneurium, as discussed previously.

Perineuriomas are benign. Long-term follow-up studies indicate that they do not recur if resected, and they do not metastasize. The treatment of choice consists only of diagnostic biopsy, followed by release of any entrapment points. Resection should be avoided to retain neurologic function for as long as possible, because nerve graft reconstruction after excision often does not result in recovery of nerve function.[14]

Malignant Peripheral Nerve Sheath Tumors

MPNSTs are nonrhabdomyosarcomatous soft-tissue tumors that arise from the peripheral nerve sheath. Cases in children and adolescents are not common and account for only 13% of all MPNSTs[8] and 12% of all peripheral neurogenic tumors of childhood.[6] The association of MPNST with NF1 is well established, with MPNSTs occurring in the setting of NF1 in 50% of cases.[25] Pediatric MPNST case series reveal that 29% to 66% of pediatric MPNSTs arise in the setting of NF1,[5,8,18] comparable to the overall NF1-related incidence.

As with other nerve sheath lesions, the most common clinical presentation is identical to that found in the adult population and consists of a progressively enlarging or painful mass, with or without associated neurologic symptoms. Pathologically, pediatric MPNSTs are identical to their counterparts in adults. A detailed discussion is found elsewhere in this book. In brief, the gross appearance of MPNST is that of globoid or fusiform, pseudoencapsulated, hard tumor that may be several centimeters in diameter at the time of diagnosis. MPNSTs grow within the nerve fascicles but commonly invade the epineurium and infiltrate the adjacent soft tissues. Microscopically, MPNSTs are highly cellular tumors that characteristically have a fascicular pattern, with spindle-shaped nuclei and scant cytoplasm.

As with MPNSTs in adults, radical surgical excision is the treatment of choice for pediatric MPNSTs. Outcome appears to be closely related to the extent of surgical removal of the primary tumor, with 75% 3-year disease-free survival[18] and 80% 10-year survival[5] in cases of gross-total resection of tumor. This compares with a 14% 10-year survival rate for patients who undergo nonradical surgical therapy.[5] MPNSTs can metastasize to lung, liver, bone, and the central nervous system (CNS), but lack of local control appears to be the major cause of treatment failure.[5,18] In recent series of pediatric MPNSTs, the 10-year survival rate was 41%,[5] whereas the overall (adult and pediatric) 10-year survival rate was 23%.[9] An initial comparison suggests that pediatric MPNSTs have a better prognosis, but direct comparison between these series is not likely to be valid, because they represent retrospective case series of disparate size taken from different decades.

Given the small number of patients in pediatric MPNST case series, it is difficult to definitively ascertain the role of radiation therapy and chemotherapy in the management of MPNSTs. Anecdotal evidence does suggest that radiation therapy decreases the rate of local recurrence in cases of nonradical resection,[5] but its role in cases of gross-total resection remains ill defined. The role of chemotherapy is even harder to define, because MPNSTs are considered a poorly responsive tumor. Chemotherapy response rates are unsatisfactory and appear to offer little efficacy, because patients with advanced disease have a poor outcome despite the use of chemotherapy regimens.[5]

TUMORS OF NEURAL ORIGIN

PNTs of neural origin are embryonal tumors that arise from migrating neuroectodermal cells derived from the neural crest and destined for the sympathetic nervous system. Because of their embryonal nature, they are exceedingly rare in adulthood but account for a significant portion of childhood peripheral neurogenic neoplasms. They are the most common solid extracranial malignant tumors of the first 2 years of life,[20] with 96% occurring in the first decade.[3] There is no sex predilection. In one large pathologic series, neuroblastic tumors made up approximately one third of all childhood PNTs.[6]

Neuroblastic tumors can arise from the abdominal (25%), thoracic (15%), cervical (5%), and pelvic (5%) sympathetic ganglia, as well as the adrenal medulla,[12] and thus commonly occur as a palpable abdominal mass, hepatomegaly, or as a thoracic mass detected on routine chest x-ray films. The International Neuroblastoma Pathology Committee has devised a classification scheme for peripheral neuroblastic tumors that consists of four types, depending on the degree and type of differentiation: neuroblastoma, ganglioneuroblastoma or intermixed, ganglioneuroblastoma or nodular, and ganglioneuroma.[12] Each of these is discussed in the following sections.

Neuroblastoma

Most neuroblastomas occur during the first 2 years of life. Neuroblastomas may be a mass at the primary site of origin and are often quite large at the time of diagnosis (see Figure 107-1) or following metastatic spread to abdominal viscera, lymph nodes, liver, or bone. CNS metastases are rare in children but when present are often dural based.[23] Although all types of peripheral neuroblastic tumors have traditionally been placed under the rubric of neuroblastoma, current recommendations suggest that the term be used to designate only the specific tumor that is microscopically characterized by groups or nests of neuroblastic (small-round-blue) cells separated by delicate stromal septa with little or no schwannian proliferation. Macroscopically, neuroblastomas are encapsulated, soft, large, gray masses. Hemorrhage and foci of calcification are often present.

Although the majority of neuroblastomas are thought to be sporadic, there have been numerous reports of familial neuroblastoma, as well as multifocal disease, suggesting a hereditary predisposition. Recent investigation has identified linkage of familial neuroblastoma to chromosome 16p, suggesting that this region may harbor a locus for neuroblastoma predisposition.[28]

The molecular genetic alterations that result in neuroblastoma formation have been the subject of intensive research over the past decade. Of most significance are (1) the status of the N-myc oncogene, located on 2p24; (2) deletion (loss of heterozygosity [LOH]) of the short arm of chromosome 1; and (3) the expression status of the neurotrophin receptor tyrosine kinase receptor (Trk)A. N-myc is amplified in approximately 25% of neuroblastomas,[4] whereas 1p deletion occurs in 30% to 40% of cases.[10] Both N-myc amplification and 1p deletion are strongly correlated with each other, with an aggressive subset of neuroblastoma, and with a subsequent poor outcome.[10] In the same manner, TrkA is also correlated with neuroblastoma prognosis because aggressive neuroblastomas are noted to lack trkA expression.[26] The status of these molecular markers is combined with the histologic stage of the neuroblastoma, as well as clinical factors (age and tumor location) to help determine the overall prognosis. Clinically, neuroblastomas have a more favorable prognosis in infants younger than 1 year, and children with intra-abdominal lesions appear to have a worse outcome than those with lesions in other anatomic compartments.

In general, if neuroblastomas are discovered before the development of metastases, complete surgical extirpation with negative margins should be the goal of treatment where anatomically possible. Patients with stage IV disease (distant metastases) are usually treated initially with chemotherapy, followed either by observation or delayed resection of tumor.[21] Recommendations for adjuvant therapy of nonmetastatic neuroblastoma depend on the stage, age, and degree of surgical resection. Patients with only microscopic residual tumor should be followed conservatively, whereas patients with gross residual disease would receive chemotherapy and radiation therapy (if older than 1 year).[21] Despite aggressive therapy, overall prognosis is poor, and survival approaches only 20% to 30% in cases with multiple negative prognostic indicators (i.e., N-myc amplification, 1p LOH, lack of trkA expression, age older than 1 year, abdominal location).[23]

Ganglioneuroma

Peripheral ganglioneuromas are more common in children during their second decade of life and usually cause symptoms secondary to mass effect. They most commonly arise in the retroperitoneal or retropleural space. Macroscopically, ganglioneuromas are well-circumscribed, firm, white, fibrous tumors, and microscopically these tumors are composed of ganglioneuromatous stroma with scattered collections of ganglion cells surrounded by satellite cells. Schwann cells are abundant, and numerous axons are observed within the tumor. Metastases from ganglioneuromas occur very seldom, and this lesion essentially behaves in a benign nature. The treatment of choice is wide local excision, and little evidence exists to support the use of adjuvant therapy.[21] Prognosis is excellent, and long-term survival after successful surgical resection is good, except in the rare cases of metastases.

Ganglioneuroblastoma (Intermixed and Nodular)

Ganglioneuroblastomas are biologically intermediate between ganglioneuromas and neuroblastomas. They most commonly occur in children younger than 6 years of age and have a distribution similar to that of ganglioneuromas. Macroscopically, ganglioneuroblastomas may resemble ganglioneuromas, but foci of calcification, necrosis, hemorrhage, and local invasion may be present. Histologically, two types of ganglioneuroblastomas are recognized. The intermixed variant contains well-defined microscopic nests of neuroblastic cells randomly distributed in a ganglioneuromatous stroma, whereas the nodular variant is characterized by the presence of grossly visible neuroblastoma nodules coexisting with intermixed ganglioneuroblastoma or ganglioneuroma components. The behavior of ganglioneuroblastomas is unpredictable, but the intermixed variant appears to have a more favorable prognosis than the nodular variant.[12] The goal of treatment should be complete surgical resection of the tumor whenever possible. Recommendations for adjuvant therapy follow those for neuroblastoma, as outlined previously. Because of their aggressive nature, the prognosis of ganglioneuroblastomas is poor and similar to that of neuroblastoma.

TUMORS OF NON-NEURAL ORIGIN

As a group, these neoplasms are exceedingly rare in childhood, with only sporadic cases reported in the literature. In general, if a non-neural lesion is suspected in the peripheral nerve of a child, the principles of management for its counterpart in adults should be followed.

The lipomatous hamartoma does deserve special mention because this is a congenital fatty-fibrous lesion that usually occurs during childhood as a mass lesion associated with sensory findings. The majority of cases are associated with the median nerve in the palm or at the wrist, although lipomatous hamartomas have been reported in the foot. The treatment of choice is decompression of the nerve (e.g., carpal tunnel release) rather than an attempt at removal of lipomatous tissue, because this tissue is interdigitated between the axons of the nerve and is not feasible to remove.[14]

References

1. Artico M, Cervoni L, Wierzbicki V, et al: Benign neural sheath tumours of major nerves: characteristics in 119 surgical cases. Acta Neurochir (Wien) 139:1108–1116, 1997.
2. Birchansky S, Altman N: Imaging the brachial plexus and peripheral nerves in infants and children. Semin Pediatr Neurol 7:15–25, 2000.
3. Brodeur GM, Castleberry RP: Neuroblastoma. In Poplack DG (ed): Principles and Practice of Pediatric Oncology, 2nd ed. Philadelphia, JB Lippincott, 1993.
4. Brodeur GM, Seeger RC, Schwab M, et al: Amplification of N-myc in untreated human neuroblastomas correlates with advanced disease stage. Science 224:1121–1124, 1984.
5. Casanova M, Ferrari A, Spreafico F, et al: Malignant peripheral nerve sheath tumors in children: a single-institution twenty-year experience. J Pediatr Hematol Oncol 21:509–513, 1999.
6. Coffin CM, Dehner LP: Peripheral neurogenic tumors of the soft tissues in children and adolescents: a clinicopathologic study of 139 cases. Pediatr Pathol 9:387–407, 1989.
7. Donner TR, Voorhies RM, Kline DG: Neural sheath tumors of major nerves. J Neurosurg 81:362–373, 1994.
8. Ducatman BS, Scheithauer BW, Piepgras DG, et al: Malignant peripheral nerve sheath tumors in childhood. J Neurooncol 2:241–248, 1984.
9. Ducatman BS, Scheithauer BW, Piepgras DG, et al: Malignant peripheral nerve sheath tumors. A clinicopathologic study of 120 cases. Cancer 57:2006–2021, 1986.
10. Fong CT, Dracopoli NC, White PS, et al: Loss of heterozygosity for the short arm of chromosome 1 in human neuroblastomas: correlation with N-myc amplification. Proc Natl Acad Sci USA 86:3753–3757, 1989.
11. Harms D: Soft tissue sarcomas in the Kiel Pediatric Tumor Registry. Curr Top Pathol 89:31–45, 1995.
12. Joshi VV: Peripheral neuroblastic tumors: pathologic classification based on recommendations of international neuroblastoma pathology committee (Modification of shimada classification). Pediatr Dev Pathol 3:184–199, 2000.
13. King AA, Debaun MR, Riccardi VM, et al: Malignant peripheral nerve sheath tumors in neurofibromatosis 1. Am J Med Genet 93:388–392, 2000.
14. Kline DG, Hudson AR: Nerve Injuries: Operative Results for Major Nerve Injuries, Entrapments, and Tumors, 1st ed. Philadelphia, WB Saunders, 1995.
15. Korf BR: Plexiform neurofibromas. Am J Med Genet 89:31–37, 1999.
16. Mautner VF, Tatagiba M, Guthoff R, et al: Neurofibromatosis 2 in the pediatric age group. Neurosurgery 33:92–96, 1993.
17. Needle MN, Cnaan A, Dattilo J, et al: Prognostic signs in the surgical management of plexiform neurofibroma: the Children's Hospital of Philadelphia experience, 1974–1994. J Pediatr 131: 678–682, 1997.
18. Raney B, Schnaufer L, Ziegler M, et al: Treatment of children with neurogenic sarcoma. Experience at the Children's Hospital of Philadelphia, 1958–1984. Cancer 59:1–5, 1987.
19. Reed RJ, Harkin JC, Armed Forces Institute of Pathology (U. S.), et al: Tumors of the peripheral nervous system. Bethesda, Md, Armed Forces Institute of Pathology under the auspices of Universities Associated for Research and Education in Pathology, 1983.
20. Ross JA, Severson RK, Pollock BH, et al: Childhood cancer in the United States. A geographical analysis of cases from the Pediatric Cooperative Clinical Trials groups. Cancer 77:201–207, 1996.
21. Saenz NC, Schnitzer JJ, Eraklis AE, et al: Posterior mediastinal masses. J Pediatr Surg 28:172–176, 1993.
22. Schorry EK, Crawford AH, Egelhoff JC, et al: Thoracic tumors in children with neurofibromatosis-1. Am J Med Genet 74:533–537, 1997.
23. Schwab M, Shimada H, Joshi VV, et al: Neuroblastic tumours of adrenal gland and sympathetic nervous system. In Cavenee WK (ed): Pathology & Genetics: Tumours of the Nervous System. Lyon, France, IARC Press, 2000.
24. Shearer P, Parham D, Kovnar E, et al: Neurofibromatosis type I and malignancy: review of 32 pediatric cases treated at a single institution. Med Pediatr Oncol 22:78–83, 1994.

25. Sorensen SA, Mulvihill JJ, Nielsen A: Long-term follow-up of von Recklinghausen neurofibromatosis. Survival and malignant neoplasms. N Engl J Med 314:1010–1015, 1986.

26. Suzuki T, Bogenmann E, Shimada H, et al: Lack of high-affinity nerve growth factor receptors in aggressive neuroblastomas. J Natl Cancer Inst 85:377–384, 1993.

27. Tonsgard JH, Kwak SM, Short MP, et al: CT imaging in adults with neurofibromatosis-1: frequent asymptomatic plexiform lesions. Neurology 50:1755–1760, 1998.

28. Weiss MJ, Guo C, Shusterman S, et al: Localization of a hereditary neuroblastoma predisposition gene to 16p12-p13. Med Pediatr Oncol 35:526–530, 2000.

29. Woodruff JM, Kourea HP, Louis DN, et al: Schwannoma. In Cavenee WK (ed): Pathology & Genetics: Tumours of the Nervous System. Lyon, France, IARC Press, 2000.

CHAPTER 108

NEUROCUTANEOUS SYNDROMES

Paul Kongkham and James T. Rutka

The neurocutaneous syndromes consist of several heterogeneous disorders grouped together because of their common involvement of the neurologic, dermatologic, and ophthalmologic systems and various other organ systems. These disorders have previously been referred to as the *phakomatoses*, a term coined by van der Hoeve in the early twentieth century. This term, derived from the Greek root *phakos* (birthmark), captured the common, visible dermatologic manifestations characteristic of these syndromes. Disorders classified as neurocutaneous syndromes include neurofibromatosis (types 1 and 2), tuberous sclerosis complex, von Hippel-Lindau disease, and Sturge-Weber syndrome. Less common disorders, also categorized as neurocutaneous syndromes, include Rendu-Osler-Weber disease, Wyburn-Mason disease, nevoid basal cell carcinoma syndrome, and Cowden's disease. In addition to the common involvement of similar organ systems with these disorders, further evidence supporting their classification together under the umbrella term *neurocutaneous syndromes* comes from the fact that these conditions are occasionally seen to overlap within affected families.

In general, these disorders are autosomal, dominantly inherited, genetic disorders, with high penetrance and variable expression. In addition, their expression is often "patchy" in nature, explained by Knudson's "two-hit" mechanism necessary for phenotype expression, characteristic of disorders secondary to abnormalities of tumor-suppressor genes.

The definitive diagnosis of these syndromes is often difficult, owing to the diversity of conditions within this category of diseases, their variable expression, and the many organ systems in which symptoms may first appear. As such, a multidisciplinary team including neurosurgeons, neurologists, dermatologists, ophthalmologists, otolaryngologists, pediatricians, and geneticists is generally required for thorough assessment of affected individuals and their families.

To date, the genes for 10 disorders classified as neurocutaneous syndromes have been identified. In fact, this number accounts for approximately one third of all cloned hereditary cancer genes. Despite the relative rarity of these disorders, the knowledge gained from this intensive study has benefited a wide range of patients, because many malignancies associated with these disorders also occur in isolation among the general population. Continued study of these disorders should increase our understanding of both normal and abnormal neural cellular proliferation and mechanisms of neuro-oncogenesis and should

suggest possible novel therapeutic strategies for those individuals affected by neurologic malignancies.

This chapter discusses the common neurocutaneous syndromes: neurofibromatosis 1 and 2, tuberous sclerosis, von Hippel-Lindau disease, and Sturge-Weber syndrome. The epidemiology, genetics, clinical manifestations, and treatment will be highlighted, with certain emphasis on their neuro-oncologic manifestations.

NEUROFIBROMATOSIS

The neurofibromatoses consist of a heterogeneous group of disorders that share abnormal pigmented cutaneous lesions and tumors of neuroectodermal origin. Most cases are represented by neurofibromatosis types 1 (NF1) and 2 (NF2).

Neurofibromatosis Type 1

NF1, also known as peripheral NF or von Recklinghausen's disease, is the most common form of NF—accounting for approximately 96% of all cases.[24] It was first thoroughly described by Friedrich Daniel von Recklinghausen in 1882. In addition to being the most common form of NF, it is also one of the most common inherited disorders to affect the nervous system, with an incidence of approximately 1 in every 4000 live births. It shows equal prevalence among the sexes and no particular preference for race.

This disorder is inherited in an autosomal dominant fashion, with nearly complete penetrance but variable expression. In only approximately 50% of cases, however, is there a positive family history of the disease. The other 50% of cases are thought to represent new mutations. The NF1 tumor-suppressor gene is located in the pericentric region on the long arm of chromosome 17 (17q11.2). It was initially identified by linkage analysis in 1990, and since then its complete DNA sequence has been determined. This gene spans approximately 335 kb pairs of genomic DNA, with a total of 60 exons. In addition, three separate genes, transcribed in the opposite direction, have been identified within the same segment of DNA. The gene product, neurofibromin, is a large, ubiquitous cytoplasmic protein of 2818 amino acids. This is thought to exist in multiple forms in various tissues because of tissue-specific alternative splicing in adults. Neurofibromin is thought to interact with intracellular cytoplasmic microtubules, exhibiting guanosine triphosphate activating protein (GAP) activity. The GTPase activating domain is believed to normally convert proto-oncogenic RAS (GTP-bound) to its inactive form (GDP-bound).

The high percentage of new mutations in NF1 may be explained by this gene's high spontaneous mutation rate—estimated to be 1×10^{-4} per gamete per generation. This is approximately 100 times greater than most other genes. More than 200 mutations affecting the NF1 gene have been identified, including insertions, deletions, point mutations, and gonadal and somatic mutations. Thus far, no specific genotype-phenotype correlations have been determined, although larger deletions seem to be associated with a more severe phenotype in general. In addition, the vast majority of mutations are unique to families, with only a few found to be recurring.

Despite this, certain genetic tests are available for the diagnosis of NF1. Recently, a commercial mutational analysis kit for NF1 (Protein Truncation Test; Boehringer Mannheim, Indianapolis, Ind.) has become available. This test utilizes ribonucleic acid (RNA) from white blood cells and reverse-transcribes it into fragments of copy-DNA for the NF1 gene. These fragments then serve as templates for in vitro synthesis of neurofibromin protein product fragments, which are subsequently analyzed on polyacrylamide gel electrophoresis to look for evidence of truncation. Abnormal fragments may then be probed further to assess for their underlying genetic mutation.[17] This test claims to be able to identify up to 70% of NF1 mutations. The utility, however, of such genetic testing remains limited. This is in part due to the fact that a positive test can determine only whether patients will be affected, not the degree to which they will be affected by the disease. In addition, conventional techniques for mutational analysis in patients with NF1 have been limited because of the gene's large size and its high spontaneous mutation rate. As such, genetic testing is rarely performed for diagnostic purposes, and therefore the diagnosis largely remains a clinical one.

Diagnostic criteria have been developed, based on the 1987 National Institutes of Health (NIH) Consensus Development Conference on Neurofibromatosis[37] (Table 108-1). Although aspects of this consensus statement have been superseded in view of continued research, these criteria are primarily valid and valuable in the diagnostic evaluation for neurofibromatosis. The clinical features of NF1 manifest, to varying degrees, in several organ systems. Among these are the cutaneous, ophthalmologic, musculoskeletal, and neurologic systems. The majority of patients show only cutaneous lesions and ocular Lisch nodules. Others, however, develop more serious complications that tend to appear as the patient ages.

One of the most common cutaneous signs of this disorder are café-au-lait macules. These lesions are areas of abnormal skin pigmentation, varying in size from a few millimeters to a few centimeters, with regular borders and an even coloration throughout. They may be more easily seen on examination by using a Wood's lamp. Often, they are present at birth and they are almost always evident by the time a child is 1 year of age. With increasing age, they may increase in size and number, with approximately 95% of adults with NF1 having at least one lesion and 78% having at least six. These lesions occur on most areas of the body, excluding the palms, soles of the feet, and scalp. The face is rarely involved. A second cutaneous sign of NF1 is skin-fold freckling. These markings may be seen in the

TABLE 108-1

Diagnostic Criteria for Neurofibromatosis 1

The patient must exhibit 2 or more of the following:

6 or more café-au-lait macules (5 mm or larger in prepubertal patient, 15 mm or larger in postpubertal patient)

2 or more neurofibromas of any kind or one plexiform neurofibroma

Axillary/inguinal freckling

Optic pathway glioma

2 or more Lisch nodules (iris hamartomas)

Distinctive osseous abnormality (sphenoid wing dysplasia, thinning of long-bone cortex, pseudoarthrosis)

A first-degree relative with NF1 as per the above criteria

Source: Modified from Neurofibromatosis. Conference Statement. National Institutes of Health Consensus Development Conference. Arch Neurol 45:575–578, 1988; Neurofibromatosis. NIH Consensus Statement Online 6:1–19, 1987, http://consensus.nih.gov/cons/064/064_statement.htm.

submammary, axillary, or inguinal regions. Unlike café-au-lait macules, these lesions may not be evident until late childhood or early puberty.

Lisch nodules are a common ophthalmologic manifestation of NF1. These lesions consist of raised, pigmented (yellow-brown), iris hamartomas, detected best by slit-lamp examination. Often absent in childhood, Lisch nodules increase in prevalence with age, with approximately 94% of postpubertal patients exhibiting them. Histopathologically, Lisch nodules consist of masses of melanocytes. Less common ophthalmologic findings in NF1 include congenital glaucoma or eyelid, conjunctival, and orbital neurofibromas. Thickened corneal, conjunctival, and ciliary nerves, as well as retinal astrocytomas and sectorial retinitis pigmentosa, may also be seen.

Musculoskeletal findings in this disorder include bone abnormalities of the spine such as vertebral body scalloping, kyphoscoliosis, and idiopathic vertebral dysplasia. Scoliosis affects between 10% and 20% of patients, often manifesting in adolescence. Short stature is estimated to affect between 25% and 35% of patients. Other bone abnormalities include thinning of long bone cortex, pseudoarthroses, and sphenoid wing dysplasia. Rarely, NF1 patients may develop musculoskeletal malignancies such as rhabdomyosarcoma.

The neurologic manifestations of NF1 can affect both the peripheral and central nervous systems (Table 108-2). In the peripheral nervous system, one finds one of the pathognomonic features of NF1: multiple cutaneous and subcutaneous neurofibromas. These lesions are often distributed in the thoracoabdominal region or around the nipple-areola complex. Although not specific to NF1, these lesions are the most common benign tumors associated with this disorder, varying in number from a few to thousands. New lesions can appear with advancing age. Malignant transformation of these tumors may occur rarely. Mainly, they pose primarily a cosmetic problem, which is somewhat amenable to treatment by local surgical excision if desired by the patient.

Another, less common peripheral lesion is the so-called *plexiform neurofibroma*. This type of neurofibroma often dif-

TABLE 108-2

Peripheral and Central Nervous System Manifestations of Neurofibromatosis 1

PNS	CNS
Cutaneous/subcutaneous neurofibroma	Optic pathway glioma
Plexiform neurofibroma	Hemispheric/posterior fossa glioma
MPNSTs (neurofibrosarcoma)	Thoracic spine meningocele
Paraspinal neurofibroma	Spinal schwannoma
	Spinal meningioma
	Learning disability/mental retardation
	Hydrocephalus/aquaductal stenosis
	Epilepsy
	Idiopathic macrocephaly

CNS, Central nervous system; MPNST, malignant peripheral nerve sheath tumor; PNS, peripheral nervous system.

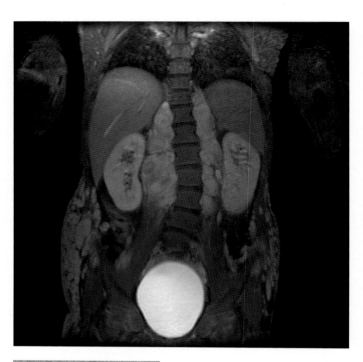

FIGURE 108-1 Gadolinium-enhanced coronal T1-weighted magnetic resonance imaging through the thoracic and lumbar spine showing extensive paraspinal neurofibromas in a 3-year-old child with neurofibromatosis 1 and scoliosis.

fusely involves a much larger peripheral nerve or part of the sympathetic chain, with potential for disfigurement or impairment of function in the involved area. Occasionally, a generalized enlargement of an affected limb (hemihypertrophy) may occur. Plexiform neurofibromas are almost always congenital lesions and are believed to be specific to NF1.[15,24] Surgical resection of plexiform neurofibromas is challenging, and recurrence at the surgical site is common. Therefore, for asymptomatic lesions, the recommended treatment is to follow conservatively. If lesions are small and symptomatic, surgical excision may be attempted with minimal resultant motor deficit. Large, symptomatic lesions often encase several neural bundles, leading to significant dysfunction if excision is attempted. Therefore the decision to operate should be individualized, with input from the surgeon, radiologist, oncologist, and pediatricians involved. Recently, trials of nonoperative management using either 13-cis retinoic acid or interferon-α 2a have begun, although definitive results are lacking at this time.

In contrast to cutaneous and subcutaneous neurofibromas, plexiform neurofibromas do have the potential to undergo malignant transformation, with the resultant formation of a malignant peripheral nerve sheath tumor (MPNST) or neurofibrosarcoma. MPNSTs are relatively rare, highly malignant tumors affecting approximately 6% of patients with NF1, often during adolescence and young adulthood. Among the general population, approximately half of patients with such tumors also have a diagnosis of NF1. These tumors are life threatening, with definite metastatic potential. Development of an MPNST is often marked by a report of new neurologic signs, persistent pain, or rapid growth of a plexiform neurofibroma. Treatment involves immediate surgical biopsy to establish the diagnosis, followed by possible limb amputation, radiation therapy, and chemotherapy. The overall 5-year survival with this lesion is reported to be approximately 40%, depending on the location, size, and invasiveness of the tumor.

Paraspinal neurofibromas are the most common tumors to affect the spine in patients with NF1 (Figure 108-1). These

generally arise from the dorsal roots in the cervical and lumbar regions. These benign tumors may grow into the spinal canal via the intervertebral foramen, resulting in a dumbbell-shaped neurofibroma. Surgical resection is indicated if this lesion causes mass effect resulting in weakness or myelopathic findings. Sensory deficits are not a common feature of this tumor.

Among the central nervous system manifestations of NF1, the optic pathway glioma is the most common (Figure 108-2). Optic pathway gliomas occur sporadically, accounting for between 2% and 5% of all childhood brain tumors. The majority, however, are seen in the context of NF1. In fact, optic pathway gliomas affect approximately 15% of NF1 patients according to neuroimaging screening studies. This tumor most commonly occurs during childhood, with the greatest risk during the first 6 years of life. Females are affected twice as often as males. These tumors are generally slow-growing, grade I pilocytic astrocytomas. They have the potential to arise at any point along the optic pathway; however, prechiasmal lesions are the most common. Approximately half of all optic pathway gliomas remain asymptomatic. When symptomatic, the particular symptoms relate to the tumor location along the optic pathway. Tumors of the optic nerve may cause diplopia, proptosis, restricted visual fields, or reduced acuity. Chiasmal lesions may also cause visual disturbances or hypothalamic-pituitary abnormalities such as accelerated growth secondary to precocious puberty. Approximately 39% of children with chiasmal lesions may show evidence of precocious puberty.

Studies of the natural history of optic pathway glioma have shown that the majority of these tumors, including symptomatic ones, rarely progress following diagnosis.[31] As such, there has been no proven role for asymptomatic radiologic screening of

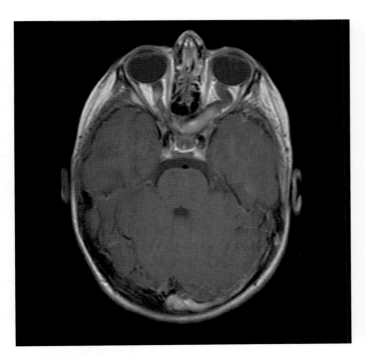

FIGURE 108-2 Gadolinium-enhanced axial T1-weighted magnetic resonance imaging through the orbits depicting left optic nerve glioma extending from the chiasm to the globe in a 4-year-old child. The nerve on the right side is less severely affected. Bilateral optic nerve gliomas are pathognomonic of neurofibromatosis 1.

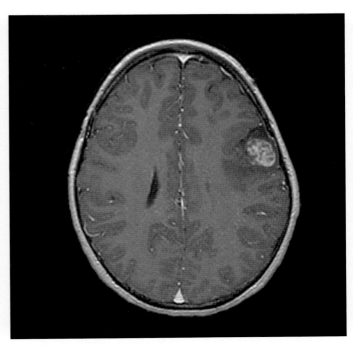

FIGURE 108-3 Contrast-enhanced axial T1-weighted magnetic resonance imaging through the insular cortex depicting an enhancing, cortically based lesion in the left hemisphere in a 7-year-old child with neurofibromatosis 1 (NF1) who presented with intractable seizures. The lesion was resected entirely, and proved to be a gangli-oglioma. Patients with NF1 are at higher risk of developing glial neo-plasms in both the supratentorial and infratentorial compartments.

children for these lesions. Those children requiring treatment for optic pathway glioma essentially all have findings on examination and are therefore clinically identifiable. Therefore recommendations suggest that asymptomatic children with NF1 have serial examinations by pediatric or neuro-ophthalmologists familiar with the disease. A complete examination, consisting of assessment of visual fields, color vision, acuity, funduscopy, slit-lamp examination, ocular alignment, papillary light reflex, and refractive status, should be performed on all newly diagnosed patients and yearly on those children younger than age 6. After that, repeat examination should be performed every 2 to 3 years or when new ophthalmologic symptoms arise. Those children with abnormalities on examination would then be referred for magnetic resonance imaging (MRI) of the brain and orbits for further assessment. Those children found to have symptomatic optic pathway glioma require careful follow-up with full ophthalmologic examinations and contrast-enhanced MRI approximately every 3 months for the first 18 months, followed by assessment at increasing intervals if the lesion remains stable.

The recommendations for treatment of optic pathway glioma depend largely on the location of the tumor. Intraorbital and prechiasmal tumors are managed based on their symptoms. Treatment for these lesions is indicated for patients with progressive proptosis, visual loss, or in certain cases with evidence of rapid radiologic progression. Treatment may involve surgery, radiation therapy, or chemotherapy. In the case of a blind eye, surgery may be performed for cosmetic purposes and to prevent spread of the tumor toward the chiasm. Chiasmatic optic pathway gliomas are generally observed for a short interval

because there is no clear evidence to suggest benefit from early intervention. The role of surgery for lesions in this location is limited. Surgery may be necessary to debulk large tumors, especially those with cystic components. This is at the risk, however, of significant visual, endocrinologic, and neurologic compromise. Radiation therapy for these lesions remains another option in the child older than 3 years. With radiation therapy, up to 80% of patients may show evidence of tumor stabilization or shrinkage, although these effects may be delayed up to 1 year. Radiation therapy poses the risks, however, of transient worsening of the patient's symptoms because of tumor enlargement, neuroendocrine and neurocognitive sequelae, and radiation-induced malignancies in the irradiated field. Recently, various data have begun to show evidence that tumor progression is delayed by using both single and multiagent chemotherapy for optic pathway glioma.[8,13,14,41,44,50] Even so, radiation therapy should still be considered the primary treatment for children with progressive optic pathway glioma.

In addition to optic pathway glioma, patients with NF1 are susceptible to hemispheric and posterior fossa gliomas (Figure 108-3). These may be either grade II pilocytic astrocytomas or a more aggressive form of tumor. Hemispheric gliomas occur in fewer than 0.5% of NF1 patients. These are rarely treated surgically. Posterior fossa gliomas (brainstem or cerebellar) affect approximately 1% of NF1 patients. For those patients who remain asymptomatic with these lesions, serial monitoring (clinical and radiologic) is appropriate. In those patients who become symptomatic, surgical excision with local radiation therapy may be required.

Less common central nervous system manifestations of NF1 include hydrocephalus, aqueductal stenosis, epilepsy, and idiopathic macrocephaly.

One common neurologic manifestation of NF1 during childhood is that of cognitive impairment. Learning disability of some degree is evident in 30% to 65% of children with NF1. In general, language skills are better preserved than visuospatial skills. Attention deficit may also be seen, as well as motor incoordination. The etiology of these deficits remains unknown. Controversy exists regarding whether focal areas of increased T2-weighted signal on MRI, known as unidentified bright objects (UBOs), represent the pathologic substrate of these deficits. These UBOs are not evident on computed tomography (CT) scanning and are isointense on T1-weighted MRI (Figure 108-4). In addition, they exhibit no mass effect, edema, or enhancement. Most often they are found within the basal ganglia, cerebellum, brainstem, and subcortical white matter. Pathologically, these regions are believed to consist of areas of spongiform myelinopathy. Over time, these lesions tend to resolve spontaneously. Whatever the etiology of these childhood deficits, any suspicion of cognitive impairment should prompt follow-up evaluation with neuropsychologic testing, neurologic examination, imaging, and the development of an appropriate rehabilitation plan to maximize the child's cognitive potential.

Despite the best medical care, the life expectancy for patients with NF1 remains approximately 15 years less than that of the general population. Malignancy is one of the primary reasons for this reduction in life expectancy among adult patients with NF1, with the overall risk of suffering from some malignant complication being approximately 3% to 15%.[5] To minimize morbidity from this disorder, multidisciplinary follow-up review is recommended. Such follow-up evaluation should include examination of the patient and all first-degree relatives, as well as a discussion regarding the natural history of the disorder and its pattern of inheritance. Annual physical and ophthalmologic examinations, by physicians knowledgeable about the disease, are recommended during the school years. These examinations should include monitoring for scoliosis, rapidly enlarging or symptomatic neurofibromas, visual problems, or alterations in the rate of linear growth.

Neurofibromatosis Type 2

NF2 is a much less common disorder, with an incidence of approximately 1 in 40,000 live births (one tenth that of NF1). This disorder shows no regard for race or sex. Previously, NF2 has been referred to as bilateral acoustic or central neurofibromatosis because of the presence of its hallmark lesion: bilateral acoustic neuromas (vestibular schwannomas). In addition to this hallmark lesion, NF2 is characterized by multiple intracranial and intraspinal tumors. Cutaneous stigmata do not figure prominently in this disease.

NF2 is an autosomal dominantly inherited disorder with the causative gene located at the 22q11 locus on the long arm of chromosome 22. This tumor-suppressor gene was first identified and cloned in 1993, and since then much work has gone into characterizing the nature of its protein product: merlin, or schwannomin. This protein is believed to function as a cytoskeletal protein. Loss of heterozygosity for the NF2 gene has been demonstrated in tumors such as vestibular schwannomas, meningiomas, and neurofibromas in NF2 patients. In general, those mutations leading to premature termination of protein translation result in a more severe phenotype. By using linkage analysis, with markers flanking the NF2 gene, a presumptive diagnosis of this disorder can be made in families with two or more affected individuals. This is relatively time consuming and expensive, however, and therefore the diagnosis of NF2 still remains largely a clinical one.

Diagnostic criteria for NF2 devised at the 1987 NIH Consensus Development Conference on Neurofibromatosis[37] were subsequently revised by the National Neurofibromatosis Foundation (NNFF) Clinical Care Advisory Board (Table 108-3). Patients with NF2 clinically may report a variety of difficulties. The majority of these are neurologic, including hearing impairment, tinnitus, imbalance, weakness, seizures, numbness or paresthesias, or impaired vision. Approximately 11% are identified while asymptomatic as a result of screening within affected families. Only 10% of patients become symptomatic before age 10.[15] In addition, new signs and symptoms may develop with increasing age, and therefore the evaluation of an NF2 patient must involve long-term, continued serial assessments.

As in NF1, patients with NF2 may suffer from a variety of ophthalmologic conditions. Juvenile posterior subcapsular lenticular opacities are the most common ocular findings in NF2, present in approximately 50% of patients. These lesions have the potential to cause visual impairment, and consideration of their surgical removal may be indicated. This is of par-

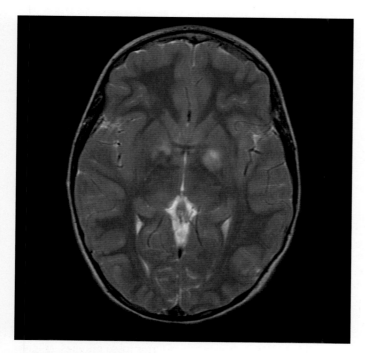

FIGURE 108-4 Axial fluid-attenuated inversion recovery magnetic resonance imaging through the basal ganglia in a 4-year-old child with neurofibromatosis 1 (NF1) showing multiple high-signal intensity lesions. These unidentified bright objects are thought to represent hamartomas or water-change in the brain and are a characteristic imaging signature of NF1.

TABLE 108-3

Diagnostic Criteria for Neurofibromatosis 2

Definite NF2

Bilateral vestibular schwannomas, or

Positive family history plus unilateral vestibular schwannoma before age 30 or two of: meningioma, schwannoma, glioma, juvenile posterior subcapsular lenticular opacity

Probable NF2

Unilateral vestibular schwannoma before age 30, plus one or more of: meningioma, schwannoma, glioma, juvenile posterior subcapsular lenticular opacity, or

Two or more meningiomas plus unilateral vestibular schwannoma before age 30 or one of: glioma, schwannoma, juvenile posterior subcapsular lenticular opacity

NF2, Neurofibromatosis 2.
Source: Modified from criteria for NF2 from the National Neurofibromatosis Foundation (NNFF) Clinical Care Advisory Board (www.nf.org).

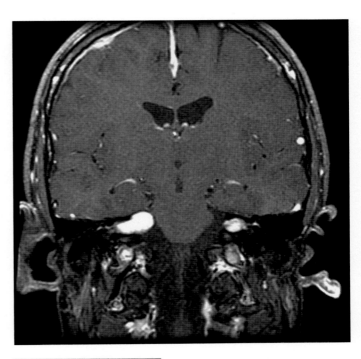

FIGURE 108-5 Gadolinium-enhanced coronal magnetic resonance imaging through the posterior fossa depicting bilateral vestibular schwannomas, the right tumor larger than the left one, in a 15-year-old boy with neurofibromatosis 2.

ticular importance, given the fact that this group of patients is also at risk for bilateral hearing loss. Additional ocular manifestations of NF2 include retinal hamartomas, epiretinal membranes, and rarely Lisch nodules. Combined, these findings hold diagnostic significance, because they may be detectable at an early age, assisting in the diagnosis of NF2 before the development of central nervous system tumors.

Aside from these ocular findings, the majority of features of NF2 involve the nervous system. As mentioned earlier, the hallmark of this disorder is bilateral vestibular schwannomas (Figure 108-5). Patients with NF2 often become symptomatic from these tumors decades earlier than those with spontaneous tumors. Sensorineural hearing loss is commonly the first complaint, although patients may also suffer from tinnitus, ataxia, headache, or facial nerve dysfunction. Diagnostic adjuvants include the use of MRI, audiometry, and brainstem auditory evoked responses (BAERs).

The standard of care for neuroimaging to detect vestibular schwannomas in NF2 patients involves thin-slice MRI of the head, with and without a contrast agent centered on the internal auditory canal. Both axial and coronal views and fat-saturation sequences should be performed. BAERs have a high positive predictive value for these tumors, showing an abnormal result in more than 95% of patients with tumors confirmed by imaging or at surgery. In contrast to the normal population, patients with vestibular schwannomas show a reversed amplitude ratio of waves I and V, as well as prolonged interpeak latencies between waves I and V. Other abnormalities include absent waveforms beyond waves I or II, and interaural differences. Pure tone audiometry provides evidence for hearing loss of a sensorineural nature.

As with spontaneous vestibular schwannomas, the growth rate of these lesions in NF2 patients is variable, with rates between 1 and 10 mm per year. Considering the often slow growth rate, following these patients conservatively, with sequential MRI to rule out continued growth, is warranted in the neurologically stable patient. Further treatment may be con-

sidered when there is evidence of symptomatic or radiologic progression. Treatment decisions must, however, weigh factors such as the patient's age and social, psychologic, and occupational circumstances against the rate of tumor progression. In addition, special consideration must be given to the possible treatment-related morbidities because these patients are at risk of possible bilateral hearing loss.

Surgery has long been considered the gold standard treatment for vestibular schwannomas. The timing and methods for surgical intervention have been well described elsewhere.[55] In general, earlier surgery on smaller lesions provides the best hope for a complete resection with maximal hearing preservation and facial nerve function. As with surgery for spontaneous vestibular schwannomas, surgery for the patient with NF2 should be limited to tertiary or quaternary care centers with neurosurgeons and otolaryngologists familiar with this disease.

Recently, the options of stereotactic fractionated radiation therapy and stereotactic radiosurgery have become available for the treatment of vestibular schwannomas in the patient with NF2. Good rates of hearing preservation and tumor control rates equal to those with surgery have been reported.[2] Tumor control rates of up to 98% have been reported in patients with NF2.[54] Long-term follow-up for these patients is still lacking, however. In addition, one must consider carefully the use of radiation as treatment in a patient population with abnormal tumor-suppressor genes because of the theoretic risk of inducing malignant tumor transformation or induction of secondary malignancies in the irradiated field.

In addition to bilateral vestibular schwannomas, patients with NF2 are susceptible to a variety of other tumors of the

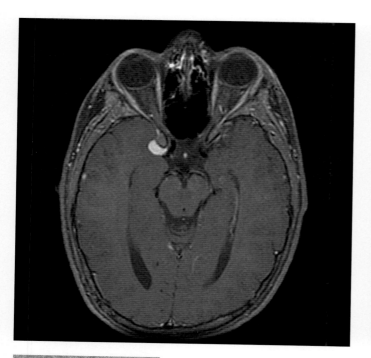

FIGURE 108-6 Right cavernous sinus, medial sphenoid wing meningioma depicted in this gadolinium-enhanced axial magnetic resonance image in a patient with neurofibromatosis 2.

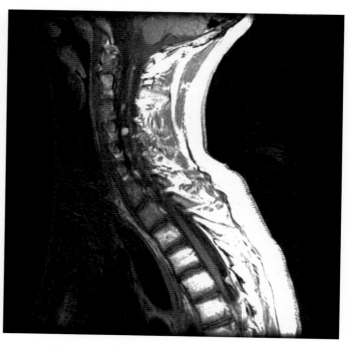

FIGURE 108-7 Gadolinium-enhanced sagittal magnetic resonance image of upper cervical spine, slightly off the midline, depicting multiple small enhancing tumors in the intraspinal space. These most likely represent intradural schwannomas, which must be followed with serial imaging studies.

neuraxis. Among these are meningiomas, ependymomas, schwannomas of other cranial or peripheral nerves, and rarely low-grade spinal cord astrocytomas. Of these, meningiomas are the next most common intracranial pathology after bilateral vestibular schwannomas (Figure 108-6). They may be single or multiple and may occur in either a synchronous or metachronous fashion. Their behavior resembles that of spontaneous intracranial meningiomas, as should their treatment. The nature and treatment of intracranial and intraspinal ependymomas in the context of NF2 also resemble those of their spontaneous counterparts (Figure 108-7). Schwannomas may affect nerves other than the vestibulocochlear nerve. The next most common cranial nerve affected by schwannomas is the trigeminal nerve. In addition, schwannomas can arise from sensory roots in the cervicothoracic region, occasionally forming "dumbbell" tumors as they extend through and expand the intervertebral foramen. Peripherally, lesions arising from cutaneous nerves in NF2 patients are often schwannomas as well, in contrast to the neurofibromas seen in NF1 patients.

The care of patients with NF2 and their families should involve the coordinated efforts of the neurosurgeon, otolaryngologist, and geneticist. At the initial diagnosis, the patient should undergo a complete neurologic and otologic assessment, followed by imaging of the entire craniospinal neuraxis, audiometry, and BAERs. Subsequently, annual or biannual evaluations are recommended between the ages of 15 and 45 years.[15] Ophthalmologic assessment should be undertaken when the patient becomes symptomatic from ocular abnormalities. For family members of a patient with NF2, either clinical, radiologic, or molecular testing may be performed. If molecular testing is positive, baseline clinical and imaging studies should follow. If no tumors are identified, serial exam-

inations and imaging studies are recommended every 3 years. Individuals with negative molecular testing or normal MRI scans at age 30 are unlikely to have inherited the disorder, and further screening in these individuals may not be justified.

TUBEROUS SCLEROSIS COMPLEX

Tuberous sclerosis complex (TSC), or Bourneville's disease, is an inherited disorder resulting in hamartomatous changes in multiple organ systems, including the brain, kidneys, heart, retina, and skin. The name refers to "tubers" (areas of swelling or protuberances) and areas of "sclerosis," or hardening, in the cortical gyri. In addition to the hamartomatous growths, true neoplasms also occur in TSC, in particular within the brain and kidneys.

This disorder was first described by von Recklinghausen in 1862 but was further characterized by Bourneville in 1880 when he correlated the presence of cortical tubers with the seizures and mental retardation seen in these patients. Vogt later described his classic triad of seizures, mental retardation, and facial angiofibroma (adenoma sebaceum) seen in this disorder, allowing premorbid diagnosis of this condition.

TSC has an incidence of approximately 1 in 6000 live births and a prevalence in the general population of approximately 1 in 10,000, affecting nearly 2,000,000 people worldwide. This makes it the second most common of the neurocutaneous syndromes, following NF1. It is an autosomal dominantly inherited condition, with 80% to 95% penetrance and variable expression, and no predilection in regard to race or sex. Up to 50% of cases, however, are thought to be due to new mutations. Therefore, affected parents have a 50% chance of having an affected child, whereas normal parents with one affected child have a risk of 2% to 3% of producing a second child with TSC.[33]

Two responsible genes have been identified (TSC1 and TSC2), with mutations in either resulting in this disorder. Both genes are transmitted in an autosomal dominant fashion. Of the sporadic cases, approximately three fourths are thought to be secondary to TSC2 mutations.[23] TSC1 mutations tend to produce disease of lesser severity than TSC2. The TSC1 gene has been localized to chromosome 9 (9q34). It includes 21 exons, encoding for a protein (hamartin) implicated in the organization of the actin cytoskeleton. The TSC2 gene is found on chromosome 16 (16p13.3), adjacent to the gene responsible for adult polycystic kidney disease. TSC2 contains 42 exons, encoding for a protein (tuberin) thought to exhibit GTPase activity. These two proteins have been shown to bind together, explaining why defects in either may result in this disorder. The exact nature of their interaction, however, is not yet fully understood. The net result from a mutation in either the TSC1 or TSC2 genes is a disorder of cellular differentiation, proliferation, and abnormal neuronal migration.[29]

Vogt's triad, long held as the diagnostic criterion for TSC, has been found to occur in only one third of patients. Part of the difficulty in diagnosing this condition stems from the fact that patients with TSC may have symptoms that result from involvement of multiple organ systems, including the skin, eyes, heart, lungs, kidneys, or nervous system. To aid in the diagnosis, criteria were set out in a recent NIH Tuberous Sclerosis Complex Consensus Conference (Table 108-4).

Many features of TSC are dermatologic in nature, and a definitive diagnosis can be made based on these findings. One of the earliest features, often present at birth, are dull-white polygonal hypopigmented macules referred to as "ash leaf spots." These lesions may also be small, round, and "confetti-like." Multiple lesions are common, often seen best with the aid of a Wood's lamp. Despite being such a common feature, these lesions are not pathognomonic for TSC, because members of the unaffected population may also have them.

A second skin lesion found in TSC is the shagreen patch—an orange-peel texture connective-tissue hamartoma most commonly seen in the lumbosacral region. Approximately 21% of TSC patients develop this lesion, usually between the ages of 2 and 6 years. Again, this lesion is not specific to TSC.

After approximately age 4, facial angiofibromas develop in approximately 75% of patients. These acne-like lesions are typically seen in a malar distribution and are composed of vascular and fibrous dermal tissue. More specific to TSC are the ungual and periungual fibromas. These flesh-colored papules are found in 19% of TSC patients, often during adolescence or adulthood.

Retinal phakomas (astrocytomas) are seen in 50% to 75% of TSC patients.[40] These mulberry-like lesions may be evident as an absent red reflex in the newborn and may be mistaken for retinoblastoma if other features of TSC are not identified. Additional ocular manifestations include achromic retinal patches. In general, these lesions do not cause impairment of vision.

Cardiac rhabdomyomas occur in up to half of TSC patients. These may be single or multiple. In most, there is little clinical impact from these lesions. Some, however, may cause

TABLE 108-4

Diagnostic Criteria for Tuberous Sclerosis Complex

Definite TSC: 2 major features or 1 major and 2 minor features
Probable TSC: 1 major feature plus 1 minor feature
Possible TSC: 1 major feature or 2 minor features

Major Features
Facial angiofibroma or forehead plaque
Atraumatic ungual/periungual fibroma
Hypomelanotic macule (more than 3)
Shagreen patch
Multiple retinal nodular hamartomas
Cortical tuber
Subependymal nodule
SEGA
Cardiac rhabdomyoma
Lymphangioleiomyomatosis
Renal angiomyolipoma

Minor Features
Multiple randomly distributed dental enamel pits
Hamartomatous rectal polyp
Bone cyst
Cerebral white matter migration lines
Gingival fibromas
Nonrenal hamartomas
Retinal achromic patch
Confetti-like skin lesions
Multiple renal cysts

Notes:
When cerebral cortical dysplasia and white matter migration tracts occur together, they count as a single minor feature.
When both lymphangioleiomyomatosis and renal angiomyolipomas are present, other features of TSC should be present before a definitive diagnosis of TSC can be made.
Histologic confirmation is suggested for rectal polyps, nonrenal hamartomas, and renal cysts.
SEGA, Subependymal giant cell astrocytoma; TSC, tuberous sclerosis complex.
Source: Modified from criteria set out at the National Institutes of Health Tuberous Sclerosis Complex Consensus Conference.

heart failure because of ventricular outflow obstruction or interference with normal contractility. Less commonly, patients may suffer from arrhythmias or thromboembolic events. In general, medical management for these sequelae is appropriate because these lesions typically decrease in size as the child ages, occasionally disappearing altogether.

One rare complication of TSC, seen only in 2% to 5% of affected females, is pulmonary lymphangioleiomyomatosis. This occurs in women during their fourth decade of life, causing dyspnea, hemoptysis, or spontaneous pneumothorax. Radiologically, it appears as a diffuse reticular pattern on chest x-ray studies. This often fatal complication may respond to hormonal therapies (progesterone, oophorectomy) or to lung transplantation in the end stages. Less common lung involvement in TSC includes multifocal micronodular pneumocyte hyperplasia, pulmonary angiomyolipoma, or clear cell tumors of the lung.

Five different renal lesions may occur in TSC. The most common symptom patients report from these lesions is pain, often secondary to hemorrhage. These renal lesions typically occur after the second decade of life. The most common is the benign angiomyolipoma, affecting between 70% and 80% of patients with TSC.[11] These lesions occur bilaterally in up to three fourths of affected patients. By age 10, the incidence of these lesions in children approaches that in adults when screening ultrasound, CT scan, or MRI is performed. Serial imaging has been recommended to follow those patients who have asymptomatic lesions. Lesions larger than 4 cm in diameter should be considered for prophylactic renal artery embolization or renal-sparing surgery because of their propensity to bleed. Symptomatic lesions may also be considered for such intervention.

Renal cysts are the second most common renal lesion, seen in 20% of TSC patients. These are often multiple and bilateral. The suggestion has been made that this phenomenon may relate to the proximity of the TSC2 gene to the gene for adult polycystic kidney disease. Renal failure resulting from parenchymal compression may result in end-stage renal disease in up to 40% of patients with TSC and renal cysts.[60]

The remaining renal lesions include malignant angiomyoliposarcoma, oncocytoma, and renal cell carcinoma. Overall, fewer than 5% of patients with TSC suffer from serious renal compromise.

Neurologic manifestations feature prominently in the clinical presentation of TSC. Although some patients remain neurologically normal, others suffer from seizure disorders, mental retardation, and behavioral disorders. Central nervous system lesions found in TSC include the characteristic cortical tubers, cortical dysplasia, radial migration tracts, subependymal nodules, and the subependymal giant cell astrocytoma (SEGA). Spinal cord involvement in TSC is rare.

Although often neurologically normal at birth, up to 85% of patients eventually develop seizures.[53,59] This may be the first sign of this disorder. Most will show evidence of seizures within the first 2 to 3 years of life, with 69% symptomatic before their first birthday.[59] Males are typically affected more than females. The initial seizure pattern is often a flexion myoclonus, with hypsarrhythmia seen on electroencephalogram (EEG) tracings. The seizure pattern may evolve into a psychomotor or general tonic-clonic form. Severely affected children may display purposeless hand movements or postures.

Cognitive dysfunction is seen in approximately 50% of patients with TSC.[59] A strong correlation between the age of onset of seizure activity, seizure control, and cognitive impairment has been established.[59]

To maximize cognitive function in these patients, aggressive seizure control is necessary. The medical treatment of seizures in TSC depends on the pattern of seizures. Children with infantile spasms may respond to adrenocorticotropic hormone (ACTH) therapy, although there is a fairly high relapse rate.[46] Patients with generalized seizures (myoclonic, absence, or generalized tonic-clonic) may benefit from treatment using benzodiazepines, with or without sodium valproate. Patients with intractable seizures may benefit from ACTH treatment or a ketogenic diet.[26] Complex partial and focal motor seizures are best treated using carbamazepine, phenytoin, or primidone.[26]

Despite aggressive medical treatment, certain patients may prove to have refractory seizures. It has been suggested that patients with five or more cortical tubers are at increased risk of being refractory to medical management. In this population, surgery for seizure control may be indicated. Good outcomes can be expected when a single cortical tuber can be identified as the epileptogenic focus, with correlation between imaging and EEG studies. When no single focus is identifiable, palliative surgery using corpus callosotomy may be an option for seizure control, in particular if the child suffers from frequent drop attacks or generalized tonic-clonic seizures.

Cortical tubers are the most common cerebral lesion seen in TSC. These cortical hamartomas are often found along the grey-white junctions of the frontal lobes; however, most patients display multiple lesions asymmetrically affecting both hemispheres, multiple lobes. Pathologically, these lesions are often 1 to 2 cm in diameter, consisting of smooth, firm, pale gliotic plaques. The normal cortical laminar organization is disrupted. An increase in number of fibrillary astrocytes, glial fibers, and eosinophilic uninucleate giant cells is seen, as is a reduction in number of neurons and myelinated fibers.[52] With age, calcification and cystic degeneration may occur. Similar collections of cells may also be seen within subcortical white matter regions.

Radiologically, cortical tubers appear as focal areas of increased attenuation on CT scans, which are rarely enhanced. MRI is a more sensitive study to detect these lesions, with the tuber appearing hyperintense on T2-weighted images, hypointense to isointense on T1-weighted images, and with minimal enhancement after intravenous administration of contrast agent (Figure 108-8).

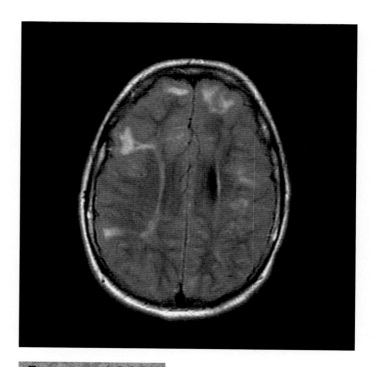

FIGURE 108-8   Axial fluid-attenuated inversion recovery magnetic resonance imaging of a 13-year-old boy with tuberous sclerosis (TS) showing multiple regions of increased signal intensity in the cortex. These lesions are cortical tubers which are hamartomas commonly found in TS.

Because these tubers are benign lesions, treatment is generally indicated only for the control of medically refractory seizure disorders.

Another lesion, pathognomonic for TSC, is a subependymal nodule—a periventricular hamartoma of 1 to 10 mm in diameter. These are typically located along the region of the head of the caudate nucleus and striothalamic zone of the lateral ventricle.

These lesions are composed histologically of abnormal glial and vascular tissues covered by a layer of ependymal cells. With the patient's increasing age, they may increase in number and show evidence of calcification. Occasionally, they may exhibit regions of hemorrhage or necrosis within them.

Because of their tendency to calcify, subependymal nodules are often best identified on CT scans, where they may resemble candle drippings along the border of the lateral ventricle. Very rarely do they enhance on CT scans. On MRI, these nodules appear heterogeneous, seen slightly more easily on T1-weighted images, where they appear isointense to white matter and hyperintense to gray matter. Peripheral enhancement with contrast agent can be seen on MRI (Figure 108-9).

Because these nodules are benign lesions, no specific treatment is necessary. These nodules do, however, have the potential for malignant transformation and as such should be followed.

SEGAs are lesions thought to be unique to TSC. They occur in approximately 6% of patients with TSC, arising along the terminal sulcus near the foramen of Monro. SEGAs are believed to arise from transformation and overgrowth of a subependymal nodule. Although the vast majority of these lesions are located within the ventricle itself, occasionally a similar lesion may be found within the brain parenchyma, secondary to degeneration of a cortical tuber.[12] Symptomatically, the presence of this lesion may be heralded by symptoms of increased intracranial pressure (secondary to mass effect or hydrocephalus) or by a change in the seizure frequency or pattern, often during the teenage years. Radiologically, SEGAs are suggested by a subependymal nodule that is either rapidly increasing in size or showing significant contrast enhancement.

SEGAs differ from other forms of astrocytoma in several ways. These tumors are not infiltrative and are found almost entirely within the lateral ventricle. In addition, features such as nuclear atypia, high mitotic indices, endothelial proliferation, or necrosis do not correlate with a worse prognosis for SEGAs. Typical features of these tumors include eosinophilic giant cells, perivascular pseudorosettes, and psammomatous calcification.

The standard of treatment for SEGA has been complete surgical excision. This may be performed via a transcortical or transcallosal approach. Studies have suggested that earlier diagnosis of SEGA by periodic radiologic surveillance, followed by early surgical excision, minimizes the degree of neurologic morbidity and the risk of tumor recurrence.[51,59] Patients in whom surgical excision is not feasible should be considered for a cerebrospinal fluid (CSF) diverting procedure, if symptomatic from hydrocephalus. For patients in whom surgical excision is possible, postoperative shunting of CSF is generally not required.

Recommendations for the assessment of patients and screening of their family members have been described.[21] In general, the initial assessment of a suspected case of TSC should include funduscopy, dermatologic screening, neurologic examination, and neurodevelopmental testing, as well as brain MRI, a cardiac echo or echocardiogram, and renal ultrasound or CT scan. Follow-up for asymptomatic patients should include imaging of the brain and kidneys every 1 to 3 years. If symptoms develop, further testing specific to that organ system should be carried out as indicated. At least one CT scan of the chest is recommended for women to rule out lymphangioleiomyomatosis.

Long-term outcomes and quality of life for patients with TSC are as variable as the disease expression itself. Patients with mild forms of the disorder can lead full lives without obvious impairment. For others, the degree of disability can be significant, with a significant reduction in life expectancy. The most serious complications are often secondary to either intracranial or renal involvement. Patients with SEGA may suffer serious neurologic compromise or death during their teenage years because of hydrocephalus, increased intracranial pressure, or hemorrhage. Older patients may suffer from renal compromise leading to end-stage renal failure.

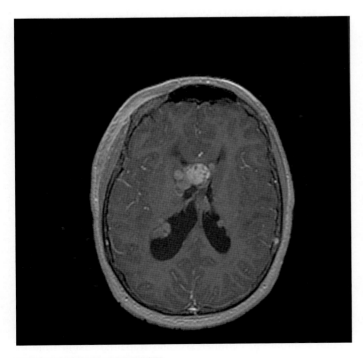

FIGURE 108-9 Axial gadolinium-enhanced magnetic resonance image showing multiple ventricular wall enhancing lesions and a midline subependymal giant cell astrocytoma (SEGA) in a patient with tuberous sclerosis.

VON HIPPEL-LINDAU DISEASE

Von Hippel-Lindau disease, or retinocerebellar angiomatosis, is an inherited disorder resulting in cystic or neoplastic changes to multiple organ systems, as well as the development of benign hemangioblastomas of the CNS. It has an incidence of approximately 1 in 40,000 live births. Similar to the other neurocutaneous syndromes, von Hippel-Lindau disease shows an autosomal dominant pattern of inheritance, high penetrance (70%), and variable expression. The cause of this disorder is thought to involve a tumor-suppressor gene or possibly a linear arrangement of genes, on the short arm of chromosome 3 (3p25-26).

One of the most common non-neurologic abnormalities seen in von Hippel-Lindau disease is retinal hemangioblastoma (HB)—present in more than 50% of patients and causing symptoms in nearly 20%. These lesions are often peripherally situated and occur bilaterally, with multiple lesions occurring within the same eye. Detection may be aided by the use of fluorescein angiography to detect small lesions. These HBs do pose a risk of hemorrhage or retinal detachment. Early detection and treatment with laser therapy helps to minimize this risk.

Other, less common lesions associated with von Hippel-Lindau disease include pancreatic cysts and islet cell tumors, renal cysts, renal cell carcinoma, and pheochromocytoma.

Cerebellar HBs are the most common finding in patients with von Hippel-Lindau disease (Figure 108-10). In this disorder, 75% of all HBs occur in the cerebellum, with most of the remaining lesions occurring within the spinal cord. Hemispheric or brainstem HBs make up only a small percentage of lesions.

Although most patients with cerebellar HBs do not have von Hippel-Lindau disease, one should always search for evidence of this disorder, because few patients will have a known positive family history of the disease. Factors suggesting von Hippel-Lindau disease include a younger age at diagnosis as well as multiple lesions.

Clinically, patients with cerebellar lesions may have headache (intermittent, suboccipital), vomiting, or rarely hemorrhage. On imaging studies these HBs appear as a hyperdense nodule with a cystic component on CT scans. This nodule often abuts the pial surface, and is brightly enhanced with contrast agent. Up to 75% are located in the cerebellar hemisphere. Commonly, a broad dural attachment is also evident. MRI shows the nodular component of these lesions to be hypointense to isointense on T1-weighted images and hyperintense on T2-weighted images. Intense contrast enhancement is also seen on MRI. For smaller lesions, angiography provides the most sensitive evaluation.

Histopathologically, these HBs are identical to the spontaneous variety. Treatment is typically surgical excision. Care must be taken to completely remove the mural nodule to prevent recurrence. The cyst wall, however, does not need to be removed in its entirety.

Spinal HBs found in von Hippel-Lindau disease are pathologically similar to the cerebellar variety. They are typically intramedullary lesions, although almost all will abut the pial surface of the cord. Compared with the cerebellar lesion, spinal HBs are less often cystic but may be associated with a syrinx. These lesions may be symptomatic, causing pain or sensorimotor abnormalities. For asymptomatic lesions, conservative treatment with serial MRI is an option. Once symptomatic, surgical excision is the treatment of choice for these lesions.[35] After complete surgical excision, recurrence of HBs is rare. New lesions are more likely to represent new primary HBs.

In the long term, patients with von Hippel-Lindau disease may suffer from blindness secondary to ophthalmologic complications. In addition, significant morbidity or mortality may result because of complications from intracranial HBs, renal cell carcinoma, pheochromocytoma, or pancreatic cancer.

STURGE-WEBER SYNDROME

Sturge-Weber syndrome, or encephalotrigeminal angiomatosis, is not a common neurocutaneous disorder. It involves the vasculature of the skin, eyes, meninges, and brain. This disorder was first characterized by Sturge in 1879, when he suggested an association between the facial cutaneous port-wine stain and contralateral neurologic deficits seen in some patients. Weber later was the first to radiographically demonstrate the cortical calcification seen in this group of patients. Little is known regarding the genetics of this disorder. No clear pattern of inheritance has been demonstrated, and therefore most investigators believe it to be secondary to new somatic mutations rather than germline mutations. In addition, no figures are available regarding the incidence of this disorder in the general population. There does not appear to be any sex or racial bias with this syndrome. A similar, related disorder is known as the Klippel-Trenaunay-Weber syndrome (spinal cutaneous angiomatosis). This variant involves extensive cutaneous hemangiomas in a dermatomal distribution, with associated spinal hemangiomas in the same dermatomal region.

The primary clinical manifestations of Sturge-Weber syndrome include a congenital, unilateral facial nevus, seizures, mental retardation, hemiparesis, and impaired vision (due to glaucoma). The characteristic facial nevus (port-wine stain or salmon patch) is often found in the V1 or V2 regions of innervation by the trigeminal nerve. This skin lesion may be the diagnostic feature of Sturge-Weber syndrome in many patients. The nevus may be a transient, midline salmon patch or a per-

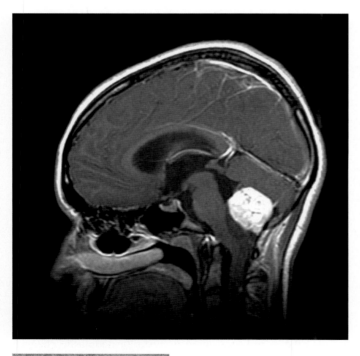

FIGURE 108-10 Gadolinium-enhanced, sagittal magnetic resonance image in a 12-year-old patient with von Hippel-Lindau disease. These lesions are extremely vascular and require stepwise elimination of the vascular feeding vessels for successful tumor extirpation.

sistent, laterally located port-wine stain. Occasionally, a bilateral distribution or extension of the nevus to the lips, neck, or trunk may occur. In addition, the nevus may be completely absent, as in the forme fruste of Sturge-Weber syndrome. Treatment of this cutaneous lesion involves selective photothermolysis using various forms of laser therapy.

Ocular defects in Sturge-Weber syndrome include glaucoma, hemangiomas of the choroid, conjunctiva, or episclera, retinal detachment, vascular tortuosity, strabismus, and buphthalmos. Of these lesions, glaucoma is the most common ophthalmologic finding, affecting between 30% and 50% of patients with Sturge-Weber syndrome. This finding is often unilateral and ipsilateral to the facial nevus. In addition, it is often congenital or develops before age 2. Trabeculotomy may be required for the treatment of this condition. Rarely, choroidal hemangiomas may cause retinal or choroidal detachment with visual loss, necessitating surgical intervention, external-beam irradiation, or photocoagulation.

Ipsilateral to the facial nevus, one often finds parietooccipital leptomeningeal venous angiomatosis. This may be bilateral in up to 15% of patients. This leptomeningeal angiomatosis consists of thin-walled veins within the pia matter. As a result, the meninges often become thickened and turn dark red-purple. The underlying brain often shows cortical atrophy, calcification, and enlarged, cystic choroid plexus. Reported associated neurologic symptoms include hemiparesis, visual field deficits, seizures, or intellectual impairment. These findings are often present to some degree by age 2 and are thought to be secondary to a vascular steal phenomenon from the overlying angioma.

The diagnosis of Sturge-Weber syndrome can often be made based on the typical cutaneous findings and the appearance of the brain and meninges on neuroimaging. CT scans of the brain often show evidence of calcification of the involved cortex. MRI with contrast may detect the leptomeningeal angiomatosis (Figure 108-11). Angiography may detect enlargement of deep cerebral or collateral veins, reduced or absent cortical veins, or early filling of enlarged veins.[49]

Seizures in Sturge-Weber syndrome occur in approximately 80% of patients, most often with an onset during the first year of life and before any evidence of hemiparesis.[49] Children with bihemispheric involvement are slightly more likely to suffer from seizures.[6] The type of seizure is often either partial motor or generalized tonic-clonic and may display a remitting and relapsing course. Up to 96% of patients have some form of abnormality evident on EEG, including attenuation of background activity or epileptiform spikes.[49]

Adequate medical seizure control is possible in up to 40% of patients with Sturge-Weber syndrome.[3] In one series, 32%

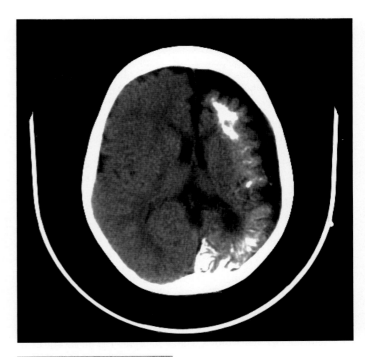

FIGURE 108-11 Axial computed tomography scan of the brain in a 4-year-old boy with severe seizure disorder and left facial port-wine stain and a clinical diagnosis of Sturge-Weber. The left hemisphere is atrophic, and calcifications are seen diffusely throughout the leptomeninges of the hemisphere.

of patients were refractory to medical therapy and required surgery for seizure control.[49] The natural history of this disorder is variable, however, and indications for surgery are not straightforward. Some recommend early surgery before any obvious motor deficit occurs, to prevent irreversible neurologic damage.[19] Others recommend surgery only for patients with intractable seizures and progressive neurologic deficits.[47] Demonstration of progressive cortical atrophy or calcification and of new neurologic signs and symptoms may also support the decision to operate in this condition.

Multiple surgical techniques have been employed, including peri-insular hemispherectomy, hemispherectomy, lobectomy, and corpus callosotomy. Following surgery, up to 65% of patients may be seizure free, with the rest reporting some reduction in seizure frequency.[49]

References

1. Al-Saleem T, Wessner LL, Scheithauer BW, et al: Malignant tumors of the kidney, brain, and soft tissues in children and young adults with tuberous sclerosis. Cancer 83:2208–2216, 1998.
2. Andrews DW, Suarez O, Goldman HW, et al: Stereotactic radiosurgery and fractionated stereotactic radiotherapy for the treatment of acoustic schwannomas: comparative observations of 125 patients treated at one institution. Int J Radiat Oncol Biol Phys 50:1265–1278, 2001.
3. Arzimanoglou A, Aicardi J: The epilepsy of Sturge-Weber syndrome: clinical features and treatment in 23 patients. Acta Neurol Scand 140:s18–s22, 1992.
4. Arzimanoglou A, Andermann F, Aicardi J, et al: Sturge-Weber syndrome. Indications and results of surgery in 20 patients. Neurology 55:1472–1479, 2000.
5. Bader JL: Neurofibromatosis and cancer: an overview. Dysmorphol Clin Genet 1:43–48, 1987.

6. Bebin EM, Gomez MR: Prognosis in Sturge-Weber disease: comparison of unihemispheric and bihemispheric involvement. J Child Neurol 3:1811–1814, 1988.

7. Bebin EM, Kelly PI, Gomez MR: Surgical treatment for epilepsy in cerebral tuberous sclerosis. Epilepsia 34:651–657, 1993.

8. Chamberlain MC, Arafe MR: Recurrent chiasmatic-hypothalamic glioma treated with oral etoposide. J Clin Oncol 13:2072–2076, 1995.

9. Committee on Genetics, American Academy of Pediatrics: Health supervision for children with neurofibromatosis. Pediatrics 96:368–372, 1995.

10. Danoff BF, Kramer S, Thompson N: The radiotherapeutic management of optic gliomas of children. Int J Radiat Oncol Biol Phys 6:45–50, 1980.

11. Ewalt DH, Sheffield E, Sparagana SP, et al: Renal lesion growth in children with tuberous sclerosis complex. J Urol 160:141–145, 1998.

12. Frerebeau P, Benezech J, Segnarbieux F, et al: Intraventricular tumors in tuberous sclerosis. Childs Nerv Syst 1:45–48, 1985.

13. Friedman HS, Krischer JP, Burger P, et al: Treatment of children with progressive or recurrent brain tumors with carboplatin or iproplatin: a Pediatric Oncology Group randomized phase II study. J Clin Oncol 10:249–256, 1992.

14. Gajjar A, Heideman RL, Kovnar EH, et al: Response of pediatric low-grade gliomas to chemotherapy. Pediatr Neurosurg 19:113–121, 1992.

15. Gutmann DH, Aylsworth A, Carey JC, et al: The diagnostic evaluation and multidisciplinary management of neurofibromatosis 1 and neurofibromatosis 2. JAMA 278:51–57, 1997.

16. Habiby R, Silverman B, Listernick R, Charrow J: Precocious puberty in children with neurofibromatosis type 1. J Pediatr 126:364–367, 1995.

17. Heim RA, Silverman LM, Farber RA, et al: Screening for truncated NF1 proteins. Nat Genet 8:218–219, 1994.

18. Hoffman HJ, Hendrick EB, Dennis M, et al: Hemispherectomy for Sturge-Weber syndrome. Childs Brain 5:233–248, 1979.

19. Hoffman HJ: Benefits of early surgery in Sturge-Weber syndrome. In Tuxhorn I, Holthausen H, Boenigk H (eds): Padiatric Epilepsy Syndromes and Their Surgical Treatment. London, John Libbey, 1997.

20. Hurst JS, Wilcoski S: Recognizing an index case of tuberous sclerosis. Am Fam Physician 61:703–708, 2000.

21. Hyman MH, Wittemore VH: National Institutes of Health Consensus Conference: tuberous sclerosis complex. Arch Neurol 57:662–665, 2000.

22. Jenkin D, Angyalfi S, Becker L, et al: Optic glioma in children: surveillance, resection or irradiation. Int J Radiat Oncol Biol Phys 25:215–225, 1993.

23. Jones AC, Danielles CE, Snell RG, et al: Molecular genetic and phenotypic analysis reveals differences between TSC1 and TSC2 associated familial and sporadic tuberous sclerosis. Hum Mol Genet 6:2155–2161, 1997.

24. Karnes PS: Neurofibromatosis: a common neurocutaneous disorder. Mayo Clin Proc 73:1071–1076, 1998.

25. Kihiczak NI, Schwartz RA, Jozwiak Sergiusz, et al: Sturge-Weber Syndrome. Cutis 65:133–136, 2000.

26. Kotagal P, Rothner AD: Epilepsy in the setting of neurocutaneous syndromes. Epilepsia 34(suppl 3):s71–s78, 1993.

27. Korf BR: Neurocutaneous syndromes: neurofibromatosis 1, neurofibromatosis 2, and tuberous sclerosis. Curr Opin Neurol 10:131–136, 1997.

28. Kretchmar CS, Linggood RM: Chemotherapeutic treatment of extensive optic pathway tumors in infants. J Neurooncol 10:263–270, 1991.

29. Kwiatkowski DJ, Short MP: Tuberous sclerosis. Arch Dermatol 130:348–354, 1994.

30. Listernick R, Charrow J, Greenwald M: Emergence of optic pathway glioma in children with neurofibromatosis type 1 after normal neuroimaging results. J Pediat 121:584–587, 1992.

31. Listernick R, Charrow J, Greenwald MJ, Mets M: Natural history of optic pathway tumors in children with neurofibromatosis type 1: a longitudinal study. J Pediatr 125:63–66, 1994.

32. Listernick R, Louis DN, Packer RJ, Gutmann DH: Optic pathway gliomas in children with neurofibromatosis 1: consensus statement from the NF1 Optic Pathway Glioma Task Force. Ann Neurol 41:143–149, 1997.

33. MacCollin M, Kwiatkowski D: Molecular genetic aspects of the phakomatoses: Tuberous sclerosis complex and neurofibromatosis 1. Curr Opin Neurol 14:163–169, 2001.

34. Mulvihill JJ, Parry DM, Sherman JL, et al: Neurofibromatosis 1 (Recklinghausen disease) and neurofibromatosis 2 (bilateral acoustic neurofibromatosis). Ann Int Med 113:39–52, 1990.

35. Neumann HPH, Eggert HR, Weigel K, et al: Hemangioblastomas of the central nervous system. A 10-year study with special reference to von Hippel-Lindau syndrome. J Neurosurg 70:24–30, 1989.

36. Neumann HPH, Eggert HR, Scheremet R, et al: Central nervous system lesions in von Hippel-Lindau syndrome. J Neurol Neurosurg Psychiatry 55:898–901, 1992.

37. Neurofibromatosis. Conference Statement. National Institutes of Health Consensus Development Conference. Arch Neurol 45:575–578, 1988; Neurofibromatosis. NIH Consensus Statement Online 6:1–19, 1987, http://consensus.nih.gov/cons/064/064_statement.htm.

38. North K: Neurofibromatosis type 1. Am J Med Genet 97:119–127, 2000.

39. Ojemann RG: Management of acoustic neuromas (vestibular schwannomas). Clin Neurosurg 40:489–535, 1993.

40. Osborne JP: Diagnosis of tuberous sclerosis. Arch Dis Child 63:1423–1425, 1988.

41. Packer RJ, Sutton LM, Bilaniuk LT, et al: Treatment of chiasmatic/hypthalmic gliomas of childhood with chemotherapy: an update. Ann Neurol 23:79–85, 1988.

42. Packer RJ, Lange B, Ater J, et al: Carboplatin and vincristine for progressive low-grade gliomas of childhood. J Clin Oncol 11:850–857, 1992.

43. Pierce SM, Barnes PD, Loeffler JS, et al: Definitive radiation therapy in the management of symptomatic patients with optic glioma: survival and long-term effects. Cancer 65:45–57, 1990.

44. Pons MA, Finlay JL, Walker RW, et al: Chemotherapy with vincristine and etoposide in children with low-grade astrocytoma. J Neurooncol 14:151–158, 1992.

45. Riccardi VM: Neurofibromatosis: Phenotype, Natural History, and Pathogenesis, 2nd ed. Baltimore, Johns Hopkins University Press, 1992.

46. Riikonen R, Simell O: Tuberous sclerosis and infantile spasms. Dev Med Child Neurol 32:203–209, 1990.

47. Roach ES, Riela AR, Chugani HT, et al: Sturge-Weber syndrome. Recommendations for surgery. J Child Neurol 9:190–192, 1994.

48. Roach ES, Gomez MR, Northrup H: Tuberous sclerosis complex consensus conference: revised clinical diagnostic criteria. J Child Neurol 13:624–628, 1998.

49. Rochkind S, Hoffman HJ, Hendrick EB: Sturge-Weber syndrome: natural history and prognosis. J Epilepsy 3(suppl):293–304, 1990.

50. Rosenstock JG, Packer RJ, Bilaniuk LT, et al: Chiasmatic optic glioma treated with chemotherapy. A preliminary report. J Neurosurg 63:862–866, 1985.

51. Roszkowski M, Drabik K, Barszcz S, Jozwiak S: Surgical treatment of intraventricular tumors associated with tuberous sclerosis. Childs Nerv Syst 11:335–339, 1995.

52. Scheithauer BW: The neuropathology of tuberous sclerosis. J Dermatol 19:897–903, 1992.

53. Sparagana SP, Roach ES: Tuberous sclerosis complex. Curr Opin Neurol 13:115–119, 2000.

54. Subach BR, Kondziolka D, Lunsford LD, et al: Stereotactic radiosurgery in the management of acoustic neuromas associated with neurofibromatosis type 2. J Neurosurg 90:815–822, 1999.

55. Tator CH: Acoustic neuromas: management of 20 cases. Can J Neuro Sci 12:353–357, 1985.

56. Torres OA, Roach ES, Delgado MR, et al: Early diagnosis of subependymal giant cell astrocytoma in patients with tuberous sclerosis. J Child Neurol 13:173–177, 1998.

57. Verhoef S, Bakker L, Tempelaars AM, et al: High rate of mosaicism in tuberous sclerosis complex. Am J Hum Genet 64:1632–1637, 1999.

58. Webb DW, Fryer AE, Osborne JP: On the incidence of fits and mental retardation in tuberous sclerosis. J Med Genet 28:395–397, 1991.

59. Webb DW, Fryer AE, Osborne JP: Morbidity associated with tuberous sclerosis: a population study. Dev Med Child Neurol 38:146–155, 1996.

60. Weiner DM, Ewalt DH, Roach ES, Hensle TW: The tuberous sclerosis complex a comprehensive review. J Am Coll Surg 187:548–561, 1998.

INDEX